Tarascon Pharmacopoeia®

2011 Edition

12TH EDITION

"Desire to take medicines ... distinguishes man from animals."
—Sir William Osler

Editor in Chief
Richard J. Hamilton, MD, FAAEM, FACMT
Professor and Chair, Department of Emergency Medicine
Drexel University College of Medicine
Philadelphia, PA

JONES & BARTLETT
L E A R N I N G

World Headquarters
Jones & Bartlett Learning
40 Tall Pine Drive
Sudbury, MA 01776
978-443-5000
info@jblearning.com
www.jblearning.com

Jones & Bartlett Learning Canada
6339 Ormindale Way
Mississauga, Ontario L5V 1J2
Canada

Jones & Bartlett Learning International
Barb House, Barb Mews
London W6 7PA
United Kingdom

Jones & Bartlett Learning books and products are available through most bookstores and online booksellers. To contact Jones & Bartlett Learning directly, call 800-832-0034, fax 978-443-8000, or visit our website, www.jblearning.com.

Substantial discounts on bulk quantities of Jones & Bartlett Learning publications are available to corporations, professional associations, and other qualified organizations. For details and specific discount information, contact the special sales department at Jones & Bartlett Learning via the above contact information or send an email to specialsales@jblearning.com.

Copyright © 2011 by Jones & Bartlett Learning, LLC

All rights reserved. No part of the material protected by this copyright may be reproduced or utilized in any form, electronic or mechanical, including photocopying, recording, or by any information storage and retrieval system, without written permission from the copyright owner.

The information in the *Pocket Pharmacopoeia* is compiled from sources believed to be reliable, and exhaustive efforts have been put forth to make the book as accurate as possible. The *Pocket Pharmacopoeia* is edited by a panel of drug information experts with extensive peer review and input from more than 50 practicing clinicians of multiple specialties. Our goal is to provide health professionals focused, core prescribing information in a convenient, organized, and concise fashion. We include FDA-approved dosing indications and those off-label uses that have a reasonable basis to support their use. *However the accuracy and completeness of this work cannot be guaranteed.* Despite our best efforts this book may contain typographical errors and omissions. The *Pocket Pharmacopoeia* is intended as a quick and convenient reminder of information you have already learned elsewhere. The contents are to be used as a guide only, and healthcare professionals should use sound clinical judgment and individualize therapy to each specific patient care situation. This book is not meant to be a replacement for training, experience, continuing medical education, or studying the latest drug prescribing literature. This book is sold without warranties of any kind, express or implied, and the publisher and editors disclaim any liability, loss, or damage caused by the contents. Although drug companies purchase and distribute our books as promotional items, the Tarascon editorial staff alone determines all book content.

Production Credits
Chief Executive Officer: Ty Field
President: James Homer
SVP, Chief Operating Officer: Don Jones, Jr.
SVP, Chief Technology Officer: Dean Fossella
SVP, Chief Marketing Officer: Alison M. Pendergast
SVP, Chief Financial Officer: Ruth Siporin
V.P., Design and Production: Anne Spencer
V.P., Manufacturing and Inventory Control:
  Therese Connell
Executive Publisher: Christopher Davis

Senior Acquisitions Editor: Nancy Anastasi Duffy
Editorial Assistant: Sara Cameron
Senior Production Editor: Daniel Stone
Medicine Marketing Manager: Rebecca Rockel
Composition: Newgen
Text Design: Anne Spencer
Cover Design: Kate Ternullo
Printing and Binding: Malloy Inc.
Cover Printing: Malloy Inc.

The cover woodcut is *The Apothecary* by Jost Amman, Frankfurt, 1574. Courtesy of National Library of Medicine.

Tarascon Pharmacopoeia 2011 Library Edition   ISBN: 978-1-4496-0067-9
Tarascon Pharmacopoeia 2011 Desk Reference Edition   ISBN: 978-1-4496-0069-3

6048
Printed in the United States of America
15 14 13 12 11 10 9 8 7 6 5 4 3 2 1

A number of you knew that the pill color goes this way – (using the first letter of the pills White, Blue Yellow, Green) - WBYB in the morning and then GWYG in the evening, or GYWG in the morning and then BYBW in the evening. This is a version of a problem first proposed by C. Dudley Langford, a Scottish mathematician.

We will send a free copy of next year's edition to the first 25 who can solve the following interpersonal dilemma puzzle:

An intern in a Philadelphia hospital has two girlfriends – one in Trenton and one in Delaware. On his days off, he takes the train to see one of them but he lets chance decide which one he sees. He goes to the platform at some random time and if the Trenton train arrives first he takes that one, if the Delaware train arrives first he takes that one. The trains arrive at the station equally often – every 10 minutes. After a few months, he notices that he has seen his Trenton girlfriend once in the last 10 days off. Why does chance favor the girlfriend in Delaware?

TARASCON POCKET PHARMACOPOEIA EDITORIAL STAFF*

EDITOR IN CHIEF
Richard J. Hamilton, MD, FAAEM, FACMT, Professor and Chair, Department of Emergency Medicine, Drexel University College of Medicine, Philadelphia, PA

ASSOCIATE EDITORS
Jill E. Allen, PharmD, BCPS, Pin Oak Associates, Drug Information Consultant, Salt Lake City, UT

Kimberly K. Birtcher, MS, PharmD, BCPS, Clinical Associate Professor, University of Houston College of Pharmacy, Houston, TX

Jill S. Burkiewicz, PharmD, BCPS, Professor, Pharmacy Practice, Director, Primary Care PGY1 Residency Program, Midwestern University Chicago College of Pharmacy, Downers Grove, IL

David S. Craig, PharmD, H. Lee Moffitt Cancer Center and Research Institute, Tampa, FL

Deborah Hass, PharmD, BCOP, Assistant Professor, Midwestern University Chicago College of Pharmacy, Downers Grove, IL

William A. Kehoe, PharmD, MA, BCPS, Professor of Clinical Pharmacy and Psychology, University of the Pacific, Stockton, CA

Neeta Bahal O'Mara, PharmD, BCPS, Coldstream Consulting LLC, Skillman, NJ

Jeffrey T. Sherer, MPH, PharmD, BCPS, Clinical Associate Professor, University of Houston College of Pharmacy, Houston, TX

EDITORIAL BOARD
Steven R. Abel, PharmD, FASHP, Associate Dean for Clinical Programs, Bucke Professor and Head, Department of Pharmacy Practice, Purdue University College of Pharmacy, West Lafayette, IN

David R. Adams, MD, PharmD, Department of Dermatology, Penn State College of Medicine, Penn State Milton S. Hershey Medical Center, Hershey, PA

Heath P. Adams, PharmD, Department of Pharmacy, Trover Health Systems Regional Medical Center, Madisonville, KY

Giovannina M. Anthony, MD, Obstetrics and Gynecology, Women's Health Center of Jackson, Jackson, WY

Ouida Antle, PharmD, Carewest, Calgary, Alberta, Canada

Bruce Barrett, MD, PhD, Associate Professor of Family Medicine, University of Wisconsin, Madison, WI

Sandra Harley Counts, PharmD, AHEC Associate Professor of Family Medicine (Anderson), AnMed Health Family Medicine Residency Program, Anderson, SC

Gary E. Davis, PharmD, Neuroscience Clinical Coordinator, Adjunct Assistant Professor, University of Utah Hospital and Clinics, Department of Pharmacy Services, Salt Lake City, UT

Lori M. Dickerson, PharmD, Professor of Family Medicine, Medical University of South Carolina, Charleston, SC

Joseph S. Esherick, MD, FAAFP, Family Medicine, Ventura County Medical Center, Ventura, CA

Randall L. Goodman, MD, FACS, Opthalmology, Shepard Eye Center, Santa Maria, CA

David Greenes, MD, Division of Emergency Medicine, Children's Hospital, Boston, MA

Holly Gustafson, MD, Park Nicollet Internal Medicine, St. Louis Park, MN

James R. Herman, MD, PhD, FACS, Urology Associates of Kingsport, Kingsport, TN

Jeffrey Jacobson, MD, Chief, Division of Infectious Disease and HIV Medicine, Drexel University College of Medicine, Philadelphia, PA

Arlyn J. LaBair, MD, Family Medicine, Denver, CO

*Affiliations are given for information purposes only, and no affiliation sponsorship is claimed.

EDITORIAL BOARD, cont.

Marc J. Laufgraben, MD, MBA, Endocrinology, Clinical Associate Professor of Medicine, Brown University, Providence, RI

Allen E. Lavee, MD, Anesthesiology, San Francisco, CA

Lawrence Loo, MD, Internal Medicine, Professor of Medicine, Department of Medicine, Loma Linda University School of Medicine, Loma Linda, CA

Yun Lu, PharmD, MS, BCPS, Clinical Associate Professor, University of Minnesota, Hennepin County Medical Center, Minneapolis, MN

Andrea Luisi, PharmD, BCPS, Cumberland, RI

Ian R. McNicholl, PharmD, BCPS (AQ – Infectious Diseases), AAHIVE, Associate Clinical Professor, Clinical Pharmacy Specialist, UCSF Positive Health Program, Editor, UCSF Center for HIV Information, Drug Interaction Database, San Francisco, CA

Susan M. Miller, PharmD, BCPS, Pharmacy Clinic Coordinator, Cape Fear Valley Health System, Fayetteville, NC

Melissa J. Nirenberg, MD, PhD, Assistant Professor of Neurology, Weill Cornell Medical College, New York, NY

John Noviasky, PharmD, BCPS, Associate Director of Pharmacy-Clinical Services, Upstate University Hospital, Syracuse, NY

Mary Ellis Pickett, MD, Associate Professor of Medicine, Oregon Health and Science University, Portland, OR

Joseph Saseen, PharmD, BCPS, CLS, Professor, University of Colorado, Schools of Pharmacy and Medicine, Aurora, CO

Timothy W. Smith, DPhil, MD, Associate Professor of Medicine, Washington University School of Medicine, St. Louis, MO

Ronald L. Swaab, MD, Hematology and Oncology, Pottstown Memorial Regional Cancer Center, Pottstown, PA

Andrew E. Thompson, MD, Rheumatology, Assistant Professor of Medicine, University of Western Ontario, Canada

Kristin Walter, MD, Pulmonary and Critical Care Medicine, St. Joseph Hospital, Chicago, IL

Izak F. Wessels, MMed, FRCSE, FRCOphth, FACS, Allied Eye Associates, Chattanooga, TN; and Clinical Associate Professor of Ophthalmology, Loma Linda University, Loma Linda, CA

Robert M. Wood, MD, Family Medicine, Santa Maria, CA; In Honor of Robert L. Wood, MD.

CONTENTS

ANALGESICS
Antirheumatic Agents 1
Muscle Relaxants 3
Non-Opioid Analgesic
   Combinations 5
Non-Steroidal Anti-
   Inflammatories 7
Opioid Agonist-Antagonists 12
Opioid Agonists 12
Opioid Analgesic
   Combinations 16
Opioid Antagonists 19
Other Analgesics 19

ANESTHESIA
Anesthetics and Sedatives 21
Local Anesthetics 22
Neuromuscular Blockers 23

ANTIMICROBIALS
Aminoglycosides 24
Antifungal Agents 25
Antimalarials 31
Antimycobacterial Agents 34
Antiparasitics 37
Antiviral Agents 39
Carbapenems 59
Cephalosporins 60
Macrolides 67
Penicillins 70
Quinolones 75
Sulfonamides 78
Tetracyclines 79
Other Antimicrobials 81

CARDIOVASCULAR
ACE Inhibitors 86
Aldosterone Antagonists 89
Angiotensin Receptor Blockers
   (ARBs) 90
Antiadrenergic Agents 92
Anti-Dysrhythmics/Cardiac
   Arrest 94
Anti-Hyperlipidemic Agents ... 101
Antihypertensive
   Combinations 107
Antiplatelet Drugs 113
Beta-Blockers 115
Calcium Channel Blockers
   (CCBs) 119
Diuretics 121
Nitrates 125
Pressors/Inotropes 126
Pulmonary Arterial
   Hypertension 128
Thrombolytics 130
Volume Expanders 131
Other 132

CONTRAST MEDIA
MRI Contrast 134
Radiography Contrast 134

DERMATOLOGY
Acne Preparations 135
Actinic Keratosis
   Preparations 138
Antibacterials (Topical) 139
Antifungals (Topical) 141
Antiparasitics (Topical) 143
Antipsoriatics 144
Antivirals (Topical) 145
Atopic Dermatitis
   Preparations 146
Corticosteroids (Topical) 147
Corticosteroid / Antimicrobial
   Combinations 150
Hemorrhoid Care 151
Other Dermatologic Agents 151

ENDOCRINE AND METABOLIC
Androgens / Anabolic
   Steroids 155
Bisphosphonates 157
Corticosteroids 159
Diabetes-Related 162
Diagnostic Agents 171
Gout-Related 172
Minerals 173
Nutritionals 179
Phosphate Binders 180
Thyroid Agents 181
Vitamins 183
Other 189

ENT
Antihistamines 193
Antitussives / Expectorants 195
Combination Products 196
Decongestants 206
Ear Preparations 207
Mouth and Lip Preparations ... 208
Nasal Preparations 209

GASTROENTEROLOGY
Antidiarrheals 211
Antiemetics 213
Antiulcer 217
Laxatives 225
Ulcerative Colitis 228
Other GI Agents 229

HEMATOLOGY
Anticoagulants 233
Antihemophilic Agents 237
Colony Stimulating Factors 239
Other Hematological
   Agents 241

HERBAL & ALTERNATIVE
   THERAPIES 243

IMMUNOLOGY
Immunizations 257
Immunoglobulins 263
Immunosuppression 266
Other 268

NEUROLOGY
Alzheimer's Disease 268
Anticonvulsants 269
Migraine Therapy 276
Multiple Sclerosis 278
Myasthenia Gravis 279
Parkinsonian Agents 280
Other Agents 283

OB/GYN
Contraceptives 285
Estrogens 296
GnRH Agents 299
Hormone Combinations 300
Labor Induction / Cervical
   Ripening 302
Ovulation Stimulants 302
Progestins 303
Selective Estrogen Receptor
   Modulators 305
Uterotonics 306
Vaginitis Preparations 306
Other OB/GYN Agents 308

ONCOLOGY
Alkylating agents 309
Antibiotics 312
Antimetabolites 314
Cytoprotective Agents 317
Hormones 317
Immunomodulators 320
Mitotic Inhibitors 324
Platinum-Containing Agents ... 326
Radiopharmaceuticals 326
Miscellaneous 327

OPHTHALMOLOGY
Antiallergy 332
Antibacterials 334
Antiviral Agents 337
Corticosteroid & Antibacterial
   Combinations 337
Corticosteroids 339
Glaucoma Agents 339
Macular Degeneration 343
Mydriatics & Cycloplegics 343
Non-Steroidal Anti-
   Inflammatories 344
Other Ophthalmologic Agents ... 345

PSYCHIATRY
Antidepressants 346
Antimanic (Bipolar) Agents 353
Antipsychotics 354
Anxiolytics/Hypnotics 361
Combination Drugs 365
Drug Dependence Therapy ... 365
Stimulants/ADHD/
   Anorexiants 367

PULMONARY
Beta Agonists 370
Combinations 372

Contents

Inhaled Steroids 374
Leukotriene Inhibitors 376
Other Pulmonary Medications ... 377
TOXICOLOGY 380

UROLOGY
Benign Prostatic Hyperplasia ... 383
Bladder Agents 384
Erectile Dysfunction 387

Nephrolithiasis 389
Other 390
Index 391
Appendix 413

PAGE INDEX FOR TABLES

GENERAL
Abbreviations viii
Therapeutic drug levels viii
Outpatient pediatric drugs ix
Pediatric vital signs and
  IV drugs x
Conversions x
P450 isozymes xi
Formulas xiii
Drug therapy reference sites xiii
Coronary Artery Disease 10-year
  Risk xiv
Adult Emergency Drugs 413
Cardiac Dysrhythmia
  Protocols 414
Antiviral drugs for influenza 415
ANALGESICS
Opioid equivalency 13
Fentanyl transdermal 14
NSAIDs 17
ANTIMICROBIALS
Bacterial pathogens 54
STDs/Vaginitis 62
Cephalosporins 65
Penicillins 68
SBE prophylaxis 71

Quinolones 76
C difficile infection in adult 82
CARDIOVASCULAR
HTN therapy 88
ACE inhibitors 88
QT interval drugs 93
LDL cholesterol goals 95
Lipid reduction by class 96
Statins lipid response 103
HTN Combinations 106
Cardiac parameters 124
Thrombolysis in MI 131
DERMATOLOGY
Topical corticosteroids 140
ENDOCRINE
Corticosteroids 161
Diabetes numbers 163
Insulin 166
IV solutions 173
Fluoride dose 175
Potassium forms 176
Peds rehydration 177
GASTROENTEROLOGY
H pylori treatment 219
HEMATOLOGY
Heparin dosing 236

Theraputic goals for
  anticoagulation 237
Warfarin interactions 238
IMMUNIZATIONS
Tetanus 258
Child immunizations 259
Adult immunizations 264
NEUROLOGY
Dermatomes 270
Nerve roots, LS spine 270
Glasgow coma scale 270
OB/GYN
Oral contraceptives 295
Emerg contraception 296
Drugs in pregnancy 301
OPHTHALMOLOGY
Visual acuity screen 336
PSYCHIATRY
Antipsychotics 355
Body mass index 368
PULMONARY
Peak flow 373
Inhaler colors 373
Inhaled steroids 375
TOXICOLOGY
Antidotes 382

PREFACE TO THE TARASCON POCKET PHARMACOPOEIA®

The *Tarascon Pocket Pharmacopoeia*® arranges drugs by clinical class with a comprehensive index in the back. Trade names are italicized and capitalized. Drug doses shown in mg/kg are generally intended for children, while fixed doses represent typical adult recommendations. Brackets indicate currently available formulations, although not all pharmacies stock all formulations. The availability of generic, over-the-counter, and scored formulations is mentioned. We have underlined the disease or indication for the pharmaceutical agent. It is meant to function as an aid to find information quickly. Codes are as follows:

▶ **METABOLISM & EXCRETION:** **L** = primarily liver, **K** = primarily kidney, **LK** = both, but liver > kidney, **KL** = both, but kidney > liver.

♀ **SAFETY IN PREGNANCY:** **A** = Safety established using human studies, **B** = Presumed safety based on animal studies, **C** = Uncertain safety; no human studies and animal studies show an adverse effect, **D** = Unsafe - evidence of risk that may in certain clinical circumstances be justifiable, **X** = Highly unsafe - risk of use outweighs any possible benefit. For drugs that have not been assigned a category: **+** Generally accepted as safe, **?** Safety unknown or controversial, **−** Generally regarded as unsafe.

▶ **SAFETY IN LACTATION:** **+** Generally accepted as safe, **?** Safety unknown or controversial, **−** Generally regarded as unsafe. Many of our "**+**" listings are from the AAP policy "The Transfer of Drugs and Other Chemicals Into Human Milk" (see www.aap.org) and may differ from those recommended by the manufacturer.

© **DEA CONTROLLED SUBSTANCES:** **I** = High abuse potential, no accepted use (eg, heroin, marijuana), **II** = High abuse potential and severe dependence liability (eg, morphine, codeine, hydromorphone, cocaine, amphetamines, methylphenidate, secobarbital). Some states require triplicates. **III** = Moderate dependence liability (eg, *Tylenol #3*, *Vicodin*), **IV** = Limited dependence liability (benzodiazepines, propoxyphene, phentermine), **V** = Limited abuse potential (eg, *Lomotil*).

$ **RELATIVE COST:** Cost codes used are "per month" of maintenance therapy (eg, antihypertensives) or "per course" of short-term therapy (eg, antibiotics). Codes are calculated using average wholesale prices (at press time in US dollars) for the most common indication and route of each drug at a typical adult dosage. For maintenance therapy, costs are calculated based upon a 30-day supply or the quantity that might typically be used in a given month. For short-term therapy (ie, 10 days or less), costs are calculated on a single treatment course. When multiple forms are available (eg, generics), these codes reflect the least expensive generally available product. When drugs don't neatly fit into the classification scheme above, we have assigned codes based upon the relative cost of other similar drugs. *These codes should be used as a rough guide only*, as (1) they reflect cost, not charges, (2) pricing often varies substantially from location to location and time to time, and (3) HMOs, Medicaid, and buying groups often negotiate quite different pricing. Check with your local pharmacy if you have any questions.

Code	Cost
$	< $25
$$	$25 to $49
$$$	$50 to $99
$$$$	$100 to $199
$$$$$	≥ $200

🍁 CANADIAN TRADE NAMES: Unique common Canadian trade names not used in the US are listed after a maple leaf symbol. Trade names used in both nations or only in the US are displayed without such notation.

ABBREVIATIONS IN TEXT

AAP – American Academy of Pediatrics
ac – before meals
ADHD – attention deficit hyperactivity disorder
AHA – American Heart Association
Al – aluminum
ANC – absolute neutrophil count
ASA – aspirin
bid – twice per day
BP – blood pressure
BPH – benign prostatic hyperplasia
Ca – calcium
CAD – coronary artery disease
cap – capsule
cm – centimeter
CMV – cytomegalovirus
CNS – central nervous system
COPD – chronic obstructive pulmonary disease
CrCl – creatinine clearance
CVA – stroke
CYP – cytochrome P450
D5W – 5% dextrose
dL – deciliter
DPI – dry powder inhaler
ECG – electrocardiogram
EPS – extrapyramidal symptoms
ET – endotracheal
g – gram
GERD – gastroesophageal reflux disease
gtts – drops
GU – genitourinary
h – hour
HAART – highly active antiretroviral therapy
Hb – hemoglobin
HCTZ – hydrochlorothiazide
HIT – heparin-induced thrombocytopenia
hs – bedtime
HSV – herpes simplex virus
HTN – hypertension
IM – intramuscular
INR – international normalized ratio
IU – international units
IV – intravenous
JRA – juvenile rheumatoid arthritis
kg – kilogram
lbs – pounds
LFT – liver function test
LV – left ventricular
LVEF – left ventricular ejection fraction
m^2 – sqaure meters
MAOI – monoamine oxidase inhibitor
mcg – microgram
MDI – metered dose inhaler
mEq – milliequivalent
mg – milligram
Mg – magnesium
MI – myocardial infarction
min – minute
mL – milliliter
mm – millimeter
mo – months old
MOA – Mechanism of Action
MRSA – methicillin-resistant *Staphylococcus aureus*
ng – nanogram
NHLBI – National Heart, Lung, and Blood Institute
NS – normal saline
N/V – nausea/vomiting
NYHA – New York Heart Association
OA – osteoarthritis
oz – ounces
pc – after meals
PO – by mouth
PR – by rectum
prn – as needed
q – every
qam – every morning
qhs – at bedtime
qid – four times/day
qod – every other day
qpm – every evening
RA – rheumatoid arthritis
RSV – respiratory synctial virus
SC – subcutaneous
sec – second
soln – solution
supp – suppository
susp – suspension
tab – tablet
TB – tuberculosis
TCA – tricyclic antidepressant
tid – three times/day
TNF – tumor necrosis factor
TPN – total parenteral nutrition
UTI – urinary tract infection
wt – weight
y – year
yo – years old

THERAPEUTIC DRUG LEVELS

Drug	Level	Optimal Timing
amikacin peak	20–35 mcg/mL	30 minutes after infusion
amikacin trough	<5 mcg/mL	Just prior to next dose
carbamazepine trough	4–12 mcg/mL	Just prior to next dose
cyclosporine trough	50–300 ng/mL	Just prior to next dose
digoxin	0.8–2.0 ng/mL	Just prior to next dose
ethosuximide trough	40–100 mcg/mL	Just prior to next dose
gentamicin peak	5–10 mcg/mL	30 minutes after infusion
gentamicin trough	<2 mcg/mL	Just prior to next dose
lidocaine	1.5–5 mcg/mL	12–24 hours after start of infusion
lithium trough	0.6–1.2 meq/l	Just prior to first morning dose
NAPA	10–30 mcg/mL	Just prior to next procainamide dose
phenobarbital trough	15–40 mcg/mL	Just prior to next dose
phenytoin trough	10–20 mcg/mL	Just prior to next dose
primidone trough	5–12 mcg/mL	Just prior to next dose
procainamide	4–10 mcg/mL	Just prior to next dose
quinidine	2–5 mcg/mL	Just prior to next dose
theophylline	5–15 mcg/mL	8–12 hours after once daily dose
tobramycin peak	5–10 mcg/mL	30 minutes after infusion
tobramycin trough	<2 mcg/mL	Just prior to next dose
valproate trough (epilepsy)	50–100 mcg/mL	Just prior to next dose
valproate trough (mania)	45–125 mcg/mL	Just prior to next dose
vancomycin trough[1]	10–20 mg/L	Just prior to next dose
zonisamide[2]	10–40 mcg/mL	Just prior to dose

[1]Maintain trough >10 mg/L to avoid resistance; optimal trough for complicated infections is 15–20 mg/L
[2]Ranges not firmly established but supported by clinical trial results

Outpatient Pediatric Drugs

PEDIATRIC DRUGS	Age	2mo	4mo	6mo	9mo	12mo	15mo	2yo	3yo	5yo
	Kg	5	6½	8	9	10	11	13	15	19
	Lbs	11	15	17	20	22	24	28	33	42
med / strength / freq		\multicolumn{9}{l}{*teaspoons of liquid per dose* (1 tsp= 5 mL)}
Tylenol (mg) / / q4h		80	80	120	120	160	160	200	240	280
Tylenol (tsp) / 160/t / q4h		½	½	¾	¾	1	1	1¼	1½	1¾
ibuprofen (mg) / / q6h		-	-	75†	75†	100	100	125	150	175
ibuprofen (tsp) / 100/t / q6h		-	-	¾†	¾†	1	1	1¼	1½	1¾
amoxicillin or / 125/t / bid		1	1¼	1½	1¾	1¾	2	2¼	2¾	3½
Augmentin / 200/t / bid		½	¾	1	1	1¼	1¼	1½	1¾	2¼
(not otitis media) / 250/t / bid		½	½	¾	¾	1	1	1¼	1¼	1¾
/ 400/t / bid		¼	½	½	½	¾	¾	¾	1	1
amoxicillin, / 200/t / bid		1	1¼	1¾	2	2	2¼	2¾	3	4
(otitis media)‡ / 250/t / bid		¾	1¼	1½	1½	1¾	1¾	2¼	2½	3¼
/ 400/t / bid		½	¾	¾	1	1	1¼	1½	1½	2
Augmentin ES‡ / 600/t / bid		?	½	½	¾	¾	¾	1	1¼	1½
azithromycin*§ / 100/t / qd		¼†	½†	½	½	½	½	¾	¾	1
(5-day Rx) / 200/t / qd		--	¼†	¼	¼	¼	¼	½	½	½
Bactrim/Septra / --- / bid		½	¾	1	1	1	1¼	1½	1½	2
cefaclor* / 125/t / bid		1	1	1¼	1½	1½	1¾	2	2½	3
" / 250/t / bid		½	½	¾	¾	¾	1	1	1¼	1½
cefadroxil / 125/t / bid		½	¾	1	1	1¼	1¼	1½	1¾	2¼
" / 250/t / bid		¼	½	½	½	¾	¾	¾	1	1
cefdinir / 125/t / qd		--	¾†	1	1	1	1¼	1½	1¾	2
cefixime / 100/t / qd		½	½	¾	¾	¾	1	1	1¼	1½
cefprozil* / 125/t / bid		--	¾†	1	1	1¼	1½	1½	2	2¼
" / 250/t / bid		--	½†	½	½	¾	¾	¾	1	1¼
cefuroxime / 125/t / bid		--	¾	¾	1	1	1	1½	1¾	2¼
cephalexin / 125/t / qid		--	½	¾	¾	1	1	1¼	1½	1¾
" / 250/t / qid		--	¼	¼	½	½	½	¾	¾	1
clarithromycin / 125/t / bid		½†	½†	½	½	¾	¾	¾	1	1¼
" / 250/t / bid		--	--	--	¼	½	½	½	½	¾
dicloxacillin / 62½/t / qid		½	¾	1	1	1¼	1¼	1½	1¾	2
nitrofurantoin / 25/t / qid		¼	½	½	½	½	¾	¾	¾	1
Pediazole / --- / tid		½	½	¾	¾	1	1	1	1¼	1½
penicillin V** / 250/t / bid-tid		--	1	1	1	1	1	1	1	1
cetirizine / 5/t / qd		-	-	½	½	½	½	½	½	½
Benadryl / 12.5/t / q6h		½	½	¾	¾	1	1	1¼	1½	2
prednisolone / 15/t / qd		¼	½	½	¾	¾	¾	1	1	1¼
prednisone / 5/t / qd		1	1¼	1½	1¾	2	2¼	2½	3	3¾
Robitussin / --- / q4h		-	-	¼†	¼†	½	½	¾	¾	1
Tylenol w/ codeine / / q4h		-	-	-	-	-	-	-	1	1

* Dose shown is for otitis media only; see dosing in text for alternative indications.
† Dosing at this age/weight not recommended by manufacturer.
‡ AAP now recommends high dose (80-90 mg/kg/d) for all otitis media in children; with Augmentin used as ES only.
§Give a double dose of azithromycin the first day.
**AHA dosing for streptococcal pharyngitis. Treat for 10 days.

tsp = teaspoon; t = teaspoon; q = every; h = hour; kg = kilogram; Lbs = pounds; ml = mililiter; bid = twice per day; qd = every day; qid = four times per day; tid = three times per day

PEDIATRIC VITAL SIGNS AND INTRAVENOUS DRUGS

Age		Pre-matr	New-born	2m	4m	6m	9m	12m	15m	2y	3y	5y
Weight	(Kg)	2	3½	5	6½	8	9	10	11	13	15	19
	(Lbs)	4½	7½	11	15	17	20	22	24	28	33	42
Maint fluids	(mL/h)	8	14	20	26	32	36	40	42	46	50	58
ET tube	(mm)	2½	3/3½	3½	3½	3½	4	4	4½	4½	4½	5
Defib	(Joules)	4	7	10	13	16	18	20	22	26	30	38
Systolic BP	(high)	70	80	85	90	95	100	103	104	106	109	114
	(low)	40	60	70	70	70	70	70	70	75	75	80
Pulse rate	(high)	145	145	180	180	180	160	160	160	150	150	135
	(low)	100	100	110	110	110	100	100	100	90	90	65
Resp rate	(high)	60	60	50	50	50	46	46	30	30	25	25
	(low)	35	30	30	30	24	24	20	20	20	20	20
adenosine	(mg)	0.2	0.3	0.5	0.6	0.8	0.9	1	1.1	1.3	1.5	1.9
atropine	(mg)	0.1	0.1	0.1	0.13	0.16	0.18	0.2	0.22	0.26	0.30	0.38
Benadryl	(mg)	-	-	5	6½	8	9	10	11	13	15	19
bicarbonate	(meq)	2	3½	5	6½	8	9	10	11	13	15	19
dextrose	(g)	1	2	5	6½	8	9	10	11	13	15	19
epinephrine	(mg)	.02	.04	.05	.07	.08	.09	0.1	0.11	0.13	0.15	0.19
lidocaine	(mg)	2	3½	5	6½	8	9	10	11	13	15	19
morphine	(mg)	0.2	0.3	0.5	0.6	0.8	0.9	1	1.1	1.3	1.5	1.9
mannitol	(g)	2	3½	5	6½	8	9	10	11	13	15	19
naloxone	(mg)	.02	.04	.05	.07	.08	.09	0.1	0.11	0.13	0.15	0.19
diazepam	(mg)	0.6	1	1.5	2	2.5	2.7	3	3.3	3.9	4.5	5
fosphenytoin*	(PE)	40	70	100	130	160	180	200	220	260	300	380
lorazepam	(mg)	0.1	0.2	0.3	0.35	0.4	0.5	0.5	0.6	0.7	0.8	1.0
phenobarb	(mg)	30	60	75	100	125	125	150	175	200	225	275
phenytoin*	(mg)	40	70	100	130	160	180	200	220	260	300	380
ampicillin	(mg)	100	175	250	325	400	450	500	550	650	750	1000
ceftriaxone	(mg)	-	-	250	325	400	450	500	550	650	750	1000
cefotaxime	(mg)	100	175	250	325	400	450	500	550	650	750	1000
gentamicin	(mg)	5	8	12	16	20	22	25	27	32	37	47

*Loading doses; fosphenytoin dosed in "phenytoin equivalents."

CONVERSIONS

Temperature:
F = (1.8) C + 32
C = (F – 32)/1.8

Liquid:
1 fluid ounce = 30 mL
1 teaspoon = 5 mL
1 tablespoon = 15 mL

Weight:
1 kilogram = 2.2 lbs
1 ounce = 30 g
1 grain = 65 mg

INHIBITORS, INDUCERS, AND SUBSTRATES OF CYTOCHROME P450 ISOZYMES

The cytochrome P450 (CYP) inhibitors and inducers below do not necessarily cause clinically important interactions with substrates listed. Underlined drugs have shown potential for important interactions in human case reports or clinical studies. We exclude in vitro data which can be inaccurate. Refer to the *Tarascon Pocket Pharmacopoeia* drug interactions database (PDA edition) or other resources for more information if an interaction is suspected based on this chart. A drug that inhibits CYP subfamily activity can block the metabolism of substrates of that enzyme and substrate accumulation and toxicity may result. CYP inhibitors are classified by how much they increase the area-under-the-curve (AUC) of a substrate: weak (1.25-2 fold), moderate (2–5 fold), or strong (≥5 fold). A drug is considered a sensitive substrate if a CYP inhibitor increases the AUC of that drug by ≥5-fold. While AUC increases of >50% often do not affect patient response, smaller increases can be important if the therapeutic range is narrow (eg, theophylline, warfarin, cyclosporine). A drug that induces CYP subfamily activity increases substrate metabolism and reduced substrate efficacy may result. This table may be incomplete since new evidence about drug interactions is continually being identified.

CYP1A2

Inhibitors. *Strong*: fluvoxamine. *Moderate*: ciprofloxacin, mexiletine, propafenone, zileuton. *Weak*: acyclovir, cimetidine, famotidine, norfloxacin, verapamil. *Unclassified*: amiodarone, atazanavir, citalopram, clarithromycin, erythromycin, estradiol, ipriflavone, isoniazid, paroxetine, peginterferon alfa-2a, tacrine, ziprasidone.
Inducers: barbiturates, carbamazepine, charcoal-broiled foods, rifampin, ritonavir, smoking, tipranavir/ritonavir.
Substrates. *Sensitive*: alosetron, asenapine, duloxetine, tizanidine. *Unclassified*: acetaminophen, amitriptyline, bendamustine, caffeine, cinacalcet, clomipramine, clozapine, cyclobenzaprine, estradiol, fluvoxamine, haloperidol, imipramine, lidocaine, mexiletine, mirtazapine, naproxen, olanzapine, ondansetron, propranolol, rameleton, rasagiline, riluzole, ropinirole, ropivacaine, R-warfarin, tacrine, theophylline, verapamil, zileuton, zolmitriptan.

CYP2B6

Inhibitors: clopidogrel, ticlopidine. *Weak*: prasugrel.
Inducers. *Strong*: rifampin. *Unclassified*: baicalin (ingredient of Limbrel), efavirenz, nevirapine.
Substrates: bupropion, cyclophosphamide, efavirenz, methadone, nevirapine, prasugrel.

CYP 2C8

Inhibitors. *Strong*: gemfibrozil. *Weak*: trimethoprim.
Inducers: barbiturates, carbamazepine, rifabutin, rifampin.
Substrates. *Sensitive*: repaglinide. *Unclassified*: amiodarone, carbamazepine, ibuprofen, isotretinoin, loperamide, paclitaxel, pioglitazone, rosiglitazone.

CYP 2C9

Inhibitors. *Moderate*: amiodarone, fluconazole, oxandrolone. *Weak*: ketoconazole. *Unclassified*: atazanavir, cimetidine, cotrimoxazole, delavirdine, etravirine, fenofibrate, fenofibric acid, fluorouracil, fluvoxamine, imatinib, isoniazid, leflunomide, metronidazole, miconazole, sulfamethoxazole, voriconazole, zafirlukast.
Inducers: aprepitant, barbiturates, bosentan, carbamazepine, rifampin, rifapentine, St John's wort.
Substrates. *Sensitive*: Flurbiprofen. *Unclassified*: alosetron, bosentan, celecoxib, chlorpropamide, diclofenac, etravirine, fluoxetine, fluvastatin, formoterol, glimepiride, glipizide, glyburide, ibuprofen, irbesartan, losartan, mefenamic acid, meloxicam, montelukast, naproxen, nateglinide, phenytoin, piroxicam, rameleton, rosiglitazone, rosuvastatin, sildenafil, tolbutamide, torsemide, vardenafil, voriconazole, S-warfarin, zafirlukast, zileuton.

CYP 2C19

Inhibitors. *Strong*: omeprazole. *Unclassified*: armodafinil, chloramphenicol, delavirdine, esomeprazole, etravirine, felbamate, fluconazole, fluoxetine, fluvoxamine, isoniazid, moclobamide, modafinil, oxcarbazepine, ticlopidine, voriconazole.
Inducers. *Moderate*: tipranavir/ritonavir. *Unclassified*: rifampin, St John's wort.
Substrates. *Sensitive*: omeprazole. *Unclassified*: amitriptyline, arformoterol, bortezomib, carisoprodol, cilostazol, citalopram, clomipramine, clopidogrel, clozapine, cyclophosphamide, desipramine, dexlansoprazole, diazepam, escitalopram, esomeprazole, etravirine, formoterol, imipramine, lacosamide, lansoprazole, methadone, moclobamide, nelfinavir, pantoprazole, phenytoin, progesterone, proguanil, propranolol, rabeprazole, voriconazole, R-warfarin.

CYP 2D6

Inhibitors. *Strong*: cinacalcet, fluoxetine, paroxetine, quinidine, tipranavir/ritonavir. *Moderate*: dronedarone, duloxetine, sertraline, terbinafine. *Weak*: amiodarone, asenapine, citalopram, desvenlafaxine, escitalopram, fluvoxamine, venlafaxine. *Unclassified*: chloroquine, cimetidine, clomipramine, delavirdine, diphenhydramine, fluphenazine, haloperidol, hydroxychloroquine, imatinib, lumefantrine, metoclopramide, moclobamide, perphenazine, propafenone, propoxyphene, quinine, ritonavir, tolterodine, thioridazine.
Inducers: None
Substrates. *Sensitive*: desipramine. *Unclassified*: almotriptan, amitriptyline, arformoterol, aripiprazole, atomoxetine, carvedilol, cevimeline, chlorpheniramine, chlorpromazine, cinacalcet, clomipramine, clozapine, codeine*, darifenacin, delavirdine, dextromethorphan, dihydrocodeine, dolasetron, donepezil, doxepin, duloxetine, fesoterodine, flecainide, fluoxetine, formoterol, galantamine, haloperidol, hydrocodone, iloperidone, imipramine, loratadine, maprotiline, methadone, methamphetamine, metoclopramide, metoprolol, mexiletine, mirtazapine, morphine, nebivolol, nortriptyline, ondansetron, paroxetine, perphenazine, promethazine, propafenone, propranolol, quetiapine, risperidone, ritonavir, tamoxifen, tetrabenazine, thioridazine, timolol, tolterodine, tramadol*, trazodone, venlafaxine.

CYP 3A4

Inhibitors. *Strong*: atazanavir, clarithromycin, indinavir, itraconazole, ketoconazole, nefazodone, nelfinavir, posaconazole, ritonavir, saquinavir, telithromycin, tipranavir/ritonavir, voriconazole. *Moderate*: amprenavir, aprepitant, diltiazem, dronedarone, erythromycin, fluconazole, fosamprenavir, grapefruit juice (variable), verapamil. *Weak*: cimetidine. *Unclassified*: amiodarone, conivaptan, cyclosporine, danazol, darunavir, delavirdine, ethinyl estradiol, fluoxetine, fluvoxamine, imatinib, miconazole, sertraline, quinupristin/dalfopristin, zafirlukast.
Inducers. *Strong*: efavirenz, nevirapine, rifampin. *Unclassified*: armodafinil, artemether, barbiturates, bexarotene, bosentan, carbamazepine, dexamethasone, ethosuximide, etravirine, griseofulvin, modafinil, nafcillin, oxcarbazepine, phenytoin, primidone, rifabutin, rifapentine, ritonavir, rufinamide, St Johns wort.
Substrates. *Sensitive*: budesonide, buspirone, conivaptan, eletriptan, eplerenone, felodipine, fluticasone, lovastatin, midazolam, saquinavir, sildenafil, simvastatin, triazolam, vardenafil. *Unclassified*: alfentanil, alfuzosin, aliskiren, almotriptan, alosetron, alprazolam, amiodarone, amlodipine, amprenavir, aprepitant, argatroban, aripiprazole, armodafinil, artemether-lumefantrine, atazanavir, atorvastatin, bexarotene, bortezomib, bosentan, bromocriptine, buprenorphine, carbamazepine, cevimeline, cilostazol, cinacalcet, cisapride, citalopram, clarithromycin, clomipramine, clonazepam, clopidogrel, colchicine, clozapine, corticosteroids, cyclophosphamide, cyclosporine, dapsone, darifenacin, darunavir, dasatinib, delavirdine, desogestrel, desvenlafaxine, dexamethasone, dexlansoprazole, diazepam, dienogest, dihydroergotamine, diltiazem, disopyramide, docetaxel, dofetilide, dolasetron, domperidone, donepezil, doxorubicin, dronedarone, dutasteride, efavirenz, ergotamine, erlotinib, erythromycin†, escitalopram, esomeprazole, eszopiclone, ethinyl estradiol, etoposide, etravirine, fentanyl, fesoterodine, finasteride, fluconazole, fosaprepitant, galantamine, gefitinib, glyburide, guanfacine, haloperidol, hydrocodone, ifosfamide, iloperidone, imatinib, imipramine, indinavir, irinotecan, isradipine, itraconazole, ixabepilone, ketoconazole, lansoprazole, lapatinib, letrozole, lidocaine, loperamide, lopinavir, loratadine, maraviroc, methylergonovine, mifepristone, mirtazapine, modafinil, mometasone, montelukast, nateglinide, nefazodone, nelfinavir, nevirapine, nicardipine, nifedipine, nilotinib, nimodipine, nisoldipine, ondansetron, oxybutynin, oxycodone, paclitaxel, pantoprazole, pazopanib, pimozide, pioglitazone, prasugrel, praziquantel, propoxyphene, quetiapine, quinidine, quinine, rabeprazole, ramelteon, ranolazine, repaglinide, rifabutin, rifampin, risperidone, ritonavir, romidepsin, ropivacaine, saxagliptin, sertraline, sibutramine, silodosin, sirolimus, solifenacin, sorafenib, sufentanil, sunitinib, tacrolimus, tadalafil, tamoxifen, telithromycin, temsirolimus, testosterone, tiagabine, tinidazole, tipranavir, tolterodine, tolvaptan, tramadol, trazodone, venlafaxine, verapamil, vinblastine, vincristine, vinorelbine, voriconazole, R-warfarin, zaleplon, ziprasidone, zolpidem, zonisamide.

* Metabolism by CYP2D6 required to convert to active analgesic metabolite; analgesia may be impaired by CYP2D6 inhibitors.
† Risk of sudden death may be increased in patients receiving erythromycin concurrently with CYP 3A4 inhibitors like ketoconazole, itraconazole, fluconazole, diltiazem, verapamil, and troleandomycin (*NEJM* 2004;351:1089).

FORMULAS

Alveolar-arterial oxygen gradient = A-a = 148 − 1.2(PaCO2) − PaO2
[normal = 10-20 mmHg, breathing room air at sea level]

Calculated osmolality = 2Na + glucose/18 + BUN/2.8 + ethanol/4.6
[norm 280-295 meq/L. Na in meq/L; all others in mg/dL]

Pediatric IV maintenance fluids (see table on page xi)
4 mL/kg/hr **or** 100 mL/kg/day for first 10 kg, plus
2 mL/kg/hr **or** 50 mL/kg/day for second 10 kg, plus
1 mL/kg/hr **or** 20 mL/kg/day for all further kg

$$\text{mcg/kg/min} = \frac{16.7 \times \text{drug conc [mg/mL]} \times \text{infusion rate [mL/h]}}{\text{weight [kg]}}$$

$$\text{Infusion rate [mL/h]} = \frac{\text{desired mcg/kg/min} \times \text{weight [kg]} \times 60}{\text{drug concentration [mcg/mL]}}$$

Fractional excretion of sodium = $\left[\dfrac{\text{urine Na / plasma Na}}{\text{urine creat / plasma creat}}\right] \times 100\%$
[Pre-renal, etc <1%; ATN, etc >1%]

Anion gap = Na − (Cl + HCO3)   [normal = 10-14 meq/L]

Creatinine clearance = $\dfrac{(\text{lean kg})(140 - \text{age})(0.85 \text{ if female})}{(72)(\text{stable creatinine [mg/dL]})}$
[normal >80]

Glomerular filtration rate using MDRD equation (mL/min/1.73 m^2)
= 186 × (creatinine)$^{-1.154}$ × (age)$^{-0.203}$ × (0.742 if ♀) × (1.210 if African American)

Body surface area (BSA) = square root of: $\left[\dfrac{\text{height (cm)} \times \text{weight (kg)}}{3600}\right]$
[in m^2]

DRUG THERAPY REFERENCE WEBSITES FORMULAS (selected)

Professional societies or governmental agencies with drug therapy guidelines		
AAP	American Academy of Pediatrics	www.aap.org
ACC	American College of Cardiology	www.acc.org
ACCP	American College of Chest Physicians	www.chestnet.org
ACCP	American College of Clinical Pharmacy	www.accp.com
ADA	American Diabetes Association	www.diabetes.org
AHA	American Heart Association	www.americanheart.org
AHRQ	Agency for Healthcare Research and Quality	www.ahcpr.gov
AMA	American Medical Association	www.ama-assn.org
APA	American Psychiatric Association	www.psych.org
APA	American Psychological Association	www.apa.org
ASHP	Amer. Society Health-Systems Pharmacists	www.ashp.org
ATS	American Thoracic Society	www.thoracic.org
CDC	Centers for Disease Control and Prevention	www.cdc.gov
CDC	CDC bioterrorism and radiation exposures	www.bt.cdc.gov
IDSA	Infectious Diseases Society of America	www.idsociety.org
MHA	Malignant Hyperthermia Association	www.mhaus.org
NHLBI	National Heart, Lung, and Blood Institute	www.nhlbi.nih.gov
Other therapy reference sites		
Cochrane library		www.cochrane.org
Emergency Contraception Website		www.not-2-late.com
Immunization Action Coalition		www.immunize.org
Int'l Registry for Drug-Induced Arrhythmias		www.qtdrugs.org
Managing Contraception		www.managingcontraception.com
Nephrology Pharmacy Associates		www.nephrologypharmacy.com

CORONARY ARTERY DISEASE 10-YEAR RISK

Framingham model for calculating 10-year risk for coronary artery disease (CAD) in patients without diabetes or clinically evident CAD. Diabetes is considered a CAD risk "equivalent", i.e., the prospective risk of CAD in diabetics is similar to those with established CAD. Automated calculator available at: http://hin.nhlbi.nih.gov/atpiii/calculator.asp?usertype=prof (NCEP, JAMA 2001; 285:2497)

MEN

Age	Points	Age	Points
20–34	-9	55–59	8
35–39	-4	60–64	10
40–44	0	65–69	11
45–49	3	70–74	12
50–54	6	75–79	13

Choles-terol*	20–39	40–49	50–59	60–69	70–79
<160	0	0	0	0	0
160–199	4	3	2	1	0
200–239	7	5	3	1	0
240–279	9	6	4	2	1
280+	11	8	5	3	1

Age (years)	20–39	40–49	50–59	60–69	70–79
Nonsmoker	0	0	0	0	0
Smoker	8	5	3	1	1

HDL mg/dL	Points	HDL mg/dL	Points
60+	-1	40–49	1
50–59	0	<40	2

Systolic BP	If Untreated	If Treated
<120 mmHg	0	0
120–129 mmHg	0	1
130–139 mmHg	1	2
140–159 mmHg	1	2
160+ mmHg	2	3

Point Total	10-Year Risk	Point Total	10-Year Risk
0	1%	9	5%
1	1%	10	6%
2	1%	11	8%
3	1%	12	10%
4	1%	13	12%
5	2%	14	16%
6	2%	15	20%
7	3%	16	25%
8	4%	17+	30+%

WOMEN

Age	Points	Age	Points
20–34	-7	55–59	8
35–39	-3	60–64	10
40–44	0	65–69	12
45–49	3	70–74	14
50–54	6	75–79	16

Choles-terol*	20–39	40–49	50–59	60–69	70–79
<160	0	0	0	0	0
160–199	4	3	2	1	1
200–239	8	6	4	2	1
240–279	11	8	5	3	2
280+	13	10	7	4	2

*Total in mg/dL

Age (years)	20–39	40–49	50–59	60–69	70–79
Nonsmoker	0	0	0	0	0
Smoker	9	7	4	2	1

HDL mg/dL	Points	HDL mg/dL	Points
60+	-1	40–49	1
50–59	0	<40	2

Systolic BP	If Untreated	If Treated
<120 mmHg	0	0
120–129 mmHg	1	3
130–139 mmHg	2	4
140–159 mmHg	3	5
160+ mmHg	4	6

Point Total	10-Year Risk	Point Total	10-Year Risk
<9	<1%	17	5%
9	1%	18	6%
10	1%	19	8%
11	1%	20	11%
12	1%	21	14%
13	2%	22	17%
14	2%	23	22%
15	3%	24	27%
16	4%	25+	30+%

ANALGESICS: Antirheumatic Agents

ANALGESICS: Antirheumatic Agents—Biologic Response Modifiers

NOTE: Death, sepsis, and serious infections (eg, TB and invasive fungal infections) have been reported. Do not start if current serious infection, discontinue if serious infection develops, and closely monitor for any new infection. Screening for latent TB infection is recommended. Use caution if history of recurring infections or with underlying conditions (eg, DM) that predispose to infections. Combination use of these drugs increases the risk of serious infection and is contraindicated.

ABATACEPT (*Orencia*) ▶Serum ♀C ▶? $$$$$
- WARNING — Do not use with TNF-blocking drugs such as adalimumab, etanercept, or infliximab or the IL-1 receptor antagonist anakinra.
- ADULTS — RA: Specialized dosing.
- PEDS — Juvenile idiopathic arthritis age 6 yo or greater: Specialized dosing.
- NOTES — Monitor patients with COPD for exacerbation and pulmonary infections. Avoid live vaccines.
- MOA — Inhibits production of tumor necrosis factor-alpha, interleukin-2 and interferon-gamma.
- ADVERSE EFFECTS — Serious: Infection, malignancies, hypersensitivity. Frequent: Headache, pharyngitis, nausea.

ADALIMUMAB (*Humira*) ▶Serum ♀B ▶– $$$$$
- WARNING — Hypersensitivity. Combination use with other immunomodulators increases the risk of serious infections. Aplastic anemia, thrombocytopenia and leukopenia. Rare CNS disorders (eg, multiple sclerosis, myelitis, optic neuritis) have been reported. May worsen heart failure; monitor signs/symptoms of heart failure.
- ADULTS — RA, psoriatic arthritis, ankylosing spondylitis: 40 mg SC q 2 weeks, alone or in combination with methotrexate or other disease-modifying antirheumatic drugs (DMARDs). May increase frequency to q week if not on methotrexate. Crohn's disease: 160 mg SC at weeks 0, 80 mg at week 2, then 40 mg q other week starting with week 4.
- PEDS — Not approved in children.
- FORMS — Trade only: 40 mg prefilled glass syringes or vials with needles, 2 per pack.
- NOTES — Monitor CBC. Refrigerate and protect from light. Avoid live vaccines. Do not use in combination with anakinra.
- MOA — Monoclonal antibody that blocks tumor necrosis factor - alpha.
- ADVERSE EFFECTS — Serious: Hypersensitivity, infection, lymphoma, lupus-like syndrome, aplastic anemia, thrombocytopenia, and leukopenia. Frequent: Injection site reaction.

ANAKINRA (*Kineret*) ▶K ♀B ▶? $$$$$
- WARNING — Increased incidence of serious infections. Do not use in active infection or with other immunomodulators.
- ADULTS — RA: 100 mg SC daily, alone or in combination with other disease-modifying antirheumatic drugs (DMARDs) except TNF inhibitors.
- PEDS — Not approved in children.
- FORMS — Trade only: 100 mg prefilled glass syringes with needles, 7 or 28 per box.
- NOTES — Monitor for neutropenia. Refrigerate and protect from light. Avoid live vaccines.
- MOA — Interleukin-1 receptor antagonist.
- ADVERSE EFFECTS — Serious: Infection, neutropenia. Frequent: Injection site reaction.

ETANERCEPT (*Enbrel*) ▶Serum ♀B ▶– $$$$$
- WARNING — Combination use with other immunomodulators increases the risk of serious infections. Rare nervous system disorders (eg, multiple sclerosis, myelitis, optic neuritis) have been reported. May worsen heart failure; monitor closely.
- ADULTS — RA, psoriatic arthritis, ankylosing spondylitis: 50 mg SC q week, alone or in combination with methotrexate. Plaque psoriasis: 50 mg SC twice per week for 3 months, then 50 mg SC q week.
- PEDS — JRA age 4 to 17 yo: 0.8 mg/kg SC q week, to max single dose of 50 mg.
- UNAPPROVED PEDS — Plaque psoriasis age 4 to 17 yo: 0.8 mg/kg SC q week, to max single dose of 50 mg.
- FORMS — Supplied in a carton containing four dose trays and as single-use prefilled syringes. Each dose tray contains one 25 mg single-use vial of etanercept, one syringe (1 mL sterile bacteriostatic water for injection, containing 0.9% benzyl alcohol), one plunger, and two alcohol swabs. Single-use syringes contain 50 mg/mL.
- NOTES — Appropriate SC injection sites are thigh, abdomen and upper arm. Rotate injection sites. Refrigerate. Avoid live vaccines. The needle cover contains latex; caution if allergy.
- MOA — Soluble tumor necrosis factor (TNF) receptor protein that blocks TNF-alpha and -beta.
- ADVERSE EFFECTS — Serious: Infection, CNS demyelinating disorders, lupus-like syndrome, allergic reactions. Frequent: Injection site reaction.

INFLIXIMAB (*Remicade*) ▶Serum ♀B ▶? $$$$$
- WARNING — May worsen heart failure; monitor signs/symptoms of heart failure. May increase risk of lymphoma and other malignancies; caution if history of malignancy or if malignancy develops during treatment. Hypersensitivity reactions may occur. Combination use with other immunomodulators increases the risk of serious infections. Rare CNS disorders (eg, multiple sclerosis, myelitis, optic neuritis) have been reported.
- ADULTS — RA: 3 mg/kg IV in combination with methotrexate at 0, 2 and 6 weeks. Give q 8 weeks thereafter. May increase up to 10 mg/kg or q 4 weeks if incomplete response. Ankylosing spondylitis: 5 mg/kg IV at 0, 2 and 6 weeks. Give q 6 weeks thereafter. Plaque psoriasis; psoriatic arthritis; moderately to severely active Crohn's disease, ulcerative colitis, or fistulizing disease: 5 mg/kg IV infusion at 0, 2, and 6 weeks, then q 8 weeks.
- PEDS — Moderately to severely active Crohn's disease or fistulizing disease: 5 mg/kg IV infusion at 0, 2 and 6 weeks then q 8 weeks.

(cont.)

ANALGESICS: Antirheumatic Agents

INFLIXIMAB (cont.)
UNAPPROVED ADULTS — <u>Moderate to severe ulcerative colitis:</u> Same dose as for Crohn's disease.
NOTES — Headache, dyspnea, urticaria, nausea, infections, abdominal pain, and fever. Avoid live vaccines. Three cases of toxic optic neuropathy reported. Refrigerate.

MOA — Monoclonal antibody that blocks tumor necrosis factor-alpha.
ADVERSE EFFECTS — Serious: Anaphylaxis, disseminated TB, sepsis, worsening heart failure, lupus-like syndrome, optic neuropathy. Frequent: Infusion reaction.

ANALGESICS: Antirheumatic Agents—Disease Modifying Antirheumatic Drugs (DMARDs)

AURANOFIN (*Ridaura*) ▶K ♀C ▶+ $$$$$
WARNING — Gold toxicity may manifest as marrow suppression, proteinuria, hematuria, pruritus, rash, stomatitis, or persistent diarrhea. Monitor CBC and urinary protein q 4 to 12 weeks (oral) or q 1 to 2 weeks (injectable) due to the risk of myelosuppression and proteinuria.
ADULTS — <u>RA:</u> Initial 3 mg PO bid or 6 mg PO daily. May increase to 3 mg PO tid after 6 months.
PEDS — <u>RA:</u> 0.1 to 0.15 mg/kg/day PO. Max dose 0.2 mg/kg/day. May be given daily or divided bid.
UNAPPROVED ADULTS — <u>Psoriatic arthritis:</u> 3 mg PO bid or 6 mg PO daily.
FORMS — Trade only: Caps 3 mg.
NOTES — Contraindicated in patients with a history of any of the following gold-induced disorders: Anaphylactic reactions, necrotizing enterocolitis, pulmonary fibrosis, exfoliative dermatitis, bone marrow suppression. Not recommended in pregnancy. Proteinuria has developed in 3% to 9% of patients. Diarrhea, rash, stomatitis, chrysiasis (gray-to-blue pigmentation of skin) may occur. Minimize exposure to sunlight or artificial UV light. Auranofin may increase phenytoin levels.
MOA — Decreases synovial inflammation; slows cartilage/bone destruction.
ADVERSE EFFECTS — Serious: Anaphylaxis, bone marrow suppression, proteinuria, chrysiasis (see NOTES). Frequent: Diarrhea, dermatitis, stomatitis.

AZATHIOPRINE (*Azasan, Imuran, ✽Immunoprin, Oprisine*) ▶LK ♀D ▶– $$$
WARNING — Chronic immunosuppression with azathioprine increases the risk of neoplasia. May cause marrow suppression or GI hypersensitivity reaction characterized by severe N/V.
ADULTS — <u>Severe RA:</u> Initial dose 1 mg/kg (50 to 100 mg) PO daily or divided bid. Increase by 0.5 mg/kg/day at 6 to 8 weeks; if no serious toxicity and if initial response is unsatisfactory can then increase thereafter at 4-week intervals. Max dose 2.5 mg/kg/day. In patients with clinical response, use the lowest effective dose for maintenance therapy.
PEDS — Not approved in children.
UNAPPROVED ADULTS — <u>Crohn's disease:</u> 75 to 100 mg PO daily. <u>Myasthenia gravis:</u> 2 to 3 mg/kg/day PO. <u>Behcet's syndrome,</u> <u>SLE:</u> 2.5 mg/kg/day PO. <u>Vasculitis:</u> 2 mg/kg/day PO.
UNAPPROVED PEDS — <u>JRA:</u> Initial: 1 mg/kg/day PO. Increase by 0.5 mg/kg/day q 4 weeks until response or max dose of 2.5 to 3 mg/kg/day.
FORMS — Generic/Trade: Tabs 50 mg, scored. Trade only (Azasan): 75, 100 mg, scored.
NOTES — Monitor CBC q 1 to 2 weeks with dose changes, then q 1 to 3 months. ACE inhibitors, allopurinol, and methotrexate may increase activity and toxicity. Azathioprine may decrease the activity of anticoagulants, cyclosporine, and neuromuscular blockers.
MOA — Immunosuppressant.
ADVERSE EFFECTS — Serious: Bone marrow depression, GI hypersensitivity. Frequent: Malaise, skin rash.

GOLD SODIUM THIOMALATE (*Myochrysine*) ▶K ♀C ▶+ $$$$
WARNING — Gold toxicity may manifest as marrow suppression, proteinuria, hematuria, pruritus, rash, stomatitis or persistent diarrhea. Monitor CBC and urinary protein q 4 to 12 weeks (oral) or q 1 to 2 weeks (injectable) due to the risk of myelosuppression and proteinuria.
ADULTS — <u>RA:</u> Weekly IM injections: First dose, 10 mg. Second dose, 25 mg. Third and subsequent doses, 25 to 50 mg. Continue the 25 to 50 mg dose weekly to a cumulative dose of 0.8 to 1 g. If improvement seen without toxicity, 25 to 50 mg q other week for 2 to 20 weeks. If stable, lengthen dosing intervals to q 3 to 4 weeks.
PEDS — <u>JRA:</u> Test dose 10 mg IM, then 1 mg/kg, not to exceed 50 mg for a single injection. Continue this dose weekly to a cumulative dose of 0.8 to 1 g. If improvement seen without toxicity, dose every other week for 2 to 20 weeks. If stable, lengthen dosing intervals to q 3 to 4 weeks.
UNAPPROVED ADULTS — Load as per approved, but then continue weekly up to 1 yr.
NOTES — Administer only IM, preferably intragluteally. Have patient remain recumbent for approximately 10 min after injection. Contraindicated in pregnancy and in patients who have uncontrolled DM, severe debilitation, renal disease, hepatic dysfunction or hepatitis, marked HTN, uncontrolled heart failure, SLE, blood dyscrasias, patients recently irradiated and those with severe toxicity from previous exposure to gold or other heavy metals, urticaria, eczema, and colitis. Arthralgia and dermatitis may occur.
MOA — Decreases synovial inflammation; slows cartilage/bone destruction.
ADVERSE EFFECTS — Serious: Anaphylaxis, bone marrow suppression, proteinuria. Frequent: Diarrhea, dermatitis, stomatitis.

HYDROXYCHLOROQUINE (*Plaquenil*) ▶K ♀C ▶+ $
ADULTS — RA: 400 to 600 mg PO daily to start, taken with food or milk. After clinical response, decrease to 200 to 400 mg PO daily. Discontinue if no objective improvement within 6 months. SLE: 400 mg PO daily to bid to start. Decrease to 200 to 400 PO daily for prolonged maintenance.
PEDS — Not approved in children.
UNAPPROVED PEDS — JRA or SLE: 3 to 5 mg/kg/day, up to a max of 400 mg/day PO daily or divided bid. Max dose 7 mg/kg/day. Take with food or milk.
FORMS — Generic/Trade: Tabs 200 mg, scored.
NOTES — May exacerbate psoriasis or porphyria. Irreversible retinal damage possible with long-term or high dosage (> 6.5 mg/kg/day). Baseline and periodic eye exams recommended. Anorexia, nausea and vomiting may occur. May increase digoxin and metoprolol levels.
MOA — Unclear in the treatment of RA.
ADVERSE EFFECTS — Serious: Retinopathy, angioedema, bronchospasm. Frequent: Anorexia, nausea.

LEFLUNOMIDE (*Arava*) ▶LK ♀X ▶— $$$$$
WARNING — Hepatotoxicity, interstitial lung disease. Rare reports of lymphoma, pancytopenia, agranulocytosis, thrombocytopenia, Stevens-Johnson syndrome, cutaneous necrotizing vasculitis, and severe HTN. Exclude pregnancy before starting. Women of childbearing potential must use reliable contraception.
ADULTS — RA: 100 mg PO daily for 3 days. Maintenance: 10 to 20 mg PO daily.
PEDS — Not approved in children.
UNAPPROVED ADULTS — Psoriatic arthritis: Initial: 100 mg PO daily for 3 days. Maintenance: 10 to 20 mg PO daily.
FORMS — Generic/Trade: Tabs 10, 20 mg. Trade only: Tabs 100 mg.
NOTES — Avoid in hepatic or renal insufficiency, severe immunodeficiency, bone marrow dysplasia, or severe infections. Consider interruption of therapy if serious infection occurs and administer cholestyramine (see below). Monitor LFTs, CBC, and creatinine monthly until stable, then q 1 to 2 months. Avoid in men wishing to father children or with concurrent live vaccines. May increase INR if on warfarin; check INR within 1 to 2 days of initiation, then weekly for 2 to 3 weeks and adjust the dose accordingly. Rifampin increases and cholestyramine decreases leflunomide levels. Give charcoal or cholestyramine in cases of overdose or drug toxicity. Cholestyramine: 8 g PO tid for up to 11 days. Activated charcoal: 50 g PO or NG q 6 h for 24 h. Administration on consecutive days is not necessary unless rapid elimination desired.
MOA — Immunosuppressant.
ADVERSE EFFECTS — Serious: Lymphoma, pancytopenia, Stevens-Johnson Syndrome, hepatotoxicity, interstitial lung disease, cutaneous necrotizing vasculitis. Frequent: Diarrhea.

METHOTREXATE (*Rheumatrex, Trexall*) ▶LK ♀X ▶— $$
WARNING — Deaths have occurred from hepatotoxicity, pulmonary disease, intestinal perforation and marrow suppression. According to the manufacturer, use is restricted to patients with severe, recalcitrant, disabling rheumatic disease unresponsive to other therapy. Use with extreme caution in renal insufficiency. May see diarrhea. Folate deficiency states may increase toxicity. The American College of Rheumatology recommends supplementation with 1 mg/day of folic acid.
ADULTS — Severe RA, psoriasis: 7.5 mg/week PO single dose or 2.5 mg PO q 12 h for 3 doses given as a course once weekly. May be increased gradually to a max weekly dose of 20 mg. After clinical response, reduce to lowest effective dose. Psoriasis: 10 to 25 mg weekly IV/IM until response, then decrease to lowest effective dose. Supplement with 1 mg/day of folic acid. Chemotherapy doses vary by indication.
PEDS — Severe JRA: 10 mg/meters 2 PO q week. Chemotherapy doses vary by indication.
UNAPPROVED ADULTS — Severe RA, psoriasis: 25 mg PO q week. After clinical response, reduce to lowest effective dose. Supplement with 1 mg/day of folic acid. Nonmetastatic osteosarcoma with leucovorin rescue.
FORMS — Trade only (Trexall): Tabs 5, 7.5, 10, 15 mg. Dose Pak (Rheumatrex) 2.5 mg (# 8, 12, 16, 20, 24). Generic/Trade: Tabs 2.5 mg, scored.
NOTES — Contraindicated in pregnant and lactating women, alcoholism, liver disease, immunodeficiency, blood dyscrasias. Avoid ethanol. Monitor CBC q month, liver and renal function q 1 to 3 months.
MOA — Immunosuppressant, antimetabolite.
ADVERSE EFFECTS — Serious: Hepatotoxicity, pulmonary disease, lymphoma, bone marrow suppression, intestinal perforation. Frequent: Increased LFTs, diarrhea, stomatitis, bone marrow suppression.

ANALGESICS: Muscle Relaxants

NOTE: May cause drowsiness and/or sedation, which may be enhanced by alcohol and other CNS depressants.

BACLOFEN (*Lioresal, Kemstro*) ▶K ♀C ▶+ $$
WARNING — Abrupt discontinuation of intrathecal baclofen has been associated with life-threatening sequelae and/or death.
ADULTS — Spasticity related to MS or spinal cord disease/injury: 5 mg PO tid for 3 days, 10 mg PO tid for 3 days, 15 mg PO tid for 3 days, then 20 mg PO tid for 3 days. Max dose: 20 mg PO qid. Spasticity related to spinal cord disease/injury, unresponsive to oral therapy: Specialized dosing via implantable intrathecal pump.
PEDS — Spasticity related to spinal cord disease/injury: Specialized dosing via implantable intrathecal pump.

(cont.)

ANALGESICS: Muscle Relaxants

BACLOFEN (cont.)
UNAPPROVED ADULTS — Trigeminal neuralgia: 30 to 80 mg/day PO divided tid to qid. Tardive dyskinesia: 40 to 60 mg/day PO divided tid to qid. Intractable hiccups: 15 to 45 mg PO divided tid.
UNAPPROVED PEDS — Spasticity age 2 yo or order: 10 to 15 mg/day PO divided q 8 h. Max doses 40 mg/day for age 2 to 7 yo, 60 mg/day for age 8 yo or older.
FORMS — Generic only: Tabs 10, 20 mg. Trade only (Kemstro): Tabs, orally disintegrating 10, 20 mg.
NOTES — Hallucinations and seizures with abrupt withdrawal. Administer with caution if impaired renal function. Efficacy not established for rheumatic disorders, CVA, cerebral palsy, or Parkinson's disease.
MOA — Skeletal muscle relaxant.
ADVERSE EFFECTS — Serious: Hallucinations and seizures with abrupt withdrawal. Frequent: Hypotonia, somnolence, dizziness.

CARISOPRODOL (*Soma*) ▶LK ♀? ▶– $
ADULTS — Acute musculoskeletal pain: 350 mg PO tid to qid with meals and at bedtime.
PEDS — Not approved in children.
FORMS — Generic/Trade: Tabs 350 mg. Trade only: Tabs 250 mg.
NOTES — Contraindicated in porphyria, caution in renal or hepatic insufficiency. Abuse potential. Use with caution if addiction-prone. Withdrawal and possible seizures with abrupt discontinuation. Sedative effects can result in impair driving.
MOA — Skeletal muscle relaxant.
ADVERSE EFFECTS — Serious: Idiosyncratic reaction with angioedema, hypotension, and anaphylactoid shock. Frequent: Dizziness and drowsiness.

CHLORZOXAZONE (*Parafon Forte DSC*) ▶LK ♀C ▶? $
WARNING — If signs/symptoms of liver dysfunction are observed, discontinue use.
ADULTS — Musculoskeletal pain: Start 500 mg PO tid to qid, increase prn to 750 mg tid to qid. After clinical improvement, decrease to 250 mg PO tid to qid.
PEDS — Not approved in children.
UNAPPROVED PEDS — Musculoskeletal pain: 125 to 500 mg PO tid to qid or 20 mg/kg/day divided tid to qid depending on age and wt.
FORMS — Generic/Trade: Tabs 250, 500 mg (Parafon Forte DSC 500 mg tabs, scored).
NOTES — Use with caution in patients with history of drug allergies. Discontinue if allergic drug reactions occur or for signs/symptoms of liver dysfunction. May turn urine orange or purple-red.
MOA — Skeletal muscle relaxant.
ADVERSE EFFECTS — Serious: Hypersensitivity, hepatotoxicity. Frequent: Dizziness and drowsiness.

CYCLOBENZAPRINE (*Amrix, Flexeril, Fexmid*) ▶LK ♀B ▶? $
ADULTS — Musculoskeletal pain: 5 to 10 mg PO tid up to max dose of 30 mg/day or 15 to 30 mg (extended release) PO daily. Not recommended in elderly or for use longer than 2 to 3 weeks.
PEDS — Not approved in children.

FORMS — Generic/Trade: Tab 5, 10 mg. Generic only: Tabs 7.5 mg. Trade only: (Amrix $$$$$): Extended-release caps 15, 30 mg.
NOTES — Contraindicated with recent or concomitant MAOI use, immediately post MI, in patients with arrhythmias, conduction disturbances, heart failure, and hyperthyroidism. Not effective for cerebral or spinal cord disease or in children with cerebral palsy. May have similar adverse effects and drug interactions as TCAs. Caution with urinary retention, angle-closure glaucoma, increased intraocular pressure.
MOA — Skeletal muscle relaxant.
ADVERSE EFFECTS — Serious: Arrhythmia. Frequent: Drowsiness, dizziness, dry mouth, blurred vision.

DANTROLENE (*Dantrium*) ▶LK ♀C ▶– $$$$
WARNING — Hepatotoxicity, monitor LFTs. Use the lowest possible effective dose.
ADULTS — Chronic spasticity related to spinal cord injury, CVA, cerebral palsy, MS: 25 mg PO daily to start, increase to 25 mg bid to qid, then by 25 mg up to max of 100 mg bid to qid if necessary. Maintain each dosage level for 4 to 7 days to determine response. Use the lowest possible effective dose. Malignant hyperthermia: 2.5 mg/kg rapid IV push q 5 to 10 min continuing until symptoms subside or to a max 10 mg/kg/dose. Doses of up to 40 mg/kg have been used. Follow with 4 to 8 mg/kg/day PO divided tid to qid for 1 to 3 days to prevent recurrence.
PEDS — Chronic spasticity: 0.5 mg/kg PO bid to start; increase to 0.5 mg/kg tid to qid, then by increments of 0.5 mg/kg up to 3 mg/kg bid to qid. Max dose 100 mg PO qid. Malignant hyperthermia: Use adult dose.
UNAPPROVED ADULTS — Neuroleptic malignant syndrome, heat stroke: 1 to 3 mg/kg/day PO/IV divided qid.
FORMS — Generic/Trade: Caps 25, 50, 100 mg.
NOTES — Photosensitization may occur. Warfarin may decrease protein binding of dantrolene and increase dantrolene's effect. Hyperkalemia and cardiovascular collapse has been reported with concomitant calcium channel blockers such as verapamil. The following website may be useful for malignant hyperthermia: www.mhaus.org.
MOA — Skeletal muscle relaxant.
ADVERSE EFFECTS — Serious: Hepatotoxicity. Frequent: Drowsiness, dizziness and weakness.

METAXALONE (*Skelaxin*) ▶LK ♀? ▶? $$$$
ADULTS — Musculoskeletal pain: 800 mg PO tid to qid.
PEDS — Use adult dose for age older 12 yo.
FORMS — Generic/Trade: Tabs 800 mg, scored.
NOTES — Contraindicated in serious renal or hepatic insufficiency or history of drug-induced hemolytic or other anemia. Beware of hypersensitivity reactions, leukopenia, hemolytic anemia, and jaundice. Monitor LFTs. Coadministration with food, especially a high-fat meal, enhances absorption significantly and may increase CNS depression.

(cont.)

ANALGESICS: Non-Opioid Analgesic Combinations

METAXALONE (cont.)
MOA — Skeletal muscle relaxant.
ADVERSE EFFECTS — Serious: Hypersensitivity, jaundice. Frequent: Drowsiness, dizziness, nausea.

METHOCARBAMOL (*Robaxin, Robaxin-750*) ▶LK ♀C ▶? $$
ADULTS — <u>Musculoskeletal pain,</u> acute relief: 1500 mg PO qid or 1000 mg IM/IV tid for 48 to 72 h. Maintenance: 1000 mg PO qid, 750 mg PO q 4 h, or 1500 mg PO tid. <u>Tetanus:</u> Specialized dosing.
PEDS — <u>Tetanus:</u> Specialized dosing.
FORMS — Generic/Trade: Tabs 500 and 750 mg. OTC in Canada.
NOTES — Max IV rate of undiluted drug 3 mL/min to avoid syncope, hypotension, and bradycardia. Total parenteral dosage should not exceed 3 g/day for more than 3 consecutive days, except in the treatment of tetanus. Urine may turn brown, black or green.
MOA — Skeletal muscle relaxant.
ADVERSE EFFECTS — Serious: Syncope, hypotension. Frequent: Drowsiness, dizziness, discolored urine (brown, black, green).

ORPHENADRINE (*Norflex*) ▶LK ♀C ▶? $$
ADULTS — <u>Musculoskeletal pain:</u> 100 mg PO bid. 60 mg IV/IM bid.
PEDS — Not approved in children.
UNAPPROVED ADULTS — <u>Leg cramps:</u> 100 mg PO at bedtime.
FORMS — Generic only: 100 mg extended-release. OTC in Canada.
NOTES — Contraindicated in glaucoma, pyloric or duodenal obstruction, BPH, and myasthenia gravis. Some products contain sulfites, which may cause allergic reactions. May increase anticholinergic effects of amantadine and decrease therapeutic effects of phenothiazines. Side effects include dry mouth, urinary retention and hesitancy, constipation, headache, and GI upset.
MOA — Skeletal muscle relaxant.
ADVERSE EFFECTS — Serious: Hypersensitivity, syncope. Frequent: Dry mouth, dizziness, constipation.

TIZANIDINE (*Zanaflex*) ▶LK ♀C ▶? $$$$
ADULTS — <u>Muscle spasticity due to MS or spinal cord injury:</u> 4 to 8 mg PO q 6 to 8 h prn, max dose 36 mg/day.
PEDS — Not approved in children.
FORMS — Generic/Trade: Tabs 4 mg, scored. Trade only: Caps 2, 4, 6 mg. Generic only: Tabs 2 mg.
NOTES — Monitor LFTs. Avoid in hepatic or renal insufficiency. Alcohol, oral contraceptives, fluvoxamine, and ciprofloxacin increase tizanidine levels; may cause significant decreases in BP and increased drowsiness and psychomotor impairment. Concurrent antihypertensives may exacerbate hypotension. Dry mouth, somnolence, sedation, asthenia, and dizziness most common side effects.
MOA — Skeletal muscle relaxant.
ADVERSE EFFECTS — Serious: Hypotension, hepatotoxicity. Frequent: Dry mouth, somnolence, asthenia, and dizziness.

ANALGESICS: Non-Opioid Analgesic Combinations

NOTE: Refer to individual components for further information. Carisoprodol and butalbital may be habit-forming; butalbital contraindicated with porphyria. May cause drowsiness and/or sedation, which may be enhanced by alcohol and other CNS depressants. Avoid exceeding 4 g/day of acetaminophen in combination products. Caution people who drink 3 or more alcoholic drinks/day to limit acetaminophen use to 2.5 g/day due to additive liver toxicity.

ASCRIPTIN (acetylsalicylic acid + aluminum hydroxide + magnesium hydroxide + calcium carbonate, Aspir-Mox) ▶K ♀D ▶? $
WARNING — Multiple strengths; see FORMS.
ADULTS — <u>Pain:</u> 1 to 2 tabs PO q 4 h.
PEDS — Not approved in children.
FORMS — OTC Trade only: Tabs 325 mg aspirin/50 mg Mg hydroxide/50 mg Al hydroxide/50 mg Ca carbonate (Ascriptin and Aspir-Mox). 500 mg aspirin/33 mg Mg hydroxide/33 mg Al hydroxide/ 237 mg Ca carbonate (Ascriptin Maximum Strength).
NOTES — See NSAIDs - Salicylic Acid subclass warning.
MOA — Anti-inflammatory, analgesic.
ADVERSE EFFECTS — Serious: Hypersensitivity, Reye's syndrome, GI bleeding, nephrotoxicity. Frequent: Nausea, dyspepsia.

BUFFERIN (acetylsalicylic acid + calcium carbonate + magnesium oxide + magnesium carbonate) ▶K ♀D ▶? $
ADULTS — <u>Pain:</u> 1 to 2 tabs/caps PO q 4 h while symptoms persist. Max 12 in 24 h.
PEDS — Not approved in children.
FORMS — OTC Trade only: Tabs/caps 325 mg aspirin/158 mg Ca carbonate/63 mg of Mg oxide/34 mg of Mg carbonate. Bufferin ES: 500 mg aspirin/222.3 mg Ca carbonate/88.9 mg of Mg oxide/55.6 mg of Mg carbonate.
NOTES — See NSAIDs - Salicylic Acid subclass warning.
MOA — Anti-inflammatory, analgesic.
ADVERSE EFFECTS — Serious: Hypersensitivity, Reye's syndrome, GI bleeding, nephrotoxicity. Frequent: Nausea, dyspepsia.

ESGIC (acetaminophen + butalbital + caffeine) ▶LK ♀C ▶? $
WARNING — Multiple strengths; see FORMS and write specific product on Rx.
ADULTS — <u>Tension or muscle contraction headache:</u> 1 to 2 tabs or caps PO q 4 h. Max 6 in 24 h.
PEDS — Not approved in children.
FORMS — Generic only: Tabs/caps, 325 mg acetaminophen/50 mg butalbital/40 mg caffeine. Oral soln 325/50/40 mg per 15 mL. Generic/Trade: Tabs, Esgic Plus is 500/50/40 mg.
MOA — Combination analgesic.

(cont.)

ANALGESICS: Non-Opioid Analgesic Combinations

ESGIC *(cont.)*
ADVERSE EFFECTS – Serious: Hepatotoxicity. Frequent: Drowsiness and dizziness.

EXCEDRIN MIGRAINE (acetaminophen + acetylsalicylic acid + caffeine) ▶LK ♀D ▶? $
ADULTS – Migraine headache: 2 tabs/caps/geltabs PO q 6 h while symptoms persist. Max 8 in 24 h.
PEDS – Use adult dose for age 12 or older.
FORMS – OTC Generic/Trade: Tabs/caps/geltabs 250 mg acetaminophen/250 mg aspirin/65 mg caffeine.
NOTES – See NSAIDs - Salicylic Acid subclass warning. Avoid concomitant use of other acetaminophen-containing products.
MOA – Combination analgesic.
ADVERSE EFFECTS – Serious: Hepatotoxicity, hypersensitivity, Reye's syndrome, GI bleeding, nephrotoxicity. Frequent: Dyspepsia, nervousness, insomnia.

FIORICET (acetaminophen + butalbital + caffeine) ▶LK ♀C ▶? $
ADULTS – Tension or muscle contraction headache: 1 to 2 tabs PO q 4 h. Max 6 in 24 h.
PEDS – Not approved in children.
FORMS – Generic/Trade: Tabs 325 mg acetaminophen/50 mg butalbital/40 mg caffeine.
MOA – Combination analgesic.
ADVERSE EFFECTS – Serious: Hepatotoxicity. Frequent: Drowsiness and dizziness.

FIORINAL (acetylsalicylic acid + butalbital + caffeine, ✦*Tecnal, Trianal*) ▶KL ♀D ▶– ©III $
ADULTS – Tension or muscle contraction headache: 1 to 2 tabs PO q 4 h. Max 6 tabs in 24 h.
PEDS – Not approved in children.
FORMS – Generic/Trade: Caps 325 mg aspirin/50 mg butalbital/40 mg caffeine.
NOTES – See NSAIDs - Salicylic Acid subclass warning.
MOA – Combination analgesic.
ADVERSE EFFECTS – Serious: Hypersensitivity, Reye's syndrome, GI bleeding, nephrotoxicity. Frequent: Drowsiness and dizziness.

GOODY'S EXTRA STRENGTH HEADACHE POWDER (acetaminophen + acetylsalicylic acid + caffeine) ▶LK ♀D ▶? $
ADULTS – Headache: Place 1 powder on tongue and follow with liquid, or stir powder into a glass of water or other liquid. Repeat in 4 to 6 h prn. Max 4 powders in 24 h.
PEDS – Use adult dose for age 12 or older.
FORMS – OTC trade only: 260 mg acetaminophen/520 mg aspirin/32.5 mg caffeine per powder paper.
NOTES – See NSAIDs - Salicylic Acid subclass warning.
MOA – Combination analgesic.
ADVERSE EFFECTS – Serious: Hepatotoxicity, hypersensitivity, Reye's syndrome, GI bleeding, nephrotoxicity. Frequent: Dyspepsia.

NORGESIC (orphenadrine + acetylsalicylic acid + caffeine) ▶KL ♀D ▶? $$
WARNING – Multiple strengths; see FORMS and write specific product on Rx.
ADULTS – Musculoskeletal pain: Norgesic: 1 to 2 tabs PO tid to qid. Norgesic Forte: 1 tab PO tid to qid.
PEDS – Not approved in children.
FORMS – Generic/Trade: Tabs Norgesic 25 mg orphenadrine/385 mg aspirin/30 mg caffeine. Norgesic Forte 50/770/60 mg.
NOTES – See NSAIDs - Salicylic Acid subclass warning.
MOA – Combination analgesic/muscle relaxant.
ADVERSE EFFECTS – Serious: Hypersensitivity, Reye's syndrome, GI bleeding, nephrotoxicity, syncope. Frequent: Dry mouth, dizziness, constipation.

PHRENILIN (acetaminophen + butalbital) ▶LK ♀C ▶? $
WARNING – Multiple strengths; see FORMS and write specific product on Rx.
ADULTS – Tension or muscle contraction headache: Phrenilin: 1 to 2 tabs PO q 4 h. Phrenilin Forte: 1 cap PO q 4 h. Max 6 in 24 h.
PEDS – Not approved in children.
FORMS – Generic/Trade: Tabs, Phrenilin 325 mg acetaminophen/50 mg butalbital. Caps, Phrenilin Forte 650/50 mg.
MOA – Combination analgesic/muscle relaxant.
ADVERSE EFFECTS – Serious: Hepatotoxicity. Frequent: Drowsiness and dizziness.

SEDAPAP (acetaminophen + butalbital) ▶LK ♀C ▶? $
ADULTS – Tension or muscle contraction headache: 1 to 2 tabs PO q 4 h. Max 6 tabs in 24 h.
PEDS – Not approved in children.
FORMS – Generic only: Tabs 650 mg acetaminophen/50 mg butalbital.
MOA – Combination analgesic.
ADVERSE EFFECTS – Serious: Hepatotoxicity. Frequent: Drowsiness and dizziness.

SOMA COMPOUND (carisoprodol + acetylsalicylic acid) ▶LK ♀D ▶– $$$
ADULTS – Musculoskeletal pain: 1 to 2 tabs PO qid.
PEDS – Not approved in children.
FORMS – Generic/Trade: Tabs 200 mg carisoprodol/325 mg aspirin.
NOTES – See NSAIDs - Salicylic Acid subclass warning. Carisoprodol may be habit-forming. Withdrawal with abrupt discontinuation.
MOA – Combination analgesic/muscle relaxant.
ADVERSE EFFECTS – Serious: Hypersensitivity, Reye's syndrome, GI bleeding, nephrotoxicity. Idiosyncratic reaction with angioedema, hypotension and anaphylactoid shock. Frequent: Dizziness and drowsiness.

ULTRACET (tramadol + acetaminophen, ✦*Tramacet*) ▶KL ♀C ▶– $$
ADULTS – Acute pain: 2 tabs PO q 4 to 6 h prn, (up to 8 tabs/day for no more than 5 days). If CrCl < 30 mL/min, increase the dosing interval to 12 h. Consider a similar adjustment in elderly patients and in cirrhosis.

(cont.)

ANALGESICS: Non-Steroidal Anti-Inflammatories

ULTRACET (*cont.*)
PEDS — Not approved in children.
FORMS — Generic/Trade: Tabs 37.5 mg tramadol/ 325 mg acetaminophen.
NOTES — Do not use with other acetaminophen-containing drugs due to potential for hepatotoxicity. Contraindicated in acute intoxication with alcohol, hypnotics, centrally acting analgesics, opioids, or psychotropic drugs. Seizures may occur with concurrent antidepressants or with seizure disorder. Use with great caution with MAOIs or in combination with SSRIs due to potential for serotonin syndrome; dose adjustment may be needed. Withdrawal symptoms may occur in patients dependent on opioids or with abrupt discontinuation. Overdose treated with naloxone may increase seizure risk. The most frequent side effects are somnolence and constipation.
MOA — Combination analgesic.
ADVERSE EFFECTS — Serious: Seizures, anaphylactoid reactions, hepatotoxicity. Frequent: Constipation, somnolence.

ANALGESICS: Non-Steroidal Anti-Inflammatories—COX-2 Inhibitors

NOTE: The risk of serious cardiovascular events and GI bleeding may be increased in patients taking long-term, high-dose NSAIDs, both COX-2 inhibitors as well as non-selective agents. All NSAIDs and COX-2 inhibitors are contraindicated immediately post CABG surgery. The FDA advises evaluating alternative therapy or using the lowest effective dose of these drugs. Fewer GI side effects than 1st generation NSAIDs and no effect on platelets, but other NSAID-related side effects (renal dysfunction, fluid retention, CNS) are possible. May cause fluid retention or exacerbate heart failure. May elevate BP or blunt effects of antihypertensives and loop diuretics. Not substitutes for aspirin for cardiovascular prophylaxis due to lack of antiplatelet effects. Monitor INR with warfarin. May increase lithium levels. Caution in aspirin-sensitive asthma. Use around the time of conception appears to increase the risk of miscarriage (use acetaminophen instead).

CELECOXIB (*Celebrex*) ▶L ♀C (D in 3rd trimester) ▶? $$$$$
WARNING — Increases the risk of serious cardiovascular events and GI bleeding. Contraindicated immediately post CABG surgery.
ADULTS — <u>OA, ankylosing spondylitis:</u> 200 mg PO daily or 100 mg PO bid. <u>RA:</u> 100 to 200 mg PO bid. <u>Familial adenomatous polyposis</u> (FAP), as an adjunct to usual care: 400 mg PO bid with food. <u>Acute pain, dysmenorrhea:</u> 400 mg once, then 200 mg PO bid. May take an additional 200 mg on day 1.
PEDS — <u>JRA:</u> Give 50 mg PO bid for age 2 to 17 yo and wt 10 to 25 kg, give 100 mg PO bid for wt greater than 25 kg.
FORMS — Trade only: Caps 50, 100, 200, 400 mg.
NOTES — Contraindicated in sulfonamide allergy. Decrease dose by 50% in hepatic dysfunction. Caps may be opened and sprinkled into 1 teaspoon of apple sauce and taken immediately with water. Drugs that inhibit CYP450 2C9, such as fluconazole, increase concentrations. Lithium concentrations increased.
MOA — Anti-inflammatory, analgesic.
ADVERSE EFFECTS — Serious: Nephrotoxicity, hepatotoxicity, SJS. Frequent: Fluid retention.

ANALGESICS: Non-Steroidal Anti-Inflammatories—Salicylic Acid Derivatives

NOTE: The risk of serious cardiovascular events and GI bleeding may be increased in patients taking long-term, high-dose NSAIDs, both COX-2 inhibitors as well as non-selective agents (excluding aspirin). All NSAIDs and COX-2 inhibitors are contraindicated immediately post CABG surgery. The FDA advises evaluating alternative therapy or using the lowest effective dose of these drugs. Avoid in aspirin allergy and in children younger than 17 yo with chickenpox or flu due to association with Reye's syndrome. May potentiate warfarin, heparin, valproic acid, methotrexate. Unlike aspirin, derivatives may have less GI toxicity and negligible effects on platelet aggregation and renal prostaglandins. Caution in aspirin-sensitive asthma. Ibuprofen and possibly other NSAIDs may antagonize antiplatelet effects of aspirin if given simultaneously. Use around the time of conception appears to increase the risk of miscarriage (use acetaminophen instead).

ACETYLSALICYLIC ACID (*Ecotrin, Empirin, Halfprin, Bayer, Anacin, Zorprin, Aspirin, ✦Asaphen, Entrophen, Novasen*) ▶K ♀D ▶? $
ADULTS — <u>Mild to moderate pain, fever:</u> 325 to 650 mg PO/PR q 4 h prn. <u>Acute rheumatic fever:</u> 5 to 8 g/day, initially. RA/OA: 3.2 to 6 g/day in divided doses. <u>Platelet aggregation inhibition:</u> 81 to 325 mg PO daily.
PEDS — <u>Mild to moderate pain, fever:</u> 10 to 15 mg/kg/dose PO q 4 to 6 h not to exceed 60 to 80 mg/kg/day. <u>JRA:</u> 60 to 100 mg/kg/day PO divided q 6 to 8 h. <u>Acute rheumatic fever:</u> 100 mg/kg/day PO/PR for 2 weeks, then 75 mg/kg/day for 4 to 6 weeks. <u>Kawasaki disease:</u> 80 to 100 mg/kg/day divided qid PO/PR until fever resolves, then 3 to 5 mg/kg/day PO qam for 7 weeks or longer if there is ECG evidence of coronary artery abnormalities.
UNAPPROVED ADULTS — <u>Primary prevention of cardiovascular events</u> (10 year CHD risk > 6 to 10% based on Framingham risk scoring): 75 to 325 mg PO daily. <u>Post ST-elevation MI:</u> 162 to 325 mg PO

(cont.)

ANALGESICS: Non-Steroidal Anti-Inflammatories

ACETYLSALICYLIC ACID (cont.)
on day 1, continue indefinitely at 75 to 162 mg/day. Post non-ST-elevation MI: 162 to 325 mg PO on day 1, continue indefinitely at 75 to 162 mg/day. Long-term antithrombotic therapy for chronic atrial fib/flutter in patients with low-moderate risk of CVA (age younger than 75 yo without risk factors): 325 mg PO daily. Percutaneous coronary intervention pretreatment: Already taking daily aspirin therapy: 75 to 325 mg PO before procedure. Not already taking daily aspirin therapy: 300 to 325 mg PO at least 2 to 24 h before procedure. Post percutaneous coronary intervention: 325 mg daily in combination with clopidogrel for at least 1 month after bare metal stent placement, at least 3 to 6 months after drug-eluting-stent placement; then 75 to 162 mg PO daily indefinitely. Post percutaneous coronary brachytherapy: 75 to 325 mg daily in combination with clopidogrel indefinitely.
FORMS — Generic/Trade (OTC): Tabs, 325, 500 mg; chewable 81 mg; enteric-coated 81, 162 mg (Halfprin), 81, 325, 500 mg (Ecotrin), 650, 975 mg. Trade only: Tabs, controlled-release 650, 800 mg (ZORprin, Rx). Generic only (OTC): Supps 60, 120, 200, 300, 600 mg.
NOTES — Consider discontinuation 1 week prior to surgery (except coronary bypass or in first year post coronary stent implantation) because of the possibility of postop bleeding. Aspirin intolerance occurs in 4% to 19% of asthmatics. Use caution in liver damage, renal insufficiency, peptic ulcer or bleeding tendencies. Crush or chew tabs (including enteric-coated products) in first dose with acute MI. Higher doses of aspirin (1.3 g/day) have not been shown to be superior to low doses in preventing TIAs and CVAs.
MOA — Anti-inflammatory, antipyretic, analgesic. Inhibits prostaglandin synthesis and platelet aggregation by inactivating the enzyme cyclooxygenase.
ADVERSE EFFECTS — Serious: Hypersensitivity, Reye's syndrome, GI bleeding, nephrotoxicity. Frequent: Nausea, dyspepsia, tinnitus (large doses), dizziness (large doses).

CHOLINE MAGNESIUM TRISALICYLATE (*Trilisate*) ▶K ♀C (D in 3rd trimester) ▶? $$
ADULTS — RA/OA: 1500 mg PO bid. Mild to moderate pain, fever: 1000 to 1500 mg PO bid.
PEDS — RA, mild to moderate pain: 50 mg/kg/day (up to 37 kg) PO divided bid.
FORMS — Generic only: Tabs 500, 750, 1000 mg. Soln 500 mg/5 mL.
MOA — Anti-inflammatory, antipyretic, analgesic.
ADVERSE EFFECTS — Serious: Hypersensitivity, Reye's syndrome, GI bleeding, nephrotoxicity. Frequent: Nausea, dyspepsia.

DIFLUNISAL (*Dolobid*) ▶K ♀C (D in 3rd trimester) ▶– $$$
ADULTS — Mild to moderate pain: Initially: 500 mg to 1 g PO, then 250 to 500 mg PO q 8 to 12 h. RA/OA: 500 mg to 1 g PO divided bid. Max dose 1.5 g/day.
PEDS — Not approved in children.
FORMS — Generic/Trade: Tabs 250, 500 mg.
NOTES — Do not crush or chew tabs. Increases acetaminophen levels.
MOA — Anti-inflammatory, analgesic.
ADVERSE EFFECTS — Serious: Hypersensitivity, Reye's syndrome, GI bleeding, nephrotoxicity. Frequent: Nausea, dyspepsia.

SALSALATE (*Salflex, Disalcid, Amigesic*) ▶K ♀C (D in 3rd trimester) ▶? $$
ADULTS — RA/OA: 3000 mg/day PO divided q 8 to 12 h.
PEDS — Not approved in children.
FORMS — Generic only: Tabs 500, 750 mg, scored.
MOA — Anti-inflammatory, analgesic.
ADVERSE EFFECTS — Serious: Hypersensitivity, Reye's syndrome, GI bleeding, nephrotoxicity. Frequent: Nausea, dyspepsia.

ANALGESICS: Non-Steroidal Anti-Inflammatories—Other

NOTE: The risk of serious cardiovascular events and GI bleeding may be increased in patients taking long-term, high-dose NSAIDs, both COX-2 inhibitors as well as non-selective agents. All NSAIDs and COX-2 inhibitors are contraindicated immediately post-CABG surgery. The FDA advises evaluating alternative therapy or using the lowest effective dose of these drugs. Chronic use associated with renal insufficiency, gastritis, peptic ulcer disease, GI bleeds. Caution in liver disease. May cause fluid retention or exacerbate heart failure. May elevate BP or blunt effects of antihypertensives and loop diuretics. May increase levels of methotrexate, lithium, phenytoin, digoxin, and cyclosporine. May potentiate warfarin. Caution in aspirin-sensitive asthma. Ibuprofen or other NSAIDs may antagonize antiplatelet effects of aspirin if given simultaneously. Use around the time of conception appears to increase the risk of miscarriage (use acetaminophen instead).

ARTHROTEC (diclofenac + misoprostol) ▶LK ♀X ▶– $$$$$
WARNING — Because of the abortifacient property of the misoprostol component, it is contraindicated in women who are pregnant. Caution in women with childbearing potential; effective contraception is essential.
ADULTS — OA: One 50/200 PO tid. RA: One 50/200 PO tid to qid. If intolerant, may use 50/200 or 75/200 PO bid.
PEDS — Not approved in children.
FORMS — Trade only: Tabs 50 mg/200 mcg, 75 mg/200 mcg, diclofenac/misoprostol.
NOTES — Refer to individual components. Abdominal pain and diarrhea may occur. Check LFTs at baseline, within 4 to 8 weeks of initiation, then periodically. Do not crush or chew tabs.
MOA — Anti-inflammatory/mucosal protectant, analgesic.

(cont.)

ANALGESICS: Non-Steroidal Anti-Inflammatories

***ARTHROTEC** (cont.)*
ADVERSE EFFECTS — Serious: Fetal death, nephrotoxicity, gastritis, peptic ulcer disease, GI bleeds. Frequent: Diarrhea, abdominal pain, nausea, dyspepsia.

DICLOFENAC (*Voltaren, Voltaren XR, Cataflam, Flector, Zipsor, Cambia, ✦Voltaren Rapide*) ▶L ♀B (D in 3rd trimester) ▶– $$$
WARNING — Multiple strengths; see FORMS and write specific product on Rx.
ADULTS — OA: Immediate- or delayed-release 50 mg PO bid to tid or 75 mg bid. Extended-release 100 mg PO daily. Gel: Apply 4 g to knees or 2 g to hands qid using enclosed dosing card. RA: Immediate- or delayed-release 50 mg PO tid to qid or 75 mg bid. Extended-release 100 mg PO daily to bid. Ankylosing spondylitis: Immediate- or delayed-release 25 mg PO qid and bedtime. Analgesia and primary dysmenorrhea: Immediate- or delayed-release 50 mg PO tid. Acute pain of strains, sprains, or contusions: Apply 1 patch to painful area bid. Acute migraine with or without aura: 50 mg single dose (Cambia), mix packet with 30 to 60 mL water.
PEDS — Not approved in children.
UNAPPROVED PEDS — JRA: 2 to 3 mg/kg/day PO.
FORMS — Generic/Trade: Tabs, immediate-release (Cataflam) 50 mg, extended-release (Voltaren XR) 100 mg. Generic only: Tabs, delayed-release 25, 50, 75 mg. Trade only: Patch (Flector) 1.3% diclofenac epolamine. Topical gel (Voltaren) 1% 100 g tube. Trade only: Caps, liquid-filled (Zipsor) 25 mg. Trade only: Powder for oral soln (Cambia) 50 mg.
NOTES — Check LFTs at baseline, within 4 to 8 weeks of initiation, then periodically. Do not apply patch to damaged or non-intact skin. Wash hands and avoid eye contact when handling the patch. Do not wear patch while bathing or showering.
MOA — Anti-inflammatory, analgesic.
ADVERSE EFFECTS — Serious: Hypersensitivity, GI bleeding, hepato/nephrotoxicity. Frequent: Nausea, dyspepsia, pruritus and dermatitis with patch and gel.

ETODOLAC (*✦Ultradol*) ▶L ♀C (D in 3rd trimester) ▶– $$$
WARNING — Multiple strengths; write specific product on Rx.
ADULTS — OA: 400 mg PO bid to tid. 300 mg PO bid to qid. 200 mg tid to qid. Extended release 400 to 1200 mg PO daily. Mild to moderate pain: 200 to 400 mg q 6 to 8 h. (Up to 1200 mg/day or if wt 60 kg or less, 20 mg/kg/day).
PEDS — Not approved in children.
UNAPPROVED ADULTS — RA, ankylosing spondylitis: 300 to 400 mg PO bid. Tendinitis, bursitis and acute gout: 300 to 400 mg PO bid to qid then taper.
FORMS — Generic only: Caps immediate-release 200, 300 mg, Tabs immediate-release 400, 500 mg, Tabs extended-release 400, 500, 600 mg.
NOTES — Brand name Lodine no longer marketed.
MOA — Anti-inflammatory, analgesic.
ADVERSE EFFECTS — Serious: Hypersensitivity, GI bleeding, nephrotoxicity, toxic epidermal necrolysis. Frequent: Nausea, dyspepsia.

FLURBIPROFEN (*Ansaid, ✦Froben, Froben SR*) ▶L ♀B (D in 3rd trimester) ▶+ $$$
ADULTS — RA/OA: 200 to 300 mg/day PO divided bid to qid. Max single dose 100 mg.
PEDS — Not approved in children.
UNAPPROVED ADULTS — Ankylosing spondylitis: 150 to 300 mg/day PO divided bid to qid. Mild to moderate pain: 50 mg PO q 6 h. Primary dysmenorrhea: 50 mg PO daily at onset, discontinue when pain subsides. Tendinitis, bursitis, acute gout, acute migraine: 100 mg PO at onset, then 50 mg PO qid, then taper.
UNAPPROVED PEDS — JRA: 4 mg/kg/day PO.
FORMS — Generic/Trade: Tabs immediate-release 50, 100 mg.
MOA — Anti-inflammatory, analgesic.
ADVERSE EFFECTS — Serious: Hypersensitivity, GI bleeding, nephrotoxicity. Frequent: Nausea, dyspepsia.

IBUPROFEN (*Motrin, Advil, Nuprin, Rufen, Neoprofen, Caldolor*) ▶L ♀B (D in 3rd trimester) ▶+ $
ADULTS — RA/OA: 200 to 800 mg PO tid to qid. Mild to moderate pain: 400 mg PO q 4 to 6 h. 400 to 800 mg IV (Caldolor) q 6 h prn. 400 mg IV (Caldolor) q 4 to 6 h or 100 to 200 mg q 4 h prn. Primary dysmenorrhea: 400 mg PO q 4 h prn. Fever: 200 mg PO q 4 to 6 h prn. Migraine pain: 200 to 400 mg PO not to exceed 400 mg in 24 h unless directed by a physician (OTC dosing). Max dose 3.2 g/day.
PEDS — JRA: 30 to 50 mg/kg/day PO divided q 6 h. Max dose 2400 mg/24 h. 20 mg/kg/day may be adequate for milder disease. Analgesic/antipyretic age older than 6 mo: 5 to 10 mg/kg PO q 6 to 8 h, prn. Max dose 40 mg/kg/day. Patent ductus arteriosus in neonates age 32 weeks gestational age or younger weighing 500 to 1500 g (NeoProfen): Specialized dosing.
FORMS — OTC: Caps/Liqui-Gel Caps 200 mg. Tabs 100, 200 mg. Chewable tabs 50, 100 mg. Susp (infant gtts) 50 mg/1.25 mL (with calibrated dropper), 100 mg/5 mL. Rx Generic/Trade: Tabs 300, 400, 600, 800 mg. Vials: 400 mg/4 mL or 800 mg/8 mL.
NOTES — May antagonize antiplatelet effects of aspirin if given simultaneously. Take aspirin 2 h prior to ibuprofen. Administer IV (Caldolor) over at least 30 min; hydration important.
MOA — Anti-inflammatory/antipyretic, analgesic.
ADVERSE EFFECTS — Serious: Hypersensitivity, GI bleeding, nephrotoxicity. Frequent: Nausea, dyspepsia.

INDOMETHACIN (*Indocin, Indocin SR, Indocin IV, ✦Indocid-P.D.A.*) ▶L ♀B (D in 3rd trimester) ▶+ $
WARNING — Multiple strengths; see FORMS and write specific product on Rx. Use during labor increases risk of fetal and maternal complications: Premature closure of the ductus arteriosus, fetal pulmonary HTN, oligohydramnios, higher rate of postpartum hemorrhage.

(cont.)

ANALGESICS: Non-Steroidal Anti-Inflammatories

INDOMETHACIN (cont.)
- ADULTS — <u>RA/OA, ankylosing spondylitis:</u> 25 mg PO bid to tid to start. Increase incrementally to a total daily dose of 150 to 200 mg. <u>Bursitis/tendinitis:</u> 75 to 150 mg/day PO divided tid to qid. <u>Acute gout:</u> 50 mg PO tid until pain tolerable, rapidly taper dose to D/C. Sustained-release: 75 mg PO daily to bid.
- PEDS — <u>Closure of patent ductus arteriosus in neonates:</u> Initial dose 0.2 mg/kg IV, if additional doses necessary, dose and frequency (q 12 h or q 24 h) based on neonate's age and urine output.
- UNAPPROVED ADULTS — <u>Primary dysmenorrhea:</u> 25 mg PO tid to qid. <u>Cluster headache:</u> 75 to 150 mg SR PO daily. <u>Polyhydramnios:</u> 2.2 to 3 mg/kg/day PO based on maternal wt; premature closure of the ductus arteriosus has been reported. <u>Preterm labor:</u> Initial 50 to 100 mg PO followed by 25 mg PO q 6 to 12 h up to 48 h.
- UNAPPROVED PEDS — <u>JRA:</u> 1 to 3 mg/kg/day tid to qid to start. Increase prn to max dose of 4 mg/kg/day or 200 mg/day, whichever is less.
- FORMS — Generic/Trade: Caps, sustained-release 75 mg. Generic only: Caps, immediate-release 25, 50 mg. Suppository 50 mg. Trade only: Oral susp 25 mg/5 mL (237 mL)
- NOTES — May aggravate depression or other psychiatric disturbances. Do not crush sustained-release cap.
- MOA — Anti-inflammatory, analgesic. Prostaglandin inhibition leads to closure of a patent ductus arteriosus. Tocolytic.
- ADVERSE EFFECTS — Serious: Hypersensitivity, GI bleeding, nephrotoxicity. During labor: Premature closure of the ductus arteriosus and fetal pulmonary hypertension, oligohydramnios, postpartum hemorrhage. Frequent: Nausea, dyspepsia, dizziness, drowsiness.

KETOPROFEN (*Orudis, Orudis KT, Actron, Oruvail, ♣Orudis SR*) ▶L ♀B (D in 3rd trimester) ▶– $$$
- ADULTS — <u>RA/OA:</u> 75 mg PO tid or 50 mg PO qid. Extended-release 200 mg PO daily. <u>Mild to moderate pain, primary dysmenorrhea:</u> 25 to 50 mg PO q 6 to 8 h prn.
- PEDS — Not approved in children.
- UNAPPROVED PEDS — <u>JRA:</u> 100 to 200 mg/m2/day PO. Max dose 320 mg/day.
- FORMS — OTC: Tabs, immediate-release 12.5 mg. Rx Generic only: Caps, extended-release 100, 150, 200 mg. Caps, immediate-release 25, 50, 75 mg.
- MOA — Anti-inflammatory, analgesic.
- ADVERSE EFFECTS — Serious: Hypersensitivity, GI bleeding, nephrotoxicity. Frequent: Nausea, dyspepsia.

KETOROLAC (*Toradol*) ▶L ♀C (D in 3rd trimester) ▶+ $
- WARNING — Indicated for short-term (up to 5 days) therapy only. Ketorolac is a potent NSAID and can cause serious GI and renal adverse effects. It may also increase the risk of bleeding by inhibiting platelet function. Contraindicated in patients with active peptic ulcer disease, recent GI bleeding or perforation, a history of peptic ulcer disease or GI bleeding, or advanced renal impairment.
- ADULTS — <u>Moderately severe, acute pain, single-dose treatment:</u> 30 to 60 mg IM or 15 to 30 mg IV. <u>Multiple-dose treatment:</u> 15 to 30 mg IV/IM q 6 h. IV/IM doses are not to exceed 60 mg/day for age 65 yo or older, wt less than 50 kg, and patients with moderately elevated serum creatinine. <u>Oral continuation therapy:</u> 10 mg PO q 4 to 6 h prn, max dose 40 mg/day. Combined duration IV/IM and PO is not to exceed 5 days.
- PEDS — Not approved in children.
- UNAPPROVED PEDS — <u>Pain:</u> 0.5 mg/kg/dose IM/IV q 6 h (up to 30 mg q 6 h or 120 mg/day), give 10 mg PO q 6 h prn (up to 40 mg/day) for wt greater than 50 kg.
- FORMS — Generic only: Tabs 10 mg.
- MOA — Anti-inflammatory, analgesic.
- ADVERSE EFFECTS — Serious: Hypersensitivity, GI bleeding, nephrotoxicity. Frequent: Nausea, dyspepsia.

MECLOFENAMATE ▶L ♀B (D in 3rd trimester) ▶– $$$
- ADULTS — <u>Mild to moderate pain:</u> 50 mg PO q 4 to 6 h prn. Max dose 400 mg/day. <u>Menorrhagia and primary dysmenorrhea:</u> 100 mg PO tid for up to 6 days. <u>RA/OA:</u> 200 to 400 mg/day PO divided tid to qid.
- PEDS — Not approved in children.
- UNAPPROVED PEDS — <u>JRA:</u> 3 to 7.5 mg/kg/day PO. Max dose 300 mg/day.
- FORMS — Generic only: Caps 50, 100 mg.
- NOTES — Reversible autoimmune hemolytic anemia with use for longer than 12 months.
- MOA — Anti-inflammatory, analgesic.
- ADVERSE EFFECTS — Serious: Hypersensitivity, GI bleeding, nephrotoxicity, autoimmune hemolytic anemia. Frequent: Nausea, dyspepsia.

MEFENAMIC ACID (*Ponstel, ♣Ponstan*) ▶L ♀D ▶– $$$$$
- ADULTS — <u>Mild to moderate pain, primary dysmenorrhea:</u> 500 mg PO initially, then 250 mg PO q 6 h prn for up to 1 week.
- PEDS — Use adult dose for age older than 14 yo.
- FORMS — Trade only: Caps 250 mg.
- MOA — Anti-inflammatory, analgesic.
- ADVERSE EFFECTS — Serious: Hypersensitivity, GI bleeding, nephrotoxicity, autoimmune hemolytic anemia. Frequent: Nausea, dyspepsia.

MELOXICAM (*Mobic, ♣Mobicox*) ▶L ♀C (D in 3rd trimester) ▶? $
- ADULTS — <u>RA/OA:</u> 7.5 mg PO daily. Max dose 15 mg/day.
- PEDS — <u>JRA</u> age 2 yo or older: 0.125 mg/kg PO daily to max of 7.5 mg.
- FORMS — Generic/Trade: Tabs 7.5, 15 mg. Susp 7.5 mg/5 mL (1.5 mg/mL).
- NOTES — Shake susp gently before using. This is not a selective COX-2 inhibitor.
- MOA — Anti-inflammatory, analgesic.
- ADVERSE EFFECTS — Serious: Hypersensitivity, GI bleeding, nephrotoxicity. Frequent: Nausea, dyspepsia.

ANALGESICS: Non-Steroidal Anti-Inflammatories

NABUMETONE (*Relafen*) ▶L ♀C (D in 3rd trimester) ▶− $$$
ADULTS — <u>RA/OA</u>: Initial: Two 500 mg tabs (1000 mg) PO daily. May increase to 1500 to 2000 mg PO daily or divided bid. Dosages more than 2000 mg/day have not been studied.
PEDS — Not approved in children.
FORMS — Generic only: Tabs 500, 750 mg.
MOA — Anti-inflammatory, analgesic.
ADVERSE EFFECTS — Serious: Hypersensitivity, GI bleeding, nephrotoxicity, hepatotoxicity, Stevens-Johnson syndrome, erythema multiforme, toxic epidermal necrolysis, eosinophilic pneumonia. Frequent: Nausea, dyspepsia.

NAPROXEN (*Naprosyn, Aleve, Anaprox, EC-Naprosyn, Naprelan, Prevacid, NapraPac*) ▶L ♀B (D in 3rd trimester) ▶+ $$$
WARNING — Multiple strengths; see FORMS and write specific product on Rx.
ADULTS — <u>RA/OA, ankylosing spondylitis, pain, dysmenorrhea, acute tendinitis and bursitis, fever</u>: 250 to 500 mg PO bid. Delayed-release: 375 to 500 mg PO bid (do not crush or chew). Controlled-release: 750 to 1000 mg PO daily. <u>Acute gout</u>: 750 mg PO once, then 250 mg PO q 8 h until the attack subsides. Controlled-release: 1000 to 1500 mg PO once, then 1000 mg PO daily until the attack subsides.
PEDS — <u>JRA</u>: 10 to 20 mg/kg/day PO divided bid (up to 1250 mg/24 h). <u>Pain</u> for age older than 2 yo: 5 to 7 mg/kg/dose PO q 8 to 12 h.
UNAPPROVED ADULTS — <u>Acute migraine</u>: 750 mg PO once, then 250 to 500 mg PO prn. <u>Migraine prophylaxis, menstrual migraine</u>: 500 mg PO bid beginning 1 day prior to onset of menses and ending on last day of period.
FORMS — OTC Generic/Trade (Aleve): Tabs immediate-release 200 mg. OTC Trade only (Aleve): Caps, Gelcaps immediate-release 200 mg. Rx Generic/Trade: Tabs immediate-release (Naprosyn) 250, 375, 500 mg, (Anaprox) 275, 550 mg. Tabs delayed-release enteric coated (EC-Naprosyn) 375, 500 mg. Tabs, controlled-release (Naprelan) 375, 500, 750 mg. Susp (Naprosyn) 125 mg/5 mL. Prevacid NapraPac: 7 lansoprazole 15 mg caps packaged with 14 naproxen tabs 375 mg or 500 mg.
NOTES — All dosing is based on naproxen content; 500 mg naproxen is equivalent to 550 mg naproxen sodium.
MOA — Anti-inflammatory, analgesic.
ADVERSE EFFECTS — Serious: Hypersensitivity, GI bleeding, nephrotoxicity. Frequent: Nausea, dyspepsia.

OXAPROZIN (*Daypro*) ▶L ♀C (D in 3rd trimester) ▶− $$$
ADULTS — <u>RA/OA</u>: 1200 mg PO daily. Max dose 1800 mg/day or 26 mg/kg/day, whichever is lower.
PEDS — Not approved in children.
FORMS — Generic/Trade: Tabs 600 mg, trade scored.
MOA — Anti-inflammatory, analgesic.
ADVERSE EFFECTS — Serious: Hypersensitivity, GI bleeding, nephrotoxicity. Frequent: Nausea, dyspepsia.

PIROXICAM (*Feldene, Fexicam*) ▶L ♀B (D in 3rd trimester) ▶+ $$$
ADULTS — <u>RA/OA</u>: 20 mg PO daily or divided bid.
PEDS — Not approved in children.
UNAPPROVED ADULTS — <u>Primary dysmenorrhea</u>: 20 to 40 mg PO daily for 3 days.
FORMS — Generic/Trade: Caps 10, 20 mg.
MOA — Anti-inflammatory, analgesic.
ADVERSE EFFECTS — Serious: Hypersensitivity, GI bleeding, nephrotoxicity. Frequent: Nausea, dyspepsia.

SULINDAC (*Clinoril*) ▶L ♀B (D in 3rd trimester) ▶− $$$
ADULTS — <u>RA/OA, ankylosing spondylitis</u>: 150 mg PO bid. <u>Bursitis, tendinitis, acute gout</u>: 200 mg PO bid, decrease after response. Max dose: 400 mg/day.
PEDS — Not approved in children.
UNAPPROVED PEDS — <u>JRA</u>: 4 mg/kg/day PO divided bid.
FORMS — Generic/Trade: Tabs 200 mg. Generic only: Tabs 150 mg.
NOTES — Sulindac-associated pancreatitis and a potentially fatal hypersensitivity syndrome have occurred.
MOA — Anti-inflammatory, analgesic.
ADVERSE EFFECTS — Serious: Hypersensitivity, GI bleeding, nephrotoxicity, pancreatitis. Frequent: Nausea, dyspepsia.

TIAPROFENIC ACID (✣*Surgam, Surgam SR*) ▶K ♀C (D in 3rd trimester) ▶− $$
ADULTS — Canada only. <u>RA or OA</u>: 600 mg PO daily of sustained release, or 300 mg PO bid of regular-release. Some OA patients may be maintained on 300 mg/day.
PEDS — Not approved in children.
FORMS — Generic/Trade: Tabs 300 mg. Trade only: Caps, sustained-release 300 mg. Generic only: Tabs 200 mg.
NOTES — Caution in renal insufficiency. Cystitis has been reported more frequently than with other NSAIDs.
MOA — Anti-inflammatory, analgesic.
ADVERSE EFFECTS — Serious: Gastric or duodenal ulceration. Frequent: Dyspepsia, drowsiness, rash.

TOLMETIN (*Tolectin*) ▶L ♀C (D in 3rd trimester) ▶+ $$$$
ADULTS — <u>RA/OA</u>: 400 mg PO tid to start. Range 600 to 1800 mg/day PO divided tid.
PEDS — <u>JRA</u> age 2 yo or older: 20 mg/kg/day PO divided tid to qid to start. Range 15 to 30 mg/kg/day divided tid to qid. Max dose 2 g/24 h.
UNAPPROVED PEDS — <u>Pain</u> age 2 yo or older: 5 to 7 mg/kg/dose PO q 6 to 8 h. Max dose 2 g/24 h.
FORMS — Generic/Trade: Tabs 200 (trade scored), 600 mg. Caps 400 mg.
NOTES — Rare anaphylaxis.
MOA — Anti-inflammatory, analgesic.
ADVERSE EFFECTS — Serious: Hypersensitivity, GI bleeding, nephrotoxicity. Frequent: Nausea, dyspepsia.

ANALGESICS: Opioid Agonist-Antagonists

NOTE: May cause drowsiness and/or sedation, which may be enhanced by alcohol and other CNS depressants. Opioid agonist-antagonists may result in inadequate pain control and/or withdrawal effects in the opioid-dependent. Reserve IM for when alternative routes are not feasible.

BUPRENORPHINE (*Buprenex, Subutex*) ▶L ♀C ▶– ©III $ IV, $$$$$ SL
  ADULTS — <u>Moderate to severe pain:</u> 0.3 to 0.6 mg IM or slow IV, q 6 h prn. Max single dose 0.6 mg. <u>Treatment of opioid dependence:</u> Induction 8 mg SL on day 1, 16 mg SL on day 2. Maintenance: 16 mg SL daily. Can individualize to range of 4 to 24 mg SL daily.
  PEDS — <u>Moderate to severe pain:</u> 2 to 12 yo: 2 to 6 mcg/kg/dose IM or slow IV q 4 to 6 h. Max single dose 6 mcg/kg.
  FORMS — Generic/Trade (Subutex): SL Tabs 2, 8 mg.
  NOTES — May cause bradycardia, hypotension, and respiratory depression. Concurrent use with diazepam has resulted in respiratory and cardiovascular collapse. For opioid dependence Subutex is preferred over Suboxone for induction. Suboxone preferred for maintenance. Prescribers must complete training and apply for special DEA number. See www.suboxone.com.
  MOA — Opioid agonist-antagonist analgesic.
  ADVERSE EFFECTS — Serious: Respiratory depression, hepatitis, hypersensitivity. Frequent: Sedation, dizziness, nausea, headache, constipation.

BUTORPHANOL (*Stadol, Stadol NS*) ▶LK ♀C ▶+ ©IV $$$
  WARNING — Approved as a nasal spray in 1991 and has been promoted as a safe treatment for migraine headaches. There have been numerous reports of dependence-addiction and major psychological disturbances. These problems have been documented by the FDA. Stadol NS should be used for patients with infrequent but severe migraine attacks for whom all other common abortive treatments have failed. Experts recommend restriction to no more than 2 bottles (30 sprays) per month in patients who are appropriate candidates for this medication.
  ADULTS — <u>Pain, including postop pain:</u> 0.5 to 2 mg IV q 3 to 4 h prn. 1 to 4 mg IM q 3 to 4 h prn. <u>Obstetric pain during labor:</u> 1 to 2 mg IV/IM at full term in early labor, repeat after 4 h. <u>Last resort for migraine pain:</u> 1 mg nasal spray (1 spray in 1 nostril). If no pain relief in 60 to 90 min, may give a 2nd spray in the other nostril. Additional doses q 3 to 4 h prn.
  PEDS — Not approved in children.
  FORMS — Generic only: Nasal spray 1 mg/spray, 2.5 mL bottle (14 to 15 doses/bottle).
  NOTES — May increase cardiac workload.
  MOA — Opioid agonist-antagonist analgesic.
  ADVERSE EFFECTS — Serious: Respiratory depression. Frequent: Sedation, dizziness.

NALBUPHINE (*Nubain*) ▶LK ♀? ▶? $
  ADULTS — <u>Moderate to severe pain:</u> 10 to 20 mg SC/IM/IV q 3 to 6 h prn. Max dose 160 mg/day.
  PEDS — Not approved in children.
  MOA — Opioid agonist-antagonist analgesic.
  ADVERSE EFFECTS — Serious: Respiratory depression. Frequent: Sedation, dizziness, nausea.

PENTAZOCINE (*Talwin NX*) ▶LK ♀C ▶? ©IV $$$
  WARNING — The oral form (Talwin NX) may cause fatal reactions if injected.
  ADULTS — <u>Moderate to severe pain:</u> Talwin: 30 mg IM/IV q 3 to 4 h prn, max dose 360 mg/day. Talwin NX: 1 tab PO q 3 to 4 h, max 12 tabs/day.
  PEDS — Not approved in children.
  FORMS — Generic/Trade: Tabs 50 mg with 0.5 mg naloxone, trade scored.
  NOTES — Rotate injection sites. Can cause hallucinations, disorientation, and seizures. Concomitant sibutramine may precipitate serotonin syndrome.
  MOA — Opioid agonist-antagonist analgesic.
  ADVERSE EFFECTS — Serious: Respiratory depression, seizures, hallucinations, hypersensitivity. Frequent: Sedation, dizziness, nausea.

ANALGESICS: Opioid Agonists

NOTE: May cause life-threatening respiratory depression. May cause drowsiness and/or sedation, which may be enhanced by alcohol and other CNS depressants. Patients with chronic pain may require more frequent and higher dosing. Opioids commonly cause constipation. All opioids are pregnancy class D if used for prolonged periods or in high doses at term.

CODEINE ▶LK ♀C ▶– ©II $$
  WARNING — Do not use IV in children due to large histamine-release and cardiovascular effects. Use in nursing mothers has led to infant death.
  ADULTS — <u>Mild to moderate pain:</u> 15 to 60 mg PO/IM/IV/SC q 4 to 6 h. Max dose 360 mg in 24 h. <u>Antitussive:</u> 10 to 20 mg PO q 4 to 6 h prn. Max dose 120 mg in 24 h.
  PEDS — <u>Mild to moderate pain</u> in age 1 yo or older: 0.5 to 1 mg/kg PO/SC/IM q 4 to 6 h, max dose 60 mg/dose. <u>Antitussive:</u> Give 2.5 to 5 mg PO q 4 to 6 h prn (up to 30 mg/day) for age 2 to 5 yo, give 5 to 10 mg PO q 4 to 6 h prn (up to 60 mg/day) for age 6 to 12 yo.
  FORMS — Generic only: Tabs 15, 30, 60 mg. Oral soln: 15 mg/5 mL.
  MOA — Opioid agonist analgesic.
  ADVERSE EFFECTS — Serious: Respiratory depression/arrest. Frequent: N/V, constipation, sedation.

ANALGESICS: Opioid Agonists

OPIOID EQUIVALENCY*

Opioid	PO	IV/SC/IM	Opioid	PO	IV/SC/IM
buprenorphine	n/a	0.3–0.4 mg	meperidine	300 mg	75 mg
butorphanol	n/a	2 mg	methadone	5–15 mg	2.5–10 mg
codeine	130 mg	75 mg	morphine	30 mg	10 mg
fentanyl	?	0.1 mg	nalbuphine	n/a	10 mg
hydrocodone	20 mg	n/a	oxycodone	20 mg	n/a
hydromorphone	7.5 mg	1.5 mg	oxymorphone	10 mg	1 mg
levorphanol	4 mg	2 mg	pentazocine	50 mg	30 mg

*Approximate equianalgesic doses as adapted from the 2003 American Pain Society (www.ampainsoc.org) guidelines and the 1992 AHCPR guidelines. Not available = "n/a." See drug entries themselves for starting doses. Many recommend initially using lower than equivalent doses when switching between different opioids. IV doses should be titrated slowly with appropriate monitoring. All PO dosing is with immediate-release preparations. Individualize all dosing, especially in the elderly, children, and in those with chronic pain, opioid naïve, or hepatic/renal insufficiency.

FENTANYL (*Durogesic, Actiq, Fentora, Sublimaze, IONSYS*) ▶L ♀C ▶+ ©II $$$$$
WARNING – Duragesic patches, Actiq, and Fentora are contraindicated in the management of acute or postop pain due to potentially life-threatening respiratory depression in opioid non-tolerant patients. Instruct patients and their caregivers that even used patches/lozenges on a stick can be fatal to a child or pet. Dispose via toilet. Actiq and Fentora are not interchangeable. IONSYS: For hospital use only; remove prior to discharge. Can cause life-threatening respiratory depression.
ADULTS – Duragesic Patches: Chronic pain: 12.5 to 100 mcg/h patch q 72 h. Titrate dose to the needs of the patient. Some patients require q 48 h dosing. May wear more than 1 patch to achieve the correct analgesic effect. Actiq: Breakthrough cancer pain: 200 to 1600 mcg sucked over 15 min, if 200 mcg ineffective for 6 units use higher strength. Goal is 4 lozenges on a stick/day in conjunction with long-acting opioid. Buccal tab (Fentora) for breakthrough cancer pain: 100 to 800 mcg, titrated to pain relief; may repeat once after 30 min during single episode of breakthrough pain. See PI for dose conversion from transmucosal lozenges. Buccal soluble film (Onsolis) for breakthrough cancer pain: 200 to 1200 mcg, titrated to pain relief; no more than 4 doses/day separated by at least 2 h. Postop analgesia: 50 to 100 mcg IM; repeat in 1 to 2 h prn. IONSYS: Acute postop pain: Specialized dosing.
PEDS – Transdermal (Duragesic): Not approved in children younger than 2 yo or in opioid-naive. Use adult dosing for age older than 2 yo. Children converting to a 25 mcg patch should be receiving 45 mg or more oral morphine equivalents/day. Actiq: Not approved for age younger than 16 yo. IONSYS not approved in children.
UNAPPROVED ADULTS – Analgesia/Procedural sedation: 50 to 100 mcg slow IV over 1 to 2 min; carefully titrate to effect. Analgesia: 50 to 100 mcg IM q 1 to 2 h prn.
UNAPPROVED PEDS – Analgesia: 1 to 2 mcg/kg/dose IV/IM q 30 to 60 min prn or continuous IV infusion 1 to 3 mcg/kg/h (not to exceed adult dosing). Procedural sedation: 2 to 3 mcg/kg/dose for age 1 to 3 yo; 1 to 2 mcg/kg/dose for age 3 to 12 yo, 0.5 to 1 mcg/kg/dose (not to exceed adult dosing) for age older than 12 yo, procedural sedation doses may repeated q 30 to 60 min prn.
FORMS – Generic/Trade: Transdermal patches 12.5, 25, 50, 75, 100 mcg/h. Actiq lozenges on a stick, berry flavored 200, 400, 600, 800, 1200, 1600 mcg. Trade only: IONSYS: Iontophoretic transdermal system: 40 mcg fentanyl per activation; max 6 doses/h. Max per system is eighty 40 mcg doses over 24 h. Trade only: (Fentora) buccal tab 100, 200, 300, 400, 600, 800 mcg. Trade only: (Onsolis) buccal soluble film 200, 400, 600, 800 and 1200 mcg in child-resistant, protective foil.
NOTES – Do not use patches for acute pain or in opioid-naive patients. Oral transmucosal fentanyl doses of 5 mcg/kg provide effects similar to 0.75 to 1.25 mcg/kg of fentanyl IM. Lozenges on a stick should be sucked, not chewed. Flush lozenge remnants (without stick) down the toilet. For transdermal systems: Apply patch to non-hairy skin. Clip (not shave) hair if you have to apply to hairy area. Fever or external heat sources may increase fentanyl released from patch. Patch should be removed prior to MRI and reapplied after the test. Dispose of a used patch by folding with the adhesive side of the patch adhering to itself, then flush it down the toilet immediately. Do not cut the patch in half. For Duragesic patches and Actiq lozenges on a stick: Titrate dose as high as necessary to relieve cancer pain or other types of non-malignant pain where chronic opioids are necessary. Do not suck, chew, or swallow buccal tab. IONSYS: Apply to intact skin on the chest or upper arm. Each dose, activated by the patient, is delivered over a 10 min period. Remove prior to hospital discharge. Do not allow gel to touch mucous membranes. Dispose of using gloves. Keep all forms of fentanyl out of the reach of children or pets. Concomitant use with potent CYP 3A4 inhibitors such as ritonavir, ketoconazole, itraconazole, troleandomycin, clarithromycin, nelfinavir, and nefazodone may result in an increase in fentanyl plasma concentrations, which could increase or

(cont.)

ANALGESICS: Opioid Agonists

FENTANYL (*cont.*)
prolong adverse drug effects and may cause potentially fatal respiratory depression. ONSOLIS is available only through the FOCUS Program and requires prescriber, pharmacy, and patient enrollment. Used films should be discarded into toilet.
MOA – Opioid agonist analgesic.
ADVERSE EFFECTS – Serious: Respiratory depression/arrest, chest wall rigidity. Frequent: N/V, constipation, sedation, skin irritation, dental decay with Actiq.

HYDROMORPHONE (*Dilaudid, Dilaudid-5, ✽Hydromorph Contin*) ▶L ♀C ▶? ©II $$
ADULTS – Moderate to severe pain: 2 to 4 mg PO q 4 to 6 h. Initial dose (opioid-naive) 0.5 to 2 mg SC/IM or slow IV q 4 to 6 h prn. 3 mg PR q 6 to 8 h.
PEDS – Not approved in children.
UNAPPROVED PEDS – Pain age 12 yo or younger: 0.03 to 0.08 mg/kg PO q 4 to 6 h prn. 0.015 mg/kg/dose IV q 4 to 6 h prn, use adult dose for older than 12 yo.
FORMS – Generic/Trade: Tabs 2, 4, 8 mg (8 mg trade scored). Oral soln 5 mg/5 mL. Suppository 3 mg.
NOTES – In opioid-naive patients, consider an initial dose of 0.5 mg or less IM/SC/IV. SC/IM/IV doses after initial dose should be individualized. May be given by slow IV injection over 2 to 5 min. Titrate dose as high as necessary to relieve cancer pain or other types of non-malignant pain where chronic opioids are necessary. 1.5 mg IV = 7.5 mg PO.
MOA – Opioid agonist analgesic.
ADVERSE EFFECTS – Serious: Respiratory depression/arrest. Frequent: N/V, constipation, sedation.

LEVORPHANOL (*Levo-Dromoran*) ▶L ♀C ▶? ©II $$$$
ADULTS – Moderate to severe pain: 2 mg PO q 6 to 8 h prn. Increase to 4 mg if necessary.
PEDS – Not approved in children.
FORMS – Generic only: Tabs 2 mg, scored.
MOA – Opioid agonist analgesic.
ADVERSE EFFECTS – Serious: Respiratory depression/arrest. Frequent: N/V, constipation, sedation.

MEPERIDINE (*Demerol, pethidine*) ▶LK ♀C but + ▶+ ©II $$$
ADULTS – Moderate to severe pain: 50 to 150 mg IM/SC/PO q 3 to 4 h prn. OB analgesia: When pains become regular, 50 to 100 mg IM/SC q 1 to 3 h. May also be given slow IV diluted to 10 mg/mL, or by continuous IV infusion diluted to 1 mg/mL.
PEDS – Moderate to severe pain: 1 to 1.8 mg/kg IM/SC/PO or slow IV (see adult dosing) up to adult dose, q 3 to 4 h prn.
FORMS – Generic/Trade: Tabs 50 (trade scored), 100 mg. Syrup 50 mg/5 mL (trade banana flavored).
NOTES – Avoid in renal insufficiency and in elderly due to risk of metabolite accumulation and increased risk of CNS disturbance and seizures. Multiple drug interactions including MAOIs and SSRIs. Poor oral absorption/efficacy. 75 mg meperidine IV/IM/SC = 300 mg meperidine PO. Take syrup with ½ glass (4 oz) water. Due to the risk of seizures at high doses, meperidine is not a good choice for treatment of chronic pain. Not recommended in children.
MOA – Opioid agonist analgesic.
ADVERSE EFFECTS – Serious: Respiratory depression/arrest, seizures, anaphylaxis. Frequent: N/V, constipation, sedation.

METHADONE (*Diskets, Dolophine, Methadose, ✽Metadol*) ▶L ♀C ▶? ©II $
WARNING – High doses (mean approximately 200 mg/day) have been inconclusively associated with arrhythmia (torsade de pointes), particularly in those with preexisting risk factors. Caution in opioid-naive patients. Elimination half-life (8 to 59 h) far longer than its duration of analgesic action (4 to 8 h); monitor for respiratory depression and titrate accordingly. Use caution with escalating doses.
ADULTS – Severe pain in opioid-tolerant patients: 2.5 to 10 mg IM/SC/PO q 3 to 4 h prn. Opioid dependence: 20 to 100 mg PO daily.
PEDS – Not approved in children.
UNAPPROVED PEDS – Pain age 12 yo or younger: 0.7 mg/kg/24 h divided q 4 to 6 h PO/SC/IM/IV prn. Max 10 mg/dose.
FORMS – Generic/Trade: Tabs 5, 10 mg. Dispersible tabs 40 mg (for opioid dependence only). Oral concentrate (Intensol): 10 mg/mL. Generic only: Oral soln 5, 10 mg/5 mL.
NOTES – Titrate dose as high as necessary to relieve cancer pain or other types of non-malignant Pain where chronic opioids are necessary. Every 8 to 12 h dosing may decrease the risk of drug accumulation and overdose. Treatment for opioid dependence longer than 3 weeks is maintenance and only permitted in approved treatment programs. Drug interactions leading to decreased methadone levels with enzyme-inducing HIV drugs (eg, efavirenz, nevirapine) and other potent inducers such as rifampin. Monitor for opiate withdrawal symptoms and increase methadone if necessary. Rapid metabolizers may require more frequent daily dosing.
MOA – Opioid agonist analgesic.
ADVERSE EFFECTS – Serious: Respiratory depression/cardiorespiratory arrest, dependence, withdrawal, seizures, bradycardia. Frequent: N/V, constipation, sedation, dry mouth, urinary retention, rash.

FENTANYL TRANSDERMAL DOSE (Dosing based on ongoing morphine requirement.)

Morphine* (IV/IM)	Morphine* (PO)	Transdermal fentanyl*
10–22 mg/d	60–134 mg/d	25 mcg/h
23–37 mg/d	135–224 mg/d	50 mcg/h
38–52 mg/d	225–314 mg/d	75 mcg/h
53–67 mg/d	315–404 mg/d	100 mcg/h

*For higher morphine doses, see product insert for transdermal fentanyl equivalencies.

ANALGESICS: Opioid Agonists

MORPHINE (*MS Contin, Kadian, Avinza, Roxanol, Oramorph SR, MSIR, DepoDur, ♦Statex, M.O.S., Doloral*) ▶LK ♀C ▶+ ©II $$$$
- WARNING – Multiple strengths; see FORMS and write specific product on Rx. Drinking alcohol while taking Avinza may result in a rapid release of a potentially fatal dose of morphine.
- ADULTS – Moderate to severe pain: 10 to 30 mg PO q 4 h (immediate-release tabs, or oral soln). Controlled-release (MS Contin, Oramorph SR): 30 mg PO q 8 to 12 h. (Kadian): 20 mg PO q 12 to 24 h. Extended-release caps (Avinza): 30 mg PO daily. 10 mg q 4 h IM/SC. 2.5 to 15 mg/70 kg IV over 4 to 5 min. 10 to 20 mg PR q 4 h. Pain with major surgery (DepoDur): 10 to 15 mg once epidurally at the lumbar level prior to surgery (max dose 20 mg), or 10 mg epidurally after clamping of the umbilical cord with cesarean section.
- PEDS – Moderate to severe pain: 0.1 to 0.2 mg/kg up to 15 mg IM/SC/IV q 2 to 4 h.
- UNAPPROVED PEDS – Moderate to severe pain: 0.2 to 0.5 mg/kg/dose PO (immediate-release) q 4 to 6 h. 0.3 to 0.6 mg/kg/dose PO (controlled release) q 12 h.
- FORMS – Generic/Trade: Tabs, immediate-release 15, 30 mg. Oral soln: 10 mg/5 mL, 20 mg/5 mL, 20 mg/mL (concentrate). Rectal supps 5, 10, 20, 30 mg. Controlled-release tabs (MS Contin) 15, 30, 60, 100, 200 mg. Trade only: Controlled-release caps (Kadian) 10, 20, 30, 50, 60, 80, 100, 200 mg, Controlled-release tabs (Oramorph SR) 15, 30, 60, 100 mg. Extended-release caps (Avinza) 30, 45, 60, 75, 90, 120 mg. Generic only: Tabs, immediate-release 10 mg.
- NOTES – Titrate dose as high as necessary to relieve cancer pain or other types of non-malignant pain where chronic opioids are necessary. The active metabolites may accumulate in hepatic/renal insufficiency and the elderly leading to increased analgesic and sedative effects. Do not break, chew, or crush MS Contin or Oramorph SR. Kadian and Avinza caps may be opened and sprinkled in applesauce for easier administration; however, the pellets should not be crushed or chewed. Doses more than 1600 mg/day of Avinza contain a potentially nephrotoxic quantity of fumaric acid. Do not mix DepoDur with other medications; do not administer any other medications into epidural space for for at least 48 h. Severe opiate overdose with respiratory depression has occurred with intrathecal leakage of DepoDur.
- MOA – Opioid agonist analgesic.
- ADVERSE EFFECTS – Serious: Respiratory depression/arrest. Frequent: N/V, constipation, sedation, hypotension.

OXYCODONE (*Roxicodone, OxyContin, Percolone, OxyIR, OxyFAST, ♦Endocodone, Supeudol*) ▶L ♀B ▶– ©II $$$$$
- WARNING – Do not Rx OxyContin tabs on a prn basis. 80 mg tabs for use in opioid-tolerant patients only. Multiple strengths; see FORMS and write specific product on Rx. Do not break, chew, or crush controlled-release preparations.
- ADULTS – Moderate to severe pain: 5 mg PO q 4 to 6 h prn. Controlled-release tabs: 10 to 40 mg PO q 12 h (no supporting data for shorter dosing intervals for controlled-release tabs).
- PEDS – Not approved in children.
- UNAPPROVED PEDS – Pain age 12 yo or younger: 0.05 to 0.3 mg/kg/dose q 4 to 6 h PO prn to max of 10 mg/dose.
- FORMS – Generic/Trade: Immediate-release: Tabs 5 mg, scored. Caps 5 mg. Tabs 15, 30 mg. Oral soln 5 mg/5 mL. Oral concentrate 20 mg/mL. Generic only: Immediate-release tabs 10, 20 mg. Trade only: Controlled-release tabs: 10, 15, 20, 30, 40, 60, 80 mg.
- NOTES – Titrate dose as high as necessary to relieve cancer pain or other types of non-malignant pain where chronic opioids are necessary.
- MOA – Opioid agonist analgesic.
- ADVERSE EFFECTS – Serious: Respiratory depression/arrest. Frequent: N/V, constipation, sedation.

OXYMORPHONE (*Opana*) ▶L ♀C ▶? ©II $$$$
- WARNING – Do not break, chew, dissolve, or crush extended-release tabs due to a rapid release and absorption of a potentially fatal dose of oxymorphone.
- ADULTS – Moderate to severe pain: 10 to 20 mg PO q 4 to 6 h (immediate-release) or 5 mg q 12 h (extended-release) 1 h before or 2 h after meals. Titrate q 3 to 7 days until adequate pain relief. 1 to 1.5 mg IM/SC q 4 to 6 h prn. 0.5 mg IV initial dose in healthy patients then q 4 to 6 h prn, increase dose until pain adequately controlled.
- PEDS – Not approved in children.
- FORMS – Trade only: Extended-release tabs (Opana ER) 5, 7.5, 10, 15, 20, 30, 40 mg. Immediate-release tabs (Opana IR) 5, 10 mg.
- NOTES – Contraindicated in moderate to severe hepatic dysfunction. Decrease dose in elderly and with CrCl < 50 mL/min. Avoid alcohol.
- MOA – Opioid agonist analgesic.
- ADVERSE EFFECTS – Serious: Respiratory depression/arrest. Frequent: N/V, constipation, sedation.

PROPOXYPHENE (*Darvon-N, Darvon Pulvules*) ▶L ♀C ▶+ ©IV $$
- ADULTS – Mild to moderate pain: 65 mg (Darvon) to 100 mg (Darvon-N) PO q 4 h prn. Max dose 6 caps/day.
- PEDS – Not approved in children.
- FORMS – Generic/Trade: Caps 65 mg. Trade only: Tabs 100 mg (Darvon-N).
- NOTES – Caution in renal and hepatic dysfunction. Avoid in renal insufficiency and in elderly due to risk of metabolite accumulation, and increased risk of CNS disturbance, seizures, and QRS prolongation.
- MOA – Opioid agonist analgesic.
- ADVERSE EFFECTS – Serious: Respiratory depression/arrest, seizures. Frequent: N/V, constipation, sedation.

ANALGESICS: Opioid Analgesic Combinations

NOTE: Refer to individual components for further information. May cause drowsiness and/or sedation, which may be enhanced by alcohol and other CNS depressants. Opioids, carisoprodol, and butalbital may be habit-forming. Avoid exceeding 4 g/day of acetaminophen in combination products. Caution people who drink 3 or more alcoholic drinks/day to limit acetaminophen use to 2.5 g/day due to additive liver toxicity. Opioids commonly cause constipation; concurrent laxatives are recommended. All opioids are pregnancy class D if used for prolonged periods or in high doses at term.

ANEXSIA (hydrocodone + acetaminophen) ▶LK ♀C ▶– ©III $$
 WARNING – Multiple strengths; see FORMS and write specific product on Rx.
 ADULTS – Moderate pain: 1 tab PO q 4 to 6 h prn.
 PEDS – Not approved in children.
 FORMS – Generic/Trade: Tabs 5/325, 5/500, 7.5/325, 7.5/650, 10/750 mg hydrocodone/mg acetaminophen, scored.
 MOA – Combination analgesic.
 ADVERSE EFFECTS – Serious: Respiratory depression/arrest, hepatotoxicity. Frequent: N/V, constipation, sedation.

CAPITAL WITH CODEINE SUSPENSION (acetaminophen + codeine) ▶LK ♀C ▶? ©V $
 ADULTS – Moderate pain: 15 mL PO q 4 h prn.
 PEDS – Moderate pain: Give 5 mL PO q 4 to 6 h prn for age 3 to 6 yo, give 10 mL PO q 4 to 6 h prn for age 7 to 12 yo, use adult dose for age older than 12 yo.
 FORMS – Generic equivalent to oral soln. Trade equivalent to susp. Both codeine 12 mg and acetaminophen 120 mg per 5 mL (trade, fruit punch flavor).
 MOA – Combination analgesic.
 ADVERSE EFFECTS – Serious: Respiratory depression/arrest, hepatotoxicity. Frequent: N/V, constipation, sedation.

COMBUNOX (oxycodone + ibuprofen) ▶L ♀C (D in 3rd trimester) ▶? ©II $$$
 ADULTS – Moderate to severe pain: 1 tab PO q 6 h prn for no more than 7 days. Max dose 4 tabs/24 h.
 PEDS – Moderate to severe pain for age 14 yo or older: Use adult dose.
 FORMS – Generic/Trade: Tabs 5 mg oxycodone/ 400 mg ibuprofen.
 NOTES – For short-term (no more than 7 days) management of pain. See NSAIDs-Other subclass warning and individual components.
 MOA – Combination analgesic.
 ADVERSE EFFECTS – Serious: Respiratory depression/arrest, hypersensitivity, GI bleeding, nephrotoxicity. Frequent: N/V, constipation, dyspepsia, sedation.

DARVOCET (propoxyphene + acetaminophen) ▶L ♀C ▶+ ©IV $$
 WARNING – Multiple strengths; see Forms below and write specific product on Rx.
 ADULTS – Moderate pain: 1 tab (100/650 or 100/500) or 2 tabs (50/325) PO q 4 h prn.
 PEDS – Not approved in children.
 FORMS – Generic/Trade: Tabs 50/325 (Darvocet N-50), 100/650 (Darvocet N-100), 100/500 (Darvocet A-500), mg propoxyphene/mg acetaminophen.

 NOTES – Avoid in renal insufficiency and in elderly due to risk of metabolite accumulation, and increased risk of CNS disturbance, seizures, and QRS prolongation.
 MOA – Combination analgesic.
 ADVERSE EFFECTS – Serious: Respiratory depression/arrest, hepatotoxicity, seizures. Frequent: N/V, constipation, sedation.

EMPIRIN WITH CODEINE (acetylsalicylic acid + codeine, ✱292 tab) ▶LK ♀D ▶– ©III $
 WARNING – Multiple strengths; see FORMS and write specific product on Rx.
 ADULTS – Moderate pain: 1 to 2 tabs PO q 4 h prn.
 PEDS – Not approved in children.
 FORMS – Generic only: Tabs 325/30, 325/60 mg aspirin/mg codeine. Empirin brand no longer made.
 MOA – Combination analgesic.
 ADVERSE EFFECTS – Serious: Respiratory depression/arrest, hypersensitivity, Reye's syndrome, GI bleeding, nephrotoxicity. Frequent: N/V, dyspepsia, constipation, sedation.

FIORICET WITH CODEINE (acetaminophen + butalbital + caffeine + codeine) ▶LK ♀C ▶– ©III $$$
 ADULTS – Moderate pain: 1 to 2 caps PO q 4 h prn, max dose 6 caps/day.
 PEDS – Not approved in children.
 FORMS – Generic/Trade: Caps 325 mg acetaminophen/50 mg butalbital/40 mg caffeine/ 30 mg codeine.
 MOA – Combination analgesic.
 ADVERSE EFFECTS – Serious: Respiratory depression/arrest, hepatotoxicity. Frequent: N/V, constipation, sedation.

FIORINAL WITH CODEINE (acetylsalicylic acid + butalbital + caffeine + codeine, ✱Fiorinal C-1/4, Fiorinal C-1/2, Tecnal C-1/4, Tecnal C-1/2) ▶LK ♀D ▶– ©III $$$
 ADULTS – Moderate pain: 1 to 2 caps PO q 4 h prn, max dose 6 caps/day.
 PEDS – Not approved in children.
 FORMS – Generic/Trade: Caps 325 mg aspirin/50 mg butalbital/40 mg caffeine/30 mg codeine.
 MOA – Combination analgesic.
 ADVERSE EFFECTS – Serious: Respiratory depression/arrest, hypersensitivity, Reye's syndrome, GI bleeding, nephrotoxicity. Frequent: N/V, dyspepsia, constipation, sedation.

IBUDONE (hydrocodone + ibuprofen) ▶LK ♀– ▶? ©III $$$
 ADULTS – Moderate pain: 1 tab PO q 4 to 6 h prn, max dose 5 tabs/day.
 PEDS – Not approved in children.

(cont.)

> **ANALGESICS—NSAIDs**
> - *Salicylic acid derivatives*: ASA, diflunisal, salsalate, Trilisate.
> - *Propionic acids*: flurbiprofen, ibuprofen, ketoprofen, naproxen, oxaprozin.
> - *Acetic acids*: diclofenac, etodolac, indomethacin, ketorolac, nabumetone, sulindac, tolmetin.
> - *Fenamates*: meclofenamate.
> - *Oxicams*: meloxicam, piroxicam.
> - *COX-2 inhibitors*: celecoxib.

Note: If one class fails, consider another.

IBUDONE (cont.)
FORMS — Generic/Trade: Tabs 5/200 mg and 10/200 mg hydrocodone/ibuprofen.
NOTES — See NSAIDs-Other subclass warning.
MOA — Combination analgesic.
ADVERSE EFFECTS — Serious: Respiratory depression/arrest, hypersensitivity, GI bleeding, nephrotoxicity. Frequent: N/V, constipation, dyspepsia, sedation.

LORCET (hydrocodone + acetaminophen) ▶LK ♀C ▶– ©III $
WARNING — Multiple strengths; see FORMS and write specific product on Rx.
ADULTS — Moderate pain: 1 to 2 caps (5/500) PO q 4 to 6 h prn, max dose 8 caps/day. 1 tab PO q 4 to 6 h prn (7.5/650 and 10/650), max dose 6 tabs/day.
PEDS — Not approved in children.
FORMS — Generic/Trade: Caps 5/500 mg, Tabs 7.5/650, 10/650 mg hydrocodone/acetaminophen.
MOA — Combination analgesic.
ADVERSE EFFECTS — Serious: Respiratory depression/arrest, hepatotoxicity. Frequent: N/V, constipation, sedation.

LORTAB (hydrocodone + acetaminophen) ▶LK ♀C ▶– ©III $$
WARNING — Multiple strengths; see FORMS and write specific product on Rx.
ADULTS — Moderate pain: 1 to 2 tabs 2.5/500 and 5/500 PO q 4 to 6 h prn, max dose 8 tabs/day. 1 tab 7.5/500 and 10/500 PO q 4 to 6 h prn, max dose 5 tabs/day. Elixir 15 mL PO q 4 to 6 h prn, max 6 doses/day.
PEDS — Not approved in children.
FORMS — Generic/Trade: Lortab 5/500 (scored), Lortab 7.5/500 (trade scored), Lortab 10/500 mg hydrocodone/mg acetaminophen. Elixir: 7.5/500 mg hydrocodone/mg acetaminophen/15 mL. Trade only: Tabs 2.5/500 mg.
MOA — Combination analgesic.
ADVERSE EFFECTS — Serious: Respiratory depression/arrest, hepatotoxicity. Frequent: N/V, constipation, sedation.

MAGNACET (oxycodone + acetaminophen) ▶L ♀C ▶– ©II $$$$
WARNING — Multiple strengths; see FORMS and write specific product on Rx.
ADULTS — Moderate-severe pain: 1 to 2 tabs PO q 6 h prn (2.5/400). 1 tab PO q 6 h prn (5/400, 7.5/400, 10/400).
PEDS — Not approved in children.
FORMS — Trade only: Tabs 2.5/400, 5/400, 7.5/400, 10/400 mg oxycodone/acetaminophen.
MOA — Combination analgesic.
ADVERSE EFFECTS — Serious: Respiratory depression/arrest, hepatotoxicity. Frequent: N/V, constipation, sedation.

MAXIDONE (hydrocodone + acetaminophen) ▶LK ♀C ▶– ©III $$$
ADULTS — Moderate pain: 1 tab PO q 4 to 6 h prn, max dose 5 tabs/day.
PEDS — Not approved in children.
FORMS — Trade only: Tabs 10/750 mg hydrocodone/mg acetaminophen.
MOA — Combination analgesic.
ADVERSE EFFECTS — Serious: Respiratory depression/arrest, hepatotoxicity. Frequent: N/V, constipation, sedation.

MERSYNDOL WITH CODEINE (acetaminophen + codeine + doxylamine) ▶LK ♀C ▶? $
ADULTS — Canada only. Headaches, cold symptoms, muscle aches, neuralgia: 1 to 2 tabs PO q 4 to 6 h prn. Maximum 12 tabs/24 h.
PEDS — Not approved in children.
FORMS — Canada Trade only: OTC tab 325 mg acetaminophen/8 mg codeine phosphate/5 mg doxylamine.
NOTES — May be habit-forming. Hepatotoxicity may be increased with acetaminophen overdose and may be enhanced with concomitant chronic alcohol ingestion.
MOA — Combination analgesic.
ADVERSE EFFECTS — See components.

NORCO (hydrocodone + acetaminophen) ▶L ♀C ▶? ©III $$$
WARNING — Multiple strengths; see FORMS and write specific product on Rx.
ADULTS — Moderate to severe pain: 1 to 2 tabs PO q 4 to 6 h prn (5/325), max dose 12 tabs/day. 1 tab (7.5/325 and 10/325) PO q 4 to 6 h prn, max dose 8 and 6 tabs/day, respectively.
PEDS — Not approved in children.
FORMS — Trade only: Tabs 5/325, 7.5/325, 10/325 mg hydrocodone/acetaminophen, scored.
MOA — Combination analgesic.
ADVERSE EFFECTS — Serious: Respiratory depression/arrest, hepatotoxicity. Frequent: N/V, constipation, sedation.

ANALGESICS: Opioid Analgesic Combinations

PERCOCET (oxycodone + acetaminophen, ✦*Percocet-demi, Oxycocet, Endocet*) ▶L ♀C ▶– ©II $
WARNING – Multiple strengths; see FORMS and write specific product on Rx.
ADULTS – <u>Moderate-severe pain:</u> 1 to 2 tabs PO q 4 to 6 h prn (2.5/325 and 5/325). 1 tab PO q 4 to 6 h prn (7.5/325, 7.5/500, 10/325 and 10/650).
PEDS – Not approved in children.
FORMS – Trade only: Tabs 2.5/325 oxycodone/acetaminophen. Generic/Trade: Tabs 5/325, 7.5/325, 7.5/500, 10/325, 10/650 mg. Generic only: 2.5/300, 5/300, 7.5/300, 10/300, 2.5/400, 5/400, 7.5/400, 10/400, 10/500 mg.
MOA – Combination analgesic.
ADVERSE EFFECTS – Serious: Respiratory depression/arrest, hepatotoxicity. Frequent: N/V, constipation, sedation.

PERCODAN (oxycodone + acetylsalicylic acid, ✦*Oxycodan, Endodan*) ▶LK ♀D ▶– ©II $$
ADULTS – <u>Moderate to severe pain:</u> 1 tab PO q 6 h prn.
PEDS – Not approved in children.
FORMS – Generic/Trade: Tabs 4.88/325 mg oxycodone/aspirin (trade scored).
MOA – Combination analgesic.
ADVERSE EFFECTS – Serious: Respiratory depression/arrest, hypersensitivity, Reye's syndrome, GI bleeding, nephrotoxicity. Frequent: N/V, dyspepsia, constipation, sedation.

ROXICET (oxycodone + acetaminophen) ▶L ♀C ▶– ©II $
WARNING – Multiple strengths; see FORMS and write specific product on Rx.
ADULTS – <u>Moderate to severe pain:</u> 1 tab PO q 6 h prn. Oral soln: 5 mL PO q 6 h prn.
PEDS – Not approved in children.
FORMS – Generic/Trade: Tabs 5/325 mg. Caps/Caplets 5/500 mg. Soln 5/325 per 5 mL, mg oxycodone/acetaminophen.
MOA – Combination analgesic.
ADVERSE EFFECTS – Serious: Respiratory depression/arrest, hepatotoxicity. Frequent: N/V, constipation, sedation.

SOMA COMPOUND WITH CODEINE (carisoprodol + acetylsalicylic acid + codeine) ▶L ♀D ▶– ©III $$$
ADULTS – <u>Moderate to severe musculoskeletal pain:</u> 1 to 2 tabs PO qid prn.
PEDS – Not approved in children.
FORMS – Generic/Trade: Tabs 200 mg carisoprodol/325 mg aspirin/16 mg codeine.
NOTES – Refer to individual components. Withdrawal with abrupt discontinuation.
MOA – Combination analgesic.
ADVERSE EFFECTS – Serious: Respiratory depression/arrest, hypersensitivity, Reye's syndrome, GI bleeding, nephrotoxicity, idiosyncratic reaction with angioedema, hypotension, and anaphylactoid shock. Frequent: N/V, dyspepsia, constipation, sedation.

SYNALGOS-DC (dihydrocodeine + acetylsalicylic acid + caffeine) ▶L ♀C ▶– ©III $
WARNING – Case reports of prolonged erections when taken concomitantly with sildenafil.
ADULTS – <u>Moderate-severe pain:</u> 2 caps PO q 4 h prn.
PEDS – Not approved in children.
FORMS – Trade only: Caps 16 mg dihydrocodeine/356.4 mg aspirin/30 mg caffeine. "Painpack" = 12 caps.
NOTES – Most common use is dental pain. Refer to individual components.
MOA – Combination analgesic.
ADVERSE EFFECTS – Serious: Respiratory depression/arrest. Frequent: N/V, constipation, sedation.

TALACEN (pentazocine + acetaminophen) ▶L ♀C ▶? ©IV $$$
ADULTS – <u>Moderate pain:</u> 1 tab PO q 4 h prn.
PEDS – Not approved in children.
FORMS – Generic/Trade: Tabs 25 mg pentazocine/650 mg acetaminophen, trade scored.
NOTES – Serious skin reactions, including erythema multiforme and Stevens-Johnson syndrome have been reported.
MOA – Combination opioid agonist-antagonist analgesic.
ADVERSE EFFECTS – Serious: Respiratory depression, hepatotoxicity. Frequent: Sedation and dizziness.

TYLENOL WITH CODEINE (codeine + acetaminophen, ✦*Lenoltec, Emtec, Triatec*) ▶LK ♀C ▶? ©III (Tabs), V(elixir) $
WARNING – Multiple strengths; see FORMS and write specific product on Rx.
ADULTS – <u>Moderate pain:</u> 1 to 2 tabs PO q 4 h prn.
PEDS – <u>Moderate pain:</u> Elixir: Give 5 mL q 4 to 6 h prn for age 3 to 6 yo, give 10 mL q 4 to 6 h prn for age 7 to 12 yo, use adult dose for age older than 12 yo.
FORMS – Generic only: Tabs Tylenol #2 (15/300). Tylenol with Codeine Elixir 12/120 per 5 mL, mg codeine/mg acetaminophen. Generic/Trade: Tabs Tylenol #3 (30/300), Tylenol #4 (60/300). Canadian forms come with (Lenoltec, Tylenol) or without (Empracet, Emtec) caffeine.
MOA – Combination analgesic.
ADVERSE EFFECTS – Serious: Respiratory depression/arrest, hepatotoxicity. Frequent: N/V, constipation, sedation.

TYLOX (oxycodone + acetaminophen) ▶L ♀C ▶– ©II $
ADULTS – <u>Moderate-severe pain:</u> 1 cap PO q 6 h prn.
PEDS – Not approved in children.
FORMS – Generic/Trade: Caps 5 mg oxycodone/500 mg acetaminophen.
MOA – Combination analgesic.
ADVERSE EFFECTS – Serious: Respiratory depression/arrest, hepatotoxicity. Frequent: N/V, constipation, sedation.

VICODIN (hydrocodone + acetaminophen) ▶LK ♀C ▶? ©III $
WARNING – Multiple strengths; see FORMS and write specific product on Rx.
ADULTS – <u>Moderate pain:</u> 5/500 (max dose 8 tabs/day) and 7.5/750 (max dose of 5 tabs/day): 1 to 2 tabs PO q 4 to 6 h prn. 10/660: 1 tab PO q 4 to 6 h prn (max of 6 tabs/day).

(cont.)

ANALGESICS: Other Analgesics

VICODIN (cont.)
PEDS — Not approved in children.
FORMS — Generic/Trade: Tabs Vicodin (5/500), Vicodin ES (7.5/750), Vicodin HP (10/660), scored, mg hydrocodone/mg acetaminophen.
MOA — Combination analgesic.
ADVERSE EFFECTS — Serious: Respiratory depression/arrest, hepatotoxicity. Frequent: N/V, constipation, sedation.

VICOPROFEN (hydrocodone + ibuprofen) ▶LK ♀– ▶? ©III $$$
ADULTS — Moderate pain: 1 tab PO q 4 to 6 h prn, max dose 5 tabs/day.
PEDS — Not approved in children.
FORMS — Generic/Trade: Tabs 7.5/200 mg hydrocodone/ibuprofen. Generic only: Tabs 2.5/200, 5/200, 10/200 mg.
NOTES — See NSAIDs-Other subclass warning.
MOA — Combination analgesic.
ADVERSE EFFECTS — Serious: Respiratory depression/arrest, hypersensitivity, GI bleeding, nephrotoxicity. Frequent: N/V, constipation, dyspepsia, sedation.

WYGESIC (propoxyphene + acetaminophen) ▶L ♀C ▶? ©IV $
ADULTS — Moderate pain: 1 tab PO q 4 h prn.
PEDS — Not approved in children.
FORMS — Generic only: Tabs 65 mg propoxyphene/650 mg acetaminophen.
NOTES — Avoid in renal insufficiency and in elderly due to risk of metabolite accumulation, and increased risk of CNS disturbance, seizures, and QRS prolongation.
MOA — Combination analgesic.
ADVERSE EFFECTS — Serious: Respiratory depression/arrest, hepatotoxicity. Frequent: N/V, constipation, sedation.

XODOL (hydrocodone + acetaminophen) ▶LK ♀C ▶– ©III $$
ADULTS — Moderate pain: 1 tab PO q 4 to 6 h prn, max 6 doses/day.
PEDS — Not approved in children.
FORMS — Trade only: Tabs 5/300, 7.5/300, 10/300 mg hydrocodone/acetaminophen.
MOA — Combination analgesic.
ADVERSE EFFECTS — Serious: Respiratory depression/arrest, hepatotoxicity. Frequent: N/V, constipation, sedation.

ZYDONE (hydrocodone + acetaminophen) ▶LK ♀C ▶? ©III $$
WARNING — Multiple strengths; see FORMS and write specific product on Rx.
ADULTS — Moderate pain: 1 to 2 tabs (5/400) PO q 4 to 6 h prn, max dose 8 tabs/day. 1 tab (7.5/400, 10/400) q 4 to 6 h prn, max dose 6 tabs/day.
PEDS — Not approved in children.
FORMS — Trade only: Tabs 5/400, 7.5/400, 10/400 mg hydrocodone/mg acetaminophen.
MOA — Combination analgesic.
ADVERSE EFFECTS — Serious: Respiratory depression/arrest, hepatotoxicity. Frequent: N/V, constipation, sedation.

ANALGESICS: Opioid Antagonists

NOTE: May result in withdrawal in the opioid-dependent, including life-threatening withdrawal if administered to neonates born to opioid-dependent mothers. Rare pulmonary edema, cardiovascular instability, hypotension, HTN, ventricular tachycardia, and ventricular fibrillation have been reported in connection with opioid reversal.

NALOXONE (Narcan) ▶LK ♀B ▶? $
ADULTS — Management of opioid overdose: 0.4 to 2 mg IV. May repeat IV at 2 to 3 min intervals up to 10 mg. Use IM/SC/ET if IV not available. IV infusion: 2 mg in 500 mL D5W or NS (0.004 mg/mL); titrate according to response. Partial postop opioid reversal: 0.1 to 0.2 mg IV at 2 to 3 min intervals; repeat IM doses may be required at 1 to 2 h intervals.
PEDS — Management of opioid overdose: 0.01 mg/kg IV. Give a subsequent dose of 0.1 mg/kg if inadequate response. Use IM/SC/ET if IV not available. Partial postop opioid reversal: 0.005 to 0.01 mg IV at 2 to 3 min intervals.
NOTES — Watch patients for re-emergence of opioid effects.
MOA — Opioid antagonist.
ADVERSE EFFECTS — Serious: Pulmonary edema, cardiovascular instability, hypo/hypertension, ventricular tachycardia and fibrillation, opioid withdrawal. Frequent: Nausea and tachycardia.

ANALGESICS: Other Analgesics

ACETAMINOPHEN (Tylenol, Panadol, Tempra, paracetamol, ✦Abenol, Atasol, Pediatrix) ▶LK ♀B ▶+ $
ADULTS — Analgesic/antipyretic: 325 to 1000 mg PO q 4 to 6 h prn. 650 mg PR q 4 to 6 h prn. Max dose 4 g/day. OA: Extended-release: 2 caps PO q 8 h around the clock. Max dose 6 caps/day.
PEDS — Analgesic/antipyretic: 10 to 15 mg/kg q 4 to 6 h PO/PR prn. Max 5 doses/day.
UNAPPROVED ADULTS — OA: 1000 mg PO qid.
FORMS — OTC: Tabs 325, 500, 650 mg. Chewable Tabs 80 mg. Oral disintegrating Tabs 80, 160 mg. Caps/Gelcaps/Caps 500 mg. Extended-release caplets 650 mg. Liquid 160 mg/5 mL, 500 mg/15 mL. Infant gtts 80 mg/0.8 mL. Supps 80, 120, 325, 650 mg.
NOTES — Risk of hepatotoxicity with chronic use, especially in alcoholics. Caution in those who drink 3 or more drinks/day. Rectal administration may produce lower/less reliable plasma levels.
MOA — Analgesic/antipyretic.
ADVERSE EFFECTS — Serious: Hepatotoxicity. Frequent: None.

CANNIBIS SATIVA L. EXTRACT (*♣Sativex*) ▶LK ♀X ▶– $$$$
ADULTS — Canada only. <u>Adjunctive treatment for the symptomatic relief of neuropathic pain in multiple sclerosis:</u> Start: 1 spray q 4 h (max 4 times per day), and titrated upwards as tolerated. Limited experience with more than 12 sprays/day.
PEDS — Not approved in children.
FORMS — Canada Trade only: Buccal spray, 27 mg/mL delta-9-tetrahydrocannabinol and 25 mg/mL cannabidiol, delivers 100 mcL per actuation, 5.5 mL vials containing up to 51 actuations per vial.
NOTES — Contraindicated in pregnancy, childbearing potential without birth control, history of psychosis, serious heart disease. Contains ethanol. Use cautiously if history of substance abuse.
MOA — Acts at cannabinoid receptors in the CNS and peripheral tissues to mediate cannabinoid-induced analgesia.
ADVERSE EFFECTS — Serious: orthostatic hypotension, syncope. Frequent: Administration site irritation, headache, depression, dizziness.

HYALURONATE (*Hyalgan, Supartz, ♣Neovisc, Orthovisc*) ▶KL ♀? ▶? $$$$$
WARNING — Do not inject extra-articularly; avoid the synovial tissues and cap. Do not use disinfectants containing benzalkonium chloride for skin preparation.
ADULTS — <u>OA (knee):</u> Hyalgan: 2 mL intra-articular injection q week for 3 to 5 weeks. Supartz: 2.5 mL intra-articular injection q week for 5 weeks. Orthovisc and Neovisc (Canada): 2 mL intra-articular injection q week for 3 weeks. Inject a local anesthetic SC prior to injections.
PEDS — Not approved in children.
FORMS — Trade only: Hyalgan, Neovisc, Orthovisc: 2 mL vials, prefilled syringes. Supartz: 2.5 mL prefilled syringes.
NOTES — For those who have failed conservative therapy. Caution in allergy to eggs, avian proteins or feathers (except Neovisc - synthetic). Remove synovial fluid or effusion before each injection. Knee pain and swelling most common side effects.
MOA — Improves viscosity/elasticity of synovial fluid.
ADVERSE EFFECTS — Serious: Anaphylactoid reactions. Frequent: Knee pain and swelling, joint pain, back pain, injection site pain.

HYLAN GF-20 (*Synvisc*) ▶KL ♀? ▶? $$$$$
WARNING — Do not inject extra-articularly; avoid the synovial tissues and cap. Do not use disinfectants containing benzalkonium chloride for skin preparation.
ADULTS — <u>OA (knee):</u> 2 mL intra-articular injection q week for 3 weeks.
PEDS — Not approved in children.
FORMS — Trade only: 2.25 mL glass syringe with 2 mL drug; 3/pack.
NOTES — For those who have failed conservative therapy. Caution in allergy to eggs, avian proteins or feathers. Remove synovial fluid or effusion before each injection. Knee pain and swelling most common side effects.
MOA — Improves viscosity/elasticity of synovial fluid.
ADVERSE EFFECTS — Serious: Anaphylactoid reactions. Frequent: Knee pain and swelling.

TAPENTADOL (*Nucynta*) ▶LK ♀C ▶– ©II $$$$
WARNING — Abuse potential.
ADULTS — <u>Moderate to severe acute pain:</u> 50 to 100 mg PO q 4 to 6 h prn. Max dose 600 mg/day. If moderate hepatic impairment, decrease dose to 50 mg PO q 8 h. Do not use in severe renal or hepatic impairment.
PEDS — Not approved in children younger than 18 yo.
FORMS — Trade only: Tabs 50, 75, 100 mg.
NOTES — Contraindicated in acute intoxication with alcohol, hypnotics, centrally acting analgesics, opioids, or psychotropic drugs and with respiratory depression. Use with caution in patients with known seizure disorders. Seizures and/or serotonin syndrome may occur with concurrent antidepressants, triptans, linezolid, lithium, St John's wort.
MOA — Opioid agonist/norepinephrine reuptake inhibitor.
ADVERSE EFFECTS — Serious: Seizures, anaphylactoid reactions, respiratory depression. Frequent: Nausea, dizziness, vomiting, somnolence.

TRAMADOL (*Ultram, Ultram ER, Ryzolt*) ▶KL ♀C ▶– $$$
ADULTS — <u>Moderate to moderately severe pain:</u> 50 to 100 mg PO q 4 to 6 h prn. Max dose 400 mg/day. If older than 75 yo, use less than 300 mg/day PO in divided doses. If CrCl < 30 mL/min, increase the dosing interval to 12 h. If cirrhosis, decrease dose to 50 mg PO q 12 h. <u>Chronic pain, extended-release:</u> 100 to 300 mg PO daily. Do not use if CrCl < 30 mL/min or with severe hepatic dysfunction.
PEDS — Not approved in children younger than 16 yo.
FORMS — Generic/Trade: Tabs, immediate-release 50 mg. Trade only (Ultram ER, Ryzolt): Extended-release tabs 100, 200, 300 mg.
NOTES — Contraindicated in acute intoxication with alcohol, hypnotics, centrally acting analgesics, opioids, or psychotropic drugs. Seizures and/or serotonin syndrome may occur with concurrent antidepressants, triptans, linezolid, lithium, St John's wort, or enzyme inducing drugs such as ketoconazole and erythromycin; use with caution and adjust dose. Withdrawal symptoms may occur in patients dependent on opioids or with abrupt discontinuation. Overdose treated with naloxone may increase seizures. Carbamazepine decreases tramadol levels. The most frequent side effects are nausea and constipation. ER tabs cannot be crushed, chewed, or split.
MOA — Opioid agonist/norepinephrine and serotonin reuptake inhibitor.
ADVERSE EFFECTS — Serious: Seizures, anaphylactoid reactions. Frequent: Constipation, nausea, somnolence.

WOMEN'S TYLENOL MENSTRUAL RELIEF (acetaminophen + pamabrom) ▶LK ♀B ▶+ $
ADULTS — <u>Menstrual cramps:</u> 2 caps PO q 4 to 6 h.
PEDS — Use adult dose for age older than 12 yo.
FORMS — OTC: Caps 500 mg acetaminophen/ 25 mg pamabrom (diuretic).
NOTES — Hepatotoxicity with chronic use, especially in alcoholics.
MOA — Analgesic/diuretic.
ADVERSE EFFECTS — Serious: Hepatotoxicity. Frequent: None.

ANESTHESIA: Anesthetics and Sedatives

ALFENTANIL (*Alfenta*) ▶L ♀C ▶? ©II $
ADULTS — IV <u>general anesthesia adjunct;</u> specialized dosing.
PEDS — Not approved in children.
MOA — Opioid agonist.
ADVERSE EFFECTS — Serious: Respiratory depression, hypotension, bradycardia, chest wall rigidity, increased intracranial pressure, opiate dependence, hypersensitivity. Frequent: Sedation, N/V.

DEXMEDETOMIDINE (*Precedex*) ▶LK ♀C ▶? $$$$
ADULTS — <u>ICU sedation</u> less than 24 h: Load 1 mcg/kg over 10 min followed by infusion 0.2 to 0.7 mcg/kg/h titrated to desired sedation endpoint.
PEDS — Not recommended age younger than 18 yo.
NOTES — Alpha 2 adrenergic agonist with sedative properties. Beware of bradycardia and hypotension. Avoid in advanced heart block.
MOA — Alpha-2 adrenergic agonist with sedative properties.
ADVERSE EFFECTS — Serious: Bradycardia, heart block, hypotension. Frequent: Sedation.

ETOMIDATE (*Amidate*) ▶L ♀C ▶? $
ADULTS — <u>Anesthesia induction/rapid sequence intubation:</u> 0.3 mg/kg IV.
PEDS — Age younger than 10 yo: Not approved. Age 10 or older: Use adult dosing.
UNAPPROVED PEDS — <u>Anesthesia induction/rapid sequence intubation:</u> 0.3 mg/kg IV.
NOTES — Adrenocortical suppression, but rarely of clinical significance.
MOA — Nonbarbiturate hypnotic without analgesic properties.
ADVERSE EFFECTS — Serious: Respiratory depression, hypotension, adrenal suppression. Frequent: Myoclonus, N/V.

FOSPROPOFOL (*Lusedra*) ▶L ♀– ▶? $$$$
WARNING — Beware of respiratory depression/apnea. Administer with appropriate monitoring.
ADULTS — <u>Deep sedation</u> (age younger than 65 yo): 6.5 mg/kg IV (not to exceed 16.5 mL), 1.6 mg/kg supplemental dose q 4 min (not to exceed 4 mL). Age older than 65 yo or severe systemic disease (aspirin P3 or P4) use 75% of initial and supplemental doses. Wt greater than 90 kg, dose at 90 kg; wt less than 60 kg, dose at 60 kg.
PEDS — Not recommended.
NOTES — Prodrug which is compatible with standard IV fluids.
MOA — Metabolized to propofol by alkaline phosphatase, and then functions as nonbarbiturate hypnotic without analgesic properties.
ADVERSE EFFECTS — Serious: Respiratory depression, hypotension, hypersensitivity. Frequent: Injection site pain, sedation.

KETAMINE (*Ketalar*) ▶L ♀? ▶? ©III $
WARNING — Emergence delirium limits value of ketamine in adults; such reactions are rare in children.
ADULTS — <u>Dissociative sedation:</u> 1 to 2 mg/kg IV over 1 to 2 min or 4 to 5 mg/kg IM.
PEDS — <u>Dissociative sedation:</u> 1 to 2 mg/kg IV over 1 to 2 min or 4 to 5 mg/kg IM.
NOTES — Raises BP and intracranial pressure; avoid if CAD, HTN, head or eye injury. Concurrent atropine minimizes hypersalivation; can be combined in same syringe with ketamine for IM use.
MOA — Dissociative agent.
ADVERSE EFFECTS — Serious: Laryngospasm, hallucinatory emergence reactions, hypersalivation. Frequent: Nystagmus, hypertension, tachycardia, N/V, muscular hypertonicity, myoclonus.

METHOHEXITAL (*Brevital*) ▶L ♀B ▶? ©IV $
ADULTS — <u>Anesthesia induction:</u> 1 to 1.5 mg/kg IV.
PEDS — <u>Anesthesia induction:</u> 6.6 to 10 mg/kg IM or 25 mg/kg PR.
UNAPPROVED PEDS — <u>Sedation for diagnostic imaging:</u> 25 mg/kg PR.
MOA — Ultra-short acting barbiturate sedative/hypnotic.
ADVERSE EFFECTS — Serious: Respiratory depression, hypotension, bronchospasm. Frequent: Respiratory depression, hypotension.

MIDAZOLAM (*Versed*) ▶LK ♀D ▶– ©IV $
WARNING — Beware of respiratory depression/apnea. Administer with appropriate monitoring.
ADULTS — <u>Sedation/anxiolysis:</u> 0.07 to 0.08 mg/kg IM (5 mg in average adult); or 1 mg IV slowly q 2 to 3 min up to 5 mg. <u>Anesthesia induction:</u> 0.3 to 0.35 mg/kg IV over 20 to 30 sec.
PEDS — <u>Sedation/anxiolysis:</u> Oral route 0.25 to 1 mg/kg (0.5 mg/kg most effective) to maximum of 20 mg PO, IM route 0.1 to 0.15 mg/kg IM. IV route initial dose 0.05 to 0.1 mg/kg IV, then titrated to max 0.6 mg/kg for age 6 mo to 5 yo, initial dose 0.025 to 0.05 mg/kg IV, then titrated to max 0.4 mg/kg for age 6 to 12 yo.
UNAPPROVED PEDS — <u>Sedation/anxiolysis:</u> Intranasal 0.2 to 0.4 mg/kg. Rectal: 0.25 to 0.5 mg/kg PR. <u>Status epilepticus:</u> Load 0.15 mg/kg IV followed by infusion 1 mcg/kg/min and titrate dose upward q 5 min prn.
FORMS — Generic only: Oral liquid 2 mg/mL.

(cont.)

ANESTHESIA: Local Anesthetics

MIDAZOLAM (cont.)
NOTES — Use lower doses in the elderly, chronically ill, and those receiving concurrent CNS depressants.
MOA — Short-acting benzodiazepine sedative.
ADVERSE EFFECTS — Serious: Respiratory depression. Frequent: Sedation.

PENTOBARBITAL (*Nembutal*) ▶LK ♀D ▶? ©II $$
ADULTS — Rarely used; other drugs preferred. Hypnotic: 150 to 200 mg IM or 100 mg IV at a rate of 50 mg/min, maximum dose is 500 mg.
PEDS — FDA approved for active seizing, but other agents preferred.
UNAPPROVED PEDS — Procedural sedation: 1 to 6 mg/kg IV, adjusted in increments of 1 to 2 mg/kg to desired effect, or 2 to 6 mg/kg IM, max 100 mg. Do not exceed 50 mg/min.
MOA — Nonselective CNS depressant.
ADVERSE EFFECTS — Serious: Respiratory depression, blood dyscrasias, anemia, thrombocytopenia, Stevens-Johnson syndrome, angioedema, dependence, withdrawal reactions. Frequent: Drowsiness, fatigue, N/V bradycardia, paradoxical CNS excitation.

PROPOFOL (*Diprivan*) ▶L ♀B ▶– $$$
WARNING — Beware of respiratory depression/apnea. Administer with appropriate monitoring.
ADULTS — Anesthesia (age younger than 55 yo): 40 mg IV q 10 sec until induction onset (typical 2 to 2.5 mg/kg). Follow with maintenance infusion generally 100 to 200 mcg/kg/min. Lower doses in elderly or for sedation. ICU ventilator sedation: Infusion 5 to 50 mcg/kg/min.
PEDS — Anesthesia age 3 yo or older: 2.5 to 3.5 mg/kg IV over 20 to 30 sec, followed with infusion 125 to 300 mcg/kg/min. Not recommended if age younger than 3 yo or for prolonged ICU use.
UNAPPROVED ADULTS — Deep sedation: 1 mg/kg IV over 20 to 30 sec. Repeat 0.5 mg/kg IV prn. Intubation adjunct: 2.0 to 2.5 mg/kg IV.
UNAPPROVED PEDS — Deep sedation: 1 mg/kg IV (max 40 mg) over 20 to 30 sec. Repeat 0.5 mg/kg (max 20 mg) IV prn.

NOTES — Avoid with egg or soy allergies. Prolonged infusions may lead to hypertriglyceridemia. Injection pain can be treated or pretreated with lidocaine 40 to 50 mg IV.
MOA — Nonbarbiturate hypnotic without analgesic properties.
ADVERSE EFFECTS — Serious: Respiratory depression, hypotension, hypersensitivity. Frequent: Injection site pain, sedation.

REMIFENTANIL (*Ultiva*) ▶L ♀C ▶? ©II $$
ADULTS — IV general anesthesia adjunct; specialized dosing.
PEDS — IV general anesthesia adjunct; specialized dosing.
MOA — Opioid agonist.
ADVERSE EFFECTS — Serious: Respiratory depression, hypotension, bradycardia, chest wall rigidity, opiate dependence, hypersensitivity. Frequent: Sedation, N/V.

SUFENTANIL (*Sufenta*) ▶L ♀C ▶? ©II $$
ADULTS — IV anesthesia adjunct: Specialized dosing.
PEDS — IV anesthesia adjunct: Specialized dosing.
MOA — Opioid agonist.
ADVERSE EFFECTS — Serious: Respiratory depression, hypotension, bradycardia, chest wall rigidity, opiate dependence, hypersensitivity. Frequent: Sedation, N/V.

THIOPENTAL (*Pentothal*) ▶L ♀C ▶? ©III $
ADULTS — Anesthesia induction: 3 to 5 mg/kg IV.
PEDS — Anesthesia induction: 3 to 5 mg/kg IV.
UNAPPROVED PEDS — Sedation for diagnostic imaging: 25 mg/kg PR.
NOTES — Duration 5 min. Hypotension, histamine-release, tissue necrosis with extravasation.
MOA — Ultra-short acting barbiturate sedative/hypnotic.
ADVERSE EFFECTS — Serious: Respiratory depression, hypotension, bronchospasm. Frequent: Respiratory depression, hypotension.

ANESTHESIA: Local Anesthetics

NOTE: Risk of chondrolysis in patients receiving intra-articular infusions of local anesthetics following arthroscopic and other surgical procedures

ARTICAINE (*Septocaine, Zorcaine*) ▶LK ♀C ▶? $
ADULTS — Dental local anesthesia: 4% injection.
PEDS — Dental local anesthesia age 4 yo or older: 4% injection.
FORMS — 4% (includes epinephrine 1:100,000).
NOTES — Do not exceed 7 mg/kg total dose.
MOA — Amide local anesthetic.
ADVERSE EFFECTS — Serious: Seizures, cardiovascular depression, bradycardia, hypersensitivity, methemoglobinemia. Frequent: None.

BUPIVACAINE (*Marcaine, Sensorcaine*) ▶LK ♀C ▶? $
ADULTS — Local anesthesia, nerve block: 0.25% injection.
PEDS — Not recommended in children age younger than 12 yo.
FORMS — 0.25%, 0.5%, 0.75%, all with or without epinephrine.
NOTES — Onset 5 min, duration 2 to 4 h (longer with epi). Amide group. Max dose 2.5 mg/kg alone, or 3.0 mg/kg with epinephrine.
MOA — Amide local anesthetic.
ADVERSE EFFECTS — Serious: Seizures, cardiovascular depression, bradycardia, hypersensitivity, methemoglobinemia. Frequent: None.

DUOCAINE (bupivacaine + lidocaine - local anesthetic) ▶LK ♀C ▶? $
ADULTS — Local anesthesia, nerve block for eye surgery.
PEDS — Not recommended in children age younger than 12 yo.
FORMS — Vials contain bupivacaine 0.375% + lidocaine 1%.
NOTES — Use standard precautions including maximum dosing without epi for both bupivacaine and lidocaine.
MOA — Amide local anesthetic combination.
ADVERSE EFFECTS — Serious: Seizures, cardiovascular depression, bradycardia, heart block, hypotension, hypersensitivity, methemoglobinemia. Frequent: None.

LIDOCAINE—LOCAL ANESTHETIC (Xylocaine) ▶LK ♀B ▶? $
ADULTS — Local anesthesia: 0.5 to 1% injection.
PEDS — Local anesthesia: 0.5 to 1% injection.
FORMS — 0.5, 1, 1.5, 2%. With epi: 0.5, 1, 1.5, 2%.
NOTES — Onset within 2 min, duration 30 to 60 min (longer with epi). Amide group. Potentially toxic dose 3 to 5 mg/kg without epinephrine, and 5 to 7 mg/kg with epinephrine. Use "cardiac lidocaine" (ie, IV formulation) for Bier blocks at maximum dose of 3 mg/kg so that neither epinephrine nor methylparaben are injected IV.
MOA — Amide local anesthetic.
ADVERSE EFFECTS — Serious: Seizures, cardiovascular depression, bradycardia, hypersensitivity, methemoglobinemia. Frequent: None.

MEPIVACAINE (Carbocaine, Polocaine) ▶LK ♀C ▶? $
ADULTS — Nerve block: 1% to 2% injection.
PEDS — Nerve block: 1% to 2% injection. Use less than 2% concentration if age younger than 3 yo or wt less than 30 pounds.
FORMS — 1, 1.5, 2, 3%.
NOTES — Onset 3 to 5 min, duration 45 to 90 min. Amide group. Max local dose 5 to 6 mg/kg.
MOA — Amide local anesthetic.
ADVERSE EFFECTS — Serious: Seizures, cardiovascular depression, bradycardia, hypersensitivity, methemoglobinemia, nephrotoxicity. Frequent: None.

ORAQUIX (prilocaine + lidocaine - Local anesthetic) ▶LK ♀B ▶? $$
ADULTS — Local anesthetic gel applied to periodontal pockets using blunt-tipped applicator: 4% injection.
PEDS — Not approved in children.
FORMS — Gel 2.5% + 2.5% with applicator.
NOTES — Do not exceed maximum dose for lidocaine or prilocaine.
MOA — Amide local anesthetic combination.
ADVERSE EFFECTS — Serious: Seizures, cardiovascular depression, bradycardia, hypersensitivity, methemoglobinemia. Frequent: None.

ANESTHESIA: Neuromuscular Blockers

NOTE: Should be administered only by those skilled in airway management and respiratory support.

ATRACURIUM (Tracrium) ▶Plasma ♀C ▶? $
ADULTS — Paralysis: 0.4 to 0.5 mg/kg IV.
PEDS — Paralysis age 2 yo or older: 0.4 to 0.5 mg/kg IV.
NOTES — Duration 15 to 30 min. Hoffman degradation.
MOA — Nondepolarizing skeletal muscle relaxant.
ADVERSE EFFECTS — Serious: Apnea, bronchospasm, hypersensitivity. Frequent: Apnea, rash.

CISATRACURIUM (Nimbex) ▶Plasma ♀B ▶? $$
ADULTS — Paralysis: 0.15 to 0.2 mg/kg IV.
PEDS — Paralysis: 0.1 mg/kg IV over 5 to 10 sec.
NOTES — Duration 30 to 60 min. Hoffman degradation.
MOA — Nondepolarizing skeletal muscle relaxant.
ADVERSE EFFECTS — Serious: Apnea, bradycardia, bronchospasm. Frequent: Apnea.

PANCURONIUM (Pavulon) ▶LK ♀C ▶? $
ADULTS — Paralysis: 0.04 to 0.1 mg/kg IV.
PEDS — Paralysis (beyond neonatal age): 0.04 to 0.1 mg/kg IV.
NOTES — Duration 45 min. Decrease dose if renal disease.
MOA — Nondepolarizing skeletal muscle relaxant.
ADVERSE EFFECTS — Serious: Apnea, hypersensitivity, bronchospasm. Frequent: Apnea, tachycardia.

ROCURONIUM (Zemuron) ▶L ♀B ▶? $$
ADULTS — Paralysis: 0.6 mg/kg IV. Rapid sequence intubation: 0.6 to 1.2 mg/kg IV. Continuous infusion: 10 to 12 mcg/kg/min; first verify spontaneous recovery from bolus dose.
PEDS — Paralysis (age older than 3 mo): 0.6 mg/kg IV. Continuous infusion: 12 mcg/kg/min; first verify spontaneous recovery from bolus dose.
NOTES — Duration 30 min. Decrease dose if severe liver disease.
MOA — Nondepolarizing skeletal muscle relaxant.
ADVERSE EFFECTS — Serious: Apnea, bronchospasm. Frequent: Apnea.

SUCCINYLCHOLINE (Anectine, Quelicin) ▶Plasma ♀C ▶? $
ADULTS — Paralysis: 0.6 to 1.1 mg/kg IV.
PEDS — Paralysis age younger than 5 yo: 2 mg/kg IV. Paralysis age 5 yo or older: 1 mg/kg IV.
NOTES — Avoid in hyperkalemia, myopathies, eye injuries, rhabdomyolysis, subacute burn, and syndromes of denervated or disused musculature (eg, Paralysis from spinal cord injury or major CVA). If immediate cardiac arrest and ET tube is in correct place and no tension pneumothorax evident, strongly consider empiric treatment for hyperkalemia. Succinylcholine can trigger malignant hyperthermia; see www.mhaus.org.

(cont.)

ANTIMICROBIALS: Aminoglycosides

SUCCINYLCHOLINE (cont.)
  MOA – Ultra-short acting depolarizing skeletal muscle relaxant.
  ADVERSE EFFECTS – Serious: Apnea, bradycardia, hyperkalemia, malignant hyperthermia. Frequent: Apnea, fasciculations, muscle pain.

VECURONIUM (Norcuron) ▶LK ♀C ▶? $
  ADULTS – Paralysis: 0.08 to 0.1 mg/kg IV bolus. Continuous infusion: 0.8 to 1.2 mcg/kg/min; first verify spontaneous recovery from bolus dose.
  PEDS – Age younger than 7 weeks: Safety has not been established. Age 7 weeks to 1 yo: Moderately more sensitive on a mg/kg dose compared to adults and take 1.5 for longer to recover. Age 1 to 10 yo: May require a slightly higher initial dose and may also require supplementation slightly more often than older patients. Paralysis age 10 yo or older: 0.08 to 0.1 mg/kg IV bolus. Continuous infusion: 0.8 to 1.2 mcg/kg/min; first verify spontaneous recovery from bolus dose.
  NOTES – Duration 15 to 30 min. Decrease dose in severe liver disease.
  MOA – Nondepolarizing skeletal muscle relaxant.
  ADVERSE EFFECTS – Serious: Apnea. Frequent: Apnea.

ANTIMICROBIALS: Aminoglycosides

NOTE: See also dermatology and ophthalmology.

AMIKACIN (Amikin) ▶K ♀D ▶? $$$
  WARNING – Nephrotoxicity, ototoxicity.
  ADULTS – Gram negative infections: 15 mg/kg/day (up to 1500 mg/day) IM/IV divided q 8 to 12 h.
  PEDS – Gram negative infections: 15 mg/kg/day (up to 1500 mg/day) IM/IV divided q 8 to 12 h. Neonates: 10 mg/kg load, then 7.5 mg/kg IM/IV q 12 h.
  UNAPPROVED ADULTS – Once daily dosing: 15 mg/kg IV q 24 h. TB (2nd line treatment): 15 mg/kg (up to 1 g) IM/IV daily. 10 mg/kg (up to 750 mg) IM/IV daily for age older than 59 yo.
  UNAPPROVED PEDS – Severe infections: 15 to 22.5 mg/kg/day IV divided q 8 h. Some experts recommend 30 mg/kg/day. Once daily: 15 mg/kg IV q 24 h. Some experts consider once daily of aminoglycosides investigational in children. TB (2nd line treatment): 15 to 30 mg/kg (up to 1 g) IM/IV daily.
  NOTES – May enhance effects of neuromuscular blockers. Avoid other ototoxic/nephrotoxic drugs. Individualize dose in renal dysfunction, burn patients. Base dose on average of actual and ideal body wt in obesity. Peak 20 to 35 mcg/mL, trough < 5 mcg/mL.
  MOA – Inhibits bacterial protein synthesis by interfering with function of ribosomal 30S subunit. Bactericidal.
  ADVERSE EFFECTS – Serious and frequent: Nephrotoxicity, neuromuscular blockade, ototoxicity. Serious and rare: Vestibular toxicity.

GENTAMICIN (Garamycin) ▶K ♀D ▶+ $
  WARNING – Nephrotoxicity, ototoxicity.
  ADULTS – Gram negative infections: 3 to 5 mg/kg/day IM/IV divided q 8 h. See table for prophylaxis of bacterial endocarditis.
  PEDS – Gram negative infections: 2.5 mg/kg IM/IV q 12 h for age younger than 1 week old and wt greater than 2 kg; 2 to 2.5 mg/kg IM/IV q 8 h for age 1 week old or older and wt greater than 2 kg. Cystic fibrosis: 9 mg/kg/day IV in divided doses with target peak of 8 to 12 mcg/mL.
  UNAPPROVED ADULTS – Once daily for gram negative infections: 5 to 7 mg/kg IV q 24 h. Endocarditis: 3 mg/kg/day for synergy with another agent. Give once daily for viridans streptococci, 2 to 3 divided doses for staphylococci, 3 divided doses for enterococci.
  UNAPPROVED PEDS – Once daily dosing: 5 to 7 mg/kg IV q 24 h. Give 4 mg/kg IV q 24 h for age younger than 1 week old and full-term. Some experts consider once daily of aminoglycosides investigational in children.
  NOTES – May enhance effects of neuromuscular blockers. Avoid other ototoxic/nephrotoxic drugs. Individualize dose in renal dysfunction, burn patients. Base dose on average of actual and ideal body wt in obesity. Peak 5 to 10 mcg/mL, trough < 2 mcg/mL.
  MOA – Inhibits bacterial protein synthesis by interfering with function of ribosomal 30S subunit. Bactericidal.
  ADVERSE EFFECTS – Serious and frequent: Nephrotoxicity, neuromuscular blockade, ototoxicity. Serious and rare: Vestibular toxicity.

STREPTOMYCIN ▶K ♀D ▶+ $$$$$
  WARNING – Nephrotoxicity, ototoxicity. Monitor audiometry, renal function, and electrolytes.
  ADULTS – Combined therapy for TB: 15 mg/kg (up to 1 g) IM/IV daily. 10 mg/kg (up to 750 mg) IM/IV daily if age 60 yo or older.
  PEDS – Combined therapy for TB: 20 to 40 mg/kg (up to 1 g) IM daily.
  UNAPPROVED ADULTS – Same IM dosing can be given IV. Streptococcal endocarditis: 7.5 mg/kg IV/IM bid. Go to www.americanheart.org for further info.
  NOTES – Contraindicated in pregnancy. Obtain baseline audiogram, vestibular, and Romberg testing, and renal function. Monitor renal function and vestibular and auditory symptoms monthly. May enhance effects of neuromuscular blockers. Avoid other ototoxic/nephrotoxic drugs. Individualize dose in renal dysfunction.
  MOA – Inhibits bacterial protein synthesis by interfering with function of ribosomal 30S subunit. Bactericidal.
  ADVERSE EFFECTS – Serious and frequent: Ototoxicity, vestibular toxicity. Serious and rare:

(cont.)

STREPTOMYCIN (cont.)

Nephrotoxicity, neuromuscular blockade. Frequent: Circumoral paresthesias immediately after injection.

TOBRAMYCIN (*Nebcin, TOBI*) ▶K ♀D ▶? $$
- WARNING – Nephrotoxicity, ototoxicity.
- ADULTS – <u>Gram negative infections:</u> 3 to 5 mg/kg/day IM/IV divided q 8 h. Parenteral for <u>cystic fibrosis:</u> 10 mg/kg/day IV divided q 6 h with target peak of 8 to 12 mcg/mL. Nebulized for cystic fibrosis (TOBI): 300 mg neb bid 28 days on, then 28 days off.
- PEDS – <u>Gram negative infections:</u> 2 to 2.5 mg/kg IV q 8 h or 1.5 to 1.9 mg/kg IV q 6 h. Give 4 mg/kg/day divided q 12 h for premature/full-term neonates age 1 week old or less. Parenteral for <u>cystic fibrosis:</u> 10 mg/kg/day IV divided q 6 h with target peak of 8 to 12 mcg/mL. Nebulized for cystic fibrosis (TOBI) age 6 yo or older: 300 mg neb bid 28 days on, then 28 days off.
- UNAPPROVED ADULTS – Once daily dosing: 5 to 7 mg/kg IV q 24 h.
- UNAPPROVED PEDS – Once daily dosing: 5 to 7 mg/kg IV q 24 h. Some experts consider once daily dosing of aminoglycosides investigational in children.
- FORMS – Trade only: TOBI 300 mg ampules for nebulizer.
- NOTES – May enhance effects of neuromuscular blockers. Avoid other ototoxic/nephrotoxic drugs. Individualize dose in renal dysfunction, burn patients. Base dose on average of actual and ideal body wt in obesity. Routine monitoring of tobramycin levels not required with nebulized TOBI. Peak 5 to 10 mcg/mL, trough < 2 mcg/mL.
- MOA – Inhibits bacterial protein synthesis by interfering with function of ribosomal 30S subunit. Bactericidal.
- ADVERSE EFFECTS – Serious and frequent: Nephrotoxicity, neuromuscular blockade, ototoxicity. Serious and rare: Vestibular toxicity.

ANTIMICROBIALS: Antifungal Agents—Azoles

NOTE: See www.idsociety.org for guidelines on the management of fungal infections. See www.aidsinfo.nih.gov for management of fungal infections in HIV-infected patients.

CLOTRIMAZOLE (*Mycelex, ♣Canesten, Clotrimaderm*) ▶L ♀C ▶? $$$$
- ADULTS – <u>Oropharyngeal candidiasis:</u> 1 troche dissolved slowly in mouth 5 times per day for 14 days. Prevention of <u>oropharyngeal candidiasis in immunocompromised patients:</u> 1 troche dissolved slowly in mouth tid until end of chemotherapy or high-dose corticosteroids.
- PEDS – <u>Oropharyngeal candidiasis</u> age 3 yo or older: Use adult dose.
- FORMS – Generic/Trade: Oral troches 10 mg.
- MOA – Imidazole that inhibits the synthesis of ergosterol (a sterol required for normal fungal cytoplasmic membrane).
- ADVERSE EFFECTS – Serious: None.

FLUCONAZOLE (*Diflucan*) ▶K ♀C ▶+ $$$$
- ADULTS – <u>Vaginal candidiasis:</u> 150 mg PO single dose ($). All other dosing regimens IV/PO. <u>Oropharyngeal candidiasis:</u> 200 mg first day, then 100 mg daily for at least 2 weeks. <u>Esophageal candidiasis:</u> 200 mg first day, then 100 mg daily (up to 400 mg/day) for at least 3 weeks and continuing for 2 weeks past symptom resolution. <u>Systemic candidiasis:</u> Up to 400 mg daily. <u>Candidal UTI, peritonitis:</u> 50 to 200 mg daily. See UNAPPROVED ADULT for IDSA regimens for Candida infections. <u>Cryptococcal meningitis:</u> 400 mg daily until 10 to 12 weeks after cerebrospinal fluid is culture negative (see UNAPPROVED ADULT for first line regimen). <u>Suppression of cryptococcal meningitis relapse in AIDS:</u> 200 mg daily until immune system reconstitution. <u>Prevention of candidiasis after bone marrow transplant:</u> 400 mg daily starting several days before neutropenia and continuing until ANC >1000 cells/mm3 for 7 days.
- PEDS – All dosing regimens IV/PO. <u>Oropharyngeal candidiasis:</u> 6 mg/kg first day, then 3 mg/kg daily for at least 2 weeks. <u>Esophageal candidiasis:</u> 6 mg/kg first day, then 3 mg/kg daily (up to 12 mg/kg daily) for at least 3 weeks and continuing for 2 weeks past symptom resolution. <u>Systemic candidiasis:</u> 6 to 12 mg/kg daily. See UNAPPROVED PEDS for alternative regimens for Candida infections. <u>Cryptococcal meningitis:</u> 12 mg/kg on first day, then 6 to 12 mg/kg daily until 10 to 12 weeks after cerebrospinal fluid is culture negative. <u>Suppression of cryptococcal meningitis relapse in AIDS:</u> 6 mg/kg daily. Peds/adult dose equivalents: 3 mg/kg peds equivalent to 100 mg adult; 6 mg/kg peds equivalent to 200 mg adult; 12 mg/kg peds equivalent to 400 mg adult; max peds dose is 600 mg/day.
- UNAPPROVED ADULTS – <u>Onychomycosis, fingernail:</u> 150 to 300 mg PO q week for 3 to 6 months. <u>Onychomycosis, toenail:</u> 150 to 300 mg PO q week for 6 to 12 months. <u>Recurrent vaginal candidiasis:</u> 150 mg PO q 3rd day for 3 doses, then 100 to 150 mg PO q week for 6 months. <u>Oropharyngeal candidiasis:</u> 100 to 200 mg daily for 7 to 14 days. <u>Esophageal candidiasis:</u> 200 to 400 mg daily for 14 to 21 days. <u>Candidemia:</u> 800 mg first day, then 400 mg once a day. Treat for 14 days after first negative blood culture and resolution of signs/symptoms. <u>Candida pyelonephritis:</u> 200 to 400 mg (3 to 6 mg/kg) daily for 14 days. <u>Prevention of candidal infections in high-risk neutropenic pts:</u> 400 mg/day during period of risk for neutropenia. <u>Cryptococcal meningitis:</u> Amphotericin B preferably in combo with flucytosine for at least 2 weeks (induction), followed by fluconazole 400 mg PO once daily for 8 weeks

(cont.)

FLUCONAZOLE (cont.)

(consolidation), then chronic suppression with fluconazole 200 mg PO once daily until immune system reconstitution. <u>Treatment/suppression of coccidioidomycosis in HIV infection</u>: 400 mg PO once daily.

UNAPPROVED PEDS — <u>Oropharyngeal candidiasis</u>: 6 mg/kg first day, then 3 mg/kg once daily for 7 to 14 days. <u>Esophageal candidiasis</u>: 12 mg/kg first day, then 6 mg/kg once daily for 14 to 21 days. <u>Systemic Candida infection</u>: 12 mg/kg on first day, then 6 to 12 mg/kg once daily. <u>Cryptococcal meningitis</u>: Amphotericin B preferably in combo with flucytosine for 2 weeks (induction), followed by fluconazole 12 mg/kg on first day, then 6 to 12 mg/kg (max 800 mg) IV/PO once a day for at least 8 weeks (consolidation), then chronic suppression with lower dose of fluconazole.

FORMS — Generic/Trade: Tabs 50, 100, 150, 200 mg. 150 mg tab in single-dose blister pack. Susp 10, 40 mg/mL (35 mL).

NOTES — Many drug interactions, including increased levels of cyclosporine, phenytoin, theophylline, and increased INR with warfarin. May inhibit metabolism of fluvastatin, and possibly simvastatin/lovastatin at higher doses. Dosing in renal dysfunction: Reduce maintenance dose by 50% for CrCl 11 to 50 mL/min. Hemodialysis: Give recommended dose after each dialysis. Single dose during first trimester of pregnancy does not appear to increase risk of congenital birth defects.

MOA — Triazole that inhibits the synthesis of ergosterol (a sterol required for normal fungal cytoplasmic membrane).

ADVERSE EFFECTS — Serious: Hepatotoxicity (rare), anaphylaxis (rare), exfoliative skin disorders (rare). Frequent: Increased transaminase levels. Single-dose for vaginal candidiasis: Headache, nausea, abdominal pain.

ITRACONAZOLE (*Hyphanox, Sporanox*) ▶L ♀C ▶– $$$$$

WARNING — Inhibition of CYP3A4 metabolism by itraconazole can lead to dangerously high levels of some drugs. High levels of some can prolong QT interval (see QT drugs table). Contraindicated with dofetilide, ergot alkaloids, lovastatin, PO midazolam, nisoldipine, pimozide, quinidine, simvastatin, triazolam. Negative inotrope (may be additive with calcium channel blockers); stop treatment if signs/symptoms of heart failure. Not for onychomycosis if heart failure; use for other indications in heart failure only if benefit exceeds risk.

ADULTS — Caps: Take caps or tabs with full meal. <u>Onychomycosis, toenails</u>: 200 mg PO daily for 12 weeks. <u>Onychomycosis "pulse dosing" for fingernails</u>: 200 mg PO bid for first week of month for 2 months. Test nail specimen to confirm diagnosis before prescribing. <u>Aspergillosis in patients intolerant/refractory to amphotericin, blastomycosis, histoplasmosis</u>: 200 mg PO bid or daily. Treat for at least 3 months. For <u>life-threatening infections</u>, load with 200 mg PO tid for 3 days. Oral soln: Swish and swallow in 10 mL increments on empty stomach. <u>Oropharyngeal candidiasis</u>: 200 mg PO daily for 1 to 2 weeks. <u>Oropharyngeal candidiasis unresponsive to fluconazole</u>: 100 mg PO bid. <u>Esophageal candidiasis</u>: 100 to 200 mg PO daily for at least 3 weeks and continuing for 2 weeks past symptom resolution.

PEDS — Not approved in children.

UNAPPROVED ADULTS — Caps: <u>Onychomycosis "pulse dosing" for toenails</u>: 200 mg PO bid for first week of mo for 3 to 4 months. Confirm diagnosis with nail specimen lab testing before prescribing. <u>Prevention of histoplasmosis in HIV infection</u>: 200 mg PO once daily. <u>Treatment/suppression of coccidioidomycosis in HIV infection</u>: 200 mg PO bid. <u>Fluconazole-refractory oropharyngeal or esophageal candidiasis</u>: 200 mg PO of oral soln daily for 14 to 21 days.

UNAPPROVED PEDS — <u>Oropharyngeal candidiasis, age 5 yo or older</u>: Oral soln 2.5 mg/kg PO bid (max 200 to 400 mg/day) for 7 to 14 days. <u>Esophageal candidiasis, age 5 yo or older</u>: Oral soln 2.5 mg/kg PO bid or 5 mg/kg PO once daily for minimum of 14 to 21 days. Caps usually ineffective for esophageal candidiasis.

FORMS — Trade: Tabs 200 mg. Oral soln 10 mg/mL (150 mL). Generic/Trade: Caps 100 mg. Oral soln 10 mg/mL (150 mL).

NOTES — Hepatotoxicity, even during first weeks of therapy. Monitor LFTs if baseline abnormal LFTs or history of drug-induced hepatotoxicity; consider monitoring in all patients. Decreased absorption of itraconazole with antacids, buffered didanosine, H2 blockers, proton pump inhibitors, or achlorhydria. Itraconazole levels reduced by carbamazepine, isoniazid, nevirapine, phenobarbital, phenytoin, rifabutin and rifampin, and potentially efavirenz. Itraconazole inhibits CYP3A4 metabolism of many drugs. Not more than 200 mg bid of itraconazole with unboosted indinavir. May increase adverse effects of trazodone; consider reducing trazodone dose. May increase QT interval with disopyramide. Caps and oral soln not interchangeable. Oral soln may be preferred in serious infections due to greater absorption. Oral soln may not achieve adequate levels in cystic fibrosis patients; consider alternative if no response. Start therapy for onychomycosis on day 1 to 2 of menses in women of childbearing potential and advise against pregnancy until 2 months after therapy ends.

MOA — Triazole that inhibits the synthesis of ergosterol (a sterol required for normal fungal cytoplasmic membrane).

ADVERSE EFFECTS — Serious: Negative inotrope, hepatotoxicity (even early in therapy), hypokalemia (with high doses). Frequent: GI complaints, allergic rash.

KETOCONAZOLE (*Nizoral*) ▶L ♀C ▶?+ $$$

WARNING — Hepatotoxicity: Inform patients of risk and monitor. Do not use with midazolam, pimozide, triazolam.

ADULTS — <u>Systemic fungal infections</u>: 200 to 400 mg PO daily.

(cont.)

KETOCONAZOLE (cont.)
- PEDS — <u>Systemic fungal infections</u>, age 2 yo or older: 3.3 to 6.6 mg/kg PO daily.
- UNAPPROVED ADULTS — <u>Tinea versicolor:</u> 400 mg PO single dose or 200 mg PO daily for 7 days.
- FORMS — Generic/Trade: Tabs 200 m.
- NOTES — Decreased absorption of ketoconazole by antacids, H2 blockers, proton pump inhibitors, buffered didanosine, and achlorhydria. Ketoconazole levels reduced by isoniazid, rifampin, and potentially efavirenz. Do not exceed 200 mg/day of ketoconazole with ritonavir or Kaletra. Ketoconazole inhibits CYP3A4 metabolism of many drugs. May increase adverse effects of trazodone; consider reducing trazodone dose.
- MOA — Triazole that inhibits the synthesis of ergosterol (a sterol required for normal fungal cytoplasmic membrane).
- ADVERSE EFFECTS — Serious: Hepatotoxicity (even early in therapy). Frequent: Dose-dependent N/V.

MICONAZOLE—BUCCAL (*Oravig*) ▶L ♀C ▶?
- ADULTS — <u>Oropharyngeal candidiasis:</u> Apply 50 mg buccal tab to gums once daily for 14 days. Apply rounded side of tab to upper gum above incisor in the morning after brushing teeth. Hold in place for 30 seconds. Tab can be used if it sticks to cheek, inside of lip or gum. Apply to new site each day.
- PEDS — Not approved in children. Not recommended for younger children due to potential risk of choking.
- FORMS — Trade: Buccal tabs, 50 mg.
- NOTES — Contraindicated if hypersensitivity to milk protein concentrate. Increased INR with warfarin. Buccal tab is intended to remain in place until it dissolves. If it falls off within 6 hours of application, reposition tab. If it does not stay in place, apply a new tab. If tab is swallowed within first 6 hours, drink a glass of water and apply a new tab. No action is needed if tab falls off or is swallowed after it has been in place for at least 6 hours. Do not to chew gum while tab is in place.
- MOA — Triazole that inhibits the synthesis of ergosterol (a sterol required for normal fungal cytoplasmic membrane).
- ADVERSE EFFECTS — Severe: Hypersensitivity.

POSACONAZOLE (*Noxafil*) ▶Glucuronidation ♀C ▶– $$$$$
- ADULTS — <u>Prevention of invasive Aspergillus or Candida infection:</u> 200 mg (5 mL) PO tid. <u>Oropharyngeal candidiasis:</u> 100 mg (2.5 mL) PO bid on day 1, then 100 mg PO once daily for 13 days. <u>Oropharyngeal candidiasis resistant to itraconazole/fluconazole:</u> 400 mg (10 mL) PO bid; duration of therapy based on severity of underlying disease and clinical response. Take during or within 20 min of full meal or liquid nutritional supplement.
- PEDS — <u>Prevention of invasive Aspergillus or Candida infection,</u> age 13 yo or older: 200 mg (5 mL) PO tid. <u>Oropharyngeal candidiasis,</u> age 13 yo or older: 100 mg (2.5 mL) PO bid on day 1, then 100 mg PO once daily for 13 days. <u>Oropharyngeal candidiasis resistant to itraconazole/fluconazole,</u> age 13 yo or older: 400 mg (10 mL) PO bid; duration of therapy based on severity of underlying disease and clinical response. Take during or within 20 min of full meal or liquid nutritional supplement.
- UNAPPROVED ADULTS — <u>Invasive pulmonary aspergillosis:</u> 200 mg PO qid, then 400 mg PO bid when stable. Treat invasive pulmonary aspergillosis for at least 6 to 12 weeks; treat immunosuppressed patients throughout immunosuppression and until lesions resolved. <u>Fluconazole-refractory oropharyngeal candidiasis:</u> 400 mg PO bid for 3 days, then 400 mg PO once daily for up to 28 days. <u>Fluconazole-refractory esophageal candidiasis:</u> 400 mg PO bid for 14 to 21 days.
- FORMS — Trade only: Oral susp 40 mg/mL, 105 mL bottle.
- NOTES — Consider alternative or monitor for breakthrough fungal infection if patient cannot take during or within 20 min of a full meal or liquid nutritional supplement. If meal or liquid supplement not tolerated, consider giving with acidic carbonated drink (eg, ginger ale). Monitor for breakthrough fungal infection if severe vomiting/diarrhea, posaconazole is given by NG tube, or proton pump inhibitor or metoclopramide is coadministered. Posaconazole is a CYP3A4 inhibitor. Contraindicated with ergot alkaloids, sirolimus, and CYP3A4 substrates that prolong the QT interval, including pimozide and quinidine. Consider dosage reduction of vinca alkaloids, calcium channel blockers, lovastatin, simvastatin. Posaconazole levels reduced by efavirenz, rifabutin, phenytoin, and cimetidine; phenytoin and rifabutin levels increased by posaconazole. Do not coadminister unless benefit exceeds risk. Monitor for rifabutin adverse effects. Reduce cyclosporine dose by 25% and tacrolimus dose by 66% when posaconazole started. Monitor levels of cyclosporine, tacrolimus. Monitor for benzodiazepine adverse effects and consider dosage reduction.
- MOA — Triazole that inhibits the synthesis of ergosterol (a sterol required for normal fungal cytoplasmic membrane).
- ADVERSE EFFECTS — Possible hepatotoxicity.

VORICONAZOLE (*Vfend*) ▶L ♀D ▶? $$$$$
- ADULTS — <u>Invasive aspergillosis:</u> 6 mg/kg IV q 12 h for 2 doses, then 4 mg/kg IV q 12 h. <u>Systemic candidiasis:</u> 6 mg/kg IV q 12 h for 2 doses, then 3 to 4 mg/kg IV q 12 h. Treat until at least 14 days past resolution of signs/symptoms or last positive blood culture. <u>Maintenance therapy, aspergillosis or candidiasis:</u> 200 mg PO bid. For wt less than 40 kg, reduce to 100 mg PO bid. See package insert for dosage adjustments for poor response/adverse effects. <u>Esophageal candidiasis:</u> 200 mg PO q 12 h for at least 14 days and 7 days past resolution of signs/symptoms. For wt less than 40 kg, reduce to 100 mg PO bid. <u>Dosage adjustment for efavirenz:</u> Voriconazole 400 mg PO bid with efavirenz 300 mg (use caps) PO once daily. Take tabs or suspension 1 h before or after meals.

(cont.)

ANTIMICROBIALS: Antifungal Agents

VORICONAZOLE (cont.)

PEDS — Safety and efficacy not established in children younger than 12 yo. Use adult dose age 12 yo or older.

UNAPPROVED ADULTS — <u>Fluconazole-refractory oropharyngeal or esophageal candidiasis:</u> 200 mg PO bid for 14 to 21 days. For wt less than 40 kg, reduce to 100 mg PO bid.

UNAPPROVED PEDS — In children younger than 12 yo, 7 mg/kg IV q 12 h is comparable to 4 mg/kg IV q 12 h in adults. <u>Invasive aspergillosis:</u> 7 mg/kg (max 400 mg) IV q 12 h for 2 doses, then 7 mg/kg (max 200 mg) IV/PO q 12 h. <u>AAP oral regimen for fungal infections:</u> 10 mg/kg PO q 12 h for 2 doses, then 7 mg/kg PO q 12 h.

FORMS — Trade only: Tabs 50, 200 mg (contains lactose). Susp 40 mg/mL (75 mL).

NOTES — Anaphylactoid reactions (IV only), QT interval prolongation, severe skin reactions and photosensitivity, hepatotoxicity rarely. Transient visual disturbances common; advise against hazardous tasks (if vision impaired), night driving and strong, direct sunlight. Monitor visual (if treated for more than 28 days), liver, and renal function. Monitor pancreatic function if at risk for acute pancreatitis (recent chemotherapy/bone marrow transplant). Many drug interactions. Substrate and inhibitor of CYP2C9, 2C19, and 3A4. Do not use with carbamazepine, ergot alkaloids, lopinavir-ritonavir (Kaletra), phenobarbital, pimozide, quinidine, rifabutin, rifampin, ritonavir 400 mg bid, sirolimus, or St John's wort. Ritonavir decreases voriconazole levels; avoid together unless benefit exceeds risk. Dosage adjustments for drug interactions with cyclosporine, omeprazole, phenytoin, tacrolimus in package insert. Increased INR with warfarin. Could inhibit metabolism of benzodiazepines, calcium channel blockers, statins, and methadone. When combining voriconazole with oral contraceptives monitor for adverse effects from increased levels of voriconazole, estrogen, and progestin. Dilute IV to 5 mg/mL or less; max infusion rate is 3 mg/kg/h over 1 to 2 h. Do not infuse IV voriconazole at same time as a blood product/concentrated electrolytes even if given by separate IV lines. IV voriconazole can be infused at the same time as non-concentrated electrolytes/total parenteral nutrition if given by separate lines; give TPN by different port if multilumen catheter is used. Vehicle in IV form may accumulate in renal impairment; oral preferred if CrCl less than 50 mL/min. <u>Mild/moderate cirrhosis</u> (Child-Pugh class A/B): Same loading dose and reduce maintenance dose by 50%. Oral susp stable for 14 days at room temperature.

MOA — Triazole that inhibits the synthesis of ergosterol (a sterol required for normal fungal cytoplasmic membrane).

ADVERSE EFFECTS — Serious: Anaphylactoid reactions (IV only), QT interval prolongation, hepatotoxicity (rare), severe skin reactions & photosensitivity rarely, pancreatitis. Frequent: Mild transient visual disturbances, rash, elevated LFTs. Other: Hallucinations, confusion.

ANTIMICROBIALS: Antifungal Agents—Echinocandins

NOTE: See www.idsociety.org for guidelines on the management of fungal infections. See www.aidsinfo.nih.gov for management of fungal infections in HIV-infected patients.

ANIDULAFUNGIN (*Eraxis*) ▶Degraded chemically ♀C ▶? $$$$$

ADULTS — <u>Candidemia, other systemic candidal infections:</u> 200 mg IV load on day 1, then 100 mg IV once daily until at least 14 days after last positive culture. <u>Esophageal candidiasis:</u> 100 mg IV load on day 1, then 50 mg IV once daily for at least 14 days, and continuing for at least 7 days after symptoms resolved.

PEDS — Not approved in children.

UNAPPROVED PEDS — 0.75 to 1.5 mg/kg IV once daily. <u>Systemic Candida infections,</u> age 2 yo or older: 1.5 mg/kg IV once daily.

NOTES — Max infusion rate of 1.1 mg/min to prevent histamine reactions. Diluent contains dehydrated alcohol.

MOA — Echinocandin that blocks the synthesis of glucan, a fungal cell wall polysaccharide.

ADVERSE EFFECTS — Hepatotoxicity (rare). Histamine reactions (rash, urticaria, flushing pruritus, dyspnea, hypotension) minimized by infusion rate less than 1.1 mg/min. Diarrhea, hypokalemia.

CASPOFUNGIN (*Cancidas*) ▶KL ♀C ▶? $$$$$

ADULTS — Infuse IV over 1 h. <u>Aspergillosis, candidemia, empiric therapy in febrile neutropenia:</u> 70 mg loading dose on day 1, then 50 mg once daily. Patients taking rifampin: 70 mg once daily. Consider this dose with other enzyme inducers (such as carbamazepine, dexamethasone, efavirenz, nevirapine, phenytoin) or if inadequate response to lower dose in febrile neutropenia or aspergillosis. <u>Esophageal candidiasis:</u> 50 mg daily. Duration of therapy in invasive aspergillosis is based on severity, treatment response, and resolution of immunosuppression. Treat candidal infections for at least 14 days after last positive culture. <u>Empiric therapy of febrile neutropenia:</u> Treat until neutropenia resolved. If fungal infection confirmed, treat for at least 14 days and continue treatment for at least 7 days after symptoms and neutropenia resolved.

PEDS — Infuse IV over 1 h. <u>Aspergillosis, candidemia, esophageal candidiasis, empiric therapy in febrile neutropenia,</u> 3 mo to 17 yo: 70 mg/m2 loading dose on day 1, then 50 mg/m2 once daily. Consider increasing daily dose to 70 mg/m2 up to max of 70 mg once daily if coadministered with

(cont.)

CASPOFUNGIN (cont.)
enzyme inducers (such as carbamazepine, dexamethasone, efavirenz, nevirapine, phenytoin, or rifampin) or if inadequate response to lower dose in febrile neutropenia or aspergillosis. Duration of therapy in invasive aspergillosis is based on severity, treatment response, and resolution of immunosuppression. Treat Candidal infections for at least 14 days after last positive culture. Empiric therapy of febrile neutropenia: Treat until neutropenia resolved. If fungal infection confirmed, treat for at least 14 days and continue treatment for at least 7 days after symptoms and neutropenia resolved. If vial strength is available, in order to improve dosing accuracy, use 50 mg vial (5 mg/mL) for pediatric dose less than 50 mg and 70 mg vial (7 mg/mL) for pediatric dose greater than 50 mg.
NOTES — Abnormal LFTs reported; possible risk of hepatitis. Monitor hepatic function if abnormal LFTs. Administration with cyclosporine increases caspofungin levels and hepatic transaminases; risk of concomitant use unclear. Caspofungin decreases tacrolimus levels. Dosage adjustment in adults with moderate liver dysfunction (Child-Pugh score 7 to 9): 35 mg IV daily (after 70 mg loading dose in patients with invasive aspergillosis).
MOA — Echinocandin that blocks the synthesis of glucan, a fungal cell wall polysaccharide.
ADVERSE EFFECTS — Serious: Anaphylaxis (rare). Abnormal LFTs reported; possible risk of hepatitis. Frequent: Fever, rash, N/V, diarrhea, hypokalemia, phlebitis at injection site. Some infusion reactions (like facial flushing) caused by histamine release.

MICAFUNGIN (*Mycamine*) ▶L, feces ♀C ▶? $$$$$
ADULTS — Esophageal candidiasis: 150 mg IV once daily. Candidemia, acute disseminated candidiasis, Candida peritonitis/abscess: 100 mg IV once daily. Prevention of candidal infections in bone marrow transplant patients: 50 mg IV once daily. Infuse over 1 h. Histamine-mediated reactions possible with more rapid infusion. Flush existing IV lines with NS before micafungin infusion.
PEDS — Not approved in children.
UNAPPROVED ADULTS — Prophylaxis of invasive aspergillosis: 50 mg IV once daily. Infuse IV over 1 h.
UNAPPROVED PEDS — Esophageal candidiasis: 3 mg/kg up to 150 mg IV once daily for wt less than 50 kg; 150 mg IV once daily for wt greater than 50 kg. Systemic candidiasis: 2 to 3 mg/kg up to 150 mg IV once daily for wt less than 40 kg; 100 to 150 mg IV once daily for wt 40 kg or greater. Higher doses may be needed in infants, but specific dose is not established.
NOTES — Increases levels of sirolimus and nifedipine. Not dialyzed. Protect diluted soln from light. Do not mix with other meds; it may precipitate.
MOA — Echinocandin that blocks the synthesis of glucan, a fungal cell wall polysaccharide.
ADVERSE EFFECTS — Serious: Anaphylaxis/anaphylactoid reactions (rare); renal/hepatic dysfunction; hemolysis/hemolytic anemia. Frequent: Rash. Injection site reactions more common with peripheral infusion.

ANTIMICROBIALS: Antifungal Agents—Polyenes

NOTE: See www.idsociety.org for guidelines on the management of fungal infections. See www.aidsinfo.nih.gov for management of fungal infections in HIV-infected patients.

AMPHOTERICIN B DEOXYCHOLATE (*Fungizone*) ▶Tissues ♀B ▶? $$$$
WARNING — Do not use IV route for noninvasive fungal infections (oral thrush, vaginal or esophageal candidiasis) in patients with normal neutrophil counts.
ADULTS — Life-threatening systemic fungal infections: Test dose 1 mg slow IV. Wait 2 to 4 h, and if tolerated start 0.25 mg/kg IV daily. Advance to 0.5 to 1.5 mg/kg/day depending on fungal type. Maximum dose 1.5 mg/kg/day. Infuse over 2 to 6 h. Hydrate with 500 mL NS before and after infusion to decrease risk of nephrotoxicity.
PEDS — No remaining FDA approved indications.
UNAPPROVED ADULTS — Alternative regimen, life-threatening systemic fungal infections: 1 mg test dose as part of first infusion (no need for separate IV bag); if tolerated continue infusion, giving target dose of 0.5 to 1.5 mg/kg on first day. Candidemia: 0.5 to 1 mg/kg IV daily. Treat until 14 days after first negative blood culture and resolution of signs/symptoms. Symptomatic Candida cystitis: 0.3 to 0.6 mg/kg IV for 1 to 7 days. Candida pyelonephritis: 0.5 to 0.7 mg/kg IV daily (± flucytosine). Cryptococcal meningitis in HIV infection: 0.7 mg/kg/day IV preferably in combo with flucytosine 25 mg/kg PO q 6 h for 2 weeks. Follow with fluconazole consolidation, then fluconazole chronic suppression until immune reconstitution.
UNAPPROVED PEDS — Systemic life-threatening fungal infections: Test dose 0.1 mg/kg (max of 1 mg) slow IV. Wait 2 to 4 h, and if tolerated start 0.25 mg/kg IV once daily. Advance to 0.5 to 1.5 mg/kg/day depending on fungal type. Maximum dose 1.5 mg/kg/day. Infuse over 2 to 6 h. Hydrate with 10 to 15 mL/kg NS before infusion to decrease risk of nephrotoxicity. Alternative dosing regimen: Give test dose as part of first infusion (separate IV bag not needed); if tolerated continue infusion, giving target dose of 0.5 to 1.5 mg/kg on first day. Cryptococcal infection in HIV-infected patients: 0.7 to 1 mg/kg IV once daily may add flucytosine depending on site and severity of infection.

(cont.)

ANTIMICROBIALS: Antifungal Agents

AMPHOTERICIN B DEOXYCHOLATE (cont.)
- NOTES — Acute infusion reactions, anaphylaxis, nephrotoxicity, hypokalemia, hypomagnesemia, acidosis, anemia. Monitor renal and hepatic function, CBC, serum electrolytes. Lipid formulations better tolerated, preferred in renal dysfunction.
- MOA — Polyene antifungal, Insertion into fungal cytoplasmic membrane increases membrane permeability.
- ADVERSE EFFECTS — Serious for IV Fungizone: Anaphylaxis, anemia, nephrotoxicity. Frequent: Acute infusion reactions, nephrotoxicity (hypokalemia, hypomagnesemia, renal tubular acidosis).

AMPHOTERICIN B LIPID FORMULATIONS (*Amphotec, Abelcet, AmBisome*) ▶? ♀B ▶? $$$$$
- ADULTS — Lipid formulations used primarily in patients refractory/intolerant to amphotericin deoxycholate. Abelcet: Invasive fungal infections: 5 mg/kg/day IV at 2.5 mg/kg/h. Shake infusion bag q 2 h. AmBisome: Infuse IV over 2 h. Empiric therapy of fungal infections in febrile neutropenia: 3 mg/kg/day. Aspergillus, candidal, cryptococcal infections: 3 to 5 mg/kg/day. Cryptococcal meningitis in HIV infection: 6 mg/kg/day. Amphotec: Test dose of 10 mL over 15 to 30 min, observe for 30 min, then 3 to 4 mg/kg/day IV at 1 mg/kg/h.
- PEDS — Lipid formulations used primarily in patients refractory/intolerant to amphotericin deoxycholate. Abelcet: Invasive fungal infections: 5 mg/kg/day IV at 2.5 mg/kg/h. Shake infusion bag q 2 h. AmBisome: Infuse IV over 2 h. Empiric therapy of fungal infections in febrile neutropenia: 3 mg/kg/day. Aspergillus, candidal, cryptococcal infections: 3 to 5 mg/kg/day. Cryptococcal meningitis in HIV infection: 6 mg/kg/day. Amphotec: Aspergillosis: Test dose of 10 mL over 15 to 30 min, observe for 30 min, then 3 to 4 mg/kg/day IV at 1 mg/kg/h.
- NOTES — Acute infusion reactions, anaphylaxis, nephrotoxicity, hypokalemia, hypomagnesemia, acidosis. Lipid formulations better tolerated than amphotericin deoxycholate, preferred in renal dysfunction. Monitor renal and hepatic function, CBC, electrolytes.
- MOA — Polyene antifungal, Insertion into fungal cytoplasmic membrane increases membrane permeability.
- ADVERSE EFFECTS — Serious: Anaphylaxis. Frequent: Acute infusion reactions, nephrotoxicity (hypokalemia, hypomagnesemia, renal tubular acidosis). Lipid formulations better tolerated than amphotericin deoxycholate.

ANTIMICROBIALS: Antifungal Agents—Other

NOTE: See www.idsociety.org for guidelines on the management of fungal infections. See www.aidsinfo.nih.gov for management of fungal infections in HIV-infected patients.

FLUCYTOSINE (*Ancobon*) ▶K ♀C ▶— $$$$$
- WARNING — Extreme caution in renal or bone marrow impairment. Monitor hematologic, hepatic, renal function in all patients.
- ADULTS — Candidal/cryptococcal infections: 50 to 150 mg/kg/day PO divided qid. Candida UTI: 100 mg/kg/day PO divided qid for 7 to 10 days for symptomatic cystitis, for 14 days (± amphotericin deoxycholate) for pyelonephritis. Initial therapy for cryptococcal meningitis: 100 mg/kg/day PO divided qid.
- PEDS — Not approved in children.
- UNAPPROVED PEDS — Candidal/cryptococcal infections: 50 to 150 mg/kg/day PO divided qid.
- FORMS — Trade only: Caps 250, 500 mg.
- NOTES — Flucytosine is given with other antifungal agents. Myelosuppression. Reduce nausea by taking caps a few at a time over 15 min. Monitor flucytosine levels. Peak 70 to 80 mg/L, trough 30 to 40 mg/L. Reduce dose in renal dysfunction. Avoid in children with severe renal dysfunction.
- MOA — Deaminated to inhibitor of thymidylate synthetase, which interferes with DNA synthesis.
- ADVERSE EFFECTS — Serious: Myelosuppression (frequent); anaphylaxis; hepatic, renal, cardiac and CNS toxicity (all rare). Frequent: N/V, diarrhea, rash.

GRISEOFULVIN (*Grifulvin V, ♣Fulvicin*) ▶Skin ♀C ▶? $$$$
- ADULTS — Tinea: 500 mg PO daily for 4 to 6 weeks for capitis, 2 to 4 weeks for corporis, 4 to 8 weeks for pedis, 4 months for fingernails, 6 months for toenails. Can use 1 g/day for pedis and unguium.
- PEDS — Tinea: 11 mg/kg PO daily for 4 to 6 weeks for capitis, 2 to 4 weeks for corporis, 4 to 8 weeks for pedis, 4 months for fingernails, 6 months for toenails.
- UNAPPROVED PEDS — Tinea capitis: AAP recommends 10 to 20 mg/kg (max 1 g) PO daily for 4 to 6 weeks, continuing for 2 weeks past symptom resolution. Some infections may require 20 to 25 mg/kg/day or ultramicrosize griseofulvin 5 to 10 mg/kg (max 750 mg) PO daily.
- FORMS — Generic/Trade: Susp 125 mg/5 mL (120 mL). Trade only: Tabs 250, 500 mg.
- NOTES — Do not use in liver failure, porphyria. May cause photosensitivity, lupus-like syndrome/exacerbation of lupus. Decreased INR with warfarin, decreased efficacy of oral contraceptives. Ultramicrosize formulations have greater GI absorption, and are available with different strengths and dosing.
- MOA — Inhibits fungal mitosis by disrupting mitotic spindle.
- ADVERSE EFFECTS — Serious: Photosensitivity, lupus-like syndrome/exacerbation of lupus, increased porphyrins (not for use by patients with porphyria). Frequent: Allergic skin reactions, headache.

ANTIMICROBIALS: Antimalarials

GRISEOFULVIN ULTRAMICROSIZE (*Gris-PEG*) ▶Skin ♀C ▶? $$$$
ADULTS — Tinea: 375 mg PO daily for 4 to 6 weeks for capitis, 2 to 4 weeks for corporis, 4 to 8 weeks for pedis, 4 months for fingernails, 6 months for toenails. Can use 750 mg/day for pedis and unguium. Best absorption when given after meal containing fat.
PEDS — Tinea, age 2 yo or older: 7.3 mg/kg PO daily for 4 to 6 weeks for capitis, 2 to 4 weeks for corporis, 4 to 8 weeks for pedis, 4 months for fingernails, 6 months for toenails. Give 82.5 to 165 mg PO daily for 13.6 to 22.6 kg. Give 165 to 330 mg for wt greater than 22.6 kg. Tinea capitis: AAP recommends 5 to 15 mg/kg (up to 750 mg) PO daily for 4 to 6 weeks, continuing for 2 weeks past symptom resolution. Best absorption when given after meal containing fat.
FORMS — Trade only: Tabs 125, 250 mg.
NOTES — Do not use in liver failure, porphyria. May cause photosensitivity, lupus-like syndrome/exacerbation of lupus. Decreased INR with warfarin, decreased efficacy of oral contraceptives. Microsize formulations, which have lower GI absorption, are available with different strengths and dosing.
MOA — Inhibits fungal mitosis by disrupting mitotic spindle.
ADVERSE EFFECTS — Serious: Photosensitivity, lupus-like syndrome/exacerbation of lupus, increased porphyrins (not for use by patients with porphyria). Frequent: Allergic skin reactions, headache.

NYSTATIN (*Mycostatin*, *✦Nilstat*, *Nyaderm*, *Candistatin*) ▶Not absorbed ♀B ▶? $$
ADULTS — Thrush: 4 to 6 mL PO swish and swallow qid or suck on 1 to 2 troches 4 to 5 times per day.
PEDS — Thrush, infants: 2 mL/dose PO with 1 mL in each cheek qid. Premature and low wt infants: 0.5 mL PO in each cheek qid. Thrush, older children: 4 to 6 mL PO swish and swallow qid or suck on 1 to 2 troches 4 to 5 times per day.
FORMS — Generic only: Susp 100,000 units/mL (60, 480 mL). Troches 500,00 units/tab.
MOA — Polyene antifungal that is not absorbed from the GI tract. Same mechanism of action as amphotericin, insertion into fungal cytoplasmic membrane increases membrane permeability.
ADVERSE EFFECTS — Serious: None. Frequent: None.

TERBINAFINE (*Lamisil*) ▶LK ♀B ▶− $
ADULTS — Onychomycosis: 250 mg PO daily for 6 weeks for fingernails, for 12 weeks for toenails.
PEDS — Tinea capitis, age 4 yo or older: Give granules once daily with food for 6 weeks: 125 mg for wt less than 25 kg, 187.5 mg for wt 25 to 35 kg, 250 mg for wt greater than 35 kg.
UNAPPROVED PEDS — Onychomycosis: 67.5 mg PO daily for wt less than 20 kg, 125 mg PO once daily for wt 20 to 40 kg, 250 mg PO once daily for wt greater than 40 kg. Treat for 6 weeks for fingernails, for 12 weeks for toenails.
FORMS — Generic/Trade: Tabs 250 mg. Trade only: Oral granules 125, 187.5 mg/packet.
NOTES — Hepatotoxicity; monitor AST and ALT at baseline. Neutropenia. May rarely cause or exacerbate lupus. Do not use in liver disease or CrCl less than 50 mL/min. Test nail specimen to confirm diagnosis before prescribing. Inhibitor of CYP2D6.
MOA — Inhibits squalene epoxidase, an enzyme involved in the synthesis of ergosterol (a sterol required for normal fungal cytoplasmic membrane).
ADVERSE EFFECTS — Serious: Hepatotoxicity, neutropenia. May rarely cause or exacerbate lupus. Frequent: N/V, rash.

ANTIMICROBIALS: Antimalarials

NOTE: For help treating malaria or getting antimalarials, see www.cdc.gov/malaria or call the CDC "malaria hotline" (770) 488–7788 Monday-Friday 9 am to 5 pm EST; after hours/weekend (770) 488–7100. Pediatric doses of antimalarials should never exceed adult doses.

CHLOROQUINE (*Aralen*) ▶KL ♀C but + ▶+ $
WARNING — Review product labeling for precautions and adverse effects before prescribing.
ADULTS — Doses as chloroquine phosphate. Malaria prophylaxis, chloroquine-sensitive areas: 500 mg PO q week from 1 to 2 weeks before exposure to 4 weeks after. Malaria treatment, chloroquine-sensitive areas: 1 g PO once, then 500 mg PO at 6, 24, and 48 h. Total dose is 2.5 g. Extraintestinal amebiasis: 1 g PO daily for 2 days, then 500 mg PO daily for 2 to 3 weeks.
PEDS — Doses as chloroquine phosphate. Malaria prophylaxis, chloroquine-sensitive areas: 8.3 mg/kg (up to 500 mg) PO week from 1 to 2 weeks before exposure to 4 weeks after. Malaria treatment, chloroquine-sensitive areas: 16.7 mg/kg PO once, then 8.3 mg/kg at 6, 24, and 48 h. Do not exceed adult dose. Chloroquine phosphate 8.3 mg/kg is equivalent to chloroquine base 5 mg/kg.
FORMS — Generic only: Tabs 250 mg. Generic/Trade: Tabs 500 mg (500 mg phosphate equivalent to 300 mg base).
NOTES — Can prolong QT interval and cause torsades. Retinopathy with chronic/high doses; eye exams required. May cause seizures (caution advised if epilepsy); ototoxicity (caution advised if hearing loss); myopathy (discontinue if muscle weakness develops); bone marrow toxicity (monitor CBC if long-term use); exacerbation of psoriasis. Concentrates in liver; caution advised if hepatic disease, alcoholism, or hepatotoxic drugs. Antacids reduce absorption; give at least 4 h apart. Chloroquine reduces ampicillin absorption; give at least 2 h apart. May increase cyclosporine levels. As little as 1 g can cause fatal overdose in a child. Fatal malaria reported after chloroquine used as malaria prophylaxis in areas with chloroquine resistance; use only in areas without resistance.

(cont.)

CHLOROQUINE (cont.)
Other agents are superior for severe chloroquine-sensitive malaria. Maternal antimalarial prophylaxis doesn't harm breastfed infant or protect infant from malaria. Use with primaquine phosphate for treatment of P. vivax or P. ovale.
MOA — Plasmodicidal mechanism of action unknown, may inhibit heme polymerase or interact with DNA.
ADVERSE EFFECTS — Serious: Retinopathy with chronic/high doses; can cause torsades. Fatal malaria in patients receiving chloroquine prophylaxis in areas with chloroquine resistance.

COARTEM (artemether + lumefantrine, Coartemether) ▶L ♀C ▶? $$$
ADULTS — Uncomplicated malaria, wt 35 kg or greater: 4 tabs PO bid for 3 days. On day 1, give second dose 8 h after first dose. Take with food.
PEDS — Uncomplicated malaria, wt greater than 5 kg and age 2 mo or older: Take with food bid for 3 days. On day 1, give second dose 8 h after first dose. Dose based on wt: 1 tab for 5 to 14 kg; 2 tabs for 15 to 24 kg; 3 tabs for 25 to 34 kg; 4 tab for 35 kg or greater.
FORMS — Trade only: Tabs, artemether 20 mg + lumefantrine 120 mg.
NOTES — Can prolong QT interval; avoid using in proarrhythmic conditions or with drugs that prolong QT interval. May inhibit CYP2D6; avoid with drugs metabolized by CYP2D6 that have cardiac effects and caution with CYP3A4 inhibitors as both interactions may prolong QT interval. Do not use Coartem and halofantrine within 1 month of each other. Repeat the dose if vomiting occurs within 1 to 2 h; use another antimalarial if second dose is vomited. Can crush tabs and mix with 1 to 2 tsp water immediately before the dose.
MOA — Artemether and lumefantrine are blood schizonticides.
ADVERSE EFFECTS — Serious: Urticaria/angioedema. Can prolong QT interval. Frequent: Headache, anorexia, dizziness, asthenia in adults. Fever, cough, vomiting, anorexia, headache in children.

FANSIDAR (sulfadoxine + pyrimethamine) ▶KL ♀C ▶– $
WARNING — Can cause life-threatening Stevens-Johnson syndrome and toxic epidermal necrolysis. Stop treatment at first sign of rash, bacterial/fungal infection, or change in CBC.
ADULTS — CDC does not recommend Fansidar for treatment of malaria.
PEDS — CDC does not recommend Fansidar for treatment of malaria.
FORMS — Trade only: Tabs sulfadoxine 500 mg + pyrimethamine 25 mg.
NOTES — CDC does not recommend Fansidar for treatment of malaria due to drug resistance and adverse effects. Do not use in sulfonamide allergy; megaloblastic anemia due to folate deficiency; or for prolonged period in hepatic/renal failure or blood dyscrasia. Can cause hemolytic anemia in G6PD deficiency. Fansidar resistance is common in many malarious regions. Avoid excessive sun exposure.
MOA — Pyrimethamine is a folic acid antagonist. Sulfadoxine is a sulfonamide (structural analog of PABA that binds with dihydropteroate synthetase and prevents nucleic acid synthesis).
ADVERSE EFFECTS — Serious: Life-threatening Stevens-Johnson syndrome & toxic epidermal necrolysis, hemolytic anemia in G6PD deficiency.

MALARONE (atovaquone + proguanil) ▶Fecal excretion; LK ♀C ▶? $$$$$
ADULTS — Malaria prophylaxis: 1 adult tab PO once daily from 1 to 2 days before exposure until 7 days after. Malaria treatment: 4 adult tabs PO once daily for 3 days. Take with food/milky drink at same time each day. Repeat dose if vomiting within 1 h after the dose. CDC recommends for presumptive self-treatment of malaria (same dose as for treatment, but not to be used by patients currently taking it for prophylaxis).
PEDS — Safety and efficacy established in children with wt 11 kg or greater for prevention, and 5 kg or greater for treatment. Prevention of malaria: Give following dose based on wt PO once daily from 1 to 2 days before exposure until 7 days after: 1 ped tab for 11 to 20 kg; 2 ped tabs for 21 to 30 kg; 3 ped tabs for 31 to 40 kg; 1 adult tab for greater than 40 kg. Treatment of malaria: Give following dose based on wt PO once daily for 3 days, 2 ped tabs for 5 to 8 kg; 3 ped tabs for 9 to 10 kg; 1 adult tab for 11 to 20 kg; 2 adult tabs for 21 to 30 kg; 3 adult tabs for 31 to 40 kg; 4 adult tabs for greater than 40 kg. Take with food or milky drink at same time each day. Repeat dose if vomiting occurs within 1 h after dose.
UNAPPROVED PEDS — CDC doses for prevention of malaria: Give PO daily from 1 to 2 days before exposure until 7 days after: ½ ped tab for wt 5 to 8 kg; ¾ ped tab for wt 9 to 10 kg. Not advised for infants less than 5 kg.
FORMS — Trade only: Adult tabs atovaquone 250 mg + proguanil 100 mg; pediatric tabs 62.5 mg + 25 mg.
NOTES — Vomiting common with malaria treatment doses (consider antiemetic). Monitor parasitemia. Atovaquone levels may be decreased by tetracycline, metoclopramide (use another antiemetic if possible), and rifampin (avoid). Atovaquone can reduce indinavir trough levels. Proguanil may increase the INR with warfarin. If CrCl < 30 mL/min avoid for malaria prophylaxis and use cautiously for treatment. CDC recommends against use by women breastfeeding infant weighing less than 5 kg.
MOA — Atovaquone and proguanil interfere with two different pyrimidine biosynthesis pathways. Atovaquone inhibits parasitic mitochondrial electron transport. A proguanil metabolite, cycloguanil, inhibits dihydrofolate reductase.
ADVERSE EFFECTS — Serious: Hepatitis/increased LFTs, anaphylaxis, Stevens-Johnson syndrome, photosensitivity. Frequent: Vomiting with malaria treatment doses, GI complaints, headache, asthenia, dizziness.

ANTIMICROBIALS: Antimalarials

MEFLOQUINE (*Lariam*) ▶L ♀C ▶? $$
- ADULTS — Malaria prophylaxis, chloroquine-resistant areas: 250 mg PO once weekly from 1 week before exposure to 4 weeks after. Malaria treatment: 1250 mg PO single dose. Take on full stomach with at least 8 oz water.
- PEDS — Malaria treatment: 20 to 25 mg/kg PO; given in 1 to 2 divided doses 6 to 8 h apart to reduce risk of vomiting. Repeat full dose if vomiting within 30 min after dose; repeat ½ dose if vomiting within 30 to 60 min after dose. Experience limited in infants age younger than 3 mo or wt less than 5 kg. Malaria prophylaxis: Give the following dose based on wt PO once a week starting 1 week before exposure to 4 weeks after. For 9 kg or less give 5 mg/kg; for wt greater than 9 to 19 kg give ¼ tablet; for wt greater than 19 to 30 kg give ½ tab; for wt greater than 31 to 45 kg give ¾ tab; for wt 45 kg or greater give 1 tab. Take on full stomach. Pharmacist needs to compound 5 mg/kg dose.
- UNAPPROVED ADULTS — CDC regimen for malaria: 750 mg PO followed by 500 mg PO 6 to 12 h later, for total of 1250 mg. Quinine + doxycycline/tetracycline/clindamycin or atovaquone-proguanil preferred over mefloquine because of high rate of neuropsychiatric adverse effects with malaria treatment doses of mefloquine.
- UNAPPROVED PEDS — Malaria prophylaxis, chloroquine-resistant areas: CDC recommends these PO doses once weekly starting 1 week before exposure to 4 weeks after: 5 mg/kg for wt 15 kg or less; ¼ tab for 15 to 19 kg; ½ tab for 20 to 30 kg; ¾ tab for 31 to 45 kg; 1 tab for 45 kg or greater. Malaria treatment for wt less than 45 kg: 15 mg/kg PO, then 10 mg/kg PO given 8 to 12 h after first dose. Take on full stomach with at least 8 oz water.
- FORMS — Generic only: Tabs 250 mg.
- NOTES — Cardiac conduction disturbances. Do not use with ziprasidone. Do not give until 12 h after the last dose of quinidine, quinine, or chloroquine; may cause ECG changes and seizures. Contraindicated for prophylaxis if depression (active/recent), generalized anxiety disorder, psychosis, schizophrenia, other major psychiatric disorder, or history of seizures. Tell patients to discontinue if psychiatric symptoms occur during prophylaxis. May cause drowsiness (warn about hazardous tasks). Can crush tabs and mix with a little water, milk, or other liquid. Pharmacists can put small doses into caps to mask bitter taste. Decreases valproate levels. Rifampin decreases mefloquine levels. Maternal use of antimalarial prophylaxis doesn't harm or protect breastfed infant from malaria.
- MOA — Acts as blood schizonticide, exact mechanism of action is unknown.
- ADVERSE EFFECTS — Serious: Cardiac conduction disturbances including QT prolongation, psychiatric reactions. Frequent: Dizziness, loss of balance, sleep disturbances (especially early in therapy and in women). Early vomiting in children with malaria treatment dose.

PRIMAQUINE ▶L ♀– ▶– $$
- WARNING — Review product labeling for precautions and adverse effects and document normal G6PD level before prescribing.
- ADULTS — Prevention of relapse, P vivax/ovale malaria: 30 mg base PO daily for 14 days.
- PEDS — Not approved in children.
- UNAPPROVED ADULTS — Pneumocystis in patients intolerant to trimethoprim/sulfamethoxazole: 15 to 30 mg primaquine base PO daily plus clindamycin 600 to 900 mg IV q 6 to 8 h or 300 to 450 mg PO q 6 to 8 h for 21 days. Primary prevention of malaria in special circumstances: 30 mg base PO once daily beginning 1 to 2 days before exposure until 7 days after (consult with malaria expert; contact CDC at 770–488–7788 for info).
- UNAPPROVED PEDS — Prevention of relapse, P vivax/ovale malaria: 0.5 mg/kg (up to 30 mg) base PO once daily for 14 days. Primary prevention of malaria in special circumstances: 0.5 mg/kg (up to 30 mg) base PO once daily beginning 1 to 2 days before exposure until 7 days after (consult with malaria expert; contact CDC at 770-488-7788 for info).
- FORMS — Generic only: Tabs 26.3 mg (equiv to 15 mg base).
- NOTES — Causes hemolytic anemia in G6PD deficiency, methemoglobinemia in NADH methemoglobin reductase deficiency. Contraindicated in pregnancy and G6PD deficiency; screen for deficiency before prescribing. Stop if dark urine or anemia. Avoid in patients with RA or SLE, recent quinacrine use, or use of other bone marrow suppressants.
- MOA — Unknown. May affect mitochondrial electron transport chain or pyrimidine synthesis. Active against all forms of malaria; only drug active against latent parasites in liver.
- ADVERSE EFFECTS — Serious: Hemolytic anemia with G6PD deficiency, methemoglobinemia with NADH methemoglobin reductase deficiency.

QUININE (*Qualaquin*) ▶L ♀C ▶+? $$$$
- WARNING — FDA has repeatedly warned that the risks of using quinine for management of nocturnal leg cramps (an unapproved indication) exceed any potential benefit. Risks include life-threatening hematological reactions, especially thrombocytopenia and hemolytic-uremic syndrome/thrombotic thrombocytopenic purpura (HUS/TTP). HUS/TTP can cause chronic renal impairment.
- ADULTS — Malaria: 648 mg PO tid for 3 days (Africa/South America) or 7 days (Southeast Asia). Also give 7-day course of doxycycline, tetracycline, or clindamycin.
- PEDS — Not approved in children.
- UNAPPROVED ADULTS — Nocturnal leg cramps: 260 to 325 mg PO at bedtime. FDA warns that risks outweigh benefits for this indication.
- UNAPPROVED PEDS — Malaria: 25 to 30 mg/kg/day (up to 2 g/day) PO divided q 8 h for 3 days (Africa/South America) or 7 days (Southeast Asia). Also give 7-day course of doxycycline, tetracycline, or clindamycin.

(cont.)

QUININE (cont.)
FORMS — Trade only: Caps 324 mg.
NOTES — Thrombocytopenia, hemolytic uremic syndrome/thrombotic thrombocytopenic purpura, cinchonism, hemolytic anemia with G6PD deficiency, cardiac conduction disturbances, hearing impairment. Contraindicated if prolonged QT interval, optic neuritis, myasthenia gravis, or hypersensitivity to quinine, quinidine, or mefloquine. Many drug interactions. Do not use with clarithromycin, erythromycin, rifampin, neuromuscular blockers. May increase digoxin levels. May decrease theophylline levels. Monitor INR with warfarin. Antacids decrease quinine absorption. Rule out G6PD deficiency in breastfed at-risk infant before giving quinine to mother.
MOA — Unknown, may have similar mechanism of action as chloroquine.
ADVERSE EFFECTS — Serious: Thrombocytopenia, hemolytic uremic syndrome/thrombotic thrombocytopenic purpura, cinchonism, hemolytic anemia with G6PD deficiency, cardiac conduction disturbances, hearing impairment with high levels, hypoglycemia (especially in pregnant women).

ANTIMICROBIALS: Antimycobacterial Agents

NOTE: Treat active mycobacterial infection with at least 2 drugs. See guidelines at www.thoracic.org/statements/index.php and www.aidsinfo.nih.gov. See www.aidsinfo.nih.gov for use of rifamycins with antiretrovirals. Get baseline LFTs, creatinine, and platelet count before treating TB. Evaluate at least monthly for adverse drug reactions. Routine liver and renal function tests not needed unless baseline dysfunction or increased risk of hepatotoxicity.

CLOFAZIMINE (*Lamprene*) ▶Fecal excretion ♀C ▶?- $
ADULTS — Approved for leprosy therapy.
PEDS — Not approved in children.
UNAPPROVED ADULTS — Mycobacterium avium complex in immunocompetent patients: 100 to 200 mg PO daily until "tan," then 50 mg PO daily or 100 mg PO 3 times a week. Use in combination with other antimycobacterial agents. Not for general use in AIDS patients due to increased mortality.
FORMS — Trade only: Caps 50 mg. Distributed only through investigational new drug application. For leprosy, contact National Hansen's Disease Program (phone 800-642-2477). For nonleprosy indications, contact FDA Division of Special Pathogen and Immunologic Drugs Program (phone 301-796-1600).
NOTES — Abdominal pain common; rare reports of splenic infarction, bowel obstruction, and GI bleeding. Pink to brownish-black skin pigmentation that may persist for months to years after drug is discontinued. Discoloration of urine, body secretions.
MOA — Unknown.
ADVERSE EFFECTS — Serious: Rare reports of splenic infarction, bowel obstruction, and GI bleeding. Frequent: Abdominal pain, discoloration of urine and body secretions, pink to brownish-black skin pigmentation that may persist for months to years.

DAPSONE (*Aczone*) ▶LK ♀C ▶- $
ADULTS — Leprosy: 100 mg PO daily with rifampin ± clofazimine or ethionamide. Acne (Aczone): Apply bid.
PEDS — Leprosy: 1 mg/kg (up to 100 mg) PO daily with other antimycobacterial agents. Acne (12 to 17 yo, Aczone): Apply bid.
UNAPPROVED ADULTS — Pneumocystis prophylaxis: 100 mg PO daily. Pneumocystis treatment: 100 mg PO daily with trimethoprim 5 mg/kg PO tid for 21 days.
UNAPPROVED PEDS — Pneumocystis prophylaxis, age 1 mo or older: 2 mg/kg (up to 100 mg/day) PO once daily or 4 mg/kg/week (up to 200 mg/week) PO once weekly.
FORMS — Generic only: Tabs 25, 100 mg. Trade only (Aczone): Topical gel 5% 30 g.
NOTES — Blood dyscrasias, severe allergic skin reactions, sulfone syndrome, hemolysis in G6PD deficiency, hepatotoxicity, neuropathy, photosensitivity, leprosy reactional states. Monitor CBC weekly for 4 weeks, then monthly for 6 months, then twice a year. Monitor LFTs.
MOA — Sulfone that inhibits dihydropteroate synthase and prevents bacterial folic acid synthesis.
ADVERSE EFFECTS — Serious: Blood dyscrasias, allergic skin reactions, sulfone syndrome, hemolysis in G6PD deficiency, hepatotoxicity, neuropathy, photosensitivity, leprosy reactional states. Frequent: Rash, headache, GI complaints, mononucleosis-like syndrome. Topical, frequent: dryness, pruritus, erythema, scaling.

ETHAMBUTOL (*Myambutol*, ✦*Etibi*) ▶LK ♀C but + ▶+ $$$$
ADULTS — TB: ATS and CDC recommend 15 to 20 mg/kg PO daily. Dose with whole tabs: 800 mg PO daily for wt 40 to 55 kg, 1200 mg PO daily for wt 56 to 75 kg, 1600 mg PO daily for wt 76 to 90 kg. Base dose on estimated lean body wt. Max dose regardless of wt is 1600 mg/day.
PEDS — TB: ATS and CDC recommend 15 to 20 mg/kg (up to 1 g) PO daily. Use cautiously if visual acuity cannot be monitored. Manufacturer recommends against use in children younger than 13 yo.
UNAPPROVED ADULTS — Treatment or prevention of recurrent Mycobacterium avium complex disease in HIV infection: 15 to 25 mg/kg (up to 1600 mg) PO daily with clarithromycin/azithromycin ± rifabutin.
UNAPPROVED PEDS — Treatment or prevention of recurrent Mycobacterium avium complex disease in HIV infection: 15 mg/kg (up to 900 mg) PO daily with clarithromycin/azithromycin ± rifabutin.
FORMS — Generic/Trade: Tabs 100, 400 mg.
NOTES — Can cause retrobulbar neuritis. Avoid, if possible, in patients with optic neuritis. Test

(cont.)

ETHAMBUTOL (cont.)
visual acuity and color discrimination at baseline. Ask about visual disturbances monthly. Monitor visual acuity and color discrimination monthly if dose is greater than 15 to 20 mg/kg, duration is longer than 2 months, or renal dysfunction. Advise patients to report any change in vision immediately; do not use in those who cannot report visual symptoms (eg, children, unconscious). Do not give aluminum hydroxide antacid until at least 4 h after ethambutol dose. Reduce dose in renal impairment.
MOA − Inhibits arabinosyl transferase enzymes involved in synthesis of mycobacterial cell wall.
ADVERSE EFFECTS − Serious: Retrobulbar neuritis, peripheral neuropathy, anaphylactoid reactions.

ISONIAZID (*INH*, ✤*Isotamine*) ▶LK ♀C but + ▶+ $
WARNING − Hepatotoxicity. Obtain baseline LFTs. Monitor LFTs monthly in high-risk patients (HIV, signs/history of liver disease, abnormal LFTs at baseline, pregnancy/postpartum, alcoholism/regular alcohol use, some patients older than 35 yo). Tell all patients to stop isoniazid and call at once if hepatotoxicity symptoms develop. Discontinue if ALT at least 3 times the upper limit of normal with hepatotoxicity symptoms or ALT at least 5 times the upper limit of normal without hepatotoxicity symptoms.
ADULTS − <u>TB treatment:</u> 5 mg/kg (up to 300 mg) PO daily or 15 mg/kg (up to 900 mg) twice a week. <u>Latent TB:</u> 300 mg PO daily.
PEDS − <u>TB treatment:</u> 10 to 15 mg/kg (up to 300 mg) PO daily. <u>Latent TB:</u> 10 mg/kg (up to 300 mg) PO daily.
UNAPPROVED ADULTS − <u>American Thoracic Society regimen, latent TB:</u> 5 mg/kg (up to 300 mg) PO daily for 9 months (6 months OK if HIV-negative, but less effective than 9 months).
UNAPPROVED PEDS − <u>American Thoracic Society regimen for latent TB:</u> 10 to 20 mg/kg (up to 300 mg) PO daily for 9 months.
FORMS − Generic only: Tabs 100, 300 mg. Syrup 50 mg/5 mL.
NOTES − To reduce risk of peripheral neuropathy, give pyridoxine if alcoholism, diabetes, HIV, uremia, malnutrition, seizure disorder, pregnant/breastfeeding woman, breast-fed infant of INH-treated mother. Many drug interactions.
MOA − Inhibits synthesis of mycolic acid, a component of mycobacterial cell walls.
ADVERSE EFFECTS − Serious: Hepatotoxicity, peripheral neuropathy, lupus. Frequent: Increased LFTs, positive ANA.

PYRAZINAMIDE (*PZA*, ✤*Tebrazid*) ▶LK ♀C ▶? $$$$
WARNING − The ATS and CDC recommend against general use of 2-month regimen of rifampin + pyrazinamide for latent TB due to reports of fatal hepatotoxicity.
ADULTS − <u>TB:</u> ATS and CDC recommend 20 to 25 mg/kg PO daily. Dose with whole tabs: Give 1000 mg PO daily for wt 40 to 55 kg, 1500 mg daily for wt 56 to 75 kg, 2000 mg for wt 76 to 90 kg. Base dose on estimated lean body wt. Max dose regardless of wt is 2000 mg PO daily.
PEDS − <u>TB:</u> 15 to 30 mg/kg (up to 2000 mg) PO daily.
FORMS − Generic only: Tabs 500 mg.
NOTES − Hepatotoxicity, hyperuricemia (avoid in acute gout). Obtain LFTs at baseline. Monitor periodically in high-risk patients (HIV infection, alcoholism, pregnancy, signs/history of liver disease, abnormal LFTs at baseline). Discontinue if ALT is at least 3 times the upper limit of normal with hepatotoxicity symptoms or ALT is at least 5 times upper limit of normal without hepatotoxicity symptoms. Consider reduced dose in renal dysfunction.
MOA − Unknown.
ADVERSE EFFECTS − Serious: Hepatotoxicity. Frequent: Hyperuricemia, polyarthralgia, myalgia, mild anorexia, nausea.

RIFABUTIN (*Mycobutin*) ▶L ♀B ▶? $$$$$
ADULTS − <u>Prevention of disseminated Mycobacterium avium complex disease in AIDS:</u> 300 mg PO daily; can give 150 mg PO bid if GI upset. Reduce dose for ritonavir, atazanavir, or ritonavir-boosted darunavir, fosamprenavir, indinavir, lopinavir (Kaletra), or tipranavir: 150 mg PO every other day. Reduce dose for nelfinavir (use nelfinavir 1250 mg PO bid), unboosted indinavir (increase indinavir to 1000 mg PO q 8 h), or unboosted fosamprenavir: 150 mg PO daily. Dosage increase for efavirenz: 450 to 600 mg PO daily or 600 mg PO 3 times a week. Use standard rifabutin dose with etravirine (without ritonavir-boosted protease inhibitor) or nevirapine. Avoid rifabutin in patients receiving etravirine with a protease inhibitor. Monitor CBC at least weekly. Consider dosage adjustment based on rifabutin levels for patients receiving antiretroviral drugs.
PEDS − Not approved in children.
UNAPPROVED ADULTS − <u>TB or Mycobacterium avium complex disease treatment in AIDS:</u> 300 mg PO daily. Dosage reduction for ritonavir-boosted protease inhibitors: 150 mg every other day or three times weekly. Consider dosage adjustment based on rifabutin levels for patients receiving antiretroviral drugs.
UNAPPROVED PEDS − <u>Mycobacterium avium complex disease.</u> Prophylaxis: Give 5 mg/kg (up to 300 mg) PO daily for age younger than 6 yo; give 300 mg PO daily for age 6 yo or older. Treatment: 10 to 20 mg/kg (max 300 mg/day) PO once daily. <u>TB:</u> 10 to 20 mg/kg (up to 300 mg/day) PO once daily.
FORMS − Trade only: Caps 150 mg.
NOTES − Uveitis (with high doses or if metabolism inhibited by other drugs), hepatotoxicity, thrombocytopenia, neutropenia. Obtain CBC and LFTs at baseline. Monitor periodically in high-risk patients (HIV infection, alcoholism, pregnancy, signs/history of liver disease, abnormal LFTs at baseline). May induce liver metabolism of other drugs including oral contraceptives, protease inhibitors, and azole antifungals. Substrate of CYP3A4; azole

(cont.)

ANTIMICROBIALS: Antimycobacterial Agents

RIFABUTIN (cont.)
antifungals, clarithromycin, and protease inhibitors increase rifabutin levels. Urine, body secretion, soft contact lenses may turn orange-brown. Consider dosage reduction for hepatic dysfunction.
MOA – Rifamycin derivative that inhibits bacterial RNA polymerase.
ADVERSE EFFECTS – Serious: Uveitis (with high doses or if metabolism inhibited by other drugs), hepatotoxicity, thrombocytopenia, neutropenia. Frequent: Arthralgia/myalgia; GI upset; increased LFTs; orange-brown discoloration of urine, body secretion, soft contact lenses.

RIFAMATE (isoniazid + rifampin) ▶LK ♀C but +▶+ $$$$
WARNING – Hepatotoxicity.
ADULTS – TB: 2 caps PO daily on empty stomach.
PEDS – Not approved in children.
FORMS – Generic/Trade: Caps isoniazid 150 mg + rifampin 300 mg.
NOTES – See components. Monitor LFTs at baseline and periodically during therapy.
MOA – See components.
ADVERSE EFFECTS – See components.

RIFAMPIN (*Rimactane, Rifadin, ✱Rofact*) ▶L ♀C but +▶+ $$$
WARNING – The ATS and CDC recommend against general use of 2-mo regimen of rifampin + pyrazinamide for latent TB due to reports of fatal hepatotoxicity.
ADULTS – TB: 10 mg/kg (up to 600 mg) PO/IV daily. Neisseria meningitidis carriers: 600 mg PO bid for 2 days. Take oral doses on empty stomach. IV and PO doses are the same.
PEDS – TB: 10 to 20 mg/kg (up to 600 mg) PO/IV daily. Neisseria meningitidis carriers: Age younger than 1 mo, 5 mg/kg PO bid for 2 days; age 1 mo or older, 10 mg/kg (up to 600 mg) PO bid for 2 days. Take oral doses on empty stomach. IV and PO doses are the same.
UNAPPROVED ADULTS – Prophylaxis of H influenza b infection: 20 mg/kg (up to 600 mg) PO daily for 4 days. Leprosy: 600 mg PO q month with dapsone. American Thoracic Society regimen for latent TB: 10 mg/kg up to 600 mg PO daily for 4 months. Staphylococcal prosthetic valve endocarditis: 300 mg PO q 8 h in combination with gentamicin plus nafcillin, oxacillin, or vancomycin. Community-acquired MRSA skin infection: 300 mg PO bid added to TMP-SMX or doxycycline. Take on empty stomach.
UNAPPROVED PEDS – Prophylaxis of H influenza type b infection: Age younger than 1 mo, 10 mg/kg PO daily for 4 days; age 1 mo or older, 20 mg/kg up to 600 mg PO daily for 4 days. Prophylaxis of invasive meningococcal disease: Age younger than 1 mo, 5 mg/kg PO bid for 2 days; age 1 mo or older, 10 mg/kg (up to 600 mg) PO bid for 2 days. American Thoracic Society regimen for latent tuberculosis: 10 to 20 mg/kg (up to 600 mg) PO daily for 4 months. CA MRSA skin infection: 10 to 20 mg/kg/day (up to 600 mg/day) PO divided bid added to TMP-SMX. Take on empty stomach.
FORMS – Generic/Trade: Caps 150, 300 mg. Pharmacists can make oral susp.
NOTES – Hepatotoxicity, thrombocytopenia. When treating TB, obtain baseline CBC, LFTs. Monitor periodically in high-risk patients (HIV infection, alcoholism, pregnancy, signs/history of liver disease, abnormal LFTs at baseline). Discontinue if ALT is at least 3 times the upper limit of normal with hepatotoxicity symptoms or ALT is at least 5 times the upper limit of normal without hepatotoxicity symptoms. The ATS and CDC recommend against general use of 2-month regimen of rifampin + pyrazinamide for latent TB due to reports of fatal hepatotoxicity. Induces hepatic metabolism of many drugs; check other sources for dosage adjustments before prescribing. If used with rifampin, consider increasing efavirenz to 800 mg once daily at bedtime if wt greater than 60 kg. Do not use rifampin with protease inhibitors. Decreased efficacy of oral contraceptives; use nonhormonal method. Decreased INR with warfarin; monitor daily or as needed. Adjust dose for hepatic impairment. Colors urine, body secretions, soft contact lenses red-orange. Give prophylactic vitamin K 10 mg IM single dose to newborns of women taking rifampin. IV rifampin is stable for 4 h after dilution in dextrose 5%.
MOA – Rifamycin derivative that inhibits bacterial RNA polymerase.
ADVERSE EFFECTS – Serious: Hepatotoxicity, thrombocytopenia, exacerbation of porphyria. Potential risk of hemorrhagic disease in newborns of women taking rifampin; give vitamin K 10 mg IM x 1 to newborn. Frequent: Rash, pruritus, arthralgia/myalgia; orange-brown discoloration of urine, body secretion, soft contact lenses.

RIFAPENTINE (*Priftin*) ▶Esterases, fecal ♀C ▶? $$$$
ADULTS – TB: 600 mg PO twice a week for 2 months, then once a week for 4 months. Use only for continuation therapy in selected HIV-negative patients.
PEDS – Not approved in children younger than 12 yo.
FORMS – Trade only: Tabs 150 mg.
NOTES – Hepatotoxicity, thrombocytopenia, exacerbation of porphyria. Obtain CBC and LFTs at baseline. Monitor LFTs periodically in high-risk patients (alcoholism, pregnancy, signs/history of liver disease, abnormal LFTs at baseline). Do not use in porphyria. Urine, body secretions, contact lenses, and dentures may turn red-orange. May induce liver metabolism of other drugs including oral contraceptives. Avoid with protease inhibitors or NNRTIs.
MOA – Long-acting derivative of rifampin, a rifamycin that inhibits bacterial RNA polymerase.
ADVERSE EFFECTS – Serious: Hepatotoxicity, thrombocytopenia, exacerbation of porphyria. Frequent: Hyperuricemia, orange-brown discoloration of urine, body secretion, soft contact lenses.

RIFATER (isoniazid + rifampin + pyrazinamide) ▶LK ♀C ▶? $$$$$
WARNING — Hepatotoxicity.
ADULTS — <u>TB,</u> initial 2 months of treatment: 4 tabs daily for wt less than 45 kg, 5 tabs daily for 45 to 54 kg, 6 tabs daily for 55 kg or greater. Additional pyrazinamide tabs required to provide adequate dose for wt greater than 90 kg. Take on empty stomach. Can finish treatment with Rifamate.
PEDS — Ratio of formulation may not be appropriate for children younger than 15 yo.
FORMS — Trade only: Tabs Isoniazid 50 mg + rifampin 120 mg + pyrazinamide 300 mg.
NOTES — See components. Monitor LFTs at baseline and during therapy. Do not use in patients with renal dysfunction.
MOA — See components.
ADVERSE EFFECTS — See components.

ANTIMICROBIALS: Antiparasitics

ALBENDAZOLE (*Albenza*) ▶L ♀C ▶? $$$
ADULTS — <u>Hydatid disease, neurocysticercosis:</u> 15 mg/kg/day (up to 800 mg/day) for wt less than 60 kg, 400 mg PO bid for wt 60 kg or greater. Treatment duration varies. Take with food.
PEDS — <u>Hydatid disease, neurocysticercosis:</u> 15 mg/kg/day (up to 800 mg/day) for wt less than 60 kg, 400 mg PO bid for wt 60 kg or greater. Treatment duration varies. Take with food.
UNAPPROVED ADULTS — <u>Hookworm, whipworm, pinworm, roundworm:</u> 400 mg PO single dose. Repeat in 2 weeks for pinworm. <u>Cutaneous larva migrans:</u> 200 mg PO bid for 3 days. <u>Giardia:</u> 400 mg PO daily for 5 days. <u>Intestinal/disseminated microsporidiosis in HIV infection</u> (not for ocular or caused by E bienuesi/V corneae): 400 mg PO bid until CD4 count > 200 for more than 6 months after starting antiretrovirals.
UNAPPROVED PEDS — <u>Roundworm, hookworm, pinworm, whipworm:</u> 400 mg PO single dose. Repeat in 2 weeks for pinworm. <u>Cutaneous larva migrans:</u> 200 mg PO bid for 3 days. <u>Giardia:</u> 400 mg PO daily for 5 days.
FORMS — Trade only: Tabs 200 mg.
NOTES — Associated with bone marrow suppression (especially if liver disease), increased LFTs (common with long-term use), and hepatotoxicity (rare). Monitor CBC and LFTs before starting and then every 2 weeks; discontinue if significant changes. Consider corticosteroids and anticonvulsants in neurocysticercosis. Consider diagnosis of preexisting neurocysticercosis if patient develops neurologic symptoms soon after albendazole treatment for another indication. Get negative pregnancy test before treatment and warn against getting pregnant until 1 month after treatment. Treat close contacts for pinworms. Can crush/chew tabs and swallow with water.
MOA — Antihelmintic that inhibits the formation of microtubules and causes glucose depletion.
ADVERSE EFFECTS — Serious: Nephrotoxicity, bone marrow suppression, hepatotoxicity (usually with long-term use). Increased LFTs increases risk of liver failure or bone marrow suppression. Frequent: Abnormal LFTs, abdominal pain.

ATOVAQUONE (*Mepron*) ▶Fecal ♀C ▶? $$$$$
ADULTS — <u>Pneumocystis in patients intolerant to trimethoprim/sulfamethoxazole:</u> Treatment 750 mg PO bid for 21 days. Prevention 1500 mg PO daily. Take with meals.
PEDS — <u>Pneumocystis in patients intolerant to trimethoprim/sulfamethoxazole, 13 to 16 yo:</u> Treatment, 750 mg PO bid for 21 days. Prevention, 1500 mg PO daily. Take with meals.
UNAPPROVED PEDS — <u>Prevention of recurrent Pneumocystis in HIV infection:</u> 30 mg/kg PO daily, for age 1 to 3 mo, 45 mg/kg PO daily for age 4 to 24 mo, 30 mg/kg PO daily for age 25 mo or older. Take with meals.
FORMS — Trade only: Susp 750 mg/5 mL (210 mL), foil pouch 750 mg/5 mL (5, 10 mL).
NOTES — Efficacy of atovaquone may be decreased by rifampin (consider using alternative), rifabutin, or rifapentine.
MOA — Ubiquinone analog that may inhibit nucleic acid and ATP synthesis via effects on mitochondrial electron transport.
ADVERSE EFFECTS — Serious: Hepatotoxicity (rare). Frequent: Rash, nausea, fever, headache, insomnia, increased LFTs.

IVERMECTIN (*Stromectol*) ▶L ♀C ▶+ $$
ADULTS — <u>Strongyloidiasis:</u> 200 mcg/kg PO single dose. <u>Onchocerciasis:</u> 150 mcg/kg PO single dose q 3 to 12 months. Take on empty stomach with water.
PEDS — <u>Strongyloidiasis:</u> 200 mcg/kg PO single dose. <u>Onchocerciasis:</u> 150 mcg/kg PO single dose q 3 to 12 months. Take on empty stomach with water. Safety and efficacy not established in children less than 15 kg.
UNAPPROVED ADULTS — <u>Scabies:</u> 200 mcg/kg PO repeated in 2 weeks. <u>Pubic lice:</u> 250 mcg/kg PO repeated in 2 weeks. <u>Cutaneous larva migrans:</u> 150 to 200 mcg/kg PO single dose. Take on empty stomach with water.
UNAPPROVED PEDS — <u>Scabies:</u> 200 mcg/kg PO single dose (dose may need to be repeated in 10 to 14 days). <u>Head lice:</u> 200-400 mcg/kg PO single dose; repeat in 7 days. <u>Cutaneous larva migrans:</u> 150 to 200 mcg/kg PO single dose. Take on empty stomach with water. Not for wt less than 15 kg.
FORMS — Trade only: Tabs 3 mg.
NOTES — Mazzotti and ophthalmic reactions with treatment for onchocerciasis. May need repeat/monthly treatment for strongyloidiasis in immunocompromised/HIV-infected patients. Increased INRs with warfarin reported rarely.
MOA — Binds to glutamate-gated chloride ion channels in invertebrate nerve and muscle cells; this leads to paralysis and death of the parasite.

(cont.)

ANTIMICROBIALS: Antiparasitics

IVERMECTIN (cont.)
ADVERSE EFFECTS – Serious: Mazzotti & ophthalmic reactions with treatment for onchocerciasis. Frequent: Nausea.

MEBENDAZOLE (Vermox) ▶L ♀C ▶? $$
ADULTS – Pinworm: 100 mg PO single dose; repeat in 2 weeks. Roundworm, whipworm, hookworm: 100 mg PO bid for 3 days.
PEDS – Pinworm: 100 mg PO single dose; repeat dose in 2 weeks. Roundworm, whipworm, hookworm: 100 mg PO bid for 3 days.
UNAPPROVED ADULTS – Roundworm, whipworm, hookworm: 500 mg PO single dose.
UNAPPROVED PEDS – Roundworm, whipworm, hookworm: 500 mg PO single dose.
FORMS – Generic only: Chewable tabs 100 mg.
NOTES – Treat close contacts for pinworms.
MOA – Anthelmintic that inhibits the formation of microtubules and causes glucose depletion.
ADVERSE EFFECTS – Serious: Angioedema (rare), seizures (rare). Frequent: Transient GI complaints.

NITAZOXANIDE (Alinia) ▶L ♀B ▶? $$$$
ADULTS – Cryptosporidial or Giardial diarrhea: 500 mg PO bid with food for 3 days.
PEDS – Cryptosporidial or Giardial diarrhea: 100 mg bid for 1 to 3 yo, 200 mg bid for 4 to 11 yo, 500 mg bid for 12 yo or older. Give PO with food for 3 days. Use susp if younger than 12 yo.
UNAPPROVED ADULTS – C. difficile associated diarrhea: 500 mg PO bid for 10 days. Cryptosporidiosis in HIV infection (alternative therapy in addition to concurrent HAART): 500 to 1000 mg PO bid with food for 14 days.
FORMS – Trade only: Oral susp 100 mg/5 mL, 60 mL bottle. Tabs 500 mg.
NOTES – Contains 1.5 g sucrose/5 mL. Turns urine bright yellow. Store at room temperature for up to 7 days.
MOA – Antiprotozoal agent that interferes with electron transfer reaction required for anaerobic energy metabolism.
ADVERSE EFFECTS – Mild and transient abdominal pain, diarrhea, vomiting, headache. Discolors urine bright yellow.

PAROMOMYCIN ▶Not absorbed ♀C ▶– $$$$
ADULTS – Intestinal amebiasis: 25 to 35 mg/kg/day PO divided tid with or after meals for 5 to 10 days.
PEDS – Intestinal amebiasis: 25 to 35 mg/kg/day PO divided tid with or after meals for 5 to 10 days.
UNAPPROVED ADULTS – Giardiasis: 500 mg PO tid for 7 days.
UNAPPROVED PEDS – Giardiasis: 25 to 35 mg/kg/day PO divided tid with or after meals for 7 days.
FORMS – Generic only: Caps 250 mg.
NOTES – Nephrotoxicity possible in inflammatory bowel disease due to increased systemic absorption. Not effective for extraintestinal amebiasis.
MOA – Aminoglycoside, inhibits parasitic protein synthesis by interfering with function of ribosomal 30S subunit.
ADVERSE EFFECTS – Serious: Nephrotoxicity possible with systemic absorption in inflammatory bowel disease. Frequent: GI distress.

PENTAMIDINE (Pentam, NebuPent) ▶K ♀C ▶– $$$
ADULTS – Pneumocystis treatment: 4 mg/kg IM/IV daily for 21 days. Some experts reduce to 3 mg/kg IM/IV daily if toxicity. IV infused over 60 to 90 min. NebuPent for Pneumocystis prevention: 300 mg nebulized every 4 weeks.
PEDS – Pneumocystis treatment: 4 mg/kg IM/IV daily for 21 days. NebuPent not approved in children.
UNAPPROVED PEDS – Pneumocystis prevention, age 5 yo or older: 300 mg NebuPent nebulized every 4 weeks.
FORMS – Trade only: Aerosol 300 mg.
NOTES – Contraindicated with ziprasidone. Fatalities due to severe hypotension, hypoglycemia, cardiac arrhythmias with IM/IV. Have patient lie down, check BP, and keep resuscitation equipment nearby during IM/IV injection. May cause torsades, hyperglycemia, neutropenia, nephrotoxicity, pancreatitis, and hypocalcemia. Monitor BUN, serum creatinine, blood glucose, CBC, LFTs, serum calcium, and ECG. Bronchospasm with inhalation (consider bronchodilator). Reduce IM/IV dose in renal dysfunction.
MOA – Unknown.
ADVERSE EFFECTS – Serious: Fatalities due to severe hypotension, hypoglycemia, cardiac arrhythmias with IM/IV. Extravasation of injection site. Can also cause hyperglycemia, neutropenia (frequent), nephrotoxicity, pancreatitis, torsades, & hypocalcemia. Inhaled pentamidine can cause bronchospasm.

PRAZIQUANTEL (Biltricide) ▶LK ♀B ▶– $$$
ADULTS – Schistosomiasis: 20 mg/kg PO q 4 to 6 h for 3 doses. Liver flukes: 25 mg/kg PO q 4 to 6 h for 3 doses.
PEDS – Schistosomiasis: 20 mg/kg PO q 4 to 6 h for 3 doses. Liver flukes: 25 mg/kg PO q 4 to 6 h for 3 doses.
UNAPPROVED ADULTS – Neurocysticercosis: 50 mg/kg/day PO divided tid for 15 days. Fish, dog, beef, pork intestinal tapeworms: 10 mg/kg PO single dose.
UNAPPROVED PEDS – Neurocysticercosis: 50 to 100 mg/kg/day PO divided tid for 15 days. Fish, dog, beef, pork intestinal tapeworms: 10 mg/kg PO single dose.
FORMS – Trade only: Tabs 600 mg.
NOTES – Contraindicated in ocular cysticercosis. May cause drowsiness; do not drive or operate machinery for 48 h. Phenytoin, carbamazepine, rifampin (avoid using together), and dexamethasone may lower praziquantel levels enough to cause treatment failure. Take with liquids during a meal. Do not chew tabs. Manufacturer advises against breastfeeding until 72 h after treatment.
MOA – Trematodicide that induces rapid contraction of schistosomes by affecting cell membrane permeability.
ADVERSE EFFECTS – Serious: None. Frequent: Drowsiness.

ANTIMICROBIALS: Antiviral Agents

PYRANTEL (*Antiminth, Pin-X, Pinworm, ✦Combantrin*) ▶Not absorbed ♀– ▶? $
- ADULTS — Pinworm, roundworm: 11 mg/kg (up to 1 g) PO single dose. Repeat in 2 weeks for pinworm.
- PEDS — Pinworm, roundworm: 11 mg/kg (up to 1 g) PO single dose. Repeat in 2 weeks for pinworm.
- UNAPPROVED ADULTS — Hookworm: 11 mg/kg (up to 1 g) PO daily for 3 days.
- UNAPPROVED PEDS — Hookworm: 11 mg/kg (up to 1 g) PO daily for 3 days.
- FORMS — OTC Trade only (Pin-X): Susp 144 mg/mL (equivalent to 50 mg/mL of pyrantel base) 30, 60 mL. Tabs 720.5 mg (equivalent to 250 mg of pyrantel base). OTC Generic only: Caps 180 mg (equivalent to 62.5 mg of pyrantel base).
- NOTES — Purging not necessary. Treat close contacts for pinworms.
- MOA — Acts as agonist at nicotinic acetylcholine receptors of sensitive nematodes, depolarizing neuromuscular blocker that paralyzes the worm.
- ADVERSE EFFECTS — Serious: None. Frequent: None.

PYRIMETHAMINE (*Daraprim*) ▶L ♀C ▶+ $$
- ADULTS — Toxoplasmonthsis, immunocompetent patients: 50 to 75 mg PO daily for 1 to 3 weeks, then reduce dose by 50% for 4 to 5 more weeks. Give with leucovorin (10 to 15 mg daily) and sulfadiazine. Reduce initial dose in seizure disorders.
- PEDS — Toxoplasmonthsis: 1 mg/kg/day PO divided bid for 2 to 4 days, then reduce by 50% for 1 month. Give with sulfadiazine and leucovorin. Reduce initial dose in seizure disorders.
- UNAPPROVED ADULTS — CNS toxoplasmosis in AIDS. Acute therapy: First dose 200 mg PO, then 50 mg PO daily for wt less than 60 kg; use 75 mg PO once daily for 60 kg or greater. In addition, add sulfadiazine 1000 mg PO q 6 h for wt less than 60 kg; use 1500 mg PO q 6 h for 60 kg or greater, as well as leucovorin 10 to 25 mg PO once daily (can increase to 50 mg/day). Treat for at least 6 weeks. Secondary prevention: 25 to 50 mg PO once daily + sulfadiazine 2000 to 4000 mg/day PO divided bid-qid + leucovorin 10 to 25 mg PO once daily. Reduce initial dose in seizure disorders.
- UNAPPROVED PEDS — Acquired toxoplasmonthsis: 2 mg/kg (up to 50 mg) PO once daily for 3 days, then 1 mg/kg (up to 25 mg) PO once daily + sulfadiazine 25 to 50 mg/kg PO (up to 1 to 1.5 g/dose) PO qid. Give leucovorin 10 to 25 mg/day PO. Treat at least 6 weeks followed by chronic suppressive therapy.
- FORMS — Trade only: Tabs 25 mg.
- NOTES — Hemolytic anemia in G6PD deficiency, dose-related folate deficiency, hypersensitivity. Monitor CBC.
- MOA — Folic acid antagonist.
- ADVERSE EFFECTS — Serious: Hemolytic anemia in G6PD deficiency, dose-related folate deficiency, hypersensitivity.

TINIDAZOLE (*Tindamax*) ▶KL ♀C ▶?- $
- WARNING — Metronidazole, a related drug, was carcinogenic in animal studies.
- ADULTS — Trichomoniasis or giardiasis: 2 g PO single dose. Amebiasis: 2 g PO daily for 3 days. Bacterial vaginosis: 2 g PO once daily for 2 days or 1 g PO once daily for 5 days. Take with food.
- PEDS — Giardiasis, age older than 3 yo: 50 mg/kg (up to 2 g) PO single dose. Amebiasis, age older than 3 yo: 50 mg/kg (up to 2 g) PO daily for 3 days. Take with food.
- UNAPPROVED ADULTS — Recurrent/persistent urethritis: 2 g PO single dose.
- FORMS — Trade only: Tabs 250, 500 mg. Pharmacists can compound oral susp.
- NOTES — Give iodoquinol/paromomycin after treatment for amebic dysentery or liver abscess. Disulfiram reaction; avoid alcohol at least 3 days after treatment. Can minimize infant exposure by withholding breastfeeding for 3 days after maternal single dose. May increase levels of cyclosporine, fluorouracil, lithium, phenytoin, tacrolimus. May increase INR with warfarin. Do not give at same time as cholestyramine. For patients undergoing hemodialysis: Give supplemental ½ dose after dialysis session.
- MOA — 5-Nitroimidazole derivative with amebicidal, Giardiacidal, and trichomonacidal activity.
- ADVERSE EFFECTS — Serious: Seizures, peripheral neuropathy. Frequent: Anorexia, headache, dizziness. May be better tolerated than metronidazole. Transient neutropenia, leukopenia.

ANTIMICROBIALS: Antiviral Agents—Anti-CMV

CIDOFOVIR (*Vistide*) ▶K ♀C ▶– $$$$$
- WARNING — Severe nephrotoxicity. Granulocytopenia: Monitor neutrophil counts.
- ADULTS — CMV retinitis: 5 mg/kg IV weekly for 2 weeks, then 5 mg/kg q other weeks. Give probenecid 2 g PO 3 h before and 1 g 2 h and 8 h after infusion. Give NS with each infusion.
- PEDS — Not approved in children.
- NOTES — Fanconi-like syndrome. Stop nephrotoxic drugs at least 1 week before cidofovir. Get serum creatinine, urine protein before each dose. See package insert for dosage adjustments based on renal function. Do not use if creatinine is greater than 1.5 mg/dL, CrCl 55 mL/min or less, or urine protein 100 mg/dL (2+) or greater. Hold/decrease zidovudine dose by 50% on day cidofovir is given. Tell women not to get pregnant until 1 month after and men to use barrier contraceptive until 3 months after cidofovir. Ocular hypotony: Monitor intraocular pressure.
- MOA — Selectively inhibits cytomegalovirus DNA polymerase.
- ADVERSE EFFECTS — Serious: Nephrotoxicity (also frequent), Fanconi syndrome, neutropenia (also frequent), metabolic acidosis, iritis/uveitis, ocular hypotony. Frequent: Nausea, fever, alopecia, myalgia.

ANTIMICROBIALS: Antiviral Agents

FOSCARNET (*Foscavir*) ▶K ♀C ▶? $$$$$
  WARNING — Nephrotoxicity; seizures due to mineral/electrolyte imbalance.
  ADULTS — Hydrate before infusion. <u>CMV retinitis:</u> 60 mg/kg IV (over 1 h) q 8 h or 90 mg/kg IV (over 1.5 to 2 h) q 12 h for 2 to 3 weeks, then 90 to 120 mg/kg IV daily over 2 h. <u>Acyclovir-resistant HSV infection:</u> 40 mg/kg IV (over 1 h) q 8 to 12 h for 2 to 3 weeks or until healed.
  PEDS — Not approved in children. Deposits into teeth and bone of young animals.
  UNAPPROVED PEDS — Hydrate before infusion. <u>CMV retinitis:</u> 60 mg/kg IV (over 1 h) q 8 h or 90 mg/kg IV (over 1.5 to 2 h) q 12 h for 2 to 3 weeks, then 90 to 120 mg/kg IV daily over 2 h. <u>Acyclovir-resistant HSV infection:</u> 40 mg/kg IV (over 1 h) q 8 h for 2 to 3 weeks or until healed. <u>Acyclovir-resistant varicella zoster infection:</u> 40 to 60 mg/kg IV q 8 h for 7 to 10 days.
  NOTES — Granulocytopenia, anemia, vein irritation, penile ulcers. Decreased ionized serum calcium, especially with IV pentamidine. Must use IV pump to avoid rapid administration. Monitor renal function, serum calcium, magnesium, phosphate, potassium. Reduce dose in renal impairment. Stop foscarnet if CrCl decreases to < 0.4 mL/min/kg.
  MOA — Direct inhibitor of herpesvirus DNA polymerase.
  ADVERSE EFFECTS — Serious: Nephrotoxicity (also frequent), neutropenia, penile ulcers. Electrolyte/mineral disorders. Frequent: Headache, fatigue, nausea, fever.

GANCICLOVIR (*Cytovene*) ▶K ♀C ▶– $$$$$
  WARNING — Neutropenia, anemia, thrombocytopenia. Do not use if ANC < 500/mm3 or platelets < 25,000/mm3.
  ADULTS — <u>CMV retinitis.</u> Induction: 5 mg/kg IV q 12 h for 14 to 21 days. Maintenance: 6 mg/kg IV daily for 5 days/week or 5 mg/kg IV daily. <u>Prevention of CMV disease after organ transplant:</u> 5 mg/kg IV q 12 h for 7 to 14 days, then 6 mg/kg IV daily for 5 days/week. Give IV infusion over 1 h.
  PEDS — Safety and efficacy not established in children; potential carcinogenic or reproductive adverse effects.
  UNAPPROVED PEDS — <u>CMV retinitis.</u>in immunocompromised patient: Induction 5 mg/kg IV q 12 h for 14 to 21 days. Maintenance 5 mg/kg IV daily or 6 mg/kg IV daily for 5 days/weeks. <u>Symptomatic congenital CMV infection:</u> 6 mg/kg IV q 12 h for 6 weeks.
  FORMS — Generic only: Caps 250, 500 mg.
  NOTES — Neutropenia (worsened by zidovudine), phlebitis/pain at infusion site, increased seizure risk with imipenem. Monitor CBC, renal function. Reduce dose if CrCl < 70 mL/min. Adequate hydration required. Potential teratogen. Tell women not to get pregnant during and men to use barrier contraceptive at least 3 months after treatment. Potential carcinogen. Follow guidelines for handling/disposal of cytotoxic agents.
  MOA — Inhibits viral DNA synthesis.
  ADVERSE EFFECTS — Serious: Myelosuppression (frequent), fever (frequent), hepatic and renal dysfunction, retinal detachment. Frequent: GI complaints, headache, phlebitis at injection site, rash, confusion.

VALGANCICLOVIR (*Valcyte*) ▶K ♀C ▶– $$$$$
  WARNING — Myelosuppression may occur at any time. Monitor CBC and platelet count frequently. Do not use if ANC < 500/mm3, platelets < 25,000/mm3, hemoglobin < 8 g/dL.
  ADULTS — <u>CMV retinitis:</u> 900 mg PO bid for 21 days, then 900 mg PO daily. <u>Prevention of CMV disease in high-risk transplant patients:</u> 900 mg PO daily given within 10 days post-transplant until 100 days post-transplant for heart or kidney-pancreas or 200 days for kidney transplant. Give with food.
  PEDS — <u>Prevention of CMV disease in high-risk kidney/heart transplant patients 4 months of age and older:</u> Daily dose in mg is 7 x body surface area x CrCl (calculated with modified Schwartz formula). Give PO once daily from within 10 days post-transplant to 100 days post-transplant. Max dose of 900 mg/day. Give with food.
  FORMS — Trade only: Tabs 450 mg. Oral soln 50 mg/mL.
  NOTES — Contraindicated in ganciclovir allergy. Potential teratogen. Tell women not to get pregnant until 1 month after and men to use barrier contraceptive until at least 3 months after treatment. CNS toxicity; warn against hazardous tasks. May increase serum creatinine; monitor renal function. Reduce dose if CrCl < 60 mL/min. Use ganciclovir instead in hemodialysis patients. Potential drug interactions with didanosine, mycophenolate, zidovudine. Potential carcinogen. Avoid direct contact with broken/crushed tabs; do not intentionally break/crush tabs. Follow guidelines for handling/disposal of cytotoxic agents.
  MOA — Prodrug of ganciclovir.
  ADVERSE EFFECTS — Similar to ganciclovir.

ANTIMICROBIALS: Antiviral Agents—Anti-Herpetic

ACYCLOVIR (*Zovirax*) ▶K ♀B ▶+ $
  ADULTS — <u>Genital herpes:</u> 200 mg PO q 4 h (5 times a day) for 10 days for first episode, for 5 days for recurrent episodes. <u>Chronic suppression:</u> 400 mg PO bid. <u>Zoster:</u> 800 mg PO q 4 h (5 times a day) for 7 to 10 days. <u>Chickenpox:</u> 800 mg PO qid for 5 days. IV: 5 to 10 mg/kg IV q 8 h, each dose over 1 h. <u>Zoster in immunocompromised patients:</u> 10 mg/kg IV q 8 h for 7 days. <u>Herpes simplex encephalitis:</u> 10 mg/kg IV q 8 h for 10 days. <u>Mucosal/cutaneous herpes simplex in immunocompromised patients:</u> 5 mg/kg IV q 8 h for 7 days.
  PEDS — Safety and efficacy of PO acyclovir not established in children younger than 2 yo. <u>Chickenpox:</u>

(cont.)

ACYCLOVIR (cont.)
20 mg/kg PO qid for 5 days. Use adult dose if wt greater than 40 kg. AAP does not recommend routine treatment of chickenpox with acyclovir, but it should be considered in patients older than 12 yo or with chronic cutaneous or pulmonary disease, chronic salicylate use, or short, intermittent, or inhaled courses of corticosteroid. Possibly also for secondary case-patients in same household as infected children. IV: 250 to 500 mg/m2 q 8 h, each dose over 1 h. Zoster in immunocompromised patients younger than 12 yo: 20 mg/kg IV q 8 h for 7 days. Herpes simplex encephalitis: 20 mg/kg IV q 8 h for 10 days for age 3 mo to 12 yo; adult dose for age 13 yo or older. Neonatal herpes simplex (birth to 3 mo): 10 mg/kg IV q 8 h for 10 days; CDC regimen is 20 mg/kg IV q 8 h for 21 days for disseminated/CNS disease, for 14 days for skin/mucous membranes. Mucosal/cutaneous herpes simplex in immunocompromised patients: 10 mg/kg IV q 8 h for 7 days for age younger than 12 yo, adult dose for 13 yo or older. Treat ASAP after symptom onset.
UNAPPROVED ADULTS — Genital herpes: 400 mg PO tid for 7 to 10 days for first episode, for 5 days for recurrent episodes, for 5 to 10 days for recurrent episodes in HIV+ patients. Alternative regimens for recurrent episodes in HIV-negative patients: 800 mg PO bid for 5 days or 800 mg PO tid for 2 days. Chronic suppression of genital herpes in HIV+ patients: 400 to 800 mg PO bid to tid. Orolabial herpes: 400 mg PO 5 times a day.
UNAPPROVED PEDS — Primary herpes gingivostomatitis: 15 mg/kg PO 5 times a day for 7 days. First episode Genital herpes: 80 mg/kg/day PO divided tid (max 1.2 g/day) for 7 to 10 days. Use dose in unapproved adult for adolescents. Zoster (mild) in mild immunosuppression: 20 mg/kg (max 800 mg/dose) PO qid for 7 to 10 days. Treat ASAP after symptom onset.
FORMS — Generic/Trade: Caps 200 mg. Tabs 400, 800 mg. Susp 200 mg/5 mL.
NOTES — Maintain adequate hydration. Severe drowsiness with acyclovir plus zidovudine. Consider suppressive therapy for patients with at least 6 episodes of genital herpes per year. Reduce dose in renal dysfunction and in elderly. Base IV dose on ideal body wt in obese adults.
MOA — Activated by viral thymidine kinase to become an inhibitor of viral DNA polymerase and block viral DNA synthesis.
ADVERSE EFFECTS — Serious: Encephalopathy, extravasation, crystalluria with IV. Frequent: GI distress & headache with PO.

FAMCICLOVIR (*Famvir*) ▶K ♀B ▶? $$
ADULTS — Recurrent genital herpes: 1000 mg PO bid for 2 doses. Chronic suppression of genital herpes: 250 mg PO bid. Recurrent herpes labialis: 1500 mg PO single dose. Recurrent orolabial/genital herpes in HIV patients: 500 mg PO bid for 7 days. Zoster: 500 mg PO tid for 7 days. Treat ASAP after symptom onset.
PEDS — Not approved in children.
UNAPPROVED ADULTS — First episode genital herpes: 250 mg PO tid for 7 to 10 days. Chronic suppression of genital herpes in HIV+ patients: 500 mg PO bid. Chickenpox in young adults: 500 mg PO tid for 5 days. Bell's palsy: 750 mg PO tid plus prednisone 1 mg/kg PO daily for 7 days. Treat ASAP after symptom onset.
UNAPPROVED PEDS — Chickenpox in adolescents: 500 mg PO tid for 5 days. First episode genital herpes in adolescents: Use dose in unapproved adult.
FORMS — Generic/Trade: Tabs 125, 250, 500 mg.
NOTES — Consider suppressive therapy for patients with at least 6 episodes of genital herpes per year. Reduce dose for CrCl < 60 mL/min.
MOA — Prodrug of penciclovir. Activated by viral thymidine kinase to become an inhibitor of viral DNA polymerase and block viral DNA synthesis.
ADVERSE EFFECTS — Similar to acyclovir. Frequent: Headache, nausea, diarrhea.

VALACYCLOVIR (*Valtrex*) ▶K ♀B ▶+ $$$$$
ADULTS — First episode genital herpes: 1 g PO bid for 10 days. Recurrent genital herpes: 500 mg PO bid for 3 days. Chronic suppression of genital herpes in immunocompetent patients: 1 g PO daily. Can use 500 mg PO daily if 9 or less recurrences per year; transmission of genital herpes reduced with use of this regimen by source partner, in conjunction with safer sex practices. Chronic suppression of genital herpes in HIV-infected patients: 500 mg PO bid. Herpes labialis: 2 g PO q 12 h for 2 doses. Zoster: 1 g PO tid for 7 days. Treat ASAP after symptom onset.
PEDS — Herpes labialis, age 12 yo or older: 2 g PO q 12 h for 2 doses. Chicken pox, age 2 to 17 yo: 20 mg/kg (max of 1 g) PO tid for 5 days. Treat ASAP after symptom onset.
UNAPPROVED ADULTS — Recurrent genital herpes: 1 g PO daily for 5 days. Recurrent genital herpes in HIV+ patients: 1 g PO bid for 5 to 10 days. Bell's palsy: 1 g PO bid plus prednisone 1 mg/kg PO daily for 7 days. Orolabial herpes in immunocompromised patients, including HIV infection: 1 g PO tid for 7 days. Chickenpox in young adults: 1 g PO tid for 5 days. Treat ASAP after symptom onset.
UNAPPROVED PEDS — First episode genital herpes in adolescents: Use adult dose. Treat ASAP after symptom onset.
FORMS — Generic/Trade: Tabs 500, 1000 mg.
NOTES — Consider suppressive therapy for patients with at least 6 episodes of genital herpes per year. Maintain adequate hydration. CNS and renal adverse effects more common if elderly or renal impairment; avoid inappropriately high doses in these patients. Reduce dose for CrCl < 50 mL/min. Thrombotic thrombocytopenic purpura/hemolytic uremic syndrome at dose of 8 g/day.
MOA — Prodrug of acyclovir, which is activated by viral thymidine kinase to become an inhibitor of viral DNA polymerase and block viral DNA synthesis.

(cont.)

ANTIMICROBIALS: Antiviral Agents

VALACYCLOVIR (cont.)
ADVERSE EFFECTS — Similar to acyclovir. CNS (e.g., agitation, hallucinations, confusion, encephalopathy): and renal adverse effects more common if elderly or renal impairment. Serious: Acute renal failure and anuria due to precipitation in renal tubules; may require hemodialysis to remove drug.

ANTIMICROBIALS: Antiviral Agents—Anti-HIV—CCR5 Antagonists

NOTE: AIDS treatment guidelines available online at www.aidsinfo.nih.gov. Consider monitoring LFTs in patients receiving HAART.

MARAVIROC (*Selzentry, MVC*) ▶LK ♀B ▶— $$$$$
WARNING — Hepatotoxicity with allergic features. Consider discontinuation if signs/symptoms of hepatitis, or increased LFTs with rash or other systemic symptoms. Caution if baseline liver dysfunction or coinfection with hepatitis B/C.
ADULTS — Combination therapy for HIV infection: 150 mg PO bid with strong CYP3A4 inhibitors (most protease inhibitors, ketoconazole, itraconazole, clarithromycin); 300 mg PO bid with drugs that are not strong CYP3A4 inducers/inhibitors (NRTIs, tipranavir-ritonavir, nevirapine, enfuvirtide, raltegravir; rifabutin without a strong CYP3A4 inhibitor or inducer); 600 mg PO bid with strong CYP3A4 inducers (efavirenz, etravirine, rifampin, carbamazepine, phenobarbital, phenytoin). Tropism test before treatment; not for dual/mixed or CXCR4-tropic HIV infection.
PEDS — Not recommended for age younger than 16 yo based on lack of data.
FORMS — Trade only: Tabs 150, 300 mg.
NOTES — May increase risk of myocardial ischemia or MI. Theoretical risk of infection/malignancy due to effects on immune system. Metabolized by CYP3A4; do not use with St John's wort. Contraindicated in patients with CrCl < 30 mL/min who are taking a strong CYP3A4 inhibitor or inducer. Consider dosage reduction to 150 mg bid if postural hypotension occurs in patients with CrCL < 30 mL/min.
MOA — CCR5 coreceptor antagonist prevents entry of CCR5-tropic HIV into uninfected CD4 T-cells.
ADVERSE EFFECTS — Serious: Hepatotoxicity with allergic features. May increase risk of myocardial ischemia or MI. May cause postural hypotension, esp in patients with impaired renal function. Frequent: Cough, fever, upper respiratory tract infection, rash, joint symptoms, muscle pain, abdominal pain, dizziness, increased AST.

ANTIMICROBIALS: Antiviral Agents—Anti-HIV—Combinations

NOTE: AIDS treatment guidelines available online at www.aidsinfo.nih.gov. Consider monitoring LFTs in patients receiving HAART. WARNING: Nucleoside reverse transcriptase inhibitors can cause lactic acidosis and hepatic steatosis.

ATRIPLA (efavirenz + emtricitabine + tenofovir) ▶KL ♀D ▶— $$$$$
WARNING — Emtricitabine and tenofovir: Potentially fatal lactic acidosis and hepatosteatosis; severe acute exacerbation of hepatitis B after discontinuation in patients coinfected with HIV and hepatitis B; not indicated for treatment of hepatitis B.
ADULTS — Combination therapy for HIV infection: 1 tab PO once daily on empty stomach, preferably at bedtime. Atripla can be used alone or in combo with other antiretrovirals that are not already in the tab.
PEDS — Safety and efficacy not established.
UNAPPROVED PEDS — Combination therapy for HIV infection, adolescents 40 kg or greater: 1 tab PO once daily on empty stomach, preferably at bedtime. Atripla can be used alone or in combo with other antiretrovirals.
FORMS — Trade only: Tabs efavirenz 600 mg + emtricitabine 200 mg + tenofovir 300 mg.
NOTES — See components. Do not give Atripla with lamivudine. Not for CrCl < 50 mL/min. Efavirenz induces CYP3A4, causing many drug interactions.
MOA — Emtricitabine is a nucleoside reverse transcriptase inhibitor structurally related to lamivudine; cross-resistance documented. Tenofovir is a nucleotide reverse transcriptase inhibitor. Emtricitabine and tenofovir have activity against hepatitis B. Efavirenz is a non-nucleoside reverse transcriptase inhibitor.
ADVERSE EFFECTS — Serious: Emtricitabine, tenofovir: Lactic acidosis/hepatic steatosis; severe acute exacerbation of hepatitis B after discontinuing either drug in patients coinfected with HIV and hepatitis B. Efavirenz: Depression, other psychiatric reactions, convulsions, severe rash, Stevens-Johnson syndrome. See components for other adverse effects.

COMBIVIR (lamivudine + zidovudine) ▶LK ♀C ▶— $$$$$
WARNING — Zidovudine: Bone marrow suppression, myopathy. Lamivudine: Severe acute exacerbation of hepatitis B can occur after discontinuation of lamivudine in patients coinfected with HIV + hepatitis B. Monitor closely for at least 2 months after discontinuing lamivudine in such patients; consider treating hepatitis B.
ADULTS — Combination therapy for HIV infection: 1 tab PO bid.
PEDS — Combination therapy for HIV infection, wt 30 kg or greater: 1 tab PO bid.

(cont.)

ANTIMICROBIALS: Antiviral Agents

COMBIVIR (cont.)
FORMS — Trade only: Tabs lamivudine 150 mg + zidovudine 300 mg.
NOTES — See components. Monitor CBC. Not for wt less than 30 kg, CrCl < 50 mL/min, hepatic dysfunction, or if dosage adjustment required.
MOA — See components.
ADVERSE EFFECTS — Serious: Lactic acidosis/hepatic steatosis; exacerbation of hepatitis B after discontinuation of lamivudine. See components for other adverse effects.

EPZICOM (abacavir + lamivudine) ▶LK ♀C ▶– $$$$$
WARNING — Abacavir: Potentially fatal hypersensitivity reactions. HLA-B*5701 predisposes to hypersensitivity; screen before starting abacavir and avoid if positive test. Never rechallenge with abacavir after suspected reaction. Abacavir and lamivudine: Lactic acidosis and hepatosteatosis. Lamivudine: Exacerbation of hepatitis B after discontinuation in patients coinfected with HIV and hepatitis B.
ADULTS — Combination therapy for HIV infection: 1 tab PO daily.
PEDS — Safety and efficacy not established in children.
FORMS — Trade only: Tabs abacavir 600 mg + lamivudine 300 mg.
NOTES — See components. Not for patients with CrCl < 50 mL/min, hepatic dysfunction, or if dosage adjustment required.
MOA — See components.
ADVERSE EFFECTS — Serious: Potentially fatal hypersensitivity (abacavir); lactic acidosis/hepatic steatosis (abacavir or lamivudine); exacerbation of hepatitis B after discontinuation in patients coinfected with HIV and hepatitis B (lamivudine). See components for other adverse effects.

TRIZIVIR (abacavir + lamivudine + zidovudine) ▶LK ♀C ▶– $$$$$
WARNING — Abacavir: Life-threatening hypersensitivity. HLA-B*5701 predisposes to hypersensitivity; screen before starting abacavir and avoid if positive test. Never rechallenge with abacavir after suspected reaction. Abacavir and lamivudine: Lactic acidosis and hepatosteatosis. Zidovudine: Bone marrow suppression, myopathy.
ADULTS — HIV infection, alone (not a preferred regimen) or in combo with other agents: 1 tab PO bid.
PEDS — HIV infection in adolescents 40 kg or greater, alone (not a preferred regimen) or in combo with other agents: 1 tab PO bid.
FORMS — Trade only: Tabs abacavir 300 mg + lamivudine 150 mg + zidovudine 300 mg.
NOTES — See components. Monitor CBC. Not for wt less than 40 kg, CrCl < 50 mL/min or if dosage adjustment required.
MOA — See components.
ADVERSE EFFECTS — Serious: Lactic acidosis/hepatic steatosis, see components for other adverse effects. Frequent: Hypersensitivity, N/V, fever/chills.

TRUVADA (emtricitabine + tenofovir) ▶K ♀B ▶– $$$$$
WARNING — Emtricitabine and tenofovir: Potentially fatal lactic acidosis and hepatosteatosis; severe acute exacerbation of hepatitis B after discontinuation in patients coinfected with HIV and hepatitis B.
ADULTS — Combination therapy for HIV infection: 1 tab PO daily.
PEDS — Safety and efficacy not established in children.
UNAPPROVED ADULTS — Antiviral-resistant chronic hepatitis B in HIV-coinfected patients: 1 tab PO daily.
FORMS — Trade only: Tabs emtricitabine 200 mg + tenofovir 300 mg.
NOTES — See components. Do not use in a triple nucleoside regimen. Not for patients with CrCl < 30 mL/min or hemodialysis; hepatic dysfunction; or if dosage adjustment required. Increase dosing interval to q 48 h if CrCl 30 to 49 mL/min. Use with didanosine cautiously; reduce didanosine dose to 250 mg for adults over 60 kg, monitor for adverse effects and discontinue didanosine if they occur. Dosage adjustment of didanosine unclear if wt less than 60 kg. Give Videx EC + Truvada on empty stomach or with light meal. Give buffered didanosine + Truvada on empty stomach. Atazanavir and lopinavir/ritonavir increase tenofovir levels; monitor and discontinue Truvada if tenofovir adverse effects. Tenofovir decreases atazanavir levels. If atazanavir is used with Truvada, use 300 mg atazanavir + 100 mg ritonavir. Do not use Truvada with lamivudine.
MOA — See components.
ADVERSE EFFECTS — Serious: Lactic acidosis/hepatic steatosis (emtricitabine and tenofovir); severe acute exacerbation of hepatitis B after discontinuing either drug in patients coinfected with HIV and hepatitis B. See components for other adverse effects.

ANTIMICROBIALS: Antiviral Agents—Anti-HIV—Fusion Inhibitors

NOTE: AIDS treatment guidelines available online at www.aidsinfo.nih.gov. Consider monitoring LFTs in patients receiving HAART.

ENFUVIRTIDE (*Fuzeon, T-20*) ▶Serum ♀B ▶– $$$$$
ADULTS — Combination therapy for HIV infection: 90 mg SC bid. Give each injection at new site in upper arm, anterior thigh, or abdomen, avoiding areas with current injection site reaction.
PEDS — Combination therapy for HIV infection, 6 to 16 yo: 2 mg/kg (up to 90 mg) SC bid. Give each injection at new site in upper arm, anterior thigh, or abdomen, avoiding areas with current injection site reaction.

(cont.)

ENFUVIRTIDE (cont.)
FORMS — 30-day kit with vials, diluent, syringes, alcohol wipes. Single-dose vials contain 108 mg to provide 90 mg enfuvirtide.
NOTES — Increased risk of bacterial pneumonia; monitor for signs and symptoms of pneumonia. Biojector 2000 can cause persistent nerve pain if used near large nerves, bruising, hematomas. Anticoagulants, hemophilia, or other coagulation disorder may increase risk of postinjection bleeding. Reconstitute with 1.1 mL sterile water for injection. This provides 1.2 mL of soln, of which only 1 mL (90 mg) is injected. Allow vial to stand until powder dissolves completely (up to 45 min). Do not shake. Second daily dose can be reconstituted ahead of time if stored in refrigerator in original vial and used within 24 h. Return to room temp before injecting. Discard unused soln. Patient education on administration available at 877–438–9366 or www.fuzeon.com.
MOA — Peptide that binds with glycoprotein on HIV viral envelope; prevents fusion of virus with CD4+ cells.
ADVERSE EFFECTS — Serious: Increased risk of bacterial pneumonia, hypersensitivity (may include flu-like symptoms, hypotension, increased LFTs), peripheral neuropathy, pancreatitis. Frequent: Injection site reactions (including induration, cysts, nodules), eosinophilia. Biojector 2000 can cause persistent nerve pain if used near large nerves, bruising, hematomas. Anticoagulants, hemophilia, or other coagulation disorder may increase risk of post-injection bleeding.

ANTIMICROBIALS: Antiviral Agents—Anti-HIV—Integrase Strand Transfer Inhibitor

NOTE: AIDS treatment guidelines available online at www.aidsinfo.nih.gov. Considermonitoring LFTs in patients receiving HAART.

RALTEGRAVIR (Isentress, RAL) ▶Glucuronidation ♀C ▶– $$$$$
ADULTS — Combination therapy for HIV infection: 400 mg PO bid. Increase to 800 mg PO bid if given with rifampin.
PEDS — Safety and efficacy not established in children.
FORMS — Trade only: Tabs 400 mg.
NOTES — Myopathy and rhabdomyolysis reported; caution advised for coadministration with drugs that cause myopathy.
MOA — Inhibits HIV-1 integrase, an enzyme required for insertion of virus into host genome. Inhibition of integrase prevents viral propagation.
ADVERSE EFFECTS — Serious: Myopathy and rhabdomyolysis (causality unclear), hypersensitivity. Frequent: Insomnia, headache, increased CPK.

ANTIMICROBIALS: Antiviral Agents—Anti-HIV—Non-Nucleoside Reverse Transcriptase Inhibitors

NOTE: Many serious drug interactions: Always check before prescribing. See www.aidsinfo.nih.gov for AIDS treatment guidelines and the use of rifamycins with NNRTIs. Consider monitoring LFTs in patients receiving HAART.

EFAVIRENZ (Sustiva, EFV) ▶L ♀D ▶– $$$$$
ADULTS — Combination therapy for HIV infection: 600 mg PO once daily at bedtime. Coadministration with voriconazole: Use voriconazole maintenance dose of 400 mg PO bid and reduce efavirenz to 300 mg (use caps) PO once daily. Avoid with high-fat meal. Take on empty stomach, preferably at bedtime.
PEDS — Consider antihistamine rash prophylaxis before starting. Combination therapy for HIV infection, age 3 yo or older: Give PO once daily at bedtime 200 mg for 10 kg to less than 15 kg; 250 mg for 15 kg to less than 20 kg; 300 mg for 20 kg to less than 25 kg; 350 mg for 25 kg to less than 32.5 kg; 400 mg for 32.5 kg to less than 40 kg; 600 mg for wt 40 kg or greater. Do not give with high-fat meal.
FORMS — Trade only: Caps 50, 100, 200 mg. Tabs 600 mg.
NOTES — Psychiatric/CNS reactions (warn about hazardous tasks), rash (stop treatment if severe), increased cholesterol (monitor). False-positive with Microgenics cannabinoid screening test. Monitor LFTs if given with ritonavir, hepatotoxic drugs, or to patients with hepatitis B/C. Induces CYP3A4. Many drug interactions including decreased levels of anticonvulsants, atorvastatin, diltiazem, itraconazole, methadone, posaconazole, pravastatin, simvastatin, and probably cyclosporine, ketoconazole, sirolimus, and tacrolimus. Do not give with pimozide, triazolam, ergot alkaloids, or St John's wort. Do not give with atazanavir to treatment-experienced patients. Midazolam contraindicated in labeling; but can use single dose IV cautiously with monitoring for procedural sedation. If used with rifampin, consider increasing efavirenz to 800 mg once daily at bedtime if wt 60 kg or greater. High risk of rash when taken with clarithromycin; consider alternative antimicrobial. Potentially teratogenic; get negative pregnancy test before use by women of child-bearing potential and recommend barrier contraceptive until 12 weeks after efavirenz is stopped.
MOA — Inhibits HIV reverse transcriptase by different mechanism of action from NRTIs. Cross-resistance possible between efavirenz and nevirapine.
ADVERSE EFFECTS — Serious: Depression and other psychiatric reactions, convulsions, severe rash, Stevens-Johnson syndrome, lipoatrophy,

(cont.)

EFAVIRENZ (cont.)
hepatotoxicity (rare). Frequent: Rash (especially in children), CNS symptoms (dizziness, insomnia, vivid dreams, impaired concentration; warn about hazardous tasks).

ETRAVIRINE (*Intelence, ETR*) ▶L ♀B ▶– $$$$$
ADULTS — Combination therapy for treatment-resistant HIV infection: 200 mg PO bid after meals.
PEDS — Safety and efficacy not established in children.
FORMS — Trade only: Tabs 100 mg.
NOTES — Severe skin reactions, Stevens-Johnson syndrome, hypersensitivity. Induces CYP3A4 and inhibits CYP2C9 and 2C19; substrate of CYP2C9, 2C19, and 3A4. Do not give with efavirenz, nevirapine, ritonavir 600 mg bid; ritonavir-boosted tipranavir/fosamprenavir/atazanavir; St John's wort, rifampin, rifapentine, carbamazepine, phenobarbital, phenytoin. Give rifabutin 300 mg once daily with etravirine (without ritonavir-boosted protease inhibitor). Avoid rifabutin in patients receiving etravirine with a protease inhibitor. Monitor INR with warfarin. Consider monitoring antiarrhythmic blood levels. Can disperse tabs in water and take immediately if swallowing difficulty.
MOA — Inhibits HIV reverse transcriptase by different mechanism of action from NRTIs.
ADVERSE EFFECTS — Serious: Severe rash (rare) including Stevens-Johnson syndrome, toxic epidermal necrolysis, and hypersensitivity with hepatic failure. Frequent: Mild/moderate rash between weeks 2-4 of therapy; nausea.

NEVIRAPINE (*Viramune, NVP*) ▶LK ♀C ▶– $$$$$
WARNING — Life-threatening skin reactions, hypersensitivity, and hepatotoxicity. Monitor clinical and lab status intensively during first 18 weeks of therapy (risk of rash and/or hepatotoxicity greatest during first 6 weeks of therapy) and frequently thereafter. Consider LFTs at baseline, before and 2 weeks after dose increase, and at least once a month. Rapidly progressive liver failure can occur after only a few weeks of therapy. Stop nevirapine and never rechallenge if clinical hepatitis, severe rash, or rash with constitutional symptoms/increased LFTs. Obtain LFTs if rash occurs. Risk of hepatotoxicity with rash high in women or high CD4 count (women with CD4 count greater than 250 especially high risk, including pregnant women). Do not use if CD4 count greater than 250 in women or greater than 400 in men unless benefit clearly outweighs risk. Elevated LFTs or hepatitis B/C infection at baseline increases risk of hepatotoxicity. Hepatotoxicity not reported after single doses of nevirapine or in children.
ADULTS — Combination therapy for HIV infection: 200 mg PO daily for 14 days, then 200 mg PO bid. Dose titration reduces risk of rash. If rash develops, do not increase dose until it resolves. If stopped for more than 7 days, restart with initial dose.
PEDS — Combination therapy for HIV infection, age 15 days old or older: 150 mg/m2 PO once daily for 14 days, then 150 mg/m2 bid (max dose 200 mg bid). Dose titration reduces risk of rash. If rash develops, do not increase dose until it resolves. If stopped for more than 7 days, restart with initial dose. Per HIV guidelines, children 8 yo or less may require up to 200 mg/m2 PO bid (max dose 200 mg bid).
UNAPPROVED ADULTS — Combination therapy for HIV infection: 200 mg PO daily for 14 days, then 400 mg PO daily. Prevention of maternal-fetal HIV transmission, maternal dosing: 200 mg PO single dose at onset of labor.
UNAPPROVED PEDS — Prevention of maternal-fetal HIV transmission, neonatal dose: 2 mg/kg PO single dose within 3 days of birth.
FORMS — Trade only: Tabs 200 mg, susp 50 mg/5 mL (240 mL).
NOTES — CYP3A4 inducer. May require increased methadone dose. Do not give with atazanavir, ketoconazole, hormonal contraceptives, St. John's wort. Granulocytopenia more common in children receiving zidovudine and nevirapine. Contraindicated if Child-Pugh Class B/C liver failure.
MOA — Inhibits HIV reverse transcriptase by different mechanism of action from NRTIs. Cross-resistance possible between efavirenz and nevirapine.
ADVERSE EFFECTS — Serious: Life-threatening rash (including Stevens-Johnson syndrome, toxic epidermal necrolysis, exfoliative dermatitis) hypersensitivity, hepatotoxicity. Risk of severe rash and/or hepatotoxicity (they can occur together) is greatest in first 6 weeks of therapy and is especially high in women with CD4 count greater than 250. Rhabdomyolysis can occur with skin reaction or hepatotoxicity. Granulocytopenia more common in children receiving zidovudine and nevirapine. Frequent: Increased LFTs, erythema, pruritus, maculopapular rash, dry desquamation.

ANTIMICROBIALS: Antiviral Agents—Anti-HIV—Nucleoside/Nucleotide Reverse Transcriptase Inhibitors

NOTE: See www.aidsinfo.nih.gov for AIDS treatment guidelines and use of rifamycins with NRTIs. Consider monitoring LFTs with HAART. Can cause lactic acidosis and hepatic steatosis.

ABACAVIR (*Ziagen, ABC*) ▶L ♀C ▶– $$$$$
WARNING — Potentially fatal hypersensitivity (look for fever, rash, GI symptoms, cough, dyspnea, pharyngitis, or other respiratory symptoms). Stop at once and never rechallenge after suspected reaction. Fatal reactions can recur within hours of rechallenge in patients with previously unrecognized reaction. HLA-B*5701 predisposes to hypersensitivity; screen

(cont.)

ABACAVIR (cont.)

before starting abacavir and avoid if positive test. Label HLA-B*5701-positive patients as abacavir-allergic in medical record.

ADULTS – <u>Combination therapy for HIV infection:</u> 300 mg PO bid or 600 mg PO daily. Severe hypersensitivity may be more common with single daily dose.

PEDS – <u>Combination therapy for HIV.</u> Oral soln, age 3 mo or greater: 8 mg/kg PO bid (up to 300 mg) PO bid. Tabs: 150 mg PO bid for wt 14 to 21 kg, 150 mg PO q am and 300 mg PO q pm for wt 22 kg to 29 kg, 300 mg PO bid for wt 30 kg or greater.

FORMS – Trade only: Tabs 300 mg scored. Oral soln 20 mg/mL (240 mL).

NOTES – Reduce dose for mild hepatic dysfunction (Child-Pugh score 5 to 6): 200 mg (10 mL of oral soln) PO bid. Possible increased risk of MI with abacavir.

MOA – Reduces HIV replication within infected cells by inhibiting HIV reverse transcriptase.

ADVERSE EFFECTS – Serious: Life-threatening hypersensitivity, lactic acidosis/hepatic steatosis, bone marrow suppression. As of Feb 2008, FDA is investigating possible increased risk of myocardial infarction with abacavir. Frequent: GI complaints.

DIDANOSINE (*Videx, Videx EC, DDI*) ▶LK ♀B ▶– $$$$$

WARNING – Potentially fatal pancreatitis; avoid use with other drugs that can cause pancreatitis. Avoid didanosine + stavudine in pregnancy due to reports of fatal lactic acidosis with pancreatitis or hepatic steatosis.

ADULTS – <u>Combination therapy for HIV infection:</u> Buffered powder: 167 mg PO bid for wt less than 60 kg, 250 mg PO bid for 60 kg or greater. Videx EC: 250 mg PO daily for wt less than 60 kg. 400 mg PO daily for wt 60 kg or greater. All formulations usually taken on empty stomach. Reduce dose if used with tenofovir to 200 mg for wt less than 60 kg and 250 mg for 60 kg or greater. Dosage reduction unclear with tenofovir if CrCl < 60 mL/min. Give tenofovir + Videx EC on empty stomach or with light meal; give tenofovir + buffered didanosine on empty stomach.

PEDS – <u>Combination therapy for HIV infection:</u> 100 mg/m2 PO bid for age 2 weeks to 8 mo. 120 mg/m2 PO bid for age older than 8 mo. Videx EC: 200 mg PO once daily for wt 20 to 24 kg, 250 mg for wt 25 to 59 kg, 400 mg for wt 60 kg or greater.

FORMS – Generic/Trade: Pediatric powder for oral soln 10 mg/mL (buffered with antacid). Delayed-release caps (Videx EC): 125, 200, 250, 400 mg.

NOTES – As of Feb 2008, FDA is investigating possible increased risk of MI with didanosine. Peripheral neuropathy (use cautiously with other neurotoxic drugs), retinal changes, optic neuritis, retinal depigmentation in children, hyperuricemia. Risk of lactic acidosis, pancreatitis, and peripheral neuropathy increased by concomitant stavudine. Diarrhea with buffered powder. See package insert for reduced dose if CrCl < 60 mL/min. Do not use with allopurinol. Give some medications at least 1 h (indinavir), 2 h (atazanavir, ciprofloxacin, levofloxacin, norfloxacin, ofloxacin, itraconazole, ketoconazole, ritonavir, dapsone, tetracyclines), or 4 h (moxifloxacin, gatifloxacin) before buffered didanosine. Contraindicated with ribavirin due to risk of didanosine toxicity. Methadone may reduce efficacy of didanosine, especially with buffered pediatric powder; use Videx EC instead of powder with methadone and monitor for reduced didanosine efficacy.

MOA – Reduces HIV replication within infected cells by inhibiting HIV reverse transcriptase.

ADVERSE EFFECTS – Serious: Lactic acidosis/hepatic steatosis, symptomatic hyperlactatemia, fatal lactic acidosis with stavudine plus didanosine in pregnant women (avoid concomitant use), retinal toxicity, pancreatitis (frequent; risk increased by stavudine), peripheral neuropathy (frequent; risk increased by stavudine), non-cirrhotic portal hypertension (rare). As of Feb 2008, FDA is investigating possible increased risk of myocardial infarction with didanosine. Frequent: Fever, GI complaints, headache, rash.

EMTRICITABINE (*Emtriva, FTC*) ▶K ♀B ▶– $$$$$

WARNING – Severe acute exacerbation of hepatitis B can occur after discontinuation in patients coinfected with HIV and hepatitis B. Monitor closely for at least 2 months; consider treating hepatitis B.

ADULTS – <u>Combination therapy for HIV infection:</u> 200 mg cap PO daily. Oral soln: 240 mg (24 mL) PO daily.

PEDS – <u>Combination therapy for HIV:</u> Give 3 mg/kg oral soln PO once daily for age birth to 3 mo; 6 mg/kg PO once daily (up to 240 mg) for age greater than 3 mo. Give 200 mg cap PO once daily for wt greater than 33 kg.

FORMS – Trade only: Caps 200 mg. Oral soln 10 mg/mL (170 mL).

NOTES – Lactic acidosis/hepatic steatosis. Exacerbation of hepatitis B after discontinuation. Reduce dose in adults with renal dysfunction. Caps: Give 200 mg PO q 96 h if CrCl less than 15 mL/min or hemodialysis; 200 mg PO q 72 h if CrCl 15 to 29 mL/min; 200 mg PO q 48 h if CrCl 30 to 49 mL/min. Oral soln: 60 mg q 24 h if CrCl less than 15 mL/min or hemodialysis; 80 mg q 24 h if CrCl 15 to 29 mL/min; 120 mg q 24 h if CrCl 30 to 49 mL/min; Refrigerate oral soln if possible; stable for 3 months at room temp.

MOA – Reduces HIV replication within infected cells by inhibiting HIV reverse transcriptase. Structurally related to lamivudine; cross-resistance documented. Has activity against hepatitis B.

ADVERSE EFFECTS – Serious: Lactic acidosis/hepatic steatosis. Frequent: Headache, diarrhea, nausea, rash. Other: Hyperpigmentation on palms/soles primarily in non-Caucasians.

LAMIVUDINE (*Epivir, Epivir-HBV, 3TC, ✦Heptovir*) ▶K ♀C ▶– $$$$$

WARNING – Lower dose of lamivudine in Epivir-HBV can cause HIV resistance; test for HIV before prescribing Epivir-HBV. Severe acute exacerbation of hepatitis

(cont.)

ANTIMICROBIALS: Antiviral Agents

LAMIVUDINE (cont.)
B can occur after discontinuation of lamivudine in patients coinfected with HIV and hepatitis B. Monitor closely for at least 2 months after discontinuing lamivudine in such patients; consider treating hepatitis B.
ADULTS — Epivir for combination therapy for HIV infection: 300 mg PO daily or 150 mg PO bid. Epivir-HBV for chronic hepatitis B: 100 mg PO daily. Coinfection with HIV and hepatitis B requires higher dose of lamivudine for HIV infection.
PEDS — Epivir for HIV infection: 3 mo to 16 yo, 4 mg/kg (up to 150 mg) PO bid. Epivir tabs: 75 mg bid for 14 to 21 kg, 75 mg q am and 150 mg q pm for 22 to 29 kg; 150 mg bid for 30 kg or greater; 300 mg PO once daily or 150 mg PO bid for age 16 yo or older. Epivir-HBV for chronic hepatitis B: 3 mg/kg (up to 100 mg) PO daily for age 2 yo or older. Coinfection with HIV and hepatitis B requires higher dose of lamivudine for HIV infection.
UNAPPROVED PEDS — Epivir for combination therapy for HIV infection. Infants, age younger than 30 days old: 2 mg/kg PO bid.
FORMS — Trade only: Epivir, 3TC: Tabs 150 (scored), 300 mg, oral soln 10 mg/mL. Epivir-HBV, Heptovir: Tabs 100 mg, oral soln 5 mg/mL.
NOTES — Lamivudine-resistant hepatitis B reported. Epivir: Pancreatitis in children. Monitor for hepatic decompensation (potentially fatal), neutropenia, and anemia if also receiving interferon for hepatitis C. If hepatic decompensation occurs, consider discontinuing lamivudine, and reducing or discontinuing interferon, and/or ribavirin. Dosage reduction for CrCl less than 50 mL/min in package insert.
MOA — Nucleoside analog. Reduces HIV replication within infected cells by inhibiting HIV reverse transcriptase. Reduces hepatitis B replication by inhibiting HBV polymerase.
ADVERSE EFFECTS — Serious: Lactic acidosis/hepatic steatosis; exacerbation of hepatitis B after discontinuation of lamivudine; pancreatitis in children; hepatic decompensation in HCV/HIV coinfected patients. Frequent: Headache, fatigue, nausea, dizziness, nasal symptoms (well-tolerated compared with other NRTIs).

TENOFOVIR (*Viread, TDF*) ▶K ♀B ▶— $$$$$
WARNING — Stop tenofovir if hepatomegaly or steatosis occur, even if LFTs normal. Severe acute exacerbation of hepatitis B can occur after discontinuation of tenofovir in patients coinfected with HIV and hepatitis B. Monitor closely for at least 2 months after discontinuing tenofovir in such patients; consider treating hepatitis B.
ADULTS — Combination therapy for HIV; chronic hepatitis B: 300 mg PO daily without regard to food. High rate of virologic failure with tenofovir + didanosine + lamivudine for HIV infection; avoid this regimen.
PEDS — Combination therapy of HIV in adolescents (age 12 years old or older and wt 35 kg or greater): 300 mg PO daily without regard to food.
FORMS — Trade only: Tabs 300 mg.
NOTES — Decreased bone mineral density; consider bone mineral density monitoring if history of pathologic fracture or high risk of osteopenia. Consider calcium and vitamin D supplement. Tenofovir increases didanosine levels and possibly serious didanosine adverse effects (eg, pancreatitis, lactic acidosis, hyperlactatemia, neuropathy). Reduce dose of Videx EC to 250 mg if wt is 60 kg or greater, reduce to 200 mg if wt is less than 60 kg. Dosage adjustment of Videx EC unclear if CrCl < 60 mL/min. Give tenofovir + Videx EC on empty stomach or with light meal; give tenofovir + buffered didanosine on empty stomach. If atazanavir is used with tenofovir, use 300 mg atazanavir + 100 mg ritonavir PO once daily. Atazanavir and lopinavir/ritonavir increase tenofovir levels; monitor and discontinue tenofovir if adverse effects. Tenofovir can cause renal impairment including acute renal failure and Fanconi syndrome. Monitor CrCl before starting tenofovir. Avoid tenofovir if current/recent nephrotoxic drug use. Drugs that reduce renal function or undergo renal elimination (eg, acyclovir, adefovir, ganciclovir) may increase tenofovir levels; do not use with adefovir. Monitor CrCl and phosphate if risk/history of renal insufficiency or nephrotoxic drug. Reduce dose for dialysis patients: 300 mg once weekly (given after dialysis); 300 mg twice weekly if CrCl 10 to 29 mL/min; 300 mg q 48 h if CrCl 30 to 49 mL/min.
MOA — Nucleotide reverse transcriptase inhibitor. Similar mechanism of action as NRTIs, but does not require phosphorylation step required to activate NRTIs. Reduces HIV replication within infected cells by inhibiting HIV reverse transcriptase. Has activity against hepatitis B.
ADVERSE EFFECTS — Serious: Lactic acidosis/hepatic steatosis, renal impairment including acute renal failure and Fanconi syndrome, hypophosphatemia. Exacerbation of hepatitis B after discontinuation of tenofovir. Decreased bone mineral density in adults & children; fracture risk unknown. Reports of syncope, usually with vagal syndrome. Frequent: GI complaints, dizziness.

ZIDOVUDINE (*Retrovir, AZT, ZDV*) ▶LK ♀C ▶— $$$$$
WARNING — Bone marrow suppression, myopathy.
ADULTS — Combination therapy for HIV infection: 600 mg/day PO divided bid or tid. IV dosing: 1 mg/kg IV administered over 1 h 5 to 6 times a day. Prevention of maternal-fetal HIV transmission, maternal dosing (after 14 weeks of pregnancy): 600 mg/day PO divided bid or tid until start of labor. During labor, 2 mg/kg (total body wt) IV over 1 h, then 1 mg/kg/h until delivery.
PEDS — Combination therapy for HIV infection, age 4 weeks or older: Give 24 mg/kg/day divided bid or tid for wt 4 to 8 kg; give 18 mg/kg/day divided bid or tid for wt 9 kg to 29 kg; give 600 mg/day divided bid or tid for wt 30 kg or greater. Alternative dose: 480 mg/m2/day PO divided bid or tid. Prevention of maternal-fetal HIV transmission, infant dosing: 2 mg/kg PO q 6 h from within 12 h of birth until 6

(cont.)

ANTIMICROBIALS: Antiviral Agents

ZIDOVUDINE *(cont.)*
weeks old. Can also give infants 1.5 mg/kg IV over 30 min q 6 h.
FORMS — Generic/Trade: Caps 100 mg. Tabs 300 mg. Syrup 50 mg/5 mL (240 mL).
NOTES — Hematologic toxicity; monitor CBC. Increased bone marrow suppression with ganciclovir or valganciclovir. Granulocytopenia more common in children receiving zidovudine and nevirapine. Monitor for hepatic decompensation, neutropenia, and anemia if also receiving interferon regimen for hepatitis C. If hepatic decompensation occurs, consider discontinuing zidovudine, interferon, and/or ribavirin. See package insert for dosage adjustments for renal dysfunction or hematologic toxicity.
MOA — Decreases or inhibits HIV replication within infected cells by inhibiting HIV reverse transcriptase.
ADVERSE EFFECTS — Serious: Lactic acidosis/hepatic steatosis, lipoatrophy (possibly), hematologic toxicity, symptomatic myopathy, hepatic decompensation in HCV/HIV coinfected patients. Granulocytopenia more common in children receiving zidovudine and nevirapine. Frequent: GI intolerance, headache, insomnia, asthenia, anorexia.

ANTIMICROBIALS: Antiviral Agents—Anti-HIV—Protease Inhibitors

NOTE: See www.aidsinfo.nih.gov for AIDS treatment guidelines and use of rifamycins with protease inhibitors. Many serious drug interactions: Always check before prescribing. Protease inhibitors inhibit CYP3A4. Contraindicated with most antiarrhythmics, alfuzosin, ergot alkaloids, lovastatin, pimozide, rifampin, salmeterol, high-dose sildenafil for pulmonary hypertension, simvastatin, St. John's wort, triazolam. Midazolam contraindicated in labeling; but can use single dose IV cautiously with monitoring for procedural sedation. Monitor INR with warfarin. Avoid inhaled/nasal fluticasone with ritonavir if possible; increased fluticasone levels can cause Cushing's syndrome/adrenal suppression. Other protease inhibitors may increase fluticasone levels; find alternatives for long-term use. May need to reduce trazodone dose. Reduce colchicine dose; do not coadminister colchicine and protease inhibitors in patients with renal or hepatic dysfunction. Adjust dose of bosentan or tadalafil for pulmonary hypertension. Erectile dysfunction: Single dose of sildenafil 25 mg every 48 h, tadalafil 5 mg (not more than 10 mg) every 72 h, or vardenafil initially 2.5 mg every 72 h. Adverse effects include spontaneous bleeding in hemophiliacs, hyperglycemia, hyperlipidemia, immune reconstitution syndrome, and fat redistribution. Coinfection with hepatitis C or other liver disease increases the risk of hepatotoxicity with protease inhibitors; monitor LFTs at least twice in first month of therapy, then every 3 months.

ATAZANAVIR *(Reyataz, ATV)* ▶L ♀B ▶— $$$$$
ADULTS — Combination therapy for HIV infection. Therapy-naive patients: Atazanavir 300 mg + ritonavir 100 mg PO once daily OR atazanavir 400 mg PO once daily. With tenofovir, therapy-naive: 300 mg + ritonavir 100 mg PO once daily. With efavirenz, therapy-naive: 400 mg + ritonavir 100 mg once daily. Therapy-experienced: 300 mg + ritonavir 100 mg once daily. Do not give atazanavir with efavirenz in therapy-experienced patients. Give atazanavir with food; give 2 h before or 1 h after buffered didanosine.
PEDS — Combination therapy for HIV infection. Therapy-naive age 6 yo or older: Give atazanavir/ritonavir PO once daily 150/80 mg for wt 15 to 24 kg; 200/100 mg for 25 to 31 kg; 250/100 mg for 32 to 38 kg; 300/100 mg for 39 kg or greater. Therapy-naive, ritonavir-intolerant, age 13 yo or older and wt 39 kg or greater: 400 mg PO once daily with food. Therapy-experienced, age 6 yo or older: Give atazanavir/ritonavir PO once daily 200/100 mg for wt 25 to 31 kg; 250/100 for 32 to 38 kg; 300/100 mg for 39 kg or greater. Give atazanavir with food. Max dose for atazanavir/ritonavir of 300/100 mg. Do not use in infants; may cause kernicterus.
FORMS — Trade only: Caps 100, 150, 200, 300 mg.
NOTES — Does not appear to increase cholesterol or triglycerides. Asymptomatic increases in indirect bilirubin due to inhibition of UDP-glucuronosyl transferase (UGT); may cause jaundice/scleral icterus. Do not use with indinavir; both may increase bilirubin. Do not use with nevirapine. Reduce rifabutin to 150 mg every other day. May inhibit irinotecan metabolism. Can prolong PR interval and rare cases of 2nd degree AV block reported; caution advised for patients with AV block or on drugs that prolong PR interval, especially if metabolized by CYP3A4. Monitor ECG with calcium channel blockers; consider reducing diltiazem dose by 50%. Reduce clarithromycin dose by 50%; consider alternative therapy for indications other than Mycobacterium avium complex. Acid required for absorption; acid-suppressing drugs can cause treatment failure. Proton pump inhibitors: In treatment-naive patients do not exceed dose equivalent of omeprazole 20 mg; give PPI 12 h before atazanavir 300 mg + ritonavir 100 mg. Do not use PPIs with unboosted atazanavir or in treatment-experienced patients. H2 blockers: Give atazanavir 300 mg + ritonavir 100 mg simultaneously with H2 blocker and/or at least 10 h after H2 blocker, with max dose equivalent of famotidine 40 mg bid for treatment-naive patients and 20 mg bid for treatment experienced patients. For treatment-experienced patients receiving tenofovir and H2 blocker, give atazanavir 400 mg + ritonavir 100 mg once daily with food. If treatment-naive and ritonavir-intolerant, give atazanavir 400 mg PO once daily with food given at least 2 h before and at least 10 h after H2 blocker (max dose equivalent to famotidine 20 mg bid). Give atazanavir 2 h before or 1 h after antacids or buffered

(cont.)

ATAZANAVIR (cont.)
didanosine. Give atazanavir and EC didanosine at different times. Inhibits CYP1A2, 2C9, and 3A4. Do not use unboosted atazanavir with buprenorphine; monitor for sedation if buprenorphine given with atazanavir/ritonavir. Use lowest possible dose of atorvastatin/rosuvastatin or consider pravastatin/fluvastatin. Monitor levels of antiarrhythmics, immunosuppressants, TCAs. Use oral contraceptive with at least 35 mcg ethinyl estradiol with ritonavir-boosted atazanavir. Use oral contraceptive with 25 to 30 mcg ethinyl estradiol if atazanavir is not boosted by ritonavir. In mild to moderate hepatic impairment (Child-Pugh class B), consider dosage reduction to 300 mg PO daily with food. Do not use in Child-Pugh Class C. Dosage adjustment for hemodialysis: Atazanavir 300 mg + ritonavir 100 mg if treatment-naive; do not use atazanavir if treatment-experienced.
MOA — Prevents cleavage of protein precursors required for HIV maturation, reproduction, and infection of new cells.
ADVERSE EFFECTS — Serious: Can prolong PR interval; rare cases of second degree AV block reported. Frequent: Increased indirect bilirubin, jaundice/scleral icterus, nausea, rash. Serious: Can prolong PR interval; rare cases of second degree AV block reported. Nephrolithiasis. Class effects: Hyperglycemia, fat redistribution, spontaneous bleeding in hemophiliacs.

DARUNAVIR (*Prezista, DRV*) ▶L ♀B ▶− $$$$$
ADULTS — Combination therapy for HIV infection. Therapy-naive patients: 800 mg + ritonavir 100 mg PO once daily. Therapy-experienced patients: 600 mg + ritonavir 100 mg PO both bid. Take with food. Darunavir should always be boosted with ritonavir.
PEDS — Combination therapy for HIV infection. age 6 yo or older: 375 mg + ritonavir 50 mg PO both bid for wt 20 to 29 kg; 450 mg + ritonavir 60 mg PO both bid for wt 30 to 39 kg; 600 mg + ritonavir 100 mg PO both bid for wt 40 kg or greater. Take with food. Darunavir should always be boosted by ritonavir.
FORMS — Trade only: Tabs 75, 150, 300, 400, 600 mg.
NOTES — Cross-sensitivity with sulfonamides possible; use caution in sulfonamide-allergic patients. Hepatotoxicity; monitor AST/ALT more frequently (especially during first few months of therapy) if patient already has liver dysfunction. CYP3A4 inhibitor and substrate. Do not give with lopinavir/ritonavir or saquinavir. Monitor levels of antiarrhythmics. Reduce dose of clarithromycin if CrCl less than 60 mL/min (see clarithromycin entry for details). Do not use with more than 200 mg/day of ketoconazole or itraconazole. Ritonavir decreases voriconazole levels; do not use darunavir/ritonavir unless benefit exceeds risk. Reduce rifabutin to 150 mg PO every other day. May decrease oral contraceptive efficacy; consider additional or alternative method. Give didanosine 1 h before or 2 h after darunavir/ritonavir.

Increases pravastatin levels up to 5-fold; use lowest possible dose of pravastatin, rosuvastatin, or atorvastatin or consider using fluvastatin.
MOA — Prevents cleavage of protein precursors required for HIV maturation, reproduction, and infection of new cells.
ADVERSE EFFECTS — Severe: Stevens-Johnson syndrome. Hepatotoxicity (esp if hepatitis B/C or baseline elevated transaminases). Frequent: Rash, diarrhea, nausea, headache, nasopharyngitis. Class effects: Hyperglycemia, fat redistribution, lipid abnormalities, spontaneous bleeding in hemophiliacs.

FOSAMPRENAVIR (*Lexiva, FPV, ✦Telzir*) ▶L ♀C
▶− $$$$$
ADULTS — Combination therapy for HIV infection. Therapy-naive patients: Fosamprenavir 1400 mg PO bid (without ritonavir) OR fosamprenavir 1400 mg PO once daily + ritonavir 100 to 200 mg PO once daily OR fosamprenavir 700 mg PO bid + ritonavir 100 mg PO bid. Protease inhibitor- experienced patients: 700 mg fosamprenavir + 100 mg ritonavir PO both bid. Do not use once-daily regimen. If once-daily ritonavir-boosted regimen given with efavirenz, increase ritonavir to 300 mg/day; no increase of ritonavir dose needed for bid regimen with efavirenz. Can give nevirapine with fosamprenavir only if bid ritonavir-boosted regimen used. No meal restrictions for tabs; advise adults to take susp with food. Re-dose if vomiting occurs within 30 min of giving oral susp.
PEDS — Combination therapy for HIV infection. Do not use once daily dosing of fosamprenavir in children. Therapy-naive: 30 mg/kg susp (up to 1400 mg) PO bid for age 2 to 5 yo; 30 mg/kg susp (up to 1400 mg) PO bid OR 18 mg/kg susp (up to 700 mg) PO bid + ritonavir 3 mg/kg (up to 100 mg) PO bid for age 6 yo or older. Can use fosamprenavir 2 tabs bid if wt 47 kg or greater. Therapy experienced: 18 mg/kg susp (up to 700 mg) PO bid + ritonavir 3 mg/kg (up to 100 mg) PO bid for age 6 yo or older. For fosamprenavir + ritonavir, can use fosamprenavir tabs if wt 39 kg or greater and ritonavir caps if wt 33 kg or greater. Do not use in infants; may cause kernicterus. Advise children to take susp with food. Take tabs without regard to meals. Re-dose if vomiting occurs within 30 min of giving oral susp.
FORMS — Trade only: Tabs 700 mg. Susp 50 mg/mL.
NOTES — Life-threatening skin reactions possible (reported with amprenavir). Cross-sensitivity with sulfonamides possible; use caution in sulfonamide-allergic patients. Increased cholesterol and triglycerides; monitor lipids. Fosamprenavir is inhibitor and substrate of CYP3A4. Do not use fosamprenavir + ritonavir with flecainide or propafenone. Use lowest possible dose of atorvastatin or rosuvastatin with monitoring for myopathy or consider fluvastatin/pravastatin. Monitor CBC at least weekly if taking rifabutin. Monitor levels of antiarrhythmics, immunosuppressants, TCAs. May need to increase dose of methadone. Do not use more than 200 mg/day ketoconazole/itraconazole with fosamprenavir +

(cont.)

FOSAMPRENAVIR (cont.)

ritonavir; may need to reduce antifungal dose if patient is receiving more than 400 mg/day itraconazole or ketoconazole with unboosted fosamprenavir. Do not use more than 2.5 mg vardenafil q 24 h with unboosted fosamprenavir or q 72 h for fosamprenavir + ritonavir. Do not use hormonal contraceptives. More adverse reactions when fosamprenavir is given with Kaletra; appropriate dose for combination therapy unclear. Mild hepatic dysfunction (Child-Pugh score 5 to 6): 700 mg PO bid unboosted (for treatment-naive) or 700 mg PO bid plus ritonavir 100 mg PO once daily (for treatment-naive or -experienced). Moderate hepatic dysfunction (Child-Pugh score 7 to 9): 700 mg PO bid unboosted (for treatment- naive) or 450 mg PO bid plus ritonavir 100 mg PO once daily (for treatment-naive or -experienced). Refrigeration not required, but may improve taste of oral susp.
MOA — Prodrug of amprenavir. Prevents cleavage of protein precursors required for HIV maturation, reproduction, and infection of new cells.
ADVERSE EFFECTS — Severe: Life-threatening rash possible. Nephrolithiasis. Frequent: Diarrhea, N/V, headache, rash, pruritus, fatigue. GI intolerance more frequent with once-daily dosing. Class effects: Hyperglycemia, fat redistribution, lipid abnormalities, spontaneous bleeding in hemophiliacs.

INDINAVIR (*Crixivan, IDV*) ▶LK ♀C ▶– $$$$$
ADULTS — Combination therapy for HIV infection: 800 mg PO q 8 h between meals with water (at least 48 oz/day).
PEDS — Not approved in children. Do not use in infants; may cause kernicterus.
UNAPPROVED ADULTS — Combination therapy for HIV infection: Indinavir 800 mg PO bid with ritonavir 100 to 200 mg PO bid; or indinavir 400 mg bid with ritonavir 400 mg bid; or indinavir 600 mg PO bid with Kaletra 400/100 mg PO bid. Can be given without regard to meals when given with ritonavir.
UNAPPROVED PEDS — Combination therapy for HIV infection: 350 to 500 mg/m2/dose (max of 800 mg/dose) PO q 8 h for children; 800 mg PO q 8 h between meals with water (at least 48 oz/day) for adolescents.
FORMS — Trade only: Caps 100, 200, 400 mg.
NOTES — Nephrolithiasis (especially in children), hemolytic anemia, indirect hyperbilirubinemia, possible hepatitis, interstitial nephritis with asymptomatic pyuria. Do not use with atazanavir; both may increase bilirubin. Inhibits CYP3A4. Avoid using with carbamazepine if possible. Give indinavir and buffered didanosine 1 h apart on empty stomach. Reduce indinavir dose to 600 mg PO q 8 h when given with ketoconazole or itraconazole 200 mg bid. Increase indinavir dose to 1000 mg PO q 8 h when given with efavirenz or nevirapine. Do not use with rosuvastatin. Give rifabutin 150 mg once daily with indinavir 1000 mg q 8 h. With ritonavir-boosted indinavir, reduce rifabutin to 150 mg every other day without increasing indinavir dose. For mild to moderate hepatic cirrhosis, give 600 mg PO q 8 h. Indinavir not recommended in pregnancy because of dramatic reduction in blood levels.
MOA — Prevents cleavage of protein precursors required for HIV maturation, reproduction, and infection of new cells.
ADVERSE EFFECTS — Serious: Nephrolithiasis, hematuria, and sterile leukocyturia (most frequent in children), interstitial nephritis with asymptomatic pyuria, hemolytic anemia. Frequent: GI complaints, headache, asthenia, blurred vision, dizziness, rash, metallic taste, indirect hyperbilirubinemia. Class effects: Hyperglycemia, fat redistribution, lipid abnormalities, spontaneous bleeding in hemophiliacs.

LOPINAVIR-RITONAVIR (*Kaletra, LPV/r*) ▶L ♀C ▶– $$$$$
ADULTS — Combination therapy for HIV infection: 400/100 mg PO bid (tabs or oral soln). Can use 800/200 mg PO once daily in patients with less than 3 lopinavir resistance-associated substitutions. Coadministration with efavirenz, nevirapine, fosamprenavir, or nelfinavir: 500/125 mg tabs (use two 200/50 mg + one 100/25 mg tab) or 533/133 mg oral soln (6.5 mL) PO bid. No once-daily dosing for pregnant patients; coadministration with carbamazepine, phenobarbital, phenytoin, efavirenz, nevirapine, fosamprenavir, or nelfinavir; or in patients with 3 or more lopinavir resistance-associated substitutions (L10F/I/R/V, K20M/N/R, L24I, L33F, M36I, I47V, G48V, I54L/T/V, V82A/C/F/S/T, and I84V). Give tabs without regard to meals; give oral soln with food.
PEDS — Combination therapy for HIV infection, age 14 days to 6 mo: Lopinavir 300 mg/m2 or 16 mg/kg PO bid. Age 6 mo to 12 yo: Lopinavir 230 mg/m2 or 12 mg/kg PO bid if wt less than 15 kg; 10 mg/kg PO bid if wt 15 to 40 kg. When coadministered with efavirenz, nevirapine, fosamprenavir, or nelfinavir give lopinavir 300 mg/m2 PO bid or 13 mg/kg PO bid for wt less than15 kg; 11 mg/kg PO bid for wt 15 to 45 kg. Do not exceed adult dose. Give tabs without regard to meals; give oral soln with food. Beware of medication errors with oral soln; fatal overdose reported in infant given excessive volume of soln.
FORMS — Trade only: Tabs 200/50 mg, 100/25 mg. Oral soln 80/20 mg/mL (160 mL).
NOTES — Medication errors can occur if Keppra (levetiracetam) confused with Kaletra. May cause pancreatitis. Ritonavir (inhibits CYP3A4 and 2D6) included in formulation to inhibit metabolism and boost levels of lopinavir. Increases tenofovir levels; monitor for adverse reactions. Many other drug interactions including decreased efficacy of oral contraceptives. Ritonavir decreases voriconazole levels; do not give with voriconazole unless benefit exceeds risk. Reduce rifabutin to 150 mg every other day. Expected to increase fentanyl exposure. May require higher methadone dose. Reduce dose of clarithromycin if CrCl less than 60 mL/min (see clarithromycin

(cont.)

ANTIMICROBIALS: Antiviral Agents

LOPINAVIR-RITONAVIR *(cont.)*
entry for details). Give buffered didanosine 1 h before or 2 h after Kaletra oral soln. Kaletra tabs can be given at same time as didanosine without food. Do not give Kaletra with tipranavir 500 mg + ritonavir 200 mg both bid. Do not give Kaletra once daily with phenytoin, phenobarbital, or carbamazepine; monitor for reduced phenytoin levels. Oral soln contains alcohol. Use oral soln within 2 months if stored at room temperature. Tabs do not require refrigeration. Do not crush, cut, or chew tabs.
MOA — Prevents cleavage of protein precursors required for HIV maturation, reproduction, and infection of new cells.
ADVERSE EFFECTS — Serious: Hepatitis, pancreatitis. Increased risk of MI possible with cumulative use of Kaletra. PR and QT interval prolongation reported; caution advised for patients at risk of cardiac conduction abnormalities or coadministration of other drugs that prolong PR or QT interval. Frequent: GI complaints (more common with once daily regimen), transaminase elevation. Class effects: Hyperglycemia, fat redistribution, lipid abnormalities, spontaneous bleeding in hemophiliacs.

NELFINAVIR (*Viracept, NFV*) ▶L ♀B ▶– $$$$$
ADULTS — Combination therapy for HIV infection: 750 mg PO tid or 1250 mg PO bid with meals. Absorption improved when meal contains at least 500 calories with 11 to 28 g of fat.
PEDS — Combination therapy for HIV infection: 45 to 55 mg/kg PO bid or 25 to 35 mg/kg PO tid (up to 2500 mg/day) for age 2 yo or older. Take with meals. Absorption improved when meal contains at least 500 calories with 11 to 28 g of fat. Use powder or 250 mg tabs which can be crushed and mixed with water or other liquids. Do not mix with acidic foods/juice; will taste bitter.
FORMS — Trade only: Tabs 250, 625 mg. Oral powder 50 mg/g (114 g).
NOTES — Diarrhea common. Inhibits CYP3A4. Use lowest possible dose of atorvastatin/rosuvastatin or consider pravastatin/fluvastatin. Decreases efficacy of oral contraceptives. May require higher methadone dose. Do not use with proton pump inhibitors. Give rifabutin 150 mg once daily with nelfinavir 1250 mg bid. Give nelfinavir 2 h before or 1 h after buffered didanosine. Oral powder stable for 6 h after mixing if refrigerated. No dosage adjustment for mild hepatic impairment (Child-Pugh Class A); not recommended for more severe hepatic failure (Child-Pugh B/C).
MOA — Prevents cleavage of protein precursors required for HIV maturation, reproduction, and infection of new cells.
ADVERSE EFFECTS — Frequent: Diarrhea, transaminase elevation. Class effects: Hyperglycemia, fat redistribution, lipid abnormalities, spontaneous bleeding in hemophiliacs.

RITONAVIR (*Norvir, RTV*) ▶L ♀B ▶– $$$$$
WARNING — Contraindicated with many drugs due to risk of drug interactions.
ADULTS — Adult doses of 100 mg PO daily to 400 mg PO bid used to boost levels of other protease inhibitors. Full-dose regimen (600 mg PO bid) poorly tolerated. Best tolerated regimen with saquinavir may be ritonavir 400 mg + saquinavir 400 mg both bid. Saquinavir 1000 mg + ritonavir 100 mg both bid also used. Take tabs with meals.
PEDS — Combination therapy for HIV infection: Start with 250 mg/m2 and increase every 2 to 3 days by 50 mg/m2 twice daily to achieve usual dose of 350 to 400 mg/m2 (up to 600 mg/dose) PO bid for age older than 1 mo. If 400 mg/m2 twice daily not tolerated, consider other alternatives. Give with meals.
UNAPPROVED ADULTS — Combination therapy for HIV infection: Ritonavir 100 to 200 mg PO bid with indinavir 800 mg PO bid or ritonavir 400 mg + indinavir 400 mg both bid.
UNAPPROVED PEDS — Used at lower than labeled doses to boost levels of other protease inhibitors.
FORMS — Trade only: Caps 100 mg, tabs 100 mg. Oral soln 80 mg/mL (240 mL).
NOTES — Nausea and vomiting, pancreatitis, alterations in AST, ALT, GGT, CPK, uric acid. Inhibits CYP3A4.
MOA — Prevents cleavage of protein precursors required for HIV maturation, reproduction, and infection of new cells.
ADVERSE EFFECTS — Serious: Greater than 200% increase in triglycerides; hepatitis, pancreatitis. Can prolong PR interval; rare cases of second/third degree AV block reported. Frequent: GI complaints, paresthesias, asthenia, taste perversion, increased CPK & uric acid. Class effects: Hyperglycemia, fat redistribution, lipid abnormalities, spontaneous bleeding in hemophiliacs.

SAQUINAVIR (*Invirase, SQV*) ▶L ♀B ▶? $$$$$
ADULTS — Combination therapy for HIV infection. Regimen must contain ritonavir. Saquinavir 1000 mg + ritonavir 100 mg PO both bid taken within 2 h after meals. Saquinavir 1000 mg + lopinavir-ritonavir (Kaletra) 400/100 mg PO both bid. If serious toxicity occurs, do not reduce Invirase dose; efficacy unclear for lower doses.
PEDS — Combination therapy for HIV, for age 16 yo or older: Use adult dose.
FORMS — Trade only: Invirase (hard gel) Caps 200 mg. Tabs 500 mg.
NOTES — In Feb 2010, FDA initiated safety review to evaluate risk of PR and QT interval prolongation with saquinavir/ritonavir. Do not use saquinavir/ritonavir with drugs that prolong the QT interval, including Class Ia or Class III antiarrhythmic drugs, or in patients with a history of QT interval prolongation. Do not use saquinavir with garlic supplements or tipranavir/ritonavir. Proton pump inhibitors may increase saquinavir levels. Do not exceed 200 mg/day ketoconazole. Reduce rifabutin to 150 mg every other day. Monitor for increased digoxin levels. May reduce methadone levels. Reduce dose of clarithromycin if CrCl less than 60 mL/min (see clarithromycin entry for details).

(cont.)

ANTIMICROBIALS: Antiviral Agents

SAQUINAVIR *(cont.)*
MOA — Prevents cleavage of protein precursors required for HIV maturation, reproduction, and infection of new cells.
ADVERSE EFFECTS — Frequent: GI complaints, headache, LFT elevation. Class effects: hyperglycemia, fat redistribution, lipid abnormalities, spontaneous bleeding in hemophiliacs.

TIPRANAVIR (*Aptivus, TPV*) ▶Feces ♀C ▶– $$$$$
WARNING — Potentially fatal hepatotoxicity. Monitor clinical status and LFTs frequently. Risk increased by coinfection with hepatitis B/C. Contraindicated in moderate to severe (Child Pugh B/C) hepatic failure. Intracranial hemorrhage can occur with tipranavir + ritonavir; caution if at risk of bleeding from trauma, surgery, other medical conditions, or receiving antiplatelet agents or anticoagulants.
ADULTS — HIV infection, boosted by ritonavir in treatment-experienced patients with strains resistant to multiple protease inhibitors: 500 mg + ritonavir 200 mg PO both bid with food.
PEDS — HIV infection, boosted by ritonavir in treatment-experienced patients age 2 yo or older with strains resistant to multiple protease inhibitors: 14 mg/kg with 6 mg/kg ritonavir (375 mg/m2 with ritonavir 150 mg/m2) PO bid to max of 500 mg with ritonavir 200 mg bid. Dosage reduction for toxicity in patients infected with virus that is not resistant to multiple protease inhibitors: 12 mg/kg with 5 mg/kg ritonavir (290 mg/m2 with 115 mg/m2 ritonavir) PO bid.
FORMS — Trade only: Caps 250 mg. Oral soln 100 mg/mL (95 mL in unit-of-use amber glass bottle).
NOTES — Contains sulfonamide moiety; potential for cross-sensitivity unknown. Al/Mg antacids may decrease absorption of tipranavir; separate doses. Ritonavir-boosted tipranavir inhibits CYP3A4 and 2D6. Contraindicated with CYP3A4 substrates that can cause life-threatening toxicity at high concentrations. Monitor levels of immunosuppressants, TCAs. May need higher methadone dose. Ritonavir decreases voriconazole levels; do not give together unless benefit exceeds risk. Do not use tipranavir/ritonavir with Kaletra or saquinavir. Decreases ethinyl estradiol levels; consider nonhormonal contraception. Reduce rifabutin to 150 mg PO every other day. Reduce clarithromycin dose if CrCl less than 60 mL/min (see clarithromycin entry for details). Caps contain alcohol. Refrigerate bottle of caps before opening. Use caps and oral soln within 60 days of opening container. Oral soln contains 116 international units/mL of vitamin E; advise patients not to take supplemental vitamin E other than a multivitamin.
MOA — Non-peptidic protease inhibitor. Prevents cleavage of protein precursors required for HIV maturation, reproduction, and infection of new cells.
ADVERSE EFFECTS — Serious: Life-threatening hepatotoxicity, intracranial hemorrhage. Frequent: Rash (high rate in women, especially those receiving ethinyl estradiol), diarrhea, N/V, fatigue, headache; increased LFTs, total cholesterol, and triglycerides. Class effects: Hyperglycemia, fat redistribution, lipid abnormalities, spontaneous bleeding in hemophiliacs.

ANTIMICROBIALS: Antiviral Agents—Anti-Influenza

NOTE: Whenever possible, immunization is the preferred method of prophylaxis. Avoid anti-influenza antivirals from 48 hours before until 2 weeks after a dose of live influenza vaccine (FluMist) unless medically necessary. Patients with suspected influenza may have primary/concomitant bacterial pneumonia; antibiotics may be indicated.

AMANTADINE (*Symmetrel, ♦Endantadine*) ▶K ♀C ▶? $$
ADULTS — Influenza A: 100 mg PO bid; reduce dose to 100 mg PO daily for age 65 yo or older. The CDC generally recommends against amantadine or rimantadine for treatment or prevention of influenza A in the United States due to high levels of resistance. Parkinsonism: 100 mg PO bid. Max 400 mg/day divided tid to qid. Drug-induced extrapyramidal disorders: 100 mg PO bid. Max 300 mg/day divided tid to qid.
PEDS — Safety and efficacy not established in infants age younger than 1 yo. Influenza A, treatment or prophylaxis: 5 mg/kg/day (up to 150 mg/day) PO divided bid for age 1 to 9 yo and any child wt less than 40 kg. 100 mg PO bid for age 10 yo or older. The CDC generally recommends against amantadine or rimantadine for treatment or prevention of influenza A in the United States due to high levels of resistance.
FORMS — Generic only: Caps 100 mg. Tabs 100 mg. Syrup 50 mg/5 mL (480 mL).
NOTES — CNS toxicity, suicide attempts, neuroleptic malignant syndrome with dosage reduction/withdrawal, anticholinergic effects, orthostatic hypotension. Do not stop abruptly in Parkinson's disease. Dosage reduction in adults with renal dysfunction: 200 mg PO once a week for CrCl less than 15 mL/min or hemodialysis. 200 mg PO first day, then 100 mg PO every other day for CrCl 15 to 29 mL/min. 200 mg PO first day, then 100 mg PO daily for CrCl 30 to 50 mL/min.
MOA — Appears to prevent viral replication by interfering with the function of the M2 protein in influenza virus. May facilitate dopamine release, and act as an NMDA receptor antagonist.
ADVERSE EFFECTS — Serious: Depression, suicidal ideation, seizures, orthostatic hypotension, neuroleptic malignant syndrome with dosage reduction/withdrawal (rare). Frequent: Anorexia, nausea, peripheral edema, CNS effects (esp. if elderly, renal

(cont.)

ANTIMICROBIALS: Antiviral Agents

AMANTADINE (cont.)
dysfunction, seizure disorders, anticholinergics, or psychiatric disorder).

OSELTAMIVIR (*Tamiflu*) ▶LK ♀C ▶? $$$
ADULTS — Influenza A/B, treatment: 75 mg PO bid for 5 days starting within 2 days of symptom onset. Prophylaxis: 75 mg PO daily. Start within 2 days of exposure and continue for 10 days. Take with food to improve tolerability.
PEDS — Influenza A/B: Dose is 30 mg for age 1 yo or older and wt 15 kg or less, 45 mg for wt 16 to 23 kg, 60 mg for wt 24 to 40 kg, 75 mg for wt greater than 40 kg or age 13 yo and older. For treatment, give dose twice daily for 5 days starting within 2 days of symptoms onset. For prophylaxis, give once daily for 10 days starting within 2 days of exposure. Can take with food to improve tolerability. Susp comes with graduated syringe calibrated to 30, 45, and 60 mg; use 30 mg plus 45 mg to measure 75 mg dose. Make sure the unit of measure on prescription matches the dosing device provided to the patient.
UNAPPROVED PEDS — Influenza treatment in infants younger than 1 yo: 3 mg/kg/dose PO bid for 5 days starting within 2 days of symptoms onset. Influenza prophylaxis in infants 3 to 11 mo: 3 mg/kg/dose PO once daily for 10 days starting within 2 days of exposure. Due to limited data, prophylaxis is not recommended for infants younger than 3 mo unless the situation is critical. These doses are not for premature infants. Take with food to improve tolerability. For infants younger than 1 year old, remove oral dosing syringe included in package and replace with a device that measures doses less than 30 mg.
FORMS — Trade only: Caps 30, 45, 75 mg. Susp 12 mg/mL (25 mL). Pharmacist can compound suspension (15 mg/mL).
NOTES — Previously not used in children younger than 1 yo; immature blood brain barrier could lead to high oseltamivir levels in CNS. Increased INR with warfarin. Postmarketing reports (mostly from Japan) of self-injury and delirium, primarily among children and adolescents; monitor for abnormal behavior. Dosage adjustment for adults with CrCl 10 to 30 mL/min: 75 mg PO daily for 5 days for treatment, 75 mg PO every other day or 30 mg PO once daily for prophylaxis. Susp stable for 10 days at room temperature.
MOA — Oral neuraminidase inhibitor.
ADVERSE EFFECTS — Serious: Anaphylaxis, erythema multiforme, toxic epidermal necrolysis (these reactions rare). Frequent: N/V, headache. Post-marketing reports (mostly from Japan) of self-injury and delirium, primarily among children and adolescents.

RIMANTADINE (*Flumadine*) ▶LK ♀C ▶– $$
ADULTS — Prophylaxis/treatment of influenza A: 100 mg PO bid. Start treatment within 2 days of symptom onset and continue for 7 days. Reduce dose to 100 mg PO once daily if severe hepatic dysfunction, CrCl less than 30 mL/min, or age older than 65 yo. The CDC generally recommends against amantadine/rimantadine for treatment/prevention of influenza A in the United States due to high levels of resistance.
PEDS — Influenza A prophylaxis: 5 mg/kg (up to 150 mg/day) PO once daily for age 1 to 9 yo; 100 mg PO bid for age 10 yo and older. The CDC generally recommends against amantadine/rimantadine for treatment/prevention of influenza A in the United States due to high levels of resistance.
UNAPPROVED PEDS — Influenza A treatment: 6.6 mg/kg (up to 150 mg/day) PO divided bid for age 1 to 9 yo; 100 mg PO bid for age 10 yo and older. Start treatment within 2 days of symptom onset and continue for 7 days.
FORMS — Generic/Trade: Tabs 100 mg. Pharmacist can compound suspension.
MOA — Appears to prevent viral replication by interfering with the function of the M2 protein in influenza virus.
ADVERSE EFFECTS — GI effects similar to amantadine, but less CNS toxicity.

ZANAMIVIR (*Relenza*) ▶K ♀C ▶? $$$
ADULTS — Influenza A/B treatment: 2 puffs bid for 5 days. Take 2 doses on day 1 at least 2 h apart. Start within 2 days of symptom onset. Influenza A/B prevention: 2 puffs once daily for 10 days, starting within 2 days of exposure.
PEDS — Influenza A/B treatment: 2 puffs bid for 5 days for age 7 yo or older. Take 2 doses on day 1 at least 2 h apart. Start within 2 days of symptom onset. Influenza A/B prevention: 2 puffs once daily for 10 days for age 5 yo or older, starting within 2 days of exposure.
FORMS — Trade only: Rotadisk inhaler 5 mg/puff (20 puffs).
NOTES — May cause bronchospasm and worsen pulmonary function in asthma or COPD; avoid if underlying airways disease. Stop if bronchospasm/decline in respiratory function. Show patient how to use inhaler.
MOA — Inhaled neuraminidase inhibitor.
ADVERSE EFFECTS — Serious: Bronchospasm in patients with reactive airway disease. Possible abnormal behavior and short-term delerium in children and adolescents; monitor for abnormal behavior. Frequent: Nasal and throat irritation.

ANTIMICROBIALS: Antiviral Agents—Other

ADEFOVIR (*Hepsera*) ▶K ♀C ▶– $$$$$
WARNING — Nephrotoxic; monitor renal function. May result in HIV resistance in untreated HIV infection; test for HIV before prescribing. Lactic acidosis with hepatic steatosis. Severe acute exacerbation of hepatitis B can occur after discontinuation of

ANTIMICROBIALS: Antiviral Agents

OVERVIEW OF BACTERIAL PATHOGENS (Selected)

By bacterial class

Gram Positive Aerobic Cocci: *Staph epidermidis* (coagulase negative), *Staph aureus* (coagulase positive), Streptococci: *S pneumoniae* (pneumococcus), *S pyogenes* (Group A), *S agalactiae* (Group B), enterococcus

Gram Positive Aerobic/Facultatively Anaerobic Bacilli: *Bacillus*, *Corynebacterium diphtheriae*, *Erysipelothrix rhusiopathiae*, *Listeria monocytogenes*, *Nocardia*

Gram Negative Aerobic Diplococci: *Moraxella catarrhalis*, *Neisseria gonorrhoeae*, *Neisseria meningitidis*

Gram Negative Aerobic Coccobacilli: *Haemophilus ducreyi*, *Haemoph. Influenzae*

Gram Negative Aerobic Bacilli: *Acinetobacter*, *Bartonella* species, *Bordetella pertussis*, *Brucella*, *Burkholderia cepacia*, *Campylobacter*, *Francisella tularensis*, *Helicobacter pylori*, *Legionella pneumophila*, *Pseudomonas aeruginosa*, *Stenotrophomonas maltophilia*, *Vibrio cholerae*, *Yersinia*

Gram Negative Facultatively Anaerobic Bacilli: *Aeromonas hydrophila*, *Eikenella corrodens*, *Pasteurella multocida*, Enterobacteriaceae: *E coli*, *Citrobacter*, *Shigella*, *Salmonella*, *Klebsiella*, *Enterobacter*, *Hafnia*, *Serratia*, *Proteus*, *Providencia*

Anaerobes: *Actinomyces*, *Bacteroides fragilis*, *Clostridium botulinum*, *Clostridium difficile*, *Clostridium perfringens*, *Clostridium tetani*, *Fusobacterium*, *Lactobacillus*, *Peptostreptococcus*

Defective Cell Wall Bacteria: *Chlamydia pneumoniae*, *Chlamydia psittaci*, *Chlamydia trachomatis*, *Coxiella burnetii*, *Mycoplasma pneumoniae*, *Rickettsia prowazekii*, *Rickettsia rickettsii*, *Rickettsia typhi*, *Ureaplasma urealyticum*

Spirochetes: *Borrelia burgdorferi*, *Leptospira*, *Treponema pallidum*

Mycobacteria: *M avium* complex, *M kansasii*, *M leprae*, *M TB*

By bacterial name

Acinetobacter   Gram Negative Aerobic Bacilli
Actinomyces   Anaerobes
Aeromonas hydrophila   Gram Negative Facultatively Anaerobic Bacilli
Bacillus   Gram Positive Aerobic/Facultatively Anaerobic Bacilli
Bacteroides fragilis   Anaerobes
Bartonella species   Gram Negative Aerobic Bacilli
Bordetella pertussis   Gram Negative Aerobic Bacilli
Borrelia burgdorferi   Spirochetes
Brucella   Gram Negative Aerobic Bacilli
Burkholderia cepacia   Gram Negative Aerobic Bacilli
Campylobacter   Gram Negative Aerobic Bacilli
Chlamydia pneumoniae   Defective Cell Wall Bacteria
Chlamydia psittaci   Defective Cell Wall Bacteria
Chlamydia trachomatis   Defective Cell Wall Bacteria
Citrobacter   Gram Negative Facultatively Anaerobic Bacilli
Clostridium botulinum   Anaerobes
Clostridium difficile   Anaerobes
Clostridium perfringens   Anaerobes
Clostridium tetani   Anaerobes
Corynebacterium diphtheriae   Gram Positive Aerobic/Facultatively Anaerobic Bacilli
Coxiella burnetii   Defective Cell Wall Bacteria
E coli   Gram Negative Facultatively Anaerobic Bacilli
Eikenella corrodens   Gram Negative Facultatively Anaerobic Bacilli
Enterobacter   Gram Negative Facultatively Anaerobic Bacilli
Enterobacteriaceae   Gram Negative Facultatively Anaerobic Bacilli
Enterococcus   Gram Positive Aerobic Cocci
Erysipelothrix rhusiopathiae   Gram Positive Aerobic/Facultatively Anaerobic Bacilli
Francisella tularensis   Gram Negative Aerobic Bacilli
Fusobacterium   Anaerobes

(cont.)

OVERVIEW OF BACTERIAL PATHOGENS (Selected)
By bacterial name, (cont.)

Haemophilus ducreyi   Gram Negative Aerobic Coccobacilli
Haemophilus influenzae   Gram Negative Aerobic Coccobacilli
Hafnia   Gram Negative Facultatively Anaerobic Bacilli
Helicobacter pylori   Gram Negative Aerobic Bacilli
Klebsiella   Gram Negative Facultatively Anaerobic Bacilli
Lactobacillus   Anaerobes
Legionella pneumophila   Gram Negative Aerobic Bacilli
Leptospira   Spirochetes
Listeria monocytogenes   Gram Positive Aerobic/Facultatively Anaerobic Bacilli
M avium complex   Mycobacteria
M kansasii   Mycobacteria
M leprae   Mycobacteria
M tuberculosis   Mycobacteria
Moraxella catarrhalis   Gram Negative Aerobic Diplococci
Myocoplasma pneumoniae   Defective Cell Wall Bacteria
Neisseria gonorrhoeae   Gram Negative Aerobic Diplococci
Neisseria meningitidis   Gram Negative Aerobic Diplococci
Nocardia   Gram Positive Aerobic/Facultatively Anaerobic Bacilli
Pasteurella multocida   Gram Negative Facultatively Anaerobic Bacilli
Peptostreptococcus   Anaerobes
Pneumococcus   Gram Positive Aerobic Cocci
Proteus   Gram Negative Facultatively Anaerobic Bacilli
Providencia   Gram Negative Facultatively Anaerobic Bacilli
Pseudomonas aeruginosa   Gram Negative Aerobic Bacilli
Rickettsia prowazekii   Defective Cell Wall Bacteria
Rickettsia rickettsii   Defective Cell Wall Bacteria
Rickettsia typhi   Defective Cell Wall Bacteria
Salmonella   Gram Negative Facultatively Anaerobic Bacilli
Serratia   Gram Negative Facultatively Anaerobic Bacilli
Shigella   Gram Negative Facultatively Anaerobic Bacilli
Staph aureus (coagulase positive)   Gram Positive Aerobic Cocci
Staph epidermidis (coagulase negative)   Gram Positive Aerobic Cocci
Stenotrophomonas maltophilia   Gram Negative Aerobic Bacilli
Strep agalactiae (Group B)   Gram Positive Aerobic Cocci
Strep pneumoniae (pneumococcus)   Gram Positive Aerobic Cocci
Strep pyogenes (Group A)   Gram Positive Aerobic Cocci
Streptococci   Gram Positive Aerobic Cocci
Treponema pallidum   Spirochetes
Ureaplasma urealyticum   Defective Cell Wall Bacteria
Vibrio cholerae   Gram Negative Aerobic Bacilli
Yersinia   Gram Negative Aerobic Bacilli

ADEFOVIR (*cont.*)
adefovir in patients with HIV and hepatitis B coinfection. Monitor closely for at least 2 months after discontinuing adefovir in such patients; consider retreating hepatitis B.
ADULTS − <u>Chronic hepatitis B:</u> 10 mg PO daily.
PEDS − <u>Chronic hepatitis B:</u> 10 mg PO daily for age 12 yo or older.
FORMS − Trade only: Tabs 10 mg.
NOTES − Monitor renal function. See package insert for dosage reduction if CrCl < 50 mL/min. Other nephrotoxic drugs may increase risk of nephrotoxicity; do not use with tenofovir. Use adefovir plus lamivudine instead of adefovir alone in patients with lamivudine-resistant hepatitis B. Adefovir resistance can cause viral load rebound. Consider change in therapy if persistent serum hepatitis B DNA > 1000 copies/mL.
MOA − Nucleotide reverse transcriptase inhibitor, similar mechanism of action as NRTIs. Negligible activity against HIV virus at 10 mg dose.

(cont.)

ANTIMICROBIALS: Antiviral Agents

ADEFOVIR (cont.)
ADVERSE EFFECTS — Serious: Lactic acidosis/hepatic steatosis, nephrotoxicity, exacerbation of hepatitis B after discontinuation. Frequent: None.

ENTECAVIR (Baraclude) ▶K ♀C ▶– $$$$$
WARNING — Nucleoside analogues can cause lactic acidosis with hepatic steatosis. Severe acute exacerbation of hepatitis B can occur after discontinuation. Monitor closely for at least 2 months after discontinuation. Patients coinfected with HIV and hepatitis B should not receive entecavir for hepatitis B unless they also receive HAART for HIV; failure to treat HIV in such patients could lead to HIV resistance to NRTIs.
ADULTS — Chronic hepatitis B: 0.5 mg PO once daily if treatment-naive; 1 mg if lamivudine-resistant, history of viremia despite lamivudine treatment, or HIV coinfected. Give on empty stomach (2 h after last meal and 2 h before next meal).
PEDS — Chronic hepatitis B, age 16 yo or older: 0.5 mg PO once daily if treatment-naive; 1 mg if lamivudine-resistant, history of viremia despite lamivudine treatment, or HIV coinfected. Give on empty stomach (2 h after last meal and 2 h before next meal).
FORMS — Trade only: Tabs 0.5, 1 mg.
NOTES — Entecavir treatment of coinfected patients not receiving HIV treatment may increase the risk of resistance to lamivudine or emtricitabine. Do not mix oral soln with water or other liquid. Reduce dose if CrCl less than 50 mL/min or dialysis. Give dose after dialysis sessions.
MOA — Guanosine nucleoside analogue that inhibits hepatitis B polymerase. Partial inhibitor of HIV replication may select for lamivudine-resistant mutation.
ADVERSE EFFECTS — Serious: Nucleoside analogues can cause lactic acidosis/hepatic steatosis. Frequent: Headache, fatigue, dizziness, nausea.

INTERFERON ALFA-2B (Intron A) ▶K ♀C ▶?+ $$$$$
WARNING — May cause or worsen serious neuropsychiatric, autoimmune, ischemic, and infectious diseases. Frequent clinical and lab monitoring required. Stop interferon if signs/symptoms of these conditions are persistently severe or worsen.
ADULTS — Chronic hepatitis B: 5 million units/day or 10 million units 3 times a week SC/IM for 16 weeks if HBeAg positive. Chronic hepatitis C: 3 million units SC/IM 3 times a week for 16 weeks. Continue for 18 to 24 months if ALT normalized. In combination with ribavirin for hepatitis C, peginterferon is preferred over interferon alfa 2b because of substantially higher response rate. Other indications: Condylomata acuminata, AIDS-related Kaposi's sarcoma, hairy-cell leukemia, melanoma, and follicular lymphoma - see package insert for specific dose.
PEDS — Chronic hepatitis B: 3 million units/m2 three times/week for first week, then 6 million units/m2 (max 10 million units/dose) SC three times/week for age 1 yo or older. Chronic hepatitis C: Interferon alfa-2b 3 million units/m2 SC 3 times/week for age 3 yo or older with PO ribavirin according to wt. Ribavirin: 200 mg bid for wt 25 to 36 kg; 200 mg q am and 400 mg q pm for wt 37 to 49 kg; 400 mg bid for wt 50 to 61 kg. Use adult dose for wt greater than 61 kg. If ribavirin contraindicated use interferon 3 to 5 million units/m2 (max 3 million units/dose) SC/IM 3 times/week.
UNAPPROVED ADULTS — Prevention of chronic hepatitis C in acute hepatitis C: 5 million units SC daily for 4 weeks then 5 million units SC 3 times a week for 20 weeks. Other indications: superficial bladder tumors, chronic myelogenous leukemia, cutaneous T-cell lymphoma, essential thrombocythemia, non-Hodgkin's lymphoma, and chronic granulocytic leukemia.
FORMS — Trade only: Powder/soln for injection 10, 18, 50 million units/vial. Soln for injection 18, 25 million units/multidose vial. Multidose injection pens 3, 5, 10 million units/0.2 mL (1.5 mL), 6 doses/pen.
NOTES — Monitor for depression, suicidal behavior (especially in adolescents), other severe neuropsychiatric effects. Thyroid abnormalities, hepatotoxicity, flu-like symptoms, pulmonary and cardiovascular reactions, retinal damage, neutropenia, thrombocytopenia, hypertriglyceridemia (consider monitoring). Increases theophylline levels. Monitor CBC, TSH, LFTs, electrolytes. Dosage adjustments for hematologic toxicity in package insert.
MOA — Interferons enhance phagocytic activity of macrophages and cytotoxicity of lymphocytes, and inhibit viral replication.
ADVERSE EFFECTS — Serious: May cause or worsen serious neuropsychiatric, autoimmune, ischemic, & infectious diseases (including thyroid abnormalities, hepatotoxicity, pulmonary & cardiovascular reactions, retinal damage, neutropenia, thrombocytopenia, hypertriglyceridemia, myelosuppression, psychiatric syndromes). Frequent: Flu-like syndrome, anorexia, dizziness, rash, depression.

INTERFERON ALFA-N3 (Alferon N) ▶K ♀C ▶– $$$$$
WARNING — Flu-like syndrome, myalgias, alopecia. Contraindicated in egg protein allergy.
ADULTS — Doses vary by indication. Condylomata acuminata, intralesional.
PEDS — Not approved in children.
MOA — Interferons exert their cellular activities by binding to specific membrane receptors on the cell surface. Once bound to the cell membrane, interferons initiate a complex sequence of intracellular events. In vitro studies demonstrated that these include the induction of certain enzymes, suppression of cell proliferation, immunomodulating activities such as enhancement of the phagocytic activity of macrophages and augmentation of the specific cytotoxicity of lymphocytes for target cells, and inhibition of virus replication in virus-infected cells.
ADVERSE EFFECTS — Serious: Hypersensitivity. Frequent: Flu-like syndrome, myalgias.

INTERFERON ALFACON-1 (Infergen) ▶Plasma ♀C ▶? $$$$$
WARNING — May cause or worsen serious neuropsychiatric, autoimmune, ischemic, and infectious diseases. Frequent clinical and lab monitoring required. Stop interferon if signs/symptoms of these conditions are persistently severe or worsen.
ADULTS — Chronic hepatitis C, monotherapy: 9 to 15 mcg SC 3 times a week. Chronic hepatitis C, with

(cont.)

INTERFERON ALFACON-1 *(cont.)*
ribavirin: 15 mcg SC daily with weight-based PO ribavirin. Optimal therapy for chronic HCV infection is combination peginterferon alfa and ribavirin.
PEDS — Not approved in children.
FORMS — Trade only: Vials injectable soln 30 mcg/mL (0.3 mL, 0.5 mL).
NOTES — Monitor for depression, suicidal behavior, or other severe neuropsychiatric effects. Thyroid dysfunction, cardiovascular reactions, retinal damage, flu-like symptoms, thrombocytopenia, neutropenia, exacerbation of autoimmune disorders, hypertriglyceridemia (consider monitoring). Monitor CBC, thyroid function. Refrigerate injectable soln.
MOA — Binding to cell surface receptors initiates intracellular events that enhances the phagocytic activity of macrophages and cytotoxicity of lymphocytes, and inhibits viral replication.
ADVERSE EFFECTS — Serious: May cause or worsen serious neuropsychiatric, autoimmune, ischemic, & infectious diseases (including thyroid abnormalities, hepatotoxicity, pulmonary & cardiovascular reactions, retinal damage, neutropenia, thrombocytopenia, hypertriglyceridemia, myelosuppression, psychiatric syndromes). Frequent: Flu-like syndrome, anorexia, dizziness, rash, depression.

PALIVIZUMAB (*Synagis*) ▶L ♀C ▶? $$$$$
PEDS — Prevention of respiratory syncytial virus pulmonary disease in high-risk infants: 15 mg/kg IM monthly during RSV season with first injection before season starts (November to April in northern hemisphere). See aappolicy.aappublications.org for eligibility criteria. Give a dose ASAP after cardiopulmonary bypass (due to decreased palivizumab levels) even if less than 1 month after last dose.
NOTES — Preservative-free; use within 6 h of reconstitution. Not more than 1 mL per injection site.
MOA — Monoclonal antibody against F glycoprotein on surface of respiratory syncytial virus.
ADVERSE EFFECTS — Serious: Acute hypersensitivity reactions (rare); anaphylaxis after re-exposure (rare). Frequent: Increases aminotransferase activity, otherwise well-tolerated.

PEGINTERFERON ALFA-2A (*Pegasys*) ▶LK ♀C ▶– $$$$$
WARNING — May cause or worsen serious neuropsychiatric, autoimmune, ischemic, and infectious diseases. Frequent clinical and lab monitoring recommended. Discontinue if signs/symptoms of these conditions are persistently severe or worsen.
ADULTS — Chronic hepatitis C not previously treated with alfa-interferon: 180 mcg SC in abdomen or thigh once a week for 48 weeks with or without PO ribavirin 800 to 1200 mg/day. Ribavirin dose and duration depends on genotype and body wt (see PO ribavirin entry). Hepatitis B: 180 mcg SC in abdomen or thigh once a week for 48 weeks.
PEDS — Not approved in children.
FORMS — Trade only: 180 mcg/1 mL soln in single-use vial, 180 mcg/0.5 mL prefilled syringe.
NOTES — Contraindicated in autoimmune hepatitis; hepatic decompensation in cirrhotic patients (Child-Pugh score > 6 if HCV only; score > 5 if HIV coinfected). Monitor for depression, suicidal behavior, relapse of drug addiction, or other severe neuropsychiatric effects. Interferons can cause thrombocytopenia, neutropenia, thyroid dysfunction, hyperglycemia, hypoglycemia, cardiovascular events, colitis, pancreatitis, hypersensitivity, flu-like symptoms, pulmonary and ophthalmologic disorders. Risk of severe neutropenia/thrombocytopenia greater in HIV-infected patients. Monitor CBC, blood chemistry. Interferons increase risk of hepatic decompensation in hepatitis C/HIV coinfected patients receiving HAART with NRTI. Monitor LFTs and clinical status; discontinue peginterferon if Child-Pugh score 6 or greater. Exacerbation of hepatitis during treatment of hepatitis B; monitor LFTs more often and consider dosage reduction if ALT flares. Discontinue treatment if ALT increase is progressive despite dosage reduction or if flares accompanied by hepatic decompensation or bilirubin increase. CYP1A2 inhibitor; may increase theophylline levels (monitor). May increase methadone levels. Use cautiously if CrCl less than 50 mL/min. Dosage adjustments for adverse effects, hepatic dysfunction, or hemodialysis in package insert. Store in refrigerator.
MOA — Interferon alfa-2a that is conjugated to polyethylene glycol to increase duration of action. Interferons enhance phagocytic activity of macrophages and cytotoxicity of lymphocytes, and inhibit viral replication.
ADVERSE EFFECTS — Serious: Alpha interferons may cause or worsen serious neuropsychiatric, autoimmune, ischemic, & infectious diseases (including thyroid dysfunction, hyperglycemia, hypoglycemia, hepatotoxicity, colitis, pulmonary & cardiovascular reactions, neutropenia, thrombocytopenia, hypertriglyceridemia, myelosuppression, psychiatric syndromes, ophthalmologic disorders). Interferons increase risk of hepatic decompensation in hep C/HIV coinfected patients receiving HAART with NRTI. Exacerbation of hepatitis during treatment of hepatitis B. Acute hypersensitivity. Frequent: Psychiatric reactions, flu-like syndrome, hematologic toxicity, fatigue, injection site reactions, dizziness, pruritus, dermatitis, headache, alopecia, anorexia.

PEGINTERFERON ALFA-2B (*PEG-Intron*) ▶K? ♀C ▶– $$$$$
WARNING — May cause or worsen serious neuropsychiatric, autoimmune, ischemic, and infectious diseases. Frequent clinical and lab monitoring recommended. Discontinue if signs/symptoms of these conditions are persistently severe or worsen.
ADULTS — Chronic hepatitis C not previously treated with alfa-interferon. Monotherapy: 1 mcg/kg/week SC for 1 year given on same day each week. To control volume of injection, use vial strength based on wt; give 40 mcg (0.4 mL, 50 mcg/0.5 mL vial) for wt 45 kg or less, give 50 mcg (0.5 mL, 50 mcg/0.5 mL vial) for 46 to 56 kg, give 64 mcg (0.4 mL, 80 mcg/0.5 mL vial) for 57 to 72 kg, give 80 mcg (0.5 mL, 80 mcg/0.5 mL vial) for 73 to 88 kg, give 96 mcg (0.4 mL, 120 mcg/0.5 mL vial) for 89 to 106 kg, give 120 mcg (0.5 mL, 120 mcg/0.5 mL vial) for 107 to 136 kg, give 150 mcg (0.5 mL, 150 mcg/0.5 mL

(cont.)

PEGINTERFERON ALFA-2B (*cont.*)

vial) for 137 to 160 kg. Combination therapy with oral ribavirin (see Rebetol entry): 1.5 mcg/kg/week given on the same day each week. Treat genotype 1 for 48 weeks; treat genotype 2 or 3 for 24 weeks. To control amount injected, use vial strength based on wt: give 50 mcg (0.5 mL, 50 mcg/0.5 mL vial) for wt less than 40 kg, give 64 mcg (0.4 mL, 80 mcg/0.5 mL vial) for 40 to 50 kg, give 80 mcg (0.5 mL, 80 mcg/0.5 mL vial) for 51 to 60 kg, give 96 mcg (0.4 mL, 120 mcg/0.5 mL vial) for 61 to 75 kg, give 120 mcg (0.5 mL, 120 mcg/0.5 mL vial) for 76 to 85 kg, give 150 mcg (0.5 mL, 150 mcg/0.5 mL vial) for 86 kg or greater. Give at bedtime or with antipyretic to minimize flu-like symptoms. Consider stopping if HCV RNA is not below limit of detection after 24 weeks of therapy.

PEDS — Chronic hepatitis C not previously treated with alfa-interferon, age 3 yo or older: 60 mcg/m2 SC once a week with ribavirin 15 mg/kg/day PO divided bid (see Rebetol entry for dosing of caps). Discontinue if HCV-RNA reduction is less than 2 log10 after 12 weeks or is still detectable after 24 weeks.

FORMS — Trade only: 50, 80, 120, 150 mcg/ 0.5 mL single-use vials with diluent, 2 syringes, and alcohol swabs. Disposable single-dose Redipen 50, 80, 120, 150 mcg.

NOTES — Contraindicated in autoimmune hepatitis; hepatic decompensation in cirrhotic patients (Child-Pugh score > 6). Coadministration with ribavirin contraindicated if CrCl less than 50 mL/min. Monitor for depression, suicidal behavior, other severe neuropsychiatric effects. Thrombocytopenia, neutropenia, thyroid dysfunction, hyperglycemia, cardiovascular events, colitis, pancreatitis, hypersensitivity, flu-like symptoms, pulmonary damage. Monitor CBC, blood chemistry. May increase methadone levels. Dosage adjustments for adverse effects or renal dysfunction in package insert. Peginterferon should be used immediately after reconstitution, but can be refrigerated for up to 24 h.

MOA — Interferon alfa-2b that is conjugated to polyethylene glycol. Binding of alpha interferon to cell surface receptors initiates intracellular events that enhances the phagocytic activity of macrophages and cytotoxicity of lymphocytes, and inhibits viral replication.

ADVERSE EFFECTS — Serious: May cause or worsen serious neuropsychiatric, autoimmune, ischemic, & infectious diseases (including thyroid abnormalities, hepatotoxicity, pulmonary & cardiovascular reactions, stroke, retinal damage, neutropenia, thrombocytopenia, hypertriglyceridemia, myelosuppression, psychiatric syndromes). Weight loss/impaired growth possible in children during peginterferon-ribavirin therapy. Frequent: Flu-like syndrome, anorexia, dizziness, rash, depression.

RIBAVIRIN—INHALED (*Virazole*) ▶Lung ♀X ▶– $$$$$
WARNING — Beware of sudden pulmonary deterioration with ribavirin. Drug precipitation may cause ventilator dysfunction.

PEDS — Severe respiratory syncytial virus infection: Aerosol 12 to 18 h/day for 3 to 7 days.

NOTES — Minimize exposure to health care workers, especially pregnant women.

MOA — Inhaled synthetic nucleoside that interferes with viral nucleic acid synthesis.

ADVERSE EFFECTS — Serious: Sudden pulmonary deterioration, ventilator dysfunction due to drug precipitation.

RIBAVIRIN—ORAL (*Rebetol, Copegus, Ribasphere*)
▶Cellular, K ♀X ▶– $$$$$

WARNING — Teratogen with extremely long half-life; contraindicated if pregnancy possible in patient/partner. Female patients and female partners of male patients must avoid pregnancy by using 2 forms of birth control during and for 6 months after stopping ribavirin. Obtain pregnancy test at baseline and monthly. Hemolytic anemia that may worsen cardiac disease. Assess for underlying heart disease before treatment with ribavirin. Do not use in significant/unstable heart disease. Baseline ECG if preexisting cardiac dysfunction.

ADULTS — In combination with ribavirin for hepatitis C, peginterferon is preferred over interferon alfa 2b because of substantially higher response rate. Rebetol in combo with peginterferon alfa 2b (PegIntron): 400 mg PO bid for wt 65 kg or less, 400 mg PO q am and 600 mg PO q pm for 66 to 85 kg, 600 mg PO bid for wt 86 to 105 kg, 600 mg PO q am and 800 mg PO q pm for wt greater than 105 kg. Treat genotype 1 for 48 weeks, genotypes 2 and 3 for 24 weeks. Copegus in combo with peginterferon alfa 2a (Pegasys): For genotypes 1 and 4, treat for 48 weeks with 1000 mg/day for wt less than 75kg, 1200 mg/day for wt 75 kg or greater. For genotypes 2 and 3, treat for 24 weeks with 800 mg/day. Divide daily dose of ribavirin bid and give with food. See package inserts for dosage reductions if Hb declines.

PEDS — In combination with ribavirin for chronic hepatitis C, peginterferon is preferred over interferon alfa because of substantially higher response rate. Rebetol in combination with peginterferon alfa-2b (PegIntron): For wt less than 47 kg or patients who cannot swallow caps: 15 mg/kg/day of soln PO divided bid. Caps: 400 mg PO bid for wt 47 to 59 kg, 400 mg PO q am and 600 mg q pm for wt 60 to 73 kg, 600 mg PO bid for wt greater than 73 kg. Take with food. Treat genotype 1 for 48 weeks, genotypes 2 and 3 for 24 weeks.

UNAPPROVED ADULTS — In combo therapy with ribavirin for chronic hepatitis C, peginterferon is preferred over interferon alfa because of substantially higher response rate. Regimen and duration of treatment is based on genotype. Divide daily dose of ribavirin bid and give with food. Chronic hepatitis C, genotypes 1 and 4: Treat for 48 weeks, evaluating response after 12 weeks. Ribavirin in combo with peginterferon alfa-2b (PegIntron): 800 mg/day PO for wt 65 kg or less, 1000 mg/day for wt 66 kg to 85 kg, 1200 mg/day for wt 86 kg

(cont.)

RIBAVIRIN—ORAL *(cont.)*
to 105 kg, 1400 mg/day for greater than 105 kg. Ribavirin in combo with peginterferon alfa-2a (Pegasys): 1000 mg/day PO for wt less than 75 kg, 1200 mg/day for wt 75 kg or greater. Chronic hepatitis C, genotypes 2 and 3: Treat for 24 weeks with ribavirin 800 mg/day in combo with peginterferon. Regimens provided here are from guideline for the management of chronic hepatitis C; they may vary from regimens in product labeling.
UNAPPROVED PEDS – Chronic hepatitis C, age 2 years old and older: Treat for 48 weeks with peginterferon alfa-2b (PegIntron) in combo with ribavirin 15 mg/kg/day PO divided bid. The regimen provided here is from guideline for the management of chronic hepatitis C; it may vary from regimens in product labeling.
FORMS – Generic/Trade: Caps 200 mg, Tabs 200, 500 mg. Generic only: Tabs 400, 600 mg. Trade only (Rebetol): Oral soln 40 mg/mL (100 mL).
NOTES – Contraindicated in hemoglobinopathies; autoimmune hepatitis; hepatic decompensation in cirrhotic patients (Child-Pugh score greater than 6 if HCV only; score greater than 5 if HIV coinfected). Get CBC at baseline, week 2 and 4, and periodically. Risk of anemia increased if age older than 50 yo or if renal dysfunction. Do not use if CrCl less than 50 mL/min. Decreased INR with warfarin; monitor INR weekly for 4 weeks after ribavirin started/stopped. May increase risk of lactic acidosis with nucleoside reverse transcriptase inhibitors. Avoid didanosine or zidovudine. Coadministration with azathioprine can cause neutropenia; monitor CBC weekly for first month, every other week for next 2 months, then monthly or more frequently if doses are adjusted.

MOA – Oral synthetic nucleoside that interferes with viral nucleic acid synthesis.
ADVERSE EFFECTS – Serious and frequent: Hemolytic anemia (especially if older than 50 yo or if renal dysfunction). Frequent: Therapy with interferon plus ribavirin causes more cough, pruritus, and rash than interferon alone. Serious and rare: Severe acute hypersensitivity during co-therapy with interferon. Possible growth delay in children.

TELBIVUDINE (*Tyzeka*) ▶K ♀B ▶– $$$$$
WARNING – Nucleoside analogues can cause lactic acidosis with hepatic steatosis. Severe acute exacerbation of hepatitis B can occur after discontinuation. Monitor closely for at least 2 months after discontinuation.
ADULTS – Chronic hepatitis B: 600 mg PO once daily.
PEDS – Chronic hepatitis B, age 16 yo or older: 600 mg PO once daily.
FORMS – Trade only: Tabs 600 mg. Oral soln 100 mg/5 mL (300 mL).
NOTES – No dosage adjustment needed for hepatic dysfunction. Renal dysfunction: 600 mg PO q 96 h for ESRD, q 72 h for CrCl less than 30 mL/min but not hemodialysis, q 48 h for CrCl 30 to 49 mL/min. Give dose after hemodialysis session. Contains 47 mg sodium/30 mL of oral soln.
MOA – Thymidine nucleoside analogue that inhibits hepatitis B polymerase. It has no activity against HIV-1.
ADVERSE EFFECTS – Serious: Myopathy. Peripheral neuropathy (incidence and severity increased by peginterferon alfa 2a or other interferon). Nucleoside analogues can cause lactic acidosis/hepatic steatosis. Frequent: Headache, dizziness, fatigue, URI/nasopharyngitis/influenza/flu-like symptoms, cough, abdominal pain, increased CK levels, N/V, dyspepsia, diarrhea.

ANTIMICROBIALS: Carbapenems

NOTE: Carbapenems can dramatically reduce valproic acid levels; use another antibiotic (preferred) or add a supplemental anticonvulsant.

DORIPENEM (*Doribax*) ▶K ♀B ▶? $$$$$
ADULTS – Complicated intra-abdominal infection: 500 mg IV q 8 h for 5 to 14 days. Complicated UTI or pyelonephritis: 500 mg IV q 8 h for 10 to 14 days.
PEDS – Not approved in children.
NOTES – Possible cross-sensitivity with other beta-lactams; C. difficile-associated diarrhea; superinfection. Dose reduction in renal dysfunction: 250 mg q 12 h for CrCl 10 to 30 mL/min, 250 mg q 8 h for CrCl 30 to 50 mL/min.
MOA – Beta-lactam resistant to hydrolysis by most beta-lactamases, including extended-spectrum beta-lactamases.
ADVERSE EFFECTS – Serious: Cross-sensitivity with other beta-lactams, C. difficile associated diarrhea, superinfection. Frequent: Headache, nausea, diarrhea, rash, phlebitis.

ERTAPENEM (*Invanz*) ▶K ♀B ▶? $$$$$
ADULTS – Community-acquired pneumonia, diabetic foot, complicated intra-abdominal, skin, urinary tract, acute pelvic infections: 1 g IM/IV over 30 min q 24 h for up to 14 days for IV, up to 7 days for IM. Prophylaxis, elective colorectal surgery: 1 g IV 1 h before incision.
PEDS – Community-acquired pneumonia, complicated intra-abdominal, skin, urinary tract, acute pelvic infections (3 mo to 12 yo): 15 mg/kg IV/IM q 12 h (up to 1 g/day). Use adult dose for age 13 yo or older. Infuse IV over 30 min. Can give IV for up to 14 days, IM for up to 7 days.
NOTES – Possible cross-sensitivity with other beta-lactams; C. difficile-associated diarrhea; superinfection; seizures (especially if renal dysfunction or CNS disorder). Not active against Pseudomonas

(cont.)

ERTAPENEM (*cont.*)

and Acinetobacter species. IM diluted with lidocaine; contraindicated if allergic to amide-type local anesthetics. For adults with renal dysfunction: 500 mg q 24 h for CrCl 30 mL/min or less or hemodialysis. Give 150 mg supplemental dose if daily dose given within 6 h before hemodialysis session. Do not dilute in dextrose.
MOA – Beta-lactam resistant to hydrolysis by most beta-lactamases, including extended-spectrum beta-lactamases.
ADVERSE EFFECTS – Serious: Cross-sensitivity with other beta-lactams, C. difficile-associated diarrhea, superinfection, seizures (0.5% of patients). Frequent: Diarrhea, N/V, infusion site reactions. Lidocaine diluent can cause allergy.

IMIPENEM-CILASTATIN (*Primaxin*) ▶K ♀C ▶? $$$$$
ADULTS – Pneumonia, sepsis, endocarditis, polymicrobic, intra-abdominal, gynecologic, bone and joint, skin infections. Normal renal function, 70 kg or greater: mild infection: 250 to 500 mg IV q 6 h; moderate infection: 500 mg IV q 6 to 8 h or 1 g IV q 8 h; severe infection: 500 mg IV q 6 h to 1 g IV q 6 to 8 h. Complicated UTI: 500 mg IV q 6 h. See product labeling for doses in adults wt less than 70 kg. Can give up to 1.5 g/day IM for mild/moderate infections.
PEDS – Pneumonia, sepsis, endocarditis, polymicrobic, intra-abdominal, bone and joint, skin infections. 25 mg/kg IV q 12 h for age younger than 1 week old; 25 mg/kg IV q 8 h for age 1 to 4 weeks old; 25 mg/kg IV q 6 h for age 1 to 3 mo; 15 to 25 mg/kg IV q 6 h for older than 3 mo. Not for children with CNS infections, or wt less than 30 kg with renal dysfunction.
UNAPPROVED ADULTS – Malignant otitis externa, empiric therapy for neutropenic fever: 500 mg IV q 6 h.
NOTES – Possible cross-sensitivity with other beta-lactams, C. difficile-associated diarrhea, superinfection, seizures (especially if given with ganciclovir, elderly with renal dysfunction, or cerebrovascular or seizure disorder). See product labeling for dose if CrCl less than 70 mL/min. Not for CrCl less than 5 mL/min unless dialysis started within 48 h.
MOA – Beta-lactam resistant to hydrolysis by most beta-lactamases, including extended-spectrum beta-lactamases. Cilastatin inhibits renal tubular metabolism of imipenem.
ADVERSE EFFECTS – Serious: Cross-sensitivity with other beta-lactams (50% in patients with anaphylaxis to penicillin), C. difficile-associated diarrhea, superinfection. Frequent: Seizures in patients with risk factors (ganciclovir, elderly with renal dysfunction, cerebrovascular or seizure disorder).

MEROPENEM (*Merrem IV*) ▶K ♀B ▶? $$$$$
ADULTS – Intra-abdominal infections: 1 g IV q 8 h. Complicated skin infections: 500 mg IV q 8 h.
PEDS – Meningitis: 40 mg/kg IV q 8 h for age 3 mo or older; 2 g IV q 8 h for wt greater than 50 kg. Intra-abdominal infection: 20 mg/kg IV q 8 h for age 3 mo or older; 1 g IV q 8 h for wt greater than 50 kg. Complicated skin infections: 10 mg/kg IV q 8 h for age 3 mo or older; 500 mg IV q 8 h for wt greater than 50 kg.
UNAPPROVED ADULTS – Meningitis: 40 mg/kg (max 2 g) IV q 8 h. Hospital-acquired pneumonia, complicated UTI, malignant otitis externa: 1 g IV q 8 h.
UNAPPROVED PEDS – Infant wt greater than 2 kg: 20 mg/kg IV q 12 h for age younger than 1 week old, q 8 h for 1 to 4 weeks old.
NOTES – Possible cross-sensitivity with other beta-lactams; C. difficile-associated diarrhea; superinfection; seizures; thrombocytopenia in renal dysfunction. For adults with renal dysfunction: Give 50% of normal dose q 24 h for CrCl < 10 mL/min, 50% of normal dose q 12 h for CrCl 10 to 25 mL/min, normal dose q 12 h for CrCl 26 to 50 mL/min.
MOA – Beta-lactam resistant to hydrolysis by most beta-lactamases, including extended-spectrum beta-lactamases.
ADVERSE EFFECTS – Serious: Cross-sensitivity with other beta-lactams, C. difficile-associated diarrhea, superinfection, seizures, thrombocytopenia in renal dysfunction. Frequent: Diarrhea.

ANTIMICROBIALS: Cephalosporins—1st Generation

NOTE: Cephalosporins are second-line to penicillins for group A strep pharyngitis, can be cross-sensitive with penicillins, and can cause C. difficile associated diarrhea.

CEFADROXIL (*Duricef*) ▶K ♀B ▶+ $$$
ADULTS – Simple UTI: 1 to 2 g/day PO divided once daily to bid. Other UTIs: 1 g PO bid. Skin infections: 1 g/day PO divided once daily to bid. Group A strep pharyngitis: 1 g/day PO divided once daily to bid for 10 days.
PEDS – UTIs, Skin infections: 30 mg/kg/day PO divided bid. Group A streptococcal pharyngitis/tonsillitis, impetigo: 30 mg/kg/day PO divided once daily to bid. Treat pharyngitis for 10 days.
FORMS – Generic/Trade: Tabs 1 g. Caps 500 mg. Susp 125, 250, 500 mg/5 mL.
NOTES – Renal dysfunction in adults: 500 mg PO q 36 h for CrCl < 10 mL/min; 500 mg PO q 24 h for CrCl 11 to 25 mL/min; 1 g load then 500 mg PO q 12 h for CrCl 26 to 50 mL/min.
MOA – Beta-lactam antibiotic that inhibits the biosynthesis of cell wall mucopeptide. (Beta-lactam fused to different ring structure from penicillins.)
ADVERSE EFFECTS – Serious: Cross-sensitivity with penicillins, C. difficile-associated diarrhea. Frequent: diarrhea.

CEFAZOLIN (*Ancef*) ▶K ♀B ▶+ $$
ADULTS – Pneumonia, sepsis, endocarditis, skin, bone and joint, genital infections. Mild infections due to gram-positive cocci: 250 to 500 mg IM/IV q 8 h. Moderate/severe infections: 0.5 to 1 g IM/IV q

(cont.)

ANTIMICROBIALS: Cephalosporins

CEFAZOLIN (cont.)
6 to 8 h. Life-threatening infections: 1 to 1.5 g IV q 6 h. Simple UTI: 1 g IM/IV q 12 h. Pneumococcal pneumonia: 500 mg IM/IV q 12 h. Surgical prophylaxis: 1 g IM/IV 30 to 60 min preop, additional 0.5 to 1 g during surgery longer than 2 h, and 0.5 to 1 g q 6 to 8 h for 24 h postop. See table for prophylaxis of bacterial endocarditis.
PEDS — Pneumonia, sepsis, endocarditis, skin, bone and joint infections. Mild/moderate infections: 25 to 50 mg/kg/day IM/IV divided q 6 to 8 h for age 1 mo or older. Severe infections: 100 mg/kg/day IV divided q 6 to 8 h for age 1 mo or older. See table for prophylaxis of bacterial endocarditis.
NOTES — Dose reduction for renal dysfunction in adults: Usual first dose, then 50% of usual dose q 18 to 24 h for CrCl < 10 mL/min; 50% of usual dose q 12 h for CrCl 11 to 34 mL/min; usual dose q 8 h for CrCl 35 to 54 mL/min. Dose reduction for renal dysfunction in children: Usual first dose, then 10% of usual dose q 24 h for CrCl 5 to 20 mL/min; 25% of usual dose q 12 h for CrCl 20 to 40 mL/min; 60% of usual dose q 12 h for CrCl 40 to 70 mL/min.
MOA — Beta-lactam antibiotic that inhibits the biosynthesis of cell wall mucopeptide. (Beta-lactam fused to different ring structure from penicillins.)
ADVERSE EFFECTS — Serious: Cross-sensitivity with penicillins, C. difficile-associated diarrhea. Frequent: Hypersensitivity.

CEPHALEXIN (*Keflex, Panixine DisperDose*) ▶K ♀B ▶? $$$
ADULTS — Pneumonia, bone, GU infections. Usual dose: 250 to 500 mg PO qid. Max: 4 g/day. Group A strep pharyngitis, skin infections, simple UTI: 500 mg PO bid. Treat pharyngitis for 10 days. See table for prophylaxis of bacterial endocarditis.
PEDS — Pneumonia, GU, bone, skin infections, group A strep pharyngitis. Usual dose: 25 to 50 mg/kg/day PO in divided doses. Max dose: 100 mg/kg/day. Can give bid for strep pharyngitis in children older than 1 yo, skin infections. Group A strep pharyngitis, skin infections, simple UTI in patients older than 15 yo: 500 mg PO bid. Treat pharyngitis for 10 days. Not for otitis media, sinusitis.
FORMS — Generic/Trade: Caps 250, 500 mg. Generic only: Tabs 250, 500 mg. Susp 125, 250 mg/5 mL. Panixine DisperDose 125, 250 mg scored tabs for oral susp. Trade only: Caps 333, 750 mg.
NOTES — Mix Panixine tab with 2 tsp water and drink mixture, then rinse container with a little water and drink that. Do not chew or swallow tab whole. Use only for doses that can be delivered by half or whole tabs.
MOA — Beta-lactam antibiotic that inhibits the biosynthesis of cell wall mucopeptide. (Beta-lactam fused to different ring structure from penicillins.)
ADVERSE EFFECTS — Serious: Cross-sensitivity with penicillins, C. difficile-associated diarrhea. Frequent: Eosinophilia.

ANTIMICROBIALS: Cephalosporins—2nd Generation

NOTE: Cephalosporins are second-line to penicillins for group A strep pharyngitis, can be cross-sensitive with penicillins, and can cause C. difficile associated diarrhea.

CEFACLOR (*Ceclor, Raniclor*) ▶K ♀B ▶? $$$$
ADULTS — Otitis media, pneumonia, group A strep pharyngitis, UTI, skin infections: 250 to 500 mg PO tid. Treat pharyngitis for 10 days.
PEDS — Pneumonia, group A streptococcal pharyngitis, UTI, skin infections: 20 to 40 mg/kg/day (up to 1 g/day) PO divided bid for pharyngitis, tid for other infections. Treat pharyngitis for 10 days. Otitis media: 40 mg/kg/day PO divided bid.
FORMS — Generic only: Caps 250, 500 mg, Susp, Chewable tabs 125, 187, 250, 375 mg per 5 mL or tab.
MOA — Beta-lactam antibiotic that inhibits the biosynthesis of cell wall mucopeptide. (Beta-lactam fused to different ring structure from penicillins.)
ADVERSE EFFECTS — Serious: Cross-sensitivity with penicillins, C. difficile-associated diarrhea; serum sickness-like reactions with repeated use. Frequent: Headache.

CEFOTETAN ▶K/Bile ♀B ▶??
ADULTS — Usual dose: 1 to 2 g IM/IV q 12 h. UTI: 0.5 to 2 g IM/IV q 12 h or 1 to 2 g IM/IV q 24 h. Pneumonia, gynecologic, intra-abdominal, bone and joint infections: 1 to 3 g IM/IV q 12 h. Skin infections: 1 to 2 g IM/IV q 12 h or 2 g IV q 24 h. Surgical prophylaxis: 1 to 2 g IV 30 to 60 min preop. Give after cord clamp for C-section.
PEDS — Not approved in children.
UNAPPROVED PEDS — Usual dose: 40 to 80 mg/kg/day IV divided q 12 h.
NOTES — Hemolytic anemia (higher risk than other cephalosporins), clotting impairment rarely. Disulfiram-like reaction with alcohol. Dosing reduction in adults with renal dysfunction: Usual dose q 48 h for CrCl < 10 mL/min; usual dose q 24 h for CrCl 10 to 30 mL/min.
MOA — Beta-lactam antibiotic that inhibits the biosynthesis of cell wall mucopeptide. (Beta-lactam fused to different ring structure from penicillins.) Cefotetan has MTT side-chain.
ADVERSE EFFECTS — Serious: Cross-sensitivity with penicillins, C. difficile-associated diarrhea, hemolytic anemia, clotting impairment rarely, disulfiram-like reaction with alcohol.

CEFOXITIN (*Mefoxin*) ▶K ♀B ▶+ $$$$$
ADULTS — Pneumonia, UTI, sepsis, intra-abdominal, gynecologic, skin, bone and joint infections: Uncomplicated, 1 g IV q 6 to 8 h. Moderate to severe, 1 g IV q 4 h or 2 g IV q 6 to 8 h. Infections requiring high doses, 2 g IV q 4 h or 3 g IV q 6 h.

(cont.)

ANTIMICROBIALS: Cephalosporins

SEXUALLY TRANSMITTED DISEASES & VAGINITIS*

Bacterial vaginosis: (1) metronidazole 5 g of 0.75% gel intravaginally daily for 5 days OR 500 mg PO bid for 7 days. (2) clindamycin 5 g of 2% cream intravaginally at bedtime for 7 days. In pregnancy: (1) metronidazole 500 mg PO bid for 7 days OR 250 mg PO tid for 7 days. (2) clindamycin 300 mg PO bid for 7 days.

Candidal vaginitis: (1) intravaginal clotrimazole, miconazole, terconazole, nystatin, tioconazole, or butoconazole. (2) fluconazole 150 mg PO single dose.

Chancroid: Single dose of: (1) azithromycin 1 g PO or (2) ceftriaxone 250 mg IM.

Chlamydia: First line either azithromycin 1 g PO single dose or doxycycline 100 mg PO bid for 7 days. Second line fluoroquinolones or erythromycin. In pregnancy: (1) azithromycin 1 g PO single dose. (2) amoxicillin 500 mg PO tid for 7 days. Repeat NAAT[‡] 3 weeks after treatment.

Epididymitis: (1) ceftriaxone 250 mg IM single dose + doxycycline 100 mg PO bid for 10 days. (2) ofloxacin 300 mg PO bid or levofloxacin 500 mg PO daily for 10 days if enteric organisms suspected, or negative gonococcal culture or NAAT.[†]

Gonorrhea: Single dose of: (1) ceftriaxone 125 mg IM (2) cefixime 400 mg PO (not for pharyngeal).[§,†] Treat chlamydia empirically.

Gonorrhea, disseminated: Initially treat with ceftriaxone 1 g IM/IV q 24 h until 24 to 48 h after improvement. Second-line alternatives: (1) cefotaxime 1 g IV q 8 h. (2) ceftizoxime 1 g IV q 8 h.[§] Complete 1 week of treatment with: (1) cefixime tabs 400 mg PO bid. (2) cefixime susp 500 mg PO bid. (3) cefpodoxime 400 mg PO bid.[†]

Gonorrhea, meningitis: ceftriaxone 1 to 2 g IV q 12 h for 10 to 14 days.[§]

Gonorrhea, endocarditis: ceftriaxone 1 to 2 g IV q 12 h for at least 4 weeks.[§]

Granuloma inguinale: doxycycline 100 mg PO bid for at least 3 weeks and until lesions completely healed. Alternative azithromycin 1 g PO once weekly for 3 weeks.

Herpes simplex (genital, first episode): (1) acyclovir 400 mg PO tid for 7 to 10 days. (2) famciclovir 250 mg PO tid for 7 to 10 days. (3) valacyclovir 1 g PO bid for 7 to 10 days.

Herpes simplex (genital, recurrent): (1) acyclovir 400 mg PO tid for 5 days. (2) acyclovir 800 mg PO tid for 2 days or bid for 5 days. (3) famciclovir 125 mg PO bid for 5 days. (4) famciclovir 1 g PO bid for 1 day. (5) valacyclovir 500 mg PO bid for 3 days. (6) valacyclovir 1 g PO daily for 5 days.

Herpes simplex (suppressive therapy): (1) acyclovir 400 mg PO bid. (2) famciclovir 250 mg PO bid. (3) valacyclovir 500 to 1000 mg PO daily.

Herpes simplex (genital, recurrent in HIV infection): (1) Acyclovir 400 mg PO tid for 5 to 10 days. (2) famciclovir 500 mg PO bid for 5 to 10 days. (3) Valacyclovir 1 g PO bid for 5 to 10 days.

Herpes simplex (suppressive therapy in HIV infection): (1) Acyclovir 400 to 800 mg PO bid to tid. (2) Famciclovir 500 mg PO bid. (3) Valacyclovir 500 mg PO bid.

Herpes simplex (prevention of transmission in immunocompetent patients with not more than 9 recurrences/year): Valacyclovir 500 mg PO daily by source partner, in conjunction with safer sex practices.

Lymphogranuloma venereum: (1) doxycycline 100 mg PO bid for 21 days. Alternative: erythromycin base 500 mg PO qid for 21 days.

Pelvic inflammatory disease (PID), inpatient regimens: (1) cefoxitin 2 g IV q6h + doxycycline 100 mg IV/PO q 12 h. (2) clindamycin 900 mg IV q 8 h + gentamicin 2 mg/kg IM/IV loading dose, then 1.5 mg/kg IM/IV q 8 h (See gentamicin entry for alternative daily dosing). Can switch to PO therapy within 24 h of improvement.

Pelvic inflammatory disease (PID), outpatient treatment: (1) ceftriaxone 250 mg IM single dose + doxycycline 100 mg PO bid +/− metronidazole 500 mg PO bid for 14 days.

Proctitis, proctocolitis, enteritis: ceftriaxone 125 mg IM single dose + doxycycline 100 mg PO bid for 7 days.

Sexual assault prophylaxis: ceftriaxone 125 mg IM single dose + metronidazole 2 g PO single dose + azithromycin 1 g PO single dose/doxycycline 100 mg PO bid for 7 days. Consider giving antiemetic.

Syphilis (primary and secondary): (1) benzathine penicillin 2.4 million units IM single dose. (2) doxycycline 100 mg PO bid for 2 weeks if penicillin-allergic.

Syphilis (early latent, i.e. duration less than 1 year): (1) benzathine penicillin 2.4 million units IM single dose. (2) doxycycline 100 mg PO bid for 2 weeks if penicillin-allergic.

Syphilis (late latent or unknown duration): (1) benzathine penicillin 2.4 million units IM q week for 3 doses. (2) doxycycline 100 mg PO bid for 4 weeks if penicillin-allergic.

Syphilis (tertiary): (1) benzathine penicillin 2.4 million units IM q week for 3 doses. (2) doxycycline 100 mg PO bid for 4 weeks if penicillin-allergic.

Syphilis (neuro): (1) penicillin G 18 to 24 million units/day continuous IV infusion or 3 to 4 million units IV q 4 h for 10 to 14 days. (2) procaine penicillin 2.4 million units IM daily + probenecid 500 mg PO qid, both for 10 to 14 days.

Syphilis in pregnancy: Treat only with penicillin regimen for stage of syphilis as noted above. Use penicillin desensitization protocol if penicillin-allergic.

(cont.)

ANTIMICROBIALS: Cephalosporins

SEXUALLY TRANSMITTED DISEASES & VAGINITIS* (cont.)

Trichomoniasis: metronidazole (can use in pregnancy) or tinidazole, each 2 g PO single dose.
Urethritis, Cervicitis: Test for Chlamydia and gonorrhea with NAAT.[‡] Treat based on test results or treat presumptively if high-risk of infection (Chlamydia: age 25 yo or younger, new/multiple sex partners, or unprotected sex. Gonorrhea: population prevalence greater than 5%), esp. if NAAT[‡] unavailable or patient unlikely to return for follow-up.
Urethritis (persistent/recurrent): metronidazole/ tinidazole 2 g PO single dose + azithromycin 2 g PO single dose (if not used in first episode).

*MMWR 2006;55:RR-11 or http://www.cdc.gov/STD/treatment/. Treat sexual partners for all except herpes, candida, and bacterial vaginosis.
[†]As of April 2007, the CDC no longer recommends fluoroquinolones for gonorrhea because of high resistance rates. Do not consider fluoroquinolone unless antimicrobial susceptibility can be documented by culture. If parenteral cephalosporin not feasible for PID (and NAAT is negative or culture documents fluoroquinolone susceptibility), can consider levofloxacin 500 mg PO once daily or ofloxacin 400 mg PO bid +/− metronidazole 500 mg PO bid for 14 days.
[‡]NAAT = nucleic acid amplification test.
§Cephalosporin desensitization advised for cephalosporin-allergic patients (e.g. pregnant women).

CEFOXITIN (cont.)
Uncontaminated GI surgery, vaginal/abdominal hysterectomy: 2 g IV 30 to 60 min preop, then 2 g IV q 6 h for 24 h. C-section: 2 g IV after cord clamped or 2 g IV q 4 h for 3 doses with first dose given after cord clamped.
PEDS — Pneumonia, UTI, sepsis, intra-abdominal, skin, bone and joint infections: 80 to 160 mg/kg/day (up to 12 g/day) IV divided into 4 to 6 doses for age 3 mo or older. Mild-moderate infections: 80 to 100 mg/kg/day IV divided into 3 to 4 doses. Surgical prophylaxis: 30 to 40 mg/kg IV 30 to 60 min preop; additional doses can be given q 6 h up to 24 h postop.
NOTES — Eosinophilia and increased AST with high doses in children. Dosing reduction in adults with renal dysfunction: Load with 1 to 2 g IV then 0.5 g IV q 24 to 48 h for CrCl < 5 mL/min, 0.5 to 1 g IV q 12 to 24 h for CrCl 5 to 9 mL/min, 1 to 2 g IV q 12 to 24 h for CrCl 10 to 29 mL/min, 1 to 2 g IV q 8 to 12 h for CrCl 30 to 50 mL/min. Give 1 to 2 g supplemental dose after each hemodialysis.
MOA — Beta-lactam antibiotic that inhibits the biosynthesis of cell wall mucopeptide. (Beta-lactam fused to different ring structure from penicillins.)
ADVERSE EFFECTS — Serious: Cross-sensitivity with penicillins, C. difficile-associated diarrhea, eosinophilia & increased AST with high doses in children.

CEFPROZIL (*Cefzil*) ▶K ♀B ▶+ $$$$
ADULTS — Group A strep pharyngitis: 500 mg PO once daily for 10 days. Sinusitis: 250 to 500 mg PO bid. Acute exacerbation of chronic/secondary infection of acute bronchitis: 500 mg PO bid. Skin infections: 250 to 500 mg PO bid or 500 mg PO once daily.
PEDS — Otitis media: 15 mg/kg/dose PO bid. Group A strep pharyngitis: 7.5 mg/kg/dose PO bid for 10 days. Sinusitis: 7.5 to 15 mg/kg/dose PO bid. Skin infections: 20 mg/kg PO once daily. Use adult dose for age 13 yo or older.
FORMS — Generic/Trade: Tabs 250, 500 mg. Susp 125, 250 mg/5 mL.
NOTES — Give 50% of usual dose at usual interval for CrCl < 30 mL/min.

MOA — Beta-lactam antibiotic that inhibits the biosynthesis of cell wall mucopeptide. (Beta-lactam fused to different ring structure from penicillins.)
ADVERSE EFFECTS — Serious: Cross-sensitivity with penicillins, C. difficile-associated diarrhea, may cause serum sickness reaction. Frequent: None.

CEFUROXIME (*Zinacef, Ceftin*) ▶K ♀B ▶? $$$
ADULTS — Uncomplicated pneumonia, simple UTI, skin infections, disseminated Gonorrhea: 750 mg IM/IV q 8 h. Bone and joint or severe/complicated infections: 1.5 g IV q 8 h. Sepsis: 1.5 g IV q 6 h to 3 g IV q 8 h. Gonorrhea: 1.5 g IM single dose split into 2 injections, given with probenecid 1 g PO. Surgical prophylaxis: 1.5 g IV 30 to 60 min preop, then 750 mg IM/IV q 8 h for prolonged procedures. Open heart surgery: 1.5 g IV q 12 h for 4 doses with first dose at induction of anesthesia. Cefuroxime axetil tabs: Group A strep pharyngitis, acute sinusitis: 250 mg PO bid for 10 days. Acute exacerbation of chronic/secondary infection of acute bronchitis, skin infections: 250 to 500 mg PO bid. Lyme disease: 500 mg PO bid for 14 days for early disease, for 28 days for Lyme arthritis. Simple UTI: 125 to 250 mg PO bid. Gonorrhea: 1 g PO single dose.
PEDS — Most infections: 50 to 100 mg/kg/day IM/IV divided q 6 to 8 h. Bone and joint infections: 150 mg/kg/day IM/IV divided q 8 h (up to adult dose). Cefuroxime axetil tabs: Group A strep pharyngitis: 125 mg PO bid for 10 days. Otitis media, sinusitis: 250 mg PO bid for 10 days. Cefuroxime axetil oral susp. Group A strep pharyngitis: 20 mg/kg/day (up to 500 mg/day) PO divided bid for 10 days. Otitis media, sinusitis, impetigo: 30 mg/kg/day (up to 1 g/day) PO divided bid for 10 days. Use adult dose for age 13 yo or older.
UNAPPROVED PEDS — Lyme disease: 30 mg/kg/day PO divided bid (max 500 mg/dose) for 14 days for early disease, for 28 days for Lyme arthritis. Community-acquired pneumonia: 150 mg/kg/day IV divided q 8 h.

(cont.)

CEFUROXIME (cont.)
  FORMS — Generic/Trade: Tabs 125, 250, 500 mg. Susp 125, 250 mg/5 mL.
  NOTES — AAP recommends 5 to 7 days of therapy for children age 6 yo or older with nonsevere otitis media, and 10 days for younger children and those with severe disease. Dosage reduction for renal dysfunction in adults: 750 mg IM/IV q 24 h for CrCl < 10 mL/min, 750 mg IM/IV q 12 h for CrCl 10 to 20 mL/min. Give supplemental dose after hemodialysis. Tabs and susp not bioequivalent on mg/mg basis. Do not crush tabs.
  MOA — Beta-lactam antibiotic that inhibits the biosynthesis of cell wall mucopeptide. (Beta-lactam fused to different ring structure from penicillins.)
  ADVERSE EFFECTS — Serious: Cross-sensitivity with penicillins, C. difficile-associated diarrhea. Frequent: Anemia, eosinophilia.

ANTIMICROBIALS: Cephalosporins—3rd Generation

NOTE: Cephalosporins are second-line to penicillins for group A strep pharyngitis, can be cross-sensitive with penicillins, and can cause C. difficile associated diarrhea.

CEFDINIR (*Omnicef*) ▶K ♀B ▶? $$$$
  ADULTS — Community-acquired pneumonia, skin infections: 300 mg PO bid for 10 days. Sinusitis: 600 mg PO once daily or 300 mg PO bid for 10 days. Group A strep pharyngitis, acute exacerbation of chronic bronchitis: 600 mg PO once daily for 10 days or 300 mg PO bid for 5 to 10 days.
  PEDS — Group A strep pharyngitis, otitis media: 14 mg/kg/day PO divided bid for 5 to 10 days or once daily for 10 days. Sinusitis: 14 mg/kg/day PO divided once daily or bid for 10 days. Skin infections: 14 mg/kg/day PO divided bid for 10 days. Use adult dose for age 13 yo or older.
  FORMS — Generic/Trade: Caps 300 mg. Susp 125, 250 mg/5 mL.
  NOTES — AAP recommends 5 to 7 days of therapy for children age 6 yo or older with non-severe otitis media, and 10 days for younger children and those with severe disease. Give iron, multivitamins with iron, or antacids at least 2 h before or after cefdinir. Complexation of cefdinir with iron may turn stools red. Reduce dose for renal dysfunction: 300 mg PO daily for adults with CrCl < 30 mL/min. 7 mg/kg/day PO once daily up to 300 mg/day for children with CrCl < 30 mL/min. Hemodialysis: 300 mg or 7 mg/kg PO after hemodialysis, then 300 mg or 7 mg/kg PO q 48 h.
  MOA — Beta-lactam antibiotic that inhibits the biosynthesis of cell wall mucopeptide. (Beta-lactam fused to different ring structure from penicillins.)
  ADVERSE EFFECTS — Serious: Cross-sensitivity with penicillins, C. difficile-associated diarrhea. Frequent: Diarrhea.

CEFDITOREN (*Spectracef*) ▶K ♀B ▶? $$$$$
  ADULTS — Skin infections, group A strep pharyngitis: 200 mg PO bid for 10 days. Give 400 mg bid for 10 days for acute exacerbation of chronic bronchitis, for 14 days for community-acquired pneumonia. Take with food.
  PEDS — Not approved for children younger than 12 yo. Skin infections, group A strep pharyngitis, adolescents age 12 yo or older: 200 mg PO bid with food for 10 days.
  FORMS — Trade only: Tabs 200, 400 mg.
  NOTES — Contraindicated if milk protein allergy or carnitine deficiency. Not for long-term use due to potential risk of carnitine deficiency. Do not take with drugs that reduce gastric acid (antacids, H2 blockers, etc). Dosage adjustment for renal dysfunction: Max 200 mg bid if CrCl 30 to 49 mL/min; max 200 mg once daily if CrCl < 30 mL/min.
  MOA — Beta-lactam antibiotic that inhibits the biosynthesis of cell wall mucopeptide. (Beta-lactam fused to different ring structure from penicillins.)
  ADVERSE EFFECTS — Serious: Cross-sensitivity with penicillins, C. difficile-associated diarrhea. Frequent: N/V, diarrhea.

CEFIXIME (*Suprax*) ▶K/Bile ♀B ▶? $$
  ADULTS — Simple UTI, pharyngitis, acute bacterial bronchitis, acute exacerbation of chronic bronchitis: 400 mg PO once daily. Gonorrhea: 400 mg PO single dose.
  PEDS — Otitis media: 8 mg/kg/day susp PO divided once daily to bid. Pharyngitis: 8 mg/kg/day PO divided once daily to bid for 10 days. Use adult dose for wt greater than 50 kg or age 13 yo or older.
  UNAPPROVED ADULTS — Disseminated gonorrhea, CDC regimen: 500 mg PO bid of susp or 400 mg PO bid of tabs. See STD table.
  UNAPPROVED PEDS — Febrile UTI (3 to 24 mo): 16 mg/kg PO on first day, then 8 mg/kg PO daily to complete 14 days. Gonorrhea: 8 mg/kg (max 400 mg) PO single dose for wt less than 45 kg, 400 mg PO single dose for 45 kg or greater.
  FORMS — Trade only: Susp 100, 200 mg/5 mL. Tabs 400 mg.
  NOTES — Poor activity against S aureus. Increased INR with warfarin. May increase carbamazepine levels. Susp stable at room temp or refrigerated for 14 days. Reduce dose in renal dysfunction: 75% of usual dose at usual interval for CrCl 21 to 60 mL/min or hemodialysis. 50% of usual dose at usual interval for CrCl < 20 mL/min or continuous peritoneal dialysis.
  MOA — Beta-lactam antibiotic that inhibits the biosynthesis of cell wall mucopeptide. (Beta-lactam fused to different ring structure from penicillins.)
  ADVERSE EFFECTS — Serious: Cross-sensitivity with penicillins, C. difficile-associated diarrhea. Frequent: N/V, diarrhea.

ANTIMICROBIALS: Cephalosporins

CEPHALOSPORINS – GENERAL ANTIMICROBIAL SPECTRUM

1st generation: gram positive (including Staph aureus); basic gram neg. coverage
2nd generation: diminished Staph aureus, improved gram negative coverage compared to 1st generation; some with anaerobic coverage
3rd generation: further diminished Staph aureus, further improved gram negative coverage compared to 1st & 2nd generation; some with Pseudomonal coverage & diminished gram positive coverage
4th generation: same as 3rd generation plus coverage against Pseudomonas

CEFOTAXIME (Claforan) ▶KL ♀B ▶+ $$$$$
ADULTS – Pneumonia, sepsis, GU and gynecologic, skin, intra-abdominal, bone and joint infections: Uncomplicated, 1 g IM/IV q 12 h. Moderate/severe, 1 to 2 g IM/IV q 8 h. Infections usually requiring high doses, 2 g IV q 6 to 8 h. Life-threatening, 2 g IV q 4 h. Meningitis: 2 g IV q 4 to 6 h. Gonorrhea: 0.5 to 1 g IM single dose.
PEDS – Pneumonia, sepsis, GU, skin, intra-abdominal, bone/joint, CNS infections: Labeled dose: 50 mg/kg/dose IV q 12 h for age younger than 1 week old; 50 mg/kg/dose IV q 8 h for age 1 to 4 weeks, 50 to 180 mg/kg/day IM/IV divided q 4 to 6 h for age 1 mo to 12 yo. AAP recommends 225 to 300 mg/kg/day IV divided q 6 to 8 h for S pneumoniae meningitis. Mild to moderate infections: 75 to 100 mg/kg/day IV/IM divided q 6 to 8 h. Severe infections: 150 to 200 mg/kg/day IV/IM divided q 6 to 8 h.
UNAPPROVED ADULTS – Disseminated gonorrhea, CDC regimen: 1 g IV q 8 h.
NOTES – Bolus injection through central venous catheter can cause arrhythmias. Decrease dose by 50% for CrCl < 20 mL/min.
MOA – Beta-lactam antibiotic that inhibits the biosynthesis of cell wall mucopeptide. (Beta-lactam fused to different ring structure from penicillins.)
ADVERSE EFFECTS – Serious: Cross-sensitivity with penicillins, C. difficile-associated diarrhea. Frequent: Coombs + anemia, phlebitis.

CEFPODOXIME (Vantin) ▶K ♀B ▶? $$$$
ADULTS – Acute exacerbation of chronic bronchitis, acute sinusitis: 200 mg PO bid for 10 days. Community-acquired pneumonia: 200 mg PO bid for 14 days. Group A strep pharyngitis: 100 mg PO bid for 5 to 10 days. Skin infections: 400 mg PO bid for 7 to 14 days. Simple UTI: 100 mg PO bid for 7 days. Gonorrhea: 200 mg PO single dose. Give tabs with food.
PEDS – 5 mg/kg PO bid for 5 days for otitis media, for 5 to 10 days for group A strep pharyngitis, for 10 days for sinusitis. Use adult dose for age 12 yo or older.
FORMS – Generic/Trade: Tabs 100, 200 mg. Susp 50, 100 mg/5 mL.
NOTES – AAP recommends 5 to 7 days of therapy for children age 6 yo or older with nonsevere otitis media, and 10 days for younger children and those with severe disease. Do not give antacids within 2 h before/after cefpodoxime. Reduce dose in renal dysfunction: Increase dosing interval to q 24 h for CrCl < 30 mL/min. Give 3 times a week after dialysis session for hemodialysis patients. Susp stable for 14 days refrigerated.
MOA – Beta-lactam antibiotic that inhibits the biosynthesis of cell wall mucopeptide. (Beta-lactam fused to different ring structure from penicillins.)
ADVERSE EFFECTS – Serious: Cross-sensitivity with penicillins; C. difficile-associated diarrhea; acute hepatitis, bloody diarrhea, and pulmonary infiltrates (rare). Frequent: Diarrhea.

CEFTAZIDIME (Ceptaz, Fortaz, Tazicef) ▶K ♀B ▶+ $$$$$
ADULTS – Simple UTI: 250 mg IM/IV q 12 h. Complicated UTI: 500 mg IM/IV q 8 to 12 h. Uncomplicated pneumonia, mild skin infections: 500 mg to 1 g IM/IV q 8 h. Serious gynecologic, intra-abdominal, bone and joint, life-threatening infections, meningitis, empiric therapy of neutropenic fever: 2 g IV q 8 h. Pseudomonas lung infections in cystic fibrosis: 30 to 50 mg/kg IV q 8 h (up to 6 g/day).
PEDS – Use sodium formulations in children (Fortaz, Tazicef). UTIs, pneumonia, skin, intra-abdominal, bone and joint infections: 100 to 150 mg/kg/day (up to 6 g/day) IV divided q 8 h for age 1 mo to 12 yo. Meningitis: 150 mg/kg/day (up to 6 g/day) IV divided q 8 h for age 1 mo to 12 yo; 30 mg/kg IV q 12 h for age younger than 4 weeks old. Use adult dose and formulations for age 12 yo or older.
UNAPPROVED ADULTS – P aeruginosa osteomyelitis of the foot from nail puncture: 2 g IV q 8 h.
UNAPPROVED PEDS – AAP recommends 50 mg/kg IV q 8 to 12 h for age younger than 1 week and wt greater than 2 kg, q 8 h for age 1 week old or older.
NOTES – High levels in renal dysfunction can cause CNS toxicity. Reduce dose in adults with renal dysfunction: load with 1 g then 500 mg q 48 h for CrCl < 5 mL/min; load with 1 g then 500 mg q 24 h for CrCl 6 to 15 mL/min; 1 g IV q 24 h for CrCl 16 to 30 mL/min; 1 g IV q 12 h for CrCl 31 to 50 mL/min. 1 g IV load in hemodialysis patients, then 1 g IV after hemodialysis sessions.
MOA – Beta-lactam antibiotic that inhibits the biosynthesis of cell wall mucopeptide. (Beta-lactam fused to different ring structure from penicillins.)
ADVERSE EFFECTS – Serious: Cross-sensitivity with penicillins, C. difficile-associated diarrhea, CNS toxicity with high levels in patients with renal dysfunction. Frequent: Coombs + anemia, eosinophilia, increased LFTs.

ANTIMICROBIALS: Cephalosporins

CEFTIBUTEN (*Cedax*) ▶K ♀B ▶? $$$$$
ADULTS — Group A strep pharyngitis, acute exacerbation of chronic bronchitis, otitis media not due to S pneumoniae: 400 mg PO once daily for 10 days.
PEDS — Group A strep pharyngitis, otitis media not due to S pneumoniae, age 6 mo or older: 9 mg/kg (up to 400 mg) PO once daily. Give susp on empty stomach.
FORMS — Trade only: Caps 400 mg. Susp 90 mg/5 mL.
NOTES — Poor activity against S aureus and S pneumoniae. Reduce dose in adults with renal dysfunction: 100 mg PO daily for CrCl 5 to 29 mL/min; 200 mg PO once daily for CrCl 30 to 49 mL/min. Reduce dose in children with renal dysfunction: 2.25 mg/kg PO once daily for CrCl 5 to 29 mL/min; 4.5 mg/kg PO once daily for CrCl 30 to 49 mL/min. Hemodialysis: Adults 400 mg PO and children 9 mg/kg PO after each dialysis session. Susp stable for 14 days refrigerated.
MOA — Beta-lactam antibiotic that inhibits the biosynthesis of cell wall mucopeptide. (Beta-lactam fused to different ring structure from penicillins.)
ADVERSE EFFECTS — Serious: Cross-sensitivity with penicillins, C. difficile-associated diarrhea. Frequent: Eosinophilia, nausea.

CEFTIZOXIME (*Cefizox*) ▶K ♀B ▶? $$$$$
ADULTS — Simple UTI: 500 mg IM/IV q 12 h. Pneumonia, sepsis, intra-abdominal, skin, bone and joint infections: 1 to 2 g IM/IV q 8 to 12 h. Pelvic inflammatory disease: 2 g IV q 8 h. Life-threatening infections: 3 to 4 g IV q 8 h. Gonorrhea: 1 g IM single dose. Split 2 g IM dose into 2 injections.
PEDS — Pneumonia, sepsis, intra-abdominal, skin, bone and joint infections: 50 mg/kg/dose IV q 6 to 8 h for age 6 mo or older. Up to 200 mg/kg/day for serious infections, not to exceed max adult dose.
UNAPPROVED PEDS — Gonorrhea, CDC regimens: 500 mg IM single dose for uncomplicated; 1 g IV q 8 h for disseminated infection.
NOTES — Can cause transient rise in eosinophils, ALT, AST, CPK in children. Not for meningitis. Dosing in adults with renal dysfunction: For less severe infection load with 500 mg to 1 g IM/IV, then 500 mg q 8 h for CrCl 50 to 79 mL/min, 250 to 500 mg q 12 h for CrCl 5 to 49 mL/min, 500 mg q 48 h or 250 mg q 24 h for hemodialysis. For life-threatening infection, give loading dose, then 750 mg to 1.5 g IV q 8 h for CrCl 50 to 79 mL/min, 500 mg to 1 g q 12 h for CrCl 5 to 49 mL/min, 500 mg to 1 g q 48 h or 500 mg q 24 h for hemodialysis. For hemodialysis patients, give dose at end of dialysis.
MOA — Beta-lactam antibiotic that inhibits the biosynthesis of cell wall mucopeptide. (Beta-lactam fused to different ring structure from penicillins.)
ADVERSE EFFECTS — Serious: Cross-sensitivity with penicillins, C. difficile-associated diarrhea. Can cause transient rise in eosinophils, ALT, AST, CPK in children. Frequent: None.

CEFTRIAXONE (*Rocephin*) ▶K/Bile ♀B ▶+ $$$
WARNING — Contraindicated in neonates who require (or are expected to require) IV calcium (including calcium in TPN); fatal lung/kidney precipitation of calcium ceftriaxone has been reported in neonates. In other patients, do not give ceftriaxone and calcium-containing solns simultaneously, but sequential administration is acceptable if lines are flushed with a compatible fluid between infusions. Do not dilute with Ringers/Hartmann's soln or TPN containing calcium.
ADULTS — Pneumonia, UTI, pelvic inflammatory disease (hospitalized), sepsis, meningitis, skin, bone and joint, intra-abdominal infections: Usual dose 1 to 2 g IM/IV q 24 h (max 4 g/day divided q 12 h). Gonorrhea: Single dose 125 mg IM (250 mg if ambulatory treatment of PID).
PEDS — Meningitis: 100 mg/kg/day (up to 4 g/day) IV divided q 12 to 24 h. Skin, pneumonia, other serious infections: 50 to 75 mg/kg/day (up to 2 g/day) IM/IV divided q 12 to 24 h. Otitis media: 50 mg/kg (up to 1 g) IM single dose.
UNAPPROVED ADULTS — Lyme disease carditis, meningitis: 2 g IV once daily for 14 days. Chancroid: 250 mg IM single dose. Disseminated gonorrhea: 1 g IM/IV q 24 h. Prophylaxis, invasive meningococcal disease: 250 mg IM single dose.
UNAPPROVED PEDS — Refractory otitis media (no response after 3 days of antibiotics): 50 mg/kg IM q 24 h for 3 doses. Lyme disease carditis, meningitis: 50 to 75 mg/kg IM/IV once daily (up to 2 g/day) for 14 days. Prophylaxis, invasive meningococcal disease: Single IM dose of 125 mg for age younger than 16 yo, 250 mg for age 16 yo or older. Gonorrhea: 125 mg IM single dose; use adult regimens in STD table if wt 45 kg or greater. Gonococcal bacteremia/arthritis: 50 mg/kg (max 1 g for wt 45 kg or less) IM/IV once daily for 7 days. Gonococcal ophthalmia neonatorum/gonorrhea prophylaxis in newborn: 25 to 50 mg/kg up to 125 mg IM/IV single dose at birth. Disseminated gonorrhea, infants: 25 to 50 mg/kg/day IM/IV once daily for 7 days. Typhoid fever: 50 to 75 mg/kg IM/IV once daily for 14 days.
NOTES — Literature supports use of 250 mg dose for uncomplicated gonorrhea. Can cause prolonged prothrombin time (due to vitamin K deficiency), biliary sludging/symptoms of gallbladder disease. Do not give to neonates with hyperbilirubinemia. Dilute in 1% lidocaine for IM use. Do not exceed 2 g/day in patients with both hepatic and renal dysfunction.
MOA — Beta-lactam antibiotic that inhibits the biosynthesis of cell wall mucopeptide. (Beta-lactam fused to different ring structure from penicillins.)
ADVERSE EFFECTS — Serious: Cross-sensitivity with penicillins, C. difficile-associated diarrhea, prolonged prothrombin time due to vitamin K deficiency, biliary sludging/symptoms of gallbladder disease, hemolytic anemia. Fatal precipitation with calcium in lungs/kidneys of neonates. Frequent: Eosinophilia.

ANTIMICROBIALS: Cephalosporins—4th Generation

NOTE: Cross-sensitivity with penicillins possible. May cause C. difficile-associated diarrhea.

CEFEPIME (*Maxipime*) ▶K ♀B ▶? $$$$$
- ADULTS – Mild, moderate UTI: 0.5 to 1 g IM/IV q 12 h. Severe UTI, skin, complicated intra-abdominal infections: 2 g IV q 12 h. Pneumonia: 1 to 2 g IV q 12 h. Empiric therapy of febrile neutropenia: 2 g IV q 8 h.
- PEDS – UTI, skin infections, pneumonia: 50 mg/kg IV q 12 h for wt 40 kg or less. Empiric therapy for febrile neutropenia: 50 mg/kg IV q 8 h for wt 40 kg or less. Do not exceed adult dose.
- UNAPPROVED ADULTS – P aeruginosa osteomyelitis of the foot from nail puncture: 2 g IV q 12 h. Meningitis: 2 g IV q 8 h.
- UNAPPROVED PEDS – Meningitis, cystic fibrosis, other serious infections: 50 mg/kg IV q 8 h up to 6 g/day).
- NOTES – An FDA safety review did not find higher mortality with cefepime than with other beta-lactams. High levels in renal dysfunction can cause CNS toxicity; dosing for CrCl < 60 mL/min in package insert.
- MOA – Beta-lactam antibiotic that inhibits the biosynthesis of cell wall mucopeptide. (Beta-lactam fused to different ring structure from penicillins.)
- ADVERSE EFFECTS – Serious: Cross-sensitivity with penicillins, C. difficile-associated diarrhea, CNS toxicity (encephalopathy, myoclonus, seizures) due to high levels of cefepime, especially in patients with renal dysfunction. An FDA safety review did not find higher mortality with cefepime than with other beta lactams. Frequent: Coombs + anemia.

ANTIMICROBIALS: Macrolides

NOTE: Macrolides can aggravate/precipitate myasthenia gravis. Contraindicated with pimozide. Monitor INR with warfarin.

AZITHROMYCIN (*Zithromax, Zmax*) ▶L ♀B ▶? $$
- ADULTS – Community-acquired pneumonia, inpatient: 500 mg IV over 1 h daily for at least 2 days, then 500 mg PO daily for 7 to 10 days total. Pelvic inflammatory disease: 500 mg IV daily for 1 to 2 days, then 250 mg PO daily to complete 7 days. Oral for acute exacerbation of chronic bronchitis, community-acquired pneumonia, Group A streptococcal pharyngitis (2nd line to penicillin), skin infections: 500 mg PO on first day, then 250 mg PO daily for 4 days. Acute sinusitis, alternative for acute exacerbation of chronic bronchitis: 500 mg PO daily for 3 days. Zmax for community-acquired pneumonia, acute sinusitis: 2 g PO single dose (contents of full bottle) on empty stomach. Chlamydia, chancroid: 1 g PO single dose. Gonorrhea: 2 g PO single dose. Observe patient for at least 30 min for poor GI tolerability. Prevention of disseminated Mycobacterium avium complex disease: 1200 mg PO once per week.
- PEDS – Oral for otitis media, community-acquired pneumonia: 10 mg/kg up to 500 mg PO on first day, then 5 mg/kg up to 250 mg PO daily for 4 days. Acute sinusitis: 10 mg/kg PO daily for 3 days. Zmax for community-acquired pneumonia or acute sinusitis: 60 mg/kg (max 2 g) PO single dose on empty stomach for age 6 mo or older; give adult dose of 2 g for wt 34 kg or greater. Otitis media: 30 mg/kg PO single dose or 10 mg/kg PO daily for 3 days. Group A streptococcal pharyngitis (2nd line to penicillin): 12 mg/kg up to 500 mg PO daily for 5 days. Take susp on empty stomach.
- UNAPPROVED ADULTS – See table for prophylaxis of bacterial endocarditis. Nongonococcal urethritis: 1 g PO single dose. See STD table for recurrent/persistent urethritis. Chlamydia in pregnancy: 1 g PO single dose. Campylobacter gastroenteritis: 500 mg PO daily for 3 days; for HIV-infected patients, treat for 7 days for mild/moderate disease, at least 14 days for bacteremia. Traveler's diarrhea: 500 mg PO on first day, then 250 mg PO daily for 4 days; or 1 g PO single dose. Mycobacterium avium complex disease treatment in AIDS: 500 mg PO daily (use at least 2 drugs for active infection). Pertussis treatment/postexposure prophylaxis: 500 mg PO on first day, then 250 mg PO daily for 4 days. Early primary/latent syphilis: 2 g PO single dose (CDC recommends only for penicillin-allergic nonpregnant patients; azithromycin treatment failures reported in the United States).
- UNAPPROVED PEDS – Prevention of disseminated Mycobacterium avium complex disease: 20 mg/kg PO once per week not to exceed adult dose. Mycobacterium avium complex disease treatment: 5 mg/kg PO daily (use at least 2 drugs for active infection). Cystic fibrosis and colonized with P aeruginosa, age 6 yo and older: 250 mg three times weekly for 24 weeks for wt less than 40 kg, 500 mg PO three times weekly for 24 weeks for wt 40 kg or greater. Chlamydia trachomatis: 1 g PO single dose for age younger than 8 yo and wt greater than 44 kg, and for age 8 yo or older for any wt. Pertussis treatment/postexposure prophylaxis: 10 mg/kg PO once daily for 5 days for infants younger than 6 mo; 10 mg/kg (max 500 mg) PO single dose on day 1, then 5 mg/kg (up to 250 mg) PO once daily for 4 days for age 6 mo or older. See table for bacterial endocarditis prophylaxis. Traveler's diarrhea: 5 to 10 mg/kg PO single dose. Cholera: 20 mg/kg up to 1 g PO single dose.
- FORMS – Generic/Trade: Tabs 250, 500, 600 mg. Susp 100, 200 mg/5 mL. Trade only: Packet 1000 mg. Z-Pak: #6, 250 mg tab. Tri-Pak: #3, 500 mg tab. Zmax extended-release oral susp: 2 g in 60 mL single-dose bottle.
- NOTES – Severe allergic/skin reactions rarely, IV site reactions, hearing loss with prolonged use. Potential for QT interval prolongation and torsades cannot be excluded in patients at risk for prolonged cardiac

(cont.)

ANTIMICROBIALS: Macrolides

AZITHROMYCIN (cont.)
repolarization. Does not inhibit CYP enzymes. Do not take at the same time as Al/Mg antacids (except Zmax which can be taken with antacids). Single dose and 3-day regimens cause more vomiting than 5-day regimen for otitis media. Zmax: Store at room temperature and use within 12 h of reconstitution. Additional treatment required if vomiting occurs within 5 min of dose; consider for vomiting within 1 h of dose; unnecessary for vomiting more than 1 h after dose.
MOA − Inhibits protein synthesis in susceptible organisms by interfering with function of ribosomal 50s subunit. Mechanism of action in cystic fibrosis is unknown; macrolides may inhibit P aeruginosa virulence factors or reduce inflammation.
ADVERSE EFFECTS − Serious: Allergic/skin reactions (rare), IV site reactions, hearing loss with prolonged use. Frequent: GI complaints, diarrhea, N/V most common with single-dose and 3-day regimens.

CLARITHROMYCIN (*Biaxin, Biaxin XL*) ▶KL ♀C ▶? $$$
ADULTS − Group A streptococcal pharyngitis (2nd line to penicillin): 250 mg PO bid for 10 days. Acute sinusitis: 500 mg PO bid for 14 days. Acute exacerbation of chronic bronchitis (S pneumoniae/M catarrhalis), community-acquired pneumonia, skin infections: 250 mg PO bid for 7 to 14 days. Acute exacerbation of chronic bronchitis (H influenzae): 500 mg PO bid for 7 to 14 days. H pylori: See table in GI section. Mycobacterium avium complex disease prevention/treatment: 500 mg PO bid. Treat active mycobacterial infections with at least 2 drugs. Biaxin XL: Acute sinusitis: 1000 mg PO daily for 14 days. Acute exacerbation of chronic bronchitis, Community-acquired pneumonia: 1000 mg PO daily for 7 days. Take Biaxin XL with food.
PEDS − Group A streptococcal pharyngitis (2nd line to penicillin), community-acquired pneumonia, sinusitis, otitis media, skin infections: 7.5 mg/kg PO bid for 10 days. Mycobacterium avium complex prevention/treatment: 7.5 mg/kg up to 500 mg PO bid. Two or more drugs are needed for the treatment of active mycobacterial infections.
UNAPPROVED ADULTS − See table for prophylaxis of bacterial endocarditis. Pertussis treatment/postexposure prophylaxis: 500 mg PO bid for 7 days. Community-acquired pneumonia: 500 mg PO bid.
UNAPPROVED PEDS − See table for prophylaxis of bacterial endocarditis. Pertussis treatment/postexposure prophylaxis (age 1 mo or older): 7.5 mg/kg (up to 500 mg) PO bid for 7 days.
FORMS − Generic/Trade: Tabs 250, 500 mg. Extended-release tab 500 mg. Susp 125, 250 mg/5 mL. Trade only: Biaxin XL-Pak: #14, 500 mg tabs. Generic only: Extended-release tab 1000 mg.
NOTES − Rare arrhythmias in patients with prolonged QT. Strong CYP3A4 inhibitor. Many drug interactions including increased levels of carbamazepine, cyclosporine, digoxin, disopyramide, lovastatin, rifabutin, simvastatin (avoid), tacrolimus,

---

PENICILLINS—GENERAL ANTIMICROBIAL SPECTRUM
1st **generation:** Most streptococci; oral anaerobic coverage
2nd **generation:** Most streptococci; *Staph aureus* (but not MRSA)
3rd **generation:** Most streptococci; basic gram negative coverage
4th **generation:** *Pseudomonas*

---

theophylline. Toxicity with ergotamine, dihydroergotamine, or colchicine (reduce colchicine dose). Clarithromycin levels decreased by efavirenz (avoid concomitant use) and nevirapine enough to impair efficacy in Mycobacterium avium complex disease. AAP recommends 5 to 7 days of therapy for children age 6 yo or older with nonsevere otitis media, and 10 days for younger children and those with severe disease. Dosage reduction for renal insufficiency in patients taking ritonavir, lopinavir/ritonavir (Kaletra), or ritonavir-boosted tipranavir or darunavir: decrease dose by 75% for CrCl < 30 mL/min, decrease dose by 50% for CrCl 30 to 60 mL/min. Reduce clarithromycin dose by 50% if given with atazanavir; consider alternative for indications other than Mycobacterium avium complex. Do not refrigerate susp.
MOA − Inhibits protein synthesis in susceptible organisms by interfering with function of ribosomal 50s subunit.
ADVERSE EFFECTS − Serious: Rare arrhythmias in patients with prolonged QT. Increased mortality reported 1 year after 2-week course of clarithromycin for prevention of cardiovascular mortality in patients with stable CHD. Frequent: Diarrhea, metallic taste.

ERYTHROMYCIN BASE (*Eryc, E-mycin, Ery-Tab, ✦Erybid, Erythromid, P.C.E.*) ▶L ♀B ▶+ $
ADULTS − Respiratory, skin infections: 250 to 500 mg PO qid or 333 mg PO tid. Pertussis, treatment/postexposure prophylaxis: 500 mg PO q 6 h for 14 days. S aureus skin infections: 250 mg PO q 6 h or 500 mg PO q 12 h. Secondary prevention of rheumatic fever: 250 mg PO bid. Chlamydia in pregnancy, nongonococcal urethritis: 500 mg PO qid for 7 days. Alternative for chlamydia in pregnancy if high dose not tolerated: 250 mg PO qid for 14 days. Erythrasma: 250 mg PO tid for 21 days. Legionnaires' disease: 2 g/day PO in divided doses for 14 to 21 days.
PEDS − Usual dose: 30 to 50 mg/kg/day PO divided qid for 10 days. Can double dose for severe infections. Pertussis: 40 to 50 mg/kg/day PO divided qid for 14 days (azithromycin preferred for age younger than 1 mo due to risk of hypertrophic pyloric stenosis with erythromycin). Chlamydia: 50 mg/kg/day PO divided qid for 14 days for wt less than 45 kg.
UNAPPROVED ADULTS − Chancroid: 500 mg PO tid for 7 days. Campylobacter gastroenteritis: 500 mg PO bid for 5 days.

(cont.)

ERYTHROMYCIN BASE (cont.)

FORMS — Generic/Trade: Tabs 250, 333, 500 mg, delayed-release cap 250 mg.
NOTES — Rare arrhythmias in patients with prolonged QT. Incidence of sudden death may be increased when erythromycin is combined with potent CYP3A4 inhibitors. Hypertrophic pyloric stenosis in infants primarily younger than 2 weeks old. CYP 3A4 and 1A2 inhibitor. Many drug interactions including increased levels of carbamazepine, cyclosporine, digoxin, disopyramide, tacrolimus, theophylline, some benzodiazepines and statins (avoid simvastatin).
MOA — Inhibits protein synthesis in susceptible organisms by interfering with function of ribosomal 50s subunit.
ADVERSE EFFECTS — Serious: Arrhythmias in patients with prolonged QT (rare), aggravation of myasthenia gravis, hypertrophic pyloric stenosis in infants primarily at least 2 weeks of age. Incidence of sudden death may be increased when erythromycin is combined with potent CYP 3A4 inhibitors. Frequent: N/V, diarrhea.

ERYTHROMYCIN ETHYL SUCCINATE (EES, Eryped) ▶L ♀B ▶+ $

ADULTS — Usual dose: 400 mg PO qid. Nongonococcal urethritis: 800 mg PO qid for 7 days. Chlamydia in pregnancy: 800 mg PO qid for 7 days or 400 mg PO qid for 14 days if high dose not tolerated. Secondary prevention of rheumatic fever: 400 mg PO bid. Legionnaires' disease: 3.2 g/day PO in divided doses for 14 to 21 days.
PEDS — Usual dose: 30 to 50 mg/kg/day PO divided qid. Maximum dose: 100 mg/kg/day. Group A streptococcal pharyngitis: 40 mg/kg/day (up to 1 g/day) PO divided bid to qid for 10 days. Secondary prevention of rheumatic fever: 400 mg PO bid. Pertussis: 40 to 50 mg/kg/day (up to 2 g/day) PO divided qid for 14 days.
FORMS — Generic/Trade: Tabs 400. Susp 200, 400 mg/5 mL. Trade only (EryPed): Susp 100 mg/2.5 mL (50 mL).
NOTES — Rare arrhythmias in patients with prolonged QT. Coadministration of strong CYP3A4 inhibitor with erythromycin may increase risk of sudden death. May aggravate myasthenia gravis. Hypertrophic pyloric stenosis primarily in infants younger than 2 weeks old. CYP3A4 inhibitor. Many drug interactions including increased levels of carbamazepine, cyclosporine, digoxin, disopyramide, tacrolimus, theophylline, some benzodiazepines and statins (avoid simvastatin).
MOA — Inhibits protein synthesis in susceptible organisms by interfering with function of ribosomal 50s subunit.
ADVERSE EFFECTS — Serious: Arrhythmias in patients with prolonged QT (rare), aggravation of myasthenia gravis, hypertrophic pyloric stenosis primarily in infants age 2 weeks or younger. Coadministration of strong CYP 3A4 inhibitor with erythromycin may increase risk of sudden death. Frequent: N/V, diarrhea.

ERYTHROMYCIN LACTOBIONATE (✦Erythrocin IV) ▶L ♀B ▶+ $$$$$

ADULTS — For severe infections/PO not possible: 15 to 20 mg/kg/day (up to 4 g/day) IV divided q 6 h. Legionnaires' disease: 4 g/day IV divided q 6 h.
PEDS — For severe infections/PO not possible: 15 to 20 mg/kg/day (up to 4 g/day) IV divided q 6 h.
UNAPPROVED PEDS — 20 to 50 mg/kg/day IV divided q 6 h.
NOTES — Dilute and give slowly to minimize venous irritation. Reversible hearing loss (increased risk in elderly given 4 g or more per day), allergic reactions, arrhythmias in patients with prolonged QT, exacerbation of myasthenia gravis. Incidence of sudden death may be increased when erythromycin is combined with potent CYP3A4 inhibitors. Hypertrophic pyloric stenosis primarily in infants younger than 2 weeks old. CYP3A4 inhibitor. Many drug interactions including increased levels of carbamazepine, cyclosporine, digoxin, disopyramide, tacrolimus, theophylline, some benzodiazepines and statins (avoid simvastatin).
MOA — Inhibits protein synthesis in susceptible organisms by interfering with function of ribosomal 50s subunit.
ADVERSE EFFECTS — Serious: Arrhythmias in patients with prolonged QT (rare), aggravation of myasthenia gravis, hypertrophic pyloric stenosis in infants primarily at least 2 weeks of age, reversible hearing loss with high doses (increased risk in elderly given >=4 g/day), allergic reactions, venous irritation. Incidence of sudden death may be increased when erythromycin is combined with potent CYP3A4 inhibitors. Frequent: N/V, diarrhea.

PEDIAZOLE (erythromycin ethyl succinate + sulfisoxazole) ▶KL ♀C ▶— $$

PEDS — Otitis media: 50 mg/kg/day (based on EES dose) PO divided tid to qid for age older than 2 mo.
FORMS — Generic/Trade: Susp, erythromycin ethyl succinate 200 mg + sulfisoxazole 600 mg/5 mL.
NOTES — Sulfisoxazole: Stevens-Johnson syndrome, toxic epidermal necrolysis, hepatotoxicity, blood dyscrasia, hemolysis in G6PD deficiency. Increased INR with warfarin. Erythromycin: Rare arrhythmias in patients with prolonged QT. Incidence of sudden death may be increased when erythromycin is combined with potent CYP3A4 inhibitors. May aggravate myasthenia gravis. CYP3A4 inhibitor. Many drug interactions including increased levels of carbamazepine, cyclosporine, digoxin, disopyramide, tacrolimus, theophylline, some benzodiazepines and statins. AAP recommends 5 to 7 days of therapy for children age 6 yo or older with nonsevere otitis media, and 10 days for younger children and those with severe disease.
MOA — See components.
ADVERSE EFFECTS — See components.

ANTIMICROBIALS: Penicillins—1st generation—Natural

NOTE: Anaphylaxis occurs rarely with penicillins; cross-sensitivity with cephalosporins is possible.

BENZATHINE PENICILLIN (*Bicillin L-A*, ✦*Megacillin*) ▶K ♀B ▶? $$
- WARNING — Not for IV administration, which can cause cardiorespiratory arrest and death.
- ADULTS — <u>Group A streptococcal pharyngitis</u>: 1.2 million units IM single dose. <u>Secondary prevention of rheumatic fever</u>: 1.2 million units IM q month (q 3 weeks for high-risk patients) or 600,000 units IM q 2 weeks. <u>Primary, secondary, early latent syphilis</u>: 2.4 million units IM single dose. <u>Tertiary, late latent syphilis</u>: 2.4 million units IM q week for 3 doses.
- PEDS — <u>Group A streptococcal pharyngitis</u> (AHA regimen): 600,000 units IM for wt 27 kg or less, 1.2 million units IM for wt greater than 27 kg. <u>Secondary prevention of rheumatic fever</u>: 600,000 units IM for wt 27 kg or less; 1.2 million units IM for wt greater than 27 kg; give q month (q 3 weeks for high-risk patients). <u>Primary, secondary, early latent syphilis</u>: 50,000 units/kg (up to 2.4 million units) IM single dose. <u>Late latent syphilis</u>: 50,000 units/kg (up to 2.4 million units) IM for 3 weekly doses.
- UNAPPROVED ADULTS — <u>Prophylaxis of diphtheria/treatment of carriers</u>: 1.2 million units IM single dose.
- UNAPPROVED PEDS — <u>Prophylaxis of diphtheria/treatment of carriers</u>: 1.2 million units IM single dose for wt 30 kg or greater. 600,000 units IM single dose for wt less than 30 kg.
- FORMS — Trade only: For IM use, 600,000 units/mL; 1, 2, 4 mL syringes.
- NOTES — Do not give IV. Doses last 2 to 4 weeks. Not for neurosyphilis. IM injection less painful if warmed to room temp before giving.
- MOA — Beta-lactam antibiotic that inhibits the biosynthesis of cell wall mucopeptide.
- ADVERSE EFFECTS — Serious: Anaphylaxis (rare), cross-sensitivity with cephalosporins, transient CNS reactions (Hoigne's syndrome), Coombs + hemolytic anemia. Frequent: Allergy.

BICILLIN C-R (procaine penicillin + benzathine penicillin) ▶K ♀B ▶? $$$
- WARNING — Not for IV administration, which can cause cardiorespiratory arrest and death.
- ADULTS — <u>Scarlet fever, erysipelas, upper-respiratory, skin, and soft-tissue infections due to group A strep</u>: 2.4 million units IM single dose. <u>Pneumococcal infections other than meningitis</u>: 1.2 million units IM q 2 to 3 days until temperature normal for 48 h. Not for treatment of syphilis.
- PEDS — <u>Scarlet fever, erysipelas, upper-respiratory, skin and soft-tissue infections due to group A strep</u>: 600,000 units IM for wt less than 13.6 kg, 900,000 to 1.2 million units IM for wt 13.6 to 27 kg, 2.4 million units IM for wt greater than 27 kg. <u>Pneumococcal infections other than meningitis</u>: 600,000 units IM q 2 to 3 days until temperature normal for 48 h. Not for treatment of syphilis.
- FORMS — Trade only: For IM use 300/300 thousand units/mL procaine/benzathine penicillin; 1, 2, 4 mL syringes.
- NOTES — Contraindicated if allergic to procaine. Do not give IV. Do not substitute Bicillin CR for Bicillin LA in treatment of syphilis.
- MOA — Beta-lactam antibiotic that inhibits the biosynthesis of cell wall mucopeptide.
- ADVERSE EFFECTS — Serious: Anaphylaxis (rare), cross-sensitivity with cephalosporins, Coombs + hemolytic anemia. Frequent: Allergy.

PENICILLIN G ▶K ♀B ▶? $$$$
- ADULTS — <u>Penicillin-sensitive pneumococcal pneumonia</u>: 8 to 12 million units/day IV divided q 4 to 6 h. <u>Penicillin-sensitive pneumococcal meningitis</u>: 24 million units/day IV divided q 2 to 4 h. <u>Empiric therapy, native valve endocarditis</u>: 20 million units/day IV continuous infusion or divided q 4 h plus nafcillin/oxacillin and gentamicin. <u>Neurosyphilis</u>: 18 to 24 million units/day continuous IV infusion or 3 to 4 million units IV q 4 h for 10 to 14 days. <u>Bioterrorism anthrax</u>: See www.idsociety.org/BT/ToC.htm.
- PEDS — <u>Mild to moderate infections</u>: 25,000 to 50,000 units/kg/day IV divided q 6 h. <u>Severe infections including pneumococcal and meningococcal meningitis</u>: 250,000 to 400,000 units/kg/day IV divided q 4 to 6 h. Neonates age younger than 1 week and wt greater than 2 kg: 25,000 to 50,000 units/kg IV q 8 h. Neonates age 1 week or older and wt greater than 2 kg: 25,000 to 50,000 units/kg IV q 6 h. <u>Group B streptococcal meningitis</u>: 250,000 to 450,000 units/kg/day IV divided q 8 h for age 1 week or younger; 450,000 to 500,000 units/kg/day IV divided q 4 to 6 h for age older than 1 week. <u>Congenital syphilis</u>: 50,000 units/kg/dose IV q 12 h during first 7 days of life, then q 8 h thereafter to complete 10 days. <u>Congenital syphilis or neurosyphilis</u>: 50,000 units/kg IV q 4 to 6 h for 10 days for age older than 1 mo.
- UNAPPROVED ADULTS — <u>Prevention of perinatal group B streptococcal disease</u>: Give to mother 5 million units IV at onset of labor/after membrane rupture, then 2.5 million units IV q 4 h until delivery. <u>Diphtheria</u>: 100,000 to 150,000 units/kg/day IV divided q 6 h for 14 days.
- UNAPPROVED PEDS — <u>Diphtheria</u>: 100,000 to 150,000 units/kg/day IV divided q 6 h for 14 days.
- NOTES — Reduce dose in renal dysfunction.
- MOA — Beta-lactam antibiotic that inhibits the biosynthesis of cell wall mucopeptide.
- ADVERSE EFFECTS — Serious: Anaphylaxis (rare); cross-sensitivity with cephalosporins; hematologic and renal toxicity, and seizures with doses greater than 20 million units/day; Coombs + hemolytic anemia. Frequent: Allergy.

PENICILLIN V (*Veetids*, ✦*PVF-K, Nadopen-V*) ▶K ♀B ▶? $
- ADULTS — Usual dose: 250 to 500 mg PO qid. AHA dosing for <u>group A streptococcal pharyngitis</u>: 500 mg

(cont.)

ANTIMICROBIALS: Penicillins

PROPHYLAXIS FOR BACTERIAL ENDOCARDITIS*	
Limited to dental or respiratory tract procedures in patients at highest risk. All regimens are single doses administered 30-60 minutes prior to procedure.	
Standard regimen	amoxicillin 2 g PO
Unable to take oral meds	ampicillin 2 g IM/IV; or cefazolin† or ceftriaxone† 1 g IM/IV
Allergic to penicillin	clindamycin 600 mg PO; or cephalexin† 2 g PO; or azithromycin or clarithromycin 500 mg PO
Allergic to penicillin and unable to take oral meds	clindamycin 600 mg IM/IV; or cefazolin† or ceftriaxone† 1 g IM/IV
Pediatric drug doses	Pediatric dose should not exceed adult dose. Amoxicillin 50 mg/kg, ampicillin 50 mg/kg, azithromycin 15 mg/kg, cephalexin† 50 mg/kg, cefazolin† 50 mg/kg, ceftriaxone† 50 mg/kg, clarithromycin 15 mg/kg, clindamycin 20 mg/kg.

*For additional details of the 2007 AHA guidelines, see http://www.americanheart.org.
†Avoid cephalosporins if prior penicillin-associated anaphylaxis, angioedema, or urticaria.

PENICILLIN V (cont.)
PO bid or tid for 10 days. Secondary prevention of rheumatic fever: 250 mg PO bid. Vincent's infection: 250 mg PO q 6 to 8 h.
PEDS — Usual dose: 25 to 50 mg/kg/day PO divided tid or qid. Use adult dose for age 12 yo or older. AHA dosing for group A streptococcal pharyngitis: 250 mg (for wt 27 kg or less) or 500 mg (wt greater than 27 kg) PO bid or tid for 10 days. Secondary prevention of rheumatic fever: 250 mg PO bid.
UNAPPROVED PEDS — Prevention of pneumococcal infections in functional/anatomic asplenia: 125 mg PO bid for age younger than 3 yo, 250 mg PO bid for age 3 yo or older.
FORMS — Generic/Trade: Tabs 250, 500 mg, oral soln 125, 250 mg/5 mL.
NOTES — Oral soln stable in refrigerator for 14 days.
MOA — Beta-lactam antibiotic that inhibits the biosynthesis of cell wall mucopeptide.
ADVERSE EFFECTS — Serious: Anaphylaxis (rare), cross-sensitivity with cephalosporins, Coombs + hemolytic anemia. Frequent: Allergy.
PROCAINE PENICILLIN (Wycillin) ▶K ♀B ▶? $$$$$
ADULTS — Pneumococcal and streptococcal infections, Vincent's infection, erysipeloid: 0.6 to 1 million units IM daily. Neurosyphilis: 2.4 million units IM daily plus probenecid 500 mg PO q 6 h, both for 10 to 14 days.
PEDS — Pneumococcal and streptococcal infections, Vincent's infection, erysipeloid, for wt less than 27 kg: 300,000 units IM daily. AAP dose for mild-moderate infections, age older than 1 mo: 25,000 to 50,000 units/kg/day IM divided once daily to bid. Congenital syphilis: 50,000 units/kg IM once daily for 10 days.
FORMS — Generic: For IM use, 600,000 units/mL; 1, 2 mL syringes.
NOTES — Peak 4 h, lasts 24 h. Contraindicated if procaine allergy; skin test if allergy suspected. Transient CNS reactions with high doses.
MOA — Beta-lactam antibiotic that inhibits the biosynthesis of cell wall mucopeptide.
ADVERSE EFFECTS — Serious: Anaphylaxis (rare), cross-sensitivity with cephalosporins, transient CNS reactions (Hoigne's syndrome), Coombs + hemolytic anemia. Frequent: Allergy.

ANTIMICROBIALS: Penicillins—2nd generation—Penicillinase-Resistant

NOTE: Anaphylaxis occurs rarely with penicillins; cross-sensitivity with cephalosporins is possible.

DICLOXACILLIN (Dynapen) ▶KL ♀B ▶? $$
ADULTS — Usual dose: 250 to 500 mg PO qid. Take on empty stomach.
PEDS — Mild to moderate upper respiratory, skin, and soft-tissue infections: 12.5 mg/kg/day PO divided qid for age older than 1 mo. Pneumonia, disseminated infections: 25 mg/kg/day PO divided qid for age older than 1 mo. Follow-up therapy after IV antibiotics for staph osteomyelitis: 50 to 100 mg/kg/day PO divided qid. Use adult dose for wt 40 kg or greater. Give on empty stomach.
FORMS — Generic only: Caps 250, 500 mg.
NOTES — Oral susp stable at room temperature for 7 days, in refrigerator for 14 days.
MOA — Beta-lactam antibiotic that inhibits the biosynthesis of cell wall mucopeptide.
Penicillinase-resistant penicillins are resistant to hydrolysis by the beta-lactamase, penicillinase.
ADVERSE EFFECTS — Serious: Anaphylaxis (rare), cross-sensitivity with cephalosporins.
NAFCILLIN ▶L ♀B ▶? $$$$$
ADULTS — Staph infections, usual dose: 500 mg IM q 4 to 6 h or 500 to 2000 mg IV q 4 h. Osteomyelitis: 1 to 2 g IV q 4 h. Empiric therapy, native valve endocarditis: 2 g IV q 4 h plus penicillin/ampicillin and gentamicin.
PEDS — Staph infections, usual dose: 25 mg/kg IM bid for pediatric patients who weigh less than 40 kg; give 10 mg/kg for neonates.
UNAPPROVED PEDS — Mild to moderate infections: 50 to 100 mg/kg/day IM/IV divided q 6 h. Severe infections: 100 to 200 mg/kg/day IM/IV divided q

(cont.)

ANTIMICROBIALS: Penicillins

NAFCILLIN (cont.)
4 to 6 h. Neonates, wt greater than 2 kg: 25 mg/kg IM/IV q 8 h for age younger than 1 week old; 25 to 35 mg/kg IM/IV q 6 h for age 1 week or older.
NOTES — Reversible neutropenia with prolonged use. Decreased INR with warfarin. Decreased cyclosporine levels.
MOA — Beta-lactam antibiotic that inhibits the biosynthesis of cell wall mucopeptide. Penicillinase-resistant penicillins are resistant to hydrolysis by the beta-lactamase, penicillinase.
ADVERSE EFFECTS — Serious: Anaphylaxis (rare), cross-sensitivity with cephalosporins, extravasation, hypokalemia with dose of 200 mg/kg/day or greater. Frequent: Reversible neutropenia with duration of therapy longer than 21 days, eosinophilia.

OXACILLIN (*Bactocill*) ▶KL ♀B ▶? $$$$$
ADULTS — Staph infections: 250 mg to 2 g IM/IV q 4 to 6 h. Osteomyelitis: 1.5 to 2 g IV q 4 h. Empiric therapy, native valve endocarditis: 2 g IV q 4 h with penicillin/ampicillin and gentamicin.
PEDS — Mild to moderate infections: 100 to 150 mg/kg/day IM/IV divided q 6 h. Severe infections: 150 to 200 mg/kg/day IM/IV divided q 4 to 6 h. Use adult dose for wt 40 kg or greater. Newborns, wt greater than 2 kg: 25 to 50 mg/kg IV q 8 h for age younger than 1 week old, increasing to q 6 h for age 1 week or older.
NOTES — Hepatic dysfunction possible with doses greater than 12 g/day; monitor LFTs.
MOA — Beta-lactam antibiotic that inhibits the biosynthesis of cell wall mucopeptide. Penicillinase-resistant penicillins are resistant to hydrolysis by the beta-lactamase, penicillinase.
ADVERSE EFFECTS — Serious: Anaphylaxis (rare), cross-sensitivity with cephalosporins, hepatic dysfunction possible with doses greater then 12 g/day. Frequent: Eosinophilia.

ANTIMICROBIALS: Penicillins—3rd generation—Aminopenicillins

NOTE: Anaphylaxis occurs rarely with penicillins; cross-sensitivity with cephalosporins is possible.

AMOXICILLIN (*Amoxil, DisperMox, Moxatag, Trimox, ✦Novamoxin*) ▶K ♀B ▶+ $
ADULTS — ENT, skin, genitourinary infections: 250 to 500 mg PO tid or 500 to 875 mg PO bid. Pneumonia: 500 mg PO tid or 875 mg PO bid. AHA dosing for group A streptococcal pharyngitis: 50 mg/kg (max 1 g) PO once daily for 10 days. Group A streptococcal pharyngitis/tonsillitis, for age 12 yo or older: 775 mg ER tab (Moxatag) PO once daily for 10 days. Do not chew/crush Moxatag tabs. H pylori: See table in GI section. See table for prophylaxis of bacterial endocarditis.
PEDS — ENT, skin, GU infections: 20 to 40 mg/kg/day PO divided tid or 25 to 45 mg/kg/day PO divided bid. See "unapproved" for AAP acute otitis media dosing. Pneumonia: 40 mg/kg/day PO divided tid or 45 mg/kg/day PO divided bid. Infants, age younger than 3 mo: 30 mg/kg/day PO divided q 12 h. AHA dosing for group A streptococcal pharyngitis: 50 mg/kg (max 1 g) PO once daily for 10 days. Group A streptococcal pharyngitis/tonsillitis, for age 12 yo or older: 775 mg ER tab (Moxatag) PO once daily for 10 days. Do not chew/crush Moxatag tabs. See table for bacterial endocarditis prophylaxis.
UNAPPROVED ADULTS — High-dose for community-acquired pneumonia: 1 g PO tid. Lyme disease: 500 mg PO tid for 14 days for early disease, for 28 days for Lyme arthritis. Chlamydia in pregnancy: 500 mg PO tid for 7 days. Bioterrorism anthrax: See www.idsociety.org/BT/ToC.htm.
UNAPPROVED PEDS — AHA dosing for group A streptococcal pharyngitis: 50 mg/kg (max 1 g) PO once daily for 10 days. Otitis media (AAP high-dose): 90 mg/kg/day PO divided bid to tid. Community-acquired pneumonia: 80 to 100 mg/kg/day PO divided tid to qid for age 4 mo to 4 yo. Lyme disease: 50 mg/kg/day (up to 1500 mg/day) PO divided tid for 14 days for early disease, for 28 days for Lyme arthritis. Bioterrorism anthrax: See www.idsociety.org/BT/ToC.htm.
FORMS — Generic/Trade: Caps 250, 500 mg, Tabs 500, 875 mg, Chewable tabs 125, 200, 250, 400 mg. Susp 125, 250 mg/5 mL. Susp 200, 400 mg/5 mL. Trade only: Infant gtts 50 mg/mL (Amoxil). DisperMox 200, 400, 600 mg tabs for oral susp, Moxatag 775 mg extended-release tab.
NOTES — Rash in patients with mononucleosis. AAP recommends 5 to 7 days of therapy for children age 6 yo or older with nonsevere otitis media, and 10 days for younger children and those with severe disease. Reduce dose in adults with renal dysfunction: Give 250 to 500 mg PO daily for CrCl < 10 mL/min or hemodialysis, 250 to 500 mg PO bid for CrCl 10 to 30 mL/min. Do not use 875 mg tab for CrCl < 30 mL/min. Give additional dose during and at end of dialysis. Oral susp and infant gtts stable for 14 days at room temperature or in the refrigerator. Mix DisperMox tab with 2 tsp water and drink mixture, then rinse container with a little water and drink that. Do not chew or swallow tab whole. Use only for doses that can be delivered by whole tabs.
MOA — Beta-lactam antibiotic that inhibits the biosynthesis of cell wall mucopeptide. Aminopenicillins are more active than natural penicillins against gram-negative cocci and Enterobacteriaceae.
ADVERSE EFFECTS — Serious: Anaphylaxis (rare), cross-sensitivity with cephalosporins. Frequent: Rash (nonallergic in patients with mononucleosis, chronic myelogenous leukemia, or allopurinol therapy), diarrhea.

AMOXICILLIN-CLAVULANATE (*Augmentin, Augmentin ES-600, Augmentin XR, ✦Clavulin*) ▶K ♀B ▶? $$$$
ADULTS — Pneumonia, otitis media, sinusitis, skin infections, UTIs: Usual dose 500 mg PO bid or

(cont.)

ANTIMICROBIALS: Penicillins

AMOXICILLIN-CLAVULANATE (*cont.*)
250 mg PO tid. <u>More severe infections:</u> 875 mg PO bid or 500 mg PO tid. Augmentin XR: 2 tabs PO q 12 h with meals for 10 days for <u>acute sinusitis,</u> give 7 to 10 days for <u>community-acquired pneumonia.</u>
PEDS – 200, 400 mg chewables and 200, 400 mg/5 mL susp for bid administration: <u>Pneumonia, otitis media, sinusitis:</u> 45 mg/kg/day PO divided bid. Less severe infections such as skin, <u>UTIs:</u> 25 mg/kg/day PO divided bid. 125, 250 mg chewables and 125, 250 mg/ 5 mL susp for tid administration: <u>Pneumonia, otitis media, sinusitis:</u> 40 mg/kg/day PO divided tid. Less severe infections such as skin, <u>UTIs:</u> 20 mg/kg/day PO divided tid. Use 125 mg/5 mL susp and give 30 mg/kg PO q 12 hr for age younger than 3 mo. Give adult dose for wt 40 kg or greater. Augmentin ES-600 susp for age 3 mo or older and wt less than 40 kg. <u>Recurrent/ persistent otitis media with risk factors</u> (antibiotics for otitis media in past 3 months and either in daycare or age 2 yo or younger): give 90 mg/kg/day PO divided bid with food for 10 days.
UNAPPROVED ADULTS – <u>Prevention of infection after dog/cat bite:</u> 875 mg PO bid or 500 mg PO tid for 3 to 5 days. <u>Treatment of infected dog/cat bite:</u> 875 mg PO bid or 500 mg PO tid, duration of treatment based on response.
FORMS – Generic/Trade: (amoxicillin/clavulanate) Tabs 250/125, 500/125, 875/125 mg, Chewables, Susp 200/28.5, 400/57 mg per tab or 5 mL, 250/62.5 mg per 5 mL, (ES) Susp 600/42.9 mg per 5 mL. Trade only: Chewables, Susp 125/31.25 per tab or 5 mL, 250/62.5 mg per tab. Extended-release tabs (Augmentin XR) 1000/62.5 mg.
NOTES – Rash in patients with mononucleosis; diarrhea common (less diarrhea with bid dosing). AAP recommends 5 to 7 days of therapy for children age 6 yo or older with non-severe otitis media, and 10 days for those with severe disease or age younger than 6 yo. Do not interchange Augmentin products with different clavulanate content. Do not use 250 mg amoxicillin + 125 mg clavulante tab in children wt less than 40 kg. Suspensions stable in refrigerator for 10 days. See package insert for dosage reduction of Augmentin tabs if CrCl less than 30 mL/min. Augmentin XR contraindicated if CrCl less than 30 mL/min.
MOA – Beta-lactam antibiotic that inhibits the biosynthesis of cell wall mucopeptide. Aminopenicillins are more active than natural penicillins against gram-negative cocci and Enterobacteriaceae. Clavulanate is beta-lactamase inhibitor.
ADVERSE EFFECTS – Serious: Anaphylaxis (rare), cross-sensitivity with cephalosporins, clavulanate-induced cholestatic hepatitis (esp. in elderly men treated for more than 2 weeks). Frequent: Diarrhea (less with bid dosing, incidence related to clavulanate dose), rash (nonallergic in patients with mononucleosis, chronic myelogenous leukemia, or allopurinol therapy).

AMPICILLIN (*Principen, ✦Penbritin*) ▶K ♀B ▶? $ PO $$$$$ IV
ADULTS – Usual dose: 1 to 2 g IV q 4 to 6 h or 250 to 500 mg PO qid. <u>Sepsis, meningitis:</u> 150 to 200 mg/kg/day IV divided q 3 to 4 h. <u>Empiric therapy, native valve endocarditis:</u> 12 g/day IV continuous infusion or divided q 4 h plus nafcillin/oxacillin and gentamicin. See table for <u>prophylaxis of bacterial endocarditis.</u> Take oral ampicillin on an empty stomach.
PEDS – AAP recommendations: <u>Mild to moderate infections:</u> 100 to 150 mg/kg/day IM/IV divided q 6 h or 50 to 100 mg/kg/day PO divided qid. <u>Severe infections:</u> 200 to 400 mg/kg/day IM/IV divided q 6 h. Newborns, wt greater than 2 kg: 25 to 50 mg/kg IV given q 8 h for age younger than 1 week old, increase to q 6 h for age 1 week or older. Use adult doses for wt 40 kg or greater. Give oral ampicillin on an empty stomach. <u>Group B streptococcal meningitis:</u> 200 to 300 mg/kg/day IV divided q 8 h for age 7 days or younger; 300 mg/kg/day divided q 6 h for age older than 7 days. Give with gentamicin initially. See table for <u>prophylaxis of bacterial endocarditis.</u>
UNAPPROVED ADULTS – <u>Prevention of neonatal group B streptococcal disease:</u> Give to mother 2 g IV during labor, then 1 to 2 g IV q 4 to 6 h until delivery.
FORMS – Generic/Trade: Caps 250, 500 mg. Susp 125, 250 mg/5 mL.
NOTES – Rash in patients with mononucleosis or taking allopurinol; C difficile-associated diarrhea. Susp stable for 7 days at room temperature, 14 days in the refrigerator. Reduce dosing interval to q 12 to 24 h for CrCl < 10 mL/min. Give dose after hemodialysis.
MOA – Beta-lactam antibiotic that inhibits the biosynthesis of cell wall mucopeptide. Aminopenicillins are more active than natural penicillins against gram-negative cocci and Enterobacteriaceae.
ADVERSE EFFECTS – Serious: Anaphylaxis (rare), cross-sensitivity with cephalosporins, C. difficile-associated diarrhea. Frequent: Nonallergic rash in patients with mononucleosis, chronic myelogenous leukemia, or allopurinol therapy; eosinophilia; diarrhea (especially with PO).

AMPICILLIN-SULBACTAM (*Unasyn*) ▶K ♀B ▶? $$$$$
ADULTS – <u>Skin, intra-abdominal, gynecologic infections:</u> 1.5 to 3 g IM/IV q 6 h.
PEDS – <u>Skin infections,</u> for age 1 yo or older: 300 mg/kg/day IV divided q 6 h. Use adult dose for wt greater than 40 kg.
UNAPPROVED ADULTS – <u>Community-acquired pneumonia:</u> 1.5 to 3 g IM/IV q 6 h with a macrolide or doxycycline.
UNAPPROVED PEDS – AAP regimens. <u>Mild to moderate infections:</u> 100 to 150 mg/kg/day of ampicillin IM/IV divided q 6 h. <u>Severe infections:</u> 200 to 400 mg/kg/day of ampicillin IM/IV divided q 6 h.
NOTES – Rash in patients with mononucleosis or taking allopurinol; C difficile-associated diarrhea.

(*cont.*)

ANTIMICROBIALS: Penicillins

AMPICILLIN-SULBACTAM (*cont.*)
Dosing for adults with renal impairment: Give usual dose q 24 h for CrCl 5 to 14 mL/min, q 12 h for CrCl 15 to 29 mL/min, q 6 to 8 h for adults with CrCl 30 mL/min or greater.
MOA — Beta-lactam antibiotic that inhibits the biosynthesis of cell wall mucopeptide. Aminopenicillins are more active than natural penicillins against gram-negative cocci and Enterobacteriaceae. Sulbactam is beta-lactamase inhibitor.
ADVERSE EFFECTS — Serious: Anaphylaxis (rare), cross-sensitivity with cephalosporins, C. difficile-associated diarrhea. Frequent: Rash (nonallergic in patients with mononucleosis, chronic myelogenous leukemia, or allopurinol therapy), eosinophilia, increased LFTs.

ANTIMICROBIALS: Penicillins—4th generation—Extended Spectrum

NOTE: Anaphylaxis occurs rarely with penicillins; cross-sensitivity with cephalosporins is possible.

PIPERACILLIN ▶K/Bile ♀B ▶? $$$$$
ADULTS — <u>Simple UTI, community-acquired pneumonia:</u> 6 to 8 g/day IM/IV divided q 6 to 12 h. <u>Complicated UTI:</u> 8 to 16 g/day IV divided q 6 to 8 h. <u>Serious infections:</u> 12 to 18 g/day IV divided q 4 to 6 h. Max dose: 24 g/day.
PEDS — Safety and efficacy not established in age younger than 12 yo. Use adult dose for age 12 yo or older.
UNAPPROVED ADULTS — <u>Empiric therapy of neutropenic fever:</u> 3 g IV q 4 h or 4 g IV q 6 h with an aminoglycoside.
UNAPPROVED PEDS — AAP doses. <u>Mild to moderate infections:</u> 100 to 150 mg/kg/day IV divided q 6 h. Severe infections: 200 to 300 mg/kg/day IV divided q 4 to 6 h.
NOTES — Hypokalemia; bleeding and coagulation abnormalities possible especially with renal impairment. May prolong neuromuscular blockade with nondepolarizing muscle relaxants. May reduce renal excretion of methotrexate; monitor methotrexate levels and toxicity. Reduce dosing for adults with renal dysfunction: Serious infections: 4 g IV q 12 h for CrCl less than 20 mL/min, 4 g IV q 8 h for CrCl 20 to 40 mL/min. Complicated UTI: 3 g IV q 12 h for CrCl less than 20 mL/min, 3 g IV q 8 h for CrCl 20 to 40 mL/min. Simple UTI: 3 g IV q 12 h for CrCl less than 20 mL/min.
MOA — Beta-lactam antibiotic that inhibits the biosynthesis of cell wall mucopeptide.
ADVERSE EFFECTS — Serious: Anaphylaxis (rare), cross-sensitivity with cephalosporins, hypokalemia, bleeding and coagulation abnormalities (especially with renal impairment). Increased risk of rash/fever in cystic fibrosis patients. Frequent: Neutropenia.

PIPERACILLIN-TAZOBACTAM (*Zosyn, ✦Tazocin*) ▶K ♀B ▶? $$$$$
ADULTS — <u>Appendicitis, peritonitis, skin infections, postpartum endometritis, pelvic inflammatory disease, moderate community-acquired pneumonia:</u> 3.375 g IV q 6 h. <u>Nosocomial pneumonia:</u> 4.5 g IV q 6 h (with aminoglycoside initially and if P aeruginosa is cultured).
PEDS — <u>Appendicitis/peritonitis:</u> 80 mg/kg of piperacillin IV q 8 h for age 2 to 9 mo; 100 mg/kg of piperacillin IV q 8 h for age older than 9 mo; use adult dose for wt greater than 40 kg.
UNAPPROVED ADULTS — <u>Serious infections:</u> 4.5 g IV q 6 h.
UNAPPROVED PEDS — 150 to 300 mg/kg/day of piperacillin IV divided q 6 to 8 h for age younger than 6 mo, 300 to 400 mg/kg/day piperacillin IV divided q 6 to 8 h for age 6 mo or older.
NOTES — Hypokalemia; bleeding and coagulation abnormalities possible especially with renal impairment. May prolong neuromuscular blockade with nondepolarizing muscle relaxants. False-positive result possible with Bio-Rad Laboratories Platelia Aspergillus EIA test. May reduce renal excretion of methotrexate; monitor methotrexate levels and toxicity. Reduce dosing in adults with renal impairment: 2.25 g IV q 8 h for CrCl less than 20 mL/min, 2.25 g IV q 6 h for CrCl 20 to 40 mL/min. Hemodialysis: Maximum dose of 2.25 g IV q 8 h plus 0.75 g after each dialysis.
MOA — Beta-lactam antibiotic that inhibits the biosynthesis of cell wall mucopeptide. Tazobactam is beta-lactamase inhibitor.
ADVERSE EFFECTS — Serious: Anaphylaxis (rare), cross-sensitivity with cephalosporins, hypokalemia, bleeding and coagulation abnormalities (especially with renal impairment). Frequent: N/V, diarrhea, headache.

TICARCILLIN-CLAVULANATE (*Timentin*) ▶K ♀B ▶? $$$$$
ADULTS — <u>Systemic infections or UTIs:</u> 3.1 g IV q 4 to 6 h. <u>Gynecologic infections: Moderate:</u> 200 mg/kg/day IV divided q 6 h. <u>Severe:</u> 300 mg/kg/day IV divided q 4 h. Adults with wt less than 60 kg: 200 to 300 mg/kg/day (based on ticarcillin content) IV divided q 4 to 6 h. Use q 4 h dosing interval for Pseudomonas infections.
PEDS — Age 3 mo or older and wt less than 60 kg: 200 mg/kg/day (based on ticarcillin content) IV divided q 6 h for mild to moderate infections, 300 mg/kg/day IV divided q 4 h for severe infections. For wt 60 kg or greater: 3.1 g IV q 6 h for mild to moderate infections, 3.1 g IV q 4 h for severe infections.
NOTES — Timentin 3.1 g = 3 g ticarcillin and 0.1 g clavulanate. Hypokalemia; bleeding and coagulation abnormalities possible especially in patients with renal impairment. 4.75 mEq sodium per g of Timentin. Reduce dose in adults with renal dysfunction: Load with 3.1 g, then give 2 g daily for

(cont.)

TICARCILLIN-CLAVULANATE (cont.)
CrCl less than 10 mL/min and liver dysfunction, 2 g every 12 h for CrCl less than 10 mL/min, 2 g every 8 h for CrCl 10 to 30 mL/min, 2 g every 4 h for CrCl 30 to 60 mL/min. Peritoneal dialysis: 3.1 g every 12 h. Hemodialysis: 3.1 g load, then 2 g every 12 h and 3.1 g after each dialysis.

MOA — Beta-lactam antibiotic that inhibits the biosynthesis of cell wall mucopeptide. Clavulanate is beta-lactamase inhibitor.
ADVERSE EFFECTS — Serious: Anaphylaxis (rare), cross-sensitivity with cephalosporins, hypokalemia, bleeding and coagulation abnormalities (especially with renal impairment), cholestatic hepatitis (due to clavulanate). Frequent: Eosinophilia, diarrhea.

ANTIMICROBIALS: Quinolones—2nd Generation

NOTE: As of April 2007, the CDC no longer recommends fluoroquinolones for gonorrhea because of high resistance rates. Fluoroquinolones can cause tendon rupture (rare; risk increased by corticosteroids, age older than 60 yo, or organ transplant), phototoxicity (risk varies among agents), C difficile-associated diarrhea (risk may vary among agents), QT interval prolongation (risk varies among agents; see QT drugs table), exacerbation of myasthenia gravis, CNS toxicity, peripheral neuropathy (rare), and hypersensitivity. Important quinolone drug interactions with antacids, iron, zinc, magnesium, sucralfate, buffered didanosine, cimetidine, caffeine, cyclosporine, phenytoin, anticoagulants, theophylline, etc.

CIPROFLOXACIN (*Cipro, Cipro XR, ProQuin XR*) ▶LK ♀C but teratogenicity unlikely ▶?+ $
WARNING — Tendon rupture (rare; risk increased by corticosteroids, age older than 60 yo, or organ transplant). Advise patients to stop fluoroquinolone, rest affected area, and seek medical advice for tendon swelling, pain, or inflammation.
ADULTS — UTI: 250 to 500 mg PO bid or 200 to 400 mg IV q 12 h. Simple UTI: 250 mg PO bid for 3 days or Cipro XR/Proquin XR 500 mg PO once daily for 3 days. Give Proquin XR with main meal of the day, preferably dinner. Cipro XR for complicated UTI, uncomplicated pyelonephritis: 1000 mg PO once daily for 7 to 14 days. Pneumonia, skin, bone/joint infections: 400 mg IV q 8 to 12 h or 500 to 750 mg PO bid. Treat bone/joint infections for 4 to 6 weeks. Acute sinusitis: 500 mg PO bid for 10 days. Chronic bacterial prostatitis: 500 mg PO bid for 28 days. Infectious diarrhea: 500 mg PO bid for 5 to 7 days. Typhoid fever: 500 mg PO bid for 10 days. Nosocomial pneumonia: 400 mg IV q 8 h. Complicated intra-abdominal infection (with metronidazole): 400 mg IV q 12 h, then 500 mg PO bid. Empiric therapy of febrile neutropenia: 400 mg IV q 8 h with piperacillin. Bioterrorism anthrax. Inhalation or severe cutaneous anthrax treatment: 400 mg IV q 12 h with at least 1 other drug initially, then monotherapy with 500 mg PO bid to complete 60 days. Monotherapy for postexposure prophylaxis or treatment of less severe cutaneous anthrax: 500 mg PO bid for 60 days. See www.idsociety.org/BT/ToC.htm for more info.
PEDS — Safety and efficacy not established for most indications in children; arthropathy in juvenile animals. Still limited data, but case series of treated children show no evidence of arthropathy other than transient large-joint arthralgias. Musculoskeletal adverse events reported with ciprofloxacin treatment of complicated UTI in peds patients were mild to moderate in severity and resolved within 1 month after treatment. Complicated UTI, pyelonephritis, 1 to 17 yo: 6 to 10 mg/kg IV q 8 h, then 10 to 20 mg/kg PO q 12 h. Max Of 400 mg IV or 750 mg PO per dose even for peds patients wt greater than 51 kg. Bioterrorism anthrax. Treatment of inhalation anthrax, severe cutaneous anthrax, or cutaneous anthrax in age younger than 2 yo: 10 to 15 mg/kg IV q 12 h with at least 1 other drug initially, then monotherapy with 10 to 15 mg/kg up to 500 mg PO bid to complete 60 days. Monotherapy for postexposure prophylaxis or less severe cutaneous anthrax treatment: 10 to 15 mg/kg up to 500 mg PO bid for 60 days. See www.idsociety.org/BT/ToC.htm for more info.
UNAPPROVED ADULTS — Acute uncomplicated pyelonephritis: 500 mg PO bid for 7 days. Chancroid: 500 mg PO bid for 3 days. Prophylaxis, high-risk GU surgery: 500 mg PO or 400 mg IV. Prophylaxis, invasive meningococcal disease: 500 mg PO single dose. Traveler's diarrhea (treatment preferred over prophylaxis): Treatment: 500 mg PO bid for 1 to 3 days or 750 mg PO single dose. Prophylaxis: 500 mg PO daily for no more than 3 weeks. Infectious diarrhea: 500 mg PO bid for 1 to 3 days for shigella, for 5 to 7 days for non-typhi salmonella (usually not treated). Malignant otitis externa: 400 mg IV or 750 mg PO q 12 h. TB (second-line treatment): 750 to 1500 mg/day IV/PO. Salmonella gastroenteritis in HIV infection: 500 to 750 mg PO bid (400 mg IV q 12 h) for 7 to 14 days if CD4 count 200 or greater, for 2 to 6 weeks if CD4 count less than 200. Campylobacter in HIV infection: 500 mg PO bid for 7 days for mild/moderate disease, at least 14 days for bacteremia.
UNAPPROVED PEDS — Acute pulmonary exacerbation of cystic fibrosis: 10 mg/kg/dose IV q 8 h for 7 days, then 20 mg/kg/dose PO q 12 h to complete 10 to 21 days of treatment. TB (second-line treatment): 10 to 15 mg/kg PO bid (max: 1.5 g/day). Cholera: 20 mg/kg up to 750 mg PO single dose for age 2 to 15 yo.
FORMS — Generic/Trade: Tabs 100, 250, 500, 750 mg. Extended-release tabs 500, 1000 mg. Trade only (ProQuin XR): Extended-release tabs 500 mg, blister pack 500 mg (#3 tabs).
NOTES — Crystalluria if alkaline urine. Ciprofloxacin inhibits CYP1A2, an enzyme that metabolizes

(cont.)

QUINOLONES—GENERAL ANTIMICROBIAL SPECTRUM

1st generation: gram negative (excluding *Pseudomonas*), urinary tract only, no atypicals
2nd generation: gram negative (including *Pseudomonas*); *Staph aureus* (but not MRSA or *pneumococcus*); some atypicals
3rd generation: gram negative (including *Pseudomonas*); gram positive, including *pneumococcus* and *Staph aureus* (but not MRSA); expanded atypical coverage
4th generation: same as 3rd generation plus enhanced coverage of *pneumococcus*, decreased activity vs. *Pseudomonas*

CIPROFLOXACIN (*cont.*)

caffeine, clozapine, tacrine, theophylline, and warfarin. Give ciprofloxacin immediate-release or Cipro XR 2 h before or 6 h after antacids, iron, sucralfate, calcium, zinc, buffered didanosine, or other highly buffered drugs (Proquin XR is 2 h before or 4 h after these multivalent cations). Can give with meals containing dairy products, but not with yogurt, milk, or calcium-fortified fruit juice alone. Do not give Cipro XR within 2 h of calcium doses greater than 800 mg. Watch for hypoglycemia with glyburide. Do not give oral susp in feeding or nasogastric tube. Cipro XR, Proquin XR, and immediate-release tabs are not inter-changeable. Do not split, crush, or chew Cipro XR or Proquin XR. In patients with complicated UTI or acute pyelonephritis and CrCl less than 30 mL/min, reduce dose of Cipro XR to 500 mg daily. Reduce dose of immediate-release ciprofloxacin in adults with renal dysfunction: 250 to 500 mg PO q 24 h given after dialysis session for hemodialysis/peritoneal dialysis, 250 to 500 mg PO q 18 h or 200 to 400 mg IV q 18 to 24 h for CrCl 5 to 29 mL/min, 250 to 500 mg PO q 12 h for CrCl 30 to 50 mL/min.
MOA – Inhibits bacterial DNA synthesis by binding with DNA gyrase and topoisomerase IV.
ADVERSE EFFECTS – Serious: Tendon rupture (rare), phototoxicity, CNS toxicity, crystalluria if alkaline urine, peripheral neuropathy (rare), hypersensitivity. Theoretical risk of cartilage toxicity in children, but no clinical evidence of harm other than transient large-joint arthralgias. Musculoskeletal adverse events reported with ciprofloxacin treatment of complicated UTI in peds patients were mild to moderate in severity and resolved within 1 month after treatment. Frequent: N/V. More GI, neurologic, and musculoskeletal adverse reactions reported during postexposure prophylaxis of bioterrorism anthrax.

NORFLOXACIN (*Noroxin*) ▶LK ♀C ▶? $
WARNING – Tendon rupture (rare; risk increased by corticosteroids, age older than 60 yo, or organ transplant). Advise patients to stop fluoroquinolone, rest affected area, and seek medical advice for tendon swelling, pain, or inflammation.
ADULTS – Simple UTI due to E coli, K pneumoniae, P mirabilis: 400 mg PO bid for 3 days. UTI due to other organisms: 400 mg PO bid for 7 to 10 days. Complicated UTI: 400 mg PO bid for 10 to 21 days. Acute/chronic prostatitis: 400 mg PO bid for 28 days. Take on an empty stomach.
PEDS – Safety and efficacy not established in children; arthropathy in juvenile animals.
UNAPPROVED ADULTS – Traveler's diarrhea (treatment preferred over prophylaxis): Treatment: 400 mg PO bid for 1 to 3 days. Prophylaxis: 400 mg PO daily for up to 3 weeks. Infectious diarrhea: 400 mg PO bid for 5 to 7 days for non-typhi salmonella (usually not treated), for 1 to 3 days for shigella. Take on an empty stomach.
FORMS – Trade only: Tabs 400 mg.
NOTES – Crystalluria with high doses. Maintain adequate hydration. Norfloxacin inhibits CYP1A2, an enzyme that metabolizes caffeine, clozapine, ropinirole, tacrine, theophylline, tizanidine, and warfarin. Increased INR with warfarin. Do not take with dairy products. Give antacids, zinc, iron, sucralfate, multivitamins, or buffered didanosine 2 h before/after norfloxacin. Reduce dose in renal dysfunction: 400 mg PO daily for CrCl less than 30 mL/min.
MOA – Inhibits bacterial DNA synthesis by binding with DNA gyrase and topoisomerase IV.
ADVERSE EFFECTS – Serious: Tendon rupture (rare), phototoxicity, crystalluria (high doses), CNS toxicity, peripheral neuropathy (rare), and hypersensitivity. Frequent: None.

OFLOXACIN (*Floxin*) ▶LK ♀C ▶?+ $$$
WARNING – Tendon rupture (rare; risk increased by corticosteroids, age older than 60 yo, or organ transplant). Advise patients to stop fluoroquinolone, rest affected area, and seek medical advice for tendon swelling, pain, or inflammation.
ADULTS – Acute exacerbation of chronic bronchitis, community-acquired pneumonia, skin infections: 400 mg PO bid for 10 days. Simple UTI due to E coli, K pneumoniae: 200 mg PO bid for 3 days. Simple UTI due to other organisms: 200 mg PO bid for 7 days. Complicated UTI: 200 mg PO bid for 10 days. Chronic bacterial prostatitis: 300 mg PO bid for 6 weeks.
PEDS – Safety and efficacy not established in children; arthropathy in juvenile animals.
UNAPPROVED ADULTS – Epididymitis: 300 mg PO bid for 10 days. Traveler's diarrhea, treatment: 300 mg PO bid for 1 to 3 days. Infectious diarrhea: 300 mg PO bid for 1 to 3 days for shigella, 5 to 7 days for non-typhi salmonella (usually not treated). TB (2nd line treatment): 600 to 800 mg PO daily.
FORMS – Generic/Trade: Tabs 200, 300, 400 mg.
NOTES – May prolong QT interval; avoid using in proarrhythmic conditions or with drugs that prolong QT interval, including Class 1A and Class III antiarrhythmics. Give antacids, iron, sucralfate,

(cont.)

ANTIMICROBIALS: Quinolones

OFLOXACIN (*cont.*)
multivitamins containing zinc, buffered didanosine 2 h before or after ofloxacin. May decrease metabolism of theophylline, increase INR with warfarin. Monitor glucose with antidiabetic agents. Can cause false positive on opiate urine screening immunoassay; may need confirmation test. Reduce dose in renal dysfunction: 50% of usual dose q 24 h for CrCl less than 20 mL/min, usual dose given q 24 h for CrCl 20 to 50 mL/min.
MOA — Inhibits bacterial DNA synthesis by binding with DNA gyrase and topoisomerase IV.
ADVERSE EFFECTS — Serious: Tendon rupture (rare), phototoxicity (risk varies among agents), QT interval prolongation, peripheral neuropathy (rare), CNS toxicity, and hypersensitivity. Frequent: N/V.

ANTIMICROBIALS: Quinolones—3rd Generation

NOTE: As of April 2007, the CDC no longer recommends fluoroquinolones for gonorrhea because of high resistance rates. Can cause tendon rupture (rare; risk increased by corticosteroids, age older than 60 yo, or organ transplant), C difficile-associated diarrhea (risk may vary among agents), phototoxicity (risk varies among agents), CNS toxicity, peripheral neuropathy (rare), hypersensitivity, and QT interval prolongation (risk varies among agents; see QT drugs table). Avoid using in proarrhythmic conditions or with drugs that prolong QT including Class 1A and Class III antiarrhythmics. Important quinolone drug interactions with antacids, iron, zinc, magnesium, sucralfate, cimetidine, caffeine, cyclosporine, phenytoin, anticoagulants, theophylline, etc.

LEVOFLOXACIN (*Levaquin*) ▶KL ♀C ▶? $$$$
WARNING — Tendon rupture (rare; risk increased by corticosteroids, age older than 60 yo, or organ transplant). Advise patients to stop fluoroquinolone, rest affected area, and seek medical advice for tendon swelling, pain, or inflammation.
ADULTS — IV & PO doses are the same. Community-acquired pneumonia: 750 mg once daily for 5 days or 500 mg once daily for 7 to 14 days. Nosocomial pneumonia: 750 mg once daily for 7 to 14 days. Acute sinusitis: 750 mg once daily for 5 days or 500 mg once daily for 10 to 14 days. Acute exacerbation of chronic bronchitis: 500 mg once daily for 7 days. Skin infections: 500 to 750 mg once daily for 7 to 14 days. Complicated UTI or pyelonephritis: 250 mg once daily for 10 days or 750 mg once daily for 5 days. Simple UTI: 250 mg once daily for 3 days. Chronic bacterial prostatitis: 500 mg once daily for 28 days. Postexposure anthrax prophylaxis: 500 mg PO once daily for 60 days. See www.idsociety.org/BT/ToC.htm for more info. Infuse IV doses over 60 min (250 to 500 mg) to 90 min (750 mg). Take oral soln on empty stomach.
PEDS — Safety and efficacy not established in children; arthropathy in juvenile animals. Musculoskeletal disorders (primarily mild arthralgias during treatment) reported in children.
UNAPPROVED ADULTS — Legionnaires' disease: 1 g IV/PO on first day, then 500 mg IV/PO once daily. Chlamydia, epididymitis: See STD table. TB (2nd line treatment): 500 to 1000 mg/day IV/PO. Traveler's diarrhea, treatment: 500 mg PO once daily for 1 to 3 days. Infectious diarrhea: 500 mg PO once daily for 1 to 3 days for shigella, for 5 to 7 days for salmonella.
FORMS — Trade only: Tabs 250, 500, 750 mg, Oral soln 25 mg/mL. Leva-Pak: #5, 750 mg tabs.
NOTES — Give Mg/Al antacids, iron, sucralfate, multivitamins containing zinc, buffered didanosine 2 h before/after PO levofloxacin. Increased INR with warfarin. Monitor glucose with antidiabetic agents. Can cause false positive on opiate urine screening immunoassay; may need confirmation test. Reduce dose in renal dysfunction: For most indications and CrCl < 50 mL/min, load with 500 mg, then 250 mg q 48 h for CrCl 10 to 19 mL/min, hemodialysis, or peritoneal dialysis; give 250 mg daily for CrCl 20 to 49 mL/min. For complicated UTI/pyelonephritis and CrCl 10 to 19 mL/min, give 250 mg q 48 h.
MOA — Inhibits bacterial DNA synthesis by binding with DNA gyrase and topoisomerase IV.
ADVERSE EFFECTS — Serious: QT interval prolongation, tendon rupture (rare), phototoxicity (rare), peripheral neuropathy (rare), CNS toxicity, hepatotoxicity, and hypersensitivity. Frequent: Headache. Musculoskeletal disorders (primarily mild arthralgias during treatment) reported in children.

ANTIMICROBIALS: Quinolones—4th Generation

NOTE: As of April 2007, the CDC no longer recommends fluoroquinolones for gonorrhea because of high resistance rates. Can cause tendon rupture (rare; risk increased by corticosteroids, age older than 60 yo, or organ transplant), C difficile-associated diarrhea (risk may vary among agents), phototoxicity (risk varies among agents), CNS toxicity, peripheral neuropathy (rare), hypersensitivity, and QT interval prolongation (risk varies among agents; see QT drugs table). Avoid using in proarrhythmic conditions or with drugs that prolong QT interval, including Class 1A and Class III antiarrhythmics. Important quinolone drug interactions with antacids, iron, zinc, magnesium, sucralfate, cimetidine, caffeine, cyclosporine, phenytoin, anticoagulants, theophylline, etc. Monitor INR with warfarin.

GEMIFLOXACIN (*Factive*) ▶Feces, K ♀C ▶– $$$$
WARNING — Tendon rupture (rare; risk increased by corticosteroids, age older than 60 yo, or organ transplant). Advise patients to stop fluoroquinolone, rest affected area, and seek medical advice for tendon swelling, pain, or inflammation.

(cont.)

ANTIMICROBIALS: Sulfonamides

GEMIFLOXACIN *(cont.)*
  ADULTS — <u>Acute exacerbation of chronic bronchitis:</u> 320 mg PO daily for 5 days. <u>Community-acquired pneumonia:</u> 320 mg PO daily for 5 to 7 days (for 7 days for multidrug-resistant S pneumoniae).
  PEDS — Safety and efficacy not established in children; arthropathy in juvenile animals.
  FORMS — Trade only: Tabs 320 mg.
  NOTES — Maintain fluid intake to prevent crystalluria. Give 2 h before or 3 h after Al/Mg antacids, iron, multivitamins with zinc, buffered didanosine. Give at least 2 h before sucralfate. May increase INR with warfarin. Discontinue if rash develops. Reduce dose for CrCl 40 mL/min or less, hemodialysis, or CAPD: 160 mg PO daily.
  MOA — Inhibits bacterial DNA synthesis by binding with DNA gyrase and topoisomerase IV.
  ADVERSE EFFECTS — Serious: QT interval prolongation, tendon rupture (rare), phototoxicity (rare), CNS toxicity, and hypersensitivity. Frequent: Rash (esp. in women younger than 40 yo or treatment duration more than 7 days).

MOXIFLOXACIN (*Avelox*) ▶LK ♀C ▶— $$$
  WARNING — Tendon rupture (rare; risk increased by corticosteroids, age older than 60 yo, or organ transplant). Advise patients to stop fluoroquinolone, rest affected area, and seek medical advice for tendon swelling, pain, or inflammation.
  ADULTS — <u>Chronic bronchitis exacerbation:</u> 400 mg PO/IV daily for 5 days. <u>Complicated intra-abdominal infection:</u> (given IV initially) 400 mg PO/IV daily for 5 to 14 days. <u>Community-acquired pneumonia, including penicillin-resistant S pneumoniae:</u> 400 mg PO/IV daily for 7 to 14 days. <u>Acute sinusitis:</u> 400 mg PO/IV daily for 10 days. <u>Uncomplicated skin infections:</u> 400 mg PO/IV daily for 7 days. <u>Complicated skin infections:</u> 400 mg PO/IV daily for 7 to 21 days.
  PEDS — Safety and efficacy not established in children; arthropathy in juvenile animals.
  UNAPPROVED ADULTS — <u>TB (2nd line treatment):</u> 400 mg IV/PO daily.
  FORMS — Trade only: Tabs 400 mg.
  NOTES — Do not exceed recommended IV dose or infusion rate due to QT prolongation risk. Contraindicated with ziprasidone. Give tabs at least 4 h before or 8 h after Mg/Al antacids, iron, multivitamins with zinc, sucralfate, buffered didanosine. Dosage adjustment not required for hepatic insufficiency.
  MOA — Inhibits bacterial DNA synthesis by binding with DNA gyrase and topoisomerase IV.
  ADVERSE EFFECTS — Serious: QT interval prolongation, tendon rupture (rare), phototoxicity, peripheral neuropathy (rare), CNS toxicity, and hypersensitivity. Frequent: Nausea, diarrhea.

ANTIMICROBIALS: Sulfonamides

NOTE: Sulfonamides can cause Stevens-Johnson syndrome; toxic epidermal necrolysis; hepatotoxicity; blood dyscrasias; hemolysis in glucose-6-phosphate dehydrogenase (G6PD) deficiency. Avoid maternal sulfonamides when the breastfed infant is ill, stressed, premature, has hyperbilirubinemia, or has G6PD deficiency.

SULFADIAZINE ▶K ♀C ▶+ $$$$
  ADULTS — Usual dose: 2 to 4 g PO initially, then 2 to 4 g/day divided into 3 to 6 doses. <u>Secondary prevention of rheumatic fever:</u> 1 g PO daily. Toxoplasmosis treatment: 1 to 1.5 g PO qid with pyrimethamine and leucovorin.
  PEDS — Not for infants younger than 2 mo, except as adjunct to pyrimethamine for congenital toxoplasmosis. Usual dose: Give 75 mg/kg PO initially, then 150 mg/kg/day up to 6 g/day divided into 4 to 6 doses. <u>Secondary prevention of rheumatic fever, for wt 27 kg or less:</u> 500 mg PO daily. Use adult dose for wt greater than 27 kg.
  UNAPPROVED ADULTS — <u>CNS toxoplasmosis in AIDS.</u> Acute therapy: For wt less than 60 kg give pyrimethamine 200 mg PO for single dose, then 50 mg PO once daily with sulfadiazine 1000 mg PO q 6 h and leucovorin 10 to 20 mg (up to 50 mg) PO once daily. For wt 60 kg or greater give pyrimethamine 200 mg PO for single dose, then 75 mg PO once daily with sulfadiazine 1500 mg PO q 6 h and leucovorin 10 to 20 mg PO once daily (up to 50 mg). Secondary prevention: Pyrimethamine 25 to 50 mg PO once daily with sulfadiazine 2000 to 4000 mg/day PO divided bid to qid and leucovorin 10 to 25 mg PO once daily.
  UNAPPROVED PEDS — Not for age younger than 2 mo, except as adjunct to pyrimethamine for congenital toxoplasmosis. AAP regimen for <u>toxoplasmosis:</u> 100 to 200 mg/kg/day PO with pyrimethamine and leucovorin (duration varies). <u>Secondary prevention after CNS toxoplasmosis in HIV infection:</u> 85 to 120 mg/kg/day PO divided in 2 to 4 doses with pyrimethamine and leucovorin.
  FORMS — Generic only: Tabs 500 mg.
  NOTES — Not effective for streptococcal pharyngitis. Maintain fluid intake to prevent crystalluria and stone formation. Reduce dose in renal insufficiency. May increase INR with warfarin. May increase levels of methotrexate, phenytoin.
  MOA — Structural analog of PABA that binds with dihydropteroate synthetase and prevents nucleic acid synthesis. Bacteriostatic.
  ADVERSE EFFECTS — Serious: Stevens-Johnson syndrome, toxic epidermal necrolysis, hepatotoxicity, blood dyscrasias, hemolysis in G6PD deficiency, crystalluria and stone formation. Frequent: Rash, N/V, diarrhea, fever.

TRIMETHOPRIM-SULFAMETHOXAZOLE (*Bactrim, Septra, Sulfatrim, cotrimoxazole*) ▶K ♀C ▶+ $
  ADULTS — <u>UTI, shigellosis, acute exacerbation of chronic bronchitis:</u> 1 tab PO bid, double-strength

(cont.)

ANTIMICROBIALS: Tetracyclines

TRIMETHOPRIM-SULFAMETHOXAZOLE (*cont.*)
(DS, 160 TMP/800 SMX). Travelers' diarrhea: 1 DS tab PO bid for 5 days. Pneumocystis treatment: 15 to 20 mg/kg/day (based on TMP) IV divided q 6 to 8 h or PO divided tid for 21 days total; can use 2 DS tabs PO tid for mild to moderate infection. Pneumocystis prophylaxis: 1 DS tab PO daily.
PEDS — UTI, shigellosis, otitis media: 1 mL/kg/day susp PO divided BID (up to 20 mL PO bid). Pneumocystis treatment: 15 to 20 mg/kg/day (based on TMP) IV divided q 6 to 8 h or 5 mL susp/8 kg/dose PO q 6 h. Pneumocystis prophylaxis: 150 mg/m2/day (based on TMP) PO divided bid on 3 consecutive days each week. Do not use in infants younger than 2 mo; may cause kernicterus.
UNAPPROVED ADULTS — Bacterial prostatitis: 1 DS tab PO bid for 10 to 14 days for acute, for 1 to 3 months for chronic. Sinusitis: 1 DS tab PO bid for 10 days. Burkholderia cepacia pulmonary infection in cystic fibrosis: 5 mg/kg (based on TMP) IV q 6 h. Pneumocystis prophylaxis: 1 SS tab PO daily. Primary prevention of toxoplasmosis in AIDS: 1 DS tab PO daily. Pertussis: 1 DS tab PO bid for 14 days (2nd line to macrolides). Community-acquired MRSA skin infections: 1 to 2 DS tabs PO bid for 7 to 10 days.
UNAPPROVED PEDS — Community-acquired MRSA skin infections: 8 to 12 mg/kg/day (based on TMP) PO divided bid for 7 to 10 days. Pertussis: 8 mg/kg/day (based on TMP) PO divided bid for 14 days (2nd line to macrolides).
FORMS — Generic/Trade: Tabs 80 mg TMP/400 mg SMX (single strength), 160 mg TMP/800 mg SMX (double strength; DS), susp 40 mg TMP/200 mg SMX per 5 mL. 20 mL susp = 2 SS tabs = 1 DS tab.
NOTES — Not effective for streptococcal pharyngitis. No activity against penicillin-nonsusceptible pneumococci. Bone marrow depression with high IV doses. Significantly increased INR with warfarin; avoid concomitant use if possible. Increases levels of methotrexate, phenytoin. Rifampin reduces TMP/SMX levels. Can cause hyperkalemia (risk increased by high doses of trimethoprim, renal impairment, other drugs that cause hyperkalemia). AAP recommends 5 to 7 days of therapy for children age 6 yo or older with nonsevere otitis media, and 10 days for younger children and those with severe disease. Dosing in renal dysfunction: Use 50% of usual dose for CrCl 15 to 30 mL/min. Don't use for CrCl less than 15 mL/min.
MOA — Sulfonamides (bacteriostatic) are structural analogs of PABA that bind with dihydropteroate synthetase and prevent bacterial folic acid synthesis. Trimethoprim inhibits dihydrofolate reductase, the enzyme after step in folic acid synthesis inhibited by sulfonamides. Trimethoprim acts like a potassium-sparing diuretic, reducing urinary potassium excretion.
ADVERSE EFFECTS — Serious: Stevens-Johnson syndrome, toxic epidermal necrolysis, hepatotoxicity, blood dyscrasias (thrombocytopenia risk possibly increased by thiazide diuretics), hemolysis in G6PD deficiency, hyperkalemia (risk increased by high doses of trimethoprim, renal impairment, or other drugs that cause hyperkalemia). Bone marrow depression with high IV doses. Frequent: N/V, anorexia, allergic skin reactions, photosensitivity.

ANTIMICROBIALS: Tetracyclines

NOTE: Tetracyclines can cause photosensitivity and pseudotumor cerebri (avoid with isotretinoin which is also linked to pseudotumor cerebri). May decrease efficacy of oral contraceptives. Increased INR with warfarin. May increase risk of ergotism with ergot alkaloids.

DEMECLOCYCLINE (*Declomycin*) ▶K, feces ♀D ▶?+ $$$$
ADULTS — Usual dose: 150 mg PO qid or 300 mg PO bid on empty stomach.
PEDS — Avoid in age younger than 8 yo due to teeth staining. Usual dose: 6.6 to 13.2 mg/kg/day PO given in 2 to 4 divided doses on empty stomach.
UNAPPROVED ADULTS — SIADH: 600 to 1200 mg/day PO given in 3 to 4 divided doses.
FORMS — Generic/Trade: Tabs 150, 300 mg.
NOTES — Can cause diabetes insipidus, high risk of photosensitivity. Use with caution in renal dysfunction; doxycycline preferred. Absorption impaired by iron, calcium, Al/Mg antacids. Take with fluids (not milk) to decrease esophageal irritation. SIADH onset of action occurs within 5 to 14 days; do not increase dose more frequently than q 3 to 4 days. May decrease oral contraceptive effectiveness.
MOA — Inhibits bacterial protein synthesis by binding with ribosomal 30S subunit and blocking addition of amino acids to peptide chain. Active against intracellular bacteria. Bacteriostatic. Blocks action of ADH at level of collecting duct and distal tubule.
ADVERSE EFFECTS — Serious: Pseudotumor cerebri, nephrotoxicity, photosensitivity (high risk), teeth staining in children younger than 8 yo, diabetes insipidus. Frequent: N/V, heartburn, epigastric distress, diarrhea.

DOXYCYCLINE (*Adoxa, Doryx, Monodox, Oracea, Periostat, Vibramycin, Vibra-Tabs, ✦Doxycin*) ▶LK ♀D ▶?+ $
ADULTS — Usual dose: 100 mg PO bid on first day, then 100 mg/day PO daily or divided bid. Severe infections: 100 mg PO bid. Chlamydia, nongonococcal urethritis: 100 mg PO bid for 7 days. Acne vulgaris: Up to 100 mg PO bid. Community-acquired MRSA skin infections: 100 mg PO bid. Periostat ($$$$$) for periodontitis: 20 mg PO bid 1 h before breakfast and dinner. Oracea ($$$$$)

(cont.)

DOXYCYCLINE (cont.)

for <u>inflammatory rosacea (papules and pustules):</u> 40 mg PO once every morning on empty stomach. <u>Cholera:</u> 300 mg PO single dose. <u>Primary, secondary, early latent syphilis if penicillin-allergic:</u> 100 mg PO bid for 14 days. <u>Late latent or tertiary syphilis if penicillin-allergic:</u> 100 mg PO bid for 4 weeks. Not for neurosyphilis. <u>Malaria prophylaxis:</u> 100 mg PO daily starting 1 to 2 days before exposure until 4 weeks after. IV: 200 mg on first day in 1 to 2 infusions, then 100 to 200 mg/day in 1 to 2 infusions. <u>Bioterrorism anthrax:</u> 100 mg bid for 60 days. Use IV with at least 1 other drug for initial treatment of inhalation or severe cutaneous anthrax. PO monotherapy for less severe cutaneous anthrax or postexposure prophylaxis. See www.idsociety.org/BT/ToC.htm for more info.

PEDS — Avoid in age younger than 8 yo due to teeth staining. Usual dose: 4.4 mg/kg/day PO divided bid on first day, then 2.2 to 4.4 mg/kg/day PO divided daily or bid for wt 45 kg or less. Use adult dose for wt greater than 45 kg. <u>Malaria prophylaxis:</u> 2 mg/kg/day up to 100 mg PO daily starting 1 to 2 days before exposure until 4 weeks after. Most PO and IV doses are equivalent. <u>Bioterrorism anthrax:</u> 100 mg bid for age older than 8 yo and wt greater than 45 kg, 2.2 mg/kg bid for age older than 8 yo and wt 45 kg or less, or age 8 yo or younger. Treat for 60 days. Use IV with at least 1 other drug for initial treatment of inhalation anthrax, severe cutaneous anthrax, or cutaneous anthrax in age younger than 2 yo. PO monotherapy for less severe cutaneous anthrax and postexposure prophylaxis. See www.idsociety.org/BT/ToC.htm for more info.

UNAPPROVED ADULTS — See STD table for <u>granuloma inguinale, lymphogranuloma venereum, pelvic inflammatory disease treatment.</u> <u>Lyme disease:</u> 100 mg PO bid for 14 days for early disease, for 28 days for Lyme arthritis. <u>Prevention of Lyme disease in highly endemic area, with deer tick attachment at least 48 h:</u> 200 mg PO single dose with food within 72 h of tick bite. <u>Ehrlichiosis:</u> 100 mg IV/PO bid for 7 to 14 days. <u>Malaria, co-therapy with quinine/quinidine:</u> 100 mg IV/PO bid for 7 days. <u>Lymphatic filariasis:</u> 100 mg PO bid for 8 weeks.

FORMS — Generic/Trade: Tabs 20, 75, 100 mg, Caps 50, 100 mg, Susp 25 mg/5 mL (60 mL). Trade only: (Vibramycin) Syrup 50 mg/5 mL (480 mL). Delayed-release (Doryx $$$$$): Tabs 75, 100 mg, Caps 40 mg (Oracea $$$$$). Generic only: Caps 75, 150 mg, Tabs 50, 150 mg.

NOTES — Photosensitivity, pseudotumor cerebri, increased BUN, painful IV infusion. Do not use Oracea for treatment of infections. Do not give antacids or calcium supplements within 2 h of doxycycline. Barbiturates, carbamazepine, rifampin, and phenytoin may decrease doxycycline levels. Preferred over tetracycline in renal dysfunction. Take with fluids to decrease esophageal irritation; can take with food/milk. Can break Doryx tabs and give immediately in a spoonful of applesauce. Do not crush or chew delayed-release pellets in tab. Maternal antimalarial prophylaxis doesn't harm breastfed infant or protect infant from malaria.

MOA — Inhibits bacterial protein synthesis by binding with ribosomal 30S subunit and blocking addition of amino acids to peptide chain. Active against intracellular bacteria. Bacteriostatic. Subantimicrobial doses have anti-inflammatory effects.

ADVERSE EFFECTS — Serious: Pseudotumor cerebri, increased BUN, erosive esophagitis if taken lying down, teeth staining in children younger than 8 yo. Frequent: Photosensitivity, vaginitis, painful IV infusion.

MINOCYCLINE (*Minocin, Dynacin, Solodyn, ✦Enca*) ▶LK ♀D ▶?+ $$

ADULTS — Usual dose: 200 mg IV/PO first dose, then 100 mg q 12 h. IV and PO doses are the same. Not more than 400 mg/day IV. <u>Community-acquired MRSA skin infections:</u> 100 mg PO bid. <u>Solodyn ($$$$$) for inflammatory nonnodular moderate to severe acne:</u> 1 mg/kg PO once daily. Dose is 45 mg for wt 45 to 54 kg, 65 mg for wt 55 to 77 kg, 90 mg for 78 to 102 kg, 115 mg for wt 103 to 125 kg, 135 mg for 126 to 136 kg.

PEDS — Avoid in age younger than 8 yo due to teeth staining. Usual dose: 4 mg/kg PO first dose, then 2 mg/kg bid. IV and PO doses are the same. Solodyn ($$$$$) for inflammatory <u>nonnodular moderate to severe acne:</u> Give PO once daily to age 12 yo or older at dose of 45 mg for wt 45 to 54 kg, 65 mg for wt 55 to 77 kg, 90 mg for 78 to 102 kg, 115 mg for wt 103 to 125 kg, 135 mg for 126 to 136 kg.

UNAPPROVED ADULTS — <u>Acne vulgaris</u> (traditional dosing, not for Solodyn): 50 mg PO bid. RA: 100 mg PO bid.

FORMS — Generic/Trade: Caps, Tabs 50, 75, 100 mg. Tabs, extended-release (Solodyn) 45, 90, 135 mg. Trade only: Tabs, extended-release (Solodyn) 65, 115 mg.

NOTES — Dizziness, hepatotoxicity, lupus. Do not use Solodyn ($$$$$) for treatment of infections. Do not give antacids or calcium supplements within 2 h of minocycline. May cause drowsiness. Take with fluids (not milk) to decrease esophageal irritation. Use with caution in renal dysfunction; doxycycline preferred.

MOA — Inhibits bacterial protein synthesis by binding with ribosomal 30S subunit and blocking addition of amino acids to peptide chain. Active against intracellular bacteria. Bacteriostatic. Subantimicrobial doses have anti-inflammatory effects.

ADVERSE EFFECTS — Serious: Pseudotumor cerebri, increased BUN, photosensitivity, hepatotoxicity, lupus, hypersensitivity pneumonitis, hyperpigmentation, teeth staining in children younger than 8 yo. Frequent: Dizziness/vestibular toxicity.

TETRACYCLINE (*Sumycin*) ▶LK ♀D ▶?+ $

ADULTS — Usual dose: 250 to 500 mg PO qid on empty stomach. <u>H pylori:</u> See table in GI section. <u>Primary, secondary, early latent syphilis if penicillin-allergic:</u> 500 mg PO qid for 14 days. <u>Late latent</u>

(cont.)

TETRACYCLINE (cont.)
syphilis if penicillin-allergic: 500 mg PO qid for 28 days.
PEDS — Avoid in children younger than 8 yo due to teeth staining. Usual dose: 25 to 50 mg/kg/day PO divided in 2 to 4 doses on empty stomach.
UNAPPROVED ADULTS — Malaria, co-therapy with quinine: 250 mg PO qid for 7 days.
UNAPPROVED PEDS — Malaria, co-therapy with quinine: 25 mg/kg/day PO divided qid for 7 days.
FORMS — Generic only: Caps 250, 500 mg.
NOTES — Increased BUN/hepatotoxicity in patients with renal dysfunction. Do not give antacids or calcium supplements within 2 h of tetracycline. Use with caution in renal dysfunction; doxycycline preferred. Take with fluids (not milk) to decrease esophageal irritation.
MOA — Inhibits bacterial protein synthesis by binding with ribosomal 30S subunit and blocking addition of amino acids to peptide chain. Active against intracellular bacteria. Bacteriostatic.
ADVERSE EFFECTS — Serious: Pseudotumor cerebri, increased BUN/hepatotoxicity in patients with renal dysfunction, photosensitivity, teeth staining in children younger than 8 yo.

ANTIMICROBIALS: Other Antimicrobials

AZTREONAM (*Azactam*) ▶K ♀B ▶+ $$$$$
ADULTS — UTI: 500 mg to 1 g IM/IV q 8 to 12 h. Pneumonia, sepsis, skin, intra-abdominal, gynecologic: Moderate infections, 1 to 2 g IM/IV q 8 to 12 h. P aeruginosa or severe infections, 2 g IV q 6 to 8 h. Use IV route for doses greater than 1 g.
PEDS — Serious gram-negative infections, usual dose: 30 mg/kg/dose IV q 6 to 8 h.
UNAPPROVED ADULTS — Meningitis: 2 g IV q 6 to 8 h.
UNAPPROVED PEDS — P aeruginosa pulmonary infection in cystic fibrosis: 50 mg/kg/dose IV q 6 to 8 h.
NOTES — Dosing in adults with renal dysfunction: 1 to 2 g IV load, then 50% of usual dose for CrCl 10 to 30 mL/min. 0.5 to 2 g IV load, then 25% of usual dose for CrCl < 10 mL/min. For life-threatening infections, also give 12.5% of initial dose after each hemodialysis.
MOA — Monobactam (monocyclic beta-lactam) that binds only to penicillin-binding proteins in gram-negative organisms.
ADVERSE EFFECTS — Serious: Cross-sensitivity with ceftazidime possible, but unlikely, C. difficile-associated diarrhea. Frequent: Eosinophilia.

CHLORAMPHENICOL (*Chloromycetin*) ▶LK ♀C ▶− $$$$$
WARNING — Serious and fatal blood dyscrasias. Dose-dependent bone marrow suppression common.
ADULTS — Typhoid fever, rickettsial infections: 50 mg/kg/day IV divided q 6 h. Up to 75 to 100 mg/kg/day IV for serious infections untreatable with other agents.
PEDS — Severe infections including meningitis: 50 to 100 mg/kg/day IV divided q 6 h. AAP recommends 75 to 100 mg/kg/day for invasive pneumococcal infections only in patients with life-threatening beta-lactam allergy.
NOTES — Monitor CBC every 2 days. Monitor serum levels. Therapeutic peak: 10 to 20 mcg/mL. Trough: 5 to 10 mcg/mL. Use cautiously in acute intermittent porphyria/G6PD deficiency. Gray baby syndrome in preemies and newborns. Barbiturates, rifampin decrease chloramphenicol levels. Chloramphenicol increases barbiturate, phenytoin levels and may increase INR with warfarin. Dosing in adults with hepatic dysfunction: 1 g IV load, then 500 mg q 6 h.
MOA — Inhibits bacterial protein synthesis by interfering with ribosomal 50S subunit. Bacteriostatic/cidal depending on pathogen.
ADVERSE EFFECTS — Serious: Fatal blood dyscrasias, dose-dependent bone marrow suppression common. Gray baby syndrome in preemies and newborns.

CLINDAMYCIN (*Cleocin*, ✦*Dalacin C*) ▶L ♀B ▶?+ $$$
WARNING — C difficile-associated diarrhea.
ADULTS — Serious anaerobic, streptococcal, Staph infections: 600 to 900 mg IV q 8 h or 150 to 450 mg PO qid. Community-acquired MRSA skin infections: 300 mg PO tid. See tables for prophylaxis of bacterial endocarditis and treatment of STDs (pelvic inflammatory disease).
PEDS — Serious anaerobic, streptococcal, Staph infections: 20 to 40 mg/kg/day IV divided q 6 to 8 h or 8 to 20 mg/kg/day (as caps) PO divided tid to qid or 8 to 25 mg/kg/day (as palmitate oral soln) PO divided tid to qid. Community-acquired MRSA skin infections: 30 mg/kg/day PO tid. Do not use doses which are less than 37.5 mg of oral soln PO tid for children wt less than 11 kg. Infants age younger than 1 mo: 15 to 20 mg/kg/day IV divided tid to qid. See table for prophylaxis of bacterial endocarditis.
UNAPPROVED ADULTS — Bacterial vaginosis: 300 mg PO bid for 7 days. Oral/dental infection: 300 mg PO qid. Prevention of perinatal group B streptococcal disease: 900 mg IV to mother q 8 h until delivery. CNS toxoplasmosis, AIDS (with leucovorin, pyrimethamine): Acute treatment 600 mg PO/IV q 6 h; secondary prevention 300 to 450 mg PO q 6 to 8 h. AHA dose for group A streptococcal pharyngitis in penicillin-allergic patients: 20 mg/kg/day (max 1.8 g/day) PO divided tid for 10 days. Group A streptococcal pharyngitis, repeated culture-positive episodes: 20 mg/kg/day (max 1.8 g/day) PO divided tid for 10 days. Malaria, co-therapy with quinine/quinidine: 10 mg/kg base IV loading dose followed by 5 mg/kg IV q 8 h or 20 mg/kg/day base PO divided tid to complete 7 days.

(cont.)

C DIFFICILE INFECTION IN ADULTS: IDSA/SHEA TREATMENT RECOMMENDATIONS

Severity	Clinical signs	Treatment
Initial episode		
Mild to moderate	Leukocytosis with WBC count 15,000 or lower AND Serum creatinine less than 1.5 times premorbid level	Metronidazole 500 mg PO q8h for 10 to 14 days
Severe	Leukocytosis with WBC count 15,000 or higher OR Serum creatinine at least 1.5 times greater than premorbid level	Vancomycin 125 mg PO q6h for 10 to 14 days
Severe complicated	Hypotension or shock, ileus, megacolon	Vancomycin 500 mg PO/NG q6h plus metronidazole 500 mg IV q8h. Consider vancomycin 500 mg/100 mL normal saline retention enema q6h if complete ileus.
Recurrent episodes		
First recurrence	--	Same as initial episode, stratified by severity. Use vancomycin if WBC count 15,000 or higher, or serum creatinine is increasing.
Second recurrence	--	Vancomycin taper* and/or pulsed regimen

Adapted from Infect Control Hosp Epidemiol 2010; 31(5). Available online at: http://www.idsociety.org.
* Example: Vancomycin 125 mg PO QID for 10 to 14 days, then 125 mg BID for 7 days, then 125 mg once daily for 7 days, then 125 mg every 2 or 3 days for 2 to 8 weeks.

CLINDAMYCIN (cont.)

UNAPPROVED PEDS — <u>AHA dose for group A streptococcal pharyngitis in penicillin-allergic patients:</u> 20 mg/kg/day (max 1.8 g/day) PO divided tid for 10 days. <u>Group A streptococcal pharyngitis, repeated culture-positive episodes:</u> 20 to 30 mg/kg/day PO divided q 8 h for 10 days. <u>Otitis media:</u> 30 to 40 mg/kg/day PO divided tid. <u>Toxoplasmosis, substitute for sulfadiazine in sulfonamide-intolerant children:</u> 5 to 7.5 mg/kg (up to 600 mg/dose) PO/IV q 6 h + pyrimethamine + leucovorin. <u>Malaria, co-therapy with quinine/quinidine:</u> 10 mg/kg base IV loading dose followed by 5 mg/kg IV q 8 h or 20 mg/kg/day base PO divided tid to complete 7 days.
FORMS — Generic/Trade: Caps 75, 150, 300 mg. Oral soln 75 mg/5 mL (100 mL).
NOTES — Not for meningitis. Not more than 600 mg/IM injection site. Avoid if lincomycin hypersensitivity. Consider using D-test for MRSA inducible resistance.
MOA — Semisynthetic derivative of lincomycin that inhibits RNA-dependent protein synthesis in susceptible organisms by interfering with function of ribosomal 50S subunit.
ADVERSE EFFECTS — Serious: C. difficile-associated diarrhea. Frequent: Diarrhea, allergic reactions.

DAPTOMYCIN (*Cubicin, Cidecin*) ▶K ♀B ▶? $$$$$
ADULTS — <u>Complicated skin infections</u> (including MRSA): 4 mg/kg IV once daily for 7 to 14 days. <u>S aureus (including MRSA) bacteremia, including endocarditis:</u> 6 mg/kg IV once daily for at least 2 to 6 weeks. Infuse over 30 min.
PEDS — Not approved in children.
NOTES — May cause myopathy; monitor CK levels weekly. Stop if myopathy symptoms and CK more than 5 times upper limit of normal, or no symptoms and CK at least 10 times upper limit of normal. Consider withholding statins during daptomycin treatment. May cause neuropathy. Eosinophilic pneumonia (rare). Can falsely elevate PT with certain thromboplastin reagents; can minimize effect by drawing PT/INR sample just before daptomycin dose or use another reagent. Not effective for pneumonia (inactivated by surfactant). Reduce dose in adults with CrCl less than 30 mL/min: 4 mg/kg IV q 48 h. Reconstituted soln stable for up to 12 h at room temp or 48 h in refrigerator (combined time in vial and IV bag). Do not use in Readymed elastomeric infusion pump due to leaching of MBT impurity.
MOA — Cyclic lipopeptide that depolarizes bacterial membrane potential. Inhibition of DNA, RNA, and protein synthesis kills bacteria.
ADVERSE EFFECTS — Serious: Myopathy, neuropathy, eosinophilic pneumonia (rare). Frequent: Increased CK levels, constipation, nausea, headache.

DROTRECOGIN (*Xigris*) ▶Plasma ♀C ▶? $$$$$
ADULTS — <u>To reduce mortality in sepsis:</u> 24 mcg/kg/h IV for 96 h. Reduced mortality only in patients with APACHE II score 25 or greater.

(cont.)

DROTRECOGIN (cont.)

PEDS — Not approved in children, and was ineffective in a clinical trial of severe sepsis in children with a trend toward increased CNS bleeding.

NOTES — Can cause severe bleeding. Contraindicated with conditions and drugs that increase risk of bleeding; see package insert for details. Xigris may not be indicated in patients with single organ dysfunction and recent surgery; these patients do not have high-enough risk of mortality to require treatment and Xigris increased mortality. Criteria for use include systemic inflammatory response plus acute organ dysfunction. Stop infusion 2 h before invasive procedure, or if bleeding occurs. May prolong APTT. Complete IV infusion within 12 h of reconstitution. Do not expose IV soln to heat or direct sunlight.

MOA — Recombinant human activated protein C, inhibits coagulation, decreases inflammation, increases fibrinolysis, inhibits TNF synthesis.

ADVERSE EFFECTS — Severe: Major bleeding. Frequent: None.

FOSFOMYCIN (*Monurol*) ▶K ♀B ▶? $$

ADULTS — Simple UTI in women: One 3 g packet PO single dose. Dissolve granules in ½ cup of water.

PEDS — Not approved for age younger than 12 yo.

FORMS — Trade only: 3 g packet of granules.

NOTES — Metoclopramide decreases urinary excretion of fosfomycin. No additional benefit with multiple dosing. Single dose less effective than ciprofloxacin or TMP/SMX; equivalent to nitrofurantoin.

MOA — Inactivates enolpyruvyl transferase, irreversibly blocking an early step in bacterial cell wall synthesis. Also reduces bacterial adherence to uroepithelial cells. Bactericidal in urine.

ADVERSE EFFECTS — Serious: None. Frequent: Diarrhea.

LINCOMYCIN (*Lincocin*) ▶LK ♀C ▶– $$$$

WARNING — C difficile-associated diarrhea.

ADULTS — Serious gram-positive infections: 600 mg IM q 12 to 24 h. 600 to 1000 mg IV q 8 to 12 h. Max IV daily dose is 8 g. Dilute to 1 g/100 mL or less, and infuse over at least 1 h. Reserve for patients who are allergic to or do not respond to penicillins.

PEDS — Serious gram-positive infections, for age older than 1 mo: 10 to 20 mg/kg/day IV divided q 8 to 12 h. Dilute to 1 g/100 mL or less, and infuse over at least 1 h. Reserve for patients who are allergic to or do not respond to penicillins.

NOTES — Do not use in patients with clindamycin hypersensitivity. Monitor hepatic and renal function and CBC during prolonged therapy. Do not coadminister with erythromycin due to potential antagonism. May enhance effects of neuromuscular blockers. Reduce dose by 25% to 30% in patients with severe renal dysfunction and consider monitoring levels.

MOA — Inhibits RNA-dependent protein synthesis in susceptible organisms by interfering with function of ribosomal 50S subunit.

ADVERSE EFFECTS — Serious: C. difficile-associated diarrhea; severe hypersensitivity reactions; Stevens-Johnson syndrome; neutropenia; thrombocytopenia; renal dysfunction. Hypotension/cardiopulmonary arrest possible if IV infusion too rapid. Frequent: No data.

LINEZOLID (*Zyvox*, ✢*Zyvoxam*) ▶Oxidation/K ♀C ▶? $$$$$

ADULTS — IV and PO doses are the same. Vancomycin-resistant E faecium infections: 600 mg IV/PO q 12 h for 14 to 28 days. Pneumonia, complicated skin infections (including MRSA and diabetic foot): 600 mg IV/PO q 12 h for 10 to 14 days. IV infused over 30 to 120 min.

PEDS — Pneumonia, complicated skin infections (including MRSA): 10 mg/kg (up to 600 mg) IV/PO q 8 h for 10 to 14 days for age younger than 12 yo, 600 mg IV/PO q 12 h for age 12 yo or older. Vancomycin-resistant E. faecium infections: 10 mg/kg IV/PO q 8 h (up to 600 mg) for 14 to 28 days for age younger than 12 yo, 600 mg IV/PO q 12 h for age 12 yo or older. Uncomplicated skin infections: 10 mg/kg PO q 8 h for 10 to 14 days for age younger than 5 yo, 10 mg/kg PO q 12 h for age 5 to 11 yo, 600 mg PO q 12 h for age 12 yo or older. Preterm infants (less than 34 weeks gestational age): 10 mg/kg q 12 h, increase to 10 mg/kg q 8 h by 7 days of life. IV infused over 30 to 120 min.

FORMS — Trade only: Tabs 600 mg. Susp 100 mg/5 mL.

NOTES — Myelosuppression. Monitor CBC weekly, especially if more than 2 weeks of therapy, pre-existing myelosuppression, other myelosuppressive drugs, or chronic infection treated with other antibiotics. Consider stopping if myelosuppression occurs or worsens. Peripheral and optic neuropathy, primarily in those treated for more than 1 month. Ophthalmic exam recommended for visual changes at any time; monitor visual function in all patients treated for 3 months or longer. In a study comparing linezolid with vancomycin, oxacillin, or dicloxacillin for catheter-related bloodstream infections, mortality was increased in linezolid-treated patients infected only with gram-negative bacteria. Inhibits MAO; may interact with adrenergic and serotonergic drugs, high-tyramine foods. Limit tyramine to < 100 mg/meal. Reduce initial dose of dopamine/epinephrine. Serotonin syndrome reported with concomitant administration of serotonergic drugs (SSRIs). Rifampin can reduce linezolid exposure; clinical significance unclear. Store susp at room temperature; stable for 21 days. Gently turn bottle over 3 to 5 times before giving a dose; do not shake.

MOA — Oxazolidinone that inhibits bacterial protein synthesis by binding with 50S ribosome (may compete for binding with chloramphenicol). Bacteriostatic.

ADVERSE EFFECTS — Serious: Myelosuppression, reports of serotonin syndrome, peripheral and optic neuropathy (with long-term use; optic neuropathy sometimes progressing to vision loss), lactic acidosis (immediate evaluation if recurrent N/V, unexplained acidosis, low bicarbonate). In a study comparing linezolid with vancomycin, oxacillin, dicloxacillin for catheter-related bloodstream

(cont.)

ANTIMICROBIALS: Other Antimicrobials

LINEZOLID (cont.)

infections, mortality was increased in linezolid-treated patients infected only with gram-negative bacteria. Frequent: Thrombocytopenia, N/V, diarrhea. Tooth discoloration (removable with cleaning).

METRONIDAZOLE (*Flagyl, Flagyl ER, ✦Florazole ER, Trikacide, Nidazol*) ▶KL ♀B ▶?- $
- WARNING — Carcinogenic in animal studies; avoid unnecessary use.
- ADULTS — <u>Trichomoniasis:</u> Treat patient and sex partners with 2 g PO single dose (may be used in pregnancy per CDC), 250 mg PO tid for 7 days, or 375 mg PO bid for 7 days. <u>Flagyl ER for bacterial vaginosis:</u> 750 mg PO daily for 7 days on empty stomach. <u>H pylori:</u> See table in GI section. <u>Anaerobic bacterial infections:</u> Load 1 g or 15 mg/kg IV, then 500 mg or 7.5 mg/kg IV/PO q 6 to 8 h (up to 4 g/day), each IV dose over 1 h. <u>Prophylaxis, colorectal surgery:</u> 15 mg/kg IV completed 1 h preop, then 7.5 mg/kg IV q 6 h for 2 doses. <u>Acute amebic dysentery:</u> 750 mg PO tid for 5 to 10 days. <u>Amebic liver abscess:</u> 500 to 750 mg IV/PO tid for 10 days.
- PEDS — <u>Amebiasis:</u> 35 to 50 mg/kg/day PO (up to 750 mg/dose) divided tid for 10 days.
- UNAPPROVED ADULTS — <u>Bacterial vaginosis:</u> 500 mg PO bid for 7 days. <u>Bacterial vaginosis in pregnancy:</u> 500 mg PO bid or 250 mg PO tid for 7 days. <u>Trichomoniasis</u> (CDC alternative to single dose): 500 mg PO bid for 7 days. <u>Pelvic inflammatory disease and recurrent/persistent urethritis:</u> See STD table. <u>C difficile-associated diarrhea, mild/moderate:</u> 500 mg PO tid for 10 to 14 days. C difficile-associated diarrhea, severe complicated: 500 mg IV q8h with PO/PR vancomycin. See table for management of C. difficile infection in adults. <u>Giardia:</u> 250 mg PO tid for 5 to 7 days.
- UNAPPROVED PEDS — <u>C difficile-associated diarrhea:</u> 30 mg/kg/day PO divided qid for 10 to 14 days (not to exceed adult dose). <u>Trichomoniasis:</u> 5 mg/kg PO tid (max 2 g/day) for 7 days. <u>Giardia:</u> 15 mg/kg/day PO divided tid for 5 to 7 days. <u>Anaerobic bacterial infections:</u> 30 mg/kg/day IV/PO divided q 6 h, each IV dose over 1 h (up to 4 g/day).
- FORMS — Generic/Trade: Tabs 250, 500 mg, Caps 375 mg. Trade only: Tabs, extended-release 750 mg.
- NOTES — Peripheral neuropathy (chronic use), seizures. Avoid long-term use. Disulfiram reaction; avoid alcohol until at least 1 day after treatment with tabs, at least 3 days with caps/Flagyl ER. Do not give within 2 weeks of disulfiram. Interacts with barbiturates, lithium, phenytoin. Increased INR with warfarin. Darkens urine. Give iodoquinol or paromomycin after treatment for amebic dysentery or liver abscess. Can minimize infant exposure by withholding breastfeeding for 12 to 24 h after maternal single dose. Decrease dose in liver dysfunction.
- MOA — Bactericidal agent that is reduced intracellularly to toxic intermediates/free radicals that damage DNA or other macromolecules.
- ADVERSE EFFECTS — Serious: Peripheral neuropathy (chronic use), seizures. Frequent: Darkens urine, N/V, diarrhea, metallic aftertaste, disulfiram-like reaction.

NITROFURANTOIN (*Furadantin, Macrodantin, Macrobid*) ▶KL ♀B ▶+? $
- WARNING — Pulmonary fibrosis with prolonged use.
- ADULTS — <u>Acute uncomplicated cystitis:</u> 50 to 100 mg PO qid with food/milk for 7 days or until 3 days after sterile urine. <u>Long-term suppressive therapy:</u> 50 to 100 mg PO at bedtime. Macrobid: 100 mg PO bid with food/milk for 7 days.
- PEDS — <u>UTI:</u> 5 to 7 mg/kg/day PO divided qid for 7 days or until 3 days after sterile urine. <u>Long-term suppressive therapy:</u> Doses as low as 1 mg/kg/day PO divided daily to bid. Give with food/milk. Macrobid, age older than 12 yo: 100 mg PO bid with food/milk for 7 days.
- FORMS — Generic/Trade (Macrodantin): Caps 25, 50, 100 mg, Generic/Trade (Macrobid): Caps 100 mg. Trade only (Furadantin): Susp 25 mg/5 mL.
- NOTES — Contraindicated if CrCl less than 60 mL/min, pregnancy 38 weeks or greater, infant age younger than 1 mo. Hemolytic anemia in G6PD deficiency (including susceptible infants exposed through breastmilk), hepatotoxicity (monitor LFTs periodically), peripheral neuropathy. May turn urine brown. Do not use for complicated UTI or pyelonephritis.
- MOA — Appears to interact with ribosomal proteins and damage bacterial DNA.
- ADVERSE EFFECTS — Serious: Pulmonary fibrosis with prolonged use, hepatotoxicity, peripheral neuropathy, hemolytic anemia in G6PD deficiency. Frequent: N/V, allergy, brown discoloration of urine.

RIFAXIMIN (*Xifaxan*) ▶Feces, no GI absorption ♀C ▶? $$$
- ADULTS — <u>Travelers diarrhea:</u> 200 mg PO tid for 3 days. <u>Prevention of recurrent hepatic encephalopathy</u> ($$$$$): 550 mg PO bid.
- PEDS — Not approved for age younger than 12 yo.
- FORMS — Trade only: Tabs 200, 550 mg.
- NOTES — Not effective for diarrhea complicated by fever/blood in stool or caused by pathogens other than E coli. Consider switching to another agent if diarrhea persists for 24 to 48 h or worsens. Rifaximin exposure may increase in severe hepatic impairment.
- MOA — Rifamycin structurally related to rifampin. Inhibits bacterial RNA synthesis by binding with beta-subunit of bacterial DNA-dependent RNA polymerase. Active against entero-toxigenic or -aggregative E Coli.
- ADVERSE EFFECTS — Serious: None found. Frequent: None found.

SYNERCID (quinupristin + dalfopristin) ▶Bile ♀B ▶? $$$$$
- WARNING — FDA approval for vancomycin-resistant Enterococcus faecium (VREF) bacteremia is based on clearance of VREF from the bloodstream, a surrogate endpoint.
- ADULTS — <u>Vancomycin-resistant E faecium infections</u> (Not active against E faecalis): 7.5 mg/kg IV q

(cont.)

ANTIMICROBIALS: Other Antimicrobials

SYNERCID (cont.)
8 h. Complicated staphylococcal/streptococcal skin infections: 7.5 mg/kg IV q 12 h. Infuse over 1 h.
PEDS — Safety and efficacy not established in children.
UNAPPROVED ADULTS — Community-acquired MRSA: 7.5 mg/kg IV q 8 to 12 h.
UNAPPROVED PEDS — Vancomycin-resistant E faecium infections (Not active against E faecalis): 7.5 mg/kg IV q 8 h. Complicated staphylococcal/streptococcal skin infections: 7.5 mg/kg IV q 12 h. Infuse over 1 h.
NOTES — Venous irritation (flush with D5W after peripheral infusion; do not use normal saline/heparin), arthralgias/myalgias, hyperbilirubinemia. Infuse by central venous catheter to avoid dose-related vein irritation. CYP3A4 inhibitor. Increases levels of cyclosporine, midazolam, nifedipine, and others.
MOA — Streptogramin fixed-dose combination that inhibits bacterial protein synthesis by binding to different sites of the 50S ribosomal subunit and forming a stable tertiary complex with each other and the ribosome.
ADVERSE EFFECTS — Serious: None. Frequent: Venous irritation after peripheral infusion, arthralgia/myalgia, hyperbilirubinemia.

TELAVANCIN (*Vibativ*) ▶K ♀C ▶? $$$$$
WARNING — Teratogenic in animal studies. Get serum pregnancy test before use in women of childbearing potential. Do not use in pregnancy unless potential benefit outweighs risk.
ADULTS — Complicated skin infections including MRSA: 10 mg/kg IV once daily for 7-14 days. Infuse over 1 h.
PEDS — Safety and efficacy not established in children.
NOTES — QT interval prolongation; do not use in congenital long QT syndrome, uncompensated heart failure, or severe left ventricular hypertrophy. Nephrotoxicity; monitor renal function at least every 2-3 days. Efficacy may be decreased in patients with baseline CrCl of 50 mL/min or less. Cyclodextrin vehicle may accumulate in renal dysfunction. Does not interfere with coagulation, but may affect some coagulation tests. To minimize interference, draw blood for INR, aPTT, clotting time, and factor Xa right before next dose of telavancin. Use IV solution within 4 h when stored at room temp. Dosage adjustment for renal dysfunction in adults: 7.5 mg/kg IV q24h for CrCl 30 to 50 mL/min; 10 mg/kg q48h for CrCl 10-29 mL/min.
MOA — Bactericidal glycopeptide derivative of vancomycin that inhibits synthesis of cell wall peptidoglycan polymers. May also have other mechanisms of action.
ADVERSE EFFECTS — Serious: Nephrotoxicity (may be increased by NSAIDs, ACE inhibitors, loop diuretics); QT interval prolongation. Frequent: N/V, rash, foamy urine, metallic/soapy taste disturbance. May cause "Red Neck" (or "Red Man") syndrome with rapid IV administration.

TELITHROMYCIN (*Ketek*) ▶LK ♀C ▶? $$$
WARNING — Contraindicated in myasthenia gravis due to reports of exacerbation, including fatal acute respiratory depression. Warn patients about exacerbation of myasthenia gravis, hepatotoxicity, visual disturbances, and loss of consciousness.
ADULTS — Community-acquired pneumonia: 800 mg PO daily for 7 to 10 days. Indications for acute sinusitis and acute exacerbation of chronic bronchitis removed from labeling because potential benefit no longer justifies risk of adverse effects.
PEDS — Safety and efficacy not established in children.
FORMS — Trade only: Tabs 300, 400 mg. Ketek Pak: #10, 400 mg tabs.
NOTES — May prolong QT interval. Avoid in proarrhythmic conditions or with drugs that prolong QT interval. Life-threatening hepatotoxicity. Monitor for signs/symptoms of hepatitis. Contraindicated if history of hepatitis due to any macrolide or telithromycin. Contraindicated in myasthenia gravis. CYP3A4 substrate and inhibitor. Contraindicated with pimozide, rifampin, ergot alkaloids. Withhold simvastatin, lovastatin, or atorvastatin during course of telithromycin. Consider monitoring INR with warfarin. Give telithromycin and theophylline at least 1 h apart. Monitor for increased toxicity of digoxin, midazolam, metoprolol. CYP3A4 inducers (ie, phenytoin, carbamazepine) could reduce telithromycin levels. Dosage adjustment for CrCl less than 30 mL/min (including hemodialysis) is 600 mg once daily. On dialysis days, give after hemodialysis session. Dosage adjustment for CrCl less than 30 mL/min with hepatic dysfunction is 400 mg once daily.
MOA — Ketolide; structure and mechanism of action similar to macrolides. Inhibits protein synthesis in susceptible organisms by interfering with function of ribosomal 50S subunit. Methoxy and ketone groups enhance acid stability and ribosomal binding, and reduce susceptibility to drug efflux pumps.
ADVERSE EFFECTS — Serious: Exacerbation of myasthenia gravis; hepatotoxicity. Frequent: Diarrhea, nausea, dizziness, elevated LFTs. Other: Visual disturbances, esp. difficulty in accommodation (rare; most cases occur after 1st or 2nd dose in women less than 40 yo), transient loss of consciousness.

TIGECYCLINE (*Tygacil*) ▶Bile, K ♀D ▶?+ $$$$$
ADULTS — Complicated skin infections, complicated intra-abdominal infections, community-acquired pneumonia: 100 mg IV first dose, then 50 mg IV q 12 h. Infuse over 30 to 60 min.
PEDS — Not approved in children. Avoid in children age younger than 8 yo due to teeth staining.
NOTES — Consider other antibiotics for severe infection because mortality is higher with tigecycline, especially in ventilator-associated pneumonia. May decrease efficacy of oral contraceptives. Monitor INR with warfarin. Dosage adjustment for severe liver dysfunction (Child Pugh C): 100 mg IV first dose, then 25 mg IV q 12 h.

(cont.)

TIGECYCLINE *(cont.)*
MOA — Inhibits bacterial protein synthesis by binding with ribosomal 30S subunit and blocking addition of amino acids to peptide chain. Bacteriostatic.
ADVERSE EFFECTS — Serious: Higher mortality than other antibiotics, especially in ventilator-associated pneumonia. Anaphylaxis/anaphylactoid rxns, acute pancreatitis, hepatic dysfunction. Other adverse effects may be similar to tetracyclines (Serious: Pseudotumor cerebri, anti-anabolic effects, photosensitivity, teeth staining in children younger than 8 yo.) Frequent: N/V.

TRIMETHOPRIM *(Primsol, ✦Proloprim)* ▶K ♀C ▶– $
ADULTS — <u>Uncomplicated UTI:</u> 100 mg PO bid or 200 mg PO daily.
PEDS — Safety not established in age younger than 2 mo. <u>Otitis media</u> (not for M catarrhalis): 10 mg/kg/day PO divided bid for 10 days for age 6 mo or greater.
UNAPPROVED ADULTS — <u>Prophylaxis of recurrent UTI:</u> 100 mg PO at bedtime. <u>Pneumocystis treatment:</u> 5 mg/kg PO tid with dapsone 100 mg PO daily for 21 days.
FORMS — Generic only: Tabs 100 mg. Trade only (Primsol): Oral soln 50 mg/5 mL.
NOTES — Contraindicated in megaloblastic anemia due to folate deficiency. Blood dyscrasias. Trimethoprim alone not first line for otitis media. Inhibits metabolism of phenytoin. Can cause hyperkalemia (risk increased by high doses of trimethoprim, renal impairment, or other drugs that cause hyperkalemia). <u>Dosing in adults with renal dysfunction:</u> 50 mg PO q 12 h for CrCl 15 to 30 mL/min. Do not use if CrCl < 15 mL/min.
MOA — Folate antagonist; inhibits bacterial dihydrofolate reductase, the enzyme after step in folate synthesis inhibited by sulfonamides.
ADVERSE EFFECTS — Serious: Blood dyscrasias. Frequent: Rash, pruritus.

VANCOMYCIN *(Vancocin)* ▶K ♀C ▶? $$$$$
ADULTS — <u>Severe Staph infections</u> (including MRSA), <u>endocarditis:</u> 1 g IV q 12 h, each dose over 1 h or 30 mg/kg/day IV divided q 12 h. <u>Empiric therapy, native valve endocarditis:</u> 15 mg/kg (up to 2 g/day unless levels monitored) IV q 12 h with gentamicin. <u>C difficile-associated diarrhea:</u> 500 to 2000 mg/day PO divided tid to qid for 7 to 10 days. IV administration ineffective for this indication. See table for management of C. difficile infection in adults. See table for <u>prophylaxis of bacterial endocarditis.</u>
PEDS — <u>Severe Staph infections</u> (including MRSA), <u>endocarditis:</u> 15 mg/kg IV load, then 10 mg/kg q 12 h for age younger than 1 week, 15 mg/kg IV load, then 10 mg/kg q 8 h for age 1 week to 1 mo, 10 mg/kg IV q 6 h for age older than 1 mo. <u>C difficile-associated diarrhea:</u> 40 to 50 mg/kg/day (up to 500 mg/day) PO divided qid for 7 to 10 days. IV administration ineffective for this indication.
UNAPPROVED ADULTS — Usual dose: 15 to 20 mg/kg IV q 8 to 12 h. <u>Severe infection:</u> Consider loading dose of 25 to 30 mg/kg. Infuse over 1 h; infuse over 1.5 to 2 h if dose greater than 1 g. Base IV dose on absolute body wt. In obese patients, base initial dose on absolute body wt, then adjust dose based on trough levels. <u>C difficile-associated diarrhea:</u> 125 mg PO qid for 10 to 14 days. See table for management of C. difficile infection in adults.
UNAPPROVED PEDS — Newborns: 10 to 15 mg/kg IV q 8 to 12 h for age younger than 1 week; 10 to 15 mg/kg IV q 6 to 8 h for age 1 week and older. <u>Bacterial meningitis:</u> 60 mg/kg/day IV divided q 6 h. <u>Nonmeningeal pneumococcal infections:</u> 40 to 45 mg/kg/day IV divided q 6 h. <u>AAP dose for C difficile-associated diarrhea:</u> 40 mg/kg/day PO divided qid for at least 10 days (max 125 mg PO qid).
FORMS — Trade only: Caps 125, 250 mg.
NOTES — Maintain trough > 10 mg/L in all patients to avoid development of resistance; optimal trough for complicated infections is 15 to 20 mg/L. Draw trough just before the next dose after steady-state is reached (usually after 4th dose). Monitoring of peak levels no longer recommended. "Red Neck" (or "Red Man") syndrome with rapid IV administration, vein irritation with IV extravasation, reversible neutropenia, ototoxicity, or nephrotoxicity rarely. Enhanced effects of neuromuscular blockers. Use caution with other ototoxic/nephrotoxic drugs. Individualize dose if renal dysfunction. Oral vancomycin poorly absorbed; do not use for extraluminal infections.
MOA — Bactericidal glycopeptide that inhibits synthesis of cell wall peptidoglycan polymers. May also have other mechanisms of action.
ADVERSE EFFECTS — Serious: Reversible neutropenia, ototoxicity (rare and reversible with monotherapy) or nephrotoxicity (rare; risk increased by high doses or nephrotoxic drug), superinfection. Can cause C. difficile-associated diarrhea. Frequent: "Red Neck" (or "Red Man") syndrome with rapid IV administration, vein irritation with IV extravasation.

CARDIOVASCULAR: ACE Inhibitors

NOTE: See also antihypertensive combinations. Hyperkalemia possible, especially if used concomitantly with other drugs that increase K+ (including K+ containing salt substitutes) and in patients with heart failure, diabetes mellitus, or renal impairment. Monitor closely for hypoglycemia, especially during first month of treatment when combined with insulin or oral antidiabetic agents. An increase in serum creatinine up to 35% above baseline is acceptable and is not reason to withhold therapy unless hyperkalemia occurs. Coadministration with NSAIDS, including selective COX-2 inhibitors, may further deteriorate renal function (usually reversible) and decrease antihypertensive effects. ACE inhibitors are contraindicated during pregnancy. Contraindicated with a history of angioedema. Consider intestinal angioedema if abdominal pain (with or without N/V). African Americans and smokers may be at higher risk for angioedema. Swelling of tongue, glottis, or larynx may result in airway obstruction, especially with history of airway surgery. Rarely associated with syndrome starting with cholestatic jaundice or hepatitis progressing to fulminant hepatic necrosis and sometimes death. Increases risk of hypotension with volume depleted or hyponatremic patients. African Americans may need higher dose to achieve adequate response. Renoprotection and decreased cardiovascular morbidity/mortality seen with some ACE inhibitors are most likely a class effect. Anaphylactoid reactions have been reported when ACE inhibitor patients are dialyzed with high-flux membranes (eg, AN69) or undergoing low-density lipoprotein apheresis with dextran sulfate absorption. Nitroid reactions (facial flushing, N/V, hypotension) have been reported with concomitant gold injections.

BENAZEPRIL (*Lotensin*) ▶LK ♀– ▶? $$
WARNING – Do not use in pregnancy.
ADULTS – HTN: Start 10 mg PO daily, usual maintenance dose 20 to 40 mg PO daily or divided bid, max 80 mg/day, but added effect not apparent above 40 mg/day. Elderly, renal impairment, or concomitant diuretic therapy: Start 5 mg PO daily.
PEDS – HTN: Start 0.2 mg/kg/day (max 10 mg/day) as monotherapy; doses greater than 0.6 mg/kg/day or 40 mg/day have not been studied. Do not use if age younger than 6 yo or if glomerular filtration rate < 30 mL/min.
UNAPPROVED ADULTS – Renoprotective dosing: 10 mg PO daily. Heart failure: Start 5 mg PO daily, usual 5 to 20 mg/day, max 40 mg/day (in 1 to 2 doses).
FORMS – Generic/Trade: Tabs unscored 5, 10, 20, 40 mg.
NOTES – Bid dosing may be required for 24 h BP control.
MOA – Inhibits angiotensin-converting enzyme which converts angiotensin I to angiotensin II.
ADVERSE EFFECTS – Serious: Angioedema, hyperkalemia, renal impairment. Frequent: Cough.

CAPTOPRIL (*Capoten*) ▶LK ♀– ▶+ $
WARNING – Do not use in pregnancy.
ADULTS – HTN: Start 25 mg PO bid to tid, usual maintenance dose 25 to 150 mg PO bid to tid, max 450 mg/day. Elderly, renal impairment, or concomitant diuretic therapy: Start 6.25 to 12.5 mg PO bid to tid. Heart failure: Start 6.25 to 12.5 mg PO tid, usual 50 to 100 mg PO tid, max 450 mg/day. Diabetic nephropathy: 25 mg PO tid.
PEDS – Not approved in children.
UNAPPROVED ADULTS – Hypertensive urgency: 12.5 to 25 mg PO, repeated once or twice if necessary at intervals of 30 to 60 min.
UNAPPROVED PEDS – Neonates: 0.1 to 0.4 mg/kg/day PO divided q 6 to 8 h. Infants: Initial dose 0.15 to 0.3 mg/kg/dose, titrate to effective dose, max dose 6 mg/kg/day divided daily to qid. Children: Initial dose 0.3 to 0.5 mg/kg/dose PO q 8 h, titrate to effective dose, maximum dose 6 mg/kg/day (not to exceed 450 mg/day) divided bid to qid.
FORMS – Generic/Trade: Tabs scored 12.5, 25, 50, 100 mg.
NOTES – A captopril soln or susp (1 mg/mL) can be made by dissolving Tabs in distilled water or flavored syrup. The soln is stable for 7 days at room temperature.
MOA – Inhibits angiotensin-converting enzyme which converts angiotensin I to angiotensin II.
ADVERSE EFFECTS – Serious: Angioedema, hyperkalemia, renal impairment. Frequent: Cough, rash.

CILAZAPRIL (✦*Inhibace*) ▶LK ♀– ▶? $
WARNING – Do not use in pregnancy.
ADULTS – Canada only. HTN: Initial dose 2.5 mg PO daily, usual maintenance dose 2.5 to 5 mg daily, max 10 mg daily. Elderly or concomitant diuretic therapy: Initiate 1.25 mg PO daily. Heart failure adjunct: Initially 0.5 mg PO daily, increase to usual maintenance of 1 to 2.5 mg daily. Renal Impairment with CrCl 10 to 40 mL/min, initiate 0.5 mg daily, max 2.5 mg/day. CrCl < 10 mL/min 0.25 to 0.5 mg once or twice per week, adjust dose according to BP response.
PEDS – Not approved in children.
FORMS – Generic/Trade: Tabs, scored 1, 2.5, 5 mg.
NOTES – Reduce dose in hepatic/renal impairment.
MOA – Inhibits angiotensin-converting enzyme which converts angiotensin I to angiotensin II.
ADVERSE EFFECTS – Serious: Angioedema, hyperkalemia, renal impairment. Frequent: Cough.

ENALAPRIL (*enalaprilat, Vasotec*) ▶LK ♀– ▶+ $$
WARNING – Do not use in pregnancy.
ADULTS – HTN: Start 5 mg PO daily, usual maintenance dose 10 to 40 mg PO daily or divided bid, max 40 mg/day. If oral therapy not possible, can use enalaprilat 1.25 mg IV q 6 h over 5 min, and increase up to 5 mg IV q 6 h if needed. Renal impairment or concomitant diuretic therapy: Start 2.5 mg PO daily. Heart failure: Start 2.5 mg PO bid, usual 10 to 20 mg PO bid, max 40 mg/day.
PEDS – Not approved in children.
UNAPPROVED ADULTS – Hypertensive crisis: Enalaprilat 1.25 to 5 mg IV q 6 h. Renoprotective dosing: 10 to 20 mg PO daily.
UNAPPROVED PEDS – HTN: Start 0.1 mg/kg/day PO daily or divided bid, titrate to effective dose, maximum dose 0.5 mg/kg/day; 0.005 to 0.01 mg/kg/dose IV q 8 to 24 h.
FORMS – Generic/Trade: Tabs, scored 2.5, 5 mg, unscored 10, 20 mg.
NOTES – Bid dosing may be required for 24 h BP control. An enalapril oral susp (0.2 mg/mL) can be made by dissolving one 2.5 mg tab in 12.5 mL sterile water, use immediately. Enalaprilat is the active metabolite of enalapril.
MOA – Inhibits angiotensin-converting enzyme which converts angiotensin I to angiotensin II.
ADVERSE EFFECTS – Serious: Angioedema, hyperkalemia, renal impairment. Frequent: Cough.

CARDIOVASCULAR: ACE Inhibitors

HTN THERAPY[1]

Area of Concern	BP Target	Preferred Therapy[2]	Comments
General CAD prevention	<140/90 mm Hg	ACEI, ARB, CCB, thiazide, or combination	Start 2 drugs if systolic BP ≥ 160 or diastolic BP ≥ 100
High CAD risk[3]	<130/80 mm Hg		
Stable angina, unstable angina, MI	<130/80 mm Hg	Beta-blocker[4] + (ACEI or ARB)[5]	May add dihydropyridine CCB or thiazide
Left heart failure[6,7]	<120/80 mm Hg	Beta-blocker + (ACEI or ARB) + diuretic[8] + aldosterone antagonist[9]	

1. ACEI = angiotensin converting enzyme inhibitor; ARB = angiotensin-receptor blocker; CCB = calcium-channel blocker; MI = myocardial infarction. Adapted from *Circulation* 2007;115:2761–2788. 2. All patients should attempt lifestyle modifications: optimize wt, healthy diet, sodium restriction, exercise, smoking cessation, alcohol moderation. 3. Diabetes mellitus, chronic kidney disease, known CAD or risk equivalent (eg, peripheral artery disease, abdominal aortic aneurysm, carotid artery disease, and prior ischemic CVA/TIA), 10-year Framingham risk score ≥ 10%. 4. Use only if hemodynamically stable. If beta-blocker contraindications or intolerable side effects (and no bradycardia or heart failure), may substitute verapamil or diltiazem. 5. Preferred if anterior wall MI, persistent HTN, heart failure, or diabetes mellitus. 6. Avoid verapamil, diltiazem, clonidine, beta-blockers. 7. For blacks with NYHA class III or IV HF, consider adding hydralazine/isosorbide dinitrate. 8. Loop or thiazide. 9. Use if NYHA class III or IV, or if clinical heart failure + LVEF < 40%.

ACE INHIBITOR DOSING	HTN Initial	HTN Max/day	Heart Failure Initial	Heart Failure Max
benazepril (*Lotensin*)	10 mg daily*	80 mg	-	-
captopril (*Capoten*)	25 mg bid/tid	450 mg	6.25 mg tid	50 mg tid
enalapril (*Vasotec*)	5 mg daily*	40 mg	2.5 mg bid	10–20 mg bid
fosinopril (*Monopril*)	10 mg daily*	80 mg	5–10 mg daily	40 mg daily
lisinopril (*Zestril/Prinivil*)	10 mg daily	80 mg	2.5–5 mg daily	20–40 mg daily
moexipril (*Univasc*)	7.5 mg daily*	30 mg	-	-
perindopril (*Aceon*)	4 mg daily*	16 mg	2 mg daily	8–16 mg daily
quinapril (*Accupril*)	10–20 mg daily*	80 mg	5 mg bid	20 mg bid
ramipril (*Altace*)	2.5 mg daily*	20 mg	1.25–2.5 mg bid	10 mg daily
trandolapril (*Mavik*)	1–2 mg daily*	8 mg	1 mg daily	4 mg daily

Data taken from prescribing information and *Circulation* 2009;119:e391–e479.
*May require bid dosing for 24-h BP control.

FOSINOPRIL (*Monopril*) ▶LK ♀− ▶? $
 WARNING − Do not use in pregnancy.
 ADULTS − <u>HTN</u>: Start 10 mg PO daily, usual maintenance dose 20 to 40 mg PO daily or divided bid, max 80 mg/day, but added effect not apparent above 40 mg/day. <u>Elderly, renal impairment, or concomitant diuretic therapy:</u> Start 5 mg PO daily. <u>Heart failure:</u> Start 5 to 10 mg PO daily, usual 20 to 40 mg PO daily, max 40 mg/day.
 PEDS − <u>HTN</u> age 6 to 16 yo and wt greater than 50 kg: 5 to 10 mg PO daily.
 UNAPPROVED ADULTS − <u>Renoprotective dosing:</u> 10 to 20 mg PO daily.
 FORMS − Generic/Trade: Tabs scored 10, unscored 20, 40 mg.
 NOTES − Elimination 50% renal, 50% hepatic. Accumulation of drug negligible with impaired renal function.
 MOA − Inhibits angiotensin-converting enzyme which converts angiotensin I to angiotensin II.
 ADVERSE EFFECTS − Serious: Angioedema, hyperkalemia, renal impairment. Frequent: Cough.

LISINOPRIL (*Prinivil, Zestril*) ▶K ♀− ▶? $
 WARNING − Do not use in pregnancy.
 ADULTS − <u>HTN</u>: Start 10 mg PO daily, usual maintenance dose 20 to 40 mg PO daily, max 80 mg/day, but added effect not apparent above 40 mg/day. <u>Renal impairment or concomitant diuretic therapy:</u> Start 2.5 to 5 mg PO daily. <u>Heart failure, acute MI:</u> Start 2.5 to 5 mg PO daily, usual 5 to 20 mg PO daily, max 40 mg/day.
 PEDS − <u>HTN</u> age older than 6 yo: 0.07 mg/kg PO daily; 5 mg/day max. Not recommended for age younger than 6 yo or with glomerular filtration rate less than 30 mL/min/1.73 meters squared.
 UNAPPROVED ADULTS − <u>Renoprotective dosing:</u> 10 to 20 mg PO daily.
 FORMS − Generic/Trade: Tabs unscored (Zestril) 2.5, 5, 10, 20, 30, 40 mg. Tabs scored (Prinivil) 10, 20, 40 mg.

(cont.)

LISINOPRIL (cont.)
MOA – Inhibits angiotensin-converting enzyme which converts angiotensin I to angiotensin II.
ADVERSE EFFECTS – Serious: Angioedema, hyperkalemia, renal impairment. Frequent: Cough.

MOEXIPRIL (*Univasc*) ▶LK ♀- ▶? $$
WARNING – Do not use in pregnancy.
ADULTS – HTN: Start 7.5 mg PO daily, usual maintenance dose 7.5 to 30 mg PO daily or divided bid, max 30 mg/day. Renal impairment or concomitant diuretic therapy: Start 3.75 mg PO daily; max 15 mg/day with renal impairment.
PEDS – Not approved in children.
FORMS – Generic/Trade: Tabs scored 7.5, 15 mg.
NOTES – Bid dosing may be required for 24 h BP control.
MOA – Inhibits angiotensin-converting enzyme which converts angiotensin I to angiotensin II.
ADVERSE EFFECTS – Serious: Angioedema, hyperkalemia, renal impairment. Frequent: Cough.

PERINDOPRIL (*Aceon*, ✦*Coversyl*) ▶K ♀- ▶? $
WARNING – Do not use in pregnancy.
ADULTS – HTN: Start 4 mg PO daily, usual maintenance dose 4 to 8 mg PO daily or divided bid, max 16 mg/day. Renal impairment or concomitant diuretic therapy: Start 2 mg PO daily or divided bid. Reduction of cardiovascular events in stable CAD: Start 4 mg PO daily for 2 weeks, max 8 mg/day. Patients aged older than 70 yo: 2 mg PO daily for 1 week, 4 mg PO daily for 1 week, max 8 mg/day.
PEDS – Not approved in children.
UNAPPROVED ADULTS – Heart failure: Start 2 mg PO daily, max dose 16 mg daily. Recurrent CVA prevention: 4 mg PO daily with indapamide.
FORMS – Generic/Trade: Tabs scored 2, 4, 8 mg.
NOTES – Bid dosing does not provide clinically significant BP lowering compared to once daily.
MOA – Inhibits angiotensin-converting enzyme which converts angiotensin I to angiotensin II.
ADVERSE EFFECTS – Serious: Angioedema, hyperkalemia, renal impairment. Frequent: Cough.

QUINAPRIL (*Accupril*) ▶LK ♀- ▶? $$
WARNING – Do not use in pregnancy.
ADULTS – HTN: Start 10 to 20 mg PO daily (start 10 mg/day if elderly), usual maintenance dose 20 to 80 mg PO daily or divided bid, max 80 mg/day, but added effect not apparent above 40 mg/day. Renal impairment or concomitant diuretic therapy: Start 2.5 to 5 mg PO daily. Heart failure: Start 5 mg PO bid, usual maintenance dose 20 to 40 mg/day divided bid.
PEDS – Not approved in children.
FORMS – Generic/Trade: Tabs scored 5, unscored 10, 20, 40 mg.
NOTES – Bid dosing may be required for 24 h BP control.
MOA – Inhibits angiotensin-converting enzyme which converts angiotensin I to angiotensin II.
ADVERSE EFFECTS – Serious: Angioedema, hyperkalemia, renal impairment. Frequent: Cough.

RAMIPRIL (*Altace*) ▶LK ♀- ▶? $$$
WARNING – Do not use in pregnancy.
ADULTS – HTN: Start 2.5 mg PO daily, usual maintenance dose 2.5 to 20 mg PO daily or divided bid, max 20 mg/day. Renal impairment or concomitant diuretic therapy: Start 1.25 mg PO daily. Heart failure/post MI: Start 2.5 mg PO bid, usual maintenance dose 5 mg PO bid. Reduce risk of MI, CVA, death from cardiovascular causes: Start 2.5 mg PO daily for 1 week, then 5 mg daily for 3 weeks, increase as tolerated to maintenance dose 10 mg daily.
PEDS – Not approved in children.
UNAPPROVED ADULTS – Renoprotective dosing: Titrate to 10 mg PO daily.
FORMS – Generic/Trade: Caps 1.25, 2.5, 5, 10 mg.
NOTES – Bid dosing may be required for 24 h BP control. Cap contents can be sprinkled on applesauce and eaten or mixed with 120 mL of water or apple juice and swallowed. Mixtures are stable for 24 h at room temperature or 48 h refrigerated. Hypoglycemia may occur with coadministration with insulin or hypoglycemic agents.
MOA – Inhibits angiotensin-converting enzyme which converts angiotensin I to angiotensin II.
ADVERSE EFFECTS – Serious: Angioedema, hepatotoxicity, hyperkalemia, pancreatitis, renal impairment. Frequent: Cough.

TRANDOLAPRIL (*Mavik*) ▶LK ♀- ▶? $$
WARNING – Do not use in pregnancy.
ADULTS – HTN: Start 1 mg PO daily in patients not of African descent or 2 mg PO daily in patients of African descent, usual maintenance dose 2 to 4 mg PO daily or divided bid, max 8 mg/day, but added effect not apparent above 4 mg/day. Renal impairment or concomitant diuretic therapy: Start 0.5 mg PO daily. Heart failure/post MI: Start 0.5 to 1 mg PO daily, titrate to target dose 4 mg PO daily.
PEDS – Not approved in children.
FORMS – Generic/Trade: Tabs scored 1, unscored 2,4 mg.
MOA – Inhibits angiotensin-converting enzyme which converts angiotensin I to angiotensin II.
ADVERSE EFFECTS – Serious: Angioedema, hyperkalemia, renal impairment. Frequent: Cough.

CARDIOVASCULAR: Aldosterone Antagonists

NOTE: Hyperkalemia possible, especially if used concomitantly with other drugs that increase K+ and in patients with renal impairment. Adding an aldosterone antagonist is recommended in select patients with moderately severe to severe HF symptoms and reduced LVEF with careful monitoring for preserved renal function and normal K+ concentration. Serum creatinine should be < 2.5 mg/dL in men or < 2.0 mg/dL in women and K+ should be < 5.0 mEq/L. Routine combination of ACE inhibitor, ARB, and aldosterone antagonist is not recommended for patients with current/prior symptoms of HF and reduced LVEF. Coadministration with NSAIDs may further deteriorate renal function (usually reversible) and decrease antihypertensive effects.

CARDIOVASCULAR: Angiotensin Receptor Blockers (ARBs)

EPLERENONE (*Inspra*) ▶L ♀B ▶? $$$$
ADULTS — HTN: Start 50 mg PO daily, increase after 4 weeks if needed to max dose 50 mg bid. Start 25 mg daily with concomitant moderate CYP 3A4 inhibitor (eg, erythromycin, verapamil, fluconazole, saquinavir). Improve survival of stable patients with LV systolic dysfunction (LVEF 40% or less) and heart failure/post MI: Start 25 mg PO daily; titrate to target dose 50 mg PO daily within 4 weeks, if tolerated.
PEDS — Not approved in children.
FORMS — Trade only: Tabs unscored 25, 50 mg.
NOTES — Contraindicated with potassium > 5.5 mEq/L; CrCl ≤ 30 mL/min; strong CYP 3A4 inhibitors (ketoconazole, itraconazole, nefazodone, troleandomycin, clarithromycin, ritonavir, nelfinavir). For treatment of HTN, contraindications include Type 2 DM with microalbuminuria; serum creatinine > 2 mg/dL in males or > 1.8 mg/dL in females; CrCl < 50 mL/min; concomitant therapy with K+ supplements, K-sparing diuretics. Hyperkalemia more common with concomitant ACE inhibitors/ARBs. Measure serum K+ before initiating, within first week, at 1 month after starting treatment or dose adjustment, then prn. With concomitant moderate CYP 3A4 inhibitor (eg, erythromycin, fluconazole, saquinavir, verapamil) check K+ and serum creatinine within 3 to 7 days of initiating eplerenone. Monitor lithium levels with concomitant lithium therapy.
MOA — Blocks the binding of aldosterone to mineralocorticoid receptors.
ADVERSE EFFECTS — Serious: Hyperkalemia, hyponatremia (rare). Frequent: Headache, dizziness.

SPIRONOLACTONE (*Aldactone*) ▶LK ♀D ▶+ $
WARNING — Use only for approved indications. Use only if necessary. Tumorigen in rats.
ADULTS — Edema (heart failure, cirrhotic ascites, nephrotic syndrome): Start 100 mg PO daily or divided bid, maintain for 5 days, increase prn to achieve diuretic response, usual dose range 25 to 200 mg/day. Other diuretics may be needed. HTN: 50 to 100 mg PO daily or divided bid, generally used in combination with a thiazide diuretic to maintain serum potassium, increase dose as needed based on serum potassium and BP. Diuretic-induced hypokalemia: 25 to 100 mg PO daily when potassium supplements/sparing regimens inappropriate. Primary hyperaldosteronism, maintenance therapy: 100 to 400 mg/day PO until surgery or indefinitely if surgery not an option. Cirrhotic ascites: Start 100 mg once daily or in divided doses. Dose may range from 25 to 200 mg/day.
PEDS — Edema: 3.3 mg/kg PO daily or divided bid.
UNAPPROVED ADULTS — Severe heart failure: Start 12.5 to 25 mg PO daily, usual maintenance dose 25 to 50 mg daily. Hirsutism: 50 to 200 mg PO daily, maximal regression of hirsutism in 6 months. Acne: 50 to 200 mg PO daily.
UNAPPROVED PEDS — Edema/HTN: 1 to 3.3 mg/kg/day, PO daily or divided bid, max 200 mg/day.
FORMS — Generic/Trade: Tabs unscored 25 mg scored 50, 100 mg.
NOTES — Contraindicated with anuria, renal insufficiency, hyperkalemia. Dosing more frequently than bid not necessary. Hyperkalemia more likely with doses 50 mg/day or more and with concomitant ACEIs or K+ supplements. Measure serum K+ and SrCr before initiating, after 1 week, monthly for the first 3 months, quarterly for 1 year, then every 6 months after starting treatment or dose adjustment.
MOA — Blocks the binding of aldosterone to mineralocorticoid receptors.
ADVERSE EFFECTS — Serious: Agranulocytosis, hyperkalemia (rare), hypersensitivity. Frequent: Gynecomastia, headache, impotence, irregular menses.

CARDIOVASCULAR: Angiotensin Receptor Blockers (ARBs)

NOTE: See also antihypertensive combinations. An increase in serum creatinine up to 35% above baseline is acceptable and is not reason to withhold therapy unless hyperkalemia occurs. ARB use during pregnancy may cause injury or death to the developing fetus: Use reliable form of contraception in women of child bearing age; discontinue as soon as pregnancy is detected. Rare cases of angioedema and rhabdomyolysis have been reported with ARBs. African Americans and smokers may be at higher risk for angioedema. Increased risk of hypotension with volume-depleted, hyponatremic patients, or during anesthesia/major surgery. Coadministration with NSAIDS, including selective COX-2 inhibitors, may further deteriorate renal function (usually reversible) and decrease antihypertensive effects.

CANDESARTAN (*Atacand*) ▶K ♀– ▶? $$$
WARNING — Do not use in pregnancy.
ADULTS — HTN: Start 16 mg PO daily, max 32 mg/day. Volume depleted patients: Start 8 mg PO daily. Reduce cardiovascular death and hospitalizations from heart failure (NYHA II-IV and LVEF 40% or less): Start 4 mg PO daily, may double dose q 2 week; maximum 32 mg/day; has an added effect when used with ACE inhibitor.
PEDS — HTN: For age 1 to 5 yo: Start 0.20 mg/kg (oral suspension), dose range 0.05 to 0.4 mg/kg/day. For age 6 to 16 yo and wt less than 50 kg: Start 4 to 8 mg/day, range 2 to 16 mg/day. For age 6 to 16 yo, wt greater than 50 kg: Start 8 to 16 mg/day, range 4 to 32 mg/day. Doses > 0.4 mg/kg/day (in ages 1 to 5 yo) or 32 mg (ages 6 to 16 yo) have not been studied. For patients with possible depleted intravascular volume (eg, treated with diuretic, particularly with impaired renal function), initiate under close supervision and consider lower dose.
UNAPPROVED ADULTS — Reduce heart failure hospitalizations in chronic heart failure and LVEF greater

(cont.)

CARDIOVASCULAR: Angiotensin Receptor Blockers (ARBs)

CANDESARTAN (cont.)
than 40%: Start 4 mg PO daily, double dose q 2 weeks; target dose 32 mg/day.
FORMS — Trade only: Tabs unscored 4, 8, 16, 32 mg.
NOTES — May increase lithium levels. Initiate/titrate cautiously with heart failure; with symptomatic hypotension, may need to reduce dose temporarily and give fluids.
MOA — Blocks binding of angiotensin II to the angiotensin subtype 1 receptor.
ADVERSE EFFECTS — Serious: Hyperkalemia, renal impairment.

EPROSARTAN (*Teveten*) ▶Fecal excretion ♀–▶? $$$
WARNING — Do not use in pregnancy.
ADULTS — HTN: Start 600 mg PO daily, maximum 800 mg/day given daily or divided bid.
PEDS — Not approved in children.
FORMS — Trade only: Tabs unscored 400, 600 mg.
MOA — Blocks binding of angiotensin II to the angiotensin subtype 1 receptor.
ADVERSE EFFECTS — Serious: Hyperkalemia, renal impairment.

IRBESARTAN (*Avapro*) ▶L ♀–▶? $$$
WARNING — Do not use in pregnancy.
ADULTS — HTN: Start 150 mg PO daily, max 300 mg/day. Volume depleted patients: Start 75 mg PO daily. Type 2 diabetic nephropathy: Start 150 mg PO daily, target dose 300 mg daily.
PEDS — Not approved in children.
FORMS — Trade only: Tabs unscored 75, 150, 300 mg.
MOA — Blocks binding of angiotensin II to the angiotensin subtype 1 receptor.
ADVERSE EFFECTS — Serious: Hyperkalemia, renal impairment.

LOSARTAN (*Cozaar*) ▶L ♀–▶? $$$
WARNING — Do not use in pregnancy.
ADULTS — HTN: Start 50 mg PO daily, max 100 mg/day given daily or divided bid. Volume-depleted patients or history of hepatic impairment: Start 25 mg PO daily. CVA risk reduction in patients with HTN and LV hypertrophy (does not appear to apply to persons of African descent): Start 50 mg PO daily. If need more BP reduction add HCTZ 12.5 mg PO daily; then increase losartan to 100 mg/day, then increase HCTZ to 25 mg/day. Type 2 diabetic nephropathy: Start 50 mg PO daily, target dose 100 mg daily.
PEDS — HTN: Start 0.7 mg/kg/day (up to 50 mg), doses greater than 1.4 mg/kg/day or above 100 mg have not been studied. Do not use for age less than 6 yo or if glomerular filtration rate < 30 mL/min.
UNAPPROVED ADULTS — Heart failure: Start 12.5 mg PO daily, target dose 50 mg daily. Renoprotective dosing: Start 50 mg PO daily, increase to 100 mg daily prn for BP control.
FORMS — Generic/Trade: Tabs unscored 25, 50, 100 mg.
NOTES — Patients of African descent with HTN and LV hypertrophy may not have the same CVA risk reduction as non-African descent patients. Monitor BP control when adding or discontinuing rifampin, fluconazole, or erythromycin.
MOA — Blocks binding of angiotensin II to the angiotensin subtype 1 receptor.
ADVERSE EFFECTS — Serious: Hyperkalemia, renal impairment, thrombocytopenia (rare).

OLMESARTAN (*Benicar*) ▶K ♀–▶? $$$
WARNING — Do not use in pregnancy.
ADULTS — HTN: Start 20 mg PO daily, maximum 40 mg/day.
PEDS — HTN, 6 to 16 yo: Weight 20 to less than 35 kg: Start 10 mg PO daily, max 20 mg/day. Weight more than 35 kg: Start 20 mg PO daily, max 40 mg/day.
FORMS — Trade only: Tabs unscored 5, 20, 40 mg.
NOTES — The FDA is evaluating data from the ROADMAP and ORIENT studies in which patients with type 2 diabetes taking olmesartan had higher rates of death from cardiovascular cause compared to the placebo group.
MOA — Blocks binding of angiotensin II to the angiotensin subtype 1 receptor.
ADVERSE EFFECTS — Serious: Hyperkalemia, renal impairment.

TELMISARTAN (*Micardis*) ▶L ♀–▶? $$$
WARNING — Do not use in pregnancy.
ADULTS — HTN: Start 40 mg PO daily, maximum 80 mg/day. Cardiovascular risk reduction in patients more than 55 yo unable to take ACE inhibitors: Start 80 mg PO daily, max 80 mg/day.
PEDS — Not approved in children.
FORMS — Trade only: Tabs unscored 20, 40, 80 mg.
NOTES — Swallow tabs whole, do not break or crush. Caution in hepatic insufficiency. May need to monitor digoxin levels when initiating, adjusting dose, or discontinuing. Avoid concomitant use of ACE inhibitor.
MOA — Blocks binding of angiotensin II to the angiotensin subtype 1 receptor.
ADVERSE EFFECTS — Serious: Hyperkalemia, renal impairment.

VALSARTAN (*Diovan*) ▶L ♀–▶? $$$
WARNING — Do not use in pregnancy.
ADULTS — HTN: Start 80 to 160 mg PO daily, max 320 mg/day. Heart failure: Start 40 mg PO bid, target dose 160 mg bid; there is no evidence of added benefit when used with adequate dose of ACE inhibitor. Reduce mortality/morbidity post MI with LV systolic dysfunction/failure: Start 20 mg PO bid, increase to 40 mg PO bid within 7 days, target dose 160 mg bid.
PEDS — HTN: Start 1.3 mg/kg/day (up to 40 mg), max 2.7 mg/kg/day (or 160 mg). Do not use if younger than 6 yo.
UNAPPROVED ADULTS — Renoprotective dosing: 80 to 160 mg PO daily.
FORMS — Trade only: Tabs scored 40 mg, unscored 80, 160, 320 mg.
MOA — Blocks binding of angiotensin II to the angiotensin subtype 1 receptor.
ADVERSE EFFECTS — Serious: Hyperkalemia, renal impairment.

CARDIOVASCULAR: Antiadrenergic Agents

CLONIDINE (*Catapres, Catapres-TTS, ♦Dixarit*) ▶LK ♀C ▶? $$
ADULTS — HTN: Start 0.1 mg PO bid, usual maintenance dose 0.2 to 1.2 mg/day divided bid to tid, max 2.4 mg/day. Transdermal (Catapres-TTS): Start 0.1 mg/24 h patch q week, titrate to desired effect, max effective dose 0.6 mg/24 h (two 0.3 mg/24 h patches).
PEDS — HTN: Start 5 to 7 mcg/kg/day PO divided q 6 to 12 h, titrate at 5 to 7 days intervals to 5 to 25 mcg/kg/day divided q 6 h; max 0.9 mg/day. Transdermal therapy not recommended in children.
UNAPPROVED ADULTS — HTN urgency: Initially 0.1 to 0.2 mg PO, followed by 0.1 mg q 1 h prn up to a total dose of 0.5 to 0.7 mg. Menopausal flushing: 0.1 to 0.4 mg/day PO divided bid to tid; transdermal applied weekly 0.1 mg/day. Tourette's syndrome: 3 to 5 mcg/kg/day PO divided bid to qid. Opioid withdrawal, adjunct: 0.1 to 0.3 mg PO tid to qid or 0.1 to 0.2 mg PO q 4 h tapering off over days 4 to 10. Alcohol withdrawal, adjunct: 0.1 to 0.2 mg PO q 4 h prn. Smoking cessation: Start 0.1 mg PO bid, increase 0.1 mg/day at weekly intervals to 0.75 mg/day as tolerated; transdermal (Catapres TTS): 0.1 to 0.2 mg/24 h patch q week for 2 to 3 weeks after cessation. ADHD: 5 mcg/kg/day PO for 8 weeks. Posttraumatic stress disorder: Start 0.1 mg PO bedtime, max 0.6 mg/day in divided doses.
UNAPPROVED PEDS — ADHD: Start 0.05 mg PO at bedtime, titrate based on response over 8 weeks to max 0.2 mg/day (for wt less 45 kg) or to max 0.4 mg/day (wt 45 kg or greater) in 2 to 4 divided doses. Tourette's syndrome: 3 to 5 mcg/kg/day PO divided bid to qid.
FORMS — Generic/Trade: Tabs unscored 0.1, 0.2, 0.3 mg. Transdermal weekly patch 0.1 mg/day (TTS-1), 0.2 mg/day (TTS-2), 0.3 mg/day (TTS-3). Generic only: Oral Susp, Extended-release, 0.09 mg/mL (118 mL). Tabs Extended-release 0.17, 0.26 mg.
NOTES — Monitor heart rate when taking concomitant digitalis, nondihydropyridine calcium channel blockers, or beta blockers. Use cautiously with severe coronary insufficiency, conduction disturbances, recent MI, cerebrovascular disease, or chronic renal failure. Rebound HTN with abrupt discontinuation of tabs, especially at doses that exceed 0.7 mg/day. Taper therapy over 4 to 7 days to avoid rebound HTN. Dispose of used patches carefully, keep away from children. Remove patch before defibrillation, cardioversion, or MRI to avoid skin burns. Transdermal therapy should not be interrupted during the surgical period. Oral therapy should be continued within 4 hours of surgery and restarted as soon as possible afterwards. May potentiate the CNS depressive effects of alcohol, barbiturates, or other sedating drugs. Concomitant TCAs may reduce the BP lowering effects.
MOA — Centrally acting alpha-2 agonist.
ADVERSE EFFECTS — Serious: Rebound hypertension, orthostatic hypotension, depression, bradycardia, syncope. Frequent: Dry mouth, constipation, drowsiness, dizziness, sedation, sexual dysfunction, rash.

DOXAZOSIN (*Cardura, Cardura XL*) ▶L ♀C ▶? $$
WARNING — Not first line agent for HTN. Increased risk of heart failure in patients who used doxazosin compared to diuretic in treating HTN.
ADULTS — BPH, immediate-release: Start 1 mg PO at bedtime, titrate by doubling the dose over at least 1 to 2 weeks intervals up to a maximum of 8 mg PO at bedtime. Extended-release (not approved for HTN): Start 4 mg PO qam with breakfast, titrate dose in 3 to 4 weeks to max dose 8 mg PO qam. HTN: Start 1 mg PO at bedtime, max 16 mg/day. Avoid use of doxazosin alone to treat combined HTN and BPH.
PEDS — Not approved in children.
UNAPPROVED ADULTS — Promote spontaneous passage of ureteral calculi: 4 mg (XL formulation only) PO daily usually combined with an NSAID, antiemetic, and opioid of choice.
FORMS — Generic/Trade: Tabs scored 1, 2, 4, 8 mg. Trade only (Cardura XL): Tabs extended-release 4, 8 mg.
NOTES — Dizziness, drowsiness, lightheadedness, syncope. Bedtime dosing may minimize side effects. Initial 1 mg dose is used to decrease postural hypotension that may occur after the first few doses. If therapy is interrupted for several days, restart at the 1 mg dose. Monitor BP after first dose, after each dose adjustment, and periodically thereafter. Increased risk of hypotension when used with erectile dysfunction medication (ie, sildenafil, tadalafil, verdenafil); use lowest dose of erectile dysfunction medication. Intraoperative Floppy Iris Syndrome may occur during cataract surgery, if patient is on or has previously taken alpha-1 blockers.
MOA — Blocks binding of catecholamines to postsynaptic alpha-1 receptors; decreases urethral resistance.
ADVERSE EFFECTS — Serious: Postural hypotension, heart failure. Frequent: Headache, dizziness, fatigue, nausea, constipation.

GUANABENZ (*Wytensin*) ▶LK ♀C ▶– $$$
WARNING — Sedation, rebound HTN with abrupt discontinuation especially with high doses.
ADULTS — HTN: Start 2 to 4 mg PO bid, max 32 mg bid.
PEDS — Children older than 12 yo: Initial dose 0.5 to 2 mg/day divided bid, usual maintenance dose 4 to 24 mg/day divided bid.
FORMS — Generic only: Tabs, 4, 8 mg.
NOTES — Sedation. Rebound HTN with abrupt discontinuation, especially at higher doses (32 mg/day). Taper therapy over 4 to 7 days to avoid rebound HTN.
MOA — Stimulates central alpha-adrenergic receptors reducing sympathetic outflow.
ADVERSE EFFECTS — Serious: Syncope, rebound hypertension. Frequent: Sedation, dizziness, dry mouth, constipation, impotence.

SELECTED DRUGS THAT MAY PROLONG THE QT INTERVAL

alfuzosin	erythromycin*†	nicardipine	sertraline
amiodarone*†	felbamate	octreotide	sotalol*†
apomorphine	flecainide*	ofloxacin	sunitinib
arsenic trioxide*	foscarnet	ondansetron	tacrolimus
azithromycin*	fosphenytoin	pentamidine*†	tamoxifen
chloroquine*	gemifloxacin	phenothiazines‡	telithromycin*
chlorpromazine	granisetron	pimozide*†	thioridazine
cisapride*†	haloperidol*‡	polyethylene glycol (PEG-salt soln)§	tizanidine
clarithromycin*	ibutilide*†		tolterodine
clozapine	indapamide*	procainamide*	vardenafil
cocaine*	isradipine	quetiapine‡	venlafaxine
dasatinib	levofloxacin*	quinidine*†	visicol§
disopyramide*†	lithium	quinine	voriconazole*
dofetilide*	mefloquine	ranolazine	vorinostat
dolasetron	methadone*†	risperidone‡	ziprasidone‡
droperidol*	moexipril/HCTZ	salmeterol	
epirubicin	moxifloxacin		

Note. This table may not include all drugs that prolong the QT interval or cause torsades. Risk of drug-induced QT prolongation may be increased in women, elderly, hypokalemia, hypomagnesemia, bradycardia, starvation, CHF, & CNS injuries. Hepatorenal dysfunction & drug interactions can increase the concentration of QT interval-prolonging drugs. Coadministration of QT interval-prolonging drugs can have additive effects. Avoid these (and other) drugs in congenital prolonged QT syndrome (www.qtdrugs.org). *Torsades reported in product labeling/case reports. †Increased risk in women. ‡QT prolongation: thioridazine > ziprasidone > risperidone, quetiapine, haloperidol. §May be due to electrolyte imbalance.

GUANFACINE (*Tenex*) ▶K ♀B ▶? $
ADULTS — HTN: Start 1 mg PO at bedtime, increase to 2 to 3 mg at bedtime if needed after 3 to 4 weeks, max 3 mg/day.
PEDS — HTN age 12 yo and older: Use adult dosage.
UNAPPROVED PEDS — ADHD: Start 0.5 mg PO daily, titrate by 0.5 mg q 3 to 4 days as tolerated to 0.5 mg PO tid.
FORMS — Generic/Trade: Tabs unscored 1, 2 mg.
NOTES — Most of the drug's therapeutic effect is seen at 1 mg/day. Rebound HTN with abrupt discontinuation, but generally BP returns to pretreatment measurements slowly without ill effects. Less sedation and hypotension compared to clonidine.
MOA — Centrally acting alpha-2 agonist.
ADVERSE EFFECTS — Serious: Syncope, rebound hypertension. Frequent: Sedation, dizziness, dry mouth, constipation, impotence.

METHYLDOPA (*Aldomet*) ▶LK ♀B ▶+ $
ADULTS — HTN: Start 250 mg PO bid to tid, usual maintenance dose 500 to 3000 mg/day divided bid to qid, max 3000 mg/day. Hypertensive crisis: 250 to 500 mg IV q 6 h, maximum 1 g IV q 6 h, maximum 4000 mg/day.
PEDS — HTN: 10 mg/kg/day PO divided bid to qid, titrate dose to a max dose 65 mg/kg/day or 3000 mg/day, whichever is less.
FORMS — Generic only: Tabs unscored 125, 250, 500 mg.
NOTES — Alternative therapy for HTN (other agents preferred) except gestational HTN. IV form has a slow onset of effect and other agents preferred for rapid reduction of BP. Hemolytic anemia possible.
MOA — Stimulates central alpha-adrenergic receptors reducing sympathetic outflow.
ADVERSE EFFECTS — Serious: Hemolytic anemia (rare), LFT abnormalities. Frequent: Sedation, dizziness, dry mouth, constipation, impotence.

PRAZOSIN (*Minipress*) ▶L ♀C ▶? $$
WARNING — Not first line agent for HTN. Increased risk of heart failure in patients who used related drug doxazosin compared to diuretic in treating HTN.
ADULTS — HTN: Start 1 mg PO bid to tid, usual maintenance dose 20 mg/day divided bid to tid, max 40 mg/day, but doses > 20 mg/day usually do not increase efficacy.
PEDS — Not approved in children.
UNAPPROVED ADULTS — Posttraumatic stress disorder: Start 1 mg PO bedtime, increase weekly by 1 to 2 mg/day to max dose of 20 mg/day. Doses greater than 10 mg/day are divided early evening and at bedtime.
UNAPPROVED PEDS — HTN: Start 0.005 mg/kg PO single dose; increase slowly as needed up to maintenance dose 0.025 to 0.150 mg/kg/day divided q 6 h; max dose 0.4 mg/kg/day.
FORMS — Generic/Trade: Caps 1, 2, 5 mg.

(cont.)

PRAZOSIN (cont.)
NOTES − To avoid syncope, start with 1 mg at bedtime, and increase dose gradually. Increased risk of hypotension when used with erectile dysfunction medication (ie, sildenafil, tadalafil, verdenafil); use lowest dose of erectile dysfunction medication. During cataract surgery, intraoperative floppy iris syndrome has been reported in association with alpha-1-blocker therapy.
MOA − Blocks binding of catecholamines to post-synaptic alpha-1 receptors.
ADVERSE EFFECTS − Serious: Postural hypotension, heart failure. Frequent: Headache, dizziness

RESERPINE (*Serpasil*) ▶LK ♀C ▶− $
ADULTS − HTN: Start 0.05 to 0.1 mg PO daily or 0.1 mg PO every other day, max dose 0.25 mg/day.
PEDS − Not approved in children.
FORMS − Generic only: Tabs, scored 0.1, 0.25 mg
NOTES − Should be used in combination with a diuretic to counteract fluid retention and augment BP control. May cause depression at higher doses, avoid use in patients with depression or active peptic ulcer disease.
MOA − Blocks transport of norepinephrine into storage granules.
ADVERSE EFFECTS − Serious: None. Frequent: Nasal stuffiness.

TERAZOSIN (*Hytrin*) ▶LK ♀C ▶? $$
WARNING − Not first line agent for HTN. Increased risk of heart failure in patients who used related drug doxazosin compared to diuretic in treating HTN.
ADULTS − HTN: Start 1 mg PO at bedtime usual effective dose 1 to 5 mg PO daily or divided bid, max 20 mg/day. BPH: Start 1 mg PO at bedtime titrate dose in a stepwise fashion to 2, 5, or 10 mg PO at bedtime to desired effect. Treatment with 10 mg PO at bedtime for 4 to 6 weeks may be needed to assess benefit. Maximum 20 mg/day.
PEDS − Not approved in children.
FORMS − Generic/Trade: Tabs Caps 1, 2, 5, 10 mg.
NOTES − Dizziness, drowsiness, lightheadedness, syncope. Bedtime dosing may minimize side effects. Initial 1 mg dose is used to decrease postural hypotension that may occur after the first few doses. If therapy is interrupted for several days, restart at the 1 mg dose. Monitor BP after first dose, after each dose adjustment, and periodically thereafter. Increased risk of hypotension when used with erectile dysfunction medication (ie, sildenafil, tadalafil, verdenafil); use lowest dose of erectile dysfunction medication. Intraoperative Floppy Iris Syndrome may occur during cataract surgery, if patient is on or has previously taken alpha-1 blockers.
MOA − Blocks binding of catecholamines to post-synaptic alpha-1 receptors, increases urinary flow rate.
ADVERSE EFFECTS − Serious: Postural hypotension, heart failure. Frequent: Headache, dizziness.

CARDIOVASCULAR: Anti-Dysrhythmics/Cardiac Arrest

ADENOSINE (*Adenocard*) ▶Plasma ♀C ▶? $$$
ADULTS − PSVT conversion (not A-fib): 6 mg rapid IV and flush, preferably through a central line. If no response after 1 to 2 min then 12 mg. A third dose of 12 mg may be given prn.
PEDS − PSVT conversion wt less than 50 kg: Initial dose 50 to 100 mcg/kg IV, give subsequent doses q 1 to 2 min prn and increase the dose 50 to 100 mcg/kg each time, up to a max single dose of 300 mcg/kg or 12 mg (whichever is less). PST coversion wt 50 kg or greater: Use adult dosage.
UNAPPROVED PEDS − PSVT conversion: Initial dose 0.1 to 0.2 mg/kg IV bolus.
NOTES − Half-life is less than 10 sec. Give doses by rapid IV push followed by NS flush. Need higher dose if on theophylline or caffeine, lower dose if on dipyridamole or carbamazepine. May cause respiratory collapse in patients with asthma, COPD. Use in setting with cardiac resuscitation readily available. Do not confuse with adenosine phosphate used for the symptomatic relief of varicose vein complications.
MOA − Blocks cardiac conduction through the AV node.
ADVERSE EFFECTS − Serious: Arrhythmias, heart block, bronchoconstriction, seizures. Frequent: Flushing, chest tightness.

AMIODARONE (*Cordarone, Pacerone*) ▶L ♀D ▶− $$$$
WARNING − May cause potentially fatal toxicities, including pulmonary toxicity, hepatic injury, and worsened arrhythmia. Only use for adults with life-threatening ventricular arrhythmias when other treatments ineffective or not tolerated.
ADULTS − Life-threatening ventricular arrhythmia without cardiac arrest: Load 150 mg IV over 10 min, then 1 mg/min for 6 h, then 0.5 mg/min for 18 h. Mix in D5W. Oral loading dose 800 to 1600 mg PO daily for 1 to 3 weeks, reduce dose to 400 to 800 mg daily for 1 month when arrhythmia is controlled or adverse effects are prominent, then reduce to lowest effective dose, usually 200 to 400 mg daily.
PEDS − Not approved in children.
UNAPPROVED ADULTS − Refractory atrial fibrillation: Loading dose 600 to 800 mg PO daily for 7 to 14 days, then 200 to 400 mg daily. Maintain sinus rhythm with A-fib: 100 to 400 mg PO daily. Shock-refractory VF/pulseless VT: 300 mg or 5 mg/kg IV bolus followed by unsynchronized shock, additional 150 mg bolus may be given if serious arrhythmias recur. Stable monomorphic ventricular tachycardia: 150 mg IV over 10 min, repeat q 10 to 15 min prn.
UNAPPROVED PEDS − May cause death or other serious side effects in children (see NOTES); do not use in infants younger than 30 days of age and use only

(cont.)

LDL CHOLESTEROL GOALS[1]

Risk Category	LDL Goal	Lifestyle Changes[2]	Also Consider Meds at LDL (mg/dL)[3]
High risk: CHD or equivalent risk,[4,5,6] 10-year risk >20%	<100 (optional <70)[7]	LDL ≥ 100[8]	≥100 (<100: consider Rx options)[9]
Moderately high risk: 2+ risk factors,[10] 10-year risk 10–20%	<130 (optional <100)	LDL ≥ 130[8]	≥130 (100–129: consider Rx options)[11]
Moderate risk: 2+ risk factors,[10] 10-year risk <10%	<130 mg/dL	LDL ≥ 130	≥160
Lower risk: 0 to 1 risk factor[5]	<160 mg/dL	LDL ≥ 160	≥190 (160–189: Rx optional)

1. CHD=coronary heart disease. LDL=low density lipoprotein. Adapted from NCEP: *JAMA* 2001; 285:2486; NCEP Report: *Circulation* 2004;110:227–239. All 10-year risks based upon Framingham stratification; calculator available at: http://hin.nhlbi.nih.gov/atpiii/calculator.asp?usertype=prof. 2. Dietary modification, wt reduction, exercise. 3. When using LDL lowering therapy, achieve at least 30-40% LDL reduction. 4. Equivalent risk defined as diabetes, other atherosclerotic disease (peripheral artery disease, abdominal aortic aneurysm, symptomatic carotid artery disease,CKD or prior ischemic CVA/TIA), or ≥ 2 risk factors such that 10-year risk > 20%. 5. History of ischemic CVA or transient ischemic attack=CHD risk equivalents (*Stroke* 2006;37:577-617). 6. Chronic kidney disease=CHD risk equivalent [*Am J Kidney Dis* 2003 Apr;41 (4 suppl 3):I-IV,S1-91]. 7. For any patient with atherosclerotic disease, may treat to LDL < 70 mg/dL (*Circulation* 2006;113:2363-72). 8. Regardless of LDL, lifestyle changes are indicated when lifestyle-related risk factors (obesity, physical inactivity, ↑TG, ↓HDL, or metabolic syndrome) are present. 9. If baseline LDL < 100, starting LDL lowering therapy is an option based on clinical trials. With ↑TG or ↓HDL, consider combining fibrate or nicotinic acid with LDL lowering drug. 10. Risk factors: Cigarette smoking, HTN (BP ≥ 140/90 mmHg or on antihypertensive meds), low HDL (< 40 mg/dL), family hx of CHD (1° relative: ♂ < 55 yo, ♀ < 65 yo), age (♂ ≥ 45 yo, ♀ ≥ 55 yo). 11. At baseline or after lifestyle changes - initiating therapy to achieve LDL < 100 is an option based on clinical trials.

AMIODARONE *(cont.)*

if medically warranted if 30 days of age or older. Ventricular arrhythmia: IV therapy limited data; 5 mg/kg IV over 30 min; followed by 5 mcg/kg/min infusion; increase infusion as needed up to max 10 mcg/kg/min or 20 mg/kg/day. Give loading dose in 1 mg/kg aliquots with each aliquot given over 5 to 10 min; do not exceed 30 mg/min.

FORMS — Trade only (Pacerone): tabs unscored 100 mg. Generic/Trade: Tabs scored 200, 400 mg.

NOTES — Contraindicated in cardiogenic shock; severe sinus-node dysfunction with marked sinus bradycardia; 2nd/3rd degree heart block; bradycardia without pacemaker that has caused syncope. Proarrhythmic. Consider inpatient rhythm monitoring during initiation of therapy, especially when treating life-threatening arrhythmias. Consult cardiologist before using with other antiarrhythmic agents. Do not use with iodine allergy. Photosensitivity and skin discoloration (blue/gray color) with oral therapy. Hypo or hyperthyroidism possible. Monitor LFTs, TFTs, and PFTs. Baseline and regular eye exams. Prompt ophthalmic examination needed with changes in visual acuity or decreased peripheral vision. Most manufacturers of laser refractive devices contraindicate eye laser surgery when taking amiodarone. Long elimination half-life, approximately 25 to 50 days. Drug interactions may persist after discontinuance due to long half-life. May increase levels of substrates of p-glycoprotein and drugs metabolized by CYP 450 enzymes (CYP 1A2, CYP 2C9, CYP 2D6, CYP 3A4). Coadministration of fluoroquinolones, macrolides, loratadine, trazodone, or azoles may prolong QTc. May double or triple phenytoin level. May increase cyclosporine levels. May increase digoxin levels; discontinue digoxin or reduce dose by 50%. May increase INR with warfarin therapy up to 100%; reduce warfarin dose by 33 to 50%. Do not use with simvastatin doses greater than 20 mg/day, lovastatin doses greater than 40 mg/day; caution with atorvastatin (use lower doses); increases risk of myopathy and rhabdomyolysis. Coadministration with clopidogrel may result in ineffective platelet inhibition. Do not use with grapefruit juice. Use cautiously with beta-blockers and calcium channel blockers. Protease inhibitors, cimetidine may increase levels. Give bid if intolerable GI effects occur with once daily. IV therapy may cause hypotension and bradycardia in adults. Administer IV infusion using a nonevacuated glass bottle and in-line IV filter. Use central line when concentration exceeds 2 mg/mL. May cause congenital hypothyroidism and hyperthyroidism if given during pregnancy. Avoid use in children younger than 1 mo: IV form contains benzyl alcohol, which may cause gasping syndrome (gasping respirations, hypotension, bradycardia, and cardiovascular collapse). In children 1 mo to 15 yo may cause life-threatening hypotension, bradycardia, and AV block. May adversely affect male reproductive tract development in infants and toddlers from plasticizer exposure from IV tubing; use syringes instead of IV tubing to administer doses to infants and toddlers.

(cont.)

LIPID REDUCTION BY CLASS/AGENT[1]

Drug class/agent	LDL	HDL	TG
Bile acid sequestrants[2]	↓ 15–30%	↑ 3–5%	No change or ↑
Cholesterol absorption inhibitor[3]	↓ 18%	↑ 1%	↓ 8%
Fibrates[4]	↓ 5–20%	↑ 10–20%	↓ 20–50%
Lovastatin+ext'd release niacin[5]*	↓ 30–42%	↑ 20–30%	↓ 32–44%
Niacin[6]*	↓ 5–25%	↑ 15–35%	↓ 20–50%
Omega 3 fatty acids[7]	No change or ↑	↑ 9%	↓ 45%
Statins[8]	↓18–63%	↑ 5–15%	↓ 7–35%
Simvastatin+ezetimibe[9]	↓ 45–60%	↑ 6–10%	↓ 23–31%

1. LDL = low density lipoprotein. HDL = high density lipoprotein. TG = triglycerides. Adapted from NCEP: *JAMA* 2001; 285:2486 and prescribing information. 2. Cholestyramine (4–16 g), colestipol (5–20 g), colesevelam (2.6–3.8 g). 3. Ezetimibe (10 mg). When added to statin therapy, will ↓ LDL 25%, ↑ HDL 3%, ↓ TG 14% in addition to statin effects. 4. Fenofibrate (145–200 mg), gemfibrozil (600 mg BID). 5. Advicor® (20/1000–40/2000 mg). 6. Extended release nicotinic acid (Niaspan® 1–2 g), immediate release (crystalline) nicotinic acid (1.5–3 g), sustained release nicotinic acid (Slo-Niacin® 1–2 g). 7. Lovaza (4 g)
8. Atorvastatin (10–80 mg), fluvastatin (20–80 mg), lovastatin (20–80 mg), pravastatin (20–80 mg), rosuvastatin (5–40 mg), simvastatin (20–80 mg). 9. Vytorin® (10/10–10/80 mg). *Lowers lipoprotein a.

AMIODARONE (*cont.*)
MOA – Prolongs cardiac repolarization (Class III antiarrhythmic properties). Also has sodium channel blockade, beta adrenergic blockade, and calcium channel blockade effects (Class I, II, IV effects).
ADVERSE EFFECTS – Serious: Pulmonary toxicity, thyroid toxicity, bradycardia/heart block, arrhythmias, rhabdomyolysis, blindness, visual impairment, SIADH, hepatotoxicity, acute renal failure, agranulocytosis. Frequent: Hypotension, elevated LFTs, photosensitivity, GI intolerance, corneal microdeposits.

ATROPINE (*AtroPen*) ▶K ♀C ▶– $
ADULTS – Bradyarrhythmia/CPR: 0.5 to 1 mg IV q 3 to 5 min, max 0.04 mg/kg (3 mg). Treatment of muscarinic symptoms of insecticide or nerve agent poisonings: Mild symptoms: 1 injection of 2 mg auto-injector pen, 2 additional injections after 10 min may be given in rapid succession if severe symptoms develop. Severe symptoms: 3 injections of 2 mg pen in rapid succession. Administer injection in mid-lateral thigh. Max 3 injections.
PEDS – CPR: 0.02 mg/kg/dose IV q 5 min for 2 to 3 doses prn (max single dose 0.5 mg); minimum single dose, 0.1 mg; max cumulative dose 1 mg. Treatment of muscarinic symptoms of insecticide or nerve agent poisonings: Follow adult dosing instructions, but if wt less than 7 kg use 0.25 mg pen, if wt 7 to 18 kg use 0.5 mg pen, if wt 18 to 41 kg use 1 mg pen, if wt greater than 41 kg use 2 mg pen.
UNAPPROVED ADULTS – ET administration prior to IV access: 2 to 2.5 times the recommended IV dose in 10 mL of NS or distilled water.
FORMS – Trade only: Prefilled auto-injector pen: 0.25 mg (yellow), 0.5 mg (blue), 1 mg (dark red), 2 mg (green).
NOTES – Injector should be used by someone who has adequate training in recognizing and treating nerve agent or insecticide intoxication. Seek immediate medical attention after injection(s).
MOA – Blocks acetylcholine activity leading to increased cardiac chronotropic effect.
ADVERSE EFFECTS – Serious: Arrhythmias, tachycardia, paradoxical bradycardia (rare), paralysis (large doses). Frequent: Dry mouth, blurred vision, mydriasis, confusion, palpitations, urinary hesitancy, anhidrosis, constipation, injection site pain.

BICARBONATE ▶K ♀C ▶? $
ADULTS – Cardiac arrest: 1 mEq/kg/dose IV initially, followed by repeat doses up to 0.5 mEq/kg at 10 min intervals during continued arrest. Severe acidosis: 2 to 5 mEq/kg dose IV administered as a 4 to 8 h infusion. Repeat dosing based on lab values.
PEDS – Cardiac arrest: Neonates or infants age younger than 2 yo, 1 mEq/kg dose IV slow injection initially, followed by repeat doses up to 1 mEq/kg at 10 min intervals during continued arrest. To avoid intracranial hemorrhage due to hypertonicity, use a 1:1 dilution of 8.4% (1 mEq/mL) sodium bicarbonate and dextrose 5% or use the 4.2% (0.5 mEq/mL) product.
UNAPPROVED ADULTS – Prevention of contrast-induced nephropathy: Administer sodium bicarbonate 154 mEq/L soln at 3 mL/kg/h IV for 1 h before contrast, followed by infusion of 1 mL/kg/h for 6 h post procedure. If wt greater than 110 kg then dose based on 110 kg wt.
NOTES – Full correction of bicarbonate deficit should not be attempted during the first 24 h. May paradoxically exacerbate intracellular acidosis.
MOA – Replacement therapy, urinary alkalinization.
ADVERSE EFFECTS – Serious: Hypernatremia (rapid infusion), edema (rapid infusion). Frequent: None.

DIGOXIN (*Lanoxin, Lanoxicaps, Digitek*) ▶KL ♀C ▶+ $
ADULTS — <u>Systolic heart failure/rate control of chronic A-fib:</u> Give 0.25 mg PO daily for age less than 70 yo, give 0.125 mg PO daily for age 70 or older; use 0.0625 to 0.125 mg PO daily for impaired renal function and titrate based on response. <u>Rapid A-fib:</u> Load 0.5 mg IV, then 0.25 mg IV q 6 h for 2 doses, maintenance 0.125 to 0.375 mg IV/PO daily; titrate to minimum effective dose. Other agents (ie, beta blockers, diltiazem, verapamil) generally more effective in controlling ventricular rate in A-fib.
PEDS — <u>Heart failure with normal sinus rhythm:</u> IV loading based on age: Give 15 to 25 mcg/kg for premature neonate, give 20 to 30 mcg/kg for full-term neonate, give 30 to 50 mcg/kg for age 1 to 24 mo, give 25 to 35 mcg/kg for age 2 to 5 yo, give 15 to 30 mcg/kg for age 5 to 10 yo; give 8 to 12 mcg/kg for age older than 10 yo. Start by administering half of the total loading dose and then reassess in 4 to 8 h to determine need for second half of loading dose. Daily IV maintenance: Use 20 to 30% of actual IV loading dose for premature neonate; use 25 to 35% of actual IV loading dose for ages full-term to older than 10; use divided bid for age younger than 10 yo. Daily PO maintenance: Give 10 to 15 mcg/kg for age 2 to 5 yo, give 7 to 10 mcg/kg for age 6 to 10 yo; give 3 to 5 mcg/kg for age older than 10 yo. Caution - pediatric doses are in mcg, elixir product is labeled in mg/mL. <u>Atrial fibrillation:</u> Titrate to minimum dose needed to achieve desired ventricular rate without undesirable side effects.
UNAPPROVED ADULTS — <u>Reentrant PSVT</u> (after carotid massage, IV adenosine, IV beta-blocker, IV diltiazem): 8 to 15 mcg/kg IV, give 50% of total dose initially, 25% 4 to 6 h later, and then the final 25% 4 to 6 h later.
FORMS — Generic/Trade: Tabs, scored (Lanoxin, Digitek) 0.125, 0.25 mg; elixir 0.05 mg/mL. Trade only: Caps (Lanoxicaps), 0.1, 0.2 mg.
NOTES — Consider patient specific characteristics (lean/ideal wt, CrCl, age, concomitant disease states, concomitant medications, and factors likely to alter pharmacokinetic/dynamic profile of digoxin) when dosing; see package insert for alterations based on wt and renal function. Assess electrolytes, renal function, levels periodically. Elimination prolonged with renal impairment. Maintain normal potassium, magnesium, and calcium levels. Adjust dose based on response and therapeutic serum levels (range from 0.8 to 2 ng/mL); about 1/3 patients have clinical toxicity with concentrations less than 2 ng/mL. Lower serum trough levels (0.5 to 1 ng/mL) may be appropriate for heart failure; A-fib may need higher levels. 100 mcg Lanoxicaps is equivalent to 125 mcg tabs or elixir. Avoid administering IM due to severe local irritation. Many drug and herb interactions. See package insert for full information before using in patients with sinus node disease, AV block, accessory AV pathway, certain heart failure disorders with preserved LV function, hypermetabolic states, thyroid disease, beri beri heart disease, or planned cardioversion. Do not use with acute MI or myocarditis. Therapeutic doses may cause EKG changes (PR interval prolongation, ST segment depression) and false positive ST-T changes during exercise testing; these are expected and do not indicate toxicity.
MOA — Slows cardiac conduction through the AV node, increases force of myocardial contraction.
ADVERSE EFFECTS — Serious: Arrhythmias, heart block. Frequent: More frequent with higher doses. Dizziness, N/V, diarrhea.

DIGOXIN IMMUNE FAB (*Digibind, Digifab*) ▶K ♀C ▶? $$$$$
ADULTS — <u>Digoxin toxicity:</u> Dose varies. Acute ingestion of known amount: 1 vial binds approximately 0.5 mg digoxin. Acute ingestion of unknown amount: 10 vials IV, may repeat once. <u>Toxicity during chronic therapy:</u> 6 vials usually adequate; one formula is: Number vials = (serum dig level in ng/mL) × (kg)/100.
PEDS — <u>Digoxin toxicity:</u> Dose varies. Acute ingestion of known amount: One vial binds approximately 0.5 mg digoxin. Acute ingestion of unknown amount: 10 vials IV, may repeat once; monitor for volume overload. <u>Toxicity during chronic therapy:</u> 1 vial usually adequate for infants and small children (< 20 kg); one formula is: Number vials = (serum dig level in ng/mL) × (kg)/100.
NOTES — Do not draw serum digoxin concentrations after administering digoxin-immune Fab; levels will be falsely elevated for several days.
MOA — Binds digoxin preventing interaction with sodium pump receptor.
ADVERSE EFFECTS — Serious: Hypersensitivity (rare), hypokalemia.

DISOPYRAMIDE (*Norpace, Norpace CR, ✦Rythmodan, Rythmodan-LA*) ▶KL ♀C ▶+ $$$$
WARNING — Proarrhythmic. Contraindicated in preexisting/congenital QT prolongation, history of torsade de pointes, cardiogenic shock; 2nd/3rd degree heart block without pacemaker Only use for adults with life-threatening ventricular arrhythmias; increased mortality in patients with non-life-threatening ventricular arrhythmias and structural heart disease (ie, MI, LV dysfunction).
ADULTS — Rarely indicated, consult cardiologist. <u>Ventricular arrhythmia:</u> 400 to 800 mg PO daily in divided doses (immediate-release is divided q 6 h: Extended-release is divided q 12 h). With cardiomyopathy or possible cardiac decompensation, limit initial dose to 100 mg of immediate-release q 6 to 8 h; do not give a loading dose. <u>With liver disease or moderate renal impairment</u> (CrCl > 40 mg/dL): 400 mg/day PO in divided doses. Use immediate-release form when CrCl is less than 40 mg/dL: Give 100 mg q 8 h for CrCl 30 to 40 mg/dL, give 100 mg q 12 h for CrCl 15 to 30 mg/dL, give 100 mg q 24 h for CrCl < 15 mg/dL.
PEDS — <u>Ventricular arrhythmia:</u> Divide all doses q 6 h. Give 10 to 30 mg/kg/day for age younger than

(cont.)

DISOPYRAMIDE *(cont.)*
1 yo, give 10 to 20 mg/kg/day for age 1 to 4 yo, give 10 to 15 mg/kg/day for age 4 to 12 yo, give 6 to 15 mg/kg/day for age 12 to 18 yo.
UNAPPROVED ADULTS – <u>Maintain sinus rhythm with A-fib:</u> 400 to 750 mg/day in divided doses.
FORMS – Generic/Trade: Caps immediate-release 100, 150 mg; extended-release 150 mg. Trade only: Caps, extended-release 100 mg.
NOTES – Consider inpatient rhythm monitoring during initiation of therapy, especially when treating life-threatening arrhythmias. Anticholinergic side effects (dry mouth, constipation, blurred vision, urinary hesitancy) commonly occur. Reduce dose in patients with CrCl < 40 mL/min. Initiate as an outpatient with extreme caution. May start 6 to 12 h after last dose of quinidine, or 3 to 6 h after last dose of procainamide. May start extended-release form 6 h after last dose of immediate-release form.
MOA – Depresses phase 0 depolarization, prolongs cardiac action potential duration (Class 1A).
ADVERSE EFFECTS – Serious: Arrhythmias. Frequent: Dizziness, headache, hypotension, dry mouth, blurred vision, urinary retention, constipation.

DOFETILIDE (*Tikosyn*) ▶KL ♀C ▶– $$$$
WARNING – Available only to hospitals and prescribers who have received appropriate dosing and treatment initiation education. Must be initiated or re-initiated in a facility that can provide CrCl calculation, ECG monitoring, and cardiac resuscitation. Monitor on telemetry for a minimum of 3 days.
ADULTS – <u>Conversion of A-fib/flutter:</u> Specialized dosing based on CrCl and QTc interval.
PEDS – Not approved in children.
FORMS – Trade only: Caps, 0.125, 0.25, 0.5 mg.
NOTES – Rarely indicated. Contraindicated in acquired/congenital QT prolongation; CrCl < 20 mL/min; baseline QTc interval > 440 msec or > 500 msec in patients with ventricular conduction abnormalities; or with concomitant HCTZ, verapamil, cimetidine, ketoconazole, megestrol, prochlorperazine, or trimethoprim. Use with heart rate below 50 bpm has not been studied. Serum K+, Mg++ should be within normal range prior to initiating and during therapy. Monitor K+ and Mg++ (low levels increase risk of arrhythmias). Assess CrCl and QTc prior to first dose. Continuously monitor ECG during hospital initiation and adjust dose based on QTc interval. Do not discharge within 12 h after conversion to normal sinus rhythm. Effects may be increased by known CYP 3A4 inhibitors and drugs that inhibit renal elimination. Using with phenothiazines, cisapride, TCAs, macrolides, fluoroquinolones may increase QTc.
MOA – Prolongs cardiac repolarization (Class III antiarrhythmic properties).
ADVERSE EFFECTS – Serious: Arrhythmias. Common: Chest pain, headache.

DRONEDARONE (*Multaq*) ▶L ♀X ▶– $$$$
WARNING – Do not use with NYHA Class IV heart failure or NYHA Class II-III heart failure with recent decompensation requiring hospitalization or referral to heart failure clinic.
ADULTS – <u>Reduce risk of CV hospitalization with paroxysmal or persistent atrial fib/flutter, with recent episode of atrial fib/flutter and CV risk factors</u> (age older than 70, HTN, diabetes, prior CVA, left atrial diameter 50 mm or greater, or LVEF less than 40%), who are in sinus rhythm or will be converted: 400 mg PO bid with morning and evening meals.
PEDS – Not approved in children.
FORMS – Trade: Tabs unscored 400 mg.
NOTES – Do not use with 2nd or 3rd degree AV block or sick sinus syndrome without functioning pacemaker; bradycardia < 50 bpm; QTc Bazett interval > 500 ms; or severe hepatic impairment. Do not use with grapefruit juice, other antiarrhythmic agents, potent inhibitors of CYP 3A4 enzyme system (clarithromycin, erythromycin, itraconazole, ketoconazole, nefazodone, ritonavir, voriconazole); inducers of CYP 3A4 enzyme system (carbamazepine, phenytoin, phenobarbital, rifampin, St. John's wort). May increase digoxin levels; discontinue digoxin or reduce dose by 50%; monitor for digoxin toxicity. May increase levels of sirolimus, tacrolimus, and CYP 3A4 substrates with narrow therapeutic index. Use cautiously with beta-blockers (BB) and calcium channel blockers (CCB); initiate lower doses of BB or CCB; verify EKG tolerability before increasing BB or CCB dose. Correct hypo/hyperkalemia and hypomagnesium before giving. Serum creatinine may increase during first weeks, but does not reflect change in renal function. Teach patients to report symptoms of worsening heart failure (wt gain, edema, SOB).
MOA – Has sodium channel blockade, beta adrenergic blockade, cardiac repolarization, and calcium channel blockade effects (Class I, II, III, IV effects).
ADVERSE EFFECTS – Serious: New/worsening HF, bradycardia/heart block, arrhythmias. Frequent: Abdominal pain, asthenia, diarrhea, nausea.

FLECAINIDE (*Tambocor*) ▶K ♀C ▶– $$$$
WARNING – Proarrhythmic. Increased mortality in patients with non-life-threatening ventricular arrhythmias, structural heart disease (ie, MI, LV dysfunction); not recommended for use with chronic atrial fibrillation.
ADULTS – <u>Prevention of paroxysmal atrial fib/ flutter or PSVT, with symptoms and no structural heart disease:</u> Start 50 mg PO q 12 h, may increase by 50 mg bid q 4 d, max 300 mg/day. <u>Life-threatening ventricular arrhythmias without structural heart disease:</u> Start 100 mg PO q 12 h, may increase by 50 mg bid q 4 d, max 400 mg/day. With severe renal impairment (CrCl < 35 mL/min): Start 50 mg PO bid.
PEDS – Consult pediatric cardiologist.
UNAPPROVED ADULTS – <u>Cardioversion of recent onset atrial fib:</u> 200 to 300 mg PO single dose. <u>Maintain sinus rhythm with A-fib:</u> 200 to 300 mg/day in divided doses.

(cont.)

CARDIOVASCULAR: Anti-Dysrhythmics/Cardiac Arrest

FLECAINIDE (cont.)
FORMS — Generic/Trade: Tabs unscored 50, scored 100, 150 mg.
NOTES — Contraindicated in cardiogenic shock; sick sinus syndrome or significant conduction delay; 2nd/3rd degree heart block or bundle brand block without pacemaker; acquired/congenital QT prolongation; or patients with history of torsade de pointes. Consider inpatient rhythm monitoring during initiation of therapy, especially when treating life-threatening arrhythmias. Use with AV nodal slowing agent (beta-blocker, verapamil, diltiazem) to minimize risk of 1:1 atrial flutter. Reduce dose if QRS widening > 20% from baseline or if 2nd/3rd degree AV block. Correct hypo/hyperkalemia before giving. Increases digoxin level 13 to 19%. Consult cardiologist before using with other antiarrhythmic agents. Reduce dose of flecainide 50% when used with amiodarone. Quinidine, cimetidine may increase levels. Use cautiously with disopyramide, verapamil, or impaired hepatic function. Use cautiously with impaired renal function; will take > 4 days to reach new steady state level. Target trough level 0.2 to 1 mcg/mL.
MOA — Depresses phase 0 depolarization significantly, slows cardiac conduction significantly (Class 1C).
ADVERSE EFFECTS — Serious: Arrhythmias, depressed conduction/widened QRS at higher heart rates. Frequent: Dizziness, headache, nausea, dyspnea, fatigue, visual disturbances.

IBUTILIDE (*Corvert*) ▶K ♀C ▶? $$$$$
WARNING — Proarrhythmic; only administer by trained personnel with continuous ECG monitoring, capable of identifying and treating acute ventricular arrhythmias. Potentially fatal ventricular arrhythmias may occur with/without QT prolongation and can lead to torsade de pointes.
ADULTS — Recent onset A-fib/flutter: Give 0.01 mg/kg over 10 min for wt less than 60 kg, may repeat if no response after 10 additional minutes. Give 1 mg (10 mL) IV over 10 mins for wt 60 kg or greater, may repeat once if no response after 10 additional min. Useful in combination with DC cardioversion if DC cardioversion alone is unsuccessful.
PEDS — Not approved in children.
NOTES — Serum K+, Mg++ should be within normal range prior to initiating and during therapy. Monitor K+ and Mg++ (low levels increase risk of arrhythmias). Keep on cardiac monitor at least 4 h. Use with caution, if at all, when QT interval is > 500 ms, severe LV dysfunction, or in patients already using class Ia or III antiarrhythmics. Stop infusion when arrhythmia is terminated.
MOA — Prolongs cardiac repolarization (Class III antiarrhythmic properties).
ADVERSE EFFECTS — Serious: Arrhythmias.

ISOPROTERENOL (*Isuprel*) ▶LK ♀C ▶? $$$
ADULTS — Refractory bradycardia or 3rd degree AV block: Bolus method: 0.02 to 0.06 mg IV: infusion method, dilute 2 mg in 250 mL D5W (8 mcg/mL), a rate of 37.5 mL/h delivers 5 mcg/min. General dose range 2 to 20 mcg/min.
PEDS — Refractory bradycardia or 3rd degree AV block: Dilute 2 mg in 250 mL D5W (8 mcg/mL). Start IV infusion 0.05 mcg/kg/min, increase every 5 to 10 min by 0.1 mcg/kg/min until desired effect or onset of toxicity, max 2 mcg/kg/min. For a 10 kg child, a rate of 8 mL/h delivers 0.1 mcg/kg/min.
MOA — Stimulates beta-1 receptors (increases cardiac contractility and chronotropic effect), stimulates beta-2 receptors (peripheral vasodilation).
ADVERSE EFFECTS — Serious: Arrhythmias, tachycardia. Frequent: Hypertension, palpitations, flushing, sweating, dizziness.

LIDOCAINE (*Xylocaine, Xylocard*) ▶LK ♀B ▶? $
ADULTS — Ventricular arrhythmia: Load 1 mg/kg IV, then 0.5 mg/kg IV q 8 to 10 min prn to max 3 mg/kg. IV infusion: 4 g in 500 mL D5W (8 mg/mL) at 1 to 4 mg/min.
PEDS — Ventricular arrhythmia: Loading dose 1 mg/kg IV/intraosseous slowly; may repeat for 2 doses 10 to 15 min apart; max 3 to 5 mg/kg in 1 h. ET tube: Use 2 to 2.5 times IV dose. IV infusion: 4 g in 500 mL D5W (8 mg/mL) at 20 to 50 mcg/kg/min. For a 10 kg child a rate of 3 mL/h delivers 40 mcg/kg/min.
UNAPPROVED ADULTS — ET administration prior to IV access: 2 to 2.5 times the recommended IV dose in 10 mL of NS or distilled water. Shock refractory VF/pulseless VT: 1 to 1.5 mg/kg IV push once, then 0.5 to 0.75 mg/kg IV push q 5 to 10 min prn to max 3 mg/kg.
NOTES — Reduce infusion in heart failure, liver disease, elderly. Not for routine use after acute MI. Monitor for CNS side effects with prolonged infusions.
MOA — Depresses phase 0 depolarization slightly, shortens cardiac action potential duration (Class 1B).
ADVERSE EFFECTS — Serious: Arrhythmias, hypersensitivity (rare), seizures (rare). Frequent: Hypotension, dizziness, drowsiness.

MEXILETINE (*Mexitil*) ▶L ♀C ▶– $$$
WARNING — Proarrhythmic. Increased mortality in patients with non-life-threatening ventricular arrhythmias and structural heart disease (ie, MI, LV dysfunction).
ADULTS — Rarely indicated, consult cardiologist. Ventricular arrhythmia: Start 200 mg PO q 8 h with food or antacid, max dose 1200 mg/day. Patients responding to q 8 h dosing may be converted to q 12 h dosing with careful monitoring, max 450 mg/dose q 12 h.
PEDS — Not approved in children.
FORMS — Generic only: Caps 150, 200, 250 mg.
NOTES — Patients may require decreased dose with severe liver disease. CNS side effects may limit dose titration. Monitor level when given with phenytoin, rifampin, phenobarbital, cimetidine, fluvoxamine. May increase theophylline level.
MOA — Depresses phase 0 depolarization slightly, shortens cardiac action potential duration (Class 1B).

(cont.)

MEXILETINE (cont.)
ADVERSE EFFECTS – Serious: Arrhythmias, blood dyscrasias, pulmonary infiltrates/fibrosis. Frequent: N/V, diarrhea, dizziness, nervousness, headache, blurred vision, tremor, ataxia.

PROCAINAMIDE (*Pronestyl*) ▶LK ♀C ▶? $
WARNING – Proarrhythmic. Increased mortality in patients with non-life-threatening ventricular arrhythmias and structural heart disease (ie, MI, LV dysfunction). Contraindicated with systemic lupus erythematosus. Has been associated with severe bone marrow suppression.
ADULTS – <u>Ventricular Arrhythmia:</u> Loading dose: 100 mg IV q 10 min or 20 mg/min (150 mL/h) until QRS widens more than 50%, dysrhythmia suppressed, hypotension, or total of 17 mg/kg or 1000 mg delivered. Infusion: Dilute 2 g in 250 mL D5W (8 mg/mL) run at rate of 15 to 45 mL/h to deliver 2 to 6 mg/min. If rhythm unresponsive, guide therapy by serum procainamide/NAPA levels.
PEDS – Not approved in children.
UNAPPROVED ADULTS – <u>Shock responsive VF/pulseless VT:</u> up to 50 mg/min until: QRS widens > 50%, dysrhythmia suppressed, hypotension, or total of 17 mg/kg or 1000 mg delivered. <u>Maintenance of sinus rhythm with A-fib:</u> 1000 to 4000 mg/day in divided doses. <u>Restoration of sinus rhythm in atrial fibrillation with Wolf-Parkinson-White syndrome (pre-excitation):</u> 100 mg IV q 10 min or 20 mg/min. until: QRS widens > 50%, dysrhythmia suppressed, hypotension, or total of 17 mg/kg or 1000 mg delivered.
UNAPPROVED PEDS – <u>Arrhythmia:</u> 2 to 6 mg/kg IV over 5 min, max loading dose 100 mg, repeat loading dose every 5 to 10 min prn up to max 15 mg/kg; 20 to 80 mcg/kg/min IV infusion, max dose 2 g/day. Consult peds cardiologist or intensivist.
NOTES – Use lower dose or longer dosing interval with liver disease. Use cautiously with renal impairment or failure. Avoid with preexisting peripheral neuropathy. If positive antinuclear antibody (ANA) test develops, weigh risk/benefit of continued therapy. Evaluate complete blood count, including white cell, differential, and platelet counts, weekly for first 12 weeks of therapy and periodically afterwards, and if patient develops unusual bleeding/bruising or signs of infection. If hematologic disorders are identified, discontinue therapy.
MOA – Depresses phase 0 depolarization, prolongs cardiac action potential duration (Class 1A).
ADVERSE EFFECTS – Serious: Arrhythmias, blood dyscrasias (rare), SLE. Frequent: Hypotension, fever, headache.

PROPAFENONE (*Rythmol, Rythmol SR*) ▶L ♀C ▶? $$$$
WARNING – Proarrhythmic. Increased mortality in patients with non-life-threatening ventricular arrhythmias and structural heart disease (ie, MI, LV dysfunction).
ADULTS – <u>Prevention of paroxysmal atrial fib/flutter or PSVT, with symptoms and no structural heart disease; or life-threatening ventricular arrhythmias:</u> Start (immediate-release) 150 mg PO q 8 h; may increase after 3 to 4 days to 225 mg PO q 8 h; max 900 mg/day. <u>Prolong time to recurrence of symptomatic atrial fib without structural heart disease:</u> 225 mg SR PO q 12 h, may increase after 5 days to 325 mg PO q 12 h, max 425 mg q 12 h.
PEDS – Not approved in children.
UNAPPROVED ADULTS – <u>Cardioversion of recent onset atrial fib:</u> 600 mg PO single dose. <u>Outpatient prn therapy for recurrent atrial fib in highly-select patients ("pill-in-the-pocket"):</u> Single dose PO of 450 mg for wt less than 70 kg, 600 mg for wt 70 kg or greater.
FORMS – Generic/Trade: Tabs immediate-release scored 150, 225, 300 mg. Trade only: SR, Caps 225, 325, 425 mg.
NOTES – Consider inpatient rhythm monitoring during initiation of therapy, especially when treating life-threatening arrhythmias. Do not use with structural heart disease or for ventricular rate control during atrial fib. Consider using with AV nodal blocking agent (beta-blocker, verapamil, diltiazem) to minimize risk of 1:1 atrial flutter. Reduce dose if QRS widening > 20% from baseline or if 2nd/3rd degree AV block. Correct hypo/hyperkalemia and hypomagnesium before giving. Consult cardiologist before using with other antiarrhythmic agents. May increase digoxin level 35 to 85%. May increase beta-blocker, cyclosporine, desipramine, haloperidol, imipramine, theophylline, venlafaxine levels. Increases warfarin activity; monitor INR. Amiodarone, cimetidine, desipramine, erythromycin, ketoconazole, paroxetine, ritonavir, saquinavir, sertraline may increase level and risk of QT prolongation. Instruct patient to report any changes in OTC, prescription, supplement use and symptoms that may be associated with altered electrolytes (prolonged/excessive diarrhea, sweating, vomiting, thirst, appetite loss). Reduce dose 70 to 80% with impaired hepatic function. Use cautiously with impaired renal function. Bioavailability of 325 mg SR bid = 150 mg immediate-release tid. Poorly metabolized by 10% population; reduce dose and monitor for toxicity.
MOA – Depresses phase 0 depolarization significantly, slows cardiac conduction significantly (Class 1C).
ADVERSE EFFECTS – Serious: Arrhythmias, heart block. Frequent: Dizziness, headache, nausea, dyspnea, fatigue, blurred vision, metallic taste.

QUINIDINE (✦*Biquin durules*) ▶LK ♀C ▶+ $$$- gluconate, $-sulfate
WARNING – Proarrhythmic. Associated with QT prolongation and torsade de pointes. Contraindicated with complete AV block or left bundle branch block. Increased mortality in patients with non-life-threatening arrhythmias and structural heart disease (ie, MI, LV dysfunction).
ADULTS – <u>Arrhythmia:</u> Gluconate, extended-release: 324 to 648 mg PO q 8 to 12 h; sulfate, immediate-release: 200 to 400 mg PO q 6 to 8 h; sulfate, extended-release: 300 to 600 mg PO q 8 to 12 h.

(cont.)

QUINIDINE (cont.)

Consider inpatient rhythm and QT monitoring during initiation of therapy. Life-threatening malaria: Load with 10 mg/kg (max 600 mg) IV over 1 to 2 h, then 0.02 mg/kg/min for at least 24. Dose given as quinidine gluconate. When parasitemia < 1% and PO meds tolerated, convert to PO quinine to complete 3 days (Africa/South America) or 7 days (Southeast Asia). Also give doxycycline, tetracycline, or clindamycin.
- PEDS — Not approved in children.
- UNAPPROVED PEDS — Arrhythmia: Test dose (oral sulfate or IM/IV gluconate) 2 mg/kg (max 200 mg). Sulfate: 15 to 60 mg/kg/day PO divided q 6 h. Life-threatening malaria: Load with 10 mg/kg IV over 1 to 2 h, then 0.02 mg/kg/min for at least 24 h. Dose given as quinidine gluconate. When parasitemia < 1% and PO meds tolerated, convert to PO quinine to complete 3 days (Africa/South America) or 7 days (Southeast Asia). Also give doxycycline, tetracycline, or clindamycin.
- FORMS — Generic gluconate: Tabs, extended-release unscored 324 mg. Generic sulfate: Tabs, scored immediate-release 200, 300 mg, Tabs, extended-release 300 mg.
- NOTES — QRS widening, QT interval prolongation (risk increased by hypokalemia, hypomagnesemia, or bradycardia), hypotension, hypoglycemia. Use cautiously with renal impairment/failure or hepatic disease. Use extreme caution with history of QT prolongation or torsade de pointes. Contraindicated with ziprasidone. Monitor ECG and BP. Drug interactions with some antiarrhythmics, digoxin, phenytoin, phenobarbital, rifampin, verapamil. Do not chew, break, or crush extended-release tabs. Do not use with digitalis toxicity, hypotension, AV/bundle branch block, or myasthenia gravis. Quinidine gluconate 267 mg = quinidine sulfate 200 mg.
- MOA — Depresses phase 0 depolarization, prolongs cardiac action potential duration (Class 1A). Unknown antimalarial mechanism.
- ADVERSE EFFECTS — Serious: Arrhythmias, syncope (rare), hypersensitivity (rare). Frequent: Diarrhea, hypotension, N/V, cinchonism (disturbed hearing, headaches, visual changes, confusion).

SOTALOL (*Betapace, Betapace AF, ♦Rylosol*) ▶K ♀B ▶− $$$$
- WARNING — Patients should be in a facility for at least 3 days with ECG monitoring, cardiac resuscitation available, and CrCl calculated when initiating or re-initiating Betapace AF. Do not substitute Betapace for Betapace AF.
- ADULTS — Ventricular arrhythmia (Betapace), symptomatic A-fib/A-flutter (Betapace AF): Start 80 mg PO bid, usual maintenance dose 160 to 320 mg/day divided bid, max 640 mg/day.
- PEDS — Not approved in children.
- FORMS — Generic/Trade: Tabs, scored 80, 120, 160, 240 mg, Tabs, scored (Betapace AF) 80, 120, 160 mg.
- NOTES — Proarrhythmic. Caution, higher incidence of torsades de pointes with doses higher than 320 mg/day, in women, or heart failure. Adjust dose if CrCl < 60 mL/min.
- MOA — Prolongs cardiac repolarization (Class III antiarrhythmic properties).
- ADVERSE EFFECTS — Serious: Arrhythmias, bradycardia, exacerbation of heart failure.

CARDIOVASCULAR: Anti-Hyperlipidemic Agents—Bile Acid Sequestrants

CHOLESTYRAMINE (*Questran, Questran Light, Prevalite, LoCHOLEST, LoCHOLEST Light*) ▶Not absorbed ♀C ▶+ $$$
- ADULTS — Elevated LDL-C: Start 4 g PO daily to bid before meals, usual maintenance 12 to 24 g/day in divided doses bid to qid before meals, max 24 g/day.
- PEDS — Not approved in children.
- UNAPPROVED ADULTS — Cholestasis-associated pruritus: 4 to 8 g bid to tid. Diarrhea: 4 to 16 g/day.
- UNAPPROVED PEDS — Elevated LDL-C: Start 240 mg/kg/day PO divided tid before meals, usual maintenance 8 to 16 g/day divided tid.
- FORMS — Generic/Trade: Powder for oral susp, 4 g cholestyramine resin/9 g powder (Questran, LoCHOLEST), 4 g cholestyramine resin/5 g powder (Questran Light), 4 g cholestyramine resin/5.5 g powder (Prevalite, LoCHOLEST Light). Each available in bulk powder and single-dose packets.
- NOTES — Administer other drugs at least 2 h before or 4 to 6 h after cholestyramine to avoid decreased absorption of the other agent. Bid dosing recommended, but may divide up to 6 times per day. Mix powder with 60 to 180 mL of water, milk, fruit juice, or drink. Avoid carbonated liquids for mixing. GI problems common, mainly constipation. May cause elevated triglycerides; do not use when triglycerides exceed 400 mg/dL.
- MOA — Binds bile acid in the intestine preventing absorption.
- ADVERSE EFFECTS — Serious: Fecal impaction (rare). Frequent: Constipation.

COLESEVELAM (*Welchol*) ▶Not absorbed ♀B ▶+ $$$$$
- ADULTS — Glycemic control of type 2 diabetes or LDL-C reduction: 6 tabs once daily or 3 tabs PO bid, max dose 6 tabs/day; or 3.75 g powder once daily or 1.875 g powder bid, max dose 3.75 g/day. Give with meal and liquid. Mix powder in 4-8 ounces water, stir well. Same dose with statins or other agents.
- PEDS — Hyperlipidemia, 10 yo or older: 6 tabs once daily with a meal, or 3 tabs PO bid, max dose 6 tabs/day; or 3.75 g powder once daily or 1.875 g powder bid, max dose 3.75 g/day; see prescribing information for more information. Give with meal. Give tabs with liquid. Mix powder in 4-8 ounces water.

(cont.)

CARDIOVASCULAR: Anti-Hyperlipidemic Agents

COLESEVELAM (cont.)
FORMS — Trade only: Tabs unscored 625 mg. Powder single-dose packets 1.875, 3.75 g
NOTES — Take with a full glass of water or other noncarbonated liquid. GI problems common, mainly constipation. May cause elevation of triglycerides. Do not use when triglycerides exceed 500 mg/dL, or with a history of bowel obstruction or triglyceride-induced pancreatitis. Administer other drugs at least 4 h or more before colesevelam to avoid decreased absorption of the other agent; may decrease levels of glyburide, levothyroxine, oral contraceptives containing ethinyl estradiol and norethindrone, phenytoin, warfarin.
MOA — Binds bile acid in the intestine preventing absorption.
ADVERSE EFFECTS — Serious: Fecal impaction (rare). Frequent: Constipation, dyspepsia, nausea.

COLESTIPOL (*Colestid, Colestid Flavored*) ▶Not absorbed ♀B ▶+ $$$$
ADULTS — Elevated LDL-C: Tabs: Start 2 g PO daily to bid, max 16 g/day. Granules: Start 5 g PO daily-bid, increase by 5 g increments as tolerated at 1 to 2 months intervals, max 30 g/day.
PEDS — Not approved in children.
UNAPPROVED PEDS — 125 to 250 mg/kg/day PO in divided doses bid to qid, dosing range 10 to 20 g/day.
FORMS — Generic/Trade: Tabs 1 g. Granules for oral susp, 5 g/7.5 g powder.
NOTES — Administer other drugs at least 1 h before or 4 to 6 h after colestipol to avoid decreased absorption of the other agent. Mix granules in at least 90 mL of water, milk, fruit juice, or drink. Avoid carbonated liquids for mixing. Swallow tabs whole with a full glass of liquid to avoid tab disintegration in the esophagus. GI problems common, mainly constipation. May cause elevated triglycerides; do not use when triglycerides exceed 400 mg/dL.
MOA — Binds bile acid in the intestine preventing absorption.
ADVERSE EFFECTS — Serious: Fecal impaction (rare). Frequent: Constipation.

CARDIOVASCULAR: Anti-Hyperlipidemic Agents—HMG-CoA Reductase Inhibitors ("Statins") and combinations

NOTE: Hepatotoxicity: Monitor LFTs initially, approximately 12 weeks after starting/titrating therapy, then annually or more frequently if indicated. May initiate, continue, or increase dose of statin with modest LFT elevation (less than 3 times upper limit of normal). Repeat LFTs and rule out other causes with isolated, asymptomatic LFT elevation less than 3 times upper limit of normal. Consider continuing vs. discontinuing statin or reducing statin dose. Patients with chronic liver disease, nonalcoholic fatty liver, or nonalcoholic steatohepatitis may receive statins. Discontinue statin with objective evidence of liver injury; seek cause; consider referral to gastroenterologist or hepatologist. Evaluate muscle symptoms before starting therapy, 6 to 12 weeks after starting/increasing therapy and at each follow-up visit. Obtain creatine kinase when patient complains of muscle soreness, tenderness, weakness, or pain. Teach patients to report promptly unexplained muscle pain, tenderness, or weakness; rule out common causes; discontinue if myopathy diagnosed or suspected. With tolerable muscle complaints or asymptomatic creatine kinase increase < 10 times upper limit of normal, continue statin at same or reduced dose; use symptoms to guide continuing/discontinuing statin. With intolerable muscle symptoms with/without creatine kinase elevation, discontinue statin; when asymptomatic, may restart same/different statin at same/lower dose. With rhabdomyolysis, discontinue statin, provide IV hydration; weigh risk/benefit of statin therapy when recovered. Consider measurement of creatine kinase before starting therapy in patients at risk for myopathy: Advanced age (especially age older than 80 yo, women > men); multisystem disease (eg, chronic renal insufficiency, especially due to diabetes); multiple medications; perioperative periods; alcohol abuse; grapefruit juice (more than 1 quart/day); specific concomitant medications: fibrates (especially gemfibrozil), nicotinic acid (rare), cyclosporine, erythromycin, clarithromycin, itraconazole, ketoconazole, protease inhibitors, nefazodone, verapamil, amiodarone. Weigh potential risk of combination therapy against potential benefit.

ADVICOR (lovastatin + niacin) ▶LK ♀X ▶— $$$$
ADULTS — Hyperlipidemia: 1 tab PO at bedtime with a low-fat snack. Establish dose using extended-release niacin first, or if already on lovastatin substitute combo product with lowest niacin dose.
PEDS — Not approved in children.
FORMS — Trade only: Tabs, unscored extended-release lovastatin/niacin 20/500, 20/750, 20/1000, 40/1000 mg.
NOTES — Do not exceed 40/2000 mg. Do not break, chew, or crush. Swallow whole. aspirin or NSAID 30 min prior may decrease niacin flushing reaction. Niacin may worsen glucose control, peptic ulcer disease, gout, headaches, and menopausal flushing. Significantly lowers LDL-C and triglycerides, raises HDL-cholesterol. Do not use with potent inhibitors of CYP 3A4 enzyme system (clarithromycin, erythromycin, grapefruit juice > 1 quart/day, HIV protease inhibitors, itraconazole, ketoconazole, nefazodone, telithromycin); increases risk of myopathy. Do not exceed 20 mg/day of lovastatin component when used with cyclosporine, danazol, fibrates, or niacin at doses 1 g/day or greater; do not exceed 40 mg/day of lovastatin component when used with amiodarone or verapamil. With concomitant cyclosporine or danazol, start with 10 mg daily of lovastatin component.
MOA — See component drugs.
ADVERSE EFFECTS — See component drugs.

CARDIOVASCULAR: Anti-Hyperlipidemic Agents

STATINS	Minimum Dose for 30-40% LDL Reduction	LDL *	LFT Monitoring**
	atorvastatin 10 mg	-39%	Baseline, 12 weeks, semiannually
	fluvastatin 40 mg bid	-36%	Baseline, 12 weeks
	fluvastatin XL 80 mg	-35%	Baseline, 12 weeks
	lovastatin 40 mg	-31%	Baseline
	pitavastatin 2 mg	-36%	Baseline, 12 weeks
	pravastatin 40mg	-34%	Baseline
	rosuvastatin 5 mg	-45%	Baseline, 12 weeks, semiannually
	simvastatin 20 mg	-38%	Baseline for all doses; Get LFTs prior to & 3 months after dose increase to 80 mg, then semiannually for first year.

LDL=low-density lipoprotein, LFT=liver function tests. Will get ~6% decrease in LDL with every doubling of dose. National Lipid Association Statin Safety Task Force Report (*Am J Cardiol* 2006; 8A:89c-94c) schedule for LFT monitoring: baseline, ~12 weeks after starting/titrating therapy, when clinically indicated. Stop statin therapy if LFTs are >3 times upper limit of normal. *Adapted from *Circulation* 2004;110:227-239.
**From Prescribing information

ATORVASTATIN (*Lipitor*) ▶L ♀X ▶– $$$$
ADULTS — Hyperlipidemia/prevention of cardiovascular events, including Type 2 DM: Start 10 mg PO daily, 40 mg daily for LDL-C reduction > 45%, increase at intervals of 4 weeks or more to a max of 80 mg/day. Do not exceed 10 mg/day when used with cyclosporine. Use > 20 mg/day cautiously when used with clarithromycin, itraconazole, or combinations of HIV protease inhibitors that include ritonavir.
PEDS — Hyperlipidemia, 10 yo or older: Start 10 mg daily, max 20 mg/day. See package insert for more information.
UNAPPROVED ADULTS — Prevention of cardiovascular events and death post acute coronary syndrome or with stable CAD, or prevention of CVA/cardiovascular events with recent CVA/TIA and no CHD: 80 mg PO daily.
FORMS — Trade only: Tabs unscored 10, 20, 40, 80 mg.
NOTES — Metabolized by CYP 3A4 enzyme system. Concomitant administration of azole antifungals, erythromycin, clarithromycin, cyclosporine, combinations of HIV protease inhibitors, fibrates, niacin, grapefruit, and grapefruit juice increase the risk of myopathy and possible rhabdomyolysis. May increase plasma levels of digoxin. May give any time of day. Patients with recent CVA/TIA and no CHD who received atorvastatin 80 mg/day had a higher incidence of hemorrhagic stroke and nonfatal hemorrhagic stroke than placebo group in the posthoc analysis of the SPARCL trial.
MOA — Inhibits 3-hydroxy-3-methyl-glutaryl-coenzyme A (HMG-CoA) reductase which converts HMG-CoA to mevalonate in cholesterol biosynthesis.
ADVERSE EFFECTS — Serious: Hepatotoxicity (rare), myopathy/rhabdomyolysis (rare). Frequent: Headache, dyspepsia.

CADUET (amlodipine + atorvastatin) ▶L ♀X ▶– $$$$
ADULTS — Simultaneous treatment of HTN and hypercholesterolemia: Establish dose using component drugs first. Dosing interval: Daily.
PEDS — Not approved in children.
FORMS — Trade only: Tabs, 2.5/10, 2.5/20, 2.5/40, 5/10, 5/20, 5/40, 5/80, 10/10, 10/20, 10/40, 10/80 mg.
MOA — See component drugs.
ADVERSE EFFECTS — See component drugs.

FLUVASTATIN (*Lescol, Lescol XL*) ▶L ♀X ▶– $$$
ADULTS — Hyperlipidemia: Start 20 mg PO at bedtime for LDL-C reduction of < 25%, 40 to 80 mg at bedtime for LDL-C reduction of 25% or more, max 80 mg/day, give 80 mg daily (Lescol XL) or 40 mg bid. Prevention of cardiac events post percutaneous coronary intervention: 80 mg of extended-release PO daily, max 80 mg daily.
PEDS — Hyperlipidemia: Start 20 mg PO at bedtime, max 80 mg daily (XL) or divided bid. See package insert for more information.
FORMS — Trade only: Caps 20, 40 mg. Tabs extended-release unscored 80 mg.
NOTES — Mainly metabolized by the CYP 2C9, so less potential for drug interactions. Increased risk of myopathy and rhabdomyolysis when used with a fibric acid agent, niacin, or colchicine.
MOA — Inhibits 3-hydroxy-3-methyl-glutaryl-coenzyme A (HMG-CoA) reductase which converts HMG-CoA to mevalonate in cholesterol biosynthesis.
ADVERSE EFFECTS — Serious: Hepatotoxicity (rare), myopathy/rhabdomyolysis (rare). Frequent: Headache, dyspepsia.

LOVASTATIN (*Mevacor, Altoprev*) ▶L ♀X ▶– $
ADULTS — Hyperlipidemia/prevention of cardiovascular events: Start 20 mg PO daily with the evening meal, increase at intervals of 4 weeks or more to max 80 mg/day (daily or divided bid). Altocor dosed daily with max dose 60 mg/day. With concomitant cyclosporine or danazol, start 10 mg PO daily, max 20 mg/day. Do not exceed 20 mg/day when used with fibrates or niacin at doses 1 g/day or greater; do not exceed 40 mg/day when used with amiodarone or verapamil.
PEDS — Hyperlipidemia, 10 yo or older: Start 10 mg PO q pm, max 40 mg/day. See package insert for more information.

(cont.)

LOVASTATIN (cont.)
  FORMS — Generic/Trade: Tabs unscored 20, 40 mg. Trade only: Tabs extended-release (Altoprev) 20, 40, 60 mg.
  NOTES — Do not use with potent inhibitors of CYP 3A4 enzyme system (clarithromycin, erythromycin, grapefruit juice > 1 quart/day, HIV protease inhibitors, itraconazole, ketoconazole, nefazodone, telithromycin); increases risk of myopathy. Measure LFTs if using 40 mg/day or more.
  MOA — Inhibits 3-hydroxy-3-methyl-glutaryl-coenzyme A (HMG-CoA) reductase which converts HMG-CoA to mevalonate in cholesterol biosynthesis.
  ADVERSE EFFECTS — Serious: Hepatotoxicity (rare), myopathy/rhabdomyolysis (rare). Frequent: Headache, dyspepsia.

PITAVASTATIN (*Livalo*) ▶L - ♀X ▶– $$$$
  ADULTS — Hyperlipidemia: Start 2 mg PO at bedtime, max 4 mg daily. Renal impairment (GFR 30-60 mL/min) or end stage renal disease receiving hemodialysis: Max start 1 mg PO daily, max 2 mg daily. Do not exceed 1 mg daily when used with erythromycin. Do not exceed 2 mg daily when used with rifampin.
  PEDS — Not approved in children.
  FORMS — Trade only: Tabs 1, 2, 4 mg.
  NOTES — Do not use with cyclosporine, protease inhibitor combination lopinavir/ritonavir, or with severe renal impairment (GFR < 30 mL/min) not on hemodialysis. Mainly metabolized by the cytochrome P450 isoenzyme 2C9, so less potential for drug interactions. Increased risk of myopathy and rhabdomyolysis when used with a fibric acid agent or niacin.
  MOA — Inhibits 3-hydroxy-3-methyl-glutaryl-coenzyme A (HMG-CoA) reductase which converts HMG-CoA to mevalonate in cholesterol biosynthesis.
  ADVERSE EFFECTS — Serious: Hepatotoxicity (rare), myopathy/rhabdomyolysis (rare). Frequent: Constipation, diarrhea, myalgia.

PRAVASTATIN (*Pravachol*) ▶L ♀X ▶– $$$
  ADULTS — Hyperlipidemia/prevention of cardiovascular events: Start 40 mg PO daily, increase at intervals of 4 weeks or more to max 80 mg/day. Renal or hepatic impairment: Start 10 mg PO daily.
  PEDS — Hyperlipidemia, 8 to 13 yo: 20 mg PO daily; 14 to 18 yo: 40 mg PO daily. See package insert for more information.
  FORMS — Generic/Trade: Tabs unscored 10, 20, 40, 80 mg. Generic only: Tabs 30 mg.
  NOTES — Not metabolized substantially by the CYP isoenzyme system, less potential for drug interactions. Increased risk of myopathy and rhabdomyolysis when used with a fibric acid agent.
  MOA — Inhibits 3-hydroxy-3-methyl-glutaryl-coenzyme A (HMG-CoA) reductase, which converts HMG-CoA to mevalonate in cholesterol biosynthesis.
  ADVERSE EFFECTS — Serious: Hepatotoxicity (rare), myopathy/rhabdomyolysis (rare). Frequent: Headache, dyspepsia.

ROSUVASTATIN (*Crestor*) ▶L ♀X ▶– $$$$
  ADULTS — Hyperlipidemia/slow progression of atherosclerosis/primary prevention of cardiovascular disease: Start 10 to 20 mg daily, may adjust dose after 2 to 4 weeks, max 40 mg/day. Do not start with 40 mg; use 40 mg only with severe hypercholesterolemia when treatment goal not achieved with 20 mg/day. With renal impairment (CrCl < 30 mL/min and not on hemodialysis) or protease inhibitor regimens that have ritonavir: Start 5 mg PO daily, max 10 mg/day. Asians: Start 5 mg PO daily. With cyclosporine: Max 5 mg/day. Avoid using with gemfibrozil; if used concomitantly, limit rosuvastatin dose to 10 mg/day.
  PEDS — Hyperlipidemia, 10 yo or older: Start 5 to 20 mg PO daily, max 20 mg/day. See package insert for more information. Canada only: May use with age older than 8 yo with homozygous familial hypercholesterolemia. Specialist should supervise use.
  UNAPPROVED ADULTS — Primary prevention of major cardiovascular events in patients with LDL-C ≤ 130 mg/dL and high-sensitivity CRP ≥ 2 mg/dL: 20 mg PO daily.
  FORMS — Trade only: Tabs unscored 5, 10, 20, 40 mg.
  NOTES — Give aluminum- and magnesium-containing antacids > 2 h after rosuvastatin. Potentiates effects of warfarin; monitor INR. Proteinuria, with unknown clinical significance, reported with 40 mg/day; consider dose reduction when using 40 mg/day with unexplained persistent proteinuria. Use caution with other drugs that may decrease levels/activity of endogenous steroid hormones (ketoconazole, spironolactone, and cimetidine). Temporarily withhold with acute, serious condition suggestive of myopathy or predisposing to renal failure from rhabdomyolysis (eg, sepsis, hypotension, dehydration, major surgery, trauma, severe metabolic/endocrine/electrolyte disorders, uncontrolled seizures). May take anytime during the day.
  MOA — Inhibits 3-hydroxy-3-methyl-glutaryl-coenzyme A (HMG-CoA) reductase which converts HMG-CoA to mevalonate in cholesterol biosynthesis.
  ADVERSE EFFECTS — Serious: Hepatotoxicity (rare), myopathy/rhabdomyolysis (rare). Frequent: Myalgia, constipation, nausea, asthenia, abdominal pain, proteinuria (transient), hematuria (transient).

SIMCOR (simvastatin + niacin) ▶LK ♀X ▶– $$$
  ADULTS — Hyperlipidemia: 1 tab PO at bedtime with a low-fat snack. If niacin-naive or switching from immediate-release niacin, start: 20/500 mg PO q pm. If receiving extended-release niacin, do not start with more than 40/2000 mg PO q pm. Max 40/2000 mg/day.
  PEDS — Not approved in children.
  FORMS — Trade only: Tabs, unscored extended-release simvastatin/niacin 20/500, 20/750, 20/1000 mg.
  NOTES — Do not exceed 40/2000 mg. Do not break, chew, or crush. Swallow whole. aspirin or NSAID 30 min prior may decrease niacin flushing reaction. Niacin may worsen glucose control, peptic ulcer disease, gout, headaches, and menopausal flushing. Significantly lowers LDL-C and triglycerides, raises

(cont.)

SIMCOR *(cont.)*
HDL-cholesterol. Do not use with potent inhibitors of CYP 3A4 enzyme system (clarithromycin, erythromycin, grapefruit juice > 1 quart/day, HIV protease inhibitors, itraconazole, ketoconazole, nefazodone, telithromycin); increases risk of myopathy. Do not use with cyclosporine, danazol, or fibrates. Do not exceed 20 mg/day of simvastatin component when used with amiodarone or verapamil. Do not exceed 40 mg/day of simvastatin component when used with diltiazem. May increase INR when added to warfarin.
MOA — See component drugs.
ADVERSE EFFECTS — See component drugs.

SIMVASTATIN *(Zocor)* ▶L ♀X ▶– $$$$
ADULTS — Hyperlipidemia: Start 20 to 40 mg PO q pm. Reduce cardiovascular mortality/events in high risk for coronary heart disease event (existing coronary heart disease, DM, peripheral vascular disease, history of CVA or cerebrovascular disease): 40 mg q pm. Increase prn at intervals of 4 weeks or more to max 80 mg/day. Severe renal impairment: Start 5 mg/day and closely monitor. Do not exceed 10 mg/day when used with gemfibrozil, cyclosporine, danazol; or 20 mg/day when used with amiodarone or verapamil; or 40 mg/day when used with diltiazem. For Chinese patients, do not use 80 mg/day with niacin 1 gram or more daily; use simvastatin less than 80 mg/day cautiously with niacin 1 gram or more daily.
PEDS — Hyperlipidemia, 10 yo or older: Start 10 mg PO q pm, max 40 mg/day. See package insert for more information.
FORMS — Generic/Trade: Tabs unscored 5, 10, 20, 40, 80 mg. Generic only: Tabs orally disintegrating 10, 20, 40, 80 mg.
NOTES — Do not use with potent inhibitors of CYP 3A4 enzyme system (clarithromycin, erythromycin, grapefruit juice > 1 quart/day, HIV protease inhibitors, itraconazole, ketoconazole, nefazodone, telithromycin); increases risk of myopathy. Use caution with fibrates, niacin at doses of 1 g/day or greater; increases risk of myopathy. There may be higher risk of muscle injury from the 80 mg dose compared to lower doses of simvastatin and possibly other statins.
MOA — Inhibits 3-hydroxy-3-methyl-glutaryl-coenzyme A (HMG-CoA) reductase which converts HMG-CoA to mevalonate in cholesterol biosynthesis.
ADVERSE EFFECTS — Serious: Hepatotoxicity, myopathy/rhabdomyolysis (rare). Frequent: Headache, dyspepsia.

VYTORIN (ezetimibe + simvastatin) ▶L ♀X ▶– $$$$
ADULTS — Hyperlipidemia: Start 10/20 mg PO q pm, max 10/80 mg/day. Start 10/40 if goal is > 55% LDL reduction.
PEDS — Not approved in children.
FORMS — Trade only: Tabs, unscored ezetimibe/simvastatin 10/10, 10/20, 10/40, 10/80 mg.
NOTES — Do not use with fibrates, clarithromycin, erythromycin, grapefruit juice > 1 quart/day, HIV protease inhibitors, itraconazole, ketoconazole, nefazodone, telithromycin; increases risk of myopathy. Do not exceed 10 mg/day when used with cyclosporine, danazol; or 20 mg/day when used with amiodarone or verapamil; or 40 mg/day when used with diltiazem; increased risk of myopathy. For Chinese patients, do not use 80 mg/day with niacin 1 g/day or more; use simvastatin < 80 mg/day cautiously with niacin 1 g/day or more. Use caution with niacin at doses 1 g/day or more; increases risk of myopathy. Give at least 2 h before or 4 h after colestipol or cholestyramine.
MOA — See component drugs.
ADVERSE EFFECTS — See component drugs.

CARDIOVASCULAR: Anti-Hyperlipidemic Agents—Other

BEZAFIBRATE (*✽Bezalip*) ▶K ♀D ▶– $$$
ADULTS — Canada only. Hyperlipidemia/hypertriglyceridemia: 200 mg of immediate-release PO bid to tid, or 400 mg of sustained-release PO q am or q evening with or after food. Reduce dose in renal insufficiency or dialysis. The 400 mg SR tab should not be used if CrCl < 60 mL/min or creatinine > 1.5 mg/dL.
PEDS — Not approved in children.
FORMS — Canada Trade only: Sustained-release tab 400 mg.
NOTES — Increased risk of myopathy and rhabdomyolysis when used with a statin. May increase serum creatinine level without changing estimated glomerular filtration rate (eGFR). May increase the effect of warfarin; reduce oral anticoagulant dose by 50%; monitor INR. Do not use in primary biliary cirrhosis. Take either at least 2 h before or 4 h after colestipol or cholestyramine.
MOA — Triglyceride reduction — Inhibits lipolysis, decreases FFA uptake, inhibits hepatic VLDL secretion HDL increase — unknown mechanism.
ADVERSE EFFECTS — Serious: Myopathy/rhabdomyolysis (rare), hepatotoxicity (rare), cholelithiasis (rare). Frequent: Epigastric distress, nausea, diarrhea, flatulence.

EZETIMIBE *(Zetia, ✽Ezetrol)* ▶L ♀C ▶? $$$$
WARNING — May increase cyclosporine levels.
ADULTS — Hyperlipidemia: 10 mg PO daily alone or in combination with statin or fenofibrate.
PEDS — Not approved in children.
UNAPPROVED PEDS — Hyperlipidemia, 10 yo or older: 10 mg PO daily coadministered with simvastatin.
FORMS — Trade only: Tabs, unscored 10 mg.
NOTES — Take either at least 2 h before or 4 h after colestipol or cholestyramine. Monitor cyclosporine levels (may increase). When used with statin, monitor LFTs at initiation and then per statin instructions.
MOA — Selectively inhibits small intestine cholesterol absorption. Decreases lipoproteins associated with high total cholesterol, LDL-C, APO B, and triglycerides.

(cont.)

ACE Inhibitor/Diuretic: *Accuretic, Capozide, Inhibace Plus, Lotensin HCT, Monopril HCT, Prinzide, Uniretic, Vaseretic, Zestoretic.*
ACE Inhibitor/Calcium Channel Blocker: *Lexxel, Lotrel, Tarka.*
Angiotensin Receptor Blocker/Diuretic: *Atacand HCT, Avalide, Benicar HCT, Diovan HCT, Hyzaar, Micardis HCT, Teveten HCT.*
Angiotensin Receptor Blocker/Calcium Channel Blocker: *Azor, Exforge, Twynsta.*
Angiotensin Receptor Blocker/Calcium Channel Blocker/Diuretic: *Exforge HCT, Tribenzor.*
Angiotensin Receptor Blocker/Direct renin inhibitor: *Valturna.*
Beta-blocker/Diuretic: *Corzide, Inderide, Lopressor HCT, Tenoretic, Ziac.*
Direct renin inhibitor/Calcium Channel Blocker: *Tekamlo*
Diuretic combinations: *Dyazide, Maxide, Moduretic.*
Diuretic/miscellaneous antihypertensive: *Aldactazide, Aldoril, Apresazide, Clorpres, Minizide, Tekturna HCT.*
Other: *BiDil.*

EZETIMIBE *(cont.)*
ADVERSE EFFECTS — Serious: Anaphylaxis, angioedema, cholelithiasis, cholecystitis, myopathy/rhabdomyolysis (rare), pancreatitis, thrombocytopenia. Frequent: Arthralgia, back pain, diarrhea, rash.

FENOFIBRATE (*TriCor, Antara, Lipofen, Triglide, ✦Lipidil Micro, Lipidil Supra, Lipidil EZ*) ▶LK ♀C ▶– $$$
ADULTS — Hypertriglyceridemia: Tricor tabs: Start 48 to 145 mg PO daily, max 145 mg/day. Antara: 43 to 130 mg PO daily; max 130 mg daily. Fenoglide: 40 to 120 mg PO daily; max 120 mg daily. Lipofen: 50 to 150 mg PO daily, max 150 mg daily. Lofibra: 54 to 200 mg PO daily, max 200 mg daily. Triglide: 50 to 160 mg PO daily, max 160 mg daily. Generic tabs: 54 to 160 mg, max 160 mg daily. Generic caps: 67 to 200 mg PO daily, max 200 mg daily. Hypercholesterolemia/mixed dyslipidemia: Tricor tabs: 145 mg PO daily. Antara: 130 mg PO daily. Fenoglide: 120 mg daily. Lipofen: 150 mg daily. Lofibra: 160 to 200 mg daily, max 200 mg daily. Triglide: 160 mg daily. Generic tabs: 160 mg daily. Generic caps: 200 mg PO daily. Renal impairment, elderly: Tricor tabs: Start 48 mg PO daily; Antara: Start 43 mg PO daily; Fenoglide: 40 mg daily/Lipofen: Start 50 mg daily; Triglide: Start 50 mg PO daily; generic tabs: Start 40 to 54 mg PO daily; generic caps 43 mg PO daily.
PEDS — Not approved in children.
FORMS — Generic only: Tabs unscored 54, 160 mg. Generic caps 67, 134, 200 mg. Trade only: Tabs (TriCor) unscored 48, 145 mg. Caps (Antara) 43, 130 mg. Tabs (Fenoglide) unscored 40, 120 mg. Tabs (Lipofen) unscored 50, 100, 150 mg. Tabs (Lofibra) unscored 54, 160 mg. Tabs (Triglide) unscored 50, 160 mg. Caps (Lofibra) 67, 134, 200 mg.
NOTES — All formulations, except Antara, Tricor, and Triglide, should be taken with food to increase plasma concentrations. Conversion between forms: Generic 200 mg cap with food = 145 mg Tricor; Antara 130 mg = 200 mg Lofibra or generic under low-fat fed conditions; Lipofen 150 mg with food = Tricor 160 mg with food. Monitor LFTs, dose-related hepatotoxicity. Increased risk of myopathy and rhabdomyolysis when used with a statin. May increase the effect of warfarin, monitor INR. Tricor 48 mg and 145 mg replaces Tricor 54 mg and 160 mg. Contraindicated with active liver disease, gall bladder disease, and/or CrCl < 30 mL/min. May increase serum creatinine level without changing estimated glomerular filtration rate (eGFR). Pulmonary embolus and deep vein thrombosis were observed at higher rates in the fenofibrate-treated group than the placebo-treated group in the FIELD trial.
MOA — Activates lipoprotein lipase and reduces apoprotein C-III leading to elimination of triglycerides.
ADVERSE EFFECTS — Serious: Tumor (rare), hepatotoxicity (rare), myopathy/rhabdomyolysis (rare), cholelithiasis (rare).

FENOFIBRIC ACID (*Fibricor, TriLipix*) ▶LK ♀C ▶– $$$
ADULTS — Mixed dyslipidemia and CHD or CHD risk equivalent in combination with optimal statin therapy: TriLipix: 135 mg PO daily. Hypertriglyceridemia: Fibricor: 35 to 105 mg PO daily, max 105 mg daily. TriLipix: 45 to 135 mg PO daily, max 135 mg daily. Hypercholesterolemia/mixed dyslipidemia: Fibricor: 105 mg PO daily. TriLipix: 135 mg PO daily. Renal impairment: Fibricor: 35 mg PO daily. TriLipix: 45 mg PO daily.
PEDS — Not approved in children.
FORMS — Trade only: Caps (TriLipix) delayed-release 45, 135 mg. Tabs (Fibricor) 35, 105 mg.
NOTES — Monitor LFTs, dose-related hepatotoxicity. Increased risk of myopathy and rhabdomyolysis when used with a statin. May increase the effect of warfarin, monitor INR. Contraindicated with active liver disease, gall bladder disease, and/or CrCl < 30 mL/min. May increase serum creatinine level without changing estimated glomerular filtration rate (eGFR). Pulmonary embolus and deep vein thrombosis were observed at higher rates in the fenofibrate-treated group than the placebo-treated group in the FIELD trial.

(cont.)

FENOFIBRIC ACID (cont.)
 MOA — Activates lipoprotein lipase and reduces apoprotein C-III leading to elimination of triglycerides.
 ADVERSE EFFECTS — Serious: Tumor (rare), hepatotoxicity (rare), myopathy/rhabdomyolysis (rare), cholelithiasis (rare).
GEMFIBROZIL (*Lopid*) ▶LK ♀C ▶? $$$
 ADULTS — <u>Hypertriglyceridemia/primary prevention of artery heart disease:</u> 600 mg PO bid 30 min before meals.
 PEDS — Not approved in children.
 FORMS — Generic/Trade: Tabs scored 600 mg.
 NOTES — Increased risk of myopathy and rhabdomyolysis when used with a statin or with moderate/severe renal dysfunction. May increase the effect of warfarin, monitor INR. Do not use with repaglinide; increases risk of hypoglycemia. Consider alternative therapy when baseline serum creatinine > 2 mg/dL; may worsen renal insufficiency. May increase serum creatinine level without changing estimated glomerular filtration rate (eGFR).
 MOA — Activates lipoprotein lipase and reduces apoprotein C-III leading to elimination of triglycerides.
 ADVERSE EFFECTS — Serious: Hepatotoxicity (rare), myopathy/rhabdomyolysis (rare), cholelithiasis (rare), angioedema. Frequent: Dyspepsia, abdominal pain, nausea, diarrhea, headache.

CARDIOVASCULAR: Antihypertensive Combinations

NOTE: Dosage should first be adjusted by using each drug separately. See component drugs for metabolism, pregnancy, and lactation.

***ACCURETIC* (quinapril + hydrochlorothiazide)** ▶See component drugs ♀See component drugs ▶See component drugs $$
 WARNING — Do not use in pregnancy.
 ADULTS — <u>HTN:</u> Establish dose using component drugs first. Dosing interval: Daily.
 PEDS — Not approved in children.
 FORMS — Generic/Trade: Tabs, 10/12.5, 20/12.5, 20/25 mg.
 MOA — See component drugs.
 ADVERSE EFFECTS — See component drugs.
***ALDACTAZIDE* (spironolactone + hydrochlorothiazide)** ▶See component drugs ♀See component drugs ▶See component drugs $$
 WARNING — Spironolactone is a tumorigen in rats. Use only for approved indications and only if necessary. Should not be used for initial therapy of edema or HTN; these conditions require individualized dosing. Treatment of HTN and edema should be reevaluated as patient's condition warrants.
 ADULTS — <u>HTN:</u> Establish dose using component drugs first. Dosing interval: Daily to bid.
 PEDS — Not approved in children.
 FORMS — Generic/Trade: Tabs, unscored 25/25. Trade only: Tabs, scored 50/50 mg.
 MOA — See component drugs.
 ADVERSE EFFECTS — See component drugs.
***ALDORIL* (methyldopa + hydrochlorothiazide)** ▶See component drugs ♀See component drugs ▶See component drugs $$
 WARNING — Titrate component drugs first to avoid hypotension.
 ADULTS — <u>HTN:</u> Establish dose using component drugs first. Dosing interval: bid.
 PEDS — Not approved in children.
 FORMS — Generic only: Tabs, unscored, 250/15, 250/25, 500/30 mg.
 MOA — See component drugs.
 ADVERSE EFFECTS — See component drugs.

***APRESAZIDE* (hydralazine + hydrochlorothiazide)** ▶See component drugs ♀See component drugs ▶See component drugs $$
 ADULTS — <u>HTN:</u> Establish dose using component drugs first. Dosing interval: bid.
 PEDS — Not approved in children.
 FORMS — Generic only: Caps 25/25, 50/50 mg.
 MOA — See component drugs.
 ADVERSE EFFECTS — See component drugs.
***ATACAND HCT* (candesartan + hydrochlorothiazide, ✦*Atacand Plus*)** ▶See component drugs ♀See component drugs ▶See component drugs $$$
 WARNING — Do not use in pregnancy.
 ADULTS — <u>HTN:</u> Establish dose using component drugs first. Dosing interval: Daily.
 PEDS — Not approved in children.
 FORMS — Trade only: Tabs, unscored 16/12.5, 32/12.5, 32/25 mg.
 MOA — See component drugs.
 ADVERSE EFFECTS — See component drugs.
***AVALIDE* (irbesartan + hydrochlorothiazide)** ▶See component drugs ♀See component drugs ▶See component drugs $$$
 WARNING — Do not use in pregnancy.
 ADULTS — <u>HTN:</u> Establish dose using component drugs first. Dosing interval: Daily. <u>HTN, initial therapy for patients needing multiple medications:</u> Start 150/12.5 PO daily, may increase after 1 to 2 weeks, max 300/25 daily.
 PEDS — Not approved in children.
 FORMS — Trade only: Tabs, unscored 150/12.5, 300/12.5, 300/25 mg.
 MOA — See component drugs.
 ADVERSE EFFECTS — See component drugs.
***AZOR* (amlodipine + olmesartan)** ▶See component drugs ♀See component drugs ▶See component drugs $$$
 WARNING — Do not use in pregnancy.
 ADULTS — <u>HTN:</u> Establish dose using component drugs first. Dosing interval: Daily. <u>HTN, initial</u>

(cont.)

AZOR (cont.)
therapy for patients needing multiple medications: Start 5/20 mg PO daily, may increase after 1 to 2 weeks, max 10/40 daily.
PEDS — Not approved in children.
FORMS — Trade only: Tabs, unscored 5/20, 5/40, 10/20, 10/40 mg.
MOA — See component drugs.
ADVERSE EFFECTS — See component drugs.

BENICAR HCT (olmesartan + hydrochlorothiazide) ▶See component drugs ♀See component drugs ▶See component drugs $$$$
WARNING — Do not use in pregnancy.
ADULTS — HTN: Establish dose using component drugs first. Dosing interval: Daily.
PEDS — Not approved in children.
FORMS — Trade only: Tabs, unscored 20/12.5, 40/12.5, 40/25 mg.
MOA — See component drugs.
ADVERSE EFFECTS — See component drugs.

CAPOZIDE (captopril + hydrochlorothiazide) ▶See component drugs ♀See component drugs ▶See component drugs $$
WARNING — Do not use in pregnancy.
ADULTS — HTN: Establish dose using component drugs first. Dosing interval: bid to tid.
PEDS — Not approved in children.
FORMS — Generic/Trade: Tabs, scored 25/15, 25/25, 50/15, 50/25 mg.
MOA — See component drugs.
ADVERSE EFFECTS — See component drugs.

CLORPRES (clonidine + chlorthalidone) ▶See component drugs ♀See component drugs ▶See component drugs $$$$
ADULTS — HTN: Establish dose using component drugs first. Dosing interval: bid to tid.
PEDS — Not approved in children.
FORMS — Trade only: Tabs, scored 0.1/15, 0.2/15, 0.3/15 mg.
MOA — See component drugs.
ADVERSE EFFECTS — See component drugs.

CORZIDE (nadolol + bendroflumethiazide) ▶See component drugs ♀See component drugs ▶See component drugs $$$
WARNING — Avoid abrupt cessation in ischemic heart disease or HTN; may exacerbate angina and MI. Warn patients against interruption or discontinuation without physician's advice.
ADULTS — HTN: Establish dose using component drugs first. Dosing interval: Daily.
PEDS — Not approved in children.
FORMS — Generic/Trade: Tabs 40/5, 80/5 mg.
MOA — See component drugs.
ADVERSE EFFECTS — See component drugs.

DIOVAN HCT (valsartan + hydrochlorothiazide) ▶See component drugs ♀See component drugs ▶See component drugs $$$
WARNING — Do not use in pregnancy.
ADULTS — HTN: Establish dose using component drugs first. Dosing interval: Daily. HTN, initial therapy for patients needing multiple medications: Start 160/12.5 mg PO daily, may increase after 1 to 2 weeks, max 320/25 daily.
PEDS — Not approved in children.
FORMS — Trade only: Tabs, unscored 80/12.5, 160/12.5, 320/12.5, 160/25, 320/25 mg.
MOA — See component drugs.
ADVERSE EFFECTS — See component drugs.

DYAZIDE (triamterene + hydrochlorothiazide) ▶See component drugs ♀See component drugs ▶See component drugs $
ADULTS — HTN: Establish dose using component drugs first. Dosing interval: Daily.
PEDS — Not approved in children.
FORMS — Generic/Trade: Caps, (Dyazide) 37.5/25 mg. Generic only: Caps, 50/25 mg.
NOTES — Dyazide 37.5/25 cap same combination as Maxzide-25 tab.
MOA — See component drugs.
ADVERSE EFFECTS — See component drugs.

EXFORGE (amlodipine + valsartan) ▶See component drugs ♀See component drugs ▶See component drugs $$$
WARNING — Do not use in pregnancy.
ADULTS — HTN: Establish dose using component drugs first. Dosing interval: Daily. HTN, initial therapy for patients needing multiple medications: Start 5/160 PO daily, may increase after 1 to 2 weeks, max 10/320 daily.
PEDS — Not approved in children.
FORMS — Trade only: Tabs, unscored 5/160, 5/320, 10/160, 10/320 mg.
MOA — See component drugs.
ADVERSE EFFECTS — See component drugs.

EXFORGE HCT (amlodipine + valsartan + hydrochlorothiazide) ▶See component drugs ♀See component drugs ▶See component drugs $$$
WARNING — Do not use in pregnancy.
ADULTS — HTN: Establish dose using component drugs first. Dosing interval: Daily.
PEDS — Not approved in children.
FORMS — Trade only: Tabs, unscored 5/160/12.5, 5/160/25, 10/160/12.5, 10/160/25, 10/320/25 mg.
MOA — See component drugs.
ADVERSE EFFECTS — See component drugs.

HYZAAR (losartan + hydrochlorothiazide) ▶See component drugs ♀See component drugs ▶See component drugs $$$
WARNING — Do not use in pregnancy.
ADULTS — HTN: Establish dose using component drugs first. Dosing interval: Daily. Severe HTN: Start 50/12.5 PO daily, may increase to 100/25 PO daily after 2 to 4 weeks. CVA risk reduction in HTN and LV hypertrophy (CVA risk reduction may not occur in patients of African descent): Establish dose using component drugs first. Dosing interval: Daily.
PEDS — Not approved in children.
FORMS — Generic/Trade: Tabs, unscored 50/12.5, 100/12.5, 100/25 mg.
MOA — See component drugs.
ADVERSE EFFECTS — See component drugs.

CARDIOVASCULAR: Antihypertensive Combinations

INDERIDE (propranolol + hydrochlorothiazide)
▶See component drugs ♀See component drugs ▶See component drugs $$
ADULTS — HTN: Establish dose using component drugs first. Dosing interval: Daily to bid.
PEDS — Not approved in children.
FORMS — Generic/Trade: Tabs, scored 40/25, 80/25 mg.
NOTES — Do not crush or chew cap contents. Swallow whole.
MOA — See component drugs.
ADVERSE EFFECTS — See component drugs.

INHIBACE PLUS (cilazapril + hydrochlorothiazide)
▶See component drugs ♀See component drugs ▶See component drugs $$
WARNING — Do not use in pregnancy.
ADULTS — Canada only, HTN: Establish dose using component drugs first. Dosing interval daily.
PEDS — Not approved in children.
FORMS — Trade: Tabs, scored 5 mg cilazapril + 12.5 mg HCTZ.
MOA — See component drugs.
ADVERSE EFFECTS — See component drugs.

LEXXEL (enalapril + felodipine) ▶See component drugs ♀See component drugs ▶See component drugs $$
WARNING — Do not use in pregnancy.
ADULTS — HTN: Establish dose using component drugs first. Dosing interval: Daily.
PEDS — Not approved in children.
FORMS — Trade only: Tabs, unscored 5/2.5, 5/5 mg.
NOTES — Do not crush or chew, swallow whole.
MOA — See component drugs.
ADVERSE EFFECTS — See component drugs.

LOPRESSOR HCT (metoprolol + hydrochlorothiazide)
▶See component drugs ♀See component drugs ▶See component drugs $$$
WARNING — Abrupt cessation may exacerbate angina pectoris and MI. Warn patients against interruption or discontinuation without physician's advice.
ADULTS — HTN: Establish dose using component drugs first. Dosing interval: Daily to bid.
PEDS — Not approved in children.
FORMS — Generic/Trade: Tabs, scored 50/25, 100/25, 100/50 mg.
MOA — See component drugs.
ADVERSE EFFECTS — See component drugs.

LOTENSIN HCT (benazepril + hydrochlorothiazide)
▶See component drugs ♀See component drugs ▶See component drugs $$
WARNING — Do not use in pregnancy.
ADULTS — HTN: Establish dose using component drugs first. Dosing interval: Daily.
PEDS — Not approved in children.
FORMS — Generic/Trade: Tabs, scored 5/6.25, 10/12.5, 20/12.5, 20/25 mg.
MOA — See component drugs.
ADVERSE EFFECTS — See component drugs.

LOTREL (amlodipine + benazepril) ▶See component drugs ♀See component drugs ▶See component drugs $$$

WARNING — Do not use in pregnancy.
ADULTS — HTN: Establish dose using component drugs first. Dosing interval: Daily.
PEDS — Not approved in children.
FORMS — Generic/Trade: Caps, 2.5/10, 5/10, 5/20, 10/20 mg. Trade only: Caps, 5/40, 10/40 mg.
MOA — See component drugs.
ADVERSE EFFECTS — See component drugs.

MAXZIDE (triamterene + hydrochlorothiazide, ✦Triazide)
▶See component drugs ♀See component drugs ▶See component drugs $
ADULTS — HTN: Establish dose using component drugs first. Dosing interval: Daily.
PEDS — Not approved in children.
FORMS — Generic/Trade: Tabs, scored 75/50 mg.
MOA — See component drugs.
ADVERSE EFFECTS — See component drugs.

MAXZIDE-25 (triamterene + hydrochlorothiazide)
▶See component drugs ♀See component drugs ▶See component drugs $
ADULTS — HTN: Establish dose using component drugs first. Dosing interval: Daily.
PEDS — Not approved in children.
FORMS — Generic/Trade: Tabs, scored 37.5/25 mg
MOA — See component drugs.
ADVERSE EFFECTS — See component drugs.

MICARDIS HCT (telmisartan + hydrochlorothiazide, ✦Micardis Plus) ▶See component drugs ♀See component drugs ▶See component drugs $$$
WARNING — Do not use in pregnancy.
ADULTS — HTN: Establish dose using component drugs first. Dosing interval: Daily.
PEDS — Not approved in children.
FORMS — Trade only: Tabs, unscored 40/12.5, 80/12.5, 80/25 mg.
NOTES — Swallow tabs whole, do not break or crush. Caution in hepatic insufficiency.
MOA — See component drugs.
ADVERSE EFFECTS — See component drugs.

MINIZIDE (prazosin + polythiazide) ▶See component drugs ♀See component drugs ▶See component drugs $$$
ADULTS — HTN: Establish dose using component drugs first. Dosing interval: bid to tid.
PEDS — Not approved in children.
FORMS — Trade only: Caps, 1/0.5, 2/0.5, 5/0.5 mg.
MOA — See component drugs.
ADVERSE EFFECTS — See component drugs.

MODURETIC (amiloride + hydrochlorothiazide ✦Moduret) ▶See component drugs ♀See component drugs ▶See component drugs $
ADULTS — HTN: Establish dose using component drugs first. Dosing interval: Daily.
PEDS — Not approved in children.
FORMS — Generic only: Tabs, scored 5/50 mg.
MOA — See component drugs.
ADVERSE EFFECTS — See component drugs.

MONOPRIL HCT (fosinopril + hydrochlorothiazide)
▶See component drugs ♀See component drugs ▶See component drugs $$
WARNING — Do not use in pregnancy.

(cont.)

CARDIOVASCULAR: Antihypertensive Combinations

MONOPRIL HCT *(cont.)*
ADULTS — <u>HTN:</u> Establish dose using component drugs first. Dosing interval: Daily.
PEDS — Not approved in children.
FORMS — Generic/Trade: Tabs, unscored 10/12.5, scored 20/12.5 mg.
MOA — See component drugs.
ADVERSE EFFECTS — See component drugs.

PRINZIDE (lisinopril + hydrochlorothiazide) ▶See component drugs ♀See component drugs ▶See component drugs $$
WARNING — Do not use in pregnancy.
ADULTS — <u>HTN:</u> Establish dose using component drugs first. Dosing interval: Daily.
PEDS — Not approved in children.
FORMS — Generic/Trade: Tabs, unscored 10/12.5, 20/12.5, 20/25 mg.
MOA — See component drugs.
ADVERSE EFFECTS — See component drugs.

TARKA (trandolapril + verapamil) ▶See component drugs ♀See component drugs ▶See component drugs $$$
WARNING — Do not use in pregnancy.
ADULTS — <u>HTN:</u> Establish dose using component drugs first. Dosing interval: Daily.
PEDS — Not approved in children.
FORMS — Trade only: Tabs, unscored 2/180, 1/240, 2/240, 4/240 mg.
NOTES — Contains extended-release form of verapamil. Do not chew or crush, swallow whole. Hypotension, bradyarrhythmias, and lactic acidosis have occurred in patients receiving concurrent erythromycin or clarithromycin.
MOA — See component drugs.
ADVERSE EFFECTS — See component drugs.

TEKTURNA HCT (aliskiren + hydrochlorothiazide)
▶See component drugs ♀See component drugs ▶See component drugs $$$
WARNING — Avoid in pregnancy.
ADULTS — <u>HTN:</u> Establish dose using component drugs first. Dosing interval: Daily. <u>HTN, initial therapy for patients needing multiple medications:</u> Start 150/12.5 PO daily, may increase after 1 to 2 weeks, max 300/25 daily.
PEDS — Not approved in children.
FORMS — Trade only: Tabs, unscored 150/12.5, 150/25, 300/12.5, 300/25 mg.
MOA — See component drugs.
ADVERSE EFFECTS — See component drugs.

TENORETIC (atenolol + chlorthalidone) ▶See component drugs ♀See component drugs ▶See component drugs $
WARNING — Avoid abrupt cessation in coronary heart disease or HTN.
ADULTS — <u>HTN:</u> Establish dose using component drugs first. Dosing interval: Daily.
PEDS — Not approved in children.
FORMS — Generic/Trade: Tabs, scored 50/25, unscored 100/25 mg.
MOA — See component drugs.
ADVERSE EFFECTS — See component drugs.

TEVETEN HCT (eprosartan + hydrochlorothiazide)
▶See component drugs ♀See component drugs ▶See component drugs $$$
WARNING — Do not use in pregnancy.
ADULTS — <u>HTN:</u> Establish dose using component drugs first. Dosing interval: Daily.
PEDS — Not approved in children.
FORMS — Trade only: Tabs, unscored 600/12.5, 600/25 mg.
MOA — See component drugs.
ADVERSE EFFECTS — See component drugs.

TRIBENZOR (amlodipine + olmesartan + hydrochlorothiazide) ▶See component drugs - ♀D ▶- $$$$
WARNING — Do not use in pregnancy.
ADULTS — Establish dose using component drugs first. Dosing interval: Daily. May increase after 2 weeks, max 10/40/25 mg daily.
PEDS — Not approved in children.
FORMS — Trade only: Tabs, unscored 5/20/12.5, 5/40/12.5, 5/40/25, 10/40/12.5, 10/40/25 mg.
MOA — See component drugs.
ADVERSE EFFECTS — See component drugs.

TWYNSTA (amlodipine + telmisartan) ▶See component drugs $$$$
WARNING — Do not use in pregnancy.
ADULTS — <u>HTN:</u> Establish dose using component drugs first. Dosing interval: Daily. <u>HTN, initial therapy for patients needing multiple medications:</u> Start 5/40 to 5/80 mg PO daily, may increase after 2 weeks, max 10/80 mg daily. Do not use as initial therapy in patients 75 yo or older or with hepatic impairment.
PEDS — Not approved in children.
FORMS — Trade only: Tabs, unscored 5/40, 5/80, 10/40, 10/80 mg.
MOA — See component drugs.
ADVERSE EFFECTS — See component drugs.

UNIRETIC (moexipril + hydrochlorothiazide) ▶See component drugs ♀See component drugs ▶See component drugs $$
WARNING — Do not use in pregnancy.
ADULTS — <u>HTN:</u> Establish dose using component drugs first. Dosing interval: Daily to bid.
PEDS — Not approved in children.
FORMS — Generic/Trade: Tabs, scored 7.5/12.5, 15/12.5, 15/25 mg.
MOA — See component drugs.
ADVERSE EFFECTS — See component drugs.

VALTURNA (aliskiren + valsartan) ▶See component drugs - ♀D ▶- $$$$
WARNING — Do not use in pregnancy.
ADULTS — <u>HTN:</u> Establish dose using component drugs first. Dosing interval: Daily. <u>HTN, initial therapy for patients needing multiple medications or add-on therapy:</u> Start 150/160 mg PO daily, may increase after 2 weeks, max 300/320 mg daily.
PEDS — Not approved in children.
FORMS — Trade only: Tabs, unscored 150/160, 300/320 mg.
MOA — See component drugs.
ADVERSE EFFECTS — See component drugs.

CARDIOVASCULAR: Antihypertensives

VASERETIC (enalapril + hydrochlorothiazide) ▶See component drugs ♀See component drugs ▶See component drugs $$
WARNING – Do not use in pregnancy.
ADULTS – <u>HTN:</u> Establish dose using component drugs first. Dosing interval: Daily to bid.
PEDS – Not approved in children.
FORMS – Generic/Trade: Tabs, unscored 5/12.5, 10/25 mg.
MOA – See component drugs.
ADVERSE EFFECTS – See component drugs.

ZESTORETIC (lisinopril + hydrochlorothiazide) ▶See component drugs ♀See component drugs ▶See component drugs $$
WARNING – Do not use in pregnancy.
ADULTS – <u>HTN:</u> Establish dose using component drugs first. Dosing interval: Daily.
PEDS – Not approved in children.
FORMS – Generic/Trade: Tabs, unscored 10/12.5, 20/12.5, 20/25 mg.
MOA – See component drugs.
ADVERSE EFFECTS – See component drugs.

ZIAC (bisoprolol + hydrochlorothiazide) ▶See component drugs ♀See component drugs ▶See component drugs $$
WARNING – Avoid abrupt cessation.
ADULTS – <u>HTN:</u> Establish dose using component drugs first. Dosing interval: Daily.
PEDS – Not approved in children.
FORMS – Generic/Trade: Tabs, unscored 2.5/6.25, 5/6.25, 10/6.25 mg.
MOA – See component drugs.
ADVERSE EFFECTS – See component drugs.

CARDIOVASCULAR: Antihypertensives—Other

ALISKIREN (*Tekturna*) ▶LK ♀– ▶–? $$$
WARNING – Avoid in pregnancy.
ADULTS – <u>HTN:</u> 150 mg PO daily, max 300 mg/day.
PEDS – Not approved in children.
FORMS – Trade only: Tabs unscored 150, 300 mg.
NOTES – Not studied with severe renal impairment (creat 1.7 mg/dL or higher for women, 2.0 mg/dL or higher for men, and/or estimated GFR < 30 mL/min). Best absorbed on empty stomach. High-fat meals decrease absorption. May decrease effects of furosemide. Monitor potassium and renal function when given with related medications (ie, ACE inhibitors, ARBs). May increase creatine kinase, uric acid levels. Do not use with cyclosporine. Coadministration with potent P-glycoprotein inhibitors (ketoconazole or atorvastatin) increase aliskiren levels.
MOA – Direct renin inhibitor.
ADVERSE EFFECTS – Serious: Angioedema, hypotension, seizures. Frequent: Diarrhea, cough, dyspepsia, rash, GERD.

FENOLDOPAM (*Corlopam*) ▶LK ♀B ▶? $$$
ADULTS – <u>Severe HTN:</u> Dilute 10 mg in 250 mL D5W (40 mcg/mL), rate at 11 mL/h delivers 0.1 mcg/kg/min for 70 kg adult, titrate q 15 min, usual effective dose 0.1 to 1.6 mcg/kg/min. Lower initial doses (0.03 to 0.1 mcg/kg/min) associated with less reflex tachycardia.
PEDS – <u>Reduce BP:</u> Start 0.2 mcg/kg/min, increase by up to 0.3 to 0.5 mcg/kg/min q 20 to 30 min. Max infusion 0.8 mcg/kg/min. Administer in hospital by continuous infusion pump; use max 4 h; monitor BP and HR continuously. Refer to package insert for dilution instructions and infusion rates.
UNAPPROVED ADULTS – <u>Prevention of contrast nephropathy in those at risk</u> (conflicting evidence of efficacy): Start 0.03 mcg/kg/min infusion 60 min prior to dye. Titrate infusion q 15 min up to 0.1 mcg/kg/min if BP tolerates. Maintain infusion (with concurrent saline) up to 4 to 6 h after procedure.
NOTES – Avoid combined use with beta-blockers; if must be done, watch for sudden hypotension. Patients at high-risk for contrast nephropathy include age older than 70 yo, creatinine > 1.5 mg/dL, HTN, DM, heart failure. Use cautiously with glaucoma or increased intraocular HTN. Concurrent acetaminophen may increase fenoldopam levels.
MOA – Stimulates dopamine-1 receptors and alpha-2 receptors causing vasodilation.
ADVERSE EFFECTS – Serious: Hypotension, tachycardia, hypokalemia (rare). Frequent: Headache, flushing, nausea.

HYDRALAZINE (*Apresoline*) ▶LK ♀C ▶+ $
ADULTS – <u>HTN:</u> Start 10 mg PO bid to qid for 2 to 4 days, increase to 25 mg bid to qid, then 50 mg bid to qid if necessary, max 300 mg/day. <u>Hypertensive emergency:</u> 10 to 50 mg IM or 10 to 20 mg IV. Use lower doses initially and repeat prn to control BP. <u>Preeclampsia/eclampsia:</u> 5 to 10 mg IV initially, followed by 5 to 10 mg IV every 20 to 30 min prn to control BP.
PEDS – Not approved in children.
UNAPPROVED ADULTS – <u>Heart failure:</u> Start 10 to 25 mg PO tid, target dose 75 mg tid, max 100 mg tid. Use in combination with isosorbide dinitrate for patients intolerant to ACE inhibitors.
UNAPPROVED PEDS – <u>HTN:</u> Start 0.75 to 1 mg/kg/day PO divided bid to qid, increase slowly over 3 to 4 weeks up to 7.5 mg/kg/day; initial IV dose 1.7 to 3.5 mg/kg/day divided in 4 to 6 doses. <u>HTN urgency:</u> 0.1 to 0.2 mg/kg IM/IV q 4 to 6 h prn. Max single dose, 25 mg PO and 20 mg IV.
FORMS – Generic only: Tabs unscored 10, 25, 50, 100 mg.
NOTES – Headache, nausea, dizziness, tachycardia, peripheral edema, systemic lupus erythematosus-like syndrome. Usually used in combination with diuretic and beta-blocker to counter side effects.
MOA – Relaxes peripheral arterial smooth muscle (vasodilation).

(cont.)

CARDIOVASCULAR: Antihypertensives

HYDRALAZINE (cont.)
ADVERSE EFFECTS – Serious: SLE, angina exacerbation, rash. Frequent: Tachycardia, headache, edema.

MECAMYLAMINE (Inversine) ▶K ♀C ▶– $$$$$
ADULTS – Severe HTN: Start 2.5 mg PO bid, increase as needed by 2.5 mg increments no sooner than every 2 days, usual maintenance dose 25 mg/day divided bid to qid.
PEDS – Not approved in children.
FORMS – Trade only: Tabs, scored, 2.5 mg.
NOTES – Orthostatic hypotension, especially during dosage titration. Monitor BP standing and supine. Rebound, severe HTN with sudden drug withdrawal. Discontinue slowly and use other antihypertensives.
MOA – Inhibits acetylcholine at the autonomic ganglia and blocks central nicotinic cholinergic receptors.
ADVERSE EFFECTS – Serious: Syncope, rebound hypertension, ileus, tremors (rare), choreiform movements (rare). Frequent: Postural hypotension, dizziness, sedation, dry mouth, anorexia, N/V, diarrhea, constipation, urinary retention, impotence.

METYROSINE (Demser) ▶K ♀C ▶? $$$$$
ADULTS – Pheochromocytoma: Start 250 mg PO qid, increase by 250 to 500 mg/day prn, max dose 4 g/day.
PEDS – Pheochromocytoma age older than 12 yo: Use adult dosage.
FORMS – Trade only: Caps, 250 mg.
MOA – Inhibits tyrosine hydroxylase which is necessary in the biosynthesis of catecholamines.
ADVERSE EFFECTS – Serious: Crystalluria (rare). Frequent: Sedation, drooling, speech difficulty, tremor, disorientation, diarrhea.

MINOXIDIL (Loniten) ▶K ♀C ▶+ $$
WARNING – Potent vasodilator; may produce serious complications from hypotension and reflex tachycardia. Initiate in hospital; patient should remain in hospital until excessive orthostasis is minimized. Relatively contraindicated in patients with cardiac disease (ie, recent/acute MI, CAD, angina). May increase pulmonary artery pressure; relatively contraindicated with chronic congestive heart failure not secondary to hypertension. Has been associated with development of pericardial effusion and tamponade; more likely to occur in patients with renal disease.
ADULTS – Refractory HTN: Start 2.5 to 5 mg PO daily, increase at no less than 3 days intervals, usual dose 10 to 40 mg daily, max 100 mg/day.
PEDS – Not approved in children younger than 12 yo.
UNAPPROVED PEDS – HTN: Start 0.2 mg/kg PO daily, increase every 3 days prn up to 0.25 to 1 mg/kg/day daily or divided bid; max 50 mg/day.
FORMS – Generic only: Tabs, scored 2.5, 10 mg.
NOTES – Edema, wt gain, hypertrichosis, may exacerbate heart failure. Usually used in combination with a diuretic and a beta-blocker to counteract side effects.
MOA – Relaxes peripheral arterial smooth muscle (vasodilation).
ADVERSE EFFECTS – Serious: Pericardial effusion (rare), angina exacerbation. Frequent: Tachycardia, headache, edema, hair growth.

NITROPRUSSIDE (Nitropress) ▶RBCs ♀C ▶– $
WARNING – May cause significant hypotension. Reconstituted soln must be further diluted before use. Cyanide toxicity may occur, especially with high infusion rates (10 mcg/kg/min), hepatic/renal impairment, and prolonged infusions (longer than 3 to 7 days). Protect from light.
ADULTS – Hypertensive emergency: 50 mg in 250 mL D5W (200 mcg/mL), start at 0.3 mcg/kg/min (for 70 kg adult = 6 mL/h) via IV infusion, titrate slowly, usual range 0.3 to 10 mcg/kg/min, max 10 mcg/kg/min.
PEDS – Severe HTN: Use adult dosage.
NOTES – Discontinue if inadequate response to 10 mcg/kg/min after 10 min. Cyanide toxicity with high doses, hepatic/renal impairment, and prolonged infusions, check thiocyanate levels. Protect IV infusion minibag from light.
MOA – Relaxes peripheral arterial and venous smooth muscle.
ADVERSE EFFECTS – Serious: Cyanide toxicity (rare), thiocyanate toxicity (rare), methemoglobinemia (rare), severe hypotension. Frequent: N/V, sweating, flushing, weakness.

PHENOXYBENZAMINE (Dibenzyline) ▶KL ♀C ▶? $$$$$
ADULTS – Pheochromocytoma: Start 10 mg PO bid, increase slowly every other day as needed, usual dose 20 to 40 mg bid to tid, max 120 mg/day.
PEDS – Not approved in children.
UNAPPROVED PEDS – Pheochromocytoma: 0.2 mg/kg/day PO daily, initial dose no more than 10 mg, increase slowly every other day as needed, usual dose 0.4 to 1.2 mg/kg/day.
FORMS – Trade only: Caps, 10 mg.
NOTES – Patients should be observed after each dosage increase for symptomatic hypotension and other adverse effects. Do not use for essential HTN.
MOA – Blocks binding of catecholamines to pre-synaptic and postsynaptic alpha receptors.
ADVERSE EFFECTS – Serious: Hypotension. Frequent: Dizziness, nasal congestion, tachycardia, miosis.

PHENTOLAMINE (Regitine, Rogitine) ▶Plasma ♀C ▶? $$$
ADULTS – Diagnosis of pheochromocytoma: 5 mg IV/IM. Rapid IV administration is preferred. An immediate, marked decrease in BP should occur, typically, 60 mmHg SBP and 25 mmHg DBP decrease in 2 min. HTN during pheochromocytoma surgery: 5 mg IV/IM 1 to 2 h preop, 5 mg IV during surgery prn.
PEDS – Diagnosis of pheochromocytoma: 0.05 to 0.1 mg/kg IV/IM, up to 5 mg/dose. Rapid IV administration is preferred. An immediate, marked decrease in BP should occur, typically, 60 mmHg SBP and 25 mmHg DBP decrease in 2 min. HTN during pheochromocytoma surgery: 0.05 to 0.1 mg/kg IV/IM 1 to 2 h preop, repeat q 2 to 4 h prn.

(cont.)

PHENTOLAMINE (cont.)
UNAPPROVED ADULTS — IV extravasation of catecholamines: 5 to 10 mg in 10 mL NS, inject 1 to 5 mL SC (in divided doses) around extravasation site. Hypertensive crisis: 5 to 15 mg IV.
UNAPPROVED PEDS — IV extravasation of catecholamines: Neonates, 2.5 to 5 mg in 10 mL NS, inject 1 mL SC (in divided doses) around extravasation site; children, Use adult dosage.
NOTES — Weakness, flushing, hypotension; priapism with intracavernous injection. Use within 12 h of extravasation. Distributed to hospital pharmacies, at no charge, only for use in life-threatening situations. Call (888) 669-6682 for ordering.
MOA — Blocks binding of catecholamines to presynaptic and postsynaptic alpha receptors.
ADVERSE EFFECTS — Serious: Hypotension, tachycardia, arrhythmias. Frequent: Weakness, dizziness, flushing, nasal congestion.

CARDIOVASCULAR: Antiplatelet Drugs

ABCIXIMAB (*ReoPro*) ▶Plasma ♀C ▶? $$$$$
ADULTS — Platelet aggregation inhibition, prevention of acute cardiac ischemic events associated with PTCA: 0.25 mg/kg IV bolus over 1 min via separate infusion line 10 to 60 min before procedure, then 0.125 mcg/kg/min up to 10 mcg/min infusion for 12 h. Unstable angina not responding to standard therapy when percutaneous coronary intervention (PCI) is planned within 24 h: 0.25 mg/kg IV bolus over 1 min via separate infusion line, followed by 10 mcg/min IV infusion for 18 to 24 h, concluding 1 h after PCI.
PEDS — Not approved in children.
NOTES — Thrombocytopenia possible. Discontinue abciximab, heparin, and aspirin if uncontrollable bleeding occurs.
MOA — Inhibits platelet aggregation by blocking the effects of fibrinogen and other substances at platelet glycoprotein IIb/IIIa receptors.
ADVERSE EFFECTS — Serious: Bleeding, hypersensitivity (rare), thrombocytopenia (rare). Frequent: Pain.

AGGRENOX (acetylsalicylic acid + dipyridamole) ▶LK ♀D ▶? $$$$
ADULTS — Prevention of CVA after TIA/CVA: 1 cap PO bid.
PEDS — Not approved in children.
FORMS — Trade only: Caps, 25 mg aspirin/200 mg extended-release dipyridamole.
NOTES — Do not crush or chew Caps. May need supplemental aspirin for prevention of MI.
MOA — See component drugs.
ADVERSE EFFECTS — See component drugs.

CLOPIDOGREL (*Plavix*) ▶LK ♀B ▶? $$$$
WARNING — Requires activation to an active metabolite by the CYP system, mainly CYP2C19. When treated at recommended doses, poor metabolizers have higher cardiovascular event rates after acute coronary syndrome or percutaneous coronary intervention than patients with normal CYP2C19 function. Tests to determine a patient's CYP2C19 genotype may aid in determining therapeutic strategy. Consider alternative treatment or treatment strategies in patients identified as CYP2C19 poor metabolizers.
ADULTS — Reduction of thrombotic events after recent acute MI, recent CVA, established peripheral arterial disease: 75 mg PO daily. Non-ST segment elevation acute coronary syndrome: 300 mg loading dose, then 75 mg PO daily in combination with aspirin PO daily. ST segment elevation MI: Start with/without 300 mg loading dose, then 75 mg PO daily in combination with aspirin, with/without thrombolytic.
PEDS — Not approved in children.
UNAPPROVED ADULTS — Medical treatment, without stent, of unstable angina/non-ST segment elevation MI: 300 to 600 mg loading dose, then 75 mg daily in combination with aspirin for at least 1 month and up to 1 year. Medical treatment, without stent and with/without thrombolytics, of ST segment elevation MI: 300 mg loading dose, then 75 mg daily in combination with aspirin for at least 14 days and up to 1 year. Before/when percutaneous coronary intervention performed: 600 mg; consider using 300 mg if patient received thrombolytic within 12 to 24 h. Post bare metal stent placement or post drug eluting stent placement: 75 mg daily in combination with aspirin for at least 1 year (in patients not at high risk for bleeding). Post percutaneous coronary brachytherapy: 75 mg daily in combination with aspirin indefinitely. Acute coronary syndrome with aspirin allergy or reduction of thrombotic events in high-risk patient after TIA: 75 mg PO daily.
FORMS — Trade: Tabs unscored 75, 300 mg.
NOTES — Effectiveness is reduced with impaired CYP2C19 function; avoid drugs that inhibit CYP2C19 (eg, omeprazole, esomeprazole, cimetidine, etravirine, felbamate, fluconazole, fluoxetine, fluvoxamine, ketoconazole, voriconazole). Contraindicated with active pathologic bleeding (peptic ulcer or intracranial bleed). Prolongs bleeding time. Discontinue use 5 days before elective surgery, except in first year post coronary stent implantation; premature discontinuation increases risk of cardiovascular events. Concomitant aspirin increases bleeding risk. Cardiovascular (but not CVA) patients may receive additional benefit when given with aspirin. Should not be used with aspirin for primary prevention of cardiovascular events.
MOA — Inhibits platelet aggregation by blocking the effects of adenosine diphosphate at its platelet receptor.
ADVERSE EFFECTS — Serious: Acute liver failure, anaphylaxis, angioedema, aplastic anemia, agranulocytosis, bleeding, pancreatitis, thrombocytopenia (rare),

(cont.)

CARDIOVASCULAR: Antiplatelet Drugs

CLOPIDOGREL (cont.)
Stevens-Johnson syndrome. Frequent: Pruritus, purpura, diarrhea, rash.

DIPYRIDAMOLE (*Persantine*) ▶L ♀B ▶? $$$
ADULTS — <u>Prevention of thromboembolic complications of cardiac valve replacement:</u> 75 to 100 mg PO qid in combination with warfarin.
PEDS — Not approved in children younger than 12 yo.
UNAPPROVED ADULTS — <u>Platelet aggregation inhibition:</u> 150 to 400 mg/day PO divided tid to qid.
FORMS — Generic/Trade: Tabs unscored 25, 50, 75 mg.
NOTES — Not effective for angina; may cause chest pain when used in CAD.
MOA — Inhibits platelet adhesion by inhibiting phosphodiesterase. Increases coronary blood flow by selective dilation of the coronary arteries.
ADVERSE EFFECTS — Serious: Angioedema, bronchospasm, thrombocytopenia. Frequent: Headache, dizziness, abdominal discomfort, perioperative bleeding (rare).

EPTIFIBATIDE (*Integrilin*) ▶K ♀B ▶? $$$$$
ADULTS — <u>Acute coronary syndrome</u> (unstable angina/non-ST segment elevation MI): Load 180 mcg/kg IV bolus, then IV infusion 2 mcg/kg/min for up to 72 h. If percutaneous coronary intervention (PCI) occurs during the infusion, continue infusion for 18 to 24 h after procedure. <u>PCI:</u> Load 180 mcg/kg IV bolus just before procedure, followed by infusion 2 mcg/kg/min and a second 180 mcg/kg IV bolus 10 min after the first bolus. Continue infusion for up to 18 to 24 h (minimum 12 h) after the procedure. <u>Renal impairment</u> (CrCl < 50 mL/min): No change in bolus dose; decrease infusion to 1 mcg/kg/min. For obese patient (greater than 121 kg): max bolus dose 22.6 mg; max infusion rate 15 mg/h. <u>Renal impairment and obese:</u> max bolus dose 22.6 mg; max infusion rate 7.5 mg/h.
PEDS — Not approved in children.
NOTES — Discontinue infusion prior to CABG. Thrombocytopenia possible. Concomitant aspirin and heparin/enoxaparin use recommended, unless contraindicated. Contraindicated in dialysis patients.
MOA — Inhibits platelet aggregation by blocking the effects of fibrinogen and other substances at platelet glycoprotein IIb/IIIa receptors.
ADVERSE EFFECTS — Serious: Bleeding, thrombocytopenia (rare). Frequent: Pain.

PRASUGREL (*Effient*) ▶LK ♀B ▶? $$$$
WARNING — May cause significant, fatal bleeding. Do not use with active bleeding or history of TIA or CVA. Generally not recommend for patients 75 yo and older. Do not start in patients likely to need urgent CABG. When possible, discontinue 7 days prior to any surgery. Risk factors for bleeding: Body wt less than 60 kg, propensity to bleed, concomitant medications that increase bleeding risk. Suspect bleeding with hypotension and recent coronary angiography, PCI, CABG, or other surgical procedure. Premature discontinuation increases risk of stent thrombosis, MI, and death.
ADULTS — <u>Reduction of thrombotic events, including stent thrombosis, after acute coronary syndrome managed with percutaneous coronary intervention (PCI):</u> 60 mg loading dose, then 10 mg PO daily in combination with aspirin. Patients wt less than 60 kg consider lowering maintenance dose to 5 mg PO daily.
PEDS — Not approved in children.
FORMS — Trade: Tabs unscored 5, 10 mg.
NOTES — Concomitant warfarin or NSAID increases bleeding risk.
MOA — Inhibits platelet activation and aggregation by blocking the effects of adenosine diphosphate at its platelet receptor.
ADVERSE EFFECTS — Serious: Bleeding.

TICLOPIDINE (*Ticlid*) ▶L ♀B ▶? $$$$
WARNING — May cause life-threatening neutropenia, agranulocytosis, and thrombotic thrombocytopenia purpura (TTP). During first 3 months of treatment, monitor patient clinically and hematologically for neutropenia or TTP; discontinue if evidence is seen.
ADULTS — Due to adverse effects, clopidogrel preferred. <u>Platelet aggregation inhibition/reduction of thrombotic CVA:</u> 250 mg PO bid with food. <u>Prevention of cardiac stent occlusion:</u> 250 mg PO bid in combo with aspirin 325 mg PO daily for up to 30 days post stent implantation.
PEDS — Not approved in children.
UNAPPROVED ADULTS — <u>Prevention of graft occlusion with CABG:</u> 250 mg PO bid.
FORMS — Generic/Trade: Tabs unscored 250 mg.
NOTES — Check CBC every 2 weeks during the first 3 months of therapy. Neutrophil counts usually return to normal within 1 to 3 weeks following discontinuation. Loading dose 500 mg PO on day 1 may be used for prevention of cardiac stent occlusion.
MOA — Inhibits platelet aggregation by blocking the effects of adenosine diphosphate at its platelet receptor.
ADVERSE EFFECTS — Serious: Bleeding, thrombocytopenia (rare), neutropenia (rare). Frequent: Diarrhea, nausea, dyspepsia.

TIROFIBAN (*Aggrastat*) ▶K ♀B ▶? $$$$$
ADULTS — <u>Acute coronary syndromes</u> (unstable angina and non-Q-wave MI): Start 0.4 mcg/kg/min IV infusion for 30 min, then decrease to 0.1 mcg/kg/min for 48 to 108 h or until 12 to 24 h after coronary intervention.
PEDS — Not approved in children.
NOTES — Thrombocytopenia possible. Concomitant aspirin and heparin/enoxaparin use recommended, unless contraindicated. Dose heparin to keep PTT 2 times normal. Decrease bolus dose and rate of infusion by 50% in patients with CrCl < 30 mL/min. Dilute concentrate soln before using.
MOA — Inhibits platelet aggregation by blocking the effects of fibrinogen and other substances at platelet glycoprotein IIb/IIIa receptors.
ADVERSE EFFECTS — Serious: Bleeding, thrombocytopenia (rare). Frequent: Pain.

CARDIOVASCULAR: Beta-Blockers

NOTE: See also antihypertensive combinations. Not first line for HTN (unless to treat angina, post MI, LV dysfunction or heart failure). Atenolol may be less effective for HTN than other beta-blockers. Abrupt discontinuation may precipitate angina, MI, arrhythmias, or rebound HTN; discontinue by tapering over 1 to 2 weeks. Discontinue beta-blocker several days before discontinuing concomitant clonidine to minimize the risk of rebound HTN. Avoid use of nonselective beta-blockers in patients with asthma/COPD. For patients with asthma/COPD, use agents with beta-1 selectivity and monitor cautiously; bronchodilators, including beta-2 agonists, should be readily available or administered concomitantly. Beta-1 selectivity diminishes at high doses. Avoid initiating beta-blocker therapy in acute decompensated heart failure, sick sinus syndrome without pacer, and severe peripheral artery disease. Agents with intrinsic sympathomimetic activity are contraindicated post acute MI. Patients with diabetes should be aware that beta-blockers may mask symptoms of hypoglycemic response. Cross-sensitivity between beta-blockers can occur. With pheochromocytoma, give beta-blocker only after initiating alpha-blocker; using beta-blocker alone may increase BP due to the attenuation of beta-mediated vasodilatation in skeletal muscle (unopposed alpha stimulation). Do not routinely stop chronic beta blocker therapy prior to surgery. Some inhalation anesthetics may increase the cardiodepressant effect of beta-blockers. Concomitant amiodarone, clonidine, digoxin, or nondihydropyridine calcium channel blockers may increase risk of bradycardia. Concomitant disopyramide may increase risk of bradycardia, asystole, and HF. Patients actively using cocaine should avoid beta-blockers with unopposed alpha-adrenergic vasoconstriction, because this will promote coronary artery vasoconstriction/spasm (carvedilol or labetalol have additional alpha-1-blocking effects and are, therefore, safe). Beta-blockers may aggravate psoriasis.

ACEBUTOLOL (Sectral, ✦Rhotral) ▶LK ♀B ▶– $$
ADULTS – HTN: Start 400 mg PO daily or 200 mg PO bid, usual maintenance 400 to 800 mg/day, max 1200 mg/day. Twice daily dosing appears to be more effective than daily dosing.
PEDS – Not approved in children age younger than 12 yo.
UNAPPROVED ADULTS – Angina: Start 200 mg PO bid, increase as needed up to 800 mg/day.
FORMS – Generic/Trade: Caps 200, 400 mg.
NOTES – Has mild intrinsic sympathomimetic activity (partial beta-agonist activity). Beta-1 receptor selective.
MOA – Blocks binding of catecholamines to beta-1 receptors.
ADVERSE EFFECTS – Serious: Bronchoconstriction (high doses), masks hypoglycemic response and slow recovery, rebound hypertension/angina. Frequent: Bradycardia, fatigue, impotence.

ATENOLOL (Tenormin) ▶K ♀D ▶– $
WARNING – Avoid abrupt cessation in coronary heart disease or HTN.
ADULTS – Acute MI: 50 to 100 mg PO daily or in divided doses; or 5 mg IV over 5 min, repeat in 10 min, follow with 50 mg PO 10 min after IV dosing in patients tolerating the total IV dose, increase as tolerated to 100 mg/day given daily or divided bid. HTN: Start 25 to 50 mg PO daily or divided bid, maximum 100 mg/day. Renal impairment, elderly: Start 25 mg PO daily, increase prn. Angina: Start 50 mg PO daily or divided bid, increase prn to max of 200 mg/day.
PEDS – Not approved in children.
UNAPPROVED ADULTS – Reduce perioperative cardiac events (death) in high-risk patients undergoing noncardiac surgery: Start 5 to 10 mg IV prior to anesthesia, then 50 to 100 mg PO daily during hospitalization (max 7 days). Maintain HR between 55 to 65 bpm. Hold dose for HR < 55 bpm and SBP < 100 mmHg. Reentrant PSVT associated with ST-elevation MI (after carotid massage, IV adenosine): 2.5 to 5 mg over 2 min to 10 mg max over 10 to 15 min. Rate control of atrial fibrillation/flutter: Start 25 mg PO daily, titrate to desired heart rate.
UNAPPROVED PEDS – HTN: 1 to 1.2 mg/kg/dose PO daily, max 2 mg/kg/day.
FORMS – Generic/Trade: Tabs unscored 25, 100 mg; scored, 50 mg.
NOTES – Doses greater than 100 mg/day usually do not provide further BP lowering. Beta-1 receptor selective. Risk of hypoglycemia to neonates born to mothers using atenolol at parturition or while breastfeeding. May be less effective for HTN than other beta-blockers.
MOA – Blocks binding of catecholamines to beta-1 receptors.
ADVERSE EFFECTS – Serious: Bronchoconstriction (high doses), masks hypoglycemic response and slow recovery, rebound hypertension/angina. Frequent: Bradycardia, fatigue, impotence.

BETAXOLOL (Kerlone) ▶LK ♀C ▶? $$
ADULTS – HTN: Start 5 to 10 mg PO daily, max 20 mg/day. Renal impairment, elderly: Start 5 mg PO daily, increase as needed.
PEDS – Not approved in children.
FORMS – Generic: Tabs scored 10 mg, unscored 20 mg.
NOTES – Beta-1 receptor selective.
MOA – Blocks binding of catecholamines to beta-1 receptors.
ADVERSE EFFECTS – Serious: Bronchoconstriction (high doses), masks hypoglycemic response and slow recovery, rebound hypertension/angina. Frequent: Bradycardia, fatigue, impotence.

BISOPROLOL (Zebeta, ✦Monocor) ▶LK ♀C ▶? $$
WARNING – Avoid abrupt cessation.
ADULTS – HTN: Start 2.5 to 5 mg PO daily, max 20 mg/day. Renal impairment: Start 2.5 mg PO daily, increase as needed.
PEDS – Not approved in children.
UNAPPROVED ADULTS – Compensated heart failure: Start 1.25 mg PO daily, double dose every 2 weeks as tolerated to goal 10 mg/day. Reduce perioperative

(cont.)

CARDIOVASCULAR: Beta-Blockers

BISOPROLOL (cont.)
cardiac events (death, MI) in high-risk patients undergoing noncardiac surgery: Start 5 mg PO daily, at least 1 week prior to surgery, increase to 10 mg daily to maintain HR < 60 bpm, continue for 30 days postop. Hold dose for HR < 50 bpm or SBP < 100 mmHg.
FORMS — Generic/Trade: Tabs scored 5 mg, unscored 10 mg.
NOTES — Monitor closely for heart failure exacerbation and hypotension when titrating dose. Avoid in decompensated heart failure (ie, NYHA class IV heart failure or pulmonary edema). Stabilize dose of digoxin, diuretics, and ACE inhibitor before starting bisoprolol. Beta-1 receptor selective.
MOA — Blocks binding of catecholamines to beta-1 receptors.
ADVERSE EFFECTS — Serious: Bronchoconstriction (high doses), masks hypoglycemic response and slow recovery, rebound hypertension/angina. Frequent: Bradycardia, fatigue, impotence.

CARVEDILOL (*Coreg, Coreg CR*) ▶L ♀C ▶? $$$$
ADULTS — Heart failure: Immediate-release: Start 3.125 mg PO bid, double dose q 2 weeks as tolerated up to max of 25 mg bid (for wt 85 kg or less) or 50 mg bid (for wt 85 kg or greater). Heart failure, sustained-release: Start 10 mg PO daily, double dose q 2 weeks as tolerated up to max of 80 mg/day. Reduce cardiovascular risk in post MI with LV dysfunction, immediate-release: Start 3.125 to 6.25 mg PO bid, double dose q 3 to 10 days as tolerated to max of 25 mg bid. LV dysfunction post MI, sustained-release: Start 10 to 20 mg PO daily, double dose q 3 to 10 days as tolerated to max of 80 mg/day. HTN, immediate-release: Start 6.25 mg PO bid, double dose q 7 to 14 days as tolerated to max 50 mg/day. HTN, sustained-release: Start 20 mg PO daily, double dose q 7 to 14 days as tolerated to max 80 mg/day.
PEDS — Not approved in children.
FORMS — Generic/Trade: Tabs immediate-release unscored 3.125, 6.25, 12.5, 25 mg. Trade only: Caps extended-release 10, 20, 40, 80 mg.
NOTES — Avoid in asthma, hepatic impairment, and acute decompensated heart failure (ie, requiring IV inotropes or pulmonary edema). Monitor closely for heart failure exacerbation and hypotension (particularly orthostatic) when titrating dose. Stabilize dose of diuretics and ACE inhibitor before starting carvedilol. Amiodarone may increase carvedilol levels. May increase digoxin levels. Reduce the dose with bradycardia (< 55 bpm). May reversibly elevate LFTs. Take with food to decrease orthostatic hypotension. Separate Coreg CR and alcohol (including medications containing alcohol) by at least 2 h. Give Coreg CR in the morning. The contents of Coreg CR may be sprinkled over applesauce and consumed immediately. Dosing conversion from immediate-release to sustained-release: 3.125 mg bid = 10 mg CR; 6.25 mg bid = 20 mg CR; 12.5 mg bid = 40 mg CR; 25 mg bid = 80 mg CR.
MOA — Blocks binding of catecholamines to post-synaptic alpha-1, beta-1, and beta-2 receptors.
ADVERSE EFFECTS — Serious: Anaphylaxis, angioedema, bronchoconstriction, masks hypoglycemic response and slow recovery, rebound hypertension/angina. Frequent: Bradycardia, fatigue, impotence, hypotension.

ESMOLOL (*Brevibloc*) ▶K ♀C ▶? $
ADULTS — SVT/HTN emergency: Load 500 mcg/kg over 1 min (dilute 5 g in 500 mL (10 mg/mL) and give 3.5 mL to deliver 35 g bolus for 70 kg patient) then start infusion 50 to 200 mcg/kg/min (40 mL/h delivers 100 mcg/kg/min for 70 kg patient). If optimal response is not attained, repeat IV load and increase IV infusion to 100 mcg/kg/min for 4 min. If necessary, additional boluses (500 mcg/kg/min over 1 min) may be given followed by IV infusion with increased dose by 50 mcg/kg/min for 4 min. Max IV infusion rate 200 mcg/kg/min.
PEDS — Not approved in children.
UNAPPROVED PEDS — Same schedule as adult except loading dose 100 to 500 mcg/kg IV over 1 min and IV infusion 25 to 100 mcg/kg/min. IV infusions may be increased by 25 to 50 mcg/kg/min every 5 to 10 min. Titrate dose based on patient response.
NOTES — Hypotension. Beta-1 receptor selective. Half-life is 9 min.
MOA — Blocks binding of catecholamines to beta-1 receptors.
ADVERSE EFFECTS — Serious: Bronchoconstriction (high doses), masks hypoglycemic response and slow recovery, rebound hypertension/angina. Frequent: Bradycardia, fatigue.

LABETALOL (*Trandate*) ▶LK ♀C ▶+ $$$
WARNING — Avoid abrupt cessation.
ADULTS — HTN: Start 100 mg PO bid, usual maintenance dose 200 to 600 mg bid, max 2400 mg/day. HTN emergency: Start 20 mg slow IV injection, then 40 to 80 mg IV q 10 min prn up to 300 mg total cumulative dose or start 0.5 to 2 mg/min IV infusion, adjust rate as needed up to total cumulative dose 300 mg.
PEDS — Not approved in children.
UNAPPROVED PEDS — HTN: 4 mg/kg/day PO divided bid, increase prn up to 40 mg/kg/day. IV: Start 0.3 to 1 mg/kg/dose (max 20 mg) slow IV injection q 10 min or 0.4 to 1 mg/kg/h IV infusion up to 3 mg/kg/h.
FORMS — Generic/Trade: Tabs scored 100, 200, 300 mg.
NOTES — Hypotension. Contraindicated in asthma/COPD. Alpha-1, beta-1, and beta-2 receptor blocker.
MOA — Blocks binding of catecholamines to post-synaptic alpha-1, beta-1, and beta-2 receptors.
ADVERSE EFFECTS — Serious: Bronchoconstriction, hepatotoxicity, masks hypoglycemic response and slow recovery, rebound hypertension/angina. Frequent: Bradycardia, fatigue, impotence, hypotension.

METOPROLOL (*Lopressor, Toprol-XL, ✦Betaloc*) ▶L ♀C ▶? $$
WARNING — Abrupt cessation may exacerbate angina pectoris and MI. Warn patients against interruption or discontinuation without physician's advice.

(cont.)

CARDIOVASCULAR: Beta-Blockers

METOPROLOL (cont.)

ADULTS — <u>Acute MI</u>: 50 to 100 mg PO q 12 h; or 5 mg IV q 5 to 15 min up to 15 mg, then start 50 mg PO q 6 h for 48 h, then 100 mg PO bid as tolerated. If usual IV dose is not tolerated, start 25 to 50 mg PO q 6 h. If early IV therapy is contraindicated, patient should be titrated to 100 mg PO bid as soon as possible. <u>HTN</u> (immediate-release): Start 100 mg PO daily or in divided doses, increase prn up to 450 mg/day; may require multiple daily doses to maintain 24 h BP control. <u>HTN</u> (extended-release): Start 25 to 100 mg PO daily, increase prn q 1 week up to 400 mg/day. <u>Heart failure:</u> Start 12.5 to 25 mg (extended-release) PO daily, double dose every 2 weeks as tolerated up to max 200 mg/day. <u>Angina:</u> Start 50 mg PO bid (immediate-release) or 100 mg PO daily (extended-release), increase prn up to 400 mg/day. Take with food.

PEDS — <u>HTN</u> 6 yo or greater: Start 1 mg/kg, max 50 mg/daily. Not recommended for younger than 6 yo.

UNAPPROVED ADULTS — <u>Heart failure:</u> Start 6.25 PO bid, max 75 mg bid. <u>Atrial tachyarrhythmia, except with Wolff-Parkinson-White syndrome:</u> 2.5 to 5 mg IV q 2 to 5 min prn to control rapid ventricular response, max 15 mg over 10 to 15 min. <u>Reentrant PSVT</u> (after carotid massage, IV adenosine): 2.5 to 5 mg q 2 to 5 min to 15 mg max over 10 to 15 min. <u>Reduce perioperative cardiac events (death) in high-risk patients undergoing noncardiac surgery:</u> Start 100 mg (extended-release) 2 h prior to anesthesia, then 50 to 100 mg (extended-release) PO daily or 2.5 to 5 mg IV q 6 h during hospitalization (max 7 days). Maintain HR between 55 to 65 bpm. Hold dose for HR < 55 bpm and SBP < 100 mmHg. <u>Rate control of atrial fibrillation/flutter:</u> Start 25 mg PO bid, titrate to desired heart rate.

FORMS — Generic/Trade: Tabs scored 50, 100 mg, extended-release 25, 50, 100, 200 mg. Generic only: Tabs scored 25 mg.

NOTES — Immediate-release form is metoprolol tartrate; extended-release form is metoprolol succinate. When switching from immediate-release to extended-release product, use same total daily dose. The immediate and extended-release products may not give same clinical response on mg:mg basis; monitor response and side effects when interchanging between metoprolol products. Do not start high-dose extended-release form in patients undergoing noncardiac surgery; has been associated with bradycardia, low BP, CVA, death. Monitor closely for heart failure exacerbation and hypotension when titrating dose. Avoid use in patients with decompensated heart failure (ie, NYHA class IV heart failure or pulmonary edema. Stabilize dose of diuretics and ACE inhibitor before starting metoprolol. Beta-1 receptor selective. Extended-release tabs may be broken in half, but do not chew or crush. Avoid using extended-release tabs with verapamil, diltiazem, or peripheral vascular disease. May need lower doses in elderly and in patients with liver impairment. Monitor BP with potent CYP 2D6 inhibitors that may increase levels (eg, bupropion, cimetidine, diphenhydramine, fluoxetine, hydroxychloroquine, paroxetine, propafenone, quinidine, thioridazine, ritonavir, terbinafine).

MOA — Blocks binding of catecholamines to beta-1 receptors.

ADVERSE EFFECTS — Serious: Bronchoconstriction (high doses), masks hypoglycemic response and slow recovery, rebound hypertension/angina. Frequent: Bradycardia, fatigue, impotence.

NADOLOL (*Corgard*) ▶K ♀C ▶− $$

WARNING — Avoid abrupt cessation in ischemic heart disease or HTN; may exacerbate angina and MI. Warn patients against interruption or discontinuation without physician's advice.

ADULTS — <u>HTN:</u> Start 20 to 40 mg PO daily, usual maintenance dose 40 to 80 mg/day, max 320 mg/day. <u>Renal impairment:</u> Start 20 mg PO daily, adjust dosage interval based on severity of renal impairment: For CrCl < 10 mL/min give q 40 to 60 h; for CrCl 10 to 30 mL/min give q 24 to 48 h; for CrCl 31 to 50 mL/min give q 24 to 36 h. <u>Angina:</u> Start 40 mg PO daily, usual maintenance dose 40 to 80 mg/day, max 240 mg/day.

PEDS — Not approved in children.

UNAPPROVED ADULTS — <u>Prevent rebleeding esophageal varices:</u> 40 to 160 mg/day PO. Titrate dose to reduce heart rate to 25% below baseline. <u>Ventricular arrhythmia:</u> 10 to 640 mg/day PO.

FORMS — Generic/Trade: Tabs scored 20, 40, 80, 120, 160 mg.

NOTES — Beta-1 and beta-2 receptor blocker.

MOA — Blocks binding of catecholamines to beta-1 and beta-2 receptors.

ADVERSE EFFECTS — Serious: Bronchoconstriction, masks hypoglycemic response and slow recovery, rebound hypertension/angina. Frequent: Bradycardia, fatigue, impotence.

NEBIVOLOL (*Bystolic*) ▶L ♀C ▶− $$$

ADULTS — <u>HTN:</u> Start 5 mg PO daily, maximum 40 mg/day. <u>Severe renal impairment</u> (CrCl < 30 mL/min), <u>moderate hepatic impairment:</u> Start 2.5 mg PO daily, increase cautiously.

PEDS — Not approved in children.

FORMS — Trade only: Tabs unscored 2.5, 5, 10, 20 mg.

NOTES — Do not use with severe liver impairment.

MOA — Blocks binding of catecholamines to beta-1 receptors at doses of 10 mg or less and in patients who extensively metabolize CYP 2D6; otherwise, inhibits both beta-1 and beta-2 receptors.

ADVERSE EFFECTS — Serious: Bronchoconstriction. Frequent: Dizziness, fatigue, headache.

OXPRENOLOL (✦*Trasicor, Slow-Trasicor*) ▶L ♀D ▶− $$

ADULTS — Canada only. <u>Mild to moderate HTN,</u> usually in combination with a thiazide-type diuretic: Regular-release: Initially 20 mg PO tid, titrate upwards prn to usual maintenance 120 to 320 mg/day divided bid to tid. Alternatively, may substitute an equivalent daily dose of sustained-release product; do not exceed 480 mg/day.

PEDS — Not approved in children.

(cont.)

OXPRENOLOL (cont.)
FORMS — Trade only: Regular-release tabs: 40, 80 mg. Sustained-release tabs: 80, 160 mg.
NOTES — Caution in bronchospasm, diabetes, or heart failure. Has mild intrinsic sympathomimetic activity (partial beta-agonist activity). No dose adjustment in impaired renal function. Empty matrix of sustained-release tab may be excreted and found in the feces.
MOA — Blocks binding of catecholamines to beta-1 and beta-2 receptors.
ADVERSE EFFECTS — Serious: Bronchoconstriction, masks hypoglycemic response and slow recovery, rebound hypertension/angina. Frequent: Bradycardia, fatigue, dizziness, impotence.

PENBUTOLOL (Levatol) ▶LK ♀C ▶? $$$$
WARNING — Abrupt cessation may exacerbate angina pectoris and MI. Warn patients against interruption or discontinuation without physician's advice.
ADULTS — HTN: Start 20 mg PO daily, usual maintenance dose 20 to 40 mg, max 80 mg/day.
PEDS — Not approved in children.
FORMS — Trade only: Tabs, scored 20 mg.
NOTES — Has mild intrinsic sympathomimetic activity (partial beta-agonist activity). Beta-1 and beta-2 receptor blocker.
MOA — Blocks binding of catecholamines to beta-1 and beta-2 receptors.
ADVERSE EFFECTS — Serious: Bronchoconstriction, masks hypoglycemic response and slow recovery, rebound hypertension/angina. Frequent: Bradycardia, fatigue, dizziness, impotence.

PINDOLOL (✱Visken) ▶K ♀B ▶? $$$
WARNING — Abrupt cessation may exacerbate angina pectoris and MI. Warn patients against interruption or discontinuation without physician's advice.
ADULTS — HTN: Start 5 mg PO bid, usual maintenance dose 10 to 30 mg/day, max 60 mg/day.
PEDS — Not approved in children.
UNAPPROVED ADULTS — Angina: 15 to 40 mg/day PO in divided doses tid to qid.
FORMS — Generic only: Tabs, scored 5, 10 mg.
NOTES — Has intrinsic sympathomimetic activity (partial beta-agonist activity). Beta-1 and beta-2 receptor blocker. Contraindicated with thioridazine.
MOA — Blocks binding of catecholamines to beta-1 and beta-2 receptors.
ADVERSE EFFECTS — Serious: Bronchoconstriction, masks hypoglycemic response and slow recovery, rebound hypertension/angina. Frequent: Bradycardia, fatigue, impotence.

PROPRANOLOL (Inderal, Inderal LA, InnoPran XL) ▶L ♀C ▶+ $$
WARNING — Avoid abrupt cessation in ischemic heart disease or HTN; may exacerbate angina and MI. Warn patients against interruption or discontinuation without physician's advice.
ADULTS — HTN: Start 20 to 40 mg PO bid, usual maintenance dose 160 to 480 mg/day, max 640 mg/day; extended-release (Inderal LA): Start 60 to 80 mg PO daily, usual maintenance dose 120 to 160 mg/day, max 640 mg/day; extended-release (InnoPran XL): Start 80 mg at bedtime (10 pm), max 120 mg at bedtime. Angina: Start 10 to 20 mg PO tid/qid, usual maintenance 160 to 240 mg/day, max 320 mg/day; extended-release (Inderal LA): Start 80 mg PO daily, same usual dosage range and max for HTN. Migraine prophylaxis: Start 40 mg PO bid or 80 mg PO daily (extended-release), max 240 mg/day. Supraventricular tachycardia or rapid atrial fibrillation/flutter: 10 to 30 mg PO tid to qid. MI: 180 to 240 mg/day PO in divided doses bid to qid. Pheochromocytoma surgery: 60 mg PO in divided doses bid to tid beginning 3 days before surgery, use in combination with an alpha-blocking agent. IV: Reserved for life-threatening arrhythmia, 1 to 3 mg IV, repeat dose in 2 min if needed, additional doses only after 4 h. Not for use in hypertensive emergency. Essential tremor: Start 40 mg PO bid, titrate prn to 120 to 320 mg/day.
PEDS — HTN: Start 1 mg/kg/day PO divided bid, usual maintenance dose 2 to 4 mg/kg/day PO divided bid, max 16 mg/kg/day.
UNAPPROVED ADULTS — Prevent rebleeding esophageal varices: 20 to 180 mg PO bid. Titrate dose to reduce heart rate to 25% below baseline. Control heart rate with A-fib: 80 to 240 mg/day daily or in divided doses.
UNAPPROVED PEDS — Arrhythmia: 0.01 to 0.1 mg/kg/dose (max 1 mg/dose) by slow IV push. Manufacturer does not recommend IV propranolol in children.
FORMS — Generic/Trade: Tabs, scored 40, 60, 80. Caps, extended-release 60, 80, 120, 160 mg. Generic only: Soln 20, 40 mg/5 mL. Tabs, 10, 20 mg. Trade only: (InnoPran XL at bedtime) 80, 120 mg.
NOTES — Beta-1 and beta-2 receptor blocker. Do not substitute extended-release product for immediate-release product on mg-for-mg basis. Dosage titration may be necessary with extended-release product when converting from immediate-release Tabs. Extended-release caps (Inderal LA) may be opened, and the contents sprinkled on food for administration. Cap contents should be swallowed whole without crushing or chewing. Contraindicated with thioridazine. InnoPran XL is a chronotherapeutic product; give at bedtime to blunt early morning surge in BP. Concomitant use of alcohol may increase propranolol levels.
MOA — Blocks binding of catecholamines to beta-1 and beta-2 receptors.
ADVERSE EFFECTS — Serious: Anaphylaxis, agranulocytosis, bronchoconstriction, masks hypoglycemic response and slows recovery, rebound hypertension/angina, Stevens-Johnson syndrome. Frequent: Bradycardia, fatigue, dizziness, impotence.

TIMOLOL (Blocadren) ▶LK ♀C ▶+ $$$
WARNING — Avoid abrupt cessation in ischemic heart disease or HTN; may exacerbate angina and MI. Warn patients against interruption or discontinuation without physician's advice.
ADULTS — HTN: Start 10 mg PO bid, usual maintenance 20 to 40 mg/day, max 60 mg/day. MI: 10 mg PO bid, started 1 to 4 weeks post MI. Migraine headaches:

(cont.)

TIMOLOL (cont.)
Start 10 mg PO bid, use 20 mg/day daily or divided bid for prophylaxis, increase prn up to max 60 mg/day. Stop therapy if satisfactory response not obtained after 6 to 8 weeks of max dose.
PEDS — Not approved in children.
UNAPPROVED ADULTS — Angina: 15 to 45 mg/day PO divided tid to qid.
FORMS — Generic only: Tabs, 5, 10, 20 mg.
NOTES — Beta-1 and beta-2 receptor blocker.
MOA — Blocks binding of catecholamines to beta-1 and beta-2 receptors.
ADVERSE EFFECTS — Serious: Bronchoconstriction, masks hypoglycemic response and slow recovery, rebound hypertension/angina. Frequent: Bradycardia, fatigue, impotence.

CARDIOVASCULAR: Calcium Channel Blockers (CCBs)—Dihydropyridines

NOTE: See also antihypertensive combinations. Peripheral edema, especially with higher doses. Extended/controlled/sustained-release tabs should be swallowed whole; do not chew or crush. Avoid concomitant grapefruit juice, which may enhance effect. Avoid in decompensated heart failure.

AMLODIPINE (*Norvasc*) ▶L ♀C ▶? $$$
ADULTS — HTN, CAD: Start 5 mg PO daily, max 10 daily. Elderly, small, frail, or with hepatic insufficiency: Start 2.5 mg PO daily.
PEDS — HTN (6 to 17 yo): 2.5 to 5 mg PO daily.
UNAPPROVED PEDS — HTN: Start 0.1 to 0.2 mg/kg/day PO daily, max 0.3 mg/kg/day (max 10 mg daily).
FORMS — Generic/Trade: Tabs unscored 2.5, 5, 10 mg. Generic only: Orally disintegrating tabs 2.5, 5, 10 mg.
NOTES — Angina may worsen and acute MI can develop after starting or increasing amlodipine, particularly in patients with severe obstructive CAD.
MOA — Blocks calcium-dependent contractions in cardiac and peripheral smooth muscle leading to vasodilation.
ADVERSE EFFECTS — Serious: None. Frequent: Peripheral edema, headache, palpitations.

CLEVIDIPINE (*Cleviprex*) ▶KL ♀C ▶? $$$
ADULTS — HTN: Start 1 to 2 mg/h IV, double dose q 1.5 min as approaches BP goal, then titrate at smaller increments q 5 to 10 min to desired bp, usual maintenance dose 4 to 6 mg/h, max 32 mg/h IV. An increase of 1 to 2 mg/h will decrease SBP approximately 2 to 4 mmHg.
PEDS — Not approved in children.
NOTES — Contraindicated with egg or soy allergy, defective lipid metabolism, or severe aortic stenosis. May exacerbate HF.
MOA — Blocks calcium-dependent contractions in cardiac and peripheral smooth muscle leading to vasodilation.
ADVERSE EFFECTS — Serious: Acute renal failure, atrial fib. Frequent: Headache, nausea, vomiting.

FELODIPINE (*Plendil*, ✦*Renedil*) ▶L ♀C ▶? $$
ADULTS — HTN: Start 2.5 to 5 mg PO daily, usual maintenance dose 5 to 10 mg/day, max 10 mg/day.
PEDS — Not approved in children.
FORMS — Generic/Trade: Tabs extended-release, unscored 2.5, 5, 10 mg.
NOTES — Extended-release tab. May increase tacrolimus concentration; monitor level.
MOA — Blocks calcium-dependent contractions in cardiac and peripheral smooth muscle leading to vasodilation.
ADVERSE EFFECTS — Serious: None. Frequent: Peripheral edema, headache, palpitations.

ISRADIPINE (*DynaCirc, DynaCirc CR*) ▶L ♀C ▶? $$$$
ADULTS — HTN: Start 2.5 mg PO bid, usual maintenance 5 to 10 mg/day, max 20 mg/day divided bid (max 10 mg/day in elderly). Controlled-release (DynaCirc CR): Start 5 mg PO daily, usual maintenance dose 5 to 10 mg/day, max 20 mg/day.
PEDS — Not approved in children.
FORMS — Trade only: Tabs controlled-release 5, 10 mg. Generic only: Immediate-release caps 2.5, 5 mg.
MOA — Blocks calcium-dependent contractions in cardiac and peripheral smooth muscle leading to vasodilation.
ADVERSE EFFECTS — Serious: Angioedema. Frequent: Peripheral edema, headache, palpitations.

NICARDIPINE (*Cardene, Cardene SR*) ▶L ♀C ▶? $$
ADULTS — HTN: Sustained-release (Cardene SR), Start 30 mg PO bid, usual maintenance dose 30 to 60 mg PO bid, max 120 mg/day; immediate-release, Start 20 mg PO tid, usual maintenance dose 20 to 40 mg PO tid, max 120 mg/day. Angina: Immediate-release, Start 20 mg PO tid, usual maintenance dose 20 to 40 mg tid. Short-term management of HTN, patient not receiving PO nicardipine: Begin IV infusion at 5 mg/h, titrate infusion rate by 2.5 mg/h q 5 to 15 min as needed, max 15 mg/h. Short-term management of HTN, patient receiving PO nicardipine: If using 20 mg PO q8h, give 0.5 mg/h IV; if using 30 mg PO q8h, give 1.2 mg/h IV; if using 40 mg PO q8h, give 2.2 mg/h. When discontinuing IV nicardipine and transitioning to an oral BP regimen: Administer first dose of nicardipine PO 1 h prior to discontinuing IV infusion; or initiate BP lowering agent other than nicardipine upon discontinuation of IV infusion.
PEDS — Not approved in children.
UNAPPROVED PEDS — HTN: 0.5 to 3 mcg/kg/min IV infusion.
FORMS — Generic/Trade: Caps immediate-release 20, 30 mg. Trade only: Caps sustained-release 30, 45, 60 mg.
NOTES — Hypotension, especially with immediate-release Caps and IV. Decrease dose if hepatically impaired. Titrate carefully if renally impaired. Use sustained-release Caps for HTN only, not for angina. Frequency, duration, or severity of angina has increased with chronic therapy.

(cont.)

NICARDIPINE (cont.)

MOA — Blocks calcium-dependent contractions in cardiac and peripheral smooth muscle leading to vasodilation.
ADVERSE EFFECTS — Serious: None. Frequent: Peripheral edema, headache, palpitations.

NIFEDIPINE (*Procardia, Adalat, Procardia XL, Adalat CC, Afeditab CR, ✦Adalat XL, Adalat PA*) ▶L ♀C ▶– $$

ADULTS — <u>HTN:</u> Extended-release, Start 30 to 60 mg PO daily, max 120 mg/day. <u>Angina:</u> Extended-release, Start 30 to 60 mg PO daily, max 120 mg/day; immediate-release, Start 10 mg PO tid, usual maintenance dose 10 to 20 mg tid, max 120 mg/day.
PEDS — Not approved in children.
UNAPPROVED ADULTS — <u>Preterm labor:</u> Loading dose 10 mg PO q 20 to 30 min if contractions persist up to 40 mg within the first h. After contractions are controlled, maintenance dose: 10 to 20 mg PO q 4 to 6 h or 60 to 160 mg extended-release PO daily. Duration of treatment has not been established. <u>Promotes spontaneous passage of ureteral calculi:</u> Extended-release, 30 mg PO daily for 10 to 28 days.
UNAPPROVED PEDS — <u>HTN:</u> 0.25 to 0.5 mg/kg/dose PO q 4 to 6 h as needed, max 10 mg/dose or 3 mg/kg/day. Doses less than 0.25 mg/kg may be effective.
FORMS — Generic/Trade: Caps 10, 20 mg. Tabs extended-release (Adalat CC, Afeditab CR, Procardia XL) 30, 60 mg, (Adalat CC, Procardia XL) 90 mg.
NOTES — Immediate-release cap should not be chewed and swallowed or given sublingually; may cause excessive hypotension, CVA. Do not use immediate-release caps for treating HTN, hypertensive emergencies, or ST-elevation MI. Extended-release tabs can be substituted for immediate-release caps at the same dose in patients whose angina is controlled. May increase blood sugar levels. Metabolized by the CYP 3A4 enzyme system. Use alternative BP lowering medication when patient on carbamazepine, phenobarbital, phenytoin, rifampin, or St John's Wort; these reduce levels of nifedipine significantly. Fluoxetine, nefazodone, protease inhibitors, or valproic acid increases nifedipine levels; monitor BP and reduce nifedipine dose. Increases tacrolimus levels. Stop grapefruit juice intake at least 3 days prior to starting nifedipine.
MOA — Blocks calcium-dependent contractions in cardiac and peripheral smooth muscle leading to vasodilation. Tocolytic.
ADVERSE EFFECTS — Serious: Hypotension. Frequent: Peripheral edema, headache, palpitations, flushing.

NISOLDIPINE (*Sular*) ▶L ♀C ▶? $$$

ADULTS — <u>HTN:</u> Start 17 mg PO daily, may increase by 8.5 mg weekly, max 34 mg/day. Impaired hepatic function, elderly: Start 8.5 mg PO daily, titrate as needed.
PEDS — Not approved in children.
UNAPPROVED ADULTS — Not approved in children.
FORMS — Trade only: Tabs extended-release 8.5, 17, 25.5, 34 mg. These replace the former 10, 20, 30, 40 mg tabs. Generic only: Tabs extended-release 20, 30, 40 mg.
NOTES — Take on an empty stomach. Sular 8.5, 17, 25.5, 34 mg replace 10, 20, 30, 40 mg respectively.
MOA — Blocks calcium-dependent contractions in cardiac and peripheral smooth muscle leading to vasodilation.
ADVERSE EFFECTS — Serious: None. Frequent: Peripheral edema, headache, palpitations.

CARDIOVASCULAR: Calcium Channel Blockers (CCBs)—Non-Dihydropyridines

NOTE: See also antihypertensive combinations. Avoid in decompensated heart failure or 2nd/3rd degree heart block.

DILTIAZEM (*Cardizem, Cardizem LA, Cardizem CD, Cartia XT, Dilacor XR, Diltiazem CD, Diltzac, Diltia XT, Tiazac, Taztia XT*) ▶L ♀C ▶+ $$

ADULTS — <u>Atrial fibrillation/flutter, PSVT:</u> 20 mg (0.25 mg/kg) IV bolus over 2 min. If needed and patient tolerated IV bolus with no hypotension, rebolus 15 min later with 25 mg (0.35 mg/kg). IV infusion: Start 10 mg/h, increase by 5 mg/h (usual range 5 to 15 mg/h). once a day, extended- release (Cardizem CD, Cartia XT, Dilacor XR, Diltia XT, Taztia XT, Tiazac), <u>HTN:</u> Start 120 to 240 mg PO daily, usual maintenance range 240 to 360 mg/day, max 540 mg/day. once at day, graded extended-release (Cardizem LA), <u>HTN:</u> Start 180 to 240 mg, max 540 mg/day. Twice a day, sustained-release (Cardizem SR), <u>HTN:</u> Start 60 to 120 mg PO bid, max 360 mg/day. <u>Immediate-release, angina:</u> Start 30 mg PO qid, max 360 mg/day divided tid to qid. <u>Extended-release, angina:</u> 120 to 180 mg PO daily, max 540 mg/day. once a day, graded extended-release (Cardizem LA), angina: Start 180 mg PO daily, doses greater than 360 mg may provide no additional benefit.
PEDS — Not approved in children. Diltiazem injection should be avoided in neonates due to potential toxicity from benzyl alcohol in the injectable product.
UNAPPROVED ADULTS — <u>Control heart rate with A-fib:</u> 120 to 360 mg/day daily or in divided doses.
UNAPPROVED PEDS — <u>HTN:</u> Start 1.5 to 2 mg/kg/day PO divided tid to qid, max 3.5 mg/kg/day.
FORMS — Generic/Trade: Tabs immediate-release, unscored (Cardizem) 30, scored 60, 90, 120 mg; Caps extended-release (Cardizem CD, Cartia XT daily) 120, 180, 240, 300, 360 mg, (Diltzac, Taztia XT, Tiazac daily) 120, 180, 240, 300, 360, 420 mg, (Dilacor XR, Diltia XT) 120, 180, 240 mg. Trade only: Tabs extended-release graded (Cardizem LA daily) 120, 180, 240, 300, 360, 420 mg.
NOTES — Contraindicated in acute MI and pulmonary congestion, hypotension (systolic BP< 90), sick sinus

(cont.)

DILTIAZEM (cont.)
syndrome without pacemaker, 2nd or 3rd degree AV block without pacemaker. Sinus bradycardia resulting in hospitalization and pacemaker insertion has been reported with concomitant clonidine; monitor heart rate. May increase levels of buspirone, quinidine. Contents of extended-release caps may be sprinkled over food. Do not chew or crush cap contents. May accumulate with hepatic impairment; dose based on clinical response. Monitor response and side effects when interchanging between diltiazem products; many are not equivalent on mg:mg basis. Cardizem LA is a chronotherapeutic product; give at bedtime to blunt early morning surge in BP.
MOA — Blocks calcium-dependent contractions in cardiac and peripheral smooth muscle leading to vasodilation; slows cardiac conduction through the AV node.
ADVERSE EFFECTS — Serious: Bradycardia, heart block (rare). Frequent: Peripheral edema, headache.

VERAPAMIL (*Isoptin SR, Calan, Covera-HS, Verelan, Verelan PM, ♦Veramil*) ▶L ♀C ▶– $$
ADULTS — <u>SVT:</u> 5 to 10 mg (0.075 to 0.15 mg/kg) IV over 2 min. A second dose of 10 mg IV may be given 15 to 30 min later if needed. <u>PSVT/rate control with atrial fibrillation:</u> 240 to 480 mg/day PO divided tid to qid. <u>Angina:</u> Start 40 to 80 mg PO tid to qid, max 480 mg/day; sustained-release (Isoptin SR, Calan SR, Verelan), start 120 to 240 mg PO daily, max 480 mg/day (use bid dosing for doses greater than 240 mg/day with Isoptin SR and Calan SR); extended-release (Covera-HS), start 180 mg PO at bedtime max 480 mg/day. <u>HTN:</u> Same as angina, except (Verelan PM) start 100 to 200 mg PO at bedtime max 400 mg/day; (Covera-HS) start 180 mg PO at bedtime max 480 mg/day; immediate-release tabs should be avoided in treating HTN.
PEDS — <u>SVT</u> age 1 to 15 yo: 2 to 5 mg (0.1 to 0.3 mg/kg) IV, max dose 5 mg. Repeat dose once in 30 min if needed, max second dose 10 mg. Immediate-release and sustained-release tabs not approved in children.
FORMS — Generic/Trade: Tabs, immediate-release, scored (Calan) 40, 80, 120 mg; Tabs, sustained-release, unscored (Isoptin SR) 120, scored 180, 240 mg; Caps, sustained-release (Verelan) 120, 180, 240, 360 mg; Caps, extended-release (Verelan PM) 100, 200, 300 mg. Trade only: Tabs, extended-release (Covera-HS) 180, 240 mg.
NOTES — Contraindicated in severe LV dysfunction, hypotension (systolic BP < 90 mm Hg), cardiogenic shock, sick sinus syndrome without pacemaker, 2nd or 3rd degree AV block without pacemaker, A-fib/flutter conducted via accessory pathway (ie, Wolff-Parkinson-White). Avoid concomitant grapefruit juice (enhances effect). Hypotension, bradyarrhythmias, and lactic acidosis have been reported with concomitant telithromycin. Sinus bradycardia resulting in hospitalization and pacemaker insertion has been reported with concomitant clonidine; monitor heart rate. Digoxin level may increase 50 to 75% when used concomitantly; consider reducing digoxin dose; monitor digoxin level. May increase doxorubicin levels. May change the level of certain chemotherapeutic agents; may get reduced absorption of verapamil with some chemotherapeutic regimens; see package insert for complete list. Scored, sustained-release tabs (Calan SR, Isoptin SR) may be broken and each piece swallowed whole, do not chew or crush. Other extended-release tabs (Covera-HS) should be swallowed whole. Monitor response and side effects when interchanging between verapamil products; many are not equivalent on mg:mg basis. Contents of sustained-release caps may be sprinkled on food (eg, apple sauce). Do not chew or crush cap contents. Use cautiously with impaired renal/hepatic function. Covera-HS and Verelan PM are chronotherapeutic products; give at bedtime to blunt early morning surge in BP.
MOA — Blocks calcium-dependent contractions in cardiac and peripheral smooth muscle leading to vasodilation; slows cardiac conduction through the SA node.
ADVERSE EFFECTS — Serious: Bradycardia, heart block (rare). Frequent: Constipation, headache.

CARDIOVASCULAR: Diuretics—Carbonic Anhydrase Inhibitors

ACETAZOLAMIDE (*Diamox, Diamox Sequels*) ▶LK ♀C ▶+ $
ADULTS — <u>Glaucoma:</u> 250 mg PO up to qid (immediate-release) or 500 mg PO up to bid (sustained-release). Max 1 g/day. <u>Acute glaucoma:</u> 250 mg IV q 4 h or 500 mg IV initially with 125 to 250 mg q 4 h, followed by oral therapy. <u>Mountain sickness prophylaxis:</u> 125 to 250 mg PO bid to tid, beginning 1 to 2 days prior to ascent and continuing at least 5 days at higher altitude. <u>Edema:</u> Rarely used, start 250 to 375 mg IV/PO qam given intermittently (every other day or 2 consecutive days followed by none for 1 to 2 days) to avoid loss of diuretic effect.
PEDS — <u>Diuretic:</u> 5 mg/kg PO/IV qam.
UNAPPROVED PEDS — <u>Glaucoma:</u> 8 to 30 mg/kg/day PO, divided tid. <u>Acute glaucoma:</u> 5 to 10 mg/kg IV every 6 h.
FORMS — Generic only: Tabs 125, 250 mg. Generic/Trade: Caps extended-release 500 mg.
NOTES — A susp (250 mg/5 mL) can be made by crushing and mixing tabs in flavored syrup. The susp is stable for 7 days at room temperature. 1 tab may be softened in 2 teaspoons of hot water, then add to 2 teaspoons of honey or syrup, and swallowed at once. Tabs and compounded susp may have a bitter taste. Use cautiously in sulfa allergy. Prompt descent is necessary if severe forms of high-altitude sickness occur (eg, pulmonary or cerebral edema). Test the drug for tolerance/allergies 1 to 2 weeks before initial dosing prior to ascent.
MOA — Inhibition of carbonic anhydrase.
ADVERSE EFFECTS — Serious: Metabolic acidosis, electrolyte imbalance, sulfonamide hypersensitivity (rare). Frequent: Nausea, diarrhea, drowsiness, numbness, tingling, altered taste, loss of appetite, tinnitus.

CARDIOVASCULAR: Diuretics—Loop

NOTE: Give second dose of bid schedule in mid afternoon to avoid nocturia when treating edema. Thiazides are preferred diuretics for HTN. Rare hypersensitivity in patients allergic to sulfa-containing drugs, except ethacrynic acid.

BUMETANIDE (*Bumex,* ✦*Burinex*) ▶K ♀C ▶? $
ADULTS — Edema: 0.5 to 2 mg PO daily, repeat doses at 4 to 5 h intervals as needed until desired response is attained, max 10 mg/day; 0.5 to 1 mg IV/IM, repeat doses at 2 to 3 h intervals as needed until desired response is attained, max 10 mg/day. Dosing for 3 to 4 consecutive days followed by no drug for 1 to 2 days is acceptable. Bid dosing may enhance diuretic effect. IV injections should be over 1 to 2 min. An IV infusion may be used, change bag every 24 h.
PEDS — Not approved in children.
UNAPPROVED PEDS — Edema: 0.015 to 0.1 mg/kg/dose PO/IV/IM daily or every other day.
FORMS — Generic/Trade: Tabs scored 0.5, 1, 2 mg.
NOTES — 1 mg bumetanide is roughly equivalent to 40 mg oral furosemide. IV administration is preferred when GI absorption is impaired.
MOA — Block chloride reabsorption by inhibiting the Na+/K+/Cl- cotransport system in the thick ascending limb of the loop of Henle.
ADVERSE EFFECTS — Serious: Electrolyte imbalances (hypokalemia, hyponatremia, hypochloremic alkalosis, hypomagnesemia, hypocalcemia, hyperuricemia), dehydration, ototoxicity (rare), skin reactions. Frequent: Dizziness, headache, fatigue, muscle cramps, impotence.

ETHACRYNIC ACID (*Edecrin*) ▶K ♀B ▶? $$$
ADULTS — Edema: 0.5 to 1 mg/kg IV, max 100 mg/dose; 25 mg PO daily on day 1, followed by 50 mg PO bid on day 2, followed by 100 mg PO in the morning and 50 to 100 mg PO in the evening depending on the response to the morning dose, max 400 mg/day.
PEDS — Not approved in children.
UNAPPROVED ADULTS — HTN: 25 mg PO daily, max 100 mg/day divided bid to tid.
UNAPPROVED PEDS — Edema: 1 mg/kg IV; 25 mg PO daily, increase slowly by 25 mg increments as needed. Ethacrynic acid should not be administered to infants.
FORMS — Trade only: Tabs scored 25 mg.
NOTES — Rarely used. Ototoxicity possible. Does not contain a sulfonamide group; may be useful in sulfonamide-allergic patients. Do not administer SC or IM due to local irritation. IV ethacrynic acid should be reconstituted to a concentration of 50 mg/mL and given slowly by IV infusion over 20 to 30 min. May increase lithium levels.
MOA — Block chloride reabsorption by inhibiting the Na+/K+/Cl- cotransport system in the thick ascending limb of the loop of Henle.
ADVERSE EFFECTS — Serious: Electrolyte imbalances (hypokalemia, hyponatremia, hypochloremic alkalosis, hypomagnesemia, hypocalcemia, hyperuricemia), dehydration, pancreatitis (rare), photosensitivity (rare), ototoxicity (rare). Frequent: Dizziness, headache, fatigue, muscle cramps, impotence.

FUROSEMIDE (*Lasix*) ▶K ♀C ▶? $
ADULTS — Edema: Start 20 to 80 mg IV/IM/PO, increase dose by 20 to 40 mg every 6 to 8 h until desired response is achieved, max 600 mg/day. Give maintenance dose daily or divided bid. IV infusion: 0.05 mg/kg/h, titrate rate to desired response.
HTN: Start 20 to 40 mg bid, adjust dose as needed based on BP response. Use lower doses in elderly.
PEDS — Edema: 0.5 to 2 mg/kg/dose IV/IM/PO q 6 to 12 h, max 6 mg/kg/dose. IV infusion: 0.05 mg/kg/h, titrate rate to achieve desired response.
FORMS — Generic/Trade: Tabs unscored 20, scored 40, 80 mg. Generic only: Oral soln 10 mg/mL, 40 mg/5 mL.
NOTES — Loops are diuretic of choice with decreased renal function (CrCl less than 30 mL/min or creatinine more than 2.5 mg/dL). Oral absorption may decrease in acute heart failure exacerbation. Bioequivalence of oral form is 50% of IV dose. Monitor renal function in elderly.
MOA — Block chloride reabsorption by inhibiting the Na+/K+/Cl- cotransport system in the thick ascending limb of the loop of Henle.
ADVERSE EFFECTS — Serious: Electrolyte imbalances (hypokalemia, hyponatremia, hypochloremic alkalosis, hypomagnesemia, hypocalcemia, hyperuricemia), dehydration, pancreatitis (rare), photosensitivity (rare), hypersensitivity (rare), ototoxicity (rare). Frequent: Dizziness, headache, fatigue, muscle cramps, impotence.

TORSEMIDE (*Demadex*) ▶LK ♀B ▶? $
ADULTS — Edema: Start 5 to 20 mg IV/PO daily, double dose as needed to desired response, max 200 mg as a single dose. HTN: Start 5 mg PO daily, increase as needed every 4 to 6 weeks, max 100 mg PO daily or divided bid.
PEDS — Not approved in children.
FORMS — Generic/Trade: Tabs scored 5, 10, 20, 100 mg.
NOTES — Loop diuretics are agent of choice for edema with decreased renal function (CrCl less than 30 mL/min or creatinine more than 2.5 mg/dL).
MOA — Block chloride reabsorption by inhibiting the Na+/K+/Cl- cotransport system in the thick ascending limb of the loop of Henle.
ADVERSE EFFECTS — Serious: Electrolyte imbalances (hypokalemia, hyponatremia, hypochloremic alkalosis, hypomagnesemia, hypocalcemia, hyperuricemia), dehydration, pancreatitis (rare), photosensitivity (rare), hypersensitivity (rare). Frequent: Dizziness, headache, fatigue, muscle cramps, impotence.

CARDIOVASCULAR: Diuretics—Potassium Sparing

NOTE: See also antihypertensive combinations and aldosterone antagonists. Beware of hyperkalemia. Use cautiously with other agents that may cause hyperkalemia (ie, ACE inhibitors, ARBs, aliskiren).

AMILORIDE (*Midamor*) ▶LK ♀B ▶? $$$
 WARNING — May cause hyperkalemia. Incidence is greater with renal impairment, diabetes, or elderly. Monitor potassium levels before initiating therapy, when adjusting diuretic doses, and with illness that may alter renal function.
 ADULTS — Diuretic-induced hypokalemia: Start 5 mg PO daily, increase prn, max 20 mg/day. Edema/HTN: Start 5 mg PO daily in combination with another diuretic, usually a thiazide for HTN, increase prn, max 20 mg/day. Other diuretics may need to be added when treating edema.
 PEDS — Not approved in children.
 UNAPPROVED ADULTS — Hyperaldosteronism: 10 to 40 mg PO daily. Do not use combination product (Moduretic) for treatment of hyperaldosteronism.
 UNAPPROVED PEDS — Edema: 0.625 mg/kg daily for children weighing 6 to 20 kg.
 FORMS — Generic only: Tabs, unscored 5 mg.
 NOTES — Spironolactone is generally preferred for treating primary hyperaldosteronism.
 MOA — Block sodium reabsorption and potassium excretion in the distal tubule.
 ADVERSE EFFECTS — Serious: Hyperkalemia (rare). Frequent: Headache.

TRIAMTERENE (*Dyrenium*) ▶LK ♀B ▶– $$$
 WARNING — May cause hyperkalemia. Incidence is greater with renal impairment, diabetes, or elderly. Monitor potassium frequently, before initiation, when adjusting diuretic doses, and with illness that may alter renal function.
 ADULTS — Edema (cirrhosis, nephrotic syndrome, heart failure): Start 100 mg PO bid, max 300 mg/day. Most patients can be maintained on 100 mg PO daily or every other day after edema is controlled. Other diuretics may be needed.
 PEDS — Not approved in children.
 UNAPPROVED PEDS — Edema: 4 mg/kg/day divided bid after meals, increase to 6 mg/kg/day if needed, max 300 mg/day.
 FORMS — Trade only: Caps 50, 100 mg.
 NOTES — Combo product with HCTZ (eg, Dyazide, Maxzide) available for HTN.
 MOA — Block sodium reabsorption and potassium excretion in the distal tubule.
 ADVERSE EFFECTS — Serious: Hyperkalemia (rare). Frequent: Headache.

CARDIOVASCULAR: Diuretics—Thiazide Type

NOTE: See also antihypertensive combinations. Possible hypersensitivity in sulfa allergy. Should be used for most patients with HTN, alone or combined with other antihypertensive agents. Thiazides are not recommended for gestational HTN. Coadministration with NSAIDs, including selective COX-2 inhibitors, may reduce the antihypertensive, diuretic, and natriuretic effects of thiazides. Thiazide-induced hypokalemia is associated with increased fasting blood glucose and new onset diabetes; keep potassium 4.0 mg/dL or greater to minimize risk; may use thiazide in combination with oral potassium supplementation, ACE inhibitor, ARB, or potassium-sparing diuretic to maintain K+ level.

CHLOROTHIAZIDE (*Diuril*) ▶L ♀C, D if used in pregnancy-induced HTN ▶+ $
 ADULTS — HTN: Start 125 to 250 mg PO daily or divided bid, max 1000 mg/day divided bid. Edema: 500 to 2000 mg PO/IV daily or divided bid. Dosing on alternate days or for 3 to 4 consecutive days followed by no drug for 1 to 2 days is acceptable.
 PEDS — Edema: Infants: Start 10 to 20 mg/kg/day PO daily or divided bid, up to 30 mg/kg/day divided bid. Children 6 mo to 2 yo: 10 to 20 mg/kg/day PO daily or divided bid, max 375 mg/day. Children 2 to 12 yo: Start 10 to 20 mg/kg/day PO daily or divided bid, up to 1 g/day. IV formulation not recommended for infants or children.
 FORMS — Trade only: Susp 250 mg/5 mL. Generic only: Tabs, scored 250, 500 mg.
 NOTES — Do not administer SC or IM.
 MOA — Blocks sodium and chloride reabsorption in the distal tubules.
 ADVERSE EFFECTS — Serious: Electrolyte imbalances (hypokalemia, hyponatremia, hypomagnesemia, hypercalcemia, hyperuricemia), pancreatitis (rare), photosensitivity (rare), hypersensitivity (rare). Frequent: Dizziness, headache, fatigue, muscle cramps, impotence.

CHLORTHALIDONE (*Thalitone*) ▶L ♀B, D if used in pregnancy-induced HTN ▶+ $
 ADULTS — HTN: For generics, start 12.5 to 25 mg PO daily, usual maintenance dose 12.5 to 50 mg/day, max 50 mg/day. For Thalitone, start 15 mg PO daily, usual maintenance 30 to 45 mg/day, max 50 mg/day. Edema: For generics, start 50 to 100 mg PO daily after breakfast or 100 mg every other day or 100 mg 3 times a week, usual maintenance dose 150 to 200 mg/day, max 200 mg/day. For Thalitone, start 30 to 60 mg PO daily or 60 mg every other day, usual maintenance dose 90 to 120 mg PO daily or every other day.
 PEDS — Not approved in children.
 UNAPPROVED ADULTS — Nephrolithiasis: 25 to 50 mg PO daily.
 UNAPPROVED PEDS — Edema: 2 mg/kg PO 3 times a week.
 FORMS — Trade only: Tabs unscored (Thalitone) 15 mg. Generic only: Tabs unscored 25, 50 mg.

(cont.)

CARDIAC PARAMETERS AND FORMULAS

Cardiac output (CO) = heart rate × CVA volume [normal 4-8 l/min]
Cardiac index (CI) = CO/BSA [normal 2.8-4.2 l/min/m^2]
MAP (mean arterial press) = [(SBP - DBP)/3] + DBP [normal 80-100 mmHg]
SVR (systemic vasc resis) = (MAP - CVP) x (80)/CO [normal 800-1200 dyne/sec/cm5]
PVR (pulm vasc resis) = (PAM - PCWP) x (80)/CO [normal 45-120 dyne/sec/cm5]
QTc = QT/square root of RR [normal 0.38-0.42]
Right atrial pressure (central venous pressure) [normal 0-8 mmHg]
Pulmonary artery systolic pressure (PAS) [normal 20-30 mmHg]
Pulmonary artery diastolic pressure (PAD) [normal 10-15 mmHg]
Pulmonary capillary wedge pressure (PCWP) [normal 8-12 mmHg (post-MI ~16 mmHg)]

CHLORTHALIDONE *(cont.)*
 NOTES — Thalitone has greater bioavailability than generic forms, do not interchange. Doses greater than 50 mg/day for HTN are usually associated with hypokalemia with little added BP control.
 MOA — Blocks sodium and chloride reabsorption in the distal tubules and decreases urinary calcium excretion.
 ADVERSE EFFECTS — Serious: Agranulocytosis, aplastic anemia, electrolyte imbalances (hypokalemia, hyponatremia, hypomagnesemia, hypercalcemia, hyperuricemia), pancreatitis (rare), photosensitivity (rare), hypersensitivity (rare), thrombocytopenia. Frequent: Dizziness, headache, fatigue, muscle cramps, impotence.

HYDROCHLOROTHIAZIDE (*HCTZ, Esidrix, Oretic, Microzide, HydroDiuril*) ▶L ♀B, D if used in pregnancy-induced HTN ▶+ $
 ADULTS — HTN: Start 12.5 to 25 mg PO daily, usual maintenance dose 12.5 to 25 mg/day, max 50 mg/day. Edema: 25 to 100 mg PO daily or in divided doses or 50 to 100 mg PO every other day or 3 to 5 days/week, max 200 mg/day.
 PEDS — Edema: 1 to 2 mg/kg/day PO daily or divided bid, max 37.5 mg/day in infants up to 2 yo, max 100 mg/day in children 2 to 12 yo.
 UNAPPROVED ADULTS — Nephrolithiasis: 50 to 100 mg PO daily.
 FORMS — Generic/Trade: Tabs scored 25, 50 mg; Caps 12.5 mg.
 NOTES — Doses as low as 6.25 mg daily may be effective in combination with other antihypertensives. Doses 50 mg/day or greater may cause hypokalemia with little added BP control.
 MOA — Blocks sodium and chloride reabsorption in the distal tubules and decreases urinary calcium excretion.
 ADVERSE EFFECTS — Serious: Agranulocytosis, aplastic anemia, electrolyte imbalances (hypokalemia, hyponatremia, hypomagnesemia, hypercalcemia, hyperuricemia), pancreatitis (rare), photosensitivity (rare), hypersensitivity (rare), thrombocytopenia. Frequent: Dizziness, headache, fatigue, muscle cramps, impotence.

INDAPAMIDE (*Lozol, ✦Lozide*) ▶L ♀B, D if used in pregnancy-induced HTN ▶? $
 ADULTS — HTN: Start 1.25 to 2.5 mg PO daily, max 5 mg/day. Edema/Heart failure: 2.5 to 5 mg PO qam.
 PEDS — Not approved in children.
 FORMS — Generic only: Tabs unscored 1.25, 2.5 mg.
 MOA — Blocks sodium and chloride reabsorption in the distal tubules.
 ADVERSE EFFECTS — Serious: Electrolyte imbalances (hypokalemia, hyponatremia, hypomagnesemia, hypercalcemia, hyperuricemia), pancreatitis (rare), photosensitivity (rare), hypersensitivity (rare). Frequent: Dizziness, headache, fatigue, muscle cramps, impotence.

METHYCLOTHIAZIDE (*Enduron*) ▶L ♀B, D if used in pregnancy-induced HTN ▶? $
 ADULTS — HTN: Start 2.5 mg PO daily, usual maintenance dose 2.5 to 5 mg/day. Edema: Start 2.5 mg PO daily, usual maintenance dose 2.5 to 10 mg/day.
 PEDS — Not approved in children.
 FORMS — Generic/Trade: Tabs, scored, 2.5, 5 mg.
 NOTES — May dose every other day or 3 to 5 days/week as maintenance therapy to control edema.
 MOA — Blocks sodium and chloride reabsorption in the distal tubules.
 ADVERSE EFFECTS — Serious: Electrolyte imbalances (hypokalemia, hyponatremia, hypomagnesemia, hypercalcemia, hyperuricemia), pancreatitis (rare), photosensitivity (rare), hypersensitivity (rare). Frequent: Dizziness, headache, fatigue, muscle cramps, impotence.

METOLAZONE (*Zaroxolyn*) ▶L ♀B, D if used in pregnancy-induced HTN ▶? $$$
 ADULTS — Edema (heart failure, renal disease): 5 to 10 mg PO daily, max 10 mg/day in heart failure, 20 mg/day in renal disease. If used with loop diuretic, start with 2.5 mg PO daily. Reduce to lowest effective dose as edema resolves. May be given every other day as edema resolves.
 PEDS — Not approved in children.
 UNAPPROVED PEDS — Edema: 0.2 to 0.4 mg/kg/day daily or divided bid.
 FORMS — Generic/Trade: Tabs 2.5, 5, 10 mg.
 NOTES — Generally used for heart failure, not HTN. When used with furosemide or other loop diuretics, administer metolazone 30 min before IV loop diuretic. Cross-allergy may occur if allergic to sulfonamides or thiazides. Correct electrolyte imbalances before initiating therapy. Electrolyte imbalances can occur at any time while taking metolazone; teach patients

(cont.)

METOLAZONE (cont.)
to report signs (ex. confusion, dizziness, headache, anorexia, thirst, nausea, vomiting, paresthesia). Combination diuretic therapy may increase the risk of electrolyte disturbances.
MOA — Blocks sodium and chloride reabsorption in the distal tubules.
ADVERSE EFFECTS — Serious: Electrolyte imbalances (hypokalemia, hyponatremia, hypomagnesemia, hypercalcemia, hyperuricemia), pancreatitis (rare), photosensitivity (rare), hypersensitivity (rare). Frequent: Dizziness, headache, fatigue, muscle cramps, impotence.

CARDIOVASCULAR: Nitrates

NOTE: Avoid if systolic BP < 90 mmHg or more than 30 mmHg below baseline, severe bradycardia (< 50 bpm), tachycardia (> 100 bpm) or right ventricular infarction. Avoid in those who have received erectile dysfunction therapy in the last 24 (sildenafil, vardenafil) to 48 (tadalafil) h.

ISOSORBIDE DINITRATE (*Isordil, Dilatrate-SR, ♣Cedocard SR, Coronex*) ▶L ♀C ▶? $
ADULTS — Acute angina: 2.5 to 10 mg SL or chewed immediately, repeat as needed every 5 to 10 min up to 3 doses in 30 min. SL and chew Tabs may be used prior to events likely to provoke angina. Angina prophylaxis: Start 5 to 20 mg PO tid (7 am, noon, and 5 pm), max 40 mg tid. Sustained-release (Dilatrate SR): Start 40 mg PO bid, max 80 mg PO bid (8 am and 2 pm).
PEDS — Not approved in children.
UNAPPROVED ADULTS — Heart failure: 10 to 40 mg PO tid, max 80 mg tid. Use in combination with hydralazine.
FORMS — Generic/Trade: Tabs, scored 5, 10, 20, 30 mg. Trade only: Tabs, (Isordil) 40 mg, Caps, extended-release (Dilatrate-SR) 40 mg. Generic only: Tabs, sustained-release 40 mg, Tabs, sublingual 2.5, 5 mg.
NOTES — Headache possible. Use SL or chew Tabs for an acute angina attack. Extended-release tab may be broken, but do not chew or crush, swallow whole; do not use for acute angina. Allow for a nitrate-free period of 10 to 14 h each day to avoid nitrate tolerance.
MOA — Relaxes cardiac and peripheral smooth muscle (venous greater than arterial).
ADVERSE EFFECTS — Serious: Hypotension, methemoglobinemia (rare). Frequent: Headache, tachycardia, dizziness, flushing.

ISOSORBIDE MONONITRATE (*ISMO, Monoket, Imdur*) ▶L ♀C ▶? $$
ADULTS — Angina: 20 mg PO bid (8 am and 3 pm). Extended-release (Imdur): Start 30 to 60 mg PO daily, max 240 mg/day.
PEDS — Not approved in children.
FORMS — Generic/Trade: Tabs unscored (ISMO, bid dosing) 20 mg, scored (Monoket, bid dosing) 10, 20 mg extended-release, scored (Imdur, daily dosing) 30, 60, unscored 120 mg.
NOTES — Headache. Extended-release tab may be broken, but do not chew or crush, swallow whole. Do not use for acute angina.
MOA — Relaxes cardiac and peripheral smooth muscle (venous greater than arterial).
ADVERSE EFFECTS — Serious: Hypotension, methemoglobinemia (rare). Frequent: Headache, tachycardia, dizziness, flushing.

NITROGLYCERIN INTRAVENOUS INFUSION (*Tridil*) ▶L ♀C ▶? $
ADULTS — Perioperative HTN, acute MI/heart failure, acute angina: Mix 50 mg in 250 mL D5W (200 mcg/mL), start at 10 to 20 mcg/min IV (3 to 6 mL/h), then titrate upward by 10 to 20 mcg/min every 3 to 5 min until desired effect is achieved.
PEDS — Not approved in children.
UNAPPROVED ADULTS — Hypertensive emergency: Start 10 to 20 mcg/min IV infusion, titrate up to 100 mcg/min. Antihypertensive effect is usually evident in 2 to 5 min. Effect may persist for only 3 to 5 min after infusion is stopped.
UNAPPROVED PEDS — IV infusion: Start 0.25 to 0.5 mcg/kg/min, increase by 0.5 to 1 mcg/kg/min q 3 to 5 min as needed, max 5 mcg/kg/min.
FORMS — Brand name "Tridil" no longer manufactured but retained herein for name recognition.
NOTES — Nitroglycerin migrates into polyvinyl chloride (PVC) tubing. Use lower initial doses (5 mcg/min) with nonPVC tubing. Use with caution in inferior/right ventricular MI. Nitroglycerin-induced venodilation can cause severe hypotension.
MOA — Relaxes cardiac and peripheral smooth muscle (venous greater than arterial).
ADVERSE EFFECTS — Serious: Hypotension, methemoglobinemia (rare). Frequent: Headache, tachycardia, dizziness, flushing.

NITROGLYCERIN OINTMENT (*Nitro-BID*) ▶L ♀C ▶? $
ADULTS — Angina prophylaxis: Start 0.5 in q 8 h applied to nonhairy skin area, maintenance 1 to 2 in q 8 h, maximum 4 in q 4 to 6 h.
PEDS — Not approved in children.
FORMS — Trade only: Ointment, 2%, tubes 1, 30, 60 g (Nitro-BID).
NOTES — 1 in ointment is about 15 mg nitroglycerin. Allow for a nitrate-free period of 10 to 14 h each day to avoid nitrate tolerance. Generally change to oral tabs or transdermal patch for long-term therapy. Do not use topical therapy (ointment, transdermal system) for acute angina.
MOA — Relaxes cardiac and peripheral smooth muscle (venous greater than arterial).
ADVERSE EFFECTS — Serious: Hypotension, methemoglobinemia (rare). Frequent: Headache, tachycardia, dizziness, flushing.

CARDIOVASCULAR: Pressors/Inotropes

NITROGLYCERIN SPRAY (*Nitrolingual, NitroMist*) ▶L ♀C ▶? $$$$
ADULTS — <u>Acute angina:</u> 1 to 2 sprays under the tongue at the onset of attack, repeat as needed, max 3 sprays in 15 min. A dose may be given 5 to 10 min before activities that might provoke angina.
PEDS — Not approved in children.
FORMS — Trade only: Nitrolingual soln, 4.9, 12 mL. 0.4 mg/spray (60 or 200 sprays/canister); NitroMist aerosol 0.4 mg/spray (230 sprays/canister).
NOTES — AHA guidelines recommend calling 911 if chest pain not relieved or gets worse after using 1 dose of nitroglycerin. May be preferred over SL tabs in patients with dry mouth. Patient can see how much medicine is left in the upright bottle. Nitrolingual: Replace bottle when fluid is below level of center tube; NitroMist: Replace bottle when fluid reaches the bottom of the hole in the side of the container. Before initial use, prime pump: Nitrolingual, spray 5 times into air (away from self and others); NitroMist, spray 10 times into air (away from self and others). Prime at least once every 6 weeks if not used: Nitrolingual spray 1 time into the air (away from self and others); NitroMist spray twice into the air (away from self and others). Do not shake NitroMist before using.
MOA — Relaxes cardiac and peripheral smooth muscle (venous greater than arterial).
ADVERSE EFFECTS — Serious: Hypotension. Frequent: Headache, tingling/mouth burning, tachycardia, dizziness, flushing.

NITROGLYCERIN SUBLINGUAL (*Nitrostat, NitroQuick*) ▶L ♀C ▶? $
ADULTS — <u>Acute angina:</u> 0.4 mg under tongue or between the cheek and gum, repeat dose every 5 min as needed up to 3 doses in 15 min. A dose may be given 5 to 10 min before activities that might provoke angina.
PEDS — Not approved in children.
FORMS — Generic/Trade: Sublingual tabs unscored 0.3, 0.4, 0.6 mg; in bottles of 100 or package of 4 bottles with 25 tabs each.
NOTES — AHA guidelines recommend calling 911 if chest pain not relieved or gets worse after using 1 dose of nitroglycerin. May produce a burning/tingling sensation when administered, although this should not be used to assess potency. Store in original glass bottle to maintain potency/stability. Traditionally, unused tabs should be discarded 6 months after the original bottle is opened; however, the Nitrostat product is stable for 24 months after the bottle is opened or until the expiration date on the bottle, whichever is earlier. If used rarely, prescribe package with 4 bottles with 25 Tabs each.
MOA — Relaxes cardiac and peripheral smooth muscle (venous greater than arterial).
ADVERSE EFFECTS — Serious: Hypotension. Frequent: Headache, tingling/mouth burning, tachycardia, dizziness, flushing.

NITROGLYCERIN SUSTAINED RELEASE ▶L ♀C ▶? $
ADULTS — <u>Angina prophylaxis:</u> Start 2.5 mg PO bid to tid, then titrate upward as needed.
PEDS — Not approved in children.
FORMS — Generic only: Caps, extended-release 2.5, 6.5, 9 mg.
NOTES — Headache. Extended-release tab may be broken, but do not chew or crush, swallow whole. Caps should be swallowed whole. Do not use extended-release Tabs or Caps for acute angina attack. Allow for a nitrate-free period of 10 to 14 h each day to avoid nitrate tolerance.
MOA — Relaxes cardiac and peripheral smooth muscle (venous greater than arterial).
ADVERSE EFFECTS — Serious: Hypotension, methemoglobinemia (rare). Frequent: Headache, tachycardia, dizziness, flushing.

NITROGLYCERIN TRANSDERMAL (*Minitran, Nitro-Dur, ✣Trinipatch*) ▶L ♀C ▶? $$
ADULTS — <u>Angina prophylaxis:</u> Start with lowest dose and apply 1 patch for 12 to 14 h each day to nonhairy skin.
PEDS — Not approved in children.
FORMS — Generic/Trade: Transdermal system 0.1, 0.2, 0.4, 0.6 mg/h. Trade only: (Nitro-Dur) 0.3, 0.8 mg/h.
NOTES — Do not use topical therapy (ointment, transdermal system) for acute angina attack. Allow for a nitrate-free period of 10 to 14 h each day to avoid nitrate tolerance. Elderly are more risk of hypotension and falling; start at lower doses.
MOA — Relaxes cardiac and peripheral smooth muscle (venous greater than arterial).
ADVERSE EFFECTS — Serious: Hypotension, methemoglobinemia (rare). Frequent: Headache, rash, tachycardia, dizziness, drug tolerance, flushing.

CARDIOVASCULAR: Pressors/Inotropes

DOBUTAMINE (*Dobutrex*) ▶Plasma ♀D ▶— $
ADULTS — <u>Inotropic support in cardiac decompensation</u> (heart failure, surgical procedures): 2 to 20 mcg/kg/min. Mix 250 mg in 250 mL D5W (1 mg/mL); a rate of 21 mL/h delivers 5 mcg/kg/min for a 70 kg patient; alternatively mix 200 mg in 100 mL D5W (2 mg/mL) set at a rate of 10.5 mL/h delivers 5 mcg/kg/min for a 70 kg patient.
PEDS — Not approved in children.
UNAPPROVED PEDS — Use adult dosage. Use lowest effective dose.
NOTES — For short-term use, up to 72 h.
MOA — Stimulates beta-1 receptors (primarily increases cardiac contractility) and stimulates beta-2 receptors (mild peripheral vasodilation).
ADVERSE EFFECTS — Serious: Arrhythmias, tachycardia. Frequent: Hypertension or hypotension.

CARDIOVASCULAR: Pressors/Inotropes

DOPAMINE (*Intropin*) ▶Plasma ♀C ▶– $
WARNING — Avoid extravasation; peripheral ischemia, necrosis, gangrene may occur. If extravasation occurs, infiltrate the area as soon as possible with a solution of phentolamine and normal saline.
ADULTS — Pressor: Start 5 mcg/kg/min, increase as needed by 5 to 10 mcg/kg/min increments at 10 min intervals, max 50 mcg/kg/min. Mix 400 mg in 250 mL D5W (1600 mcg/mL); a rate of 13 mL/h delivers 5 mcg/kg/min in a 70 kg patient. Alternatively, mix 320 mg in 100 mL D5W (3200 mcg/mL) set at a rate of 6.5 mL/h delivers 5 mcg/kg/min in a 70 kg patient.
PEDS — Not approved in children.
UNAPPROVED ADULTS — Symptomatic bradycardia unresponsive to atropine: 5 to 20 mcg/kg/min IV infusion.
UNAPPROVED PEDS — Pressor: Use adult dosage.
NOTES — Doses in mcg/kg/min: 2 to 4 is the traditional renal dose; recent evidence suggests ineffective and active at dopaminergic receptors; 5 to 10 is the cardiac dose: Active at dopaminergic and beta-1 receptors; greater than 10 is active at the dopaminergic, beta-1, and alpha-1 receptors.
MOA — Stimulates beta-1 receptors (increases cardiac contractility and chronotropic effect), stimulates alpha receptors (peripheral vasoconstriction), and stimulates renal dopaminergic receptors (increases renal perfusion).
ADVERSE EFFECTS — Serious: Arrhythmias, tachycardia. Frequent: Hypotension, N/V, palpitations, headache, dyspnea.

EPHEDRINE ▶K ♀C ▶? $
ADULTS — Pressor: 10 to 25 mg IV slow injection, with repeat doses every 5 to 10 min as needed, max 150 mg/day. Orthostatic hypotension: 25 mg PO daily to qid. Bronchospasm: 25 to 50 mg PO q 3 to 4 h prn.
PEDS — Not approved in children.
UNAPPROVED PEDS — Pressor: 3 mg/kg/day SC or IV in 4 to 6 divided doses.
FORMS — Generic only: Caps, 50 mg.
MOA — Stimulates beta-1 receptors (increases cardiac contractility and chronotropic effect), stimulates alpha receptors (peripheral vasoconstriction), stimulates beta-2 receptors (mild peripheral vasodilation).
ADVERSE EFFECTS — Serious: Arrhythmias, tachycardia. Frequent: Hypertension, headache, palpitations, flushing, sweating, dizziness.

EPINEPHRINE (*EpiPen, EpiPen Jr, Twinject, adrenalin*) ▶Plasma ♀C ▶– $
ADULTS — Cardiac arrest: 1 mg (1:10,000 soln) IV, repeat every 3 to 5 min if needed; infusion 1 mg in 250 mL D5W (4 mcg/mL) at rate of 15 to 60 mL/h delivers 1 to 4 mcg/min. Anaphylaxis: 0.1 to 0.5 mg SC/IM (1:1000 soln), may repeat SC dose every 10 to 15 min for anaphylactic shock. Acute asthma and Hypersensitivity reactions: 0.1 to 0.3 mg of 1:1000 soln SC or IM. Hypersensitivity reactions: 0.01 mg/kg SC autoinjector.
PEDS — Cardiac arrest: 0.01 mg/kg IV/intraosseous (IO) (max 1 mg/dose) or 0.1 mg/kg ET (max 10 mg/dose), repeat 0.1 to 0.2 mg/kg IV/IO/ET every 3 to 5 min if needed. Neonates: 0.01 to 0.03 mg/kg IV (preferred) or up to 0.1 mg/kg ET, repeat every 3 to 5 min if needed; IV infusion start 0.1 mcg/kg/min, increase in increments of 0.1 mcg/kg/min if needed, max 1 mcg/kg/min. Anaphylaxis: 0.01 mg/kg (0.01 mL/kg of 1:1000 injection) SC, may repeat SC dose at 20 min to 4 h intervals depending on severity of condition. Acute asthma: 0.01 mL/kg (up to 0.5 mL) of 1:1000 soln SC or IM; repeat q 15 min for 3 to 4 doses prn. Hypersensitivity reactions: 0.01 mg/kg SC autoinjector.
UNAPPROVED ADULTS — Symptomatic bradycardia unresponsive to atropine: 2 to 10 mcg/kg/min IV infusion. ET administration prior to IV access: 2 to 2.5 times the recommended IV dose in 10 mL of NS or distilled water.
FORMS — Soln for injection: 1:1000 (1 mg/mL in 1 mL amps or 10 mL vial). Trade only: EpiPen Autoinjector delivers one 0.3 mg (1:1000, 0.3 mL) IM dose. EpiPen Jr. Autoinjector delivers one 0.15 mg (1:2000, 0.3 mL) IM dose. Twinject Auto-injector delivers one 0.15 mg (1:1000, 0.15 mL) or 0.3 mg (1:1000, 0.3 mL) IM/SQ dose.
NOTES — Cardiac arrest: ADULT: Use the 1:10,000 injectable soln for IV use in cardiac arrest (10 mL = 1 mg); PEDS: Use 1:10,000 for initial IV dose, then 1:1000 for subsequent dosing or ET doses. Anaphylaxis: Use the 1:1000 injectable soln for SC/IM (0.1 mL = 0.1 mg);. consider EpiPen Jr. in patients weighing less than 30 kg. Directions for injectable kit use: Remove cap. Place black tip end on thigh and push down to inject. Hold in place for 10 sec. May be injected directly through clothing.
MOA — Stimulates beta-1 receptors (increases cardiac contractility and chronotropic effect), stimulates alpha receptors (peripheral vasoconstriction), stimulates beta-2 receptors (peripheral vasodilation).
ADVERSE EFFECTS — Serious: Arrhythmias, tachycardia. Frequent: Hypertension, headache, palpitations, flushing, sweating, dizziness.

INAMRINONE ▶K ♀C ▶? $$$$$
ADULTS — Heart failure (NYHA class III, IV): 0.75 mg/kg bolus IV over 2 to 3 min, then infusion 100 mg in 100 mL NS (1 mg/mL); a rate of 21 mL/h delivers 5 mcg/kg/min for a 70 kg patient. An additional IV bolus of 0.75 mg/kg may be given 30 min after initiating therapy if needed. Total daily dose should not exceed 10 mg/kg.
PEDS — Not approved in children.
UNAPPROVED ADULTS — CPR: 0.75 mg/kg bolus IV over 2 to 3 min, followed by 5 to 15 mcg/kg/min.
UNAPPROVED PEDS — Inotropic support: 0.75 mg/kg IV bolus over 2 to 3 min, followed by 3 to 5 mcg/kg/min (neonates) or 5 to 10 mcg/kg/min (children) maintenance infusion.
NOTES — Thrombocytopenia possible. Children may require higher bolus doses, 3 to 4.5 mg/kg. Name changed from "amrinone" to avoid medication errors.

(cont.)

INAMRINONE (cont.)
MOA – Inhibits phosphodiesterase enzyme leading to increased intracellular cAMP (positive inotropic effect).
ADVERSE EFFECTS – Serious: Arrhythmias, hepatotoxicity, thrombocytopenia (prolonged therapy). Frequent: None.

MIDODRINE (*Orvaten, ProAmatine, ♦Amatine*) ▶LK ♀C ▶? $$$$$
WARNING – May cause significant supine HTN. Contraindicated with severe cardiac disease or persistent/excessive supine HTN. Clinical benefits (ie, improved activities of daily living) have not been verified. Use in patients when nonpharmacological treatment fails.
ADULTS – Orthostatic hypotension: Start 10 mg PO tid while awake, increase dose as needed to max 40 mg/day. Renal impairment: Start 2.5 mg tid while awake, increase dose as needed.
PEDS – Not approved in children.
FORMS – Generic/Trade: Tabs, scored 2.5, 5, 10 mg.
NOTES – The last daily dose should be no later than 6 pm to avoid supine HTN during sleep.
MOA – Stimulates alpha receptors (peripheral vasoconstriction).
ADVERSE EFFECTS – Serious: Hypertension. Frequent: Paresthesia, piloerection, pruritus, dysuria, chills.

MILRINONE (*Primacor*) ▶K ♀C ▶? $$
ADULTS – Systolic heart failure (NYHA class III, IV): Load 50 mcg/kg IV over 10 min, then begin IV infusion of 0.375 to 0.75 mcg/kg/min. Renal impairment: Reduce IV infusion rate (mcg/kg/min) as follows: Give 0.2 for CrCl 5 mL/min or less, give 0.23 for CrCl 10 to 6 mL/min, give 0.28 for CrCl 20 to 11 mL/min, give 0.33 for CrCl 30 to 21 mL/min, give 0.38 for CrCl 40 to 31 mL/min, give 0.43 for CrCl 50 to 41 mL/min.
PEDS – Not approved in children.
UNAPPROVED PEDS – Inotropic support: Limited data, 50 mcg/kg IV bolus over 10 min, followed by 0.5 to 1 mcg/kg/min IV infusion, titrate to effect within dosing range.
MOA – Inhibits phosphodiesterase enzyme leading to increased intracellular cAMP (positive inotropic effect).
ADVERSE EFFECTS – Serious: Arrhythmias. Frequent: None.

NOREPINEPHRINE (*Levophed*) ▶Plasma ♀C ▶? $
WARNING – Avoid extravasation; tissue ischemia, necrosis, gangrene may occur. If extravasation occurs, infiltrate area as soon as possible with solution of normal saline and phentolamine.
ADULTS – Acute hypotension: Start 8 to 12 mcg/min, adjust to maintain BP, average maintenance rate 2 to 4 mcg/min, mix 4 mg in 500 mL D5W (8 mcg/mL); a rate of 22.5 mL/h delivers 3 mcg/min. Ideally through central line.
PEDS – Not approved in children.
UNAPPROVED PEDS – Acute hypotension: Start 0.05 to 0.1 mcg/kg/min IV infusion, titrate to desired effect, max dose 2 mcg/kg/min.
NOTES – Avoid extravasation, do not administer IV push or IM.
MOA – Stimulates beta-1 receptors (increases cardiac contractility and chronotropic effect) and stimulates alpha receptors (peripheral vasoconstriction).
ADVERSE EFFECTS – Serious: Arrhythmias, tissue hypoxia. Frequent: Hypertension, headache.

PHENYLEPHRINE—INTRAVENOUS (*Neo-Synephrine*) ▶Plasma ♀C ▶– $
WARNING – Avoid with severe organic cardiac disease, including CAD and dilated cardiomyopathy. Avoid extravasation; peripheral ischemia, necrosis, gangrene can occur. If extravasation occurs, infiltrate as soon as possible with solution of phentolamine and normal saline.
ADULTS – Mild to moderate hypotension: 0.1 to 0.2 mg slow IV injection, do not exceed 0.5 mg in initial dose, repeat dose as needed no less than every 10 to 15 min; 1 to 10 mg SC/IM, initial dose should not exceed 5 mg. Infusion for severe hypotension: 20 mg in 250 mL D5W (80 mcg/mL), start 100 to 180 mcg/min (75 to 135 mL/h), usual dose once BP is stabilized 40 to 60 mcg/min.
PEDS – Not approved in children.
UNAPPROVED PEDS – Mild to moderate hypotension: 5 to 20 mcg/kg IV bolus every 10 to 15 min as needed; 0.1 to 0.5 mcg/kg/min IV infusion, titrate to desired effect.
NOTES – Avoid SC or IM administration during shock, use IV route to ensure drug absorption.
MOA – Stimulates alpha receptors (peripheral vasoconstriction).
ADVERSE EFFECTS – Serious: Arrhythmias. Frequent: Hypertension, headache, N/V, sweating, dizziness.

CARDIOVASCULAR: Pulmonary Arterial Hypertension

BOSENTAN (*Tracleer*) ▶L ♀X ▶–? $$$$$
WARNING – Hepatotoxicity; monitor LFTs prior to starting therapy and monthly thereafter. Contraindicated in pregnancy due to birth defects; women of child bearing age must use reliable contraception and have monthly pregnancy tests. Oral, injectable, transdermal, and implanted contraception must be supplemented with another method. Women of childbearing age need pregnancy test before each refill.
ADULTS – Pulmonary arterial hypertension (PAH): Start 62.5 mg PO bid for 4 weeks, increase to 125 mg bid maintenance dose. With low body weight (< 40 kg) and > 12 years old: 62.5 mg PO bid. Stop bosentan > 36 hr prior to initiating ritonavir; when on ritonavir > 10 days, give bosentan 62.5 mg PO daily or every other day.
PEDS – Not approved in children.
FORMS – Trade only: Tabs, unscored 62.5, 125 mg.

(cont.)

BOSENTAN (cont.)

NOTES — Available only through access program by calling 866-228-3546. Concomitant glyburide or cyclosporine is contraindicated. Induces metabolism of other drugs (eg, contraceptives, simvastatin, lovastatin, atorvastatin). Do not use with both CYP2C9 inhibitor (eg, amiodarone, fluconazole) and strong CYP3A4 inhibitor (eg, ketoconazole, itraconazole, ritonavir) or moderate CYP3A4 inhibitor (eg, amprenavir, erythromycin, fluconazole, diltiazem); will increase levels of bosentan. May decrease warfarin plasma concentration; monitor INR. Rifampin alters bosentan levels; monitor LFTs weekly x 4 wk, followed by normal monitoring. Discontinue with signs of pulmonary edema. Monitor hemoglobin after 1 and 3 months of therapy, then q3 months. May reduce sperm count in some men.

MOA — Blocks binding of endothelin-1 at both endothelin receptors.

ADVERSE EFFECTS — Serious: Hepatotoxicity, pulmonary veno-occlusive disease. Frequent: Anemia, flushing, rash.

EPOPROSTENOL (*Flolan*) ▶Plasma ♀B ▶? $$$$$

ADULTS — <u>Pulmonary arterial hypertension (PAH):</u> Acute dose ranging, 2 ng/kg/min increments via IV infusion until the patient develops symptomatic intolerance (mean maximal dose without symptoms 8.6 ng/kg/min), start continuous IV infusion at 4 ng/kg/min or less than the patient's maximum-tolerated infusion (MTI) rate for acute dose ranging. If the MTI rate is less than 5 ng/kg/min, start chronic IV infusion at ½ the MTI.

PEDS — Not approved in children.

NOTES — Administer by continuous IV infusion via a central venous catheter. Temporary peripheral IV infusions may be used until central access is established. Inhibits platelet aggregation; may increase bleeding risk.

MOA — Stimulates dopamine-1 receptors and alpha-2 receptors (vasodilation).

ADVERSE EFFECTS — Serious: Hypotension, tachycardia, hypokalemia (rare). Frequent: Headache.

ILOPROST (*Ventavis*) ▶L ♀C ▶? $$$$$

ADULTS — <u>Pulmonary arterial hypertension:</u> Start 2.5 mcg/dose by inhalation (as delivered at mouthpiece); if well tolerated increase to 5 mcg/dose by inhalation (as delivered at mouthpiece). Use 6 to 9 times a day (minimum of 2 h between doses) during waking h.

PEDS — Not approved in children.

NOTES — Only administer with Prodose or I-neb AAD Systems. Each single-use ampule delivers 20 mcg to medication chamber of nebulizer and 2.5 or 5 mcg to the mouthpiece; discard remaining soln after each inhalation. Do not mix with other medications. Avoid contact with skin/eyes or oral ingestion. Monitor vital signs when initiating therapy. Do not initiate therapy if SBP less than 85 mmHg. With Child Pugh Class B or C hepatic impairment, consider increasing the dosing interval (eg, 3 to 4 h between doses) depending on patient's response at end of dosing interval. Do not use in patients with moderate to severe hepatic impairment and/or 3 times the upper limit of transaminase or patients on dialysis. May potentiate bleeding risk for patients on anticoagulants. May potentiate hypotensive effects of other medications. Discontinue therapy if pulmonary edema occurs; this may be sign of pulmonary venous hypertension. May induce bronchospasm; carefully monitor patients with COPD, severe asthma, or acute pulmonary infection. Epistaxis and gingival bleeding may occur during first month of therapy.

MOA — Prostacyclin analog. Dilates systemic and pulmonary arteries. Inhibit platelet function.

ADVERSE EFFECTS — Serious: Bronchospasm, hepatotoxicity, hypotension, syncope, thrombosis. Frequent: Cough, flushing, headache, hemoptysis, insomnia, myalgia, N/V, tongue pain, trismus.

SILDENAFIL (*Revatio*) ▶LK ♀B ▶– $$$$

ADULTS — <u>Pulmonary arterial hypertension:</u> 20 mg PO tid, approximately 4 to 6 h apart; or 10 mg IV tid.

PEDS — Not approved in children.

FORMS — Trade only (Revatio): Tabs 20 mg.

NOTES — Do not use with nitrates. Coadministration is not recommended with ritonavir, potent CYP3A inhibitors, or other phosphodiesterase-5 inhibitors. Alpha-blockers may potentiate hypotension. Use not recommended for patients with pulmonary veno-occlusive disease. Sudden vision loss due to nonarteritic ischemic optic neuropathy (NAION) has been reported; patients with prior NAION are at higher risk. Discontinue with sudden decrease/loss of hearing. Teach patients to seek medical attention for vision loss, hearing loss, or erections lasting longer than 4 h.

MOA — Selectively inhibits phosphodiesterase-5 resulting in relaxation of pulmonary vascular smooth muscle bed.

ADVERSE EFFECTS — Serious: MI, CVA, hypotension, syncope, cerebral thrombosis, retinal hemorrhage, vision loss (nonarteritic ischemic optic neuropathy). Frequent: Dyspepsia, dyspnea, erythema, epistaxis, flushing, headache, insomnia, rhinitis.

TADALAFIL (*Adcirca*) ▶L ♀B ▶– $$$$

ADULTS — <u>Pulmonary arterial hypertension:</u> 40 mg PO daily, 20 mg if CrCl less than 80 mL/min or mild to moderate hepatic impairment. Avoid with CrCl less than 30 mL/min or severe hepatic impairment.

PEDS — Not approved in children.

FORMS — Trade only (Adcirca): Tabs 20 mg.

NOTES — Do not use with nitrates; if nitrates needed give no sooner than 48 h after the last tadalafil dose. Coadministration is not recommended with potent CYP3A inhibitors (itraconazole, ketoconazole), potent CYP3A inducers (rifampin), or other phosphodiesterase-5 inhibitors. Caution with ritonavir, see PI for specific dose adjustments. Alpha-blockers or alcohol may potentiate hypotension. Use not recommended for patients with pulmonary veno-occlusive disease. Sudden vision loss due to nonarteritic ischemic optic neuropathy (NAION)

(cont.)

TADALAFIL (cont.)
has been reported; patients with prior NAION are at higher risk. Retinal artery occlusion has been reported. Discontinue with sudden decrease/loss of hearing. Transient global amnesia. Teach patients to seek medical attention for vision loss, hearing loss, or erections lasting longer than 4 h.
MOA — Selectively inhibits phosphodiesterase-5 resulting in relaxation of pulmonary vascular smooth muscle bed.
ADVERSE EFFECTS — Serious: Priapism, hypotension, myocardial infarction, vision loss (nonarteritic ischemic optic neuropathy), retinal artery occlusion. Frequent: Headache, flushing, dyspepsia, back pain.

TREPROSTINIL (*Tyvaso*) ▶KL - ♀B ▶? $$$$$
ADULTS — Pulmonary arterial hypertension: Start 3 breaths (18 mcg) per treatment session qid during waking hours; treatments should be at least 4 hours apart; may reduce initial dose to 1 to 2 breaths per treatment session if 3 breaths not tolerated. May increase by 3 breaths every 1 to 2 weeks as tolerated, max 9 breaths (54 mcg) per treatment qid.
PEDS — Not approved in children.
FORMS — 1.74 mg in 2.9 mL inhalation solution
NOTES — Administer undiluted with the Tyvaso Inhalation System. A single breath delivers about 6 mcg treprostinil; discard remaining solution at the end of each day. Do not mix with other medications. Avoid contact with skin/eyes or oral ingestion. Safety and efficacy not established with existing lung disease (asthma, COPD). Carefully monitor patients with acute pulmonary infection. May need to adjust doses if CYP2C8 inducers (rifampin) or CYP2C8 inhibitors (gemfibrozil). Use cautiously in the elderly and those with liver or renal dysfunction. May potentiate bleeding risk for patients on anticoagulants. May potentiate hypotensive effects of other medications.
MOA — Endothelin receptor antagonist. Vasodilates pulmonary and systemic arteries and inhibits platelet aggregation.
ADVERSE EFFECTS — Serious: Hypotension, may increase risk of bleeding. Frequent: Cough, flushing, headache, diarrhea, nausea, rash, pharyngollaryngeal pain.

TREPROSTINIL SODIUM (*Remodulin*) ▶KL ♀B ▶? $$$$$
ADULTS — Continuous SC (preferred) or central IV infusion in pulmonary arterial HTN with NYHA Class II to IV symptoms: 1 Start 1.25 ng/kg/min based on ideal body wt. Reduce to 0.625 ng/kg/min if initial dose not tolerated. Dose based on clinical response and tolerance. Increase by no more than 1.25 ng/kg/min/week in first 4 weeks, then increase by no more than 2.5 ng/kg/min/week. Max 40 ng/kg/min. Mild to moderate hepatic insufficiency: Start 0.625 ng/kg/min based on ideal body wt; increase cautiously. Not studied with severe hepatic insufficiency. Transitioning from epoprostenol: Must be done in hospital; initiate at 10% epoprostenol dose; gradually increase dose as epoprostenol dose is decreased (see chart in package insert).
PEDS — Not approved in children.
NOTES — Use cautiously in the elderly and those with liver or renal dysfunction. Initiate in setting with personnel and equipment for physiological monitoring and emergency care. Administer by continuous infusion using infusion pump. Patient must have access to backup infusion pump and infusion sets. Must dilute prior to giving IV; see package insert for details. May potentiate bleeding risk for patients on anticoagulants. May potentiate hypotensive effects of other medications.
MOA — Endothelin receptor antagonist. Vasodilates pulmonary and systemic arteries and inhibits platelet aggregation.
ADVERSE EFFECTS — Serious: Hypotension, may increase risk of bleeding, sepsis (from indwelling catheter). Frequent: Pain at infusion site, local reaction at infusion site, headache, diarrhea, nausea, rash, jaw pain, vasodilation.

CARDIOVASCULAR: Thrombolytics

ALTEPLASE (*tpa, t-PA, Activase, Cathflo, ✦Activase rt-PA*) ▶L ♀C ▶? $$$$$
ADULTS — Acute MI: 15 mg IV bolus, then 50 mg IV over 30 min, then 35 mg IV over the next 60 min for wt greater than 67 kg, 15 mg IV bolus, then 0.75 mg/kg (max 50 mg) over 30 min, then 0.5 mg/kg (max 35 mg) over the next 60 min for wt 67 kg or less. Concurrent heparin infusion. Acute ischemic CVA with symptoms 3 h or less: 0.9 mg/kg (max 90 mg); give 10% of total dose as an IV bolus, and the remainder IV over 60 min. Multiple exclusion criteria. Acute pulmonary embolism: 100 mg IV over 2 h, then restart heparin when PTT twice normal or less. Occluded central venous access device: 2 mg/mL in catheter for 2 h. May use second dose if needed.
PEDS — Occluded central venous access device: Wt at least 10 kg but less than 30 kg: Dose equal to 110% of the internal lumen volume, not to exceed 2 mg/2 mL. Other uses not approved in children.
NOTES — Must be reconstituted. Soln must be used within 8 h after reconstitution.
MOA — Enhances conversion of plasminogen to plasmin to achieve fibrinolysis.
ADVERSE EFFECTS — Serious: Bleeding, intracranial hemorrhage, hypersensitivity. Frequent: N/V, bleeding, hypotension, fever.

RETEPLASE (*Retavase*) ▶L ♀C ▶? $$$$$
ADULTS — Acute MI: 10 units IV over 2 min; repeat 1 dose in 30 min.
PEDS — Not approved in children.
NOTES — Must be reconstituted with sterile water for injection to 1 mg/mL concentration. Soln must be used within 4 h after reconstitution.

(cont.)

CARDIOVASCULAR: Volume Expanders

THROMBOLYTIC THERAPY FOR ACUTE MI

Indications (if high-volume cath lab unavailable): Clinical history & presentation strongly suggestive of MI within 12 h plus at least 1 of the following: 1 mm ST elevation in at least 2 contiguous leads; new left BBB; or 2 mm ST depression in V1-4 suggestive of true posterior MI.

Absolute contraindications: Previous cerebral hemorrhage, known cerebral aneurysm or arteriovenous malformation, known intracranial neoplasm, recent (<3 months) ischemic CVA (except acute ischemic CVA < 3 h), aortic dissection, active bleeding or bleeding diathesis (excluding menstruation), significant closed head or facial trauma (<3 months).

Relative contraindications: Severe uncontrolled HTN (>180/110 mm Hg) on presentation or chronic severe HTN; prior ischemic CVA (>3 months), dementia, other intracranial pathology; traumatic/prolonged (>10 min) cardiopulmonary resuscitation; major surgery (<3 weeks); recent (within 2–4 weeks) internal bleeding; puncture of noncompressible vessel; pregnancy; active peptic ulcer disease; current use of anticoagulants. For streptokinase/anistreplase: prior exposure (>5 days ago) or prior allergic reaction.

Reference: *Circulation* 2004;110:588–636

RETEPLASE *(cont.)*
MOA – Enhances conversion of plasminogen to plasmin.
ADVERSE EFFECTS – Serious: Bleeding. Frequent: None.

STREPTOKINASE (*Streptase, Kabikinase*) ▶L ♀C ▶? $$$$$
ADULTS – <u>Acute MI:</u> 1.5 million units IV over 60 min. <u>Pulmonary embolism:</u> 250,000 units IV loading dose over 30 min, followed by 100,000 units/h IV infusion for 24 h (maintain infusion for 72 h if concurrent DVT suspected). <u>DVT:</u> 250,000 units IV loading dose over 30 min, followed by 100,000 units/h IV infusion for 24 h. <u>Occluded arteriovenous catheter:</u> 250,000 units instilled into the catheter, remove soln containing 250,000 units of drug from catheter after 2 h using a 5 mL syringe.
PEDS – Not approved in children.
NOTES – Must be reconstituted. Soln must be used within 8 h of reconstitution. Do not shake vial. Do not repeat use in less than 1 year. Do not use with history of severe allergic reaction.
MOA – Enhances conversion of plasminogen to plasmin.
ADVERSE EFFECTS – Serious: Bleeding, hypersensitivity (rare). Frequent: None.

TENECTEPLASE (*TNKase*) ▶L ♀C ▶? $$$$$
ADULTS – <u>Acute MI:</u> Single IV bolus dose over 5 sec based on body wt; 30 mg for wt less than 60 kg, 35 mg for wt 60 to 69 kg, 40 mg for wt 70 to 79 kg, 45 mg for wt 80 to 89 kg, 50 mg for wt 90 kg or more.
PEDS – Not approved in children.
NOTES – Must be reconstituted. Soln must be used within 8 h after reconstitution.

MOA – Enhances conversion of plasminogen to plasmin.
ADVERSE EFFECTS – Serious: Bleeding. Frequent: None.

UROKINASE (*Kinlytic*) ▶L ♀B ▶? $$$$$
ADULTS – <u>Pulmonary embolism:</u> 4400 units/kg IV loading dose over 10 min, followed by IV infusion 4400 units/kg/h for 12 h. <u>Occluded IV catheter:</u> 5000 units instilled into the catheter with a tuberculin syringe, remove soln containing 5000 units of drug from catheter after 5 min using a 5 mL syringe. Aspiration attempts may be repeated q 5 min. If unsuccessful, cap catheter and allow 5000 unit soln to remain in catheter for 30 to 60 min before again attempting to aspirate soln and residual clot.
PEDS – Not approved in children.
UNAPPROVED ADULTS – <u>Acute MI:</u> 2 to 3 million units IV infusion over 45 to 90 min. Give ½ the total dose as a rapid initial IV injection over 5 min.
UNAPPROVED PEDS – <u>Arterial or venous thrombosis:</u> 4400 units/kg IV loading dose over 10 min, followed by 4400 units/kg/h for 12 to 72 h. <u>Occluded IV catheter:</u> 5000 units instilled into the catheter with a tuberculin syringe, remove solution containing 5000 units of drug from catheter after 5 min using a 5 mL syringe.
NOTES – Must be reconstituted. Do not shake vial.
MOA – Enhances conversion of plasminogen to plasmin.
ADVERSE EFFECTS – Serious: Bleeding, hypersensitivity (rare). Frequent: None.

CARDIOVASCULAR: Volume Expanders

ALBUMIN (*Albuminar, Buminate, Albumarc, ♣Plasbumin*) ▶L ♀C ▶? $$$$$
ADULTS – <u>Shock, burns:</u> 500 mL of 5% soln (50 mg/mL) infused as rapidly as tolerated. Repeat infusion in 30 min if response is inadequate. 25% soln may be used with or without dilution if necessary. Undiluted 25% soln should be infused at 1 mL/min to avoid too rapid plasma volume expansion.
PEDS – <u>Shock, burns:</u> 10 to 20 mL/kg IV infusion at 5 to 10 mL/min using 50 mL of 5% soln.

(cont.)

ALBUMIN (cont.)
UNAPPROVED PEDS – Shock/hypovolemia: 1 g/kg/dose IV rapid infusion. Hypoproteinemia: 1 g/kg/dose IV infusion over 30 to 120 min.
NOTES – Fever, chills. Monitor for plasma volume overload (dyspnea, fluid in lungs, abnormal increase in BP or CVP). Less likely to cause hypotension than plasma protein fraction, more purified. In treating burns, large volumes of crystalloid solns (0.9% sodium chloride) are used to maintain plasma volume with albumin. Use 5% soln in pediatric hypovolemic patients. Use 25% soln in pediatric patients with volume restrictions.
MOA – Expands plasma volume.
ADVERSE EFFECTS – Serious: Pulmonary edema (rapid infusion), hypersensitivity (rare), bleeding. Frequent: Hypotension (rapid infusion), fever, chills, itching.

DEXTRAN (*Rheomacrodex, Gentran, Macrodex*) ▶K ♀C ▶? $$
ADULTS – Shock/hypovolemia: Dextran 40, Dextran 70 and 75, up to 20 mL/kg during the first 24 h, up to 10 mL/kg/day thereafter, do not continue for longer than 5 days. The first 500 mL may be infused rapidly with CVP monitoring. DVT/PE prophylaxis during surgery: Dextran 40, 50 to 100 g IV infusion the day of surgery, continue for 2 to 3 days postop with 50 g/day. 50 g/day may be given every 2nd or 3rd day thereafter up to 14 days.
PEDS – Total dose should not exceed 20 mL/kg.
UNAPPROVED ADULTS – DVT/PE prophylaxis during surgery: Dextran 70 and 75 solns have been used. Other uses: To improve circulation with sickle cell crisis, prevention of nephrotoxicity with radiographic contrast media, toxemia of late pregnancy.
NOTES – Monitor for plasma volume overload (dyspnea, fluid in lungs, abnormal increase in BP or CVP) and anaphylactoid reactions. May impair platelet function. Less effective that other agents for DVT/PE prevention.
MOA – Expands plasma volume.

ADVERSE EFFECTS – Serious: Pulmonary edema (rapid infusion), anaphylaxis (rare), bleeding. Frequent: Hypotension (rapid infusion), fever, chills, itching.

HETASTARCH (*Hespan, Hextend*) ▶K ♀C ▶? $$
ADULTS – Shock/hypovolemia: 500 to 1000 mL IV infusion, total daily dose usually should not exceed 20 mL/kg (1500 mL). Renal impairment: CrCl less than 10 mL/min, usual initial dose followed by 20 to 25% of usual dose.
PEDS – Not approved in children.
UNAPPROVED PEDS – Shock/hypovolemia: 10 mL/kg/dose; do not exceed 20 mL/kg/day.
NOTES – Monitor for plasma volume overload (dyspnea, fluid in lungs, abnormal increase in BP or CVP). Little or no antigenic properties compared to dextran.
MOA – Expands plasma volume.
ADVERSE EFFECTS – Serious: Pulmonary edema (rapid infusion), hypersensitivity (rare), bleeding. Frequent: Hypotension (rapid infusion), fever, chills, itching.

PLASMA PROTEIN FRACTION (*Plasmanate, Protenate, Plasmatein*) ▶L ♀C ▶? $$$
ADULTS – Shock/hypovolemia: Adjust initial rate according to clinical response and BP, but rate should not exceed 10 mL/min. As plasma volume normalizes, infusion rate should not exceed 5 to 8 mL/min. Usual dose 250 to 500 mL. Hypoproteinemia: 1000 to 1500 mL/day IV infusion.
PEDS – Shock/hypovolemia: Initial dose 6.6 to 33 mL/kg infused at a rate of 5 to 10 mL/min.
NOTES – Fever, chills, hypotension with rapid infusion. Monitor for plasma volume overload (dyspnea, fluid in lungs, abnormal increase in BP or CVP). Less pure than albumin products.
MOA – Expands plasma volume.
ADVERSE EFFECTS – Serious: Pulmonary edema (rapid infusion), hypersensitivity (rare), bleeding. Frequent: Hypotension (rapid infusion), fever, chills, itching.

CARDIOVASCULAR: Other

BIDIL (hydralazine + isosorbide dinitrate) ▶LK ♀C ▶? $$$$$
ADULTS – Heart failure (adjunct to standard therapy in black patients): Start 1 tab PO tid, increase as tolerated to max 2 tabs tid. May decrease to ½ tab tid with intolerable side effects; try to increase dose when side effects subside.
PEDS – Not approved in children.
FORMS – Trade only: Tabs, scored 37.5/20 mg.
NOTES – See component drugs.
MOA – See component drugs.
ADVERSE EFFECTS – See component drugs

CILOSTAZOL (*Pletal*) ▶L ♀C ▶? $$$$
WARNING – Contraindicated in heart failure of any severity due to decreased survival.
ADULTS – Intermittent claudication: 100 mg PO bid on empty stomach. 50 mg PO bid with CYP 3A4 inhibitors (like ketoconazole, itraconazole, erythromycin, diltiazem) or CYP 2C19 inhibitors (like omeprazole). Beneficial effect may take up to 12 weeks.
PEDS – Not approved in children.
FORMS – Generic/Trade: Tabs 50, 100 mg.
NOTES – Caution with moderate/severe liver impairment or CrCl less than 25 mL/min. Give with other antiplatelet therapy (aspirin or clopidogrel) when treating lower extremity peripheral arterial disease to reduce cardiovascular risk. Grapefruit juice may increase levels and the risk of side effects.
MOA – Inhibits platelet aggregation and causes vasodilation by blocking the effects of phosphodiesterase III enzyme.
ADVERSE EFFECTS – Serious: Heart failure exacerbation, cerebral/pulmonary hemorrhage,

(cont.)

CARDIOVASCULAR: Other

CILOSTAZOL (cont.)
Stevens-Johnson syndrome, thrombocytopenia. Frequent: Palpitations, dizziness, nausea, diarrhea, dyspepsia, headache.

ISOXSUPRINE (Vasodilan) ▶KL ♀C ▶? $$
ADULTS — Adjunctive therapy for cerebral vascular insufficiency and PVD: 10 to 20 mg PO tid to qid.
PEDS — Not approved in children.
FORMS — Generic/Trade: Tabs, 10, 20 mg.
NOTES — Drug has questionable therapeutic effect.
MOA — Blocks alpha receptors (peripheral vasodilation) and stimulates beta receptors (peripheral vasodilation).
ADVERSE EFFECTS — Serious: Rash. Frequent: Tachycardia, hypotension, chest pain, N/V, abdominal discomfort, dizziness, weakness.

NESIRITIDE (Natrecor) ▶K, plasma ♀C ▶? $$$$$
ADULTS — Hospitalized patients with decompensated heart failure with dyspnea at rest: 2 mcg/kg IV bolus over 60 sec, then 0.01 mcg/kg/min IV infusion for up to 48 h. Do not initiate at higher doses. Limited experience with increased doses: 0.005 mcg/kg/min increments, preceded by 1 mcg/kg bolus, no more frequently than q 3 h up to max infusion dose 0.03 mcg/kg/min. Mix 1.5 mg vial in 250 mL D5W (6 mcg/mL). a bolus of 23.3 mL is 2 mcg/kg for a 70 kg patient, infusion set at rate 7 mL/h delivers a 0.01 mcg/kg/min for a 70 kg patient.
PEDS — Not approved in children.
NOTES — May increase mortality; meta-analysis showed nonstatistically significant increased risk of death within 30 days post treatment compared with noninotropic control group. Not indicated for outpatient infusion, for scheduled repetitive use, to improve renal function, or to enhance diuresis. Contraindicated as primary therapy for cardiogenic shock and when SBP less than 90 mmHg. Discontinue if dose-related symptomatic hypotension occurs and support BP prn. May restart infusion with dose reduced by 30% (no bolus dose) once BP stabilized. Do not shake reconstituted vial, and dilute vial prior to administration. Incompatible with most injectable drugs; administer agents using separate IV lines. Do not measure BNP levels while infusing; may measure BNP at least 2 to 6 h after infusion completion.
MOA — Human B-type natriuretic peptide that relaxes cardiac smooth muscle (arterial and venous vasodilation).
ADVERSE EFFECTS — Serious: Arrhythmias, altered kidney function. Frequent: Hypotension, headache, insomnia, dizziness, nausea.

PAPAVERINE ▶LK ♀C ▶? $
ADULTS — Cerebral and peripheral ischemia: Start 150 mg PO bid, increase to max 300 mg bid if needed. Start 30 mg IV/IM, dose range 30 to 120 mg q 3 h prn. Give IV doses over 1 to 2 min.
PEDS — Not approved in children.
FORMS — Generic only: Caps, extended-release, 150 mg.
MOA — Relaxes smooth muscle (vasodilation).
ADVERSE EFFECTS — Serious: Arrhythmias, hepatitis (rare). Frequent: Tachycardia, vertigo, drowsiness, headache, nausea, abdominal discomfort, flushing.

PENTOXIFYLLINE (Trental) ▶L ♀C ▶? $$$
ADULTS — Intermittent claudication: 400 mg PO tid with meals. For CNS/GI adverse effects, decrease dose to 400 mg PO bid. Beneficial effect may take up to 8 weeks. May be less effective in relieving cramps, tiredness, tightness, and pain during exercise.
PEDS — Not approved in children.
FORMS — Generic/Trade: Tabs, extended-release 400 mg.
NOTES — Contraindicated with recent cerebral/retinal bleed. Increases theophylline levels. Increases INR with warfarin.
MOA — Decreases blood viscosity and improves erythrocyte flexibility.
ADVERSE EFFECTS — None.

RANOLAZINE (Ranexa) ▶LK ♀C ▶? $$$$
ADULTS — Chronic angina: 500 mg PO bid, increase to 1000 mg PO bid prn based on clinical symptoms, max 2000 mg daily. Max 500 mg bid, if used with diltiazem, verapamil, or moderate CYP3A inhibitors.
PEDS — Not approved in children.
FORMS — Trade only: Tabs extended-release 500, 1000 mg.
NOTES — Baseline and follow-up ECGs; may prolong QT interval. Contraindicated with hepatic clinically significant impairment, potent CYP 3A4 inhibitors (eg, clarithromycin, protease inhibitors, itraconazole, ketoconazole, nefazodone), CYP3A inducers (eg, carbamazepine, phenobarbital, phenytoin, rifabutin, rifapentine, rifampin, St John's wort). Limit dose of ranolazine to max 500 mg bid with moderate CYP3A inhibitors (eg, aprepitant, diltiazem, erythromycin, fluconazole, grapefruit juice-containing products, verapamil), Down-titrate ranolazine based on clinical response when given with concomitant P-gp inhibitors (eg, cyclosporin). Increases levels of digoxin; monitor and adjust dose of digoxin. May increase levels of antipsychotics, simvastatin, tricyclic antidepressants. Swallow whole; do not crush, break, or chew. May be less effective in women. Instruct patients to report palpitations or fainting spells.
MOA — Unknown; inhibits late sodium current at therapeutic levels. Antianginal and anti-ischemic effects not dependent on HR or BP.
ADVERSE EFFECTS — Serious: QT prolongation. Frequent: Constipation, dizziness, headache, nausea.

CONTRAST MEDIA: MRI Contrast—Gadolinium-based

NOTE: Avoid gadolinium-based contrast agents if severe renal insufficiency (GFR less than 30 mL/min/1.73 m2) due to risk of nephrogenic systemic fibrosis/nephrogenic fibrosing dermopathy. Similarly avoid in acute renal insufficiency of any severity due to hepatorenal syndrome or during the perioperative phase of liver transplant.

GADOBENATE (*MultiHance*) ▶K ♀C ▶? $$$$
ADULTS — Noniodinated, nonionic IV contrast for MRI.
PEDS — Not approved in children.
MOA — Gadolinium-based noniodinated, nonionic IV contrast for MRI.
ADVERSE EFFECTS — Serious: Hypersensitivity, nephropathy. Frequent: None.

GADODIAMIDE (*Omniscan*) ▶K ♀C ▶? $$$$
ADULTS — Noniodinated, no-ionic IV contrast for MRI.
PEDS — Noniodinated, nonionic IV contrast for MRI.
NOTES — Use caution if renal disease. May falsely lower serum calcium. Not for intrathecal use.
MOA — Gadolinium-based noniodinated, nonionic IV contrast for MRI.
ADVERSE EFFECTS — Serious: Hypersensitivity, nephropathy. Frequent: None.

GADOPENTETATE (*Magnevist*) ▶K ♀C ▶? $$$
ADULTS — Noniodinated IV contrast for MRI.
PEDS — Age older than 2 yo: Noniodinated IV contrast for MRI.
NOTES — Use caution in sickle cell and renal disease.
MOA — Gadolinium-based noniodinated IV contrast for MRI.

ADVERSE EFFECTS — Serious: Hypersensitivity, nephropathy. Frequent: None.

GADOTERIDOL (*Prohance*) ▶K ♀C ▶? $$$$
ADULTS — Noniodinated, nonionic IV contrast for MRI.
PEDS — Age older than 2 yo: Noniodinated, nonionic IV contrast for MRI.
NOTES — Use caution in sickle cell and renal disease.
MOA — Gadolinium-based noniodinated, nonionic IV contrast for MRI.
ADVERSE EFFECTS — Serious: Hypersensitivity, nephropathy. Frequent: None.

GADOVERSETAMIDE (*OptiMARK*) ▶K ♀C ▶– $$$$
ADULTS — Noniodinated IV contrast for MRI.
PEDS — Not approved in children.
NOTES — Use caution in sickle cell and renal disease.
MOA — Gadolinium-based noniodinated IV contrast for MRI.
ADVERSE EFFECTS — Serious: Hypersensitivity, nephropathy. Frequent: None.

CONTRAST MEDIA: MRI Contrast—Other

FERUMOXIDES (*Feridex*) ▶L ♀C ▶? $$$$
ADULTS — Noniodinated, nonionic, iron-based IV contrast for hepatic MRI.
PEDS — Not approved in children.
NOTES — Contains dextran.
MOA — Noniodinated, nonionic, iron-based IV contrast for hepatic MRI.
ADVERSE EFFECTS — Serious: Hypersensitivity. Frequent: None.

FERUMOXSIL (*GastroMARK*) ▶L ♀B ▶? $$$$
ADULTS — Noniodinated, nonionic, iron-based, oral GI contrast for MRI.
PEDS — Not approved in children younger than 16 yo.
MOA — Noniodinated, nonionic, iron-based, oral GI contrast for MRI.
ADVERSE EFFECTS — Serious: Hypersensitivity. Frequent: Abdominal pain, N/V.

MANGAFODIPIR (*Teslascan*) ▶L ♀– ▶– $$$$
ADULTS — Noniodinated IV contrast for MRI.
PEDS — Not approved in children.
NOTES — Contains manganese.
MOA — Noniodinated IV contrast for MRI.
ADVERSE EFFECTS — Serious: Hypersensitivity. Frequent: Headache.

CONTRAST MEDIA: Radiography Contrast

NOTE: Beware of allergic or anaphylactoid reactions. Avoid IV contrast in renal insufficiency or dehydration. Hold metformin (Glucophage) prior to or at the time of iodinated contrast dye use and for 48 h after procedure. Restart after procedure only if renal function is normal.

BARIUM SULFATE ▶Not absorbed ♀? ▶+ $
ADULTS — Noniodinated GI (eg, oral, rectal) contrast.
PEDS — Noniodinated GI (eg, oral, rectal) contrast.
NOTES — Contraindicated if suspected esophageal, gastric, or intestinal perforation. Use with caution in GI obstruction. May cause abdominal distention, cramping, and constipation with oral use.
MOA — Noniodinated GI contrast.
ADVERSE EFFECTS — Serious: Hypersensitivity, worsening of bowel obstruction. Frequent: Constipation. None.

DIATRIZOATE (*Cystografin, Gastrografin, Hypaque, MD-Gastroview, RenoCal, Reno-DIP, Reno-60, Renografin*) ▶K ♀C ▶? $
WARNING — Not for intrathecal or epidural use.
ADULTS — Iodinated, ionic, high osmolality IV or GI contrast.
PEDS — Iodinated, ionic, high osmolality IV or GI contrast.
NOTES — High osmolality contrast may cause tissue damage if infiltrated/extravasated. IV: Hypaque,

(cont.)

DIATRIZOATE (cont.)
Renografin, Reno-DIP, RenoCal. GI: Gastrografin, MD-Gastroview.
MOA — Iodinated, ionic, high-osmolality IV or GI contrast.
ADVERSE EFFECTS — Serious: Hypersensitivity. Frequent: None.

IODIXANOL (*Visipaque*) ▶K ♀B ▶? $$$
ADULTS — Iodinated, nonionic, iso-osmolar IV contrast.
PEDS — Iodinated, nonionic, iso-osmolar IV contrast.
NOTES — Not for intrathecal use.
MOA — Iodinated, nonionic, low osmolality IV contrast.
ADVERSE EFFECTS — Serious: Hypersensitivity. Frequent: None.

IOHEXOL (*Omnipaque*) ▶K ♀B ▶? $$$
ADULTS — Iodinated, nonionic, low osmolality IV and oral/body cavity contrast.
PEDS — Iodinated, nonionic, low osmolality IV and oral/body cavity contrast.
MOA — Iodinated, nonionic, low osmolality IV and oral/body cavity contrast.
ADVERSE EFFECTS — Serious: Hypersensitivity. Frequent: None.

IOPAMIDOL (*Isovue*) ▶K ♀? ▶? $$
ADULTS — Iodinated, nonionic, low osmolality IV contrast.
PEDS — Iodinated, nonionic, low osmolality IV contrast.
MOA — Iodinated, nonionic, low osmolality IV contrast.
ADVERSE EFFECTS — Serious: Hypersensitivity. Frequent: None.

IOPROMIDE (*Ultravist*) ▶K ♀B ▶? $$$
ADULTS — Iodinated, nonionic, low osmolality IV contrast.
PEDS — Iodinated, nonionic, low osmolality IV contrast.
MOA — Iodinated, nonionic, low osmolality IV contrast.
ADVERSE EFFECTS — Serious: Hypersensitivity. Frequent: None.

IOTHALAMATE (*Conray, ✦Vascoray*) ▶K ♀B ▶– $
ADULTS — Iodinated, ionic, high osmolality IV contrast.
PEDS — Iodinated, ionic, high osmolality IV contrast.
NOTES — High osmolality contrast may cause tissue damage if infiltrated/extravasated.
MOA — Iodinated, ionic, high osmolality IV contrast.
ADVERSE EFFECTS — Serious: Hypersensitivity. Frequent: None.

IOVERSOL (*Optiray*) ▶K ♀B ▶? $$
ADULTS — Iodinated, nonionic, low osmolality IV contrast.
PEDS — Iodinated, nonionic, low osmolality IV contrast.
MOA — Iodinated, nonionic, low osmolality IV contrast.
ADVERSE EFFECTS — Serious: Hypersensitivity. Frequent: None.

IOXAGLATE (*Hexabrix*) ▶K ♀B ▶– $$$
ADULTS — Iodinated, ionic, low osmolality IV contrast.
PEDS — Iodinated, ionic, low osmolality IV contrast.
MOA — Iodinated, ionic, low osmolality IV contrast.
ADVERSE EFFECTS — Serious: Hypersensitivity. Frequent: None.

IOXILAN (*Oxilan*) ▶K ♀B ▶– $$$
ADULTS — Iodinated, nonionic, low osmolality IV contrast.
PEDS — Iodinated, nonionic, low osmolality IV contrast.
MOA — Iodinated, nonionic, low osmolality IV contrast.
ADVERSE EFFECTS — Serious: Hypersensitivity. Frequent: None.

DERMATOLOGY: Acne Preparations

NOTE: For topical agents, wash area prior to application. Wash hands before and after application; avoid eye area.

ACANYA (clindamycin + benzoyl peroxide) ▶K ♀C ▶+ $$$$
ADULTS — Acne: Apply once daily.
PEDS — Not approved in children 12 yo or younger.
FORMS — Trade only: Gel (clindamycin 1.2% + benzoyl peroxide 2.5%) 50 g.
NOTES — Expires 2 months after mixing.
MOA — Antibacterial + drying and sebostatic effects.
ADVERSE EFFECTS — Frequent: Dryness, scaling, erythema, burning, pruritus. Severe: C. difficile-associated diarrhea, anaphylaxis.

ADAPALENE (*Differin*) ▶Bile ♀C ▶? $$$$
ADULTS — Acne: Apply at bedtime.
PEDS — Not approved in children.
UNAPPROVED PEDS — Acne: Apply at bedtime.
FORMS — Generic/Trade: Gel 0.1%. Cream 0.1% (45 g). Trade only: Gel 0.3% (45 g). Soln 0.1% (30 mL). Swabs 0.1% (60 ea).
NOTES — During early weeks of therapy, acne exacerbation may occur. May cause erythema, scaling, dryness, pruritus, and burning in up to 40% of patients. Therapeutic results take 8 to 12 weeks.
MOA — Modulates cellular differentiation, inflammation, keratinization.
ADVERSE EFFECTS — Frequent: Dryness, scaling, erythema, burning, pruritus.

AZELAIC ACID (*Azelex, Finacea, Finevin*) ▶K ♀B ▶? $$$$
ADULTS — Acne (Azelex, Finevin): Apply bid. Rosacea (Finacea): Apply bid.
PEDS — Not approved in children.
UNAPPROVED ADULTS — Melasma: Apply bid.
UNAPPROVED PEDS — Acne: Apply at bedtime.
FORMS — Trade only: Cream 20%, 30, 50 g (Azelex). Gel 15% 50 g (Finacea).
NOTES — Improvement of acne occurs within 4 weeks. Monitor for hypopigmentation especially in

(cont.)

DERMATOLOGY: Acne Preparations

AZELAIC ACID (cont.)
patients with dark complexions. Avoid use of occlusive dressings.
MOA – May possess antibacterial activity.
ADVERSE EFFECTS – Frequent: Dryness, scaling, erythema, burning, stinging, tingling, pruritus.

BENZACLIN (clindamycin + benzoyl peroxide) ▶K ♀C ▶+ $$$$
ADULTS – Acne: Apply bid.
PEDS – Not approved in children.
UNAPPROVED PEDS – Acne: Apply at bedtime.
FORMS – Generic/Trade: Gel (clindamycin 1% + benzoyl peroxide 5%) 50 g (jar). Trade only: 25, 35 g (jar) and 50 g (pump).
NOTES – Expires 10 weeks after mixing.
MOA – Antibacterial + drying and sebostatic effects.
ADVERSE EFFECTS – Frequent: Dryness, scaling, erythema, burning, pruritus. Severe: C. difficile-associated diarrhea, allergic reactions/hypersensitivity.

BENZAMYCIN (erythromycin base + benzoyl peroxide) ▶LK ♀C ▶? $$$
ADULTS – Acne: Apply bid.
PEDS – Not approved in children.
UNAPPROVED PEDS – Acne: Apply at bedtime.
FORMS – Generic/Trade: Gel (erythromycin 3% + benzoyl peroxide 5%) 23.3, 46.6 g. Trade only: Benzamycin Pak, #60 gel pouches.
NOTES – Must be refrigerated, expires 3 months after pharmacy dispensing.
MOA – Antibacterial + drying and sebostatic effects.
ADVERSE EFFECTS – Frequent: Dryness, scaling, erythema, burning, pruritus.

BENZOYL PEROXIDE (Benzac, Benzagel 10%, Desquam, Clearasil, ✦Solugel, Benoxyl) ▶LK ♀C ▶? $
ADULTS – Acne: Cleansers: Wash daily to bid. Creams/gels/lotion: Apply daily initially, gradually increase to bid to tid if needed.
PEDS – Not approved in children.
UNAPPROVED PEDS – Acne: Cleansers: Wash daily to bid. Creams/gels/lotion: Apply daily initially, gradually increase to bid to tid if needed.
FORMS – OTC and Rx generic: Liquid 2.5, 5, 10%. Bar 5, 10%. Mask 5%. Lotion 4, 5, 8, 10%. Cream 5, 10%. Gel 2.5, 4, 5, 6, 10, 20%. Pad 3, 4, 6, 8, 9%. Other strengths available.
NOTES – If excessive drying or peeling occurs, reduce frequency of application. Use with PABA-containing sunscreens may cause transient skin discoloration. May bleach fabric.
MOA – Antibacterial + drying and sebostatic effects.
ADVERSE EFFECTS – Frequent: Dryness, scaling, erythema, burning, pruritus.

CLENIA (sulfacetamide + sulfur) ▶K ♀C ▶? $$$
ADULTS – Acne, rosacea, seborrheic dermatitis: Apply cream/gel daily to tid, foaming wash daily to bid.
PEDS – Not approved in children.
FORMS – Generic only: Lotion (sodium sulfacetamide 10%/sulfur 5%) 25, 30, 45, 60 g. Trade only: Cream (sodium sulfacetamide 10%/sulfur 5%) 28 g. Generic/Trade: Foaming Wash 170, 340 g.
NOTES – Avoid with sulfa allergy, renal failure.
MOA – Antibacterial.
ADVERSE EFFECTS – Frequent: Local irritation, stinging, burning.

CLINDAMYCIN—TOPICAL (Cleocin T, Clindagel, ClindaMax, Evoclin, ✦Dalacin T) ▶L ♀B ▶– $
ADULTS – Acne: Apply daily (Evoclin) or bid (Cleocin T).
PEDS – Not approved in children.
UNAPPROVED ADULTS – Rosacea: Apply lotion bid.
UNAPPROVED PEDS – Acne: Apply bid.
FORMS – Generic/Trade: Gel 1% 30, 60 g. Lotion 1% 60 mL. Soln 1% 30, 60 mL. Trade only: Foam 1% 50, 100 g (Evoclin). Gel 1% 40, 75 mL (Clindagel).
NOTES – Concomitant use with erythromycin may decrease effectiveness. Most common adverse effects dryness, erythema, burning, peeling, oiliness, and itching. C. difficile-associated diarrhea has been reported with topical use.
MOA – Antibacterial.
ADVERSE EFFECTS – Frequent: Dryness, burning, pruritus. Severe: C. difficile-associated diarrhea.

DIANE-35 (cyproterone + ethinyl estradiol) ▶L ♀X ▶– $$
WARNING – Not recommended in women who smoke. Increased risk of thromboembolism, CVA, MI, hepatic neoplasia, and gallbladder disease. Nausea, breast tenderness, and breakthrough bleeding are common, transient side effects. Nighttime dosing may minimize nausea. Effectiveness is reduced by hepatic enzyme-inducing drugs such as certain anticonvulsants and barbiturates, rifampin, rifabutin, griseofulvin, and protease inhibitors. Antibiotics or products that contain St. John's wort may reduce efficacy.
ADULTS – Canada only. In women, severe acne unresponsive to oral antibiotics and other treatments, with associated symptoms of androgenization, including seborrhea and mild hirsutism: 1 tab PO daily for 21 consecutive days, stop for 7 days, repeat cycle.
PEDS – Not approved in children.
FORMS – Canada Generic/Trade: Blister pack of 21 tabs 2 mg cyproterone acetate/0.035 mg ethinyl estradiol.
NOTES – Higher thromboembolic risk than other oral contraceptives, therefore only indicated for acne, and not solely for contraception (although effective for the latter). Same warnings, precautions, and contraindications as other oral contraceptives.
MOA – Cyproterone: Potent antiandrogenic, progestogenic and antigonadotrophic activity; blocks androgen receptors and reduces androgen synthesis. Ethinyl estradiol increases levels of sex hormone binding globulin, and decreases circulating plasma levels of androgens. The combination also prevents ovulation and possible conception.

(cont.)

DIANE-35 (cont.)
ADVERSE EFFECTS — Serious: DVT/PE, stroke, MI, hepatic neoplasia, gallbladder disease. Frequent: Nausea, breast tenderness, and breakthrough bleeding.

DUAC (clindamycin + benzoyl peroxide, ♣ *Clindoxyl*) ▶K ♀C ▶+ $$$$
ADULTS — <u>Acne:</u> Apply at bedtime.
PEDS — Not approved in children.
UNAPPROVED PEDS — <u>Acne:</u> Apply at bedtime.
FORMS — Trade only: Gel (clindamycin 1% + benzoyl peroxide 5%) 45 g.
NOTES — Expires 2 months after pharmacy dispensing.
MOA — Antibacterial + drying and sebostatic effects.
ADVERSE EFFECTS — Frequent: Dryness, scaling, erythema, burning, pruritus. Severe: C. difficile-associated diarrhea, anaphylaxis.

EPIDUO (adapalene + benzoyl peroxide) ▶Bile, K ♀C ▶? $$$$$
ADULTS — <u>Acne:</u> Apply daily.
PEDS — Not approved in children.
FORMS — Trade only: Gel (0.1% adapalene + benzoyl peroxide 2.5%) 45 g.
NOTES — During early weeks of therapy, acne exacerbation may occur. May cause erythema, scaling, dryness, pruritus, and burning.
MOA — Modulates cellular differentiation, inflammation, keratinization + drying and sebostatic effects.
ADVERSE EFFECTS — Frequent: Erythema, scaling, dryness, stinging, burning.

ERYTHROMYCIN—TOPICAL (*Eryderm, Erycette, Erygel, A/T/S* ♣ *Sans-Acne, Erysol*) ▶L ♀B ▶? $
ADULTS — <u>Acne:</u> Apply bid.
PEDS — Not approved in children.
UNAPPROVED PEDS — <u>Acne:</u> Apply bid.
FORMS — Generic/Trade: Soln 2% 60 mL. Pads 2%. Gel 2% 30, 60 g. Ointment 2% 25 g. Generic only: Soln 1.5% 60 mL.
NOTES — May be more irritating when used with other acne products. Concomitant use with clindamycin may decrease effectiveness.
MOA — Antibacterial.
ADVERSE EFFECTS — Frequent: Dryness, pruritus, erythema, scaling.

ISOTRETINOIN (*Accutane, Amnesteem, Claravis, Sotret,* ♣ *Clarus*) ▶LK ♀X ▶— $$$$$
WARNING — Contraindicated in pregnant women or in women who may become pregnant. If used in a woman of childbearing age, patient must have severe, disfiguring acne, be reliable, comply with mandatory contraceptive measures, receive written and oral instructions about hazards of taking during pregnancy, have 2 negative pregnancy tests prior to beginning therapy. Must use 2 forms of effective contraception, unless absolute abstinence is chosen or patient has undergone a hysterectomy, from 1 month prior until 1 month after discontinuation of therapy. Men should not father children. May cause depression, suicidal thought, and aggressive or violent behavior; monitor for symptoms. Obtain written informed consent. Write prescription for no more than a 1 month supply. Informed consent documents available from the manufacturer.
ADULTS — <u>Severe, recalcitrant cystic acne:</u> 0.5 to 2 mg/kg/day PO divided bid for 15 to 20 weeks. Typical target dose is 1 mg/kg/day. May repeat 2nd course of therapy after at least 2 months off therapy.
PEDS — Not approved in children.
UNAPPROVED ADULTS — <u>Prevention of 2nd primary tumors in patients treated for squamous cell carcinoma of the head and neck:</u> 50 to 100 mg/m2/day PO. Also been used in keratinization disorders.
UNAPPROVED PEDS — <u>Severe, recalcitrant cystic acne:</u> 0.5 to 2 mg/kg/day PO divided bid for 15 to 20 weeks. Typical target dose is 1 mg/kg/day. Maintenance therapy for neuroblastoma: 100 to 250 mg/m2/day PO in 2 divided doses.
FORMS — Generic: Caps 10, 20, 40 mg. Generic only (Sotret and Claravis): Caps 30 mg.
NOTES — Prescription can be for a maximum of a 1 month supply. May cause headache, cheilitis, drying of mucous membranes including eyes, nose, mouth, hair loss, abdominal pain, pyuria, joint and muscle pain/stiffness, conjunctivitis, elevated ESR, and changes in serum lipids and LFTs. Effect on bone loss unknown; use caution in patients predisposed to osteoporosis. In children in whom skeletal growth is not complete, do not exceed the recommended dose for the recommended duration of treatment. Pseudotumor cerebri has occurred during therapy; avoid concomitant vitamin A, tetracycline, minocycline. May cause corneal opacities, decreased night vision, and inflammatory bowel disease. May decrease carbamazepine concentrations. Avoid excessive exposure to sunlight.
MOA — Decreases sebaceous gland size and sebum production.
ADVERSE EFFECTS — Frequent: Dryness, burning, pruritus, inflammation, photosensitivity, xerostomia, increased triglycerides, bone pain, arthralgias, myalgias, epistaxis. Severe: Teratogenic, possible depression, aggressive or violent behavior, premature epiphyseal closure, osteoporosis, osteopenia, delayed bone healing, pseudotumor cerebri, corneal opacities, hepatitis, back pain, severe skin reactions including Stevens-Johnson syndrome.

ROSULA (sulfacetamide + sulfur) ▶K ♀C ▶? $$$$
ADULTS — <u>Acne, rosacea, seborrheic dermatitis:</u> Apply cream/gel/aqueous cleanser daily to tid, foaming wash daily to bid.
PEDS — Not approved in children.
FORMS — Trade only: Gel (sodium sulfacetamide 10%/sulfur 5%) 45 g. Aqueous cleanser (sodium sulfacetamide 10%/sulfur 5%) 355 mL. Soap (sodium sulfacetamide 10%/sulfur 4%) 473 mL.
NOTES — Avoid with sulfa allergy or renal failure.
MOA — Antibacterial.
ADVERSE EFFECTS — Frequent: Local irritation, stinging, burning.

DERMATOLOGY: Actinic Keratosis Preparations

SALICYLIC ACID (*Akurza, Clearasil Cleanser, Stridex Pads*) ▶Not absorbed ♀? ▶? $
ADULTS — Acne (OTC): Apply/wash area up to 3 times a day. Removal of excessive keratin in hyperkeratotic disorders (Rx): Apply to affected area at bedtime and cover. Hydrate skin before application.
PEDS — Acne: Apply/wash area up to 3 times a day.
FORMS — OTC Generic/Trade: Pads, Gel, Lotion, Liquid, Mask scrub, 0.5%, 1%, 2%. Rx Trade only (Akurza): Cream 6% 340 g. Lotion 6%, 355 mL.
MOA — Keratolytic.
ADVERSE EFFECTS — Frequent: Irritation, stinging, burning.

SULFACET-R (sulfacetamide + sulfur) ▶K ♀C ▶? $$$
ADULTS — Acne, rosacea, seborrheic dermatitis: Apply cream/gel daily to tid, foaming wash daily to bid.
PEDS — Not approved in children.
FORMS — Generic/Trade: Lotion (sodium sulfacetamide 10%/sulfur 5%) 25 g.
NOTES — Avoid with sulfa allergy or renal failure.
MOA — Antibacterial.
ADVERSE EFFECTS — Frequent: Local irritation, stinging, burning.

SULFACETAMIDE—TOPICAL (*Klaron, Rosula NS*) ▶K ♀C ▶? $$$$
ADULTS — Acne: Apply bid.
PEDS — Not approved in children.
FORMS — Generic/Trade (Klaron): Lotion 10% 118 mL. Trade only: Single-use pads 10%, 30 ea (Rosula NS).
NOTES — Cross-sensitivity with sulfa or sulfite allergy.
MOA — Antibacterial.
ADVERSE EFFECTS — Frequent: Irritation, stinging, burning. Severe: Stevens-Johnson syndrome, systemic lupus erythematosus.

TAZAROTENE (*Tazorac, Avage*) ▶L ♀X ▶? $$$$
ADULTS — Acne (Tazorac): Apply 0.1% cream at bedtime. Palliation of fine facial wrinkles, mottled hyper- and hypopigmentation, benign facial lentigines (Avage): Apply at bedtime. Psoriasis: Apply 0.05% cream at bedtime, increase to 0.1% prn.
PEDS — Not approved in children.
UNAPPROVED PEDS — Acne: Apply 0.1% cream at bedtime. Psoriasis: Apply 0.05% cream at bedtime.
FORMS — Trade only (Tazorac): Cream 0.05% and 0.1% 30, 60 g. Gel 0.05% and 0.1% 30, 100 g. Trade only (Avage): Cream 0.1% 15, 30 g.
NOTES — In psoriasis, may reduce irritation and improve efficacy by using topical corticosteroid in morning and tazarotene at bedtime. Desquamation, burning, dry skin, erythema, pruritus may occur in up to 30% of patients. May cause photosensitivity.
MOA — Modulates cellular differentiation, keratinization; anti-inflammatory, immunologic activity.
ADVERSE EFFECTS — Frequent: Pruritus, burning, erythema.

TRETINOIN—TOPICAL (*Retin-A, Retin-A Micro, Renova, Retisol-A, ✦Stieva-A, Rejuva-A, Vitamin A Acid Cream*) ▶LK ♀C ▶? $$$
ADULTS — Acne (Retin A, Retin-A Micro): Apply at bedtime. Wrinkles, hyperpigmentation, tactile roughness (Renova): Apply at bedtime.
PEDS — Not approved in children.
UNAPPROVED ADULTS — Used in skin cancer and lamellar ichthyosis, mollusca contagiosa, verrucae plantaris, verrucae planae juvenilis, hyperpigmented lesions in black individuals, ichthyosis vulgaris, and pityriasis rubra pilaris.
FORMS — Generic/Trade: Cream 0.025% 20, 45 g, 0.05% 20, 45 g, 0.1% 20, 45 g. Gel 0.025% 15, 45 g, 0.1% 15, 45 g. Trade only: Renova cream 0.02% 40, 60 g. Retin-A Micro gel 0.04%, 0.1% 20, 45, 50 g.
NOTES — May induce erythema, peeling. Minimize sun exposure. Concomitant use with sulfur, resorcinol, benzoyl peroxide, or salicylic acid may result in skin irritation. Gel preps are flammable.
MOA — Induces loosening of keratinocytes, inhibits microcomedone formation.
ADVERSE EFFECTS — Frequent: Dryness, erythema, scaling. Severe: Contraindicated in pregnancy.

ZIANA (clindamycin + tretinoin) ▶LK ♀C ▶? $$$$
ADULTS — Acne: Apply at bedtime.
PEDS — Use adult dose for age 12 yo or older.
FORMS — Trade only: Gel clindamycin 1.2% + tretinoin 0.025% 30, 60 g.
NOTES — May induce erythema, peeling. Minimize sun exposure.
MOA — Induces loosening of keratinocytes, inhibits microcomedone formation, antibacterial.
ADVERSE EFFECTS — Frequent: Dryness, erythema, scaling.

DERMATOLOGY: Actinic Keratosis Preparations

AMINOLEVULINIC ACID (*Levulan Kerastick*) ▶Not absorbed ♀C ▶? $$$$
ADULTS — Non-hyperkeratotic actinic keratoses: Apply soln to lesions on scalp or face; expose to special light source 14 to 18 h later.
PEDS — Not approved in children.
FORMS — Trade only: 20% soln, single-use applicator stick.
NOTES — Soln should be applied by healthcare personnel. Advise patients to avoid sunlight during 14 to 18 h period before blue light illumination.
MOA — Photosensitizer as precursor to protoporphyrin.
ADVERSE EFFECTS — Frequent: Scaling, pruritus, hypo- or hyperpigmentation, erosions, stinging, burning.

DICLOFENAC—TOPICAL (*Solaraze, Voltaren*) ▶L ♀B ▶? $$$$$
ADULTS — Solaraze: Actinic/solar keratoses: Apply bid to lesions for 60 to 90 days. Voltaren: OA of areas amenable to topical therapy: 2 grams (upper extremities) to 4 grams (lower extremities) qid.
PEDS — Not approved in children.

(cont.)

DERMATOLOGY: Antibacterials (Topical)

DICLOFENAC—TOPICAL (cont.)
FORMS — Trade only: Gel 3% 50 g (Solaraze), 100 g (Solaraze, Voltaren).
NOTES — Avoid exposure to sun and sunlamps. Use caution in aspirin-sensitive patients. When using for OA (Voltaren), maximum daily dose 16 grams to any single lower extremity joint, 8 grams to any single upper extremity joint.
MOA — Inhibits prostaglandins at level of cyclooxygenase.
ADVERSE EFFECTS — Frequent: Rash, abdominal cramps, nausea, indigestion.

FLUOROURACIL—TOPICAL (*5-FU, Carac, Efudex, Fluoroplex*) ▶L ♀X ▶− $$$
WARNING — Contraindicated in pregnant women or women who plan to get pregnant during therapy. Avoid application to mucous membranes.
ADULTS — <u>Actinic or solar keratoses:</u> Apply bid to lesions for 2 to 6 weeks. <u>Superficial basal cell carcinomas:</u> Apply 5% cream/soln bid.
PEDS — Not approved in children.
UNAPPROVED ADULTS — <u>Condylomata acuminata:</u> 1% soln in 70% ethanol and the 5% cream has been used.
FORMS — Trade only: Cream 0.5% 30 g (Carac), 5% 25 g (Efudex), 1% 30 g (Fluoroplex). Generic/Trade: Soln 2%, 5% 10 mL (Efudex). Cream 5% 40 g.
NOTES — May cause severe irritation and photosensitivity. Contraindicated in women who are or who may become pregnant during therapy. Avoid application to mucous membranes.
MOA — Pyrimidine anti-metabolite that interferes with DNA synthesis.
ADVERSE EFFECTS — Frequent: Dermatitis, pruritic maculopapular rash, alopecia, heartburn, nausea, inflammation along segments of the GI tract, diarrhea. Severe: Myelosuppression, mucositis.

METHYLAMINOLEVULINATE (*Metvix, Metvixia*) ▶Not absorbed ♀C ▶? ?
ADULTS — <u>Non-hyperkeratotic actinic keratoses of face/scalp:</u> Apply cream 1 mm thick (max 1 gram) to lesion and 5 mm surrounding area; cover with dressing for 3 h; remove dressing and cream and perform illumination therapy. Repeat in 7 days.
PEDS — Not approved in children.
FORMS — Trade only: Cream 16.8%, 2 g tube.
NOTES — Use in immunocompetent individuals. Lesion debridement should be performed prior to application of cream. Formulated in peanut and almond oil; has not been tested in patients allergic to peanuts.
MOA — Photosensitizer as precursor to photoactive porphyrin.
ADVERSE EFFECTS — Frequent: Peeling, pruritus, edema, ulceration, bleeding, blisters, stinging, burning, pain, crusting, contact sensitization.

DERMATOLOGY: Antibacterials (Topical)

BACITRACIN (*✦Baciguent*) ▶Not absorbed ♀C ▶? $
ADULTS — <u>Minor cuts, wounds, burns, or skin abrasions:</u> Apply daily to tid.
PEDS — Not approved in children.
UNAPPROVED PEDS — <u>Minor cuts, wounds, burns, or skin abrasions:</u> Apply daily to tid.
FORMS — OTC Generic/Trade: Ointment 500 units/g 1, 15, 30 g.
NOTES — May cause contact dermatitis or anaphylaxis.
MOA — Antibacterial, inhibit bacterial wall synthesis.
ADVERSE EFFECTS — Frequent: None.

FUSIDIC ACID—TOPICAL (*✦Fucidin*) ▶L ♀? ▶? $
ADULTS — Canada only. <u>Skin infections:</u> Apply tid to qid.
PEDS — Canada only. <u>Skin infections:</u> Apply tid to qid.
FORMS — Canada trade only: Cream 2% fusidic acid 5, 15, 30 g. Ointment 2% sodium fusidate 5, 15, 30 g.
NOTES — Contains lanolin; possible hypersensitivity.
MOA — Antibacterial, interferes with bacterial protein synthesis.
ADVERSE EFFECTS — Serious: Hypersensitivity. Frequent: Mild irritation, pain.

GENTAMICIN—TOPICAL (*Garamycin*) ▶K ♀D ▶? $
ADULTS — <u>Skin infections:</u> Apply tid to qid.
PEDS — <u>Skin infections</u> in children older than 1 yo: Apply tid to qid.
FORMS — Generic only: Ointment 0.1% 15, 30 g. Cream 0.1% 15, 30 g.
MOA — Antibacterial, interferes with bacterial protein synthesis.
ADVERSE EFFECTS — Frequent: Neurotoxicity (when applied to large areas), gait instability, ototoxicity, nephrotoxicity.

MAFENIDE (*Sulfamylon*) ▶LK ♀C ▶? $$
ADULTS — <u>Adjunctive treatment of burns:</u> Apply daily to bid.
PEDS — <u>Adjunctive treatment of burns:</u> Apply daily to bid.
FORMS — Trade only: Cream 5% 57, 114, 454 g. Topical soln 50 g packets.
NOTES — Can cause metabolic acidosis. Contains sulfonamides.
MOA — Antibacterial, interferes with bacterial folic acid synthesis.
ADVERSE EFFECTS — Frequent: Burning, pain, excoriation.

METRONIDAZOLE—TOPICAL (*Noritate, MetroCream, MetroGel, MetroLotion, ✦Rosasol*) ▶KL ♀B(− in 1st trimester) ▶− $$$
ADULTS — <u>Rosacea:</u> Apply daily (1%) or bid (0.75%).
PEDS — Not approved in children.

(cont.)

DERMATOLOGY: Antibacterials (Topical)

CORTICOSTEROIDS—TOPICAL

Potency*	Generic	Trade Name	Forms	Frequency
Low	alclometasone dipropionate	Aclovate	0.05% C/O	bid-tid
Low	clocortolone pivalate	Cloderm	0.1% C	tid
Low	desonide	DesOwen, Tridesilon	0.05% C/L/O	bid-tid
Low	hydrocortisone	Hytone, others	0.5% C/L/O; 1% C/L/O; 2.5% C/L/O	bid-qid
Low	hydrocortisone acetate	Cortaid, Corticaine	0.5% C/O; 1% C/O/Sp	bid-qid
Medium	betamethasone valerate	Luxiq	0.1% C/L/O; 0.12% F (Luxiq)	qd-bid
Medium	desoximetasone‡	Topicort	0.05% C	bid
Medium	fluocinolone	Synalar	0.01% C/S; 0.025% C/O	bid-qid
Medium	flurandrenolide	Cordran	0.025% C/O; 0.05% C/L/O/T	bid-qid
Medium	fluticasone propionate	Cutivate	0.005% O; 0.05% C/L	qd-bid
Medium	hydrocortisone butyrate	Locoid	0.1% C/O/S	bid-tid
Medium	hydrocortisone valerate	Westcort	0.2% C/O	bid-tid
Medium	mometasone furoate	Elocon	0.1% C/L/O	qd
Medium	triamcinolone‡	Aristocort, Kenalog	0.025% C/L/O; 0.1% C/L/O/S	bid-tid
High	amcinonide	Cyclocort	0.1% C/L/O	bid-tid
High	betamethasone dipropionate‡	Maxivate, others	0.05% C/L/O (non-Diprolene)	qd-bid
High	desoximetasone‡	Topicort	0.05% G; 0.25% C/O	bid
High	diflorasone diacetate‡	Maxiflor	0.05% C/O	bid
High	fluocinonide	Lidex	0.05% C/G/O/S	bid-qid
High	halcinonide	Halog	0.1% C/O/S	bid-tid
High	triamcinolone‡	Aristocort, Kenalog	0.5% C/O	bid-tid
Very high	betamethasone dipropionate‡	Diprolene, Diprolene AF	0.05% C/G/L/O	qd-bid
Very high	clobetasol	Temovate, Cormax, Olux	0.05% C/G/O/L/S/Sp/F (Olux)	bid
Very high	diflorasone diacetate‡	Psorcon	0.05% C/O	qd-tid
Very high	halobetasol propionate	Ultravate	0.05% C/O	qd-bid

*Potency based on vasoconstrictive assays, which may not correlate with efficacy. Not all available products are listed, including those lacking potency ratings. ‡These drugs have formulations in more than once potency category. C, cream; O, ointment; L, lotion; T, tape; F, foam; S, solution; G, gel; Sp, spray

METRONIDAZOLE—TOPICAL (cont.)

UNAPPROVED ADULTS – A 1% soln prepared from the oral tabs has been used in the treatment of infected decubitus ulcers.
FORMS – Trade only: Gel (MetroGel) 1% 45, 60 g. Cream (Noritate) 1% 60 g. Generic/Trade: Gel 0.75% 45 g. Cream 0.75% 45 g. Lotion (MetroLotion) 0.75% 59 mL.
NOTES – Results usually noted within 3 weeks, with continuing improvement through 9 weeks. Avoid using vaginal prep on face due to irritation because of formulation differences.
MOA – Antibacterial, breakage of bacterial DNA.
ADVERSE EFFECTS – Frequent: Dizziness, headache, nausea, diarrhea, anorexia, vomiting.

MUPIROCIN (Bactroban, Centany) ▶Not absorbed ♀B ▶? $$
ADULTS – Impetigo: Apply tid for 3 to 5 days. Infected wounds: Apply tid for 10 days. Nasal methicillin-resistant S aureus eradication: 0.5 g in each nostril bid for 5 days.
PEDS – Impetigo (mupirocin cream/ointment): Apply tid. Infected wounds: Apply tid for 10 days. Nasal form not approved in children younger than 12 yo.
FORMS – Generic/Trade: Ointment 2% 22 g. Nasal ointment 2% 1 g single-use tubes (for MRSA eradication). Trade only: Cream 2% 15, 30 g.
MOA – Antibacterial; inhibits bacterial protein and RNA synthesis.
ADVERSE EFFECTS – Frequent: Dryness, burning, erythema, stinging, tenderness.

NEOSPORIN CREAM (neomycin + polymyxin + bacitracin) ▶K ♀C ▶? $
ADULTS – Minor cuts, wounds, burns, or skin abrasions: Apply daily to tid.
PEDS – Not approved in children.
UNAPPROVED PEDS – Minor cuts, wounds, burns, or skin abrasions: Apply daily to tid.
FORMS – OTC Trade only: neomycin 3.5 mg/g + polymyxin 10,000 units/g 15 g and unit dose 0.94 g.
NOTES – Neomycin component can cause contact dermatitis.
MOA – Antibacterial.
ADVERSE EFFECTS – Frequent: None.

NEOSPORIN OINTMENT (bacitracin + neomycin + polymyxin) ▶K ♀C ▶? $
ADULTS — Minor cuts, wounds, burns, or skin abrasions: Apply daily to tid.
PEDS — Not approved in children.
UNAPPROVED PEDS — Minor cuts, wounds, burns, or skin abrasions: Apply daily to tid.
FORMS — OTC Generic/Trade: bacitracin 400 units/g + neomycin 3.5 mg/g + polymyxin 5000 units/g 15, 30 g and "to go" 0.9 g packets.
NOTES — Also known as triple antibiotic ointment. Neomycin component can cause contact dermatitis.
MOA — Antibacterial.
ADVERSE EFFECTS — Frequent: None.

POLYSPORIN (bacitracin + polymyxin, ♣*Polytopic*) ▶K ♀C ▶? $
ADULTS — Minor cuts, wounds, burns, or skin abrasions: Apply daily to tid.
PEDS — Not approved in children.
UNAPPROVED PEDS — Minor cuts, wounds, burns, or skin abrasions: Apply daily to tid.
FORMS — OTC Trade only: Ointment 15, 30 g and unit dose 0.9 g. Powder 10 g.
NOTES — May cause allergic contact dermatitis and rarely contact anaphylaxis.
MOA — Antibacterial.
ADVERSE EFFECTS — May cause allergic contact dermatitis and rarely contact anaphylaxis.

RETAPAMULIN (*Altabax*) ▶Not absorbed ♀B ▶? $$$
ADULTS — Impetigo: Apply bid for 5 days.
PEDS — Impetigo (9 mo or older): Apply bid for 5 days.
FORMS — Trade only: Ointment 1% 5, 10, 15 g.
MOA — Antibacterial; inhibits bacterial protein and RNA synthesis.
ADVERSE EFFECTS — Frequent: Skin irritation.

SILVER SULFADIAZINE (*Silvadene*, ♣ *Dermazin, Flamazine, SSD*) ▶LK ♀B ▶– $$
ADULTS — Burns: Apply daily to bid.
PEDS — Not approved in children.
UNAPPROVED ADULTS — Has been used for pressure ulcers.
UNAPPROVED PEDS — Burns: Apply daily to bid.
FORMS — Generic/Trade: Cream 1% 20, 50, 85, 400, 1000 g.
NOTES — Avoid in sulfa allergy. Leukopenia, primarily decreased neutrophil count in up to 20% of patients. Significant absorption may occur and serum sulfa concentrations approach therapeutic levels. Avoid in G6PD deficiency. Use caution in pregnancy nearing term, premature infants, infants 2 mo or younger and in patients with renal or hepatic dysfunction.
MOA — Antibacterial; acts on bacterial cell wall.
ADVERSE EFFECTS — Frequent: Pruritus, rash. Severe: Erythema multiforme, hemolytic anemia, leukopenia, agranulocytosis, aplastic anemia, interstitial nephritis, hepatitis.

DERMATOLOGY: Antifungals (Topical)

BUTENAFINE (*Lotrimin Ultra, Mentax*) ▶L ♀B ▶? $
ADULTS — Treatment of tinea pedis: Apply daily for 4 weeks or bid for 7 days. Tinea corporis, tinea versicolor, or tinea cruris: Apply daily for 2 weeks.
PEDS — Not approved in children.
FORMS — Rx Trade only: Cream 1% 15, 30 g (Mentax). OTC Trade only: Cream 1% 12, 24 g (Lotrimin Ultra).
NOTES — Most common adverse effects include contact dermatitis, burning, and worsening of condition. If no improvement in 4 weeks, reevaluate diagnosis.
MOA — Antifungal; binds to fungal cell membrane.
ADVERSE EFFECTS — Frequent: Burning, stinging, erythema, irritation.

CICLOPIROX (*Loprox, Penlac*, ♣*Stieprox shampoo*) ▶K ♀B ▶? $$$$
ADULTS — Tinea pedis, cruris, corporis, and versicolor, candidiasis (cream, lotion): Apply bid. Onychomycosis of fingernails/toenails (nail soln): Apply daily to affected nails; apply over previous coat; remove with alcohol every 7 days. Seborrheic dermatitis (Loprox shampoo): Shampoo twice weekly for 4 weeks.
PEDS — Onychomycosis of fingernails/toenails in children age 12 yo or older (nail soln): Apply daily to affected nails; apply over previous coat; remove with alcohol every 7 days (Penlac). Not approved in children younger than 12 yo.
FORMS — Trade only: Shampoo (Loprox) 1% 120 mL. Generic/Trade: Gel 0.77% 30, 45, 100 g. Nail soln (Penlac) 8% 6.6 mL. Cream (Loprox) 0.77% 15, 30, 90 g. Lotion (Loprox TS) 0.77% 30, 60 mL.
NOTES — Clinical improvement of tinea usually occurs within first week. Patients with tinea versicolor usually exhibit clinical and mycological clearing after 2 weeks. If no improvement in 4 weeks, reevaluate diagnosis. Do not get shampoo in eyes. No safety information available in diabetes or immunocompromise. Shampoo may affect hair color in those with light-colored hair. For nail soln, infected portion of each nail should be removed by health care professional as frequently as monthly. Oral antifungal therapy is more effective for onychomycosis than Penlac.
MOA — Antifungal; inhibits fungal DNA, RNA, protein synthesis.
ADVERSE EFFECTS — Frequent: Pruritus, erythema, burning.

CLOTRIMAZOLE—TOPICAL (*Lotrimin AF, Mycelex*, ♣*Canesten, Clotrimaderm*) ▶L ♀B ▶? $
ADULTS — Treatment of tinea pedis, cruris, corporis, and versicolor, and cutaneous candidiasis: Apply bid.
PEDS — Treatment of tinea pedis, cruris, corporis, versicolor, cutaneous candidiasis: Apply bid.
FORMS — Note that Lotrimin brand cream, lotion, soln are clotrimazole, while Lotrimin powders and liquid spray are miconazole. Rx Generic only: Cream 1% 15,

(cont.)

DERMATOLOGY: Antifungals (Topical)

CLOTRIMAZOLE—TOPICAL (*cont.*)
30, 45 g. Soln 1% 10, 30 mL. OTC Trade only (Lotrimin AF): Cream 1% 12, 24 g. Soln 1% 10 mL.
NOTES — If no improvement in 4 weeks, reevaluate diagnosis.
MOA — Antifungal; alters fungal cell wall permeability.
ADVERSE EFFECTS — Frequent: Burning, irritation, stinging.

ECONAZOLE ▶Not absorbed ♀C ▶? $$
ADULTS — Treatment of tinea pedis, cruris, corporis, and versicolor: Apply daily. Cutaneous candidiasis: Apply bid.
PEDS — Not approved in children.
FORMS — Generic only: Cream 1% 15, 30, 85 g.
NOTES — Treat candidal infections, tinea cruris and tinea corporis for 2 weeks and tinea pedis for 1 month to reduce risk of recurrence.
MOA — Antifungal; alters fungal cell wall permeability.
ADVERSE EFFECTS — Frequent: Burning, stinging, pruritus, erythema.

KETOCONAZOLE—TOPICAL (*Extina, Nizoral, Xolegel, ✽Ketoderm*) ▶L ♀C ▶? $$
ADULTS — Shampoo (2%): Tinea versicolor: Apply to affected area, leave on for 5 min, rinse. Cream: Cutaneous candidiasis, tinea corporis, cruris, and versicolor: Apply daily. Seborrheic dermatitis: Apply cream (2%) bid for 4 weeks or gel daily for 2 weeks or foam bid for 4 weeks. Dandruff: Apply shampoo (1%) twice a week.
PEDS — Not approved in children younger than 12 yo.
UNAPPROVED ADULTS — Seborrheic dermatitis: Apply cream (2%) daily.
UNAPPROVED PEDS — Shampoo (2%): Tinea versicolor: Apply to affected area, leave on for 5 min, rinse. Cream: Cutaneous candidiasis, tinea corporis, cruris, and versicolor: Apply daily. Seborrheic dermatitis: Apply cream (2%) bid. Dandruff: Apply shampoo (1%) twice a week.
FORMS — Generic/Trade: Cream 2% 15, 30, 60 g. Shampoo 2% 120 mL. Trade only: Shampoo 1% 120, 210 mL (OTC Nizoral). Gel 2% 15 g (Xolegel). Foam 2% 50, 100 g (Extina).
NOTES — Treat candidal infections, tinea cruris, corporis, and versicolor for 2 weeks. Treat seborrheic dermatitis for 4 weeks. Treat tinea pedis for 6 weeks.
MOA — Antifungal; alters fungal cell wall permeability.
ADVERSE EFFECTS — Frequent: Burning, stinging, irritation.

MICONAZOLE—TOPICAL (*Micatin, Lotrimin AF, ZeaSorb AF*) ▶L ♀+ ▶? $
ADULTS — Tinea pedis, cruris, corporis, and versicolor, cutaneous candidiasis: Apply bid.
PEDS — Not approved in children.
UNAPPROVED PEDS — Tinea pedis, cruris, corporis, and versicolor, cutaneous candidiasis: Apply bid.
FORMS — Note that Lotrimin brand cream, lotion, soln are clotrimazole, while Lotrimin powders and liquid spray are miconazole. OTC Trade only: Powder 2% 70, 160 g. Spray powder 2% 90, 100, 140 g. Spray liquid 2% 90, 105 mL. Gel 2% 24 g.
NOTES — Symptomatic relief generally occurs in 2 to 3 days. Treat candida, tinea cruris, tinea corporis for 2 weeks, tinea pedis for 1 month to reduce risk of recurrence.
MOA — Antifungal; alters fungal cell wall permeability.
ADVERSE EFFECTS — Frequent: Rash, pruritus.

NAFTIFINE (*Naftin*) ▶LK ♀B ▶? $$$
ADULTS — Tinea pedis, cruris, and corporis: Apply daily (cream) or bid (gel).
PEDS — Not approved in children.
FORMS — Trade only: Cream 1% 15, 30, 60, 90 g. Gel 1% 20, 40, 60, 90 g.
NOTES — If no improvement in 4 weeks, reevaluate diagnosis.
MOA — Antifungal; alters fungal cell wall synthesis.
ADVERSE EFFECTS — Frequent: Burning, stinging, erythema, irritation, pruritus.

NYSTATIN—TOPICAL (*Mycostatin, ✽Nilstat, Nyaderm, Candistatin*) ▶Not absorbed ♀C ▶? $
ADULTS — Cutaneous or mucocutaneous Candida infections: Apply bid to tid.
PEDS — Cutaneous or mucocutaneous Candida infections: Apply bid to tid.
FORMS — Generic/Trade: Cream, Ointment 100,000 units/g 15, 30 g. Powder 100,000 units/g 15, 30, 60 g.
NOTES — Ineffective for dermatophytes/tinea. For fungal infections of the feet, dust feet and footwear with powder.
MOA — Antifungal; alters fungal cell wall permeability.
ADVERSE EFFECTS — Frequent: Contact dermatitis, N/V, diarrhea, stomach pain. Severe: Stevens-Johnson syndrome, hypersensitivity.

OXICONAZOLE (*Oxistat, Oxizole*) ▶? ♀B ▶? $$$
ADULTS — Tinea pedis, cruris, and corporis: Apply daily to bid. Tinea versicolor (cream only): Apply daily.
PEDS — Cream: Tinea pedis, cruris, and corporis: Apply daily to bid. Tinea versicolor: Apply daily.
FORMS — Trade only: Cream 1% 15, 30, 60 g. Lotion 1% 30 mL.
MOA — Antifungal; alters fungal cell wall integrity.
ADVERSE EFFECTS — Frequent: Burning, stinging, erythema, irritation, pruritus, xeroderma.

SERTACONAZOLE (*Ertaczo*) ▶Not absorbed ♀C ▶? $$$
ADULTS — Tinea pedis: Apply bid.
PEDS — Not approved for children younger than 12 yo.
FORMS — Trade only: Cream 2% 30, 60 g.
MOA — Antifungal; alters fungal cell wall integrity.
ADVERSE EFFECTS — Frequent: Burning, dermatitis, dry skin.

TERBINAFINE—TOPICAL (*Lamisil, Lamisil AT*) ▶L ♀B ▶? $
ADULTS — Tinea pedis: Apply bid. Tinea cruris and corporis: Apply daily to bid. Tinea versicolor (soln): Apply bid.
PEDS — Not approved in children.

(cont.)

DERMATOLOGY: Antiparasitics (Topical)

TERBINAFINE—TOPICAL (cont.)
UNAPPROVED ADULTS – Cutaneous candidiasis.
UNAPPROVED PEDS – Tinea pedis: Apply bid. Tinea cruris and corporis: Apply daily to bid. Tinea versicolor (soln): Apply bid.
FORMS – OTC Trade only (Lamisil AT): Cream 1% 12, 24 g. Spray pump soln 1% 30 mL. Gel 1% 6, 12 g.
NOTES – In many patients, improvement noted within 3 to 4 days, but therapy should continue for a minimum of 1 week, maximum of 4 weeks. Topical therapy not effective for nail fungus.
MOA – Antifungal; alters fungal cell wall synthesis.
ADVERSE EFFECTS – Frequent: Contact dermatitis, burning, irritation, pruritus.

TOLNAFTATE (*Tinactin*) ▶? ♀? ▶? $
ADULTS – Tinea pedis, cruris, corporis, and versicolor: Apply bid. Prevention of tinea pedis (powder and aerosol): Apply prn.
PEDS – Tinea pedis, cruris, corporis, and versicolor: Apply bid for older than 2 yo. Prevention of tinea pedis (powder and aerosol): Apply prn.
FORMS – OTC Generic/Trade: Cream 1% 15, 30 g. Soln 1% 10 mL. Powder 1% 45 g. OTC Trade only: Gel 1% 15 g. Powder 1% 90 g. Spray powder 1% 100, 133, 150 g. Spray liquid 1% 100, 113 mL.
MOA – Antifungal; inhibits fungal cell growth.
ADVERSE EFFECTS – Frequent: Contact dermatitis, stinging, irritation, pruritus.

DERMATOLOGY: Antiparasitics (Topical)

A-200 (pyrethrins + piperonyl butoxide, ✦*R&C*) ▶L ♀C ▶? $
ADULTS – Lice: Apply shampoo, wash after 10 min. Reapply in 5 to 7 days.
PEDS – Lice: Apply shampoo, wash after 10 min. Reapply in 5 to 7 days.
FORMS – OTC Generic/Trade: Shampoo (0.33% pyrethrins, 4% piperonyl butoxide) 60, 120 mL.
NOTES – Use caution if allergic to ragweed. Avoid contact with mucous membranes.
MOA – Neuronal toxin to lice; inhibits pyrethrin metabolism.
ADVERSE EFFECTS – Frequent: Burning, stinging, pruritus.

CROTAMITON (*Eurax*) ▶? ♀C ▶? $$
ADULTS – Scabies: Massage cream/lotion into entire body from chin down, repeat 24 h later, bathe 48 h later. Pruritus: Massage into affected areas prn.
PEDS – Not approved in children.
UNAPPROVED PEDS – Scabies: Massage cream/lotion into entire body from chin down, repeat 24 h later, bathe 48 h later. Pruritus: Massage into affected areas prn.
FORMS – Trade only: Cream 10% 60 g. Lotion 10% 60, 480 mL.
NOTES – Patients with scabies should change bed linen and clothing in am after 2nd application and bathe 48 h after last application. Consider treating entire family.
MOA – Scabicidal; mechanism of action unknown.
ADVERSE EFFECTS – Frequent: None.

LINDANE (✦*Hexit*) ▶L ♀B ▶? $
WARNING – For use only in patients who have failed other agents. Seizures and deaths have been reported with repeat or prolonged use. Use caution with infants, children, elderly, those who weigh less than 50 kg. Contraindicated in premature infants and patients with uncontrolled seizures.
ADULTS – Head/crab lice: Lotion: Apply 30 to 60 mL to affected area, wash off after 12 h. Shampoo: Apply 30 to 60 mL, wash off after 4 min. Scabies (lotion): Apply 30 to 60 mL to total body from neck down, wash off after 8 to 12 h.
PEDS – Lindane penetrates human skin and has potential for CNS toxicity. Studies indicate potential toxic effects of topical lindane are greater in young. Maximum dose for age younger than 6 yo is 30 mL.
FORMS – Generic only: Lotion 1% 60, 480 mL. Shampoo 1% 60, 480 mL.
NOTES – For lice, reapply if living lice noted after 7 days. After shampooing, comb with fine tooth comb to remove nits. Consider treating entire family.
MOA – Nervous system stimulant lethal to ova and parasites.
ADVERSE EFFECTS – Frequent: None. Severe: CNS side effects—headache, restlessness, seizures, aplastic anemia, arrhythmias, hepatitis, pulmonary edema, hematuria.

MALATHION (*Ovide*) ▶? ♀B ▶? $$$$
ADULTS – Head lice: Apply to dry hair, let dry naturally, wash off in 8 to 12 h.
PEDS – Head lice in children: Apply to dry hair, let dry naturally, wash off in 8 to 12 h for 6 yo or older.
FORMS – Generic/Trade only: Lotion 0.5% 59 mL.
NOTES – Do not use hair dryer; flammable. Avoid contact with eyes. Use a fine tooth comb to remove nits and dead lice. Application may be repeated in 7 to 9 days.
MOA – Kills lice and their ova.
ADVERSE EFFECTS – Frequent: None.

PERMETHRIN (*Elimite, Acticin, Nix,* ✦*Kwellada-P*) ▶L ♀B ▶? $$
ADULTS – Scabies (cream): Massage cream into entire body (avoid mouth, eyes, nose), wash off after 8 to 14 h. 30 grams is typical adult dose. Head lice (liquid): Apply to clean, towel-dried hair, saturate hair and scalp, wash off after 10 min.
PEDS – Scabies (cream) age older than 2 mo: Massage cream into entire body (avoid mouth, eyes, nose), wash off after 8 to 14 h. Head lice (liquid) in age older than 2 yo: Saturate hair and scalp, wash off after 10 min.
FORMS – Generic/Trade: Cream (Elimite, Acticin) 5% 60 g. OTC Generic/Trade: Liquid creme rinse (Nix) 1% 60 mL.

(cont.)

PERMETHRIN (cont.)
NOTES – If necessary, may repeat application in 7 days. Consider treating entire family.
MOA – Neuronal toxin which paralyzes lice.
ADVERSE EFFECTS – Frequent: Burning, stinging, erythema, numbness, pruritus.

RID (pyrethrins + piperonyl butoxide) ▶L ♀C ▶? $
ADULTS – <u>Lice:</u> Apply shampoo/monthusse, wash after 10 min. Reapply in 5 to 10 days.
PEDS – <u>Lice:</u> Apply shampoo/monthusse, wash after 10 min. Reapply in 5 to 10 days.
FORMS – OTC Generic/Trade: Shampoo 60, 120, 240 mL. OTC Trade only: Mousse 5.5 oz.
NOTES – Use caution if allergic to ragweed. Avoid contact with mucus membranes. Available alone or as part of a RID 1-2-3 kit containing shampoo, egg, and nit comb-out gel and home lice control spray for non-washable items.
MOA – Neuronal toxin to lice; inhibits pyrethrin metabolism.
ADVERSE EFFECTS – Frequent: Burning, stinging, pruritus.

DERMATOLOGY: Antipsoriatics

ACITRETIN (Soriatane) ▶L ♀X ▶– $$$$$
WARNING – Contraindicated in pregnancy and avoid pregnancy for 3 years following medication discontinuation. Major human fetal abnormalities have been reported. Females of child bearing age must avoid alcohol while on medication and for 2 months following therapy since alcohol prolongs elimination of a teratogenic metabolite. Use in reliable females of reproductive potential only if they have severe, unresponsive psoriasis, have received written and oral warnings of the teratogenic potential, are using 2 reliable forms of contraception, and have 2 negative pregnancy tests within 1 week prior to starting therapy. Contraception should start at least 1 month prior to therapy and continue for 3 years following discontinuation. Must have negative monthly pregnancy test during treatment. Therefore, prescribe limited amount and do not allow refill until documented negative pregnancy test. Following discontinuation, repeat pregnancy test every 3 months. It is unknown whether residual acitretin in seminal fluid poses a risk to the fetus while a male patient is taking the drug or after it is discontinued.
ADULTS – <u>Severe psoriasis:</u> Initiate at 25 to 50 mg PO daily.
PEDS – Not approved in children.
UNAPPROVED ADULTS – <u>Lichen planus:</u> 30 mg/day PO for 4 weeks, then titrate to 10 to 50 mg/day for 12 weeks total. <u>Sjogren-Larsson syndrome:</u> 0.47 mg/kg/day PO. Also used in Darier's disease, palmoplantar pustulosis, nonbullous and bullous ichthyosiform erythroderma, lichen sclerosus et atrophicus of the vulva, palmoplantar lichen nitidus and chemoprevention for high-risk immunosuppressed patients with history of squamous cell carcinomas of the skin.
UNAPPROVED PEDS – Has been used in children with <u>lamellar ichthyosis.</u> Pediatric use is not recommended. Adverse effects on bone growth are suspected.
FORMS – Trade only: Caps 10, 25 mg.
NOTES – Transient worsening of psoriasis may occur, and full benefit may take 2 to 3 months. Elevated LFTs may occur in one-third of patients; monitor LFTs at 1 to 2 weeks intervals until stable and then periodically thereafter. Monitor serum lipid concentrations every 1 to 2 weeks until response to drug is established. May decrease tolerance to contact lenses due to dry eyes. Avoid prolonged exposure to sunlight. May cause hair loss. May cause depression. May cause bone changes, especially with use more than 6 months. Many adverse drug reactions.
MOA – Unknown.
ADVERSE EFFECTS – Frequent: Cheilitis, xerostomia, rhinitis, epistaxis, alopecia, skin peeling, pruritus, erythematous rash, rigors, arthralgias, xerophthalmus. Severe: Hepatitis, pancreatitis, pseudotumor cerebri.

ALEFACEPT (Amevive) ▶? ♀B ▶? $$$$$
ADULTS – <u>Moderate to severe psoriasis:</u> 7.5 mg IV or 15 mg IM once a week for 12 doses. May repeat with 1 additional 12 weeks course after 12 weeks have elapsed from last dose.
PEDS – Not approved in children.
NOTES – Monitor CD4+ T lymphocyte cells weekly; withhold therapy if count less than 250/mcL and stop altogether if less than 250/mcL for 1 month. Do not give to HIV-positive patients or with other immunosuppressive or phototherapy.
MOA – Interferes with lymphocyte activation.
ADVERSE EFFECTS – Frequent: Chills, dizziness, nausea, pruritus, myalgia, injection site pain/inflammation. Severe: Anaphylaxis/allergic reactions, malignancies, severe infections.

ANTHRALIN (Drithocreme, ✦Anthrascalp, Anthranol, Anthraforte, Dithranol) ▶? ♀C ▶– $$$
ADULTS – <u>Chronic psoriasis:</u> Apply daily.
PEDS – Not approved in children.
UNAPPROVED PEDS – <u>Chronic psoriasis:</u> Apply daily.
FORMS – Trade only: Cream 0.5, 1% 50 g.
NOTES – Short contact periods (ie, 15 to 20 min) followed by removal with an appropriate solvent (soap or petrolatum) may be preferred. May stain fabric, skin, or hair.
MOA – Inhibits proliferation of epidermal cells in psoriasis.
ADVERSE EFFECTS – Frequent: Irritation, discoloration of skin and clothing.

CALCIPOTRIENE (Dovonex) ▶L ♀C ▶? $$$$
ADULTS – <u>Moderate plaque psoriasis:</u> Apply bid.
PEDS – Not approved in children.
UNAPPROVED ADULTS – Has been used for <u>vitiligo.</u>
UNAPPROVED PEDS – <u>Moderate plaque psoriasis:</u> Apply bid. Has been used for <u>vitiligo.</u>

(cont.)

CALCIPOTRIENE (cont.)
FORMS — Trade only: Ointment 0.005% 30, 60, 100 g. Cream 0.005% 30, 60, 100 g. Generic/Trade: Scalp soln 0.005% 60 mL.
NOTES — Avoid contact with face. Do not exceed 100 g/week to minimize risk of hypercalcemia, hypercalciuria. Burning, itching, and skin irritation may occur in 10 to 15% of patients.
MOA — Regulates skin cell production and proliferation.
ADVERSE EFFECTS — Frequent: Burning, irritation, drying, rash, worsening of psoriasis, pruritus.

METHOXSALEN (*8-MOP, Oxsoralen-Ultra*) ▶Skin ♀C ▶? $$$$$
WARNING — Should only by physicians who have special training. For the treatment of patients with psoriasis, restrict to severe cases. Possibility of ocular damage, aging of the skin, and skin cancer (including melanoma).
ADULTS — Psoriasis: Dose based on wt (0.4 mg/kg/dose), 1½ to 2 h before ultraviolet light exposure.
PEDS — Not approved in children.
FORMS — Soft gelatin cap 10 mg (Oxsoralen-Ultra). Hard gelatin cap 10 mg (8-MOP).
NOTES — Oxsoralen-Ultra (soft gelatin cap) cannot be interchanged with 8-MOP (hard gelatin cap) due to significant bioavailability differences and photosensitization onset times. Take with food or milk. Wear ultraviolet light blocking glasses and avoid sun exposure after ingestion and for remainder of day.
MOA — DNA photodamage and decreased cell proliferation.
ADVERSE EFFECTS — Frequent: Nausea, pruritus, erythema, nervousness, insomnia. Severe: Depression, skin cancer with prolonged use, cataracts.

TACLONEX (calcipotriene + betamethasone) ▶L ♀C ▶? $$$$$
ADULTS — Psoriasis: Apply daily for up to 4 weeks.
PEDS — Not approved in children.
FORMS — Trade only: Ointment (calcipotriene 0.005% + betamethasone dipropionate 0.064%) 15, 30, 60, 100 g. Topical susp 15, 30, 60 g.
NOTES — Do not exceed 100 grams/week. Do not use on more than 30% of body surface area. Do not apply to face, groin, or axillae.
MOA — Vitamin D3 analog that inhibits cell proliferation, regulates skin cell production, anti-inflammatory.
ADVERSE EFFECTS — See calcipotriene and betamethasone.

USTEKINUMAB (*Stelara*) ▶L - ♀B ▶? $$$$$
WARNING — Can cause serious infections. Discontinue if serious infection. Caution if high risk of malignancy. Theoretical risk of infection from mycobacterium, salmonella, and BCG vaccine. Evaluate patients for TB prior to therapy. Risk of reversible posterior leukoencephalopathy syndrome.
ADULTS — Severe plaque psoriasis: Less than 100 kg-45 mg initially and 4 weeks later, followed by 45 mg every 12 weeks. Greater than 100 kg-90 mg initially and 4 weeks later, followed by 90 mg every 12 weeks.
PEDS — Not approved in children.
FORMS — Trade only: 45 and 90 mg prefilled syringe and vial.
MOA — Interleukin antagonist.
ADVERSE EFFECTS — Frequent: Headache, fatigue. Severe: Serious infection, malignancy, disseminated TB-reversible posterior leukoencephalopathy syndrome.

DERMATOLOGY: Antivirals (Topical)

ACYCLOVIR—TOPICAL (*Zovirax*) ▶K ♀C ▶? $$$$$
ADULTS — Initial episodes of herpes genitalis: Apply ointment q 3 h (6 times per day) for 7 days. Non-life-threatening mucocutaneous herpes simplex in immunocompromised patients: Apply ointment q 3 h (6 times per day) for 7 days. Recurrent herpes labialis: Apply cream 5 times per day for 4 days.
PEDS — Recurrent herpes labialis: Apply cream 5 times per day for 4 days for age 12 yo or older.
UNAPPROVED PEDS — Initial episodes of herpes genitalis: Apply ointment q 3 h (6 times per day) for 7 days. Non-life-threatening mucocutaneous herpes simplex in immunocompromised patients: Apply ointment q 3 h (6 times per day) for 7 days.
FORMS — Trade only: Ointment 5% 15 g. Cream 5% 2, 5 g.
NOTES — Use finger cot or rubber glove to apply ointment to avoid dissemination. Burning/stinging may occur in up to 28% of patients. Oral form more effective than topical for herpes genitalis.
MOA — Antiviral; inhibits DNA synthesis and viral replication.
ADVERSE EFFECTS — Frequent: Rash (oint). Skin irritation (cream). Severe: Cutaneous sensitization.

DOCOSANOL (*Abreva*) ▶Not absorbed ♀B ▶? $
ADULTS — Oral-facial herpes (cold sores): Apply 5 times per day until healed.
PEDS — Oral-facial herpes (cold sores): Use adult dose for age 12 yo or older.
FORMS — OTC Trade only: Cream 10% 2 g.
MOA — Inhibits entry of lipid-enveloped viruses.
ADVERSE EFFECTS — Frequent: Headache, site reaction, rash, pruritus, dry skin, ache.

IMIQUIMOD (*Aldara*) ▶Not absorbed ♀C ▶? $$$$$
ADULTS — External genital and perianal warts: Apply 3 times a week at bedtime for up to 16 weeks. Wash off after 8 h. Non-hyperkeratotic, non-hypertrophic actinic keratoses on face/scalp in immunocompetent adults: Apply to face or scalp (but not both) twice a week for up to 16 weeks. Wash off after 8 h. Primary superficial basal cell carcinoma: Apply 5 times per week for 6 weeks. Wash off after 8 h.

(cont.)

IMIQUIMOD (cont.)

PEDS — <u>External genital and perianal warts:</u> Apply 3 times per week at bedtime and wash off after 6 to 10 h for age 12 yo or older.

UNAPPROVED ADULTS — <u>Molluscum contagiosum.</u> Apply 3 times per week for 6 to 10 h.

UNAPPROVED PEDS — <u>Molluscum contagiosum.</u>

FORMS — Generic/Trade: Cream 5% single-use packets.

NOTES — May weaken condoms and diaphragms. Avoid sexual contact while cream is on when used for genital/perianal warts. Most common adverse effects include erythema, itching, erosion, burning, excoriation, edema, and pain. Discard partially used packets.

MOA — Mechanism unknown but may increase cytokine concentrations.

ADVERSE EFFECTS — Frequent: Pruritus, erythema, burning, erosion, edema, flu-like symptoms. Severe: Erythema, erosion, edema.

PENCICLOVIR (Denavir) ▶Not absorbed ♀B ▶? $$

ADULTS — <u>Recurrent herpes labialis (cold sores):</u> Apply q 2 h while awake for 4 days.

PEDS — Not approved in children.

UNAPPROVED PEDS — <u>Recurrent herpes labialis:</u> Apply q 2 h while awake for 4 days.

FORMS — Trade only: Cream 1% tube 1.5 g.

NOTES — Start therapy as soon as possible during prodrome. For moderate to severe cases of herpes labialis, systemic treatment with famciclovir or acyclovir may be preferred.

MOA — Antiviral: Inhibits viral DNA synthesis and replication.

ADVERSE EFFECTS — Frequent: Headache, erythema.

PODOFILOX (Condylox, *Condyline, Wartec) ▶? ♀C ▶? $$$$

ADULTS — <u>External genital warts (gel and soln) and perianal warts (gel only):</u> Apply bid for 3 consecutive days of a weeks and repeat for up to 4 weeks.

PEDS — Not approved in children.

FORMS — Generic/Trade: Soln 0.5% 3.5 mL. Trade only: Gel 0.5% 3.5 g.

MOA — Unknown.

ADVERSE EFFECTS — Frequent: Inflammation, burning, erosion, pain, pruritus, bleeding.

PODOPHYLLIN (Podocon-25, Podofin, Podofilm) ▶? ♀– ▶– $$$

ADULTS — <u>Genital wart removal:</u> Initial application: Apply to wart and leave on for 30 to 40 min to determine patient's sensitivity. Thereafter, use minimum contact time necessary (1 to 4 h depending on result). Remove dried podophyllin with alcohol or soap and water.

PEDS — Not approved in children.

FORMS — Not to be dispensed to patients. For hospital/clinic use; not intended for outpatient prescribing. Trade only: Liquid 25% 15 mL.

NOTES — Not to be dispensed to patients. Do not treat large areas or numerous warts all at once. Contraindicated in diabetics, pregnancy, patients using steroids or with poor circulation, and on bleeding warts.

MOA — Arrests mitosis by binding to microtubule spindle.

ADVERSE EFFECTS — Frequent: Pruritus, N/V, abdominal pain, diarrhea. Severe: Hallucination, hepatotoxicity, leukopenia, thrombocytopenia, renal failure.

SINECATECHINS (Veregen) ▶Unknown ♀C ▶? $$$$$

ADULTS — Apply tid to <u>external genital warts</u> for up to 16 weeks.

PEDS — Not approved in children.

FORMS — Trade only: Ointment 15% 15, 30 g.

NOTES — Botanical drug product. Contains a partially purified fraction of the water extract of green tea leaves. Do not use on open wounds. Do not use in immunocompromised patients. Generic name used to be kunecatechins.

MOA — Unknown, but thought to be immunomodulatory.

ADVERSE EFFECTS — Frequent: Burning, pain, erythema at application site, erosion, edema, induration, rash.

DERMATOLOGY: Atopic Dermatitis Preparations

NOTE: Potential risk of cancer. Should only be used as second-line agent for short-term and intermittent treatment of atopic dermatitis in those unresponsive to or intolerant of other treatments. Long-term safety has not been established. Avoid use in immunocompromised patients and in children younger than 2 yo. Use minimum amount to control symptoms.

PIMECROLIMUS (Elidel) ▶L ♀C ▶? $$$$

ADULTS — <u>Atopic dermatitis:</u> Apply bid.

PEDS — <u>Atopic dermatitis:</u> Apply bid for age 2 yo or older.

FORMS — Trade only: Cream 1% 30, 60, 100 g.

NOTES — Long-term safety unclear.

MOA — Unknown but binds FKBP-12 and inhibits calcium-dependent phosphatase.

ADVERSE EFFECTS — Frequent: Stinging, skin infection, folliculitis.

TACROLIMUS—TOPICAL (Protopic) ▶Minimal absorption ♀C ▶? $$$$$

ADULTS — <u>Atopic dermatitis:</u> Apply bid.

PEDS — <u>Atopic dermatitis:</u> Apply 0.03% ointment bid for age 2 to 15 yo.

UNAPPROVED ADULTS — <u>Vitiligo:</u> Apply 0.1% bid. <u>Chronic allergic contact dermatitis (ie, nickel-induced):</u> Apply 0.1% ointment bid.

FORMS — Trade only: Ointment 0.03%, 0.1% 30, 60, 100 g.

NOTES — Do not use with an occlusive dressing. Continue treatment for 1 week after clearing of symptoms.

TACROLIMUS—TOPICAL (cont.)

MOA — Topical immunomodulator that suppresses T-cell activation and cytokine release.

ADVERSE EFFECTS — Frequent: Skin burning/tingling, pruritus, flu-like symptoms, erythema, headache, urticaria, acne. Severe: LFT increase, anaphylactoid reaction, angina, angioedema.

DERMATOLOGY: Corticosteroids (Topical)

NOTE: After long-term use, do not discontinue abruptly; switch to a less potent agent or alternate use of corticosteroids and emollient products. Monitor for hyperglycemia/adrenal suppression if used for long period of time or over a large area of the body, especially in children. Chronic administration may cause skin atrophy and interfere with pediatric growth and development.

ALCLOMETASONE DIPROPIONATE (*Aclovate*) ▶L ♀C ▶? $$
ADULTS — Inflammatory and pruritic manifestations of corticosteroid-responsive dermatoses: Apply sparingly bid to tid.
PEDS — Inflammatory and pruritic manifestations of corticosteroid-responsive dermatoses: Apply sparingly bid to tid for age 1 yo or older. Safety and efficacy for more than 3 weeks have not been established.
FORMS — Generic/Trade: Ointment, Cream 0.05% 15, 45, 60 g.
MOA — Anti-inflammatory; suppresses DNA synthesis, decreases WBC influx.
ADVERSE EFFECTS — Frequent: Burning, pruritus, dryness, irritation, erythema.

AMCINONIDE (*Cyclocort*) ▶L ♀C ▶? $$
ADULTS — Inflammatory and pruritic manifestations of corticosteroid-responsive dermatoses: Apply sparingly bid to tid.
PEDS — Inflammatory and pruritic manifestations of corticosteroid-responsive dermatoses: Apply sparingly bid to tid.
FORMS — Generic only: Cream, Ointment 0.1% 15, 30, 60 g. Lotion 0.1% 60 mL.
MOA — Anti-inflammatory; suppresses DNA synthesis, decreases WBC influx.
ADVERSE EFFECTS — Frequent: Burning, pruritus, dryness, irritation, erythema. Severe: Steroid atrophy, hypothalamic axis suppression with higher potency preparations.

AUGMENTED BETAMETHASONE DIPROPIONATE (*Diprolene, Diprolene AF, ✦Topilene Glycol*) ▶L ♀C ▶? $$$
ADULTS — Inflammatory and pruritic manifestations of corticosteroid-responsive dermatoses: Apply sparingly daily to bid.
PEDS — Not approved younger than 12 yo.
FORMS — Generic/Trade: Diprolene: Ointment 0.05% 15, 50 g. Lotion 0.05% 30, 60 mL. Diprolene AF: Cream 0.05% 15, 50 g. Generic only: Gel 0.05% 15, 50 g.
NOTES — Do not use occlusive dressings. Do not use for longer than 2 consecutive week and do not exceed a total dose of 45 to 50 g per weeks or 50 mL per weeks of the lotion.
MOA — Anti-inflammatory; suppresses DNA synthesis, decreases WBC influx.
ADVERSE EFFECTS — Frequent: Burning, pruritus, dryness, irritation, erythema. Severe: Steroid atrophy, hypothalamic axis suppression with higher potency preparations.

BETAMETHASONE DIPROPIONATE (*Diprosone, Maxivate, ✦Propaderm, TARO-sone*) ▶L ♀C ▶? $
ADULTS — Inflammatory and pruritic manifestations of corticosteroid-responsive dermatoses: Apply sparingly daily to bid.
PEDS — Inflammatory and pruritic manifestations of corticosteroid-responsive dermatoses: Apply sparingly daily to bid.
FORMS — Generic only: Ointment, Cream 0.05% 15, 45 g. Lotion 0.05% 30, 60 mL.
NOTES — Do not use occlusive dressings.
MOA — Anti-inflammatory; suppresses DNA synthesis, decreases WBC influx.
ADVERSE EFFECTS — Frequent: Burning, pruritus, dryness, irritation, erythema. Severe: Steroid atrophy, hypothalamic axis suppression with higher potency preparations.

BETAMETHASONE VALERATE (*Luxiq foam, Beta-Val, ✦Betaderm*) ▶L ♀C ▶? $
ADULTS — Inflammatory and pruritic manifestations of corticosteroid-responsive dermatoses: Apply sparingly daily to bid. Dermatoses of scalp: Apply small amount of foam to scalp bid.
PEDS — Inflammatory and pruritic manifestations of corticosteroid-responsive dermatoses: Apply sparingly daily to bid.
FORMS — Generic only: Ointment, Cream 0.1% 15, 45 g. Lotion 0.1% 60 mL. Trade only: Foam (Luxiq) 0.12% 50, 100, 150 g.
MOA — Anti-inflammatory; suppresses DNA synthesis, decreases WBC influx.
ADVERSE EFFECTS — Frequent: Burning, pruritus, dryness, irritation, erythema. Severe: Steroid atrophy, hypothalamic axis suppression with higher potency preparations.

CLOBETASOL (*Temovate, Olux, Clobex, Cormax, ✦Dermasone*) ▶L ♀C ▶? $$
ADULTS — Inflammatory and pruritic manifestations of corticosteroid-responsive dermatoses: Apply sparingly bid. For scalp apply foam bid.
PEDS — Not approved in children.
FORMS — Generic/Trade: Cream, Ointment 0.05% 15, 30, 45, 60 g. Scalp application 0.05% 25, 50 mL. Gel 0.05% 15, 30, 60 g. Foam (Olux) 0.05% 50, 100 g. Lotion (Clobex) 0.05% 30, 60, 120 mL. Trade only (Clobex): Spray 0.05% 60, 125 mL. Shampoo 0.05% 118 mL.

(cont.)

DERMATOLOGY: Corticosteroids (Topical)

CLOBETASOL (cont.)
- NOTES — Adrenal suppression at doses as low as 2 g per day. Do not use occlusive dressings. Do not use for longer than 2 consecutive weeks and do not exceed a total dose of 50 g per weeks.
- MOA — Anti-inflammatory; suppresses DNA synthesis, decreases WBC influx.
- ADVERSE EFFECTS — Frequent: Burning, pruritus, dryness, irritation, erythema. Severe: Steroid atrophy, hypothalamic axis suppression with higher potency preparations.

CLOCORTOLONE PIVALATE (*Cloderm*) ▶L ♀C ▶? $$$
- ADULTS — Inflammatory and pruritic manifestations of corticosteroid-responsive dermatoses: Apply sparingly tid.
- PEDS — Inflammatory and pruritic manifestations of corticosteroid-responsive dermatoses: Apply sparingly tid.
- FORMS — Trade only: Cream 0.1% 30, 45, 75, 90 g.
- MOA — Anti-inflammatory; suppresses DNA synthesis, decreases WBC influx.
- ADVERSE EFFECTS — Frequent: Burning, pruritus, dryness, irritation, erythema. Severe: Hypothalamic axis suppression with higher potency preparations.

DESONIDE (*DesOwen, Desonate, Tridesilon, Verdeso*) ▶L ♀C ▶? $$
- ADULTS — Inflammatory and pruritic manifestations of corticosteroid-responsive dermatoses: Apply sparingly bid to tid.
- PEDS — Inflammatory and pruritic manifestations of corticosteroid-responsive dermatoses: Apply sparingly bid to tid.
- FORMS — Generic/Trade: Cream, Ointment 0.05%, 15, 60 g. Lotion 0.05%, 60, 120 mL. Trade only: Gel (Desonate) 0.05% 60 g, Foam (Verdeso) 0.05%, 50, 100 g.
- NOTES — Do not use with occlusive dressings.
- MOA — Anti-inflammatory; suppresses DNA synthesis, decreases WBC influx.
- ADVERSE EFFECTS — Frequent: Burning, pruritus, dryness, irritation, erythema.

DESOXIMETASONE (*Topicort, Topicort LP, ✦Desoxi*) ▶L ♀C ▶? $$$
- ADULTS — Inflammatory and pruritic manifestations of corticosteroid-responsive dermatoses: Apply sparingly bid.
- PEDS — Safety and efficacy have not been established for Topicort 0.25% ointment. For inflammatory and pruritic manifestations of corticosteroid-responsive dermatoses (cream and gel): Apply sparingly bid.
- FORMS — Generic/Trade: Cream, Gel 0.05% 15, 60 g. Cream, Ointment 0.25% 15, 60, 100 g.
- MOA — Anti-inflammatory; suppresses DNA synthesis, decreases WBC influx.
- ADVERSE EFFECTS — Frequent: Burning, pruritus, dryness, irritation, erythema. Severe: Steroid atrophy, hypothalamic axis suppression with higher potency preparations.

DIFLORASONE (*Psorcon E, Maxiflor*) ▶L ♀C ▶? $$$
- ADULTS — Inflammatory and pruritic manifestations of corticosteroid-responsive dermatoses: Apply sparingly daily to tid.
- PEDS — Not approved in children.
- FORMS — Generic/Trade: Cream, Ointment 0.05% 15, 30, 60 g.
- NOTES — Doses of 30 g/day of diflorasone 0.05% cream for 1 week resulted in adrenal suppression in some psoriasis patients.
- MOA — Anti-inflammatory; suppresses DNA synthesis, decreases WBC influx.
- ADVERSE EFFECTS — Frequent: Burning, pruritus, dryness, irritation, erythema. Severe: Steroid atrophy, hypothalamic axis suppression with higher potency preparations.

FLUOCINOLONE (*Synalar, Capex, Derma-Smoothe/FS, ✦Caprex*) ▶L ♀C ▶? $
- ADULTS — Inflammatory and pruritic manifestations of corticosteroid-responsive dermatoses: Apply sparingly bid to tid. Psoriasis of the scalp (Derma-Smoothe/FS): Massage into scalp, cover with shower cap and leave on 4 or more h or overnight and then wash off.
- PEDS — Inflammatory and pruritic manifestations of corticosteroid-responsive dermatoses: Apply sparingly bid to qid. Atopic dermatitis: Moisten skin and apply to affected areas bid for up to 4 weeks (Derma-Smoothe/FS).
- FORMS — Generic/Trade: Cream, Ointment 0.025% 15, 30, 60 g. Soln 0.01% 20, 60 mL. Generic only: Cream 0.01% 15, 60 g. Trade only (Derma-Smoothe/FS): Topical oil 0.01% 120 mL. (Capex) Shampoo 0.01% 120 mL.
- MOA — Anti-inflammatory; suppresses DNA synthesis, decreases WBC influx.
- ADVERSE EFFECTS — Frequent: Burning, pruritus, dryness, irritation, erythema. Severe: Hypothalamic axis suppression with higher potency preparations.

FLUOCINONIDE (*Lidex, Lidex-E, Vanos, ✦Lidemol, Topsyn, Tiamol*) ▶L ♀C ▶? $$
- ADULTS — Inflammatory and pruritic manifestations of corticosteroid-responsive dermatoses: Apply sparingly bid to qid. Plaque-type psoriasis: Apply 0.1% cream (Vanos) daily to bid for 2 consecutive weeks only; no more than 60 g per week. Atopic dermatitis: Apply 0.1% cream (Vanos) once a day.
- PEDS — Inflammatory and pruritic manifestations of corticosteroid-responsive dermatoses: Apply sparingly bid to qid.
- FORMS — Generic/Trade: Cream, Ointment, Gel 0.05% 15, 30, 60 g. Soln 0.05% 20, 60 mL. Trade only: Cream 0.1% 30, 60, 120 g (Vanos).
- MOA — Anti-inflammatory by inhibiting production of prostaglandins and leukotrienes; suppresses DNA synthesis, decreases WBC influx.
- ADVERSE EFFECTS — Frequent: Burning, pruritus, dryness, irritation, erythema. Severe: Immunosuppression (with more than 2 weeks use), steroid atrophy, hypothalamic axis suppression with higher potency preparations.

DERMATOLOGY: Corticosteroids (Topical)

FLURANDRENOLIDE (*Cordran, Cordran SP*) ▶L ♀C ▶? $$$
- ADULTS — <u>Inflammatory and pruritic manifestations of corticosteroid-responsive dermatoses:</u> Apply sparingly bid to tid.
- PEDS — <u>Inflammatory and pruritic manifestations of corticosteroid-responsive dermatoses:</u> Apply sparingly bid to tid.
- FORMS — Trade only: Ointment, Cream 0.05% 15, 30, 60 g. Lotion 0.05% 15, 60 mL. Tape 4 mcg/cm2.
- MOA — Anti-inflammatory; suppresses DNA synthesis, decreases WBC influx.
- ADVERSE EFFECTS — Frequent: Burning, pruritus, dryness, irritation, erythema. Severe: Hypothalamic axis suppression with higher potency preparations.

FLUTICASONE—TOPICAL (*Cutivate, ✽ Flixonase, Flixotide*) ▶L ♀C ▶? $$
- ADULTS — <u>Eczema:</u> Apply sparingly daily to bid. <u>Other inflammatory and pruritic manifestations of corticosteroid-responsive dermatoses:</u> Apply sparingly bid.
- PEDS — Children older than 3 mo: <u>Eczema:</u> Apply sparingly daily to bid. <u>Other inflammatory and pruritic manifestations of corticosteroid-responsive dermatoses:</u> Apply sparingly bid.
- FORMS — Generic/Trade: Cream 0.05% 15, 30, 60 g. Ointment 0.005% 15, 30, 60 g. Trade only: Lotion 0.05% 120 mL.
- NOTES — Do not use with an occlusive dressing.
- MOA — Anti-inflammatory; suppresses DNA synthesis, decreases WBC influx.
- ADVERSE EFFECTS — Frequent: Burning, pruritus, dryness, irritation, erythema. Severe: Hypothalamic axis suppression with higher potency preparations.

HALCINONIDE (*Halog*) ▶L ♀C ▶? $$
- ADULTS — <u>Inflammatory and pruritic manifestations of corticosteroid-responsive dermatoses:</u> Apply sparingly bid to tid.
- PEDS — <u>Inflammatory and pruritic manifestations of corticosteroid-responsive dermatoses:</u> Apply sparingly bid to tid.
- FORMS — Trade only: Cream, Ointment 0.1% 15, 30, 60 g. Soln 0.1% 20, 60 mL.
- MOA — Anti-inflammatory; suppresses DNA synthesis, decreases WBC influx.
- ADVERSE EFFECTS — Frequent: Burning, pruritus, dryness, irritation, erythema. Severe: Steroid atrophy, hypothalamic axis suppression with higher potency preparations.

HALOBETASOL PROPIONATE (*Ultravate*) ▶L ♀C ▶? $$
- ADULTS — <u>Inflammatory and pruritic manifestations of corticosteroid-responsive dermatoses:</u> Apply sparingly daily to bid.
- PEDS — Not approved in children.
- FORMS — Generic/Trade: Cream, Ointment 0.05% 15, 50 g.
- NOTES — Do not use occlusive dressings. Do not use for more than 2 consecutive weeks and do not exceed a total dose of 50 g/week.
- MOA — Anti-inflammatory; suppresses DNA synthesis, decreases WBC influx.
- ADVERSE EFFECTS — Frequent: Burning, pruritus, dryness, irritation, erythema. Severe: Steroid atrophy, hypothalamic axis suppression with higher potency preparations.

HYDROCORTISONE—TOPICAL (*Cortizone, Hycort, Hytone, Tegrin-HC, Dermolate, Synacort, Anusol-HC, Proctocream HC, ✽ Cortoderm, Prevex-HC, Cortate, Emo-Cort*) ▶L ♀C ▶? $
- ADULTS — <u>Inflammatory and pruritic manifestations of corticosteroid-responsive dermatoses:</u> Apply sparingly bid to qid. <u>External anal itching:</u> Apply cream tid to qid prn or suppository bid or rectal foam daily to bid.
- PEDS — <u>Inflammatory and pruritic manifestations of corticosteroid-responsive dermatoses:</u> Apply sparingly bid to qid.
- FORMS — Products available OTC and Rx depending on labeling. 2.5% preparation available Rx only. Generic/Trade: Ointment 0.5% 30 g. Ointment 1% 15, 20, 30, 60, 454 g. Ointment 2.5% 5, 20, 30, 454 g. Cream 0.5% 30 g. Cream 1% 5, 15, 20, 30, 120 g. Cream 2.5% 5, 20, 30, 454 g. Lotion 1% 120 mL. Lotion 2.5% 60 mL. Anal preparations: Generic/Trade: Cream 2.5% 30 g (Anusol HC, Proctocream HC). Suppositories 25 mg (Anusol HC).
- MOA — Anti-inflammatory; suppresses DNA synthesis, decreases WBC influx.
- ADVERSE EFFECTS — Frequent: Burning, pruritus, dryness, irritation, erythema.

HYDROCORTISONE ACETATE (*Cortaid, Corticaine, Cortifoam, Micort-HC Lipocream, ✽ Hyderm, Cortamed*) ▶L ♀C ▶? $
- ADULTS — <u>Inflammatory and pruritic manifestations of corticosteroid-responsive dermatoses:</u> Apply sparingly bid to qid.
- PEDS — <u>Inflammatory and pruritic manifestations of corticosteroid-responsive dermatoses:</u> Apply sparingly bid to qid.
- FORMS — OTC Generic/Trade: Ointment 0.5% 15 g. Ointment 1% 15, 30 g. Cream 0.5% 15 g. Cream 1% 15, 30, 60 g. Topical spray 1% 60 mL. Rx Trade only: Cream 2.5% 30 g (Micort-HC Lipocream). Rectal foam 15 g (Cortifoam).
- MOA — Anti-inflammatory; suppresses DNA synthesis, decreases WBC influx.
- ADVERSE EFFECTS — Frequent: Burning, pruritus, dryness, irritation, erythema.

HYDROCORTISONE BUTYRATE (*Locoid, Locoid Lipocream*) ▶L ♀C ▶? $$
- ADULTS — <u>Inflammatory and pruritic manifestations of corticosteroid-responsive dermatoses:</u> Apply sparingly bid to tid. <u>Seborrheic dermatitis</u> (soln only): Apply bid to tid.
- PEDS — <u>Inflammatory and pruritic manifestations of corticosteroid-responsive dermatoses:</u> Apply sparingly bid to tid. <u>Seborrheic dermatitis</u> (soln only): Apply bid to tid.
- FORMS — Generic/Trade: Cream, Ointment 0.1% 15, 45 g. Soln 0.1% 20, 60 mL. Trade only: Cream 0.1% (Lipocream) 15, 45, 60 g.
- MOA — Anti-inflammatory; suppresses DNA synthesis, decreases WBC influx.
- ADVERSE EFFECTS — Frequent: Burning, pruritus, dryness, irritation, erythema. Severe: Hypothalamic axis suppression with higher potency preparations.

DERMATOLOGY: Corticosteroid/Antimicrobial Combinations

HYDROCORTISONE PROBUTATE (*Pandel*) ▶L ♀C ▶? $$
- ADULTS — <u>Inflammatory and pruritic manifestations of corticosteroid-responsive dermatoses:</u> Apply sparingly daily to bid.
- PEDS — Not approved in children.
- FORMS — Trade only: Cream 0.1% 15, 45, 80 g.
- MOA — Anti-inflammatory; suppresses DNA synthesis, decreases WBC influx.
- ADVERSE EFFECTS — Frequent: Burning, pruritus, dryness, irritation, erythema. Severe: Hypothalamic axis suppression with higher potency preparations.

HYDROCORTISONE VALERATE (*Westcort,* ✦*Hydroval*) ▶L ♀C ▶? $$
- ADULTS — <u>Inflammatory and pruritic manifestations of corticosteroid-responsive dermatoses:</u> Apply sparingly bid to tid.
- PEDS — Safety and efficacy of Westcort ointment have not been established in children. <u>Inflammatory and pruritic manifestations of corticosteroid-responsive dermatoses</u> (cream only): Apply sparingly bid to tid.
- FORMS — Generic/Trade: Cream, Ointment 0.2% 15, 45, 60 g.
- MOA — Anti-inflammatory; suppresses DNA synthesis, decreases WBC influx.
- ADVERSE EFFECTS — Frequent: Burning, pruritus, dryness, irritation, erythema. Severe: Hypothalamic axis suppression with higher potency preparations.

MOMETASONE—TOPICAL (*Elocon,* ✦*Elocom*) ▶L ♀C ▶? $
- ADULTS — <u>Inflammatory and pruritic manifestations of corticosteroid-responsive dermatoses:</u> Apply sparingly once a day.
- PEDS — <u>Inflammatory and pruritic manifestations of corticosteroid-responsive dermatoses:</u> Apply sparingly once a day for 2 yo or older. Safety and efficacy for more than 3 weeks have not been established.
- FORMS — Generic/Trade: Cream, Ointment 0.1% 15, 45 g. Lotion 0.1% 30, 60 mL.
- NOTES — Do not use an occlusive dressing. Not for ophthalmic use.
- MOA — Anti-inflammatory; suppresses DNA synthesis, decreases WBC influx.
- ADVERSE EFFECTS — Frequent: Burning, pruritus, dryness, irritation, erythema. Severe: Hypothalamic axis suppression with higher potency preparations, skin atrophy.

PREDNICARBATE (*Dermatop*) ▶L ♀C ▶? $$
- ADULTS — <u>Inflammatory and pruritic manifestations of corticosteroid-responsive dermatoses:</u> Apply sparingly bid.
- PEDS — <u>Inflammatory and pruritic manifestations of corticosteroid-responsive dermatoses:</u> Apply sparingly bid for age 1 yo or older. Safety and efficacy for more than 3 weeks have not been established.
- FORMS — Generic/Trade: Cream, Ointment 0.1% 15, 60 g.
- MOA — Anti-inflammatory; suppresses DNA synthesis, decreases WBC influx.
- ADVERSE EFFECTS — Frequent: Burning, pruritus, dryness, irritation, erythema. Severe: Hypothalamic axis suppression with higher potency preparations.

TRIAMCINOLONE—TOPICAL (*Kenalog, Kenalog in Orabase,* ✦*Oracort, Triaderm*) ▶L ♀C ▶? $
- ADULTS — <u>Inflammatory and pruritic manifestations of corticosteroid-responsive dermatoses:</u> Apply sparingly tid to qid. <u>Oral paste: Aphthous ulcers:</u> Using finger, apply about 1 cm of paste to oral lesion and a thin film will develop. Apply paste bid to tid, ideally after meals and at bedtime.
- PEDS — <u>Inflammatory and pruritic manifestations of corticosteroid-responsive dermatoses:</u> Apply sparingly tid to qid.
- FORMS — Generic/Trade: Cream, Ointment 0.1% 15, 60, 80 g. Cream 0.5% 20 g. Lotion 0.025% and 0.1% 60 mL. Oral paste (in Orabase) 0.1% 5 g. Generic only: Cream, Ointment 0.025% 15, 80 g. Cream, Ointment 0.5% 15 g. Trade only: Aerosol topical spray 0.147 mg/g, 63 g.
- MOA — Anti-inflammatory; suppresses DNA synthesis, decreases WBC influx.
- ADVERSE EFFECTS — Frequent: Burning, pruritus, dryness, irritation, erythema. Severe: Steroid atrophy, hypothalamic axis suppression with higher potency preparations.

DERMATOLOGY: Corticosteroid/Antimicrobial Combinations

CORTISPORIN (neomycin + polymyxin + hydrocortisone) ▶LK ♀C ▶? $$$
- ADULTS — <u>Corticosteroid-responsive dermatoses with secondary infection:</u> Apply bid to qid.
- PEDS — Not approved in children.
- UNAPPROVED PEDS — <u>Corticosteroid-responsive dermatoses with secondary infection:</u> Apply bid to qid.
- FORMS — Trade only: Cream 7.5 g. Ointment 15 g.
- NOTES — Due to concerns about nephrotoxicity and ototoxicity associated with neomycin, do not use over wide areas or for prolonged periods of time.
- MOA — Antibacterial + anti-inflammatory.
- ADVERSE EFFECTS — Ocular: Frequent: Blurred vision, itching, elevation of intraocular pressure, glaucoma. Severe: Hypersensitivity, anaphylaxis.

FUCIDIN H (fusidic acid + hydrocortisone) ▶L ♀? ▶? $$
- ADULTS — Canada only. <u>Atopic dermatitis:</u> Apply tid.
- PEDS — Canada only. <u>Atopic dermatitis:</u> Apply tid for age 3 yo or older.
- FORMS — Canada Trade only: Cream (2% fusidic acid, 1% hydrocortisone acetate) 30 g.
- MOA — Antibacterial, interferes with bacterial protein synthesis + anti-inflammatory.
- ADVERSE EFFECTS — Serious: Hypersensitivity. Frequent: Mild irritation, flare of dermatitis.

DERMATOLOGY: Other Dermatologic Agents

LOCACORTEN VIOFORM (flumethasone + cloquinol) ▶? ♀? ▶? $$
ADULTS — Canada only. Skin: Apply bid to tid. Otic gtts: 2 to 3 gtts bid.
PEDS — Canada only. Skin: Apply bid to tid for age 2 yo or older. Otic gtts: 2 to 3 gtts bid.
FORMS — Canada trade only: Cream 0.02% flumethasone, 3% clioquinol 15, 50 g. Otic gtts 0.02% flumethasone, 1% clioquinol, 10 mL.
NOTES — May stain clothing.
MOA — Topical antibacterial/antifungal/corticosteroid.
ADVERSE EFFECTS — Frequent: Administration site irritation.

LOTRISONE (clotrimazole + betamethasone, ✦*Lotriderm*) ▶L ♀C ▶? $$$
ADULTS — Tinea pedis, cruris, and corporis: Apply bid.
PEDS — Not approved in children.
FORMS — Generic/Trade: Cream (clotrimazole 1% + betamethasone 0.05%) 15, 45 g. Lotion (clotrimazole 1% + betamethasone 0.05%) 30 mL.
NOTES — Treat tinea cruris and corporis for 2 weeks and tinea pedis for 4 weeks. Do not use for diaper dermatitis.
MOA — Antifungal + anti-inflammatory.
ADVERSE EFFECTS — Frequent: Erythema, stinging, blistering, peeling, edema, pruritus, urticaria, irritation, telangiectasia.

MYCOLOG II (nystatin + triamcinolone) ▶L ♀C ▶? $
ADULTS — Cutaneous candidiasis: Apply bid.
PEDS — Not approved in children.
UNAPPROVED PEDS — Sometimes used for diaper dermatitis, but not recommended due to risk of adrenal suppression.
FORMS — Generic only: Cream, Ointment 15, 30, 60, 120, 454 g.
NOTES — Avoid occlusive dressings.
MOA — Antifungal + anti-inflammatory.
ADVERSE EFFECTS — Frequent: None. Severe: Stevens-Johnson syndrome.

DERMATOLOGY: Hemorrhoid Care

DIBUCAINE (*Nupercainal*) ▶L ♀? ▶? $
ADULTS — Hemorrhoids or other anorectal disorders: Apply tid to qid prn.
PEDS — Not approved in children.
UNAPPROVED PEDS — Hemorrhoids or other anorectal disorders: Apply tid to qid prn for age older than 2 yo or wt greater than 35 lbs.
FORMS — OTC Trade only: Ointment 1% 30, 60 g.
NOTES — Do not use if younger than 2 yo or wt less than 35 pounds.
MOA — Anesthetic, anti-inflammatory.
ADVERSE EFFECTS — Frequent: None.

HYDROCORTISONE + PRAMOXINE-TOPICAL (*Analpram-HC, Epifoam, Proctofoam HC*) ▶L ♀C ▶? $$$
ADULTS — Inflammatory and pruritic manifestations of corticosteroid-responsive dermatoses of the anal region: Apply bid to qid.
PEDS — Use with caution. Inflammatory and pruritic manifestations of corticosteroid-responsive dermatoses of the anal region: Apply bid to qid.
FORMS — Trade only: Topical aerosol foam (Proctofoam HC, Epifoam 1% hydrocortisone + 1% pramoxine) 10 g. Cream (Analpram-HC 1% hydrocortisone + 1% pramoxine, 2.5% hydrocortisone + 1% pramoxine) 4 g, 30 g. Lotion (Analpram-HC 2.5% hydrocortisone + 1% pramoxine) 60 mL.
MOA — Combination of local anesthetic and anti-inflammatory; suppresses DNA synthesis, decreases WBC influx.
ADVERSE EFFECTS — Frequent: Redness, irritation, pain.

PRAMOXINE (*Tucks Hemorrhoidal Ointment, Fleet Pain Relief, Proctofoam NS*) ▶Not absorbed ♀+ ▶+ $
ADULTS — Hemorrhoids: Apply ointment, pads, or foam up to 5 times per day prn.
PEDS — Not approved in children.
FORMS — OTC Trade only: Ointment (Tucks Hemorrhoidal Ointment) 30 g. Pads (Fleet Pain Relief) 100 ea. Aerosol foam (ProctoFoam NS) 15 g.
MOA — Anesthetic.
ADVERSE EFFECTS — Frequent: Redness, irritation, swelling, pain.

STARCH (*Tucks Suppositories*) ▶Not absorbed ♀+ ▶+ $
ADULTS — Hemorrhoids: 1 suppository PR up to 6 times per day prn or after each bowel movement.
PEDS — Not approved in children.
FORMS — OTC Trade only: Suppository (51% topical starch; vegetable oil, tocopheryl acetate) 12, 24 ea.
MOA — Lubricant.
ADVERSE EFFECTS — Frequent: None.

WITCH HAZEL (*Tucks*) ▶? ♀+ ▶+ $
ADULTS — Hemorrhoids: Apply to anus/perineum up to 6 times per day prn.
PEDS — Not approved in children.
FORMS — OTC Generic/Trade: Pads 50% 12, 40, 100 ea, generically available in various quantities.
MOA — Astringent.
ADVERSE EFFECTS — Frequent: None.

DERMATOLOGY: Other Dermatologic Agents

ALITRETINOIN (*Panretin*) ▶Not absorbed ♀D ▶− $$$$$
WARNING — May cause fetal harm if significant absorption were to occur. Women of child-bearing age should be advised to avoid becoming pregnant during treatment.
ADULTS — Cutaneous lesions of AIDS-related Kaposi's sarcoma: Apply bid to qid.
PEDS — Not approved in children.
FORMS — Trade only: Gel 0.1% 60 g.

(cont.)

152   DERMATOLOGY: Other Dermatologic Agents

ALITRETINOIN (cont.)
MOA – Binds retinoid receptors to inhibit Kaposi's sarcoma.
ADVERSE EFFECTS – Frequent: Pain, rash, pruritus, paresthesia, edema, dermatitis.

ALUMINUM CHLORIDE (*Drysol, Certain Dri*) ▶K ♀? ▶? $
ADULTS – <u>Hyperhidrosis:</u> Apply at bedtime. For maximum effect, cover area with plastic wrap held in place with tight shirt and wash area following morning. Once excessive sweating stopped, use once a week or twice a week.
PEDS – Not approved in children.
FORMS – Rx Trade only: Soln 20% 37.5 mL bottle, 35, 60 mL bottle with applicator. OTC Trade only (Certain Dri): Soln 12.5% 36 mL bottle.
NOTES – To prevent irritation, apply to dry area.
MOA – Astringent.
ADVERSE EFFECTS – Frequent: Irritation, burning, prickling.

BECAPLERMIN (*Regranex*) ▶Minimal absorption ♀C ▶? $$$$$
WARNING – Increased rate of mortality due to malignancy in patients who used 3 or more tubes. Use with caution in patients with known malignancy.
ADULTS – <u>Diabetic neuropathic ulcers:</u> Apply daily and cover with saline-moistened gauze for 12 h. Rinse after 12 h and cover with saline gauze without medication.
PEDS – Not approved in children.
FORMS – Trade only: Gel 0.01%, 2, 15 g.
NOTES – Length of gel to be applied calculated by size of wound (length × width × 0.6 = amount of gel in inches). If ulcer does not decrease by 30% in size by 10 weeks or complete healing has not occurred by 20 weeks, continued therapy should be reassessed. Ineffective for stasis ulcers and pressure ulcers. Increased cancer mortality in patients who use 3 or more tubes of the product.
MOA – Recombinant human platelet-derived growth factor, which promotes cellular proliferation and angiogenesis, enhances new granulation tissue, and induces fibroblast proliferation and differentiation.
ADVERSE EFFECTS – Frequent: None Severe: Increased cancer mortality.

CALAMINE ▶? ♀? ▶? $
ADULTS – <u>Itching due to poison ivy/oak/sumac, insect bites, or minor irritation:</u> Apply up to tid to qid prn.
PEDS – <u>Itching due to poison ivy/oak/sumac, insect bites, or minor irritation:</u> Apply up to tid to qid prn for age older than 2 yo.
FORMS – OTC Generic only: Lotion 120, 240, 480 mL.
MOA – Astringent.
ADVERSE EFFECTS – Frequent: Dryness.

CAPSAICIN (*Zostrix, Zostrix-HP*) ▶? ♀? ▶? $
ADULTS – <u>Pain due to RA, OA, and neuralgias such as zoster or diabetic neuropathies:</u> Apply to affected area up to tid to qid.
PEDS – Children older than 2 yo: <u>Pain due to RA, OA, and neuralgias such as zoster or diabetic neuropathies:</u> Apply to affected area up to tid to qid.

UNAPPROVED ADULTS – <u>Psoriasis and intractable pruritus, postmastectomy/postamputation neuromas (phantom limb pain), vulvar vestibulitis, apocrine chromhidrosis, and reflex sympathetic dystrophy.</u>
FORMS – OTC Generic/Trade: Cream 0.025% 60 g, 0.075% (HP) 60 g. OTC Generic only: Lotion 0.025% 59 mL, 0.075% 59 mL.
NOTES – Burning occurs in 30% or more of patients but diminishes with continued use. Pain more commonly occurs when applied less than tid to qid. Wash hands immediately after application.
MOA – Counter-irritant, releases Substance P.
ADVERSE EFFECTS – Frequent: Burning, redness, sensation of warmth.

CARMOL HC (hydrocortisone acetate + urea) ▶L ♀C ▶? $$
ADULTS – <u>Inflammatory and pruritic manifestations of corticosteroid-responsive dermatoses:</u> Apply sparingly bid to qid.
PEDS – <u>Inflammatory and pruritic manifestations of corticosteroid-responsive dermatoses:</u> Apply sparingly bid to qid.
FORMS – Generic/Trade: Hydrocortisone acetate 1% + urea 10% cream 85 g (Trade), 30 g (U-cort).
MOA – Anti-inflammatory; suppresses DNA synthesis, decreases WBC influx.
ADVERSE EFFECTS – Frequent: Burning, pruritus, dryness, irritation, erythema.

COAL TAR (*Polytar, Tegrin, Cutar, Tarsum*) ▶? ♀? ▶? $
ADULTS – <u>Dandruff, seborrheic dermatitis:</u> Apply shampoo at least twice a week. <u>Psoriasis:</u> Apply to affected areas daily to qid or use shampoo on affected areas.
PEDS – Children older than 2 yo: <u>Dandruff, seborrheic dermatitis:</u> Apply shampoo at least twice a week. <u>Psoriasis:</u> Apply to affected areas daily to qid or use shampoo on affected areas.
FORMS – OTC Generic/Trade: Shampoo, cream, ointment, gel, lotion, liquid, oil, soap.
NOTES – May cause photosensitivity for up to 24 h after application.
MOA – Unknown.
ADVERSE EFFECTS – Frequent: folliculitis, skin and hair staining, photosensitivity, contact dermatitis.

DEET (*Off, Cutter, Repel, Ultrathon, n-n-diethyl-m-toluamide*) ▶L ♀+ ▶+ $
ADULTS – <u>Mosquito repellant:</u> 10% to 50% every 2 to 6 h. Higher concentration products do not work better, but have a longer duration of action.
PEDS – Up to 30% spray/lotion every 2 to 6 h for age 2 mo or older.
FORMS – OTC Generic/Trade: Spray, lotion, towelette 4.75% to 100%.
NOTES – Duration of action varies by concentration. For example, 23.8% DEET provides approximately 5 h of protection from mosquito bites, 20% DEET provides approximately 4 h of protection, 6.65% DEET provides approximately 2 h of protection and products with 4.75% DEET provides approximately 1.5 h of protection. Apply sunscreen prior to application of DEET-containing products.

(cont.)

DERMATOLOGY: Other Dermatologic Agents

DEET (cont.)
MOA – Repels female mosquitos; does not kill them.
ADVERSE EFFECTS – Frequent: Dermatitis.

DOXEPIN—TOPICAL (*Zonalon*) ▶L ♀B ▶– $$$$
ADULTS – <u>Pruritus associated with atopic dermatitis, lichen simplex chronicus, eczematous dermatitis:</u> Apply qid for up to 8 days.
PEDS – Not approved in children.
FORMS – Trade only: Cream 5% 30, 45 g.
NOTES – Risk of systemic toxicity increased if applied to more than 10% of body. Can cause contact dermatitis.
MOA – Inhibits pre-synaptic uptake of serotonin +/- norepinephrine.
ADVERSE EFFECTS – Frequent: None.

EFLORNITHINE (*Vaniqa*) ▶K ♀C ▶? $$$
ADULTS – <u>Reduction of facial hair:</u> Apply to face bid at least 8 h apart.
PEDS – Not approved in children.
FORMS – Trade only: Cream 13.9% 30 g.
NOTES – Takes 4 to 8 weeks or more to see an effect.
MOA – Specific, irreversible inhibition of ornithine decarboxylase, reduces length of growing cycle so hair becomes progressively shorter.
ADVERSE EFFECTS – Frequent: Stinging, burning, tingling, erythema, rash.

EMLA (prilocaine + lidocaine - topical) ▶LK ♀B ▶? $$
ADULTS – <u>Topical anesthesia for minor dermal procedures</u> (eg, IV cannulation, venipuncture) apply 2.5 g over 20 to 25 cm2 area or 1 disc at least 1 h prior to procedure, for major dermal procedures (ie, skin grafting harvesting) apply 2 g/10 cm2 area at least 2 h prior to procedure.
PEDS – <u>Prior to circumcision in infants older than 37 weeks gestation:</u> Apply a max dose 1 g over max of 10 cm2. <u>Topical anesthesia:</u> Children age 1 to 3 mo or less than 5 kg: Apply a max 1 g dose over max of 10 cm2; age 4 to 12 mo and more than 5 kg: Apply max 2 g dose over a max of 20 cm2; age 1 to 6 yo and more than 10 kg: Apply max dose 10 g over max of 100 cm2; age 7 to 12 yo and more than 20 kg: Apply max dose 20 g over max of 200 cm2.
FORMS – Generic/Trade: Cream (2.5% lidocaine + 2.5% prilocaine) 5, 30 g.
NOTES – Cover cream with an occlusive dressing. Do not use in children younger than 12 mo if child is receiving treatment with methemoglobin-inducing agents. Do not use on open wounds. Patients with glucose-6-phosphate deficiencies are more susceptible to methemoglobinemia. Use caution with amiodarone, bretylium, sotalol, dofetilide; possible additive cardiac effects. Dermal analgesia increases for up to 3 h under occlusive dressings and persists for 1 to 2 h after removal.
MOA – Anesthetic.
ADVERSE EFFECTS – Frequent: None. Severe: CNS effects, tachycardia, bronchospasm, hypotension.

HYALURONIC ACID (*Bionect, Restylane, Perlane*) ▶? ♀? ▶? $$$
ADULTS – <u>Moderate to severe facial wrinkles:</u> Inject into wrinkle/fold (Restylane). <u>Protection of dermal ulcers:</u> Apply gel/cream/spray to wound bid or tid (Bionect).
PEDS – Not approved in children.
FORMS – OTC Trade only: Cream 2% 15, 30 g. Rx Generic/Trade: Soln 3% 30 mL. Gel 4% 30 g. Cream 4% 15, 30, 60 g.
NOTES – Do not use more than 1.5 mL of injectable form per treatment area. Injectable product contains trace amounts of gram positive bacterial proteins; contraindicated if history of anaphylaxis or severe allergy.
MOA – Increases volume under skin to smooth out wrinkle.
ADVERSE EFFECTS – Frequent (injectable product): Bruising, redness, swelling, pain, tenderness, itching. Severe (injectable product): Bacterial infections, anaphylaxis, severe allergic reactions.

HYDROQUINONE (*Eldopaque, Eldoquin, Eldoquin Forte, EpiQuin Micro, Esoterica, Glyquin, Lustra, Melanex, Solaquin, Claripel, ✦Ultraquin*) ▶? ♀C ▶? $
ADULTS – <u>Temporary bleaching of hyperpigmented skin conditions (ie, chloasma, melasma, freckles, senile lentigines, ultraviolet-induced discoloration from oral contraceptives, pregnancy, or hormone therapy):</u> Apply bid to affected area.
PEDS – Not approved in children.
FORMS – OTC Trade only: Cream 2% 15, 30 g. Rx Generic/Trade: Soln 3% 30 mL. Gel 4% 30 g. Cream 4% 15, 30, 60 g.
NOTES – Responses may take 3 weeks to 6 months. Use a sunscreen on treated exposed areas.
MOA – Reversible depigmentation of skin by suppression of melanocytes.
ADVERSE EFFECTS – Frequent: None.

LACTIC ACID (*Lac-Hydrin, Amlactin, ✦Dermalac*) ▶? ♀? ▶? $$
ADULTS – <u>Ichthyosis vulgaris and xerosis</u> (dry, scaly skin): Apply bid to affected area.
PEDS – <u>Ichthyosis vulgaris and xerosis</u> (dry, scaly skin) in children older than 2 yo: Apply bid to affected area.
FORMS – Trade only: Lotion 12% 150, 360 mL. Generic/OTC: Cream 12% 140, 385 g. AmLactin AP is lactic acid (12%) with pramoxine (1%).
NOTES – Frequently causes irritation in non-intact skin. Minimize exposure to sun, artificial sunlight.
MOA – Humectant, reduce corneocyte cohesion.
ADVERSE EFFECTS – Frequent: Stinging, burning.

LIDOCAINE—TOPICAL (*Xylocaine, Lidoderm, Numby Stuff, LMX, Zingo, ✦Maxilene*) ▶LK ♀B ▶+ $$
WARNING – Contraindicated in allergy to amide-type anesthetics.
ADULTS – <u>Topical anesthesia:</u> Apply to affected area prn. Dose varies with anesthetic procedure, degree of anesthesia required and individual patient response. <u>Postherpetic neuralgia</u> (patch): Apply up

(cont.)

154 DERMATOLOGY: Other Dermatologic Agents

LIDOCAINE—TOPICAL (cont.)
to 3 patches to affected area at once for up to 12 h within a 24 h period.
PEDS − Topical anesthesia: Apply to affected area prn. Dose varies with anesthetic procedure, degree of anesthesia required and individual patient response. Max 3 mg/kg/dose, do not repeat dose within 2 h. Intradermal powder injection for venipuncture/IV cannulation, for age 3 to 18 yo (Zingo): 0.5 mg to site 1 to 10 min prior.
UNAPPROVED PEDS − Topical anesthesia prior to venipuncture: Apply 30 min prior to procedure (ELA-Max 4%).
FORMS − For membranes of mouth and pharynx: Spray 10%, Ointment 5%, Liquid 5%, Soln 2%, 4%, Dental patch. For urethral use: Jelly 2%. Patch (Lidoderm) 5%. Intradermal powder injection system: 0.5 mg (Zingo). OTC Trade only: Liposomal lidocaine 4% (ELA-Max).
NOTES − Apply patches only to intact skin to cover the most painful area. Patches may be cut into smaller sizes with scissors prior to removal of the release liner. Store and dispose out of the reach of children and pets to avoid possible toxicity from ingestion.
MOA − Anesthetic.
ADVERSE EFFECTS − Frequent: Skin irritation. Severe: CNS effects, bradycardia, bronchospasm, hypotension, allergic reactions.

MINOXIDIL—TOPICAL (*Rogaine, Women's Rogaine, Rogaine Extra Strength, Minoxidil for Men, Theroxidil Extra Strength, ✦Minox, Apo-Gain*) ▶K ♀C ▶− $
ADULTS − Androgenetic alopecia in men or women: 1 mL to dry scalp bid.
PEDS − Not approved in children.
UNAPPROVED ADULTS − Alopecia areata.
UNAPPROVED PEDS − Alopecia: Apply to dry scalp bid.
FORMS − OTC Generic/Trade: Soln 2% 60 mL (Rogaine, Womens Rogaine). Soln 5% 60 mL (Rogaine Extra Strength, Theroxidil Extra Strength - for men only). Foam 5% 60 g (Rogaine Extra Strength).
NOTES − 5% strength for men only. Alcohol content may cause burning and stinging. Evidence of hair growth usually takes at least 4 months. If treatment is stopped, new hair will be shed in a few months.
MOA − Promotes hair growth.
ADVERSE EFFECTS − None.

MONOBENZONE (*Benoquin*) ▶Minimal absorption ♀C ▶? $$$
ADULTS − Extensive vitiligo: Apply bid to tid.
PEDS − Not approved age if younger than 12 yo.
FORMS − Trade only: Cream 20% 35.4 g.
NOTES − Avoid prolonged exposure to sunlight. May take 1 to 4 months for depigmentation to occur. Depigmentation is permanent and can cause lifelong increase in photosensitivity.
MOA − Increases excretion of melanin from melanocytes.
ADVERSE EFFECTS − Frequent: Minor skin irritation.

OATMEAL (*Aveeno*) ▶Not absorbed ♀? ▶? $
ADULTS − Pruritus from poison ivy/oak, varicella: Apply lotion qid prn. Also available in packets to be added to bath.

PEDS − Pruritus from poison ivy/oak, varicella: Apply lotion qid prn. Also available in bath packets for tub.
FORMS − OTC Generic/Trade: Lotion. Bath packets.
MOA − Anti-pruritic, lubricating.
ADVERSE EFFECTS − Frequent: None.

PANAFIL (papain + urea + chlorophyllin copper complex) ▶? ♀? ▶? $$$
ADULTS − Debridement of acute or chronic lesions: Apply to clean wound and cover daily to bid.
PEDS − Not approved in children.
FORMS − Trade only: Ointment 6, 30 g. Spray 33 mL.
NOTES − Longer redressings (2 to 3 days) are acceptable. May be applied under pressure dressings. Hydrogen peroxide inactivates papain; avoid concomitant use.
MOA − Enzymatic debridement.
ADVERSE EFFECTS − Frequent: Burning, profuse exudates.

PLIAGIS (tetracaine + lidocaine - topical) ▶Minimal absorption ♀B ▶? $$
WARNING − Contraindicated in allergy to amide-type anesthetics.
ADULTS − Prior to venipuncture, intravenous cannulation, superficial dermatological procedure: Apply 20 to 30 min prior to procedure (60 min for tattoo removal).
PEDS − Not approved in children.
FORMS − Trade only: Cream lidocaine 7% + tetracaine 7%.
MOA − Topical anesthetic.
ADVERSE EFFECTS − Frequent: Skin irritation, erythema, blanching, rash. Severe: CNS effects, bradycardia, bronchospasm, hypotension.

POLY-L-LACTIC ACID (*Sculptra*) ▶Not absorbed ♀? ▶? $$$$$
ADULTS − Restoration of facial fat loss due to HIV lipoatrophy: Dose based on degree of correction needed.
PEDS − Not approved in children younger than 18 yo.
MOA − Biocompatible, biodegradable, synthetic polymer.
ADVERSE EFFECTS − Frequent: Bruising, edema, discomfort, hematoma, inflammation, erythema, injection site papule.

PRAMOSONE (pramoxine + hydrocortisone, ✦*Pramox HC*) ▶Not absorbed ♀C ▶? $$$
ADULTS − Apply tid to qid.
PEDS − Apply bid to tid.
FORMS − Trade only: 1% pramoxine/1% hydrocortisone acetate Cream 30, 60 g. Ointment 30 g. Lotion 60, 120, 240 mL. 1% pramoxine/2.5% hydrocortisone acetate Cream 30, 60 g. Ointment 30 g. Lotion 60, 120 mL.
NOTES − Monitor for hyperglycemia/adrenal suppression if used for long period of time or over a large area of the body, especially in children. Chronic administration may interfere with pediatric growth and development.
MOA − Anti-inflammatory; suppresses DNA synthesis, decreases WBC influx.
ADVERSE EFFECTS − Frequent: Burning, pruritus, dryness, irritation, erythema.

SELENIUM SULFIDE (*Selsun, Exsel, Versel*) ▶? ♀C ▶? $
ADULTS — <u>Dandruff, seborrheic dermatitis:</u> Massage 5 to 10 mL of shampoo into wet scalp, allow to remain 2 to 3 min, rinse. Apply twice a week for 2 weeks. For maintenance, less frequent administration needed. <u>Tinea versicolor:</u> Apply 2.5% shampoo/lotion to affected area, allow to remain on skin 10 min, rinse. Repeat daily for 7 days.
PEDS — <u>Dandruff, seborrheic dermatitis:</u> Massage 5 to 10 mL of shampoo into wet scalp, allow to remain 2 to 3 min, rinse. Apply twice a week for 2 weeks. For maintenance, less frequent administration needed. <u>Tinea versicolor:</u> Apply 2.5% lotion/shampoo to affected area, allow to remain on skin 10 min, rinse. Repeat daily for 7 days.
FORMS — OTC Generic/Trade: Lotion/Shampoo 1% 120, 210, 240, 325 mL, 2.5% 120 mL. Rx Generic/Trade: Lotion/Shampoo 2.5% 120 mL.
MOA — May inhibit epidermal growth enzymes.
ADVERSE EFFECTS — Frequent: Unusual dryness, oiliness of skin.

SOLAG (mequinol + tretinoin, ✦*Solage*) ▶Not absorbed ♀X ▶? $$$$
ADULTS — <u>Solar lentigines:</u> Apply bid separated by at least 8 h.
PEDS — Not approved in children.
FORMS — Trade only: Soln 30 mL (mequinol 2% + tretinoin 0.01%).
NOTES — Use in non-Caucasians has not been evaluated. Avoid in patients taking photosensitizers. Minimize exposure to sunlight.
MOA — Competitively inhibits melanin precursors.
ADVERSE EFFECTS — Frequent: Erythema, burning, stinging, pruritus, desquamation.

SYNERA (tetracaine + lidocaine - topical) ▶Minimal absorption ♀B ▶? $$
WARNING — Contraindicated in allergy to amide-type anesthetics.
ADULTS — <u>Prior to venipuncture, intravenous cannulation, superficial dermatological procedure:</u> Apply 20 to 30 min prior to procedure.
PEDS — Children 3 yo or older: <u>Prior to venipuncture, IV cannulation, superficial dermatological procedure:</u> Apply 20 to 30 min prior to procedure.
FORMS — Trade only: Topical patch (lidocaine 70 mg + tetracaine 70 mg.
NOTES — Do not cut patch or remove top cover.
MOA — Topical anesthetic.
ADVERSE EFFECTS — Frequent: Skin irritation, erythema, blanching, rash. Severe: CNS effects, bradycardia, bronchospasm, hypotension.

TRI-LUMA (fluocinolone + hydroquinone + tretinoin) ▶Minimal absorption ♀C ▶? $$$$
ADULTS — <u>Melasma of the face:</u> Apply at bedtime for 4 to 8 weeks.
PEDS — Not approved in children.
FORMS — Trade only: Cream 30 g (fluocinolone 0.01% + hydroquinone 4% + tretinoin 0.05%).
NOTES — Minimize exposure to sunlight. Not intended for melasma maintenance therapy.
MOA — Competitively inhibits melanin precursors, anti-inflammatory.
ADVERSE EFFECTS — Frequent: Erythema, desquamation, burning, dryness, pruritus, acne.

UREA (*Carmol 40*) ▶? ♀B ▶? $$$$
ADULTS — <u>Debridement of hyperkeratotic surface lesions:</u> Apply bid.
PEDS — <u>Debridement of hyperkeratotic surface lesions:</u> Apply bid.
FORMS — Trade only: Urea 40% Cream 30, 85, 200 g. Lotion 240 mL. Gel 15 mL.
MOA — Dissolves intracellular matrix thereby softening hyperkeratotic lesions.
ADVERSE EFFECTS — AWP = $101.74 for 85 g cream, RB (9/08).

VUSION (miconazole - topical + zinc oxide + white petrolatum) ▶Minimal absorption ♀C ▶? $$$$$
ADULTS — Not approved in adults.
PEDS — Apply to affected diaper area with each change for 7 days.
FORMS — Trade only: Ointment 50 g.
NOTES — Use only in documented cases of candidiasis.
MOA — Antifungal; alters fungal cell wall permeability; barrier.
ADVERSE EFFECTS — Frequent: None.

ENDOCRINE AND METABOLIC: Androgens / Anabolic Steroids

NOTE: Monitor LFTs and lipids. See OB/GYN section for other hormones.

FLUOXYMESTERONE (*Halotestin, Androxy*) ▶L ♀X ▶? ©III $$$$
ADULTS — <u>Palliative treatment of androgen-responsive recurrent breast cancer in women who are 1 to 5 years postmenopausal:</u> 5 to 10 mg PO bid to qid for 1 to 3 months. <u>Hypogonadism in men:</u> 5 to 20 mg PO daily.
PEDS — <u>Delayed puberty in males:</u> 2.5 to 10 mg PO daily for 4 to 6 months.
FORMS — Trade only: Tabs (scored) 2, 5, 10 mg. Generic only: Tabs 10 mg.
NOTES — Transdermal or injectable therapy preferred for hypogonadism. Pediatric use by specialists who monitor bone maturation q 6 months. Prolonged high-dose use may cause hepatic adenomas, hepatocellular carcinoma, and peliosis hepatitis.
MOA — Steroid with anabolic and androgenic actions.
ADVERSE EFFECTS — Serious: Peliosis hepatitis, liver tumors, cholestatic hepatitis, habituation, heart failure exacerbation, polycythemia. Frequent: Virilization, testicular atrophy, oligospermia, excitation, insomnia, anxiety, depression, paresthesia, altered libido, bladder irritability, menstrual irregularity, gynecomastia, acne, edema, lipid abnormalities.

METHYLTESTOSTERONE (*Android, Methitest, Testred, Virilon*) ▶L ♀X ▶? ©III $$$
ADULTS – Advancing inoperable breast cancer in women who are 1 to 5 years postmenopausal: 50 to 200 mg/day PO in divided doses. Hypogonadism in men: 10 to 50 mg PO daily.
PEDS – Delayed puberty in males: 10 mg PO daily for 4 to 6 months.
FORMS – Trade/Generic: Caps 10 mg, Tabs 10, 25 mg.
NOTES – Transdermal or injectable therapy preferred to oral for hypogonadism. Pediatric use by specialists who monitor bone maturation q 6 months. Prolonged high-dose use may cause hepatic adenomas, hepatocellular carcinoma, and peliosis hepatitis.
MOA – Steroid with anabolic and androgenic actions.
ADVERSE EFFECTS – Serious: Peliosis hepatitis, liver tumors, cholestatic hepatitis, habituation, heart failure exacerbation, polycythemia. Frequent: Virilization, testicular atrophy, oligospermia, excitation, insomnia, anxiety, depression, paresthesia, altered libido, bladder irritability, menstrual irregularity, gynecomastia, acne, edema, lipid abnormalities.

OXANDROLONE (*Oxandrin*) ▶L ♀X ▶? ©III $$$$$
WARNING – Peliosis hepatitis, liver cell tumors, and lipid changes have occurred secondary to anabolic steroid use.
ADULTS – To promote weight gain following extensive surgery, chronic infection, or severe trauma; in some patients who fail to gain or maintain weight without a physiologic cause; to offset protein catabolism associated with long-term corticosteroid therapy: 2.5 mg/day to 20 mg/day PO divided bid to qid for 2 to 4 weeks. May repeat therapy intermittently as indicated.
PEDS – Weight gain: Up to 0.1 mg/kg or up to 0.045 mg/pound PO divided bid to qid for 2 to 4 weeks. May repeat therapy intermittently as indicated.
FORMS – Generic/Trade: Tabs 2.5, 10 mg.
NOTES – Contraindicated in known or suspected prostate/breast cancer. Not shown to enhance athletic ability. Associated with dyslipidemia. Pediatric use by specialists who monitor bone maturation every 6 months. Long-term use may cause hepatic adenomas, hepatocellular carcinoma, and peliosis hepatitis. May increase anticoagulant effects of warfarin.
MOA – Steroid with anabolic and androgenic actions.
ADVERSE EFFECTS – Serious: Peliosis hepatitis, liver tumors, cholestatic hepatitis, habituation, heart failure exacerbation, polycythemia. Frequent: Virilization, testicular atrophy, oligospermia, excitation, insomnia, anxiety, depression, paresthesia, altered libido, bladder irritability, menstrual irregularity, gynecomastia, acne, edema, lipid abnormalities.

TESTOSTERONE (*Androderm, AndroGel, Delatestryl, Depo-Testosterone, Striant, Testim, Testopel, Testro AQ, ✦Andriol*) ▶L ♀X ▶? ©III $$$
WARNING – Risk of transfer and secondary exposure with topical products. Virilization has been reported in children after secondary exposure to gel. Women and children should avoid contact with skin areas to which gel has been applied. Advise patient to wash hands with soap and water following application and cover area with clothing once gel has dried.
ADULTS – Hypogonadism in men: Injectable enanthate or cypionate, 50 to 400 mg IM q 2 to 4 weeks. Androderm, 5 mg patch at bedtime to clean, dry area of skin on back, abdomen, upper arms, or thighs. Nonvirilized patients start with 2.5 mg patch at bedtime. AndroGel 1%: Apply 5 g from gel pack or 4 pumps (5 g) from dispenser daily to clean, dry, intact skin of the shoulders, upper arms, or abdomen. May increase dose to 7.5 to 10 g after 2 weeks. Testim: 1 tube (5 g) daily to the clean, dry intact skin of the shoulders or upper arms. May increase dose to 2 tubes (10 g) after 2 weeks. Testopel: 2 to 6 pellets (150 to 450 mg testosterone) SC q 3 to 6 months. 2 pellets for each 25 mg testosterone propionate required weekly. Buccal (Striant): 30 mg q 12 h on upper gum above the incisor tooth; alternate sides for each application.
PEDS – Not approved in children.
FORMS – Trade only: Patch 2.5, 5 mg/24 h (Androderm). Gel 1% 2.5, 5 g packet, 75 g multidose pump (AndroGel). Gel 1%, 5 g tube (Testim). Pellet 75 mg (Testopel). Buccal: Blister packs: 30 mg (Striant). Generic/Trade: Injection 100, 200 mg/mL (cypionate), 200 mg/mL (ethanate).
NOTES – Do not apply Androderm or AndroGel to scrotum. Do not apply Testim to the scrotum or abdomen. Pellet implantation is less flexible for dosage adjustment, therefore, take great care when estimating the amount of testosterone. For testosterone gel form, obtain serum testosterone level 2 weeks after initiation, then increase dose if necessary. Inject IM formulations slowly into gluteal muscle; rare reports of cough or respiratory distress following injection. Prolonged high-dose use may cause hepatic adenomas, hepatocellular carcinoma, and peliosis hepatitis. May promote the development of prostatic hyperplasia or prostate cancer. Monitor prostate exam, PSA, hemoglobin to detect polycythemia. Advise patient to regularly inspect the gum region where Striant is applied and report any abnormality; refer for dental consultation as appropriate.
MOA – Steroid with anabolic and androgenic actions.
ADVERSE EFFECTS – Serious: Peliosis hepatitis, liver tumors, cholestatic hepatitis, habituation, heart failure exacerbation, polycythemia. Frequent: Virilization, testicular atrophy, oligospermia, excitation, insomnia, anxiety, depression, paresthesia, altered libido, bladder irritability, menstrual irregularity, gynecomastia, acne, edema, gum or mouth irritation (buccal), transient cough or respiratory distress (IM).

ENDOCRINE AND METABOLIC: Bisphosphonates

NOTE: Supplemental Vitamin D and calcium are recommended for osteoporosis prevention and treatment. Osteonecrosis of the jaw has been reported with bisphosphonates; generally associated with tooth extraction and/or local infection with delayed healing. Prior to treatment, consider dental exam and appropriate preventative dentistry, particularly with risk factors (eg, cancer, chemotherapy, corticosteroids, poor oral hygiene). While on bisphosphonate therapy, avoid invasive dental procedures when possible. Severe musculoskeletal pain has been reported; may occur at any time during therapy.

ALENDRONATE (*Fosamax, Fosamax Plus D, ✦Fosavance*) ▶K ♀C ▶– $$
ADULTS — Postmenopausal osteoporosis prevention (5 mg PO daily or 35 mg PO weekly) and treatment (10 mg daily, 70 mg PO weekly, 70 mg/vit D3 2800 international units PO weekly, or 70 mg/vit D3 5600 international units PO weekly). Treatment of glucocorticoid-induced osteoporosis: 5 mg PO daily in men and women or 10 mg PO daily postmenopausal women not taking estrogen. Treatment of osteoporosis in men: 10 mg PO daily, 70 mg PO weekly, 70 mg/vit D3 2800 international units PO weekly, or 70 mg/vit D3 5600 international units PO weekly. Paget's disease in men and women: 40 mg PO daily for 6 months.
PEDS — Not approved in children.
UNAPPROVED ADULTS — Prevention of glucocorticoid-induced osteoporosis men and women: 5 mg PO daily or 35 mg PO weekly; 10 mg PO daily or 70 mg PO weekly (postmenopausal women not taking estrogen). Treatment of glucocorticoid-induced osteoporosis in men and women: 35 mg weekly or 70 mg weekly (postmenopausal women not taking estrogen).
FORMS — Generic/Trade (Fosamax): Tabs 5, 10, 35, 40, 70 mg. Trade only: Oral soln 70 mg/75 mL (single-dose bottle). Fosamax Plus D: 70 mg + either 2800 or 5600 units of vitamin D3.
NOTES — May cause esophagitis, esophageal ulcers and esophageal erosions, occasionally with bleeding and rarely followed by esophageal stricture or perforation. Monitor frequently for dysphagia, odynophagia, and retrosternal pain. Take 30 min before first food, beverage, and medication of the day with a full glass of water only. Remain in upright position for at least 30 min following dose. Caution if CrCl less than 35 mL/min. For patients requiring invasive dental procedures, discontinuation may reduce the risk for osteonecrosis of the jaw.
MOA — Inhibits osteoclast-mediated bone resorption, increases bone mineral density.
ADVERSE EFFECTS — Serious: Esophageal disease (ulcers, erosion, esophagitis, stricture, perforation), gastric/duodenal ulcer, osteonecrosis of the jaw, severe skin reactions. low-energy femoral shaft and subtrochanteric fractures. Frequent: Headache, musculoskeletal pain, abdominal pain, diarrhea, dizziness, joint swelling, rash, photosensitivity.

CLODRONATE (*✦Clasteon, Bonefos*) ▶K ♀D ▶– $$$$$
ADULTS — Canada only. Hypercalcemia of malignancy; management of osteolysis resulting from bone metastases of malignant tumors: IV single dose, 1500 mg slow infusion over at least 4 h. IV multiple dose, 300 mg slow infusion daily over 2 to 6 h up to 10 days. Oral, following IV therapy, maintenance 1600 to 2400 mg/day in single or divided doses. Max PO dose 3200 mg/day; duration of therapy is usually 6 months.
PEDS — Not approved in children.
FORMS — Generic/Trade: Caps 400 mg.
NOTES — Contraindicated if creatinine more than 5 mg/dL or if severe GI tract inflammation. Avoid rapid bolus which may cause severe local reactions, thrombophlebitis, or renal failure. Do not mix with calcium-containing infusions. Ensure adequate hydration prior to infusion. Normocalcemia usually occurs within 2 to 5 days after initiation of therapy with multiple dose infusion. Monitor serum calcium, renal function in those with renal insufficiency, LFTs and hematological parameters.
MOA — Inhibits osteoclast-mediated bone resorption without an inhibitory effect on mineralization, decreases serum calcium.
ADVERSE EFFECTS — Serious: Hypersensitivity, decreased renal function, hypocalcemia. Frequent: N/V, anorexia, abdominal pain, diarrhea (with oral form), infusion site reaction.

ETIDRONATE (*Didronel*) ▶K ♀C ▶? $$$$$
ADULTS — Paget's disease: 5 to 10 mg/kg PO daily for 6 months or 11 to 20 mg/kg daily for 3 months. Heterotopic ossification with hip replacement: 20 mg/kg/day PO for 1 month before and 3 months after surgery. Heterotopic ossification with spinal cord injury: 20 mg/kg/day PO for 2 weeks, then 10 mg/kg/day PO for 10 weeks.
PEDS — Not approved in children.
FORMS — Generic/Trade: Tabs 400 mg. Generic only: Tabs 200 mg.
NOTES — Divide dose if GI discomfort occurs. Avoid in abnormalities of the esophagus that may delay esophageal emptying (eg, stricture). Avoid food, vitamins with minerals, or antacids within 2 h of dose.
MOA — Inhibits osteoclast-mediated bone resorption, blocks growth and mineralization of hydroxyapatite crystals.
ADVERSE EFFECTS — Serious: Esophageal disease (ulcers, esophagitis, perforation), peptic ulcer disease, agranulocytosis, pancytopenia, leukopenia, fractures, osteonecrosis of the jaw. Frequent: Headache, gastritis, leg cramps, arthralgia, bone pain.

IBANDRONATE (*Boniva*) ▶K ♀C ▶? $$$$
ADULTS — Treatment/Prevention of postmenopausal osteoporosis. Oral: 2.5 mg PO daily or 150 mg PO q month. IV: 3 mg IV every 3 months.

(cont.)

IBANDRONATE (cont.)
PEDS — Not approved in children.
FORMS — Trade only: Tabs 2.5, 150 mg. IV: 3 mg.
NOTES — May cause esophagitis. Avoid in abnormalities of the esophagus that may delay esophageal emptying (eg, stricture). Avoid if CrCl less than 30 mL/min. Oral: Take 1 h before first food/beverage with a full glass of plain water; remain in upright position 1 h after taking. IV: Administer over 15 to 30 sec.
MOA — Inhibits osteoclast-mediated bone resorption, increases bone mineral density.
ADVERSE EFFECTS — Serious: Esophageal disease (ulcer, esophagitis), osteonecrosis of the jaw. Frequent: Back pain, dyspepsia, diarrhea, myalgia, headache, injection site reaction.

PAMIDRONATE (*Aredia*) ▶K ♀D ▶? $$$$$
WARNING — Single dose should not exceed 90 mg due to risk of renal impairment/failure.
ADULTS — <u>Hypercalcemia of malignancy, moderate</u> (corrected Ca is in the range of 12 to 13.5 mg/dL): 60 to 90 mg IV single dose infused over 2 to 24 h. <u>Hypercalcemia of malignancy, severe</u> (Ca more than 13.5 mg/dL): 90 mg IV single dose infused over 2 to 24 h. Wait at least 7 days before considering retreatment. <u>Paget's disease:</u> 30 mg IV over 4 h daily for 3 days. <u>Osteolytic bone lesions:</u> 90 mg IV over 4 h once a month. <u>Osteolytic bone metastases:</u> 90 mg IV over 2 h q 3 to 4 weeks.
PEDS — Not approved in children.
UNAPPROVED ADULTS — <u>Mild hypercalcemia:</u> 30 mg IV single dose over 4 h. <u>Osteoporosis treatment:</u> 30 mg IV q 3 months. <u>Prevention of bone loss during androgen deprivation treatment for prostate cancer:</u> 60 mg IV q 12 weeks.
NOTES — Fever occurs in more than 20% of patients. Monitor creatinine (prior to each dose), lytes, calcium, phosphate, magnesium and Hb (regularly). Avoid in severe renal impairment and hold dosing if worsening renal function. Longer infusions (more than 2 h) may reduce renal toxicity. Not studied in patients with SCr more than 3 mg/dL. Maintain adequate hydration.
MOA — Inhibits osteoclast-mediated bone resorption, decreases serum calcium.
ADVERSE EFFECTS — Serious: Atrial fibrillation, syncope, hypertension, tachycardia, osteonecrosis of the jaw, severe musculoskeletal pain. Frequent: Electrolyte depletion (potassium, magnesium, calcium, phosphate), fever, infusion site reaction, bone pain, dyspepsia, anorexia, nausea, diarrhea.

RISEDRONATE (*Actonel, Actonel Plus Calcium*) ▶K ♀C ▶? $$$$
ADULTS — <u>Prevention and treatment of postmenopausal osteoporosis:</u> 5 mg PO daily, 35 mg PO weekly or 150 mg once a month. <u>Treatment of osteoporosis in men:</u> 35 mg PO weekly. <u>Prevention and treatment of glucocorticoid-induced osteoporosis:</u> 5 mg PO daily. <u>Paget's disease:</u> 30 mg PO daily for 2 months.
PEDS — Not approved in children.
UNAPPROVED ADULTS — <u>Prevention and treatment of glucocorticoid-induced osteoporosis:</u> 35 mg PO weekly.
FORMS — Trade only: Tabs 5, 30, 35, 150 mg. Trade only (Actonel + Calcium): Tabs 35/1250 mg combination package.
NOTES — May cause esophagitis, monitor frequently for dysphagia, odynophagia, and retrosternal pain; take 30 min before first food, beverage, or medication of the day with a full glass of water only. Remain in upright position for at least 30 min following dose. Avoid in abnormalities of the esophagus that may delay esophageal emptying (eg, stricture).
MOA — Inhibits osteoclast-mediated bone resorption, increases bone mineral density.
ADVERSE EFFECTS — Serious: Esophageal disease (ulcers, erosion, esophagitis, stricture, perforation), gastric/duodenal ulcer, hypersensitivity. Frequent: Headache, musculoskeletal pain, abdominal pain, diarrhea.

TILUDRONATE (*Skelid*) ▶K ♀C ▶? $$$$$
ADULTS — <u>Paget's disease:</u> 400 mg PO daily for 3 months.
PEDS — Not approved in children.
FORMS — Trade only: Tabs 200 mg.
NOTES — May cause esophagitis, esophageal ulcers and esophageal erosions, occasionally with bleeding and rarely followed by esophageal stricture or perforation. Monitor frequently for dysphagia, odynophagia, and retrosternal pain. Take 30 min before first food, beverage, or medication of the day with a full glass of water only. Remain in upright position for at least 30 min following dose.
MOA — Inhibits osteoclast-mediated bone resorption, increases bone mineral density.
ADVERSE EFFECTS — Serious: Esophageal disease (ulcers, erosion, esophagitis, stricture, perforation), gastric/duodenal ulcer, hyperparathyroidism, cataract, glaucoma. Frequent: Edema, diarrhea, nausea.

ZOLEDRONIC ACID (*Reclast, Zometa, ✦Aclasta*) ▶K ♀D ▶? $$$$$
ADULTS — <u>Treatment of Osteoporosis:</u> 5 mg (Reclast) once yearly IV infusion over 15 min or longer. <u>Prevention and treatment of glucocorticoid-induced osteoporosis in patients expected to receive glucocorticoids for at least 12 months:</u> 5 mg (Reclast) once yearly IV infusion over 15 min or longer. <u>Hypercalcemia of malignancy</u> (corrected Ca at least 12 mg/dL, Zometa): 4 mg single-dose IV infusion over 15 min or longer. Wait at least 7 days before considering retreatment. <u>Paget's disease</u> (Reclast): 5 mg IV single dose. <u>Multiple myeloma and metastatic bone lesions from solid tumors</u> (Zometa): 4 mg (CrCl more than 60 mL/min), 3.5 mg (CrCl 50 to 60 mL/min), 3.3 mg (CrCl 40 to 49 mL/min) or 3 mg (CrCl 30 to 39 mL/min) IV infusion over 15 min or longer q 3 to 4 weeks.
PEDS — Not approved in children.
UNAPPROVED ADULTS — <u>Osteoporosis:</u> 4 mg (Zometa) once yearly IV infusion over 15 min or

(cont.)

ZOLEDRONIC ACID (cont.)
longer. Paget's disease (Zometa; approved in Canada): 5 mg IV single dose. Treatment of hormone-refractory prostate cancer metastatic to bone (Zometa): 4 mg IV q 3 to 4 weeks. Prevention of bone loss during androgen-deprivation treatment for non-metastatic prostate cancer (Zometa): 4 mg IV q 3 month for 1 year or 4 mg every 12 months. Prevention of bone loss during aromatase inhibitor use in breast cancer (Zometa): 4 mg IV q6 months.
NOTES — Avoid in severe renal impairment (CrCl less than 35 mL/min) and hold dosing with worsening renal function. Monitor creatinine (before each dose), lytes, calcium, phosphate, magnesium and Hb/HCT (regularly). Avoid single doses more than 4 mg (Zometa) or more than 5 mg (Reclast), infusions less than 15 min. Fever occurs in more than 15%. In treatment of Paget's disease, correct preexisting hypocalcemia with calcium and vitamin D before therapy. Maintain adequate hydration for those with hypercalcemia of malignancy, and give 500 mg calcium supplement and vitamin D 400 international units PO daily to those with multiple myeloma or metastatic bone lesions.
MOA — A bisphosphonate that inhibits osteoclast-mediated bone resorption, increases bone mineral density, decreases serum calcium.
ADVERSE EFFECTS — Serious: Hypotension, renal impairment, granulocytopenia, thrombocytopenia, pancytopenia, osteonecrosis of the jaw, severe musculoskeletal pain, ocular inflammation. Frequent: Electrolyte depletion (potassium, magnesium, calcium, phosphate), flu-like symptoms, fever, infusion site reaction, N/V, skeletal pain, constipation, diarrhea, conjunctivitis.

ENDOCRINE AND METABOLIC: Corticosteroids

NOTE: See also dermatology, ophthalmology.

BETAMETHASONE (Celestone, Celestone Soluspan, ♣Betaject) ▶L ♀C ▶– $$$$$
ADULTS — Anti-inflammatory/Immunosuppressive: 0.6 to 7.2 mg/day PO divided bid to qid or up to 9 mg/day IM. 0.25 to 2 mL intra-articular depending on location and size of joint.
PEDS — Dosing guidelines not established.
UNAPPROVED ADULTS — Fetal lung maturation, maternal antepartum between 24 and 34 weeks gestation: 12 mg IM q 24 h for 2 doses.
UNAPPROVED PEDS — Anti-inflammatory/Immunosuppressive: 0.0175 to 0.25 mg/kg/day PO divided tid to qid. Fetal lung maturation, maternal antepartum: 12 mg IM q 24 h for 2 doses.
FORMS — Trade only: Syrup 0.6 mg/5 mL.
NOTES — Avoid prolonged use in children due to possible bone growth retardation. If such therapy necessary monitor growth and development.
MOA — Long-acting glucocorticoid.
ADVERSE EFFECTS — Serious: Hypertension, diabetes, osteoporosis, immunosuppression, impaired wound healing, adrenal suppression, peptic ulcer disease, cataracts. Frequent: Cushingoid state, N/V, weight gain, myopathy, leukocytosis, skin atrophy, edema.

CORTISONE (Cortone) ▶L ♀D ▶– $
ADULTS — Adrenocortical insufficiency: 25 to 300 mg PO daily.
PEDS — Dosing guidelines not established.
UNAPPROVED PEDS — Adrenocortical insufficiency: 0.5 to 0.75 mg/kg/day PO divided q 8 h.
FORMS — Generic only: Tabs 25 mg.
MOA — Short-acting glucocorticoid with mineralocorticoid activity at higher doses.
ADVERSE EFFECTS — Serious: Hypertension, diabetes, osteoporosis, immunosuppression, impaired wound healing, adrenal suppression, peptic ulcer disease, cataracts. Frequent: Cushingoid state, N/V, weight gain, myopathy, leukocytosis, skin atrophy, edema.

DEXAMETHASONE (Decadron, Dexpak, ♣Dexasone) ▶L ♀C ▶– $
ADULTS — Anti-inflammatory/immunosuppressive: 0.5 to 9 mg/day PO/IV/IM divided bid to qid. Cerebral edema: 10 to 20 mg IV load, then 4 mg IM q 6 h (off-label IV use common) or 1 to 3 mg PO tid.
PEDS — Dosing varies by indication; start 0.02 to 0.3 mg/kg/day divided tid to qid.
UNAPPROVED ADULTS — Initial treatment of immune thrombocytopenic purpura: 40 mg PO daily for 4 days. Fetal lung maturation, maternal antepartum between 24 and 34 weeks gestation: 6 mg IM q 12 h for 4 doses. Bacterial meningitis (controversial): 0.15 mg/kg IV q 6 h for 2 to 4 days; start 10 to 15 min before the first dose of antibiotic. Antiemetic, prophylaxis: 8 mg IV or 12 mg PO prior to chemotherapy; 8 mg PO daily for 2 to 4 days. Antiemetic, treatment: 10 to 20 mg PO/IV q 4 to 6 h.
UNAPPROVED PEDS — Anti-inflammatory/immunosuppressive: 0.08 to 0.3 mg/kg/day PO/IV/IM divided q 6 to 12 h. Croup: 0.6 mg/kg PO/IV/IM for one dose. Bacterial meningitis (controversial): 0.15 mg/kg IV q 6 h for 2 to 4 days; start 10 to 15 min before the first dose of antibiotic. Bronchopulmonary dysplasia in preterm infants: 0.5 mg/kg PO/IV divided q 12 h for 3 days, then taper. Acute asthma: Older than 2 yo: 0.6 mg/kg to max 16 mg PO daily for 2 days.
FORMS — Generic/Trade: Tabs 0.5, 0.75. Generic only: Tabs 0.25, 1.0, 1.5, 2, 4, 6 mg; elixir 0.5 mg/5 mL; Soln 0.5 mg/5 mL, 1 mg/1 mL (concentrate). Trade only: Dexpak 13 day (51 total 1.5 mg tabs for a 13-day taper), Dexpak 10 day (35 total 1.5 mg tabs for 10-day taper), Dexpak 6 days (21 total 1.5 mg tabs for 6-day taper).

(cont.)

DEXAMETHASONE (cont.)
NOTES — Avoid prolonged use in children due to possible bone growth retardation. If such therapy necessary monitor growth and development.
MOA — Long-acting glucocorticoid.
ADVERSE EFFECTS — Serious: Hypertension, diabetes, osteoporosis, immunosuppression, impaired wound healing, adrenal suppression, peptic ulcer disease, cataracts. Frequent: Cushingoid state, N/V, weight gain, myopathy, leukocytosis, skin atrophy, edema.

FLUDROCORTISONE (*Florinef*) ▶L ♀C ▶? $
ADULTS — Adrenocortical insufficiency/Addison's disease: 0.1 mg PO 3 times a week to 0.2 mg PO daily. Salt-losing adrenogenital syndrome: 0.1 to 0.2 mg PO daily.
PEDS — Not approved in children.
UNAPPROVED ADULTS — Postural hypotension: 0.05 to 0.4 mg PO daily.
UNAPPROVED PEDS — Adrenocortical insufficiency: 0.05 to 0.2 mg PO daily.
FORMS — Generic only: Tabs 0.1 mg.
NOTES — Usually given in conjunction with cortisone or hydrocortisone for adrenocortical insufficiency.
MOA — Potent mineralocorticoid with high glucocorticoid activity; primarily used for its mineralocorticoid effects.
ADVERSE EFFECTS — Serious: Hypokalemic alkalosis, hypertension, diabetes, osteoporosis, immunosuppression, impaired wound healing, adrenal suppression, peptic ulcer disease, cataracts. Frequent: Edema, cushingoid state, N/V, weight gain, myopathy, leukocytosis, skin atrophy.

HYDROCORTISONE (*Cortef, Cortenema, Solu-Cortef*) ▶L ♀C ▶– $
ADULTS — Adrenocortical insufficiency: 20 to 240 mg/day PO divided tid to qid or 100 to 500 mg IV/IM q 2 to 10 h prn (sodium succinate). Ulcerative colitis: 100 mg retention enema at bedtime (laying on side for 1 h or longer) for 21 days. May use for 2 to 3 months for severe cases; when course extends more than 3 weeks then discontinue gradually by decreasing frequency to every other night for 2 to 3 weeks. Multiple sclerosis acute exacerbation: 800 mg daily then 320 mg every other day for 1 month.
PEDS — Dosing guidelines not established. Product information suggests tailoring doses to the specific disease being treated with a range of initial doses of 0.56 to 8 mg/kg/day IV/PO divided tid-qid.
UNAPPROVED PEDS — Chronic Adrenocortical insufficiency: 0.5 to 0.75 mg/kg/day PO divided q 8 h or 0.25 to 0.35 mg/kg/day IM daily. Acute adrenocortical insufficiency: Infants and young children 1 to 2 mg/kg IV bolus, then 25 to 150 mg/day divided q 6 to 8 h. Older children 1 to 2 mg/kg IV bolus, then 150 to 250 mg/day IV q 6 to 8 h.
FORMS — Generic/Trade: Tabs 5, 10, 20 mg; Enema 100 mg/60 mL.
NOTES — Agent of choice for adrenocortical insufficiency because of mixed glucocorticoid and mineralocorticoid properties at doses more than 100 mg/day.
MOA — Short-acting glucocorticoid with mineralocorticoid activity at higher doses.
ADVERSE EFFECTS — Serious: Hypertension, diabetes, osteoporosis, immunosuppression, impaired wound healing, adrenal suppression, peptic ulcer disease, cataracts. Frequent: Cushingoid state, N/V, weight gain, myopathy, leukocytosis, skin atrophy, edema.

METHYLPREDNISOLONE (*Solu-Medrol, Medrol, Depo-Medrol*) ▶L ♀C ▶– $
ADULTS — Anti-inflammatory/Immunosuppressive: Parenteral (Solu-Medrol) 10 to 250 mg IV/IM q 4 h prn. Oral (Medrol) 4 to 48 mg PO daily. Medrol Dosepak tapers 24 to 0 mg PO over 7 days. IM/joints (Depo-Medrol) 4 to 120 mg IM q 1 to 2 weeks. Multiple sclerosis flare: 200 mg PO/IV daily for 1 week followed by 80 mg PO daily for 1 month.
PEDS — Dosing guidelines not established.
UNAPPROVED ADULTS — Acute asthma exacerbation ("burst" therapy): 40 to 60 mg PO daily or divided bid for 3 to 10 days. Acute asthma exacerbation (vomiting or nonadherent): 240 mg IM once. Optic neuritis: 1 g IV daily (or in divided doses) for 3 days, then PO prednisone 1 mg/kg/day for 11 days (followed by a 3-day taper). Multiple sclerosis flare: 1 g IV daily (or in divided doses) for 3 to 5 days. May follow with PO prednisone 1 mg/kg/day for 14 days, then taper off. Spinal cord injury: 30 mg/kg IV over 15 min, followed in 45 min by 5.4 mg/kg/h IV infusion for 23 h (if initiated within 3 h of injury) or for 47 h (if initiated 3 to 8 h after injury).
UNAPPROVED PEDS — Anti-inflammatory/Immunosuppressive: 0.5 to 1.7 mg/kg/day PO/IV/IM divided q 6 to 12 h. Spinal cord injury: 30 mg/kg IV over 15 min, followed in 45 min by 5.4 mg/kg/h IV infusion for 23 h. Acute asthma exacerbation ("burst" therapy): 1 to 2 mg/kg/day PO; max 60 mg daily for 3 to 10 days. Acute asthma exacerbation (vomiting or nonadherent): Age younger than 5 yo: 7.5 mg/kg IM once; age 5-11 yo: 240 mg IM once; age at least 12: 240 mg IM once.
FORMS — Trade only: Tabs 2, 16, 32 mg. Generic/Trade: Tabs 4, 8 mg. Medrol Dosepak (4 mg, 21 tabs).
NOTES — Other dosing regimens have been used for MS and optic neuritis. Avoid initial treatment of optic neuritis with oral steroids, as it may increase the risk of new episodes. Contains benzyl alcohol, contraindicated in premature infants and for intrathecal administration. Do not use for traumatic brain injury.
MOA — Intermediate-acting glucocorticoid.
ADVERSE EFFECTS — Serious: Cardiac arrest or arrhythmia (with IV), hypertension, osteoporosis, immunosuppression, impaired wound healing, adrenal suppression, peptic ulcers, cataracts, postinjection flare, HPA axis suppression. Frequent: Cushingoid state, N/V, weight gain, edema, hyperglycemia, hypokalemia, injection site hypo/hyperpigmentation, myopathy, dermal or subdermal changes, deltoid muscle atrophy with IM injection.

ENDOCRINE AND METABOLIC: Corticosteroids

CORTICOSTEROIDS	Approximate Equivalent Dose (mg)	Relative Anti-inflammatory Potency	Relative Mineralocorticoid Potency	Biological Half-life (h)
betamethasone	0.6–0.75	20–30	0	36–54
cortisone	25	0.8	2	8–12
dexamethasone	0.75	20–30	0	36–54
fludrocortisone	n.a.	10	125	18–36
hydrocortisone	20	1	2	8–12
methylprednisolone	4	5	0	18–36
prednisolone	5	4	1	18–36
prednisone	5	4	1	18–36
triamcinolone	4	5	0	12–36

n.a., not available.

PREDNISOLONE (Flo-Pred, Prelone, Pediapred, Orapred, Orapred ODT) ▶L ♀C ▶+ $$
ADULTS — Anti-inflammatory/Immunosuppressive: 5 to 60 mg/day PO; individualize to severity of disease and response. Multiple sclerosis: 200 mg PO daily for 1 week, then 80 mg every other day for 1 month.
PEDS — Anti-inflammatory/Immunosuppressive: 0.14 to 2 mg/kg/day PO divided tid to qid (4 to 60 mg/m2/day); individualize to severity of disease and response. Acute asthma: 1 to 2 mg/kg/day daily or divided bid for 3 to 10 days. Nephrotic syndrome: 60 mg/m2/day divided tid for 4 weeks; then 40 mg/m2/day every other day for 4 weeks.
UNAPPROVED ADULTS — Acute asthma exacerbation ("burst" therapy): 40 to 60 mg PO daily or divided bid for 3 to 10 days.
UNAPPROVED PEDS — Acute asthma exacerbation ("burst" therapy): 1 to 2 mg/kg/day PO; max 60 mg daily for 3 to 10 days. Early active RA: 10 mg/day PO.
FORMS — Generic/Trade: Syrup 15 mg/5 mL (Prelone; wild cherry flavor). Soln 5 mg/5 mL (Pediapred, raspberry flavor), 15 mg/5 mL (Orapred; grape flavor). Trade only: Orally disintegrating tabs 10, 15, 30 mg (Orapred ODT); Susp 5 mg/5 mL, 15 mg/5 mL (Flo-Pred; cherry flavor). Generic only: Tabs 5 mg. Syrup 5 mg/5 mL.
MOA — Intermediate-acting glucocorticoid with mineralocorticoid activity; primarily used for its glucocorticoid effects.
ADVERSE EFFECTS — Serious: Hypertension, diabetes, osteoporosis, immunosuppression, impaired wound healing, adrenal suppression, peptic ulcer disease, cataracts. Frequent: Cushingoid state, N/V, weight gain, myopathy, leukocytosis, skin atrophy, edema.

PREDNISONE (Deltasone, Sterapred, ♦Winpred) ▶L ♀C ▶+ $
ADULTS — Anti-inflammatory/Immunosuppressive: 5 to 60 mg/day PO daily or divided bid to qid.
PEDS — Dosing guidelines not established.
UNAPPROVED ADULTS — Acute asthma exacerbation ("burst" therapy): 40 to 60 mg PO daily or divided bid for 3 to 10 days.
UNAPPROVED PEDS — Anti-inflammatory/Immunosuppressive: 0.05 to 2 mg/kg/day divided daily to qid. Acute asthma exacerbation ("burst" therapy): 1 to 2 mg/kg/day PO; max 60 mg daily for 3 to 10 days.
FORMS — Trade only: Sterapred (5 mg tabs: Tapers 30 to 5 mg PO over 6 days or 30 to 10 mg over 12 days), Sterapred DS (10 mg tabs: Tapers 60 to 10 mg over 6 days, or 60 to 20 mg PO over 12 days) taper packs. Generic only: Tabs 1, 2.5, 5, 10, 20, 50 mg. Soln 5 mg/5 mL, 5 mg/mL (Prednisone Intensol).
NOTES — Conversion to prednisolone may be impaired in liver disease.
MOA — Intermediate-acting glucocorticoid with mineralocorticoid activity; primarily used for its glucocorticoid effects.
ADVERSE EFFECTS — Serious: Hypertension, diabetes, osteoporosis, immunosuppression, impaired wound healing, adrenal suppression, peptic ulcer disease, cataracts, psychosis, depression. Frequent: Cushingoid state, N/V, weight gain, myopathy, leukocytosis, skin atrophy, edema.

TRIAMCINOLONE (Aristospan, Kenalog, Trivaris) ▶L ♀C ▶– $
ADULTS — Anti-inflammatory/Immunosuppressive: 4 to 48 mg/day PO divided daily to qid. 2.5 to 60 mg IM daily (Kenalog, Trivaris). Intra-articular: Small joints 2.5 to 5 mg (Kenalog, Trivaris), 2 to 6 mg (Aristospan); large joints 5 to 15 mg (Kenalog, Trivaris); 10 to 20 mg (Aristospan). Intravitreal: 4 mg (Trivaris).
PEDS — Dosing guidelines not established.
UNAPPROVED PEDS — Anti-inflammatory/Immunosuppressive: 0.117 to 1.66 mg/kg/day PO divided qid.
FORMS — Trade only: Injection 10 mg/mL, 40 mg/mL (Kenalog), 5 mg/mL, 20 mg/mL (Aristospan), 8 mg (80 mg/mL) syringe (Trivaris).
NOTES — Parenteral form not for IV use. Kenalog and Aristospan contain benzyl alcohol; do not use in neonates. Due to Trivaris availability in a syringe, multiple injections may be required for dose.
MOA — Intermediate-acting glucocorticoid.

(cont.)

ENDOCRINE AND METABOLIC: Diabetes-Related

TRIAMCINOLONE (cont.)
ADVERSE EFFECTS — Serious: Hypertension, diabetes, osteoporosis, immunosuppression, impaired wound healing, adrenal suppression, peptic ulcer disease, cataracts, postinjection flare. Frequent: Cushingoid state, N/V, weight gain, myopathy, leukocytosis, skin atrophy, injection site hyper/hypopigmentation, edema.

ENDOCRINE AND METABOLIC: Diabetes-Related—Alpha-Glucosidase Inhibitors

NOTE: No clinical studies have established conclusive evidence of decreased macrovascular outcomes with antidiabetic drugs.

ACARBOSE (Precose, ✦Glucobay) ▶Gut/K ♀B ▶– $$$
ADULTS — Diabetes: Initiate therapy with 25 mg PO tid with the first bite of each meal. May start with 25 mg PO daily to minimize GI adverse effects. May increase to 50 mg PO tid after 4 to 8 weeks. Usual range is 50 to 100 mg PO tid. Maximum dose for patients wt 60 kg or less is 50 mg tid, wt greater than 60 kg max is 100 mg tid.
PEDS — Not approved in children.
UNAPPROVED ADULTS — Type 2 DM prevention: 100 mg PO tid or to maximum tolerated dose.
FORMS — Generic/Trade: Tabs 25, 50, 100 mg.
NOTES — Acarbose alone should not cause hypoglycemia. If hypoglycemia occurs, treat with oral glucose rather than sucrose (table sugar). Adverse GI effects (eg, flatulence, diarrhea, abdominal pain) may occur with initial therapy.
MOA — Inhibits intestinal alpha-glucoside hydrolase and pancreatic alpha-amylase and delays glucose absorption.
ADVERSE EFFECTS — Serious: Elevated serum transaminases, hypersensitivity, ileus. Frequent: Flatulence, diarrhea, abdominal pain.

MIGLITOL (Glyset) ▶K ♀B ▶– $$$
ADULTS — Diabetes: Initiate therapy with 25 mg PO tid with the first bite of each meal. Use 25 mg PO daily to start if GI adverse effects. May increase dose to 50 mg PO tid after 4 to 8 weeks, max 300 mg/day.
PEDS — Not approved in children.
FORMS — Trade only: Tabs 25, 50, 100 mg.
NOTES — Miglitol administered alone should not cause hypoglycemia. If hypoglycemia occurs, treat with oral glucose rather than sucrose (table sugar). Adverse GI effects (ie, flatulence, diarrhea, abdominal pain) may occur with initial therapy.
MOA — Inhibits intestinal alpha-glucoside hydrolase and delays glucose absorption.
ADVERSE EFFECTS — Serious: None. Frequent: Flatulence, diarrhea, abdominal pain, rash, transient decrease in serum iron.

ENDOCRINE AND METABOLIC: Diabetes-Related—Combinations

NOTE: Metformin-containing products may cause life-threatening lactic acidosis, usually in setting of decreased tissue perfusion, hypoxia, hepatic dysfunction, or impaired renal clearance. Hold prior to IV contrast agents and for 48 h after. Avoid if ethanol abuse, heart failure (requiring treatment), hepatic or renal insufficiency (creatinine at least 1.4 mg/dL in women, at least 1.5 mg/dL in men), or hypoxic states (cardiogenic shock, septicemia, acute MI). Glitazone-containing products may cause edema, wt gain, new heart failure, or exacerbate existing heart failure (avoid in NYHA Class III or IV). Monitor for signs of heart failure (rapid wt gain, dyspnea, edema) following initiation or dose increase. If occurs, manage fluid retention and consider discontinuation or dosage decrease. Rosiglitazone (Avandia) is not recommended with nitrates or insulin, and its labeling includes boxed warning regarding increased risk of myocardial ischemic events and notes that studies are currently inconclusive. Avoid if liver disease or ALT > 2.5 times normal. Monitor LFTs before therapy and periodically thereafter. Discontinue if ALT > 3 times upper normal limit. Full effect may not be apparent for up to 12 weeks. May cause resumption of ovulation in premenopausal anovulatory women; recommend contraception use. No clinical studies have established conclusive evidence of decreased macrovascular outcomes with antidiabetic drugs.

ACTOPLUS MET (pioglitazone + metformin) ▶KL ♀C ▶? $$$$$
ADULTS — Type 2 DM: 1 tab PO daily to bid. If inadequate control with metformin monotherapy, start 15/500 or 15/850 PO daily to bid. If inadequate control with pioglitazone monotherapy, start 15/500 bid or 15/850 daily. Max 45/2550 mg/day. Extended release, start 1 tab (15/100 mg or 30/1000 mg) daily with evening meal. Max: 45/2000 mg/day.
PEDS — Not approved in children.
FORMS — Trade only: Tabs 15/500, 15/850 mg, Extended release, tabs: 15/1000 mg, 30/1000 mg.
NOTES — Initial GI upset may be minimized by starting with lower dose of metformin component.
MOA — Combination product that increases insulin sensitivity, decreases hepatic gluconeogenesis.
ADVERSE EFFECTS — Serious: Potential hepatotoxicity, heart failure exacerbation, resumption of ovulation, macular edema, lactic acidosis, decreased vitamin B12, fracture. Frequent: Asthenia, anemia, edema, weight gain or loss, headache, dyslipidemia, diarrhea, increased LFTs, N/V, flatulence, abdominal discomfort, headache, taste disturbance.

ENDOCRINE AND METABOLIC: Diabetes-Related

DIABETES NUMBERS*

Criteria for diagnosis:	*Self-monitoring glucose goals*	
Pre-diabetes: Fasting glucose 100–125 mg/dL Diabetes:† A1C ⩾ 6.5% Fasting glucose ⩾ 126 mg/dL, random glucose with symptoms: ⩾ 200 mg/dL, or ⩾ 200 mg/dL 2 h after 75 g oral glucose load	Preprandial Postprandial	70–130 mg/dL < 180 mg/dL
	A1C goal < 7%	

Critically ill glucose goal: 140–180 mg/dl
Non-critically ill glucose goal (hospitalized patients): premeal blood glucose < 140 mg/dL, random < 180 mg/dL. May consider stricter targets in stable patients.

Estimated average glucose (eAG): eAG (mg/dL) = (28.7 × A1C) − 46.7

Complications prevention & management: ASA‡ (75–162 mg/day) in Type 1 & 2 adults for primary prevention if 10-year cardiovascular risk > 10% (includes most men > 50 yo or women > 60 yo with at least one other major risk factor) and secondary prevention (those with vascular disease); statin therapy to achieve 30–40% LDL reduction regardless of baseline LDL (for those with vascular disease, those > 40 yo and additional risk factor, or those < 40 yo but LDL > 100 mg/dL); ACE inhibitor or ARB if hypertensive or micro-/macro-albuminuria; pneumococcal vaccine (revaccinate one time if age ⩾ 65 and previously received vaccine at age < 65 and > 5 yr ago). *Every visit*: Measure wt & BP (goal < 130/80 mm Hg); visual foot exam; review self-monitoring glucose record; review/adjust meds; review self-mgmt skills, dietary needs, and physical activity; smoking cessation counseling. *Twice a year*: A1C in those meeting treatment goals with stable glycemia (quarterly if not); dental exam. *Annually*: Fasting lipid profile** [goal LDL < 100 mg/dL; cardiovascular disease consider LDL < 70mg/dL, HDL > 40 mg/dL (> 50 mg/dL in women), TG < 150 mg/dL], q 2 yr with low-risk lipid values; creatinine; albumin to creatinine ratio spot collection; dilated eye exam; flu vaccine.

*See recommendations at: care.diabetesjournals.org. Reference: *Diabetes Care* 2010;33(Suppl 1):S11-61. Glucose values are plasma. †In the absence of symptoms, confirm diagnosis with glucose testing on subsequent day. ‡Avoid ASA if < 21 yo due to Reye's Syndrome risk; use if < 30 yo has not been studied. **LDL is primary target of therapy.

AVANDAMET (rosiglitazone + metformin) ▶KL ♀C ▶? $$$$$
ADULTS — Type 2 DM, initial therapy (drug-naive): Start 2/500 mg PO daily or bid. If inadequate control with metformin alone, select tab strength based on adding 4 mg/day rosiglitazone to existing metformin dose. If inadequate control with rosiglitazone alone, select tab strength based on adding 1000 mg/day metformin to existing rosiglitazone dose. Max 8/2000 mg/day.
PEDS — Not approved in children.
FORMS — Trade only: Tabs 2/500, 4/500, 2/1000, 4/1000 mg.
NOTES — May be given concomitantly with sulfonylureas. Initial GI upset may be minimized by starting with lower dose of metformin component.
MOA — Combination product that increases insulin sensitivity, decreases hepatic gluconeogenesis.
ADVERSE EFFECTS — Serious: Potential hepatotoxicity, heart failure, resumption of ovulation, lactic acidosis, decreased vitamin B12, macular edema, fracture in women, myocardial infarction. Frequent: Asthenia, anemia, edema, weight gain or loss, headache, dyslipidemia, diarrhea, increased LFTs, N/V, flatulence, abdominal discomfort, headache, taste disturbance.

AVANDARYL (rosiglitazone + glimepiride) ▶LK ♀C ▶? $$$$
ADULTS — Type 2 DM, initial therapy (drug-naive): Start 4/1 mg PO daily. If switching from monotherapy with a sulfonylurea or glitazone, consider 4/2 mg PO daily. Max 8/4 mg/day. Give with breakfast or the first main meal of the day. Use low starting dose of 4/1 mg and titrate more slowly in elderly, malnourished and in renal and hepatic impairment.
PEDS — Not approved in children.
FORMS — Trade only: Tabs 4/1, 4/2, 4/4, 8/2, 8/4 mg rosiglitazone/glimepiride.
MOA — Combination product that stimulates pancreatic beta-cell insulin release and increases insulin sensitivity in adipose tissue, skeletal muscle, and liver.
ADVERSE EFFECTS — Serious: Potential hepatotoxicity, heart failure, resumption of ovulation, macular edema, hypoglycemia, hypersensitivity, SIADH, disulfiram-like reaction, cholestatic jaundice, marrow suppression, hemolytic anemia, eosinophilia, hepatic porphyria, increased LFTs, fracture, myocardial infarction. Frequent: Edema, weight gain, upper respiratory tract infection, headache, fatigue, N/V/D, dyspepsia, rash, pruritus, blurred vision.

DUETACT (pioglitazone + glimepiride) ▶LK ♀C ▶− $$$$
ADULTS — Type 2 DM: Start 30/2 mg PO daily. Start up to 30/4 mg PO daily if prior glimepiride therapy, or 30/2 mg PO daily if prior pioglitazone therapy; max 30/4 mg/day. Give with breakfast or the first main meal of the day. In the elderly, the malnourished, or those with renal/hepatic impairment,

(cont.)

ENDOCRINE AND METABOLIC: Diabetes-Related

DUETACT (cont.)
precede therapy with trial of glimepiride 1 mg/day and then titrate Duetact more slowly.
PEDS — Not approved in children.
FORMS — Trade only: Tabs 30/2, 30/4 mg pioglitazone/glimepiride.
MOA — Combination product that stimulates pancreatic beta-cell insulin release and increases insulin sensitivity in adipose tissue, skeletal muscle, and liver.
ADVERSE EFFECTS — Serious: Potential hepatotoxicity, heart failure exacerbation, resumption of ovulation, hypoglycemia, hypersensitivity, SIADH, disulfiram-like reaction, cholestatic jaundice, marrow suppression, hemolytic anemia, eosinophilia, hepatic porphyria, increased LFTs, macular edema, fracture. Frequent: Edema, weight gain, upper respiratory tract infection, headache, fatigue, N/V/D, dyspepsia, rash, pruritus, blurred vision. Fracture risk in PI for women; in men citation is: Arch Intern Med. 2008;168(8):820-825.

GLUCOVANCE (glyburide + metformin) ▶KL ♀B ▶? $$$
ADULTS — Type 2 DM, initial therapy (drug-naive): Start 1.25/250 mg PO daily or bid with meals; maximum 10/2000 mg daily. Inadequate control with a sulfonylurea or metformin alone: Start 2.5/500 or 5/500 mg PO bid with meals; maximum 20/2000 mg daily.
PEDS — Not approved in children.
FORMS — Generic/Trade: Tabs 1.25/250, 2.5/500, 5/500 mg.
NOTES — May add thiazolidinedione if glycemic control is not obtained. Caution in patients with G6PD deficiency as may cause hemolytic anemia.
MOA — Combination product that stimulates pancreatic beta-cell insulin release, decreases hepatic gluconeogenesis, and increases insulin sensitivity.
ADVERSE EFFECTS — Serious: Hypoglycemia, hypersensitivity, SIADH, disulfiram-like reaction, cholestatic jaundice, aplastic anemia, hemolytic anemia, leukopenia, thrombocytopenia, agranulocytosis, pancytopenia, eosinophilia, hepatic porphyria, increased LFTs, hepatitis, liver failure, lactic acidosis, decreased serum vitamin B12. Frequent: Diarrhea, N/V, flatulence, abdominal discomfort, headache, fatigue, rash, weight gain or loss, taste disturbance.

JANUMET (sitagliptin + metformin) ▶K ♀B ▶? $$$$
ADULTS — Type 2 DM: Start 1 tab PO bid. Individualize based on patient's current therapy. If inadequate control with metformin monotherapy, start 50/500 or 50/1000 bid based on current metformin dose. If inadequate control on sitagliptin monotherapy, start 50/500 bid. Max 100/2000 mg daily. Give with meals.
PEDS — Not approved in children.
FORMS — Trade only: Tabs 50/500, 50/1000 mg sitagliptin/metformin.
NOTES — Not for use in Type 1 DM or DKA. Assess renal function and hematologic parameters prior to initiating and at least annually thereafter. Report pancreatitis and discontinue drug if occurs.
MOA — Combination product that decreases hepatic gluconeogenesis, increases insulin sensitivity and slows inactivation of incretin hormones.
ADVERSE EFFECTS — Serious: Lactic acidosis, hypersensitivity, decreased serum vitamin B12, pancreatitis. Frequent: Diarrhea, N/V, flatulence, abdominal discomfort, headache, weight loss, taste disturbance, URI, nasopharyngitis.

METAGLIP (glipizide + metformin) ▶KL ♀C ▶? $$$
ADULTS — Type 2 DM, initial therapy (drug-naive): Start 2.5/250 mg PO daily to 2.5/500 mg PO bid with meals; max 10/2000 mg daily. Inadequate control with a sulfonylurea or metformin alone: Start 2.5/500 or 5/500 mg PO bid with meals; max 20/2000 mg daily.
PEDS — Not approved in children.
FORMS — Generic/Trade: Tabs 2.5/250, 2.5/500, 5/500 mg.
NOTES — May add thiazolidinedione if glycemic control is not obtained.
MOA — Combination product that stimulates pancreatic beta-cell insulin release, decreases hepatic gluconeogenesis, and increases insulin sensitivity.
ADVERSE EFFECTS — Serious: Hypoglycemia, hypersensitivity, SIADH, disulfiram-like reaction, cholestatic jaundice, aplastic anemia, hemolytic anemia, leukopenia, thrombocytopenia, agranulocytosis, pancytopenia, eosinophilia, hepatic porphyria, increased LFTs, lactic acidosis, decreased serum vitamin B12. Frequent: Weight gain or loss, fatigue, diarrhea, nausea, dyspepsia, rash, vomiting, flatulence, asthenia, abdominal discomfort, headache, taste disturbance.

PRANDIMET (repaglinide + metformin) ▶KL ♀C ▶? $$$
ADULTS — Type 2 DM, initial therapy (drug-naive): Start 1/500 mg PO daily before meals; max 10/2500 mg daily or 4/1000 mg/meal. Inadequate control with metformin alone: Start 1/500 mg PO bid before meals. Inadequate control with repaglinide alone: Start 500 mg metformin component PO bid before meals. In patients taking repaglinide and metformin concomitantly: Start at current dose and titrate to achieve adequate response.
PEDS — Not approved in children.
FORMS — Trade: Tabs 1/500, 2/500 mg.
NOTES — May take dose immediately preceding meal to as long as 30 min before the meal. Patients should be advised to skip dose if skipping meal. Gemfibrozil and itraconazole increase blood repaglinide levels and may result in an increased risk of hypoglycemia. Do not use with NPH insulin.
MOA — Combination product that stimulates pancreatic beta-cell insulin release, decreases hepatic gluconeogenesis, and increases insulin sensitivity.
ADVERSE EFFECTS — Serious: Hypoglycemia, hypersensitivity, thrombocytopenia, leukopenia, increased serum transaminases, lactic acidosis, decreased serum vitamin B12. Frequent: Headache, diarrhea, arthralgia, N/V, flatulence, abdominal discomfort, weight loss, taste disturbance.

(cont.)

ENDOCRINE AND METABOLIC: Diabetes-Related—"Glitazones" (Thiazolidinediones)

NOTE: No clinical studies have established conclusive evidence of decreased macrovascular outcomes with antidiabetic drugs. May cause edema, wt gain, new heart failure, or exacerbate existing heart failure (contraindicated in NYHA Class III or IV). Monitor for signs of heart failure (rapid wt gain, dyspnea, edema) following initiation or dose increase. If occurs, manage fluid retention and consider discontinuation or dosage decrease. Avoid if liver disease or ALT > 2.5 times normal. Monitor LFTs before therapy and periodically thereafter. Discontinue if ALT > 3 times upper normal limit. Full effect may not be apparent for up to 12 weeks. May cause resumption of ovulation in premenopausal anovulatory women; recommend contraception use.

PIOGLITAZONE (*Actos*) ▶L ♀C ▶– $$$$$
ADULTS — <u>Type 2 DM:</u> Start 15 to 30 mg PO daily, may adjust dose after 3 months to max 45 mg/day.
PEDS — Not approved in children.
FORMS — Trade only: Tabs 15, 30, 45 mg.
NOTES — Reports of fracture risk.
MOA — Increases insulin sensitivity in adipose tissue, skeletal muscle, and liver.
ADVERSE EFFECTS — Serious: Potential hepatotoxicity, heart failure exacerbation, resumption of ovulation, macular edema, fracture. Frequent: Edema, weight gain, upper respiratory tract infection, headache, myalgia.

ROSIGLITAZONE (*Avandia*) ▶L ♀C ▶– $$$$
ADULTS — <u>Diabetes monotherapy or in combination with metformin or sulfonylurea:</u> Start 4 mg PO daily or divided bid, may increase after 8 to 12 weeks to max 8 mg/day.
PEDS — Not approved in children younger than 18 yo.
FORMS — Trade only (restricted access): Tabs 2, 4, 8 mg.
NOTES — Rosiglitazone (Avandia) is not recommended with nitrates or insulin, and its labeling includes boxed warning regarding increased risk of myocardial ischemic events and notes that studies are currently inconclusive. Reports of fracture risk.
MOA — Increases insulin sensitivity in adipose tissue, skeletal muscle, and liver.
ADVERSE EFFECTS — Serious: Potential hepatotoxicity, heart failure, resumption of ovulation, macular edema, fracture, myocardial infarction. Frequent: Edema, weight gain, upper respiratory tract infection, headache, back pain, dyslipidemia.

ENDOCRINE AND METABOLIC: Diabetes-Related—Insulins

NOTE: Adjust insulin dosing to achieve glycemic control. See table "diabetes numbers" for goals.

INSULIN—INJECTABLE COMBINATIONS (*Humalog Mix 75/25, Humalog Mix 50/50, Humulin 70/30, Humulin 50/50, Novolin 70/30, Novolog Mix 70/30, Novolog Mix 50/50*)) ▶LK ♀B/C ▶+ $$$$
ADULTS — Doses vary, but typically total insulin 0.3 to 1 unit/kg/day SC in divided doses (Type 1), and 0.5 to 1.5 unit/kg/day SC in divided doses (Type 2). Generally, 50% of insulin requirements are provided by basal insulin (intermediate- or long-acting) and the remainder from rapid or short-acting insulin.
PEDS — Not approved in children.
UNAPPROVED PEDS — <u>Diabetes:</u> Maintenance: Total insulin 0.5 to 1 unit/kg/day SC, but doses vary.
FORMS — Trade only: Insulin lispro protamine susp/insulin lispro (Humalog Mix 75/25, Humalog Mix 50/50). Insulin aspart protamine/insulin aspart (Novolog Mix 70/30, Novolog Mix 50/50). NPH and regular mixtures (Humulin 70/30, Novolin 70/30 or Humulin 50/50). Insulin available in pen form: Novolin 70/30 InnoLet, Novolog Mix 70/30, Novolog Mix 50/50, FlexPen, Humulin 70/30, Humalog Mix 75/25 KwikPen, Humalog Mix 50/50 KwikPen.
NOTES — Administer rapid-acting insulin mixtures (Humalog, NovoLog) within 15 min before meals. Administer regular insulin mixtures 30 min before meals. Pens for use by one person only.
MOA — Stimulates peripheral glucose uptake, and inhibits hepatic gluconeogenesis.
ADVERSE EFFECTS — Serious: Hypoglycemia, allergic reaction, hypokalemia. Frequent: Weight gain, lipoatrophy, lipohypertrophy, injection site reaction.

INSULIN—INJECTABLE INTERMEDIATE/LONG-ACTING (*Novolin N, Humulin N, Lantus, Levemir*) ▶LK ♀B/C ▶+ $$$$
ADULTS — Doses vary, but typically total insulin 0.3 to 0.5 unit/kg/day SC in divided doses (Type 1), and 1 to 1.5 unit/kg/day SC in divided doses (Type 2). Generally, 50 to 70% of insulin requirements are provided by rapid or short-acting insulin and the remainder from intermediate- or long-acting insulin. Lantus: Start 10 units SC daily (same time everyday) in insulin-naive patients, adjust to usual dose of 2 to 100 units/day. When transferring from twice a day NPH human insulin, the initial Lantus dose should be reduced by about 20% from the previous total daily NPH dose, then adjust dose based on patient response. Levemir: Type 2 DM (inadequately controlled on oral meds): Start 0.1 to 0.2 units/kg once a day; or 10 units SC daily or BID. When transferring from basal insulin (Lantus, NPH) in type 1 or 2 DM, change on a unit-to-unit basis; more Levemir may be required than NPH insulin.
PEDS — <u>Diabetes: Maintenance:</u> Total insulin 0.5 to 1 unit/kg/day SC, but doses vary. Generally, 50 to 70% of insulin requirements are provided by rapid-acting insulin and the remainder from

(cont.)

166 ENDOCRINE AND METABOLIC: Diabetes-Related

INJECTABLE INSULINS*		Onset (h)	Peak (h)	Duration (h)
Rapid/short-acting:	Insulin aspart (NovoLog)	<0.2	1–3	3–5
	Insulin glulisine (Apidra)	0.30–0.4	1	4–5
	Insulin lispro (Humalog)	0.25–0.5	0.5–2.5	≤5
	Regular (Novolin R, Humulin R)	0.5–1	2–3	3–6
Intermediate/long-acting:	NPH (Novolin N, Humulin N)	2–4	4–10	10–16
	Insulin detemir (Levemir)	n.a.	flat action profile	up to 23†
	Insulin glargine (Lantus)	2–4	peakless	24
Mixtures:	Insulin aspart protamine susp/aspart (NovoLog Mix 70/30, NovoLog Mix 50/50)	0.25	1–4 (biphasic)	up to 24
	Insulin lispro protamine susp/insulin lispro (HumaLog Mix 75/25, HumaLog Mix 50/50)	<0.25	1–3 (biphasic)	10–20
	NPH/Reg (Humulin 70/30, Humulin 50/50, Novolin 70/30)	0.5–1	2–10 (biphasic)	10–20

*These are general guidelines, as onset, peak, and duration of activity are affected by the site of injection, physical activity, body temperature, and blood supply. † Dose dependent duration of action, range from 6 to 23 h. n.a., not available.

INSULIN—INJECTABLE INTERMEDIATE/LONG-ACTING (cont.)
intermediate- or long-acting insulin. Age 6 to 15 yo (Lantus): Start 10 units SC daily (same time everyday) in insulin-naive patients, adjust to usual dose of 2 to 100 units/day. When transferring from twice a day NPH human insulin, the initial Lantus dose should be reduced by about 20% from the previous total daily NPH dose, then adjust dose based on patient response. Levemir (Type 1 DM): When transferring from NPH, change on a unit-to-unit basis; more Levemir may be required than NPH.
FORMS — Trade only: Injection NPH (Novolin N, Humulin N). Insulin glargine (Lantus). Insulin detemir (Levemir). Insulin available in pen form: Novolin N InnoLet, Humulin N Pen, Lantus OptiClik (reusable), Lantus SoloStar (prefilled-disposable), Levemir InnoLet, Levemir FlexPen. Premixed preparations of NPH and regular insulin also available.
NOTES — May mix NPH with aspart, lispro, glulisine or regular. Draw up rapid/short-acting insulin first. Do not mix Lantus (glargine) or Levemir (detemir) with other insulins. Pens for use by one person only.
MOA — Stimulates peripheral glucose uptake, and inhibits hepatic gluconeogenesis.
ADVERSE EFFECTS — Serious: Hypoglycemia, allergic reaction, hypokalemia. Frequent: Weight gain, lipoatrophy, lipohypertrophy, injection site reaction.

INSULIN—INJECTABLE SHORT/RAPID-ACTING (Apidra, Novolin R, NovoLog, Humulin R, Humalog, ✦NovoRapid) ▶LK ♀B/C ▶+ $$$
ADULTS — Doses vary, but typically total insulin 0.3 to 0.5 unit/kg/day SC in divided doses (Type 1), and 1 to 1.5 unit/kg/day SC in divided doses (Type 2). Generally, 50 to 70% of insulin requirements are provided by rapid or short-acting insulin and the remainder from intermediate- or long-acting insulin.
PEDS — Diabetes age older than 4 yo (Apidra), older than 3 yo (Humalog) or older than 2 yo (NovoLog): Doses vary, but typically total insulin maintenance dose 0.5 to 1 unit/kg/day SC in divided doses. Generally, 50 to 70% of insulin requirements are provided by rapid-acting insulin and the remainder from intermediate- or long-acting insulin.
UNAPPROVED ADULTS — Severe hyperkalemia: 5 to 10 units regular insulin plus concurrent dextrose IV. Profound hyperglycemia (eg, DKA): 0.1 unit/kg regular insulin IV bolus, then begin IV infusion 100 units in 100 mL NS (1 unit/mL) at 0.1 units/kg/h. 70 kg: 7 units/h (7 mL/h). Titrate to clinical effect.
UNAPPROVED PEDS — Profound hyperglycemia (eg, DKA): 0.1 unit/kg regular insulin IV bolus, then IV infusion 100 units in 100 mL NS (1 unit/mL) at 0.1 units/kg/h. Titrate to clinical effect. Severe hyperkalemia: 0.1 units/kg regular insulin IV with glucose over 30 min. May repeat in 30 to 60 min or start 0.1 units/kg/h.
FORMS — Trade only: Injection regular (Novolin R, Humulin R). Insulin glulisine (Apidra). Insulin lispro (Humalog). Insulin aspart (NovoLog). Insulin available in pen form: Novolin R InnoLet, Humulin R, Apidra OptiClik, Humalog KwikPen, Novolog FlexPen.
NOTES — Administer rapid-acting insulin (Humalog, NovoLog, Apidra) within 15 min before or immediately after a meal. Administer regular insulin 30 min before meals. May mix with NPH. Draw up rapid/short-acting insulin first. Pens for use by one person only.
MOA — Stimulates peripheral glucose uptake, and inhibits hepatic gluconeogenesis.
ADVERSE EFFECTS — Serious: Hypoglycemia, allergic reaction, hypokalemia. Frequent: Weight gain, lipoatrophy, lipohypertrophy, injection site reaction.

ENDOCRINE AND METABOLIC: Diabetes-Related—Meglitinides

NOTE: No clinical studies have established conclusive evidence of decreased macrovascular outcomes with antidiabetic drugs.

NATEGLINIDE (*Starlix*) ▶L ♀C ▶? $$$
ADULTS – <u>Diabetes (Type 2), monotherapy or in combination with metformin or thiazolidinedione:</u> 120 mg PO tid within 30 min before meals; use 60 mg PO tid in patients who are near goal A1C.
PEDS – Not approved in children.
FORMS – Generic/Trade: Tabs 60, 120 mg.
NOTES – Not to be used as monotherapy in patients inadequately controlled with glyburide or other antidiabetic agents previously. Patients with severe renal impairment are at risk for hypoglycemic episodes.
MOA – Stimulates pancreatic beta-cell insulin release.
ADVERSE EFFECTS – Serious: Hypoglycemia, jaundice, cholestatic hepatitis, increased LFTs. Frequent: Arthralgia, upper respiratory tract infection, hypersensitivity.

REPAGLINIDE (*Prandin*, ✦*Gluconorm*) ▶L ♀C ▶? $$$$$
ADULTS – <u>Diabetes:</u> 0.5 to 2 mg PO tid within 30 min before a meal. Allow 1 week between dosage adjustments. Usual range is 0.5 to 4 mg PO tid to qid, max 16 mg/day.
PEDS – Not approved in children.
FORMS – Trade only: Tabs 0.5, 1, 2 mg.
NOTES – May take dose immediately preceding meal to as long as 30 min before the meal. Gemfibrozil and itraconazole increase blood repaglinide levels and may result in an increased risk of hypoglycemia. Do not use with NPH insulin.
MOA – Stimulates pancreatic beta-cell insulin release.
ADVERSE EFFECTS – Serious: Hypoglycemia, hypersensitivity, thrombocytopenia, leukopenia, increased serum transaminases. Frequent: Diarrhea, arthralgia, upper respiratory tract infection.

ENDOCRINE AND METABOLIC: Diabetes-Related—Sulfonylureas—1st Generation

CHLORPROPAMIDE (*Diabinese*) ▶LK ♀C ▶– $$
ADULTS – Initiate therapy with 100 to 250 mg PO daily. Titrate after 5 to 7 days by increments of 50 to 125 mg at intervals of 3 to 5 days to obtain optimal control. Max 750 mg/day.
PEDS – Not approved in children.
FORMS – Generic/Trade: Tabs 100, 250 mg.
NOTES – Clinical use in the elderly has not been properly evaluated. Elderly are more prone to hypoglycemia and/or hyponatremia possibly from renal impairment or drug interactions. May cause disulfiram-like reaction with alcohol. No clinical studies have established conclusive evidence of decreased macrovascular outcomes with antidiabetic drugs.
MOA – Stimulates pancreatic beta-cell insulin release.
ADVERSE EFFECTS – Serious: Hypoglycemia, hypersensitivity, SIADH, disulfiram-like reaction, cholestatic jaundice, aplastic anemia, hemolytic anemia, leukopenia, thrombocytopenia, agranulocytosis, pancytopenia, eosinophilia, hepatic porphyria, increased serum transaminases. Frequent: Weight gain, fatigue, diarrhea, nausea, dyspepsia, rash.

TOLAZAMIDE (*Tolinase*) ▶LK ♀C ▶? $
ADULTS – Initiate therapy with 100 mg PO daily in patients with FBS < 200 mg/dL, and in patients who are malnourished, underweight, or elderly. Initiate therapy with 250 mg PO daily in patients with FBS more than 200 mg/dL. Give with breakfast or the first main meal of the day. If daily doses exceed 500 mg, divide the dose bid. Max 1000 mg/day.
PEDS – Not approved in children.
FORMS – Generic only: Tabs 100, 250, 500 mg.
MOA – Stimulates pancreatic beta-cell insulin release.
ADVERSE EFFECTS – Serious: Hypoglycemia, hypersensitivity, SIADH, disulfiram-like reaction, cholestatic jaundice, aplastic anemia, hemolytic anemia, leukopenia, thrombocytopenia, agranulocytosis, pancytopenia, eosinophilia, hepatic porphyria, increased serum transaminases. Frequent: Weight gain, fatigue, diarrhea, nausea, dyspepsia, rash.

TOLBUTAMIDE ▶LK ♀C ▶+ $
ADULTS – Start 1 g PO daily. Maintenance dose is usually 250 mg to 2 g PO daily. Total daily dose may be taken in the morning, divide doses if GI intolerance occurs. Max 3 g/day.
PEDS – Not approved in children.
FORMS – Generic only: Tabs 500 mg.
MOA – Stimulates pancreatic beta-cell insulin release.
ADVERSE EFFECTS – Serious: Hypoglycemia, hypersensitivity, SIADH, disulfiram-like reaction, cholestatic jaundice, aplastic anemia, hemolytic anemia, leukopenia, thrombocytopenia, agranulocytosis, pancytopenia, eosinophilia, hepatic porphyria, increased serum transaminases. Frequent: Weight gain, fatigue, diarrhea, nausea, dyspepsia, rash.

ENDOCRINE AND METABOLIC: Diabetes-Related—Sulfonylureas—2nd Generation

GLICLAZIDE (*Diamicron, Diamicron MR*) ▶KL ♀C ▶? $
ADULTS — Canada only, diabetes type 2: Immediate-release: Start 80 to 160 mg PO daily, max 320 mg PO daily (160 mg or more per day should be in divided doses). Modified-release: Start 30 mg PO daily, max 120 mg PO daily.
PEDS — Not approved in children.
FORMS — Generic/Trade: Tabs 80 mg (Diamicron). Trade only: Tabs, modified-release 30 mg (Diamicron MR).
NOTES — Immediate and modified-release not equipotent; 80 mg of immediate-release can be changed to 30 mg of modified-release.
MOA — Stimulates pancreatic beta-cell insulin release.
ADVERSE EFFECTS — Serious: Hypoglycemia, hypersensitivity, disulfiram-like reaction, cholestatic jaundice, aplastic anemia, hemolytic anemia, leukopenia, thrombocytopenia, agranulocytosis, pancytopenia, eosinophilia, hepatic porphyria, increased LFTs. Frequent: Weight gain, fatigue, diarrhea, nausea, dyspepsia, rash.

GLIMEPIRIDE (*Amaryl*) ▶LK ♀C ▶− $$
ADULTS — Diabetes: Initiate therapy with 1 to 2 mg PO daily. Start with 1 mg PO daily in elderly, malnourished patients or those with renal or hepatic insufficiency. Give with breakfast or the first main meal of the day. Titrate in increments of 1 to 2 mg at 1 to 2 weeks intervals based on response. Usual maintenance dose is 1 to 4 mg PO daily, max 8 mg/day.
PEDS — Not approved in children.
FORMS — Generic/Trade: Tabs 1, 2, 4 mg. Generic only: Tabs 3, 6, 8 mg.
NOTES — No clinical studies have established conclusive evidence of decreased macrovascular outcomes with antidiabetic drugs. Use with caution in patients with G6PD deficiency; may cause hemolytic anemia. Allergy may develop if allergic to other sulfonamide derivatives.
MOA — Stimulates pancreatic beta-cell insulin release.
ADVERSE EFFECTS — Serious: Hypoglycemia, hypersensitivity, SIADH, disulfiram-like reaction, cholestatic jaundice, aplastic anemia, hemolytic anemia, leukopenia, thrombocytopenia, agranulocytosis, pancytopenia, eosinophilia, hepatic porphyria, increased serum transaminases. Frequent: Weight gain, fatigue, diarrhea, nausea, dyspepsia, rash.

GLIPIZIDE (*Glucotrol, Glucotrol XL*) ▶LK ♀C ▶? $
ADULTS — Diabetes: Initiate therapy with 5 mg PO daily. Give 2.5 mg PO daily to geriatric patients or those with liver disease. Adjust dose in increments of 2.5 to 5 mg to a usual maintenance dose of 10 to 20 mg/day, max 40 mg/day. Doses more than 15 mg should be divided bid. Extended-release (Glucotrol XL): Initiate therapy with 5 mg PO daily. Usual dose is 5 to 10 mg PO daily, max 20 mg/day.
PEDS — Not approved in children.
FORMS — Generic/Trade: Tabs 5, 10 mg; Extended-release tabs 2.5, 5, 10 mg.
NOTES — Maximum effective dose is generally 20 mg/day. No clinical studies have established conclusive evidence of decreased macrovascular outcomes with antidiabetic drugs.
MOA — Stimulates pancreatic beta-cell insulin release.
ADVERSE EFFECTS — Serious: Hypoglycemia, hypersensitivity, SIADH, disulfiram-like reaction, cholestatic jaundice, aplastic anemia, hemolytic anemia, leukopenia, thrombocytopenia, agranulocytosis, pancytopenia, eosinophilia, hepatic porphyria, increased serum transaminases. Frequent: Weight gain, fatigue, diarrhea, nausea, dyspepsia, rash.

GLYBURIDE (*DiaBeta, Glynase PresTab, *Euglucon*) ▶LK ♀B ▶? $
ADULTS — Diabetes: Initiate therapy with 2.5 to 5 mg PO daily. Start with 1.25 mg PO daily in elderly or malnourished patients or those with renal or hepatic insufficiency. Give with breakfast or the first main meal of the day. Titrate in increments of no more than 2.5 mg at weekly intervals based on response. Usual maintenance dose is 1.25 to 20 mg PO daily or divided bid, max 20 mg/day. Micronized tabs: Initiate therapy with 1.5 to 3 mg PO daily. Start with 0.75 mg PO daily in elderly, malnourished patients or those with renal or hepatic insufficiency. Give with breakfast or the first main meal of the day. Titrate in increments of no more than 1.5 mg at weekly intervals based on response. Usual maintenance dose is 0.75 to 12 mg PO daily, max 12 mg/day. May divide dose bid if more than 6 mg/day.
PEDS — Not approved in children.
FORMS — Generic/Trade: Tabs (scored) 1.25, 2.5, 5 mg. Micronized Tabs (scored) 1.5, 3, 4.5, 6 mg.
NOTES — Maximum effective dose is generally 10 mg/day. No clinical studies have established conclusive evidence of decreased macrovascular outcomes with antidiabetic drugs.
MOA — Stimulates pancreatic beta-cell insulin release.
ADVERSE EFFECTS — Serious: Hypoglycemia, hypersensitivity, SIADH, disulfiram-like reaction, cholestatic jaundice, aplastic anemia, hemolytic anemia, leukopenia, thrombocytopenia, agranulocytosis, pancytopenia, eosinophilia, hepatic porphyria, increased serum transaminases. Frequent: Weight gain, fatigue, diarrhea, nausea, dyspepsia, rash.

ENDOCRINE AND METABOLIC: Diabetes-Related—Other

A1C HOME TESTING (*A1CNow*) ▶None ♀+ ▶+ $
ADULTS — Use for home A1C testing.
PEDS — Use for home A1C testing.
FORMS — Fingerstick blood.
NOTES — Result displays in 5 min.
MOA — Measures average glucose levels over a 90- to 120-day period.
ADVERSE EFFECTS — Serious: None. Frequent: Local pain.

DEXTROSE (*Glutose, B-D Glucose, Insta-Glucose, Dex-4*) ▶L ♀C ▶? $
ADULTS — Hypoglycemia: 0.5 to 1 g/kg (1 to 2 mL/kg) up to 25 g (50 mL) of 50% soln by slow IV injection. Hypoglycemia in conscious diabetics: 10 to 20 g PO q 10 to 20 min prn.
PEDS — Hypoglycemia in neonates: 0.25 to 0.5 g/kg/dose (5 to 10 mL of 25% dextrose in a 5 kg infant). Severe hypoglycemia or older infants may require larger doses up to 3 g (12 mL of 25% dextrose) followed by a continuous IV infusion of 10% dextrose. Non-neonates may require 0.5 to 1 g/kg.
FORMS — OTC Generic/Trade: Chewable tabs 4 g (Dex-4), 5 g (Glutose). Trade only: Oral gel 40%.
NOTES — Do not exceed an infusion rate of 0.5 g/kg/h.
MOA — Elevates blood glucose.
ADVERSE EFFECTS — Serious: None. Frequent: Nausea.

EXENATIDE (*Byetta*) ▶K ♀C ▶? $$$$$
ADULTS — Type 2 DM adjunctive therapy when inadequate control on metformin, a sulfonylurea, or a glitazone (alone or in combination): 5 mcg SC bid (within 1 h before the morning and evening meals, or 1 h before the two main meals of the day at least 6 h apart). May increase to 10 mcg SC bid after 1 month.
PEDS — Not approved in children.
FORMS — Trade only: Prefilled pen (60 doses each) 5 mcg/dose, 1.2 mL; 10 mcg/dose, 2.4 mL.
NOTES — Protect from light. Prior to initial use, keep refrigerated. After initial use, store at temperature below 78 degrees; do not freeze. Discard pen 30 days after first use. May give SC in upper arm, abdomen, or thigh. Avoid use if renal insufficiency (CrCl less than 30 mL/min) or severe GI disease, including gastroparesis. Caution recommended if increasing dose from 5 to 10 mcg in patients with CrCl 30 to 50 ml/min. Monitor for kidney dysfunction. Reports of hemorrhagic or necrotizing pancreatitis; discontinue and do not rechallenge if pancreatitis occurs. Do not substitute for insulin in the insulin-dependent. Concurrent use with insulin, meglitinides or alpha-glucosidase inhibitors has not been studied. Risk of hypoglycemia is higher when used with sulfonylurea, therefore, consider reduction in sulfonylurea dose. Take medications that require rapid GI absorption at least 1 h prior to exenatide. May promote slight wt loss. May potentiate warfarin.
MOA — Incretin analog that reduces fasting and postprandial glucose by increasing glucose-stimulated insulin secretion, decreasing glucagon secretion, slowing gastric emptying and reducing appetite.
ADVERSE EFFECTS — Serious: angioedema, hypersensitivity, anaphylaxis, pancreatitis, renal dysfunction. Frequent: hypoglycemia, N/V, diarrhea, constipation, flatulence, dizziness, headache.

GLUCAGON (*GlucaGen*) ▶LK ♀B ▶? $$$
ADULTS — Hypoglycemia in adults: 1 mg IV/IM/SC. If no response within 15 min, may repeat dose 1 to 2 times (preferred via IV for repeat). Diagnostic aid for GI tract radiography: 1 mg IV/IM/SC.
PEDS — Hypoglycemia in children wt greater 20 kg: Same as adults. Hypoglycemia in children wt less than 20 kg: 0.5 mg IV/IM/SC or 20 to 30 mcg/kg. If no response in 5 to 20 min, may repeat dose 1 to 2 times.
UNAPPROVED ADULTS — The following indications are based upon limited data. Esophageal obstruction caused by food: 1 mg IV over 1 to 3 min. Symptomatic bradycardia/hypotension, especially with beta-blocker therapy: 3 to 10 mg IV bolus (0.05 mg/kg general recommendation) may repeat in 10 min; may be followed by continuous infusion of 1 to 5 mg/h or 0.07 mg/kg/h. Infusion rate should be titrated to the desired response.
FORMS — Trade only: Injection 1 mg.
NOTES — Should be reserved for refractory/severe cases or when IV/IM dextrose cannot be administered. Advise patients to educate family members and co-workers how to administer a dose. Give supplemental carbohydrates when patient responds.
MOA — Inhibits glycogen synthesis, enhances glucose formation, and increases hepatic glycogenolysis; has relaxant effect on the GI tract; temporarily inhibits GI tract movement for diagnostic procedures.
ADVERSE EFFECTS — Serious: Generalized allergic reaction, hypotension. Frequent: N/V.

GLUCOSE HOME TESTING (*Accu-Chek Active, Accu-Check Advantage, Accu-Check Aviva, Accu-Check Compact, Accu-Check Compact Plus, Accu-Check Complete, Accu-Check Voicemate, FreeStyle Flash, FreeStyle Freedom, FreeStyle Freedom Lite, FreeStyle Lite, OneTouch Ultra, OneTouch UltraMin*) ▶None ♀+ ▶+ $$
ADULTS — Use for home glucose monitoring.
PEDS — Use for home glucose monitoring.
FORMS — Plasma: Accu-Check meters, FreeStyle meters, OneTouch meters, Precision Xtra, ReliOn, Sidekick, True Track. Urine: Clinistix, Clinitest, Diastix, Tes-Tape.
NOTES — Product list is not all-inclusive; check with manufacturers for current products. Accu-Check Active, Accu-Check Aviva, Accu-Check Compact, Accu-Check Compact Plus, FreeStyle meters, OneTouch Ultra, OneTouch UltraSmart, ReliOn

(cont.)

ENDOCRINE AND METABOLIC: Diabetes-Related

GLUCOSE HOME TESTING (cont.)

Sidekick, Precision Xtra, and True Track can be used on alternate site testing (eg, forearm) prior to or at least 2 h after meals or exercise. Accu-Check Voicemate has voice prompts for visually impaired. Precision Xtra allows for ketone testing. Sidekick is 50 strip disposable meter.
MOA − Measures plasma or whole blood glucose, varies by manufacturer.
ADVERSE EFFECTS − Serious: None. Frequent: Local pain.

LIRAGLUTIDE (*Victoza*) ♀C ▶? $$$$$
WARNING − Thyroid C-cell tumors reported in animal studies. Contraindicated if history or family history of medullary thyroid cancer or in patients with multiple endocrine neoplasia syndrome type 2. Counsel patients on risk of thyroid tumors.
ADULTS − Type 2 DM: Start 0.6 mg SC daily for 1 week, then increase to 1.2 mg SC daily. May increase to 1.8 mg SC daily.
PEDS − Not approved in children.
FORMS − Trade only: Multidose pen (18 mg/3ml) delivers doses of 0.6 mg, 1.2 mg or 1.8 mg.
NOTES − Start with low dose to increase GI tolerance. May be given any time of day, independent of meals. May give SC in abdomen, thigh or upper arm. Consider decreasing dose of sulfonylureas when initiating to reduce risk of hypoglycemia. Take medications that require rapid GI absorption at least 1 hour prior to liraglutide. Use caution in patients with renal or hepatic impairment or history of pancreatitis. Concurrent use with insulin has not been studied. May promote slight weight loss.
MOA − Incretin analog that reduces fasting and postprandial glucose by increasing glucose-stimulated insulin secretion, decreasing glucagon secretion, slowing gastric emptying and reducing appetite.
ADVERSE EFFECTS − Serious: pancreatitis, hypersensitivity. Frequent: Headache, nausea, diarrhea, anti-liraglutide antibody formation.

METFORMIN (*Glucophage, Glucophage XR, Glumetza, Fortamet, Riomet*) ▶K ♀B ▶? $
ADULTS − Diabetes, type 2: Immediate-release: Start 500 mg PO daily-bid or 850 mg PO daily with meals. Increase by 500 mg q week or 850 mg q 2 weeks to a maximum of 2550 mg/day. Higher doses may be divided tid with meals. Extended-release: Glucophage XR: 500 mg PO daily with evening meal; increase by 500 mg q week to max 2000 mg/day (may divide bid). Glumetza: 1000 mg PO daily with evening meal; increase by 500 mg q week to max 2000 mg/day (may divide bid). Fortamet: 500 to 1000 mg daily with evening meal; increase by 500 mg q week to max 2500 mg/day.
PEDS − Diabetes 10 yo or older: Start 500 mg PO daily-bid (Glucophage) with meals, increase by 500 mg q week to max 2000 mg/day in divided doses (10 to 16 yo). Glucophage XR and Fortamet are indicated for age 17 yo or older.

UNAPPROVED ADULTS − Polycystic ovary syndrome: 500 mg PO tid or 850 mg PO bid. Prevention/delay Type 2 DM (with lifestyle modifications): 850 mg PO daily for 1 month, then increase to 850 mg PO bid.
FORMS − Generic/Trade: Tabs 500, 850, 1000 mg, extended-release 500, 750 mg. Trade only, extended-release: Fortamet 500, 1000 mg; Glumetza 500, 1000 mg. Trade only: Oral soln 500 mg/5 mL (Riomet).
NOTES − May reduce the risk of progression to Type 2 diabetes in those with impaired glucose tolerance, but less effectively than intensive lifestyle modification. Metformin-containing products may cause life-threatening lactic acidosis, usually in setting of decreased tissue perfusion, hypoxia, hepatic dysfunction, unstable congestive heart failure or impaired renal clearance. Hold prior to IV contrast agents and for 48 h after. Avoid if ethanol abuse, hepatic or renal insufficiency (creatinine ≥1.4 mg/dL in women, ≥1.5 mg/dL in men), or hypoxic states (cardiogenic shock, septicemia, acute MI). No clinical studies have established conclusive evidence of decreased macrovascular outcomes with antidiabetic drugs.
MOA − Decreases hepatic gluconeogenesis and increases insulin sensitivity.
ADVERSE EFFECTS − Serious: Lactic acidosis, decreased serum vitamin B12. Frequent: Diarrhea, N/V, flatulence, abdominal discomfort, headache, weight loss, taste disturbance.

PRAMLINTIDE (*Symlin, Symlinpen*) ▶K ♀C ▶? $$$$
WARNING − May cause severe insulin-induced hypoglycemia especially in Type 1 DM, usually within 3 h. Avoid if hypoglycemic unawareness, gastroparesis, GI motility medications, alpha-glucosidase inhibitors, A1C more than 9%, poor compliance, or hypersensitivity to the metacresol preservative. Appropriate patient selection, careful patient instruction and insulin dose adjustments (reduction in premeal short-acting insulin of 50%) are critical for reducing the hypoglycemia risk.
ADULTS − Type 1 DM with mealtime insulin therapy: Initiate 15 mcg SC immediately before major meals and titrate by 15 mcg increments (if significant nausea has not occurred for at least 3 days) to maintenance 30 to 60 mcg as tolerated. If significant nausea, decrease to 30 mcg. Type 2 DM with mealtime insulin therapy: Initiate 60 mcg SC immediately before major meals and increase to 120 mcg as tolerated (if significant nausea has not occurred for 3 to 7 days). If significant nausea, decrease dose to 60 mcg.
PEDS − Not approved in children.
FORMS − Trade only: 600 mcg/mL in 5 mL vials, 1000 mcg/mL pen injector (Symlinpen) 1.5, 2.7 mL.
NOTES − Keep unopened vials refrigerated. Opened vials can be kept at room temperature or refrigerated up to 28 days. May give SC in abdomen or thigh. Take medications that require rapid onset 1 h prior or 2 h after. Careful patient selection and skilled health care supervision are critical for safe

(cont.)

PRAMLINTIDE (cont.)
and effective use. Monitor pre-/postmeal and bedtime glucose. Decrease initial premeal short-acting insulin doses by 50% including fixed-mix insulin (ie, 70/30). Do not mix with insulin. Use new needle and syringe for each dose.
MOA — Amylin analog that reduces postprandial hyperglycemia by slowing gastric emptying and decreasing postprandial glucagon secretion. It also decreases caloric intake by decreasing appetite.
ADVERSE EFFECTS — Serious: Severe hypoglycemia, systemic allergic reaction. Frequent: N/V, headache, abdominal pain, hypoglycemia, injection site reactions.

SAXAGLIPTIN (*Onglyza*) ▶LK ♀B ▶? $$$$$
WARNING — None
ADULTS — Type 2 DM: 2.5 or 5 mg PO daily. If CrCl ≤ 50 mL/min reduce dose to 2.5 mg daily.
PEDS — Not approved in children.
FORMS — Trade only: Tabs 2.5, 5 mg.
NOTES — Not for use in Type 1 DM or DKA. Assess renal function periodically. Not studied in combination with insulin. When adding to sulfonylurea therapy, consider reducing dose of sulfonylurea to decrease risk of hypoglycemia. Reduce dose when administered with strong CYP 3A4/5 inhibitors such as ketoconazole. No clinical studies have established conclusive evidence of decreased macrovascular outcomes with antidiabetic drugs.
MOA — Dipeptidyl peptidase IV (DPP-IV) inhibitor that slows inactivation of incretin hormones, resulting in increased glucose-stimulated insulin secretion and decreased glucagon secretion.
ADVERSE EFFECTS — Serious: hypersensitivity, facial edema, hypoglycemia, lympopenia, Frequent: URI, UTI, headache, GI, nasopharyngitis, peripheral edema.

SITAGLIPTIN (*Januvia*) ▶K ♀B ▶? $$$$
ADULTS — Type 2 DM: 100 mg PO daily. If CrCl 30 to 49 mL/min reduce dose to 50 mg daily; if CrCl less than 30 mL/min then 25 mg daily.
PEDS — Not approved in children.
FORMS — Trade only: Tabs 25, 50, 100 mg.
NOTES — Not for use in Type 1 DM or DKA. Assess renal function periodically. Not studied in combination with insulin. When adding to sulfonylurea therapy, consider reducing dose of sulfonylurea to decrease risk of hypoglycemia. No clinical studies have established conclusive evidence of decreased macrovascular outcomes with antidiabetic drugs. Monitor for pancreatitis at initiation of therapy and dosage increases; discontinue drug if occurs. Discontinue if signs of hypersensitivity, including anaphylaxis, angioedema and severe dermatologic reactions.
MOA — Dipeptidyl peptidase IV (DPP-IV) inhibitor that slows inactivation of incretin hormones, resulting in increased glucose-stimulated insulin secretion and decreased glucagon secretion.
ADVERSE EFFECTS — Serious: Hypersensitivity, anaphylaxis, angioedema, pancreatitis. Frequent: URI, nasopharyngitis, HA, increased serum transaminases.

ENDOCRINE AND METABOLIC: Diagnostic Agents

CORTICOTROPIN (*H.P. Acthar Gel*) ▶K ♀C ▶− $$$$$
ADULTS — Diagnostic testing of adrenocortical function: 80 units IM or SC. Acute exacerbation of multiple sclerosis: 80 to 120 units IM daily IM for 2 to 3 weeks.
UNAPPROVED PEDS — Various dosing regimens have been used for infantile spasms.
NOTES — Has limited therapeutic value in conditions responsive to corticosteroid therapy, corticosteroids should be the treatment of choice. Prolonged use in children may inhibit skeletal growth. Cosyntropin preferred for diagnostic testing as it is less allergenic and more potent.
MOA — Stimulates the adrenal cortex to secrete cortisol, corticosterone, aldosterone and weakly androgenic substances.
ADVERSE EFFECTS — Serious: Hypersensitivity, convulsions. Frequent: Electrolyte imbalances, menstrual irregularities.

COSYNTROPIN (*Cortrosyn, ✦Synacthen*) ▶L ♀C ▶? $
ADULTS — Rapid screen for adrenocortical insufficiency: 0.25 mg IM/IV over 2 min; measure serum cortisol before and 30 to 60 min after.
PEDS — Rapid screen for adrenocortical insufficiency: 0.25 mg (0.125 mg if age younger than 2 yo) IM/IV over 2 min; measure serum cortisol before and 30 to 60 min after.
MOA — Stimulates the adrenal cortex to produce and secrete hormones.
ADVERSE EFFECTS — Serious: Hypersensitivity. Frequent: None (since used diagnostically).

METYRAPONE (*Metopirone*) ▶KL ♀C ▶? $
WARNING — May cause acute adrenal insufficiency.
ADULTS — Diagnostic aid for testing hypothalamic-pituitary adrenocorticotropic hormone (ACTH) function: Specialized single- and multiple-test dose available.
PEDS — Diagnostic aid for testing hypothalamic-pituitary adrenocorticotropic hormone (ACTH) function: Specialized single- and multiple-test dose available.
UNAPPROVED ADULTS — Cushing's syndrome: Dosing varies.
FORMS — Trade only: Caps 250 mg. Only available from manufacturer due to limited supply: 1-800-988-7768.
NOTES — Ability of adrenals to respond to exogenous ACTH should be demonstrated before metyrapone is employed as a test. In the presence of hypo- or hyperthyroidism, response to the test may

(cont.)

METYRAPONE (cont.)
be subnormal. May suppress aldosterone synthesis. May cause dizziness and sedation.
MOA — Inhibits endogenous adrenal corticosteroid synthesis.
ADVERSE EFFECTS — Serious: Acute adrenal insufficiency, bone marrow suppression, neutropenia. Frequent: Sedation, dizziness, headache, rash, abdominal discomfort, vomiting.

ENDOCRINE AND METABOLIC: Gout-Related

ALLOPURINOL (*Aloprim, Zyloprim*) ▶K ♀C ▶+ $
ADULTS — <u>Mild gout or recurrent calcium oxalate stones:</u> 200 to 300 mg PO daily (start with 100 mg PO daily). <u>Moderately severe gout:</u> 400 to 600 mg PO daily. <u>Secondary hyperuricemia:</u> 600 to 800 mg PO daily. Doses in excess of 300 mg should be divided. Max 800 mg/day. Reduce dose in renal insufficiency (CrCl 10 to 20 mL/min: 200 mg/day, CrCl 3 to 10 mL/min: 100 mg/day, CrCl less than 3 mL/min: 100 mg/day at extended intervals). <u>Prevention of hyperuricemia secondary to chemotherapy and unable to tolerate PO:</u> 200 to 400 mg/m2/day as a single IV infusion or in equally divided infusions q 6 to 12 h. Max 600 mg/day. Reduce dose in renal insufficiency (CrCl 10 to 20 mL/min: 200 mg/day, CrCl 3 to 10 mL/min: 100 mg/day, CrCl less than 3 mL/min: 100 mg/day at extended intervals). Initiate 24 to 48 h before chemotherapy.
PEDS — <u>Secondary hyperuricemia:</u> Age younger than 6 yo give 150 mg PO daily; age 6 to 10 yo give 300 mg PO daily or 1 mg/kg/day divided q 6 h to a maximum of 600 mg/day. <u>Prevention of hyperuricemia secondary to chemotherapy and unable to tolerate PO:</u> Initiate with 200 mg/m2/day as a single IV infusion or in equally divided infusions q 6 to 12 h.
FORMS — Generic/Trade: Tabs 100, 300 mg.
NOTES — May precipitate acute gout; consider using NSAIDs or colchicine prophylactically. Start with 100 mg PO daily and increase weekly to target serum uric acid of less than 6 mg/dL. Incidence of rash and allopurinol hypersensitivity syndrome is increased in renal impairment. Discontinue if rash or allergic symptoms, do not restart after severe rash. Drug interaction with warfarin and azathioprine. Normal serum uric acid levels are usually achieved after 1 to 3 weeks of therapy. Ensure hydration before IV administration.
MOA — Inhibits xanthine oxidase decreasing uric acid production.
ADVERSE EFFECTS — Serious: Hepatotoxicity, hypersensitivity reaction, severe rash, renal failure, mobilization gout, bone marrow depression. Frequent: Headache, peripheral neuropathy, rash, neuritis, somnolence, N/V, diarrhea, dyspepsia, abdominal pain, fever, myopathy.

COLBENEMID (colchicine + probenecid) ▶KL ♀C ▶? $
ADULTS — <u>Chronic gouty arthritis:</u> Start 1 tab PO daily for 1 week, then 1 tab PO bid.
PEDS — Not approved in children.
FORMS — Generic only: Tabs 0.5 mg colchicine + 500 mg probenecid.
NOTES — Maintain alkaline urine.
MOA — Combination product that reduces the inflammatory response to deposited crystals, diminishes phagocytosis and inhibits tubular reabsorption of uric acid.
ADVERSE EFFECTS — Serious: Peripheral neuritis, hepatotoxicity, renal failure, bone marrow depression with aplastic anemia, thrombocytopenia, purpura, myopathy, hypersensitivity, nephrotic syndrome, hemolytic anemia, mobilization gout. Frequent: Diarrhea, N/V, abdominal pain, dermatoses, hair loss, headache, anorexia, urinary frequency, sore gums, dizziness.

COLCHICINE (*Colcrys*) ▶L ♀C ▶? $
ADULTS — <u>Acute gout:</u> 1.2 mg (2 tabs) PO at signs of attack then 0.6 mg (1 tab) 1 h later. CrCl < 30 mL/min: Do not repeat more than every 2 weeks. CrCl < 15 mL/min: 0.6 mg PO for one dose; do not repeat more than every 2 weeks. <u>Familial Mediterranean Fever:</u> 1.2 to 2.4 mg PO daily or divided bid. <u>Renal insufficiency:</u> See product information.
PEDS — <u>Familial Mediterranean Fever:</u> Age 4 to 6 yo: 0.3 to 1.8 mg PO daily or divided bid; age 6 to 12 yo: 0.9 to 1.8 mg daily or divided bid; age 12 yo or older: See adult dosing.
UNAPPROVED ADULTS — <u>Gout prophylaxis:</u> 0.6 mg PO bid if CrCl ≥ 50 mL/min, 0.6 mg PO daily if CrCl 35 to 49 mL/min, 0.6 mg PO q 2 to 3 days if CrCl 10 to 34 mL/min. <u>Primary biliary cirrhosis:</u> 0.6 mg PO bid.
FORMS — Generic/Trade: Tabs 0.6 mg.
NOTES — Contraindicated with P-glycoprotein or strong CYP 3A4 inhibitors. Lower max doses with specific concomitant drugs. For Familial Mediterranean Fever, increase or decrease by 0.3 mg/day to effect/tolerability up to max. Most effective when initiated on the first day of gouty arthritis.
MOA — Reduces the inflammatory response to deposited crystals, and diminishes phagocytosis.
ADVERSE EFFECTS — Serious: Peripheral neuritis, hepatotoxicity, renal failure, bone marrow depression, leukocytopenia, granulocytopenia, aplastic anemia, thrombocytopenia, purpura, myopathy, rhabdomyolysis, hypersensitivity. Frequent: Diarrhea, N/V, abdominal pain, dermatoses, hair loss.

FEBUXOSTAT (*Uloric*) ▶LK ♀C ▶? $$$$
ADULTS — <u>Hyperuricemia with gout:</u> Start 40 mg daily. After 2 weeks, if uric acid > 6 mg/dL may increase to 80 mg daily.
PEDS — Not approved in children.
FORMS — Trade only: Tabs 40, 80 mg.
NOTES — May precipitate acute gout; consider using NSAIDs or colchicine prophylactically for up to 6

(cont.)

ENDOCRINE AND METABOLIC: Minerals

IV SOLUTIONS								
Solution	Dextrose	Calories/Liter	Na*	K*	Ca*	Cl*	Lactate*	Osm*
0.9 NS	0 g/L	0	154	0	0	154	0	310
LR	0 g/L	9	130	4	3	109	28	273
D5 W	50 g/L	170	0	0	0	0	0	253
D5 0.2 NS	50 g/L	170	34	0	0	34	0	320
D5 0.45 NS	50 g/L	170	77	0	0	77	0	405
D5 0.9 NS	50 g/L	170	154	0	0	154	0	560
D5 LR	50 g/L	179	130	4	2.7	109	28	527

* All given in mEq/L

FEBUXOSTAT (cont.)
months. Monitor LFTs periodically. Do not use with azathioprine, mercaptopurine or theophylline. May increase risk of thromboembolic events, monitor for cardiovascular events (MI, CVA). Caution in severe renal or hepatic impairment.
MOA – Inhibits xanthine oxidase decreasing uric acid production.
ADVERSE EFFECTS – Serious: Thromboembolism. Frequent: LFT elevations, nausea, arthralgia, rash, gout flare.

PROBENECID (✦Benuryl) ▶KL ♀B ▶? $
ADULTS – <u>Gout:</u> 250 mg PO bid for 7 days, then 500 mg PO bid. May increase by 500 mg/day q 4 weeks not to exceed 2 g/day. <u>Adjunct to penicillin:</u> 2 g/day PO in divided doses. Reduce dose to 1 g/day in renal impairment.
PEDS – <u>Adjunct to penicillin in children 2 to 14 yo:</u> 25 mg/kg PO initially, then 40 mg/kg/day divided qid. For children greater than 50 kg, use adult dose. Contraindicated in children age younger than 2 yo.
FORMS – Generic only: Tabs 500 mg.
NOTES – Decrease dose if GI intolerance occurs. Maintain alkaline urine. Begin therapy 2 to 3 weeks after acute gouty attack subsides.
MOA – Inhibits tubular reabsorption of uric acid.
ADVERSE EFFECTS – Serious: Hepatotoxicity, nephrotic syndrome, hemolytic anemia, hypersensitivity, mobilization gout. Frequent: Headache, anorexia, N/V, urinary frequency, sore gums, dizziness.

ENDOCRINE AND METABOLIC: Minerals

CALCIUM ACETATE (PhosLo) ▶K ♀+ ▶? $$$$
ADULTS – <u>Hyperphosphatemia in end-stage renal failure:</u> Initially 2 tabs/caps PO tid with each meal. Titrate dose based on serum phosphorus.
PEDS – Not approved in children.
UNAPPROVED PEDS – Titrate to response.
FORMS – Generic/Trade: Gelcaps 667 mg (169 mg elem Ca).
NOTES – Higher doses more effective, but may cause hypercalcemia, especially if given with vitamin D. Most patients require 3 to 4 tabs/meal.
MOA – Binds with dietary phosphate to form a nonabsorbable complex.
ADVERSE EFFECTS – Serious: Severe hypercalcemia (with confusion, delirium, stupor, coma), renal calculi. Frequent: Mild hypercalcemia, constipation, anorexia, N/V.

CALCIUM CARBONATE (Caltrate, Mylanta Children's, Os-Cal, Oyst-Cal, Tums, Surpass, Viactiv, ✦Calsan) ▶K ♀+ (? 1st trimester) ▶? $
ADULTS – <u>Supplement:</u> 1 to 2 g elem Ca/day or more PO with meals divided bid to qid. <u>Prevention of osteoporosis:</u> 1000 to 1500 mg elem Ca/day PO divided bid to tid with meals. The adequate intake in most adults is 1000 to 1200 mg elem Ca/day. <u>Antacid:</u> 1000 to 3000 mg (2 to 4 tab) PO q 2 h prn or 1 to 2 pieces gum chewed prn, max 7000 mg/day.
PEDS – <u>Hypocalcemia:</u> Neonates: 50 to 150 mg elem Ca/kg/day PO in 4 to 6 divided doses; Children: 45 to 65 mg elem Ca/kg/day PO divided qid. <u>Adequate intake</u> for children (in elem calcium): Age younger than 6 mo: 210 mg/day when fed human milk and 315 mg/day when fed cow's milk; 6 to 12 mo: 270 mg/day when fed human milk + solid food and 335 mg/day when fed cow's milk + solid food; 1 to 3 yo: 500 mg/day; 4 to 8 yo: 800 mg/day; 9 to 18 yo 1300 mg/day.
UNAPPROVED ADULTS – <u>May lower BP in patients with HTN. May reduce PMS symptoms such as fluid retention, pain, and negative affect.</u>
FORMS – OTC Generic/Trade: Tabs 500, 650, 750, 1000, 1250, 1500 mg, Chewable tabs 400, 500, 750, 850, 1000, 1177, 1250 mg, Caps 1250 mg, Gum 300, 450 mg, Susp 1250 mg/5 mL. Calcium carbonate is 40% elem Ca and contains 20 mEq of elem Ca/g calcium carbonate. Not more than 500 to 600 mg elem Ca/dose. Available in combination with sodium fluoride, vitamin D and/or vitamin K. Trade examples: Caltrate 600 + D = 600 mg elemental Ca/200 units vit D, Os-Cal 500 + D = 500 mg elemental Ca/200 units vit D, Os-Cal Extra D = 500 mg elemental

(cont.)

CALCIUM CARBONATE (cont.)

Ca/400 units vit D, Tums (regular strength) = 200 mg elemental Ca, Tums (ultra) = 400 mg elemental Ca, Viactiv (chewable) 500 mg elemental Ca+ 100 units vit D + 40 mcg vit K.
NOTES − Decreases absorption of levothyroxine, tetracycline, and fluoroquinolones.
MOA − Antacid, mineral supplement.
ADVERSE EFFECTS − Serious: Severe hypercalcemia (with confusion, delirium, stupor, coma), renal calculi. Frequent: Mild hypercalcemia, constipation, anorexia, N/V.

CALCIUM CHLORIDE ▶K ♀+ ▶+ $
ADULTS − Hypocalcemia: 500 to 1000 mg slow IV q 1 to 3 d. Magnesium intoxication: 500 mg IV. Hyperkalemic ECG changes: Dose based on ECG.
PEDS − Hypocalcemia: 0.2 mL/kg IV up to 10 mL/day. Cardiac resuscitation: 0.2 mL/kg IV.
UNAPPROVED ADULTS − Has been used in calcium channel blocker toxicity and to treat or prevent calcium channel blocker-induced hypotension.
UNAPPROVED PEDS − Has been used in calcium channel blocker toxicity.
FORMS − Generic only: Injectable 10% (1000 mg/10 mL) 10 mL ampules, vials, syringes.
NOTES − Calcium chloride contains 14.4 mEq Ca/g versus calcium gluconate 4.7 mEq Ca/g. For IV use only; do not administer IM or SC. Avoid extravasation. Administer no faster than 0.5 to 1 mL/min. Use cautiously in patients receiving digoxin; inotropic and toxic effects are synergistic and may cause arrhythmias. Usually not recommended for hypocalcemia associated with renal insufficiency because calcium chloride is an acidifying salt.
MOA − Antagonizes the cardiotoxic effects of hyperkalemia.
ADVERSE EFFECTS − Serious: Vasodilation, hypotension. Frequent: Irritation at infusion site.

CALCIUM CITRATE (*Citracal*) ▶K ♀+ ▶+ $
ADULTS − 1 to 2 g elem Ca/day or more PO with meals divided bid to qid. Prevention of osteoporosis: 1000 to 1500 mg elem Ca/day PO divided bid to tid with meals. The adequate intake in most adults is 1000 to 1200 mg elem Ca/day.
PEDS − Not approved in children.
FORMS − OTC Trade only (mg elem Ca): 200, 250 mg with 200 units vitamin D and 250 mg with 125 units vitamin D and 80 mg of magnesium. Chewable tabs 500 mg with 200 units vitamin D. OTC Generic/Trade: Tabs 200 mg, 315 mg with 200 units vitamin D.
NOTES − Calcium citrate is 21% elem Ca. Not more than 500 to 600 mg elem Ca/dose. Decreases absorption of levothyroxine, tetracycline and fluoroquinolones.
MOA − Essential mineral that maintains the nervous, muscular, and skeletal systems and cell membrane and capillary permeability.
ADVERSE EFFECTS − Serious: Severe hypercalcemia (with confusion, delirium, stupor, coma), renal calculi. Frequent: Mild hypercalcemia, constipation, anorexia, N/V.

CALCIUM GLUCONATE ▶K ♀+ ▶+ $
ADULTS − Emergency correction of hypocalcemia: 7 to 14 mEq slow IV prn. Hypocalcemic tetany: 4.5 to 16 mEq IM prn. Hyperkalemia with cardiac toxicity: 2.25 to 14 mEq IV while monitoring ECG. May repeat after 1 to 2 min. Magnesium intoxication: 4.5 to 9 mEq IV, adjust dose based on patient response. If IV not possible, give 2 to 5 mEq IM. Exchange transfusions: 1.35 mEq calcium gluconate IV concurrent with each 100 mL of citrated blood. Oral calcium gluconate: 1 to 2 g elem Ca/day or more PO with meals divided bid to qid. Prevention of osteoporosis: 1000 to 1500 mg elem Ca/day PO with meals in divided doses.
PEDS − Emergency correction of hypocalcemia: Children: 1 to 7 mEq IV prn. Infants: 1 mEq IV prn. Hypocalcemic tetany: Children: 0.5 to 0.7 mEq/kg IV tid to qid. Neonates: 2.4 mEq/kg/day IV in divided doses. Exchange transfusions: Neonates: 0.45 mEq IV/100 mL of exchange transfusions. Oral calcium gluconate: Hypocalcemia: Neonates: 50 to 150 mg elem Ca/kg/day PO in 4 to 6 divided doses; children: 45 to 65 mg elem Ca/kg/day PO divided qid.
UNAPPROVED ADULTS − Has been used in calcium channel blocker toxicity and to treat or prevent calcium channel blocker-induced hypotension.
UNAPPROVED PEDS − Has been used in calcium channel blocker toxicity.
FORMS − Generic only: Injectable 10% (1000 mg/10 mL, 4.65 mEq/10 mL) 1, 10, 50, 100, 200 mL. OTC Generic only: Tabs 50, 500, 650, 975, 1000 mg. Chewable tabs 650 mg.
NOTES − Calcium gluconate is 9.3% elem Ca and contains 4.6 mEq elem Ca/g calcium gluconate. Administer IV calcium gluconate not faster than 0.5 to 2 mL/min. Use cautiously in patients receiving digoxin; inotropic and toxic effects are synergistic and may cause arrhythmias.
MOA − Essential mineral that maintains the nervous, muscular, and skeletal systems and cell membrane and capillary permeability; antagonizes the cardiotoxic effects of hyperkalemia.
ADVERSE EFFECTS − Serious: Severe hypercalcemia (with confusion, delirium, stupor, coma), renal calculi; with IV: vasodilation, hypotension, arrhythmia, syncope and cardiac arrest. Frequent: Mild hypercalcemia, constipation, anorexia, N/V, irritation at infusion site (for IV).

FERRIC GLUCONATE COMPLEX (*Ferrlecit*) ▶KL ♀B ▶? $$$$$
WARNING − Potentially fatal hypersensitivity reactions rarely reported with sodium ferric gluconate complex. Facilities for CPR must be available during dosing.
ADULTS − Iron deficiency in chronic hemodialysis patients: 125 mg elem iron IV over 10 min or diluted in 100 mL NS IV over 1 h. Most hemodialysis patients require 1 g of elem iron over 8 consecutive hemodialysis session.
PEDS − Iron deficiency in chronic hemodialysis age 6 yo or older: 1.5 mg/kg elem iron diluted

(cont.)

ENDOCRINE AND METABOLIC: Minerals

FLUORIDE SUPPLEMENTATION			
Age	<0.3 ppm in drinking water	0.3–0.6 ppm in drinking water	>0.6 ppm in drinking water
0–0.5 yo	none	none	none
0.5–3 yo	0.25 mg PO daily	none	none
3–6 yo	0.5 mg PO daily	0.25 mg PO daily	none
6–16 yo	1 mg PO daily	0.5 mg PO daily	none

FERRIC GLUCONATE COMPLEX (cont.)
in 25 mL NS and administered IV over 1 h at 8 sequential dialysis sessions. Max 125 mg/dose.
UNAPPROVED ADULTS − Iron deficiency in cancer- and chemotherapy-induced anemia: 125 mg elem iron IV over 60 min, repeat weekly for 8 doses, or 200 mg IV over 3 to 4 hours repeated every 3 weeks for 5 doses.
NOTES − Potentially fatal hypersensitivity reactions, including serious hypotension, reported with sodium ferric gluconate complex. Facilities for CPR must be available during dosing.
MOA − Essential mineral needed for hemoglobin, myoglobin, and enzymatic function.
ADVERSE EFFECTS − Serious: Anaphylactic reaction, chest pain, hypotension, shock, cardiac arrest, iron overdose. Frequent: Arthralgia, backache, chills, dizziness, fever, flushing, headache, infusion site reaction, malaise, myalgia, N/V.

FERROUS GLUCONATE (*Fergon*) ▶K ♀+ ▶+ $
WARNING − Severe iron toxicity possible in overdose, especially in children. Store out of reach of children and in child-resistant containers. Iron overdose is the leading cause of poisoning in children younger than 6 yo.
ADULTS − Iron deficiency: 800 to 1600 mg ferrous gluconate (100 to 200 mg elem iron) PO divided tid. RDA (elem iron): 8 mg for adult males age 19 yo or older, 18 mg for adult premenopausal females age 19 to 50 yo, 8 mg for females age 51 yo or older, 27 mg during pregnancy, 10 mg during lactation if age 14 to 18 yo and 9 mg if age 19 to 50 yo. Upper limit: 45 mg/day.
PEDS − Mild-moderate iron deficiency: 3 mg/kg/day of elem iron PO in 1 to 2 divided doses. Severe iron deficiency: 4 to 6 mg/kg/day PO in 3 divided doses. RDA (elem iron): 0.27 mg for age younger than 6 mo, 11 mg for age 7 to 12 mo, 7 mg for age 1 to 3 yo, 10 mg for age 4 to 8 yo, 8 mg for age 9 to 13 yo, 11 mg for males age 14 to 18 yo, 15 mg for females age 14 to 18 yo.
UNAPPROVED ADULTS − Adjunct to epoetin to maximize hematologic response: 200 mg elem iron/day PO.
UNAPPROVED PEDS − Adjunct to epoetin to maximize hematologic response: 2 to 3 mg/kg elem iron/day PO.
FORMS − OTC Generic/Trade: Tabs (ferrous gluconate) 240 mg (27 mg elemental iron). Generic only: Tabs 324, 325 mg.
NOTES − Ferrous gluconate is 12% elem iron. For iron deficiency, 4 to 6 months of therapy generally necessary to replete stores even after hemoglobin has returned to normal. Do not take within 2 h of antacids, tetracyclines, levothyroxine or fluoroquinolones. May cause black stools, constipation or diarrhea.
MOA − Essential mineral needed for hemoglobin, myoglobin, and enzymatic function.
ADVERSE EFFECTS − Serious: Hypersensitivity, iron overdose. Frequent: Constipation, N/V, diarrhea, black stools.

FERROUS SULFATE (*Fer-in-Sol, Feosol, Slow FE, ✦Ferodan, Slow-Fe*) ▶K ♀+ ▶+ $
WARNING − Severe iron toxicity possible in overdose, especially in children. Store out of reach of children and in child-resistant containers. Iron overdose is the leading cause of poisoning in children younger than 6 yo.
ADULTS − Iron deficiency: 500 to 1000 mg ferrous sulfate (100 to 200 mg elem iron) PO divided tid. For iron supplementation RDA see ferrous gluconate.
PEDS − Mild-moderate iron deficiency: 3 mg/kg/day of elem iron PO in 1 to 2 divided doses; Severe Iron deficiency: 4 to 6 mg/kg/day PO in 3 divided doses. For Iron supplementation RDA see ferrous gluconate.
UNAPPROVED ADULTS − Adjunct to epoetin to maximize hematologic response: 200 mg elem iron/day PO.
FORMS − OTC Generic/Trade (mg ferrous sulfate): Tabs extended-release 160 mg. Tabs 200, 324, 325 mg. OTC Generic only (mg ferrous sulfate): Soln 75 mg/0.6 mL, Elixir 220 mg/5 mL.
NOTES − Iron sulfate is 20% elem iron. For iron deficiency, 4 to 6 months of therapy generally necessary. Do not take within 2 h of antacids, tetracyclines, levothyroxine or fluoroquinolones. May cause black stools, constipation or diarrhea.
MOA − Essential mineral needed for hemoglobin, myoglobin, and enzymatic function.
ADVERSE EFFECTS − Serious: Hypersensitivity, iron overdose. Frequent: Constipation, N/V, diarrhea, black stools, tooth staining (liquid preparations).

FERUMOXYTOL (*Feraheme*) ▶KL ♀C ▶? $$$$$
ADULTS − Iron deficiency in chronic kidney disease: Give 510 mg IV push, followed by 510 mg IV push for one dose given 3 to 8 days after initial injection. May re-administer if persistent/recurrent iron deficiency anemia.
PEDS − Not studied in pediatrics.
NOTES − Administer IV push undiluted up to 30 mg/sec. Monitor Hgb and iron studies at least 1 month following second injection. Observe for

(cont.)

ENDOCRINE AND METABOLIC: Minerals

FERUMOXYTOL (cont.)
hypersensitivity for 30 min following injection. May alter MRI imaging studies.
MOA – Superparamagnetic iron oxide to provide essential mineral needed for hemoglobin, myoglobin, and enzymatic function.
ADVERSE EFFECTS – Serious: Anaphylactic reaction, hypersensitivity, hypotension, iron overdose. Frequent: Diarrhea, nausea, dizziness, hypotension, consiptaion, peripheral edema.

FLUORIDE (Luride, *Fluor-A-Day, Fluotic) ▶K ♀? ▶? $
ADULTS – Prevention of dental cavities: 10 mL of topical rinse swish and spit daily.
PEDS – Prevention of dental caries: Dose based on age and fluoride concentrations in water. See table.
FORMS – Generic only: Chewable tabs 0.5, 1 mg; Tabs 1 mg, gtts 0.125 mg, 0.25 mg, and 0.5 mg/dropperful, Lozenges 1 mg, Soln 0.2 mg/mL, Gel 0.1%, 0.5%, 1.23%, Rinse (sodium fluoride) 0.05, 0.1, 0.2%).
NOTES – In communities without fluoridated water, fluoride supplementation should be used until 13 to 16 yo. Chronic overdosage of fluorides may result in dental fluorosis (mottling of tooth enamel) and osseous changes. Use rinses and gels after brushing and flossing and before bedtime.
MOA – Trace element that promotes tooth remineralization and inhibits cariogenesis.
ADVERSE EFFECTS – Serious: Increased bone fracture, allergic rash. Frequent: Rash, eczema, gastric distress, headache, tooth staining (liquid preparations).

IRON DEXTRAN (InFed, DexFerrum, *Dexiron, Infufer) ▶KL ♀C ▶? $$$$
WARNING – Administer a test dose prior to first dose. Parenteral iron therapy has resulted in anaphylactic reactions, even with test dose and after uneventful test doses. Potentially fatal hypersensitivity reactions have been reported with iron dextran injection. Facilities for CPR must be available during dosing. Use only when clearly warranted.
ADULTS – Iron deficiency: Dose based on patient wt and hemoglobin. Total dose (mL) = 0.0442 × (desired Hgb - observed Hgb) × wt (kg) + [0.26 × wt (kg)]. For wt, use lesser of lean body wt or actual body wt. Iron replacement for blood loss: Replacement iron (mg) = blood loss (mL) × hematocrit. Maximum daily IM dose 100 mg.
PEDS – Not recommended for infants less than 4 mo of age. Iron deficiency in children greater than 5 kg: Dose based on patient wt and hemoglobin. Dose (mL) = 0.0442 × (desired Hgb - observed Hgb) × wt (kg) + [0.26 × wt (kg)]. For wt, use lesser of lean body wt or actual body wt. Iron replacement for blood loss: Replacement iron (mg) = blood loss (mL) × hematocrit. Maximum daily IM dose: Infants wt less than 5 kg give 25 mg; children 5 to 10 kg give 50 mg; children wt greater than 10 kg give 100 mg.
UNAPPROVED ADULTS – Adjunct to epoetin to maximize hematologic response. Total dose (325 to 1500 mg) as a single, slow (6 mg/min) IV infusion has been used.
UNAPPROVED PEDS – Adjunct to epoetin to maximize hematologic response.
NOTES – A 0.5 mL IV test dose (0.25 mL in infants) over 30 sec or longer should be given at least 1 h before therapy. Infuse no faster than 50 mg/min. For IM administration, use Z-track technique.
MOA – Essential mineral needed for hemoglobin, myoglobin, and enzymatic function.
ADVERSE EFFECTS – Serious: Anaphylactic reaction, chest pain, hypotension, shock, cardiac arrest, iron overdose. Frequent: Arthralgia, backache, chills, dizziness, fever, flushing, headache, infusion site reaction, malaise, myalgia, N/V.

IRON POLYSACCHARIDE (Niferex, Niferex-150, Nu-Iron 150, Ferrex 150) ▶K ♀+ ▶+ $$
WARNING – Severe iron toxicity possible in overdose, especially in children. Store out of reach of children and in child-resistant containers. Iron overdose is the leading cause of poisoning in children younger than 6 yo.
ADULTS – Iron deficiency: 50 to 200 mg PO divided daily to tid. For iron supplementation RDA see ferrous gluconate.
PEDS – Mild-moderate iron deficiency: 3 mg/kg/day of elem iron PO in 1 to 2 divided doses. Severe iron deficiency: 4 to 6 mg/kg/day PO in 3 divided doses. For iron supplementation RDA see ferrous gluconate.
UNAPPROVED ADULTS – Adjunct to epoetin to maximize hematologic response: 200 mg elem iron/day PO.
UNAPPROVED PEDS – Adjunct to epoetin to maximize hematologic response: 2 to 3 mg/kg elem iron/day PO.
FORMS – OTC Trade only: Caps 60 mg (Niferex). OTC Generic/Trade: Caps 150 mg (Niferex-150, Nu-Iron 150, Ferrex-150), Elixir 100 mg/5 mL (Niferex). 1 mg iron polysaccharide = 1 mg elemental iron.
NOTES – For iron deficiency, 4 to 6 months of therapy generally necessary. Do not take within 2 h of

POTASSIUM (oral forms)
Effervescent Granules: 20 mEq: Klorvess Effervescent, K-vescent
Effervescent Tabs: 10 mEq: Effer-K 20 mEq: Effer-K 25 mEq: Effer-K, K+Care ET, K-Lyte, K-Lyte/Cl, Klor-Con/EF 50 mEq: K-Lyte DS, K-Lyte/Cl 50
Liquids: 20 mEq/15 mL: Cena-K, Kaochlor S-F, K-G Elixir, Kaochlor 10%, Kay Ciel, Kaon, Kaylixir, Kolyum, Potasalan, Twin-K 30 mEq/15 mL: Rum-K 40 mEq/15 mL: Cena-K, Kaon-Cl 20% 45 mEq/15 mL: Tri-K
Powders: 15 mEq/pack: K+Care 20 mEq/pack: Gen-K, K+Care, Kay Ciel, K-Lor, Klor-Con 25 mEq/pack: K+Care, Klor-Con 25
Tabs/Caps: 8 mEq: K+8, Klor-Con 8, Slow-K, Micro-K 10 mEq: K+10, K-Norm, Kaon-Cl 10, Klor-Con M10 Klotrix, K-Tab, K-Dur 10, Micro-K 10 20 mEq: Klor-Con M20, K-Dur 20

(cont.)

ENDOCRINE AND METABOLIC: Minerals

PEDIATRIC REHYDRATION SOLUTIONS

Brand	Glucose	Calories/Liter	Na*	K*	Cl*	Citrate*	Phos*	Ca*	Mg*
CeraLyte 50†	0 g/L	160	50	20	40	30	0	0	0
CeraLyte 70†	0 g/L	160	70	20	60	30	0	0	0
CeraLyte 90†	0 g/L	160	90	20	80	30	0	0	0
Infalyte	30 g/L	140	50	25	45	34	0	0	0
Kao Lectrolyte†	20 g/L	90	50	20	40	30	0	0	0
Lytren (Canada)	20 g/L	80	50	25	45	30	0	0	0
Naturalyte	25 g/L	100	45	20	35	48	0	0	0
Pedialyte and Pedialyte Freezer Pops	25 g/L	100	45	20	35	30	0	0	0
Rehydralyte	25 g/L	100	75	20	65	30	0	0	0
Resol	20 g/L	80	50	20	50	34	5	4	4

* All given in mEq/L
† Premeasured powder packet

IRON POLYSACCHARIDE (*cont.*)
antacids, tetracyclines, levothyroxine, or fluoroquinolones. May cause black stools, constipation or diarrhea.
MOA — Essential mineral needed for hemoglobin, myoglobin, and enzymatic function.
ADVERSE EFFECTS — Serious: Hypersensitivity, iron overdose. Frequent: Constipation, N/V, diarrhea, black stools.

IRON SUCROSE (*Venofer*) ▶KL ♀B ▶? $$$$$
WARNING — Potentially fatal hypersensitivity reactions have been rarely reported with iron sucrose injection. Facilities for CPR must be available during dosing.
ADULTS — <u>Iron deficiency in chronic hemodialysis patients:</u> 5 mL (100 mg elem iron) IV over 5 min or diluted in 100 mL NS IV over 15 min or longer. <u>Iron deficiency in non-dialysis chronic kidney disease patients:</u> 10 mL (200 mg elem iron) IV over 5 min or 500 mg diluted in 250 mL NS IV over 4 h.
PEDS — Not approved in children.
UNAPPROVED ADULTS — <u>Iron deficiency:</u> 5 mL (100 mg elem iron) IV over 5 min or diluted in 100 mL NS IV over 15 min or longer.
NOTES — Most hemodialysis patients require 1 g of elem iron over 10 consecutive hemodialysis sessions. Non-dialysis patients require 1 g of elemental iron divided and given over 14 days.
MOA — Essential mineral needed for hemoglobin, myoglobin, and enzymatic function.
ADVERSE EFFECTS — Serious: Anaphylactic reaction, chest pain, hypotension, shock, cardiac arrest, iron overdose. Frequent: Arthralgia, backache, chills, dizziness, fever, flushing, headache, infusion site reaction, malaise, myalgia, N/V.

MAGNESIUM CHLORIDE (*Slow-Mag*) ▶K ♀A ▶+ $
ADULTS — <u>Dietary supplement:</u> 2 tabs PO daily. RDA (elem Mg): Adult males: 400 mg if 19 to 30 yo, 420 mg if older than 30 yo. Adult females: 310 mg if 19 to 30 yo, 320 mg if older than 30 yo.
PEDS — Not approved in children.
UNAPPROVED ADULTS — <u>Hypomagnesemia:</u> 300 mg elem magnesium PO divided qid.
FORMS — OTC Trade only: Enteric coated tab 64 mg. 64 mg tab Slow-Mag = 64 mg elemental magnesium.
NOTES — May cause diarrhea. May accumulate in renal insufficiency.
MOA — Essential mineral needed for muscle function, organ function, potassium and calcium absorption.
ADVERSE EFFECTS — Serious: Potential magnesium intoxication. Frequent: Diarrhea, weakness, N/V.

MAGNESIUM GLUCONATE (*Almora, Magtrate, Maganate, ♣Maglucate*) ▶K ♀A ▶+ $
ADULTS — <u>Dietary supplement:</u> 500 to 1000 mg/day PO divided tid. RDA (elem Mg): Adult males: 19 to 30 yo: 400 mg; older than 30 yo: 420 mg. Adult females: 19 to 30 yo: 310 mg; older than 30 yo: 320 mg.
PEDS — Not approved in children.
UNAPPROVED ADULTS — <u>Hypomagnesemia:</u> 300 mg elem magnesium PO divided qid. Unproven efficacy for oral tocolysis following IV magnesium sulfate.
UNAPPROVED PEDS — <u>Hypomagnesemia:</u> 10 to 20 mg elem magnesium/kg/dose PO qid. RDA (elem Mg): Age 0 to 6 mo: 30 mg/day; age 7 to 12 mo: 75 mg/day; age 1 to 3 yo: 80 mg; age 4 to 8 yo: 130 mg; age 9 to 13 yo: 240 mg; age 14 to 18 yo (males): 410 mg; age 14 to 18 yo (females): 360 mg.
FORMS — OTC Generic only: Tabs 500 mg (27 mg elemental Mg), liquid 54 mg elemental Mg/5 mL.
NOTES — May cause diarrhea. Use caution in renal failure; may accumulate.

(cont.)

ENDOCRINE AND METABOLIC: Minerals

MAGNESIUM GLUCONATE *(cont.)*
MOA — Essential mineral needed for muscle function, organ function, potassium and calcium absorption.
ADVERSE EFFECTS — Serious: Potential magnesium intoxication. Frequent: Diarrhea, weakness, N/V.

MAGNESIUM OXIDE (*Mag-200, Mag-Ox 400*) ▶K ♀A ▶+ $
ADULTS — Dietary supplement: 400 to 800 mg PO daily. RDA (elem Mg): Adult males: 19 to 30 yo: 400 mg; older than 30 yo 420 mg. Adult females: 19 to 30 yo: 310 mg; older than 30 yo: 320 mg.
PEDS — Not approved in children.
UNAPPROVED ADULTS — Hypomagnesemia: 300 mg elem magnesium PO qid. Has also been used as oral tocolysis following IV magnesium sulfate (unproven efficacy) and in the prevention of calcium-oxalate kidney stones.
FORMS — OTC Generic/Trade: Caps - 140 (84.5 mg elemental Mg), 250 (elemental), 400 (240 mg elemental Mg), 420 (253 mg elemental Mg), 500 mg (elemental).
NOTES — Take with food. Magnesium oxide is approximately 60% elemental magnesium. May accumulate in renal insufficiency.
MOA — Essential mineral needed for muscle function, organ function, potassium and calcium absorption.
ADVERSE EFFECTS — Serious: Potential magnesium intoxication. Frequent: Diarrhea, weakness, N/V.

MAGNESIUM SULFATE ▶K ♀A ▶+ $
ADULTS — Hypomagnesemia: Mild deficiency: 1 g IM q 6 h for 4 doses; severe deficiency: 2 g IV over 1 h (monitor for hypotension). Hyperalimentation: Maintenance requirements not precisely known; adults generally require 8 to 24 mEq/day. Seizure prevention in preeclampsia or eclampsia: 4 to 6 g IV over 30 min, then 1 to 2 g IV per h. 5 g in 250 mL D5W (20 mg/mL), 2 g/h = 100 mL/h. 4 to 5 g of a 50% soln IM q 4 h prn.
PEDS — Not approved in children.
UNAPPROVED ADULTS — Preterm labor: 6 g IV over 20 min, then 1 to 3 g/h titrated to decrease contractions. Has been used as an adjunctive bronchodilator in very severe acute asthma (2 g IV over 10 to 20 min), and in chronic fatigue syndrome. Torsades de pointes: 1 to 2 g IV in D5W over 5 to 60 min.
UNAPPROVED PEDS — Hypomagnesemia: 25 to 50 mg/kg IV/IM q 4 to 6 h for 3 to 4 doses, maximum single dose 2 g. Hyperalimentation: Maintenance requirements not precisely known; infants require 2 to 10 mEq/day. Acute nephritis: 20 to 40 mg/kg (in 20% soln) IM prn. Adjunctive bronchodilator in very severe acute asthma: 25 to 100 mg/kg IV over 10 to 20 min.
NOTES — 1000 mg magnesium sulfate contains 8 mEq elem magnesium. Do not give faster than 1.5 mL/min (of 10% soln) except in eclampsia or seizures. Use caution in renal insufficiency; may accumulate. Monitor urine output, patellar reflex, respiratory rate and serum magnesium level. Concomitant use with terbutaline may lead to fatal pulmonary edema. IM administration must be diluted to a 20% soln. If needed, may reverse toxicity with calcium gluconate 1 g IV.
MOA — Essential mineral needed for muscle function, organ function, potassium and calcium absorption; blocks neuromuscular transmission to prevent or control convulsions.
ADVERSE EFFECTS — Serious: Magnesium intoxication, cardiac depression, CNS depression, respiratory paralysis, hypotension, stupor, hypothermia, circulatory collapse. Frequent: Flushing, sweating, depressed reflexes.

PHOSPHORUS (*Neutra-Phos, K-Phos*) ▶K ♀C ▶? $
ADULTS — Dietary supplement: 1 cap/packet (Neutra-Phos) PO qid or 1 to 2 tab (K-Phos) PO qid after meals and at bedtime. Severe hypophosphatemia (< 1 mg/dL): 0.08 to 0.16 mmol/kg IV over 6 h. In TPN, 310 to 465 mg/day (10 to 15 mM) IV is usually adequate, although higher amounts may be necessary in hypermetabolic states. RDA for adults is 800 mg.
PEDS — RDA (elem phosphorus): 0 to 6 mo: 100 mg; 6 to 12 mo: 275 mg; 1 to 3 yo: 460 mg; 4 to 8 yo: 500 mg; 9 to 18: 1250 mg. Severe hypophosphatemia (< 1 mg/dL): 0.25 to 0.5 mmol/kg IV over 4 to 6 h. Infant TPN: 1.5 to 2 mmol/kg/day in TPN.
FORMS — OTC Trade only: (Neutra-Phos, Neutra-Phos K) tab/cap/packet 250 mg (8 mmol) phosphorus. Rx: Trade only: (K-Phos) tab 250 mg (8 mmol) phosphorus.
NOTES — Dissolve caps/tabs/powder in 75 mL water prior to ingestion.
MOA — Essential mineral needed for bone metabolism and enzymatic functions.
ADVERSE EFFECTS — Serious: Phosphate intoxication with reciprocal hypocalcemic tetany (with IV). Frequent: Laxative-like effect, nausea, abdominal pain, vomiting.

POTASSIUM (*Cena-K, Effer-K, K+8, K+10, Kaochlor, Kaon, Kaon Cl, Kay Ciel, Kaylixir, K+Care, K+Care ET, K-Dur, K-G Elixir, K-Lease, K-Lor, Klor-con, Klorvess Effervescent, Klotrix, K-Lyte, K-Lyte Cl, K-Norm, Kolyum, K-Tab, K-vescent, Micro-K, Micro-K LS, SI*) ▶K ♀C ▶? $
ADULTS — Hypokalemia: 20 to 40 mEq/day or more PO/IV. Intermittent infusion: 10 to 20 mEq/dose IV over 1 to 2 h prn. Consider monitoring for infusions > 10 mEq/h. Prevention of hypokalemia: 20 to 40 mEq/day PO daily to bid.
PEDS — Not approved in children.
UNAPPROVED ADULTS — Diuretic-induced Hypokalemia: 20 to 60 mEq/day PO.
UNAPPROVED PEDS — Hypokalemia: 2.5 mEq/kg/day given IV/PO daily to bid. Intermittent infusion: 0.5 to 1 mEq/kg/dose IV at 0.3 to 0.5 mEq/kg/h prn. Infusions faster than 0.5 mEq/kg/h require continuous monitoring.
FORMS — Injectable, many different products in a variety of salt forms (ie, chloride, bicarbonate, citrate, acetate, gluconate), available in tabs, caps,

(cont.)

ENDOCRINE AND METABOLIC: Nutritionals

POTASSIUM (*cont.*)
liquids, effervescent tabs, packets. Potassium gluconate is available OTC.
NOTES — Use potassium chloride for hypokalemia associated with alkalosis; use potassium bicarbonate, citrate, acetate, or gluconate when associated with acidosis.
MOA — Intracellular cation that participates in numerous essential physiological processes.
ADVERSE EFFECTS — Serious: Hyperkalemia, gastrointestinal toxicity (obstruction, bleed, ulcer, perforation, esophagitis). Frequent: N/V, diarrhea, abdominal pain, infusion site irritation (IV).

ZINC ACETATE (*Galzin*) ▶Minimal absorption ♀A ▶− $$$
ADULTS — RDA (elemental Zn): Adult males: 11 mg daily. Adult females: 8 to 12 mg daily. Zinc deficiency: 25 to 50 mg (elemental) daily. Wilson's disease, previously treated with chelating agent: 25 to 50 mg (elemental) PO tid.
PEDS — RDA (elem Zn): Age 7 mo to 3 yo: 3 mg; 4 to 8 yo: 5 mg; 9 to 13 yo: 8 mg; 14 to 18 yo (males): 8 mg; 14 to 18 yo (females): 9 to 14 mg. Zinc deficiency: 0.5 to 1 mg elemental zinc mg/kg/day divided bid to tid. Wilson's disease (age 10 yo or older): 25 to 50 mg (elemental) tid.
FORMS — Trade only: Caps 25, 50 mg elemental zinc.
NOTES — Poorly absorbed; take 1 h before or 2 to 3 h after meals. Decreases absorption of tetracycline and fluoroquinolones.
MOA — Nutritional supplement. Blocks intestinal absorption of copper.
ADVERSE EFFECTS — Serious: Sideroblastic anemia, pancreatitis. Frequent: N/V.

ZINC SULFATE (*Orazinc, Zincate*) ▶Minimal absorption ♀A ▶− $
ADULTS — RDA (elemental Zn): Adult males: 11 mg daily. Adult females: 8 to 12 mg daily. Zinc deficiency: 25 to 50 mg (elemental) PO daily.
PEDS — RDA (elemental Zn): Age 7 mo to 3 yo: 3 mg; 4 to 8 yo: 5 mg; 9 to 13 yo: 8 mg; 14 to 18 yo (males): 8 mg; 14 to 18 yo (females): 9 to 14 mg. Zinc deficiency: 0.5 to 1 mg elemental zinc mg/kg/day PO divided bid to tid.
UNAPPROVED ADULTS — Wound healing in zinc deficiency: 200 mg PO tid.
FORMS — OTC Generic/Trade: Tabs 66, 110, 200 mg. Rx Generic/Trade: Caps 220 mg.
NOTES — Zinc sulfate is 23% elemental Zn. Decreases absorption of tetracycline and fluoroquinolones. Poorly absorbed; increased absorption on empty stomach; however, administration with food decreases GI upset.
MOA — Nutritional supplement.
ADVERSE EFFECTS — Serious: Sideroblastic anemia, pancreatitis. Frequent: N/V.

ENDOCRINE AND METABOLIC: Nutritionals

BANANA BAG ▶KL ♀+ ▶+ $
UNAPPROVED ADULTS — Alcoholic malnutrition (one formula): Add thiamine 100 mg + folic acid 1 mg + IV multivitamins to 1 liter NS and infuse over 4 h. Magnesium sulfate 2 g may be added. "Banana bag" is jargon and not a valid drug order; also known as "rally pack"; specify individual components.
MOA — Mixture of vitamin supplements that mediates glucose utilization to prevent Wernicke-Korsakoff syndrome in alcoholism.
ADVERSE EFFECTS — Serious: Hypersensitivity, anaphylaxis, cyanosis, pulmonary edema, GI hemorrhage, cardiovascular shock. Frequent: Injection-site reaction, feeling of warmth, pruritus, sweating, N/V, restlessness, angioedema.

FAT EMULSION (*Intralipid, Liposyn*) ▶L ♀C ▶? $$$$$
WARNING — Deaths have occurred in preterm infants after infusion of IV fat emulsions. Autopsy results showed intravascular fat accumulation in the lungs. Strict adherence to total daily dose and administration rate is mandatory. Premature and small for gestational age infants have poor clearance of IV fat emulsion. Monitor infant's ability to eliminate fat (ie, triglycerides or plasma free fatty acid levels).
ADULTS — Calorie and essential fatty acids source: As part of TPN, fat emulsion should be no more than 60% of total calories; when correcting essential fatty acid deficiency, 8 to 10% of caloric intake should be supplied by lipids. Initial infusion rate 1 mL/min IV (10% fat emulsion) or 0.5 mL/min (20% fat emulsion) IV for first 15 to 30 min. If tolerated increase rate. If using 10% fat emulsion infuse no more than 500 mL first day and increase the next day. Maximum daily dose 2.5 g/kg. If using 20% fat emulsion, infuse up to 250 mL (Liposyn II) or up to 500 mL (Intralipid) first day and increase the next day. Maximum daily dose 2.5 g/kg.
PEDS — Calorie and essential fatty acids source: As part of TPN, fat emulsion should be no more than 60% of total calories; when correcting essential fatty acid deficiency, 8 to 10% of caloric intake should be supplied by lipids. Initial infusion rate 0.1 mL/min IV (10% fat emulsion) or 0.05 mL/min (20% fat emulsion) for first 10 to 15 min. If tolerated increase rate up to 1 mL/kg/h (10% fat emulsion) or 0.5 mL/kg/h (20% fat emulsion). Max daily dose 3 g/kg. For premature infants, start at 0.5 g/kg/day and increase based on infant's ability to eliminate fat. Maximum infusion rate 1 g fat/kg in 4 hours.
NOTES — Do not use in patients with severe egg allergy; contains egg yolk phospholipids. Use caution in severe liver disease, pulmonary disease, anemia, blood coagulation disorders, when there is the danger of fat embolism or in jaundiced or premature infants. Monitor CBC, blood coagulation, LFTs, plasma lipid profile and platelet count.

(cont.)

ENDOCRINE AND METABOLIC: Phosphate Binders

FAT EMULSION (cont.)
MOA — Treats or prevents nutritional deficiency by providing essential fatty acids.
ADVERSE EFFECTS — Serious: Intravascular fat accumulation in lungs (preterm infants), sepsis, hepatomegaly (long-term use). Frequent: Thrombophlebitis, hypertriglyceridemia, brown pigmentation (long-term use).

FORMULAS—INFANT (*Enfamil, Similac, Isomil, Nursoy, Prosobee, Soyalac, Alsoy, Nutramigen Lipil*) ▶L ♀+ ▶+ $
ADULTS — Not used in adults.
PEDS — Infant meals.
FORMS — OTC: Milk-based (Enfamil, Similac, SMA) or soy-based (Isomil, Nursoy, ProSobee, Soyalac, Alsoy).
MOA — Treats or prevents nutritional deficiency to sustain growth and activity.
ADVERSE EFFECTS — Serious: Dehydration, hypersensitivity. Frequent: Diarrhea, abdominal distention, abdominal cramps, vomiting.

LEVOCARNITINE (*Carnitor*) ▶KL ♀B ▶? $$$$$
ADULTS — Prevention of levocarnitine deficiency in dialysis patients: 10 to 20 mg/kg IV at each dialysis session. Titrate dose based on serum concentration.
PEDS — Prevention of deficiency in dialysis patients: 10 to 20 mg/kg IV at each dialysis session. Titrate dose based on serum concentration.
FORMS — Generic/Trade: Tabs 330 mg, Oral soln 1 g/10 mL.
NOTES — Adverse neurophysiologic effects may occur with long-term, high doses of oral levocarnitine in patients with renal dysfunction. Only the IV formulation is indicated in patients receiving hemodialysis.
MOA — Facilitates long-chain fatty acid utilization.
ADVERSE EFFECTS — Serious: Seizures. Frequent: N/V, body odor, mild myasthenia.

OMEGA-3-ACID ETHYL ESTERS (*Lovaza*, fish oil, omega 3 fatty acids) ▶L ♀C ▶? $
ADULTS — Adjunct to diet to reduce high triglycerides (500 mg/dL or above): 4 caps PO daily or divided bid.
PEDS — Not approved in children.
UNAPPROVED ADULTS — Hypertriglyceridemia: 2 to 4 g EPA + DHA content daily under physician's care. Secondary prevention of CHD: 1 to 2 g EPA + DHA content daily. Adjunctive treatment in RA: 20 g/day PO. Psoriasis: 10 to 15 g/day PO. Prevention of early restenosis after coronary angioplasty in combination with dipyridamole and aspirin: 18 g/day PO.
FORMS — Trade only: (Lovaza) 1 g cap (total 840 mg EPA + DHA).
NOTES — Lovaza is only FDA approved fish oil, previously known as Omacor. Other products available with varying EPA and DHA content. May increase LDL-cholesterol, monitor periodically. Effect on cardiovascular morbidity and mortality has not been determined. Treatment doses lower triglycerides by 30 to 50%. Prolongs bleeding time, may potentiate warfarin. Caution in seafood allergy; derived from fish oil. Monitor AST/ALT if hepatic impairment.
MOA — Fish oil supplement that decreases serum triglycerides, mechanism not completely understood. Possible mechanisms include EPA and DHA inhibition of esterification of other fatty acids.
ADVERSE EFFECTS — Serious: Bleeding (rare), hypersensitivity, infection. Frequent: Nausea, belching, taste changes (fish), diarrhea, body odor, rash.

RALLY PACK ▶KL ♀C ▶– $
UNAPPROVED ADULTS — Alcoholic malnutrition (one formula): Add thiamine 100 mg + folic acid 1 mg + IV multivitamins to 1 liter NS and infuse over 4 h. Magnesium sulfate 2 g may be added. "Rally pack" is jargon and not a valid drug order; also known as "Banana Bag"; specify individual components.
MOA — Mixture of vitamin supplements that mediates glucose utilization to prevent Wernicke-Korsakoff syndrome in alcoholism.
ADVERSE EFFECTS — Serious: Hypersensitivity, anaphylaxis, cyanosis, pulmonary edema, GI hemorrhage, cardiovascular shock. Frequent: Injection-site reaction, feeling of warmth, pruritus, sweating, N/V, restlessness, angioedema.

ENDOCRINE AND METABOLIC: Phosphate Binders

LANTHANUM CARBONATE (*Fosrenol*) ▶Not absorbed ♀C ▶? $$$$$
ADULTS — Treatment of hyperphosphatemia in end stage renal disease: Start 1500 mg/day PO in divided doses with meals. Titrate dose every 2 to 3 weeks in increments of 750 mg/day until acceptable serum phosphate is reached. Most will require 1500 to 3000 mg/day to reduce serum phosphate < 6.0 mg/dL. Chewable tabs completely before swallowing; tabs may be crushed to aid in chewing.
PEDS — Not approved in children.
FORMS — Trade only: Chewable tabs 500, 750, 1000 mg.
NOTES — Divided doses up to 3750 mg/day have been used. Caution if acute peptic ulcer, ulcerative colitis, Crohn's disease or bowel obstruction. Avoid medications known to interact with antacids within 2 h. May be radio-opaque enough to appear on abdominal x-ray.
MOA — Binds dietary phosphate forming highly insoluble complexes that are eliminated through the GI tract.
ADVERSE EFFECTS — Serious: Dialysis graft occlusion. Frequent: N/V, abdominal pain, diarrhea.

SEVELAMER (*Renagel, Renvela*) ▶Not absorbed ♀C ▶? $$$$$
ADULTS — Hyperphosphatemia in kidney disease on dialysis: Start 800 to 1600 mg PO tid with meals, adjust according to serum phosphorus concentration.

(cont.)

SEVELAMER (cont.)
PEDS — Not approved in children.
FORMS — Trade only (Renagel - sevelamer hydrochloride): Tabs 400, 800 mg. (Renvela - sevelamer carbonate): Tabs 800 mg; Powder: 800, 2400 mg packets.
NOTES — Titrate by 800 mg/meal at 2 week intervals to keep phosphorus < 5.5 mg/dL; highest daily dose in studies: Renagel, 13 g; Renvela, 14 g. Decreases absorption of ciprofloxacin; may decrease absorption of antiarrhythmic and antiseizure medications; administer these meds 1 h before or 3 h. Caution in GI motility disorders, including severe constipation.
MOA — Binds intestinal phosphate preventing absorption.
ADVERSE EFFECTS — Serious: Hypophosphatemia, intestinal obstruction. Frequent: N/V, dyspepsia, diarrhea, flatulence, constipation.

ENDOCRINE AND METABOLIC: Thyroid Agents

LEVOTHYROXINE (*L-Thyroxine, Levolet, Levo-T, Levothroid, Levoxyl, Novothyrox, Synthroid, Thyro-Tabs, Tirosint, Unithroid, T4, ✦Eltroxin, Euthyrox*) ▶L ♀A ▶+ $
WARNING — Do not use for obesity/weight loss; possible serious or life-threatening toxic effects when used in euthyroid patients.
ADULTS — Hypothyroidism: Start 100 to 200 mcg PO daily (healthy adults) or 12.5 to 50 mcg PO daily (elderly or CV disease), increase by 12.5 to 25 mcg/day at 3 to 8 weeks intervals. Usual maintenance dose 100 to 200 mcg PO daily, max 300 mcg/day.
PEDS — Hypothyroidism: 0 to 6 mo: 8 to 10 mcg/kg/day PO; 6 to 12 mo: 6 to 8 mcg/kg/day PO; 1 to 5 yo: 5 to 6 mcg/kg/day PO; 6 to 12 yo: 4 to 5 mcg/kg/day PO; older than 12 yo: 2 to 3 mcg/kg/day PO, max 300 mcg/day.
UNAPPROVED ADULTS — Hypothyroidism: 1.6 mcg/kg/day PO; start with lower doses (25 mcg PO daily) in elderly and patients with cardiac disease.
FORMS — Generic/Trade: Tabs 25, 50, 75, 88, 100, 112, 125, 137, 150, 175, 200, 300 mcg. Trade only: Caps: 25, 50, 75, 100, 125, 150 mcg in 7 days blister packs, Tabs: 13 mcg (Tirosint).
NOTES — May crush tabs for infants and children. May give IV or IM at ½ oral dose in adults and ½- ¾ oral dose in children; then adjust based on tolerance and therapeutic response. Generics are not necessarily bioequivalent to brand products; reevaluate thyroid function when switching.
MOA — Synthetic thyroid derivative that increases metabolic rate of body tissues.
ADVERSE EFFECTS — Serious: Hyperthyroidism (arrhythmia, heart failure, angina, cardiac arrest), pseudotumor cerebri. Frequent: Palpitations, tachycardia, tremor, headache, nervousness, insomnia, diarrhea, vomiting, weight loss, menstrual irregularity, sweating, heat intolerance.

LIOTHYRONINE (T3, *Cytomel, Triostat*) ▶L ♀A ▶? $$
WARNING — Do not use for obesity/weight loss; possible serious or life-threatening toxic effects when used in euthyroid patients.
ADULTS — Mild hypothyroidism: 25 mcg PO daily, increase by 12.5 to 25 mcg/day at 1 to 2 weeks intervals to desired response. Usual maintenance dose 25 to 75 mcg PO daily. Goiter: 5 mcg PO daily, increase by 5 to 10 mcg/day at 1 to 2 weeks intervals. Usual maintenance dose 75 mcg PO daily. Myxedema: 5 mcg PO daily, increase by 5 to 10 mcg/day at 1 to 2 weeks intervals. Usual maintenance dose 50 to 100 mcg/day.
PEDS — Congenital hypothyroidism: 5 mcg PO daily, increase by 5 mcg/day at 3 to 4 days intervals to desired response.
FORMS — Generic/Trade: Tabs 5, 25, 50 mcg.
NOTES — Levothyroxine is preferred maintenance treatment for hypothyroidism. Start therapy at 5 mcg/day in children and elderly and increase by 5 mcg increments only. Rapidly absorbed from the GI tract. Monitor T3 and TSH. Elderly may need lower doses due to potential decreased renal function.
MOA — Synthetic thyroid derivative that increases metabolic rate of body tissues.
ADVERSE EFFECTS — Serious: Hyperthyroidism (arrhythmia, heart failure, angina, cardiac arrest), pseudotumor cerebri. Frequent: Palpitations, tachycardia, tremor, headache, nervousness, insomnia, diarrhea, vomiting, weight loss, menstrual irregularity, sweating, heat intolerance.

METHIMAZOLE (*Tapazole*) ▶L ♀D ▶+ $$$
ADULTS — Mild Hyperthyroidism: 5 mg PO tid. Moderate Hyperthyroidism: 10 mg PO tid. Severe Hyperthyroidism: 20 mg PO tid (q 8 h intervals). Maintenance dose is 5 to 30 mg/day.
PEDS — Hyperthyroidism: 0.4 mg/kg/day PO divided q 8 h. Maintenance dose is ½ initial dose, max 30 mg/day.
UNAPPROVED ADULTS — Start 10 to 30 mg PO daily, then adjust.
FORMS — Generic/Trade: Tabs 5, 10. Generic only: Tabs 15, 20 mg.
NOTES — Monitor CBC for evidence of marrow suppression if fever, sore throat, or other signs of infection. Propylthiouracil preferred over methimazole in pregnancy.
MOA — Inhibits synthesis of thyroid hormones.
ADVERSE EFFECTS — Serious: Agranulocytosis, granulocytopenia, thrombocytopenia, aplastic anemia, leukopenia, interstitial pneumonitis, dermatitis, hepatotoxicity, periarteritis, nephritis, hypoprothrombinemia. Frequent: N/V, rash, pruritus, headache, dizziness, vertigo, drowsiness, alopecia, constipation, paresthesia, neuritis, hyperpigmentation.

POTASSIUM IODIDE (*Iosat, SSKI, Thyrosafe, Thyroshield*) ▶L ♀D ▶– $
WARNING — Do not use for obesity.
ADULTS — Thyroidectomy preparation: 50 to 250 mg PO tid for 10 to 14 days prior to surgery. Thyroid

(cont.)

ENDOCRINE AND METABOLIC: Thyroid Agents

POTASSIUM IODIDE (cont.)
storm: 1 mL (Lugol's) PO tid at least 1 h after initial propylthiouracil or methimazole dose. Thyroid blocking in radiation emergency: 130 mg PO daily for 10 days or as directed by state health officials.
PEDS — Thyroid blocking in radiation emergency age 3 to 18 yo: 65 mg (½ of a 130 mg tab) PO daily, or 130 mg PO daily in adolescents greater than 70 kg. 1 mo to 3 yo: 32 mg (¼ of a 130 mg tab) PO daily. Birth to 1 mo: 16 mg (1/8 of a 130 mg tab) PO daily. Duration is until risk of exposure to radioiodines no longer exists.
FORMS — OTC Trade only: Tabs 130 mg (Iosat). Trade only Rx: Soln 1 g/mL (30, 240 mL, SSKI). OTC Generic only: Tabs 65 mg (Thyrosafe), Soln 65 mg/mL (30 mL, Thyroshield).
MOA — Elemental substance used therapeutically to block thyroid uptake or suppress thyroid hormone synthesis and release.
ADVERSE EFFECTS — Serious: Agranulocytosis, granulocytopenia, thrombocytopenia, aplastic anemia, leukopenia, interstitial pneumonitis, exfoliative dermatitis, vasculitis, hepatotoxicity. Frequent: N/V, rash, pruritus, headache, dizziness, drowsiness, alopecia, constipation, paresthesia, neuritis, hyperpigmentation.

PROPYLTHIOURACIL (*PTU*, ✦*Propyl Thyracil*) ▶L ♀D (but preferred over methimazole in first trimester) ▶+ $
WARNING — Acute liver failure and severe liver injury reported, including fatal injury and need for liver transplantation. Use only if patient cannot tolerate methimazole or if not a candidate for radioactive iodine therapy or surgery. May be preferred just prior to or in first trimester of pregnancy.
ADULTS — Hyperthyroidism: 100 to 150 mg PO tid. Severe Hyperthyroidism and/or large goiters: 200 to 400 mg PO tid. Continue initial dose for approximately 2 months. Adjust dose to desired response. Usual maintenance dose 100 to 150 mg/day. Thyroid storm: 200 mg PO q 4 to 6 h once daily, decrease dose gradually to usual maintenance dose.
PEDS — Hyperthyroidism in children age 6 to 10 yo: 50 mg PO daily to tid. Children or older 10 yo: 50 to 100 mg PO tid. Continue initial dose for 2 months, then maintenance dose is 1/3 to 2/3 initial dose.
UNAPPROVED PEDS — Hyperthyroidism in neonates: 5 to 10 mg/kg/day PO divided q 8 h. Children: 5 to 7 mg/kg/day PO divided q 8 h.
FORMS — Generic only: Tabs 50 mg.
NOTES — Monitor CBC for marrow suppression if fever, sore throat, or other signs of infection. Vasculitic syndrome with positive antineutrophilic icytoplasmic antibodies (ANCAs) reported requiring discontinuation. Propylthiouracil preferred over methimazole in pregnancy.
MOA — Inhibits synthesis of thyroid hormones.
ADVERSE EFFECTS — Serious: Agranulocytosis, granulocytopenia, thrombocytopenia, aplastic anemia, leukopenia, interstitial pneumonitis, exfoliative dermatitis, vasculitis, hepatotoxicity. Frequent: N/V, rash, pruritus, headache, dizziness, drowsiness, alopecia, constipation, paresthesia, neuritis, hyperpigmentation.

SODIUM IODIDE I-131 (*Hicon, Iodotope, Sodium Iodide I-131 Therapeutic*) ▶K ♀X ▶– $$$$$
ADULTS — Specialized dosing for hyperthyroidism and thyroid carcinoma.
PEDS — Not approved in children.
FORMS — Generic/Trade: Caps Oral soln: Radioactivity range varies at the time of calibration. Hicon is a kit containing caps and a concentrated oral soln for dilution and cap preparation.
NOTES — Hazardous substance, handle with necessary precautions and use proper disposal. Avoid if preexisting vomiting or diarrhea. Discontinue antithyroid therapy at least 3 days before starting. Low serum chloride or nephrosis may increase uptake; renal insufficiency may decrease excretion and thus increase radiation exposure. Ensure adequate hydration before and after administration. Follow low-iodine diet for 1 to 2 weeks before treatment. Women should have negative pregnancy test prior to treatment and advise not to conceive for at least 6 months.
MOA — Radioactive iodide that is trapped by thyroid tissue; radiation exposure results in cell destruction.
ADVERSE EFFECTS — Serious: Hypersensitivity, bone marrow suppression (high doses), acute thyroid crises, chromosomal abnormalities, death, sialoadenitis. Frequent: Hypothyroidism.

THYROID—DESICCATED (*Thyroid USP, Armour Thyroid*) ▶L ♀A ▶? $
WARNING — Do not use for weight loss; possible serious or life-threatening toxic effects when used in euthyroid patients.
ADULTS — Obsolete; use thyroxine instead. Hypothyroidism: Start 30 mg PO daily, increase by 15 mg/day at 2 to 3 weeks intervals to a maximum dose of 180 mg/day.
PEDS — Congenital hypothyroidism: 15 mg PO daily. Increase at 2 weeks intervals.
FORMS — Generic/Trade: Tabs 15, 30, 60, 90, 120, 180, 300 mg. Trade only: Tabs 240 mg.
NOTES — 60 mg thyroid desiccated is roughly equivalent to 100 mcg levothyroxine. Combination of levothyroxine (T4) and liothyronine (T3); content varies (range 2:1 to 5:1).
MOA — Thyroid hormones from animal thyroid gland that increases metabolic rate of body tissues.
ADVERSE EFFECTS — Serious: Hyperthyroidism (arrhythmia, heart failure, angina, cardiac arrest), pseudotumor cerebri, hypersensitivity. Frequent: Palpitations, tachycardia, tremor, headache, nervousness, insomnia, diarrhea, vomiting, weight loss, menstrual irregularity, sweating, heat intolerance.

THYROLAR, LIOTRIX (levothyroxine + liothyronine) ▶L ♀A ▶? $
WARNING — Do not use for weight loss; possible serious or life-threatening toxic effects when used in euthyroid patients.
ADULTS — Hypothyroidism: 1 PO daily, starting with small doses initially (¼ to ½ strength), then increase at 2 week intervals.
PEDS — Not approved in children.

(cont.)

THYROLAR, LIOTRIX *(cont.)*
FORMS — Trade only: Tabs T4/T3 12.5 mcg/3.1 mcg (¼ strength), 25 mcg/6.25 mcg (half-strength), 50 mcg/12.5 mcg (#1), 100 mcg/25 mcg (#2), 150 mcg/37.5 mcg (#3).
NOTES — Combination of levothyroxine (T4) and liothyronine (T3).
MOA — Synthetic thyroid derivative that increases metabolic rate of body tissues.
ADVERSE EFFECTS — Serious: Hyperthyroidism (arrhythmia, heart failure, angina, cardiac arrest), pseudotumor cerebri. Frequent: Palpitations, tachycardia, tremor, headache, nervousness, insomnia, diarrhea, vomiting, weight loss, menstrual irregularity, sweating, heat intolerance.

ENDOCRINE AND METABOLIC: Vitamins

ASCORBIC ACID (vitamin C, ✦*Redoxon*) ▶K ♀C ▶? $
ADULTS — Prevention of scurvy: 70 to 150 mg/day PO. Treatment of scurvy: 300 to 1000 mg/day PO. RDA females: 75 mg/day; males: 90 mg/day. Smokers: Add 35 mg/day more than nonsmokers.
PEDS — Prevention of scurvy: Infants: 30 mg/day PO. Treatment of scurvy: Infants: 100 to 300 mg/day PO. Adequate daily intake for infants 0 to 6 mo: 40 mg; 7 to 12 mo: 50 mg. RDA for children: 1 to 3 yo: 15 mg; 4 to 8 yo: 25 mg; 9 to 13 yo: 45 mg; 14 to 18 yo: 75 mg (males), 65 mg (females).
UNAPPROVED ADULTS — Urinary acidification with methenamine: More than 2 g/day PO. Idiopathic methemoglobinemia: 150 mg/day or more PO. Wound healing: 300 to 500 mg/day or more PO for 7 to 10 days. Severe burns: 1 to 2 g/day PO.
FORMS — OTC Generic only: Tabs 25, 50, 100, 250, 500, 1000 mg, Chewable tabs 100, 250, 500 mg, Timed-release tabs 500, 1000, 1500 mg, Timed-release caps 500 mg, Lozenges 60 mg, Liquid 35 mg/0.6 mL, Oral soln 100 mg/mL, Syrup 500 mg/5 mL.
NOTES — Use IV/IM/SC ascorbic acid for acute deficiency or when oral absorption is uncertain. Avoid excessive doses in diabetics, patients prone to renal calculi, those undergoing stool occult blood tests (may cause false-negative), those on sodium restricted diets and those taking anticoagulants (may decrease INR). Doses in adults more than 2 g/day may cause osmotic diarrhea.
MOA — Water-soluble vitamin with antioxidant properties.
ADVERSE EFFECTS — Serious: Renal calculi, hypersensitivity. Frequent: Injection-site irritation (if IV).

CALCITRIOL (*Rocaltrol, Calcijex*) ▶L ♀C ▶? $$
ADULTS — Hypocalcemia in chronic renal dialysis: Oral: 0.25 mcg PO daily, increase by 0.25 mcg q 4 to 8 weeks until normocalcemia achieved. Most hemodialysis patients require 0.5 to 1 mcg/day PO. Hypocalcemia and/or secondary hyperparathyroidism in chronic renal dialysis IV: 1 to 2 mcg, 3 times a week; increase dose by 0.5 to 1 mcg every 2 to 4 weeks. If PTH decreased less than 30% then increase dose; if PTH decreased 30 to 60% then maintain current dose; if PTH decreased more than 60% then decrease dose; if PTH 1.5 to 3 times the upper normal limit then maintain current dose. Hypoparathyroidism: 0.25 mcg PO qam; increase dose q 2 to 4 weeks if inadequate response. Most adults respond to 0.5 to 2 mcg/day PO. Secondary hyperparathyroidism in predialysis patients: 0.25 mcg PO q am; may increase dose to 0.5 mcg q am.

PEDS — Hypoparathyroidism 1 to 5 yo: 0.25 to 0.75 mcg PO q am. If age 6 yo or older then 0.25 mcg PO qam; increase dose in 2 to 4 weeks; usually respond to 0.5 to 2 mcg/day PO. Secondary hyperparathyroidism in predialysis patients age 3 yo or older: 0.25 mcg q am; may increase dose to 0.5 mcg q am. If younger than 3 yo: 0.01 to 0.015 mcg/kg/day PO.
UNAPPROVED ADULTS — Psoriasis vulgaris: 0.5 mcg/day PO or 0.5 mcg/g petrolatum topically daily.
FORMS — Generic/Trade: Caps 0.25, 0.5 mcg. Oral soln 1 mcg/mL. Injection 1, 2 mcg/mL.
NOTES — Calcitriol is the activated form of vitamin D. During titration period, monitor serum calcium at least twice a week. Successful therapy requires an adequate daily calcium intake. Topical preparation must be compounded (not commercially available).
MOA — Vitamin D analogue that suppresses PTH secretion, bone resorption and increases gastrointestinal calcium absorption thus affecting bone homeostasis.
ADVERSE EFFECTS — Serious: Vitamin D toxicity/overdose, anaphylaxis, hypersensitivity, mild acidosis, renal toxicity, pancreatitis, arrhythmia, overt psychosis, elevated serum transaminases. Frequent: Weakness, headache, N/V, dry mouth, constipation, muscle pain, bone pain, metallic taste, irritability, weight loss, conjunctivitis, dyslipidemia, hypertension.

CEREFOLIN (L-methylfolate + riboflavin + pyridoxine + cyanocobalamin) ▶KL ♀C ▶+ $$
ADULTS — Nutritional supplement for hyperhomocysteinemia: 1 to 2 tab PO daily.
PEDS — Not approved in children.
FORMS — Trade only: Each tab contains 5.635 mg of L-methylfolate + 5 mg riboflavin + 50 mg pyridoxine + 1 mg cyanocobalamin.
NOTES — Folic acid doses > 0.1 mg may obscure pernicious anemia; preventable with the concurrent cyanocobalamin in product.
MOA — Combination product that lowers plasma homocysteine.
ADVERSE EFFECTS — Serious: Polycythemia vera, hypersensitivity. Frequent: Paresthesia, somnolence, headache, nausea, diarrhea, itching.

CEREFOLIN NAC (L-methylfolate + methylcobalamin + acetylcysteine) ▶KL ♀B ▶− $$
ADULTS — Nutritional supplement for neurovascular oxidative stress or hyperhomocysteinemia: 1 cap PO daily.
PEDS — Not approved in children.
FORMS — Trade only: L-methylfolate 5.6 mg + methylcobalamin 2 mg + N-acetylcysteine 600 mg cap.

(cont.)

ENDOCRINE AND METABOLIC: Vitamins

CEREFOLIN NAC *(cont.)*
NOTES — Folic acid doses > 0.1 mg may obscure pernicious anemia; preventable with the concurrent cyanocobalamin in product.
MOA — Combination product that lowers plasma homocysteine.
ADVERSE EFFECTS — Serious: Polycythemia vera, hypersensitivity, renal stone formation. Frequent: Paresthesia, somnolence, headache, nausea, diarrhea, itching.

CYANOCOBALAMIN (vitamin B12, *CaloMist, Nascobal*) ▶K ♀C ▶+ $
ADULTS — See also "unapproved adult" dosing. <u>Maintenance of nutritional deficiency following IM correction:</u> 500 mcg intranasal weekly (Nascobal: 1 spray 1 nostril once a week) or 50 to 100 mcg intranasal daily (CaloMist: 1 to 2 sprays each nostril daily). <u>Pernicious anemia:</u> 100 mcg IM/SC daily, for 6 to 7 days, then every other day for 7 doses, then q 3 to 4 d for 2 to 3 weeks, then q month. <u>Other patients with vitamin B12 deficiency:</u> 30 mcg IM daily for 5 to 10 d, then 100 to 200 mcg IM q month. RDA for adults is 2.4 mcg.
PEDS — <u>Nutritional deficiency:</u> 100 mcg/24 h deep IM/SC for 10 to 15 days then at least 60 mcg/month IM/deep SC. <u>Pernicious anemia:</u> 30 to 50 mcg/24 h for 14 days or more to total dose of 1000 to 5000 mcg deep IM/SC then 100 mcg/month deep IM/SC. Adequate daily intake for infants: 0 to 6 mo: 0.4 mcg; 7 to 11 mo: 0.5 mcg. RDA for children: 1 to 3 yo: 0.9 mcg; 4 to 8 yo: 1.2 mcg; 9 to 13 yo: 1.8 mcg; 14 to 18 yo: 2.4 mcg.
UNAPPROVED ADULTS — <u>Pernicious anemia and nutritional deficiency states:</u> 1000 to 2000 mcg PO daily for 1 to 2 weeks, then 1000 mcg PO daily. <u>Prevention and treatment of cyanide toxicity associated with nitroprusside.</u>
UNAPPROVED PEDS — <u>Prevention/treatment of nitroprusside-associated cyanide toxicity.</u>
FORMS — OTC Generic only: Tabs 100, 500, 1000, 5000 mcg; Lozenges 100, 250, 500 mcg. Rx Trade only: Nasal spray 500 mcg/spray (Nascobal 2.3 mL), 25 mcg/spray (CaloMist, 18 mL).
NOTES — Prime nasal pump before use per package insert directions. Although official dose for deficiency states is 100 to 200 mcg IM q month, some give 1000 mcg IM periodically. Oral supplementation is safe and effective for B12 deficiency even when intrinsic factor is not present. Monitor B12, folate, iron and CBC.
MOA — Water-soluble vitamin required for purine nucleotides synthesis and amino acid metabolism.
ADVERSE EFFECTS — Serious: Anaphylaxis (IM), angioedema (IM). Frequent: Asthenia, dizziness, headache, infection, glossitis, nausea, paresthesia, rash, rhinitis (nasal), nasopharyngitis (nasal), nasal discomfort (nasal).

DIATX ZN (folic acid + niacinamide + cobalamin + pantothenic acid + pyridoxine + d-biotin + thiamine + ascorbic acid + riboflavin + zinc oxide) ▶LK ♀? ▶? $$$
ADULTS — <u>Nutritional supplement for hyperhomocysteinemia,</u> particularly for patients with chronic kidney disease, end stage renal failure or on dialysis: 1 tab PO daily.
PEDS — Not approved in children.
FORMS — Trade only: Each tab contains folic acid 5 mg + niacinamide 20 mg + cobalamin 2 mg + pantothenic acid 10 mg + pyridoxine 50 mg + d-biotin 300 mcg + thiamine 1.5 mg + vitamin C 60 mg + riboflavin 1.5 mg + zinc (oxide) 25 mg, copper (gluconate) 1.5 mg.
NOTES — Cobalamin component appears to prevent masking of pernicious anemia by folic acid.
MOA — Combination of water-soluble vitamins.
ADVERSE EFFECTS — Serious: Hypersensitivity, possible masking of pernicious anemia, polycythemia vera, peripheral vascular thrombosis. Frequent: Mild transient diarrhea.

DOXERCALCIFEROL (*Hectorol*) ▶L ♀B ▶? $$$$$
ADULTS — <u>Secondary hyperparathyroidism on dialysis:</u> Oral: If PTH > 400 pg/mL then start 10 mcg PO 3 times a week; if PTH > 300 pg/mL then increase by 2.5 mcg/dose q 8 weeks as necessary; if PTH 150 to 300 pg/mL then maintain current dose; if PTH < 100 pg/mL then stop for 1 week, then resume at a dose at least 2.5 mcg lower. Max 60 mcg/week. IV: If PTH > 400 pg/mL then 4 mcg IV 3 times a week; if PTH decreased by < 50% and > 300 pg/mL then increase by 1 to 2 mcg q 8 weeks as necessary; if PTH decreased by > 50% and > 300 pg/mL then maintain current dose; if PTH 150 to 300 pg/mL then maintain current dose; if PTH < 100 pg/mL then stop for 1 week, then resume at a dose that is at least 1 mcg lower. Max 18 mcg/week. <u>Secondary hyperparathyroidism not on dialysis:</u> If PTH > 70 pg/mL (Stage 3) or > 110 pg/mL (Stage 4) then start 1 mcg PO daily; if PTH > 70 pg/mL (Stage 3) or > 110 pg/mL (Stage 4) then increase by 0.5 mcg/dose q 2 weeks; if PTH 35 to 70 pg/mL (Stage 3) or 70 to 110 pg/mL (Stage 4) then maintain current dose; if < 35 pg/mL (Stage 3) or < 70 pg/mL (Stage 4) then stop for 1 week, then resume at a dose that is at least 0.5 mcg lower. Max 3.5 mcg/day.
PEDS — Not approved in children.
FORMS — Trade only: Caps 0.5, 2.5 mcg.
NOTES — Monitor PTH, serum calcium and phosphorus weekly during dose titration; may need to monitor patients with hepatic insufficiency more closely.
MOA — Vitamin D analogue that suppresses PTH secretion and bone resorption thus affecting bone homeostasis.
ADVERSE EFFECTS — Serious: Vitamin D toxicity/overdose, hypersensitivity, mild acidosis, renal toxicity, pancreatitis, arrhythmia, overt psychosis, elevated serum transaminases. Frequent: Weakness, headache, N/V, dry mouth, constipation, muscle pain, bone pain, metallic taste, irritability, weight loss, conjunctivitis, dyslipidemia, hypertension.

ERGOCALCIFEROL (vitamin D2, *Calciferol, Drisdol, ✦Osteoforte*) ▶L ♀A (C if exceed RDA) ▶+ $
ADULTS — <u>Familial hypophosphatemia</u> (Vitamin D Resistant Rickets): 12,000 to 500,000 units PO daily. <u>Hypoparathyroidism:</u> 50,000 to 200,000 units PO daily. <u>Adequate daily intake adults:</u> 19 to 50 yo: 5 mcg (200

(cont.)

ERGOCALCIFEROL (cont.)
units); 51 to 70 yo: 10 mcg (400 units); older than 70 yo: 15 mcg (600 units). Max recommended daily dose in nondeficiency 50 mcg (2000 units).
PEDS — <u>Adequate daily intake infants and children:</u> 5 mcg (200 units). <u>Hypoparathyroidism:</u> 1.25 to 5 mg PO daily.
UNAPPROVED ADULTS — <u>Osteoporosis prevention and treatment</u> (age 50 or older): 800 to 1000 units PO daily with calcium supplements. <u>Fanconi syndrome:</u> 50,000 to 200,000 units PO daily. <u>Osteomalacia:</u> 1000 to 5000 units PO daily. <u>Anticonvulsant-induced osteomalacia:</u> 2000 to 50,000 units PO daily. <u>Vitamin D deficiency:</u> 50,000 units PO weekly or biweekly for 8-12 weeks.
UNAPPROVED PEDS — <u>Familial hypophosphatemia:</u> 400,000 to 800,000 units PO daily, increased by 10,000 to 20,000 units/day q 3 to 4 months as needed. <u>Hypoparathyroidism:</u> 50,000 to 200,000 units PO daily. <u>Fanconi syndrome:</u> 250 to 50,000 units PO daily.
FORMS — OTC Generic only: Caps 400, 1000, 5000 units, Soln 8000 units/mL (Calciferol). Rx Generic/Trade: Caps 50,000 units. Rx Generic only: Caps 25,000 units.
NOTES — 1 mcg ergocalciferol = 40 units vitamin D. Optimal level of 25(OH) Vitamin D is greater than 30 ng/mL. Vitamin D2 (ergocalciferol) is 30% as effective as vitamin D3 (cholecalciferol) in maintaining 25-OH vitamin D levels. IM or high-dose oral therapy may be necessary if malabsorption exists. Familial hypophosphatemia also requires phosphate supplementation; hypoparathyroidism also requires calcium supplementation.
MOA — Fat-soluble vitamin needed for calcium homeostasis (GI absorption, renal resorption, mobilization from bone).
ADVERSE EFFECTS — Serious: Vitamin D toxicity/overdose, hypersensitivity, mild acidosis, renal toxicity, pancreatitis, arrhythmia, overt psychosis, elevated serum transaminases. Frequent: Weakness, headache, N/V, dry mouth, constipation, muscle pain, bone pain, metallic taste, irritability, weight loss, conjunctivitis, dyslipidemia, hypertension.

FOLGARD (folic acid + cyanocobalamin + pyridoxine) ▶K ♀? ▶? $
ADULTS — <u>Nutritional supplement:</u> 1 tab PO daily.
PEDS — Not approved in children.
FORMS — OTC Trade only: Folic acid 0.8 mg + cyanocobalamin 0.115 mg + pyridoxine 10 mg tab.
NOTES — Folic acid doses > 0.1 mg may obscure pernicious anemia, preventable with the concurrent cyanocobalamin.
MOA — Combination product containing 3 water-soluble vitamins that lowers plasma homocysteine.
ADVERSE EFFECTS — Serious: Masking pernicious anemia, sensory neuropathic syndromes. Frequent: Unstable gait, numb feet, awkwardness of the hands, perioral numbness, decreased sensations (touch, temperature, vibrations), paresthesia, photosensitivity, ataxia, asthenia, headache, infection, glossitis, nausea, rhinitis.

FOLGARD RX (folic acid + cyanocobalamin + pyridoxine) ▶K - ▶? $
ADULTS — <u>Nutritional supplement:</u> 1 tab PO daily.
PEDS — Not approved in children.
FORMS — Trade only: Folic acid 2.2 mg + cyanocobalamin 1000 mcg + pyridoxine 25 mg tab.
NOTES — Folic acid doses > 0.1 mg may obscure pernicious anemia, preventable with the concurrent cyanocobalamin.
MOA — Combination product containing 3 water-soluble vitamins that lowers plasma homocysteine.
ADVERSE EFFECTS — Serious: Masking pernicious anemia, sensory neuropathic syndromes. Frequent: Unstable gait, numb feet, awkwardness of the hands, perioral numbness, decreased sensations (touch, temperature, vibrations), paresthesia, photosensitivity, ataxia, asthenia, headache, infection, glossitis, nausea, rhinitis.

FOLIC ACID (folate *Folvite*) ▶K ♀A ▶+ $
ADULTS — <u>Megaloblastic anemia:</u> 1 mg PO/IM/IV/SC daily. When symptoms subside and CBC normalizes, give maintenance dose of 0.4 mg PO daily and 0.8 mg PO daily in pregnant and lactating females. <u>RDA</u> for adults 0.4 mg, 0.6 mg for pregnant females, and 0.5 mg for lactating women. Max recommended daily dose 1 mg.
PEDS — <u>Megaloblastic anemia:</u> Infants: 0.05 mg PO daily, maintenance of 0.04 mg PO daily; Children: 0.5 to 1 mg PO daily, maintenance of 0.4 mg PO daily. <u>Adequate daily intake for infants:</u> 0 to 6 mo: 65 mcg; 7 to 12 mo: 80 mcg. <u>RDA</u> for children: 1 to 3 yo: 150 mcg; 4 to 8 yo: 200 mcg; 9 to 13 yo: 300 mcg, 14 to 18 yo: 400 mcg.
UNAPPROVED ADULTS — <u>Hyperhomocysteinemia:</u> 0.5 to 1 mg PO daily.
FORMS — OTC Generic only: Tabs 0.4, 0.8 mg. Rx Generic 1 mg.
NOTES — Folic acid doses > 0.1 mg/day may obscure pernicious anemia. Prior to conception all women should receive 0.4 mg/day to reduce the risk of neural tube defects in infants. Consider high dose (up to 4 mg) in women with prior history of infant with neural tube defect. Use oral route except in cases of severe intestinal absorption.
MOA — Water-soluble vitamin that stimulates red blood cell, white blood cell, and platelet production, and is a cofactor for transformylation reactions.
ADVERSE EFFECTS — Serious: Masking pernicious anemia. Frequent: None.

FOLTX (folic acid + cyanocobalamin + pyridoxine) ▶K ♀A ▶+ $$
ADULTS — <u>Nutritional supplement for end stage renal failure, dialysis, hyperhomocysteinemia, homocystinuria, nutrient malabsorption or inadequate dietary intake:</u> 1 tab PO daily.
PEDS — Not approved in children.
FORMS — Trade only: Folic acid 2.5 mg/cyanocobalamin 2 mg/pyridoxine 25 mg tab.
NOTES — Folic acid doses > 0.1 mg may obscure pernicious anemia, preventable with the concurrent cyanocobalamin.

(cont.)

FOLTX (cont.)
MOA — Combination product containing 3 water-soluble vitamins that lowers plasma homocysteine.
ADVERSE EFFECTS — Serious: Masking pernicious anemia, sensory neuropathic syndromes. Frequent: Unstable gait, numb feet, awkwardness of the hands, perioral numbness, decreased sensations (touch, temperature, vibrations), paresthesia, photosensitivity, ataxia, asthenia, headache, infection, glossitis, nausea, rhinitis.

METANX (L-methylfolate + pyridoxal phosphate + methylcobalamin) ▶K ♀C ▶? $$$
ADULTS — <u>Nutritional supplement for endothelial dysfunction or hyperhomocysteinemia:</u> 1 to 2 tab PO daily.
PEDS — Not approved in children.
FORMS — Trade only: Each tab contains 2.8 mg L-methylfolate + 25 mg pyridoxal phosphate + 2 mg methylcobalamin.
NOTES — Folic acid doses > 0.1 mg may obscure pernicious anemia; preventable with the concurrent cyanocobalamin in product.
MOA — Combination product that lowers plasma homocysteine.
ADVERSE EFFECTS — Serious: Polycythemia vera, hypersensitivity. Frequent: Paresthesia, somnolence, headache, nausea, diarrhea, itching.

MULTIVITAMINS (MVI) ▶LK ♀+ ▶+ $
WARNING — Severe iron toxicity possible in overdose, especially in children. Store out of reach of children and in child-resistant containers. Iron overdose is the leading cause of poisoning in children younger than 6 yo.
ADULTS — <u>Dietary supplement:</u> Dose varies by product.
PEDS — <u>Dietary supplement:</u> Dose varies by product.
FORMS — OTC and Rx: Many different brands and forms available with and without iron (Tabs, Caps, Chewable tabs, Gtts, liquid).
NOTES — Do not take within 2 h of antacids, tetracyclines, levothyroxine or fluoroquinolones.
MOA — Combination vitamin that usually contains vitamins A, D, E, B1, B2, B3, B5, B6, B12, and C, biotin and folic acid.
ADVERSE EFFECTS — Usually no adverse effects in recommended doses (see individual vitamins).

NEPHROCAP (ascorbic acid + folic acid + niacin + thiamine + riboflavin + pyridoxine + pantothenic acid + biotin + cyanocobalamin) ▶K ♀? ▶? $
ADULTS — Nutritional supplement for chronic renal failure, uremia, impaired metabolic functions of the kidney and to maintain levels when the dietary intake of vitamins is inadequate or excretion and loss are excessive: 1 cap PO daily. If on dialysis, take after treatment.
PEDS — Not approved in children.
FORMS — Generic/Trade: Vitamin C 100 mg/folic acid 1 mg/niacin 20 mg/thiamine 1.5 mg/riboflavin 1.7 mg/pyridoxine 10 mg/pantothenic acid 5 mg/biotin 150 mcg/cyanocobalamin 6 mcg.
NOTES — Folic acid doses > 0.1 mg/day may obscure pernicious anemia (preventable with the concurrent cyanocobalamin).
MOA — Combination product containing water-soluble vitamins.
ADVERSE EFFECTS — Serious: Masking pernicious anemia. Frequent: Mild transient diarrhea.

NEPHROVITE (ascorbic acid + folic acid + niacin + thiamine + riboflavin + pyridoxine + pantothenic acid + biotin + cyanocobalamin) ▶K ♀? ▶? $
ADULTS — <u>Nutritional supplement for chronic renal failure, dialysis, hyperhomocysteinemia or inadequate dietary vitamin intake:</u> 1 tab PO daily. If on dialysis, take after treatment.
PEDS — Not approved in children.
FORMS — Generic/Trade: Vitamin C 60 mg/folic acid 1 mg/niacin 20 mg/thiamine 1.5 mg/riboflavin 1.7 mg/pyridoxine 10 mg/pantothenic acid 10 mg/biotin 300 mcg/cyanocobalamin 6 mcg.
NOTES — Folic acid doses > 0.1 mg/day may obscure pernicious anemia (preventable with the concurrent cyanocobalamin).
MOA — Combination product containing water-soluble vitamins.
ADVERSE EFFECTS — Serious: Masking pernicious anemia. Frequent: Mild transient diarrhea.

NIACIN (vitamin B3, *nicotinic acid, Niacor, Nicolar, Slo-Niacin, Niaspan*) ▶K ♀C ▶? $
ADULTS — <u>Niacin deficiency:</u> 100 mg PO daily. RDA is 16 mg for males and 14 mg for females. <u>Hyperlipidemia:</u> Start 50 to 100 mg PO bid to tid with meals, increase slowly, usual maintenance range 1.5 to 3 g/day, max 6 g/day. Extended-release (Niaspan): Start 500 mg at bedtime with a low-fat snack for 4 weeks, increase as needed every 4 weeks to max 2000 mg.
PEDS — Safety and efficacy not established for doses which exceed nutritional requirements. <u>Adequate daily intake for infants:</u> 0 to 6 mo: 2 mg; 7 to 12 mo: 3 mg. <u>RDA</u> for children: 1 to 3 yo: 6 mg; 48 yo: 8 mg; 9 to 13 yo: 12 mg; 14 to 18 yo: 16 mg (males) and 14 mg (females).
UNAPPROVED ADULTS — <u>Pellagra:</u> 50 to 100 mg tid-qid, up to 500 mg PO daily.
FORMS — OTC Generic only: Tabs 50, 100, 250, 500 mg; Timed-release cap 125, 250, 400 mg; Timed-release tab 250, 500 mg; Liquid 50 mg/5 mL. Trade only: 250, 500, 750 mg (Slo-Niacin). Rx: Trade only: Tabs 500 mg (Niacor), Timed-release caps 500 mg, Timed-release tabs 500, 750, 1000 mg (Niaspan, $$$$).
NOTES — Start with low doses and increase slowly to minimize flushing (usually less than 2 h); 325 mg aspirin 30 to 60 min prior to niacin ingestion will minimize flushing. Use caution in diabetics, patients with gout, peptic ulcer, liver, or gallbladder disease. Extended-release formulations may have greater hepatotoxicity.
MOA — Water-soluble vitamin that serves as a coenzyme for oxidation-reduction reactions. Decreases lipoproteins associated with high LDL-cholesterol

(cont.)

NIACIN (cont.)
and triglycerides and increases lipoproteins associated with low HDL-cholesterol.
ADVERSE EFFECTS − Serious: Hepatotoxicity, diabetes, peptic ulcer disease, gout, hypotension, myopathy, creatine kinase increase, hepatitis. Frequent: Flushing, dyspepsia, vomiting, abdominal pain, rash, burning paresthesias.

PARICALCITOL (*Zemplar*) ▶L ♀C ▶? $$$$$
ADULTS − Prevention/treatment of secondary hyperparathyroidism with renal insufficiency: If PTH < 500 pg/mL then start 1 mcg PO daily or 2 mcg PO 3 times a week. If PTH > 500 pg/mL then start 2 mcg PO daily or 4 mcg PO 3 times a week. Can increase PO dose by 1 mcg daily or 2 mcg 3/week based on PTH in 2 to 4 weeks intervals. Prevention/treatment of secondary hyperparathyroidism with renal failure (CrCl < 15 mL/min): PO: To calculate initial dose divide baseline iPTH by 80 and then administer this dose in mcg 3 times a week. To titrate dose based on response, divide recent iPTH by 80 and then administer this dose in mcg 3 times a week. IV: Initially 0.04 to 0.1 mcg/kg (2.8 to 7 mcg) IV 3 times a week during dialysis. Can increase IV dose 2 to 4 mcg based on PTH in 2 to 4 weeks intervals. PO/IV: If PTH level decreased < 30% then increase dose; if PTH level decreased 30 to 60% then maintain current dose; if PTH level decreased > 60% then decrease dose.
PEDS − Prevention/treatment of secondary hyperparathyroidism with renal failure (CrCl < 15 mL/min): 0.04 to 0.1 mcg/kg (2.8 to 7 mcg) IV 3 times a week at dialysis; increase dose by 2 to 4 mcg or 0.04 mcg/kg q 2 to 4 weeks until desired PTH level is achieved. Max dose 0.24 mcg/kg (16.8 mcg).
FORMS − Trade only: Caps 1, 2, 4 mcg.
NOTES − Monitor serum PTH, calcium and phosphorous. IV doses up to 0.24 mcg/kg (16.8 mcg) have been administered. Do not initiate PO therapy in renal failure until calcium is 9.6 mg/dL or lower.
MOA − Vitamin D analogue that suppresses PTH secretion and bone resorption thus affecting bone homeostasis.
ADVERSE EFFECTS − Serious: Vitamin D toxicity/overdose, hypersensitivity, mild acidosis, renal toxicity, pancreatitis, arrhythmia, overt psychosis, elevated serum transaminases, angioedema. Frequent: Weakness, headache, N/V, dry mouth, constipation, muscle pain, bone pain, metallic taste, irritability, weight loss, conjunctivitis, dyslipidemia, hypertension.

PHYTONADIONE (vitamin K, *Mephyton, AquaMephyton*) ▶L ♀C ▶+ $
WARNING − Severe reactions, including fatalities, have occurred during and immediately after IV injection, even with diluted injection and slow administration. Restrict IV use to situations where other routes of administration are not feasible.
ADULTS − Excessive oral anticoagulation: Dose varies based on INR. INR 5 to 9: 1 to 2.5 mg PO (up to 5 mg PO may be given if rapid reversal necessary); INR > 9 with no bleeding: 5 to 10 mg PO; Serious bleeding and elevated INR: 10 mg slow IV infusion. Hypoprothrombinemia due to other causes: 2.5 to 25 mg PO/IM/SC. Adequate daily intake 120 mcg (males) and 90 mcg (females).
PEDS − Hemorrhagic disease of the newborn: Prophylaxis: 0.5 to 1 mg IM 1 h after birth; Treatment: 1 mg SC/IM.
UNAPPROVED PEDS − Nutritional deficiency: Children: 2.5 to 5 mg PO daily or 1 to 2 mg IM/SC/IV. Excessive oral anticoagulation: Infants: 1 to 2 mg IM/SC/IV q 4 to 8 h; Children: 2.5 to 10 mg PO/IM/SC/IV, may be repeated 12 to 48 h after PO dose or 6 to 8 h after IM/SC/IV dose.
FORMS − Trade only: Tabs 5 mg.
NOTES − Excessive doses of vitamin K in a patient receiving warfarin may cause warfarin resistance for up to a week. Avoid IM administration in patients with a high INR.
MOA − Fat-soluble vitamin that promotes formation of clotting factors.
ADVERSE EFFECTS − Serious: Anaphylactic reaction. Frequent: Injection-site reaction, flushing sensation, "peculiar" taste sensation.

PYRIDOXINE (vitamin B6) ▶K ♀A ▶+ $
ADULTS − Dietary deficiency: 10 to 20 mg PO daily for 3 weeks. Prevention of deficiency due to isoniazid in high-risk patients: 10 to 25 mg PO daily. Treatment of neuropathies due to INH: 50 to 200 mg PO daily. INH overdose (> 10 g): 4 g IV followed by 1 g IM over 30 min, repeat until total dose of 1 g for each g of INH ingested. RDA for adults: 19 to 50 yo: 1.3 mg; older than 50 yo: 1.7 mg (males), 1.5 mg (females). Max recommended: 100 mg/day.
PEDS − Not approved in children. Adequate daily intake for infants: 0 to 6 mo: 0.1 mg; 7 to 12 mo: 0.3 mg. RDA for children: 1 to 3 yo: 0.5 mg; 4 to 8 yo: 0.6 mg; 9 to 13 yo: 1 mg; 14 to 18 yo: 1.3 (boys) and 1.2 mg (girls).
UNAPPROVED ADULTS − PMS: 50 to 500 mg/day PO. Hyperoxaluria type I and oxalate kidney stones: 25 to 300 mg/day PO. Prevention of oral contraceptive-induced deficiency; 25 to 40 mg PO daily. Hyperemesis of pregnancy: 10 to 50 mg PO q 8 h. Has been used in hydrazine poisoning.
UNAPPROVED PEDS − Dietary deficiency: 5 to 10 mg PO daily for 3 weeks. Prevention of deficiency due to isoniazid: 1 to 2 mg/kg/day PO daily. Treatment of neuropathies due to INH: 10 to 50 mg PO daily. Pyridoxine-dependent epilepsy: Neonatal: 25 to 50 mg/dose IV; older infants and children: 100 mg/dose IV for 1 dose then 100 mg PO daily.
FORMS − OTC Generic only: Tabs 25, 50, 100 mg; Timed-release tab 100 mg.
MOA − Water-soluble vitamin that is a coenzyme involved in numerous metabolic transformations of proteins and amino acids.
ADVERSE EFFECTS − Serious: Sensory neuropathic syndromes. Frequent: Unstable gait, numb feet, awkwardness of the hands, perioral numbness, decreased sensations (touch, temperature, vibrations), paresthesia, photosensitivity, ataxia.

ENDOCRINE AND METABOLIC: Vitamins

RIBOFLAVIN (vitamin B2) ▶K ♀A ▶+ $
ADULTS — Deficiency: 5 to 25 mg/day PO. RDA for adults is 1.3 mg (males) and 1.1 mg (females), 1.4 mg for pregnant women and 1.6 mg for lactating women.
PEDS — Deficiency: 5 to 10 mg/day PO. Adequate daily intake for infants: 0 to 6 mo: 0.3 mg; 7 to 12 mo: 0.4 mg. RDA for children: 1 to 3 yo: 0.5 mg; 4 to 8 yo: 0.6 mg; 9 to 13 yo: 0.9 mg; 14 to 18 yo: 1.3 mg (males) and 1 mg (females).
UNAPPROVED ADULTS — Prevention of migraine headaches: 400 mg PO daily.
FORMS — OTC Generic only: Tabs 25, 50, 100 mg.
NOTES — May cause yellow/orange discoloration of urine.
MOA — Water-soluble vitamin that catalyzes oxidative-reduction reactions.
ADVERSE EFFECTS — Serious: None. Frequent: Yellow discoloration of urine.

THIAMINE (vitamin B1) ▶K ♀A ▶+ $
ADULTS — Beriberi: 10 to 20 mg IM 3 times per week for 2 weeks. Wet beriberi with MI: 10 to 30 mg IV tid. Wernicke encephalopathy: 50 to 100 mg IV and 50 to 100 mg IM for 1 dose then 50 to 100 mg IM daily until patient resumes normal diet. Give before starting glucose. RDA for adults is 1.2 mg (males) and 1.1 mg (females).
PEDS — Beriberi: 10 to 25 mg IM daily or 10 to 50 mg PO daily for 2 weeks then 5 to 10 mg PO daily for 1 month. Adequate daily intake infants: 0 to 6 mo: 0.2 mg; 7 to 12 mo: 0.3 mg. RDA for children: 1 to 3 yo: .5 mg; 4 to 8 yo: 0.6 mg; 9 to 13 yo: 0.9 mg; 14 to 18 yo: 1.2 mg (males), 1.0 mg (females).
FORMS — OTC Generic only: Tabs 50, 100, 250, 500 mg; Enteric-coated tab 20 mg.
MOA — Water-soluble vitamin needed for carbohydrate metabolism, normal growth maintenance, nerve impulse transmission, and acetylcholine synthesis.
ADVERSE EFFECTS — Serious: Hypersensitivity, anaphylaxis, cyanosis, pulmonary edema, GI hemorrhage, cardiovascular shock. Frequent: Injection site reaction, feeling of warmth, pruritus, sweating, N/V, restlessness, angioedema.

TOCOPHEROL (vitamin E, ✦Aquasol E) ▶L ♀A ▶? $
ADULTS — RDA is 22 units (natural, d-alpha- tocopherol) or 33 units (synthetic, d,l-alpha-tocopherol) or 15 mg (alpha-tocopherol). Max recommended 1000 mg (alpha-tocopherol).
PEDS — Adequate daily intake (alpha-tocopherol): Infants 0 to 6 mo: 4 mg; 7 to 12 mo: 6 mg. RDA for children (alpha-tocopherol): 1 to 3 yo: 6 mg; 4 to 8 yo: 7 mg; 9 to 13 yo: 11 mg; 14 to 18 yo: 15 mg.
UNAPPROVED ADULTS — Alzheimer's disease: 1000 units PO bid (controversial based on limited data and efficacy).
UNAPPROVED PEDS — Nutritional deficiency: Neonates: 25 to 50 units PO daily; Children: 1 units/kg PO daily. Cystic fibrosis: 5 to 10 units/kg PO daily (use water soluble form), max 400 units/day.
FORMS — OTC Generic only: Tabs 200, 400 units; Caps 73.5, 100, 147, 165, 200, 330, 400, 500, 600, 1000 units; Gtts 50 mg/mL.
NOTES — 1 mg alpha-tocopherol equivalents equals ~1.5 units. Natural vitamin E (d-alpha-tocopherol) recommended over synthetic (d,l-alpha-tocopherol). Higher doses may increase risk of bleeding. Large randomized trials have failed to demonstrate cardioprotective effects.
MOA — Fat-soluble vitamin that protects cellular constituents from oxidation.
ADVERSE EFFECTS — Serious: Vitamin E toxicity/overdose. Frequent: None.

VITAMIN A ▶L ♀A (C if exceed RDA, X in high doses) ▶+ $
ADULTS — Treatment of deficiency states: 100,000 units IM daily for 3 days, then 50,000 units IM daily for 2 weeks. RDA: 1000 mcg RE (males), 800 mcg RE (females). Max recommended daily dose in nondeficiency 3000 mcg (see notes).
PEDS — Treatment of deficiency states: Infants: 7500 to 15,000 units IM daily for 10 days; children 1 to 8 yo: 17,500 to 35,000 units IM daily for 10 days. Kwashiorkor: 30 mg IM of water-soluble palmitate followed by 5000 to 10,000 units PO daily for 2 months. Xerophthalmia: Older than 1 yo: 110 mg retinyl palmitate PO or 55 mg IM plus 110 mg PO next day. Administer another 110 mg PO prior to discharge. Vitamin E (40 units) should be coadministered to increase efficacy of retinol. RDA for children: 0 to 6 mo: 400 mcg (adequate intake); 7 to 12 mo: 500 mcg; 1 to 3 yo: 300 mcg; 4 to 8 yo: 400 mcg; 9 to 13 yo: 600 mcg; 14 to 18 yo: 900 mcg (males), 700 mcg (females).
UNAPPROVED ADULTS — Test for fat absorption: 7000 units/kg (2100 RE/kg) PO for one dose. Measure serum vitamin A concentrations at baseline and 4 h after ingestion. Dermatologic disorders such as follicularis keratosis: 50,000 to 500,000 units PO daily for several weeks.
UNAPPROVED PEDS — Has been tried in reduction of malaria episodes in children older than 12 mo and to reduce the mortality in HIV-infected children.
FORMS — OTC Generic only: Caps 10,000, 15,000 units. Trade only: Tabs 5000 units. Rx: Generic: 25,000 units. Trade only: Soln 50,000 units/mL.
NOTES — 1 RE (retinol equivalent) = 1 mcg retinol or 6 mcg beta-carotene. Continued Vitamin A/retinol intake of 2000 mcg/day or more may increase risk of hip fracture in postmenopausal women.
MOA — Fat-soluble vitamin needed for vision, dental development, growth, steroid synthesis, epithelial differentiation, embryonic development and reproduction.
ADVERSE EFFECTS — Serious: Vitamin A toxicity/overdose, hypersensitivity. Frequent: None.

VITAMIN D3 (cholecalciferol, DDrops) ▶L - ▶+ $
ADULTS — Familial hypophosphatemia (Vitamin D Resistant Rickets): 12,000 to 500,000 units PO daily. Hypoparathyroidism: 50,000 to 200,000 units PO daily. Adequate daily intake adults: 19 to 50 yo: 5 mcg (200 units); 51 to 70 yo: 10 mcg (400 units); older than 70 yo: 15 mcg (600 units). Max recommended daily dose in nondeficiency 50 mcg (2000 units).
PEDS — Adequate daily intake infants and children: 5 mcg (200 units). Hypoparathyroidism: 1.25 to 5 mg PO daily.
UNAPPROVED ADULTS — Osteoporosis prevention: 400 prevention and treatment (age 50 or older): 800 to 800 1000 units PO daily with calcium supplements.

(cont.)

VITAMIN D3 (*cont.*)
UNAPPROVED PEDS — Familial hypophosphatemia: 400,000 to 800,000 units PO daily, increased by 10,000 to 20,000 units/day q 3 to 4 months as needed. Hypoparathyroidism: 50,000 to 200,000 units PO daily. Fanconi syndrome: 250 to 50,000 units PO daily.
FORMS — OTC Generic: 200 units, 400 units, 800 units, 1000 units, 2000 units (cap/tab).Trade only: Soln 400 units/drop, 1000 units/drop, 2000 units/drop.
NOTES — Vitamin D2 (ergocalciferol) is 30% as effective as vitamin D3 (cholecalciferol) in maintaining 25-OH vitamin D levels. Optimal level of 25(OH) Vitamin D is greater than 30 ng/mL.
MOA — Fat-soluble vitamin needed for calcium homeostasis (GI absorption, renal resorption, mobilization from bone).
ADVERSE EFFECTS — Serious: Vitamin D toxicity/overdose, hypersensitivity, mild acidosis, renal toxicity, pancreatitis, arrhythmia, overt psychosis, elevated serum transaminases. Frequent: Weakness, headache, N/V, dry mouth, constipation, muscle pain, bone pain, metallic taste, irritability, weight loss, conjunctivitis, dyslipidemia, hypertension.

ENDOCRINE AND METABOLIC: Other

AMMONUL (**sodium phenylacetate + sodium benzoate**) ▶KL ♀C ▶? $$$$$
ADULTS — Acute hyperammonemia with encephalopathy in urea cycle enzyme deficiency: 55 mL/m2 IV over 90 to 120 min, followed by maintenance 55 mL/m2 over 24 h. Stop when hyperammonemia resolved or oral nutrition and medications are tolerated.
PEDS — Acute hyperammonemia with encephalopathy in urea cycle enzyme deficiency: If wt 20 kg or less, then 2.5 mL/kg IV over 90 to 120 min, followed by maintenance 2.5 mL/kg over 24 h. If greater than 20 kg, then 55 mL/m2 IV over 90 to 120 min, followed by maintenance 55 mL/m2 over 24 h. Consider coadministration of arginine in hyperammonemic infants. Stop when hyperammonemia resolved or oral nutrition and medications are tolerated.
FORMS — Single-use vial 50 mL (10% sodium phenylacetate/10% sodium benzoate).
NOTES — Administer through a central line. Closely monitor if renal insufficiency. Monitor plasma ammonia level, neurological status, electrolytes, blood pH, blood pCO2 and clinical response. May cause hypokalemia. Consider coadministration of antiemetic. Penicillin and probenecid may affect renal secretion.
MOA — Serves an alternative to urea which effectively reduces waste nitrogen levels via hepatic conjugation and renal secretion.
ADVERSE EFFECTS — Serious: Neurotoxicity, brain edema, convulsions, pancytopenia, cardiac arrest, metabolic acidosis. Frequent: N/V, pyrexia, hyperglycemia, hypokalemia, hypotension, mental impairment.

BROMOCRIPTINE (*Cycloset, Parlodel*) ▶L ♀B ▶– $$$$$
ADULTS — Type 2 DM: Start 0.8 mg PO q am, may increase by 0.8 weekly to max 4.8 mg. Hyperprolactinemia: Start 1.25 to 2.5 mg PO at bedtime, then increase q 3 to 7 days to usual effective dose of 2.5 to 15 mg/day, max 40 mg/day. Acromegaly: Usual effective dose is 20 to 30 mg/day, max 100 mg/day. Doses > 20 mg/day can be divided bid. Also approved for Parkinson's disease, but rarely used. Take with food to minimize dizziness and nausea.
PEDS — Not approved in children.
UNAPPROVED ADULTS — Neuroleptic malignant syndrome: 2.5 to 5 mg PO 2 to 6 times a day. Hyperprolactinemia: 2.5 to 7.5 mg/day vaginally if GI intolerance occurs with PO dosing.
FORMS — Generic/Trade: Tabs 2.5 mg. Caps 5 mg.
NOTES — Take with food to minimize dizziness and nausea. Ergots have been associated with potentially life-threatening fibrotic complications. Seizures, CVA, HTN, arrhythmias, and MI have been reported. Should not be used for postpartum lactation suppression. Contraindicated in Raynaud's syndrome. Avoid concomitant use of other ergot medications.
MOA — Dopamine agonist (ergot).
ADVERSE EFFECTS — Serious: Orthostatic hypotension, syncope, sleep attacks, shock, MI, stroke, arrhythmias, seizures, psychosis; retroperitoneal, pleural, pericardial, or cardiac valvular fibrosis, erythromelalgia, neutropenia and other blood dyscrasias, hemolytic anemia, adrenal insufficiency, hepatotoxicity. Frequent: N/V, anorexia, diarrhea, constipation, abdominal pain, headache, dizziness, drowsiness, fatigue, confusion, orthostatic hypotension, edema, hallucinations, hypothyroidism, Parkinson's disease only: abnormal involuntary movements.

CABERGOLINE (*Dostinex*) ▶L ♀B ▶– $$$$$
ADULTS — Hyperprolactinemia: Initiate therapy with 0.25 mg PO twice a week. Increase by 0.25 mg twice a week at 4 week intervals up to a maximum of 1 mg twice a week.
PEDS — Not approved in children.
UNAPPROVED ADULTS — Acromegaly: 0.5 mg PO twice a week. Increase as needed up to 3.5 mg/week based on plasma IGF-1 levels.
FORMS — Generic/Trade: Tabs 0.5 mg.
NOTES — Monitor serum prolactin levels. Use with caution in hepatic insufficiency or valvular disease. Postmarketing reports of pathological gambling, increased libido and hypersexuality.
MOA — Dopamine agonist that decreases prolactin secretion.
ADVERSE EFFECTS — Serious: Hypotension, pulmonary fibrosis, increased ESR, valvulopathy. Frequent: Nausea, headache, dizziness, fatigue, lightheadedness, vomiting, abdominal cramps, rhinorrhea.

CALCITONIN (*Miacalcin, Fortical, ✦Calcimar, Caltine*) ▶Plasma ♀C ▶? $$$$
ADULTS — Osteoporosis: 100 units SC/IM every other day or 200 units (1 spray) intranasal daily (alternate nostrils). Paget's disease: 50 to 100 units SC/IM daily or 3 times a week. Hypercalcemia: 4 units/kg SC/IM q 12 h. May increase after 2 days to maximum of 8 units/kg q 6 h.

(cont.)

CALCITONIN (cont.)
PEDS — Not approved in children.
UNAPPROVED ADULTS — <u>Acute osteoporotic vertebral fracture pain:</u> 100 units SC/IM daily or 200 units intranasal daily (alternate nostrils).
UNAPPROVED PEDS — <u>Osteogenesis imperfecta</u> age 6 mo to 15 yo: 2 units/kg SC/IM 3 times a week with oral calcium supplements.
FORMS — Generic/Trade: Nasal spray 200 units/activation in 3.7 mL bottle (minimum of 30 doses/bottle).
NOTES — Skin test before using injectable product: 1 unit intradermally and observe for local reaction. Hypocalcemic effect diminishes in 2 to 7 days, therefore, only useful during acute short-term management of hypercalcemia.
MOA — Polypeptide hormone that decreases the rate of bone resorption.
ADVERSE EFFECTS — Serious: Antibody formation, hypersensitivity, anaphylaxis, bronchospasm. Frequent: Nasal irritation, rhinitis, back pain, arthralgia, epistaxis, headache, sinusitis, dizziness, N/V, flushing, rash, abdominal pain, diarrhea, injection site irritation (for SC/IM).

CINACALCET (Sensipar) ▶LK ♀C ▶? $$$$$
ADULTS — <u>Treatment of secondary hyperparathyroidism in dialysis patients:</u> 30 mg PO daily. May titrate q 2 to 4 weeks through sequential doses of 60, 90, 120 and 180 mg daily to target intact parathyroid hormone level of 150 to 300 pg/mL. <u>Treatment of hypercalcemia in parathyroid carcinoma:</u> 30 mg PO bid. May titrate q 2 to 4 weeks through sequential does of 60 mg bid, 90 mg bid and 90 mg tid to qid as necessary to normalize serum calcium levels.
PEDS — Not approved in children.
UNAPPROVED ADULTS — <u>Primary hyperparathyroidism:</u> 30 mg PO bid. May titrate q 2 to 8 weeks up to 5 mg bid to maintain serum calcium < 10.3 mg/dL.
FORMS — Trade only: Tabs 30, 60, 90 mg.
NOTES — Monitor serum calcium and phosphorus 1 week after initiation or dose adjustment, then monthly after a maintenance dose has been established. Intact parathyroid hormone should be checked 1 to 4 weeks after initiation or dose adjustment, and then 1 to 3 months after a maintenance dose has been established. For parathyroid carcinoma, monitor serum calcium within 1 week after initiation or dose adjustment, then q 2 months after a maintenance dose has been established. Withhold if serum calcium falls below < 7.5 mg/dL or if signs and symptoms of hypocalcemia. May restart when calcium level reaches 8.0 mg/dL or when signs and symptoms of hypocalcemia resolve. Re-initiate using the next lowest dose. Use calcium-containing phosphate binder and/or vitamin D to raise calcium if it falls between 7.5 to 8.4 mg/dL. Reduce dose or discontinue if intact parathyroid hormone level is < 150 to 300 pg/mL to prevent adynamic bone disease. Do not check parathyroid hormone levels within 12 h after administration of a dose. Inhibits metabolism by CYP 2D6; may increase levels of flecainide, vinblastine, thioridazine, TCAs. Dose adjustment may be needed when initiating/discontinuing a strong CYP 3A4 inhibitor (ie, ketoconazole, erythromycin and itraconazole). Closely monitor parathyroid hormone and serum calcium if moderate to severe hepatic impairment.
MOA — Lowers parathyroid hormone levels and decreases serum calcium by increasing sensitivity of the calcium-sensing receptor to extracellular calcium.
ADVERSE EFFECTS — Serious: Seizures, adynamic bone disease, hypocalcemia, hypotension, worsening heart failure, arrhythmia, hypersensitivity. Frequent: N/V, diarrhea, myalgia, dizziness, rash.

CONIVAPTAN (Vaprisol) ▶LK ♀C ▶? $$$$$
WARNING — Avoid concurrent use of CYP 3A4 inhibitors (ketoconazole, itraconazole, clarithromycin, ritonavir, indinavir). Discontinue if hypovolemia, hypotension, or rapid rise in serum sodium (> 12 mEq/L/24 h) occurs.
ADULTS — <u>Euvolemic or hypervolemic hyponatremia:</u> Loading dose of 20 mg IV over 30 min, then continuous infusion 20 mg over 24 h for 1 to 4 days. Titrate to desired serum sodium. Max dose 40 mg daily as continuous infusion.
PEDS — Not approved in children.
NOTES — No benefit expected in anuric patients. Avoid concurrent use of CYP 3A4 inhibitors (ketoconazole, itraconazole, clarithromycin, ritonavir, indinavir). May increase digoxin levels. Discontinue if hypovolemia, hypotension, or rapid rise in serum sodium (> 12 mEq/L/24 h) occurs. Rapid correction of serum sodium may cause osmotic demyelination syndrome. Requires frequent monitoring of serum sodium, volume, and neurologic status. Administer through large veins and change infusion site daily to minimize irritation. Not approved for hyponatremia in heart failure. Increased exposure to conivaptan in renal or hepatic impairment. No recommended if CrCl < 30 ml/min.
MOA — Arginine vasopressin antagonist that promotes free water excretion to raise sodium levels.
ADVERSE EFFECTS — Serious: hypotension, hypovolemia. Frequent: Infusion site reactions, constipation, nausea, diarrhea, vomiting, infection, electrolyte changes, polyuria, erythema, hypotension, hypertension.

DENOSUMAB (Prolia) ▶? ♀C ▶? $$$$$
ADULTS — <u>Postmenopausal osteoporosis at high risk for fracture:</u> 60 mg SC q6 months.
PEDS — Not approved in children
FORMS — Trade only: 60 mg/1 mL vial, prefilled syringe.
NOTES — Must correct hypocalcemia before administration, monitor calcium especially in renal insufficiency. Administered by a health care professional SC in upper arm, upper thigh or abdomen. Give calcium 1000 mg and at least 400 International units vitamin D daily.
MOA — RANK ligand (RANKL) inhibitor that decreases bone resorption.

(cont.)

ENDOCRINE AND METABOLIC: Other

DENOSUMAB (cont.)
ADVERSE EFFECTS — Serious: Hypocalcemia, serious infections, serious dermatologic reactions, cellulitis, osteonecrosis of the jaw, pancreatitis. Frequent: Dermatitis, rash, eczema, back pain, pain in extremity, hypercholesterlemia, musculoskeletal pain, cystitis, constipation.

DESMOPRESSIN (*DDAVP, Stimate, ✦Minirin, Octostim*) ▶LK ♀B ▶? $$$$
WARNING — Adjust fluid intake downward to decrease potential water intoxication and hyponatremia; use cautiously in those at risk.
ADULTS — Diabetes insipidus: 10 to 40 mcg (0.1 to 0.4 mL) intranasally daily or divided bid to tid or 0.05 to 1.2 mg PO daily or divided bid to tid or 0.5 to 1 mL (2 to 4 mcg) SC/IV daily in 2 divided doses. Hemophilia A, von Willebrand's disease: 0.3 mcg/kg IV over 15 to 30 min; 300 mcg intranasally if wt 50 kg or more (1 spray in each nostril), 150 mcg intranasally if wt less than 50 kg (single spray in 1 nostril). Primary nocturnal enuresis: 0.2 to 0.6 mg PO at bedtime.
PEDS — Diabetes insipidus 3 mo to 12 yo: 5 to 30 mcg (0.05-0.3 mL) intranasally daily-bid or 0.05 mg PO daily. Hemophilia A, von Willebrand's disease (age 3 mo or older for IV, age 11 mo 12 yo for nasal spray): 0.3 mcg/kg IV over 15 to 30 min; 300 mcg intranasally if wt 50 kg or greater (1 spray in each nostril), 150 mcg intranasally if wt less than 50 kg (single spray in 1 nostril). Primary nocturnal enuresis age 6 yo or older: 0.2 to 0.6 mg PO at bedtime.
UNAPPROVED ADULTS — Uremic bleeding: 0.3 mcg/kg IV single dose or q 12 h (onset 1 to 2 h; duration 6 to 8 h after single dose). Intranasal is 20 mcg/day (onset 24 to 72 h; duration 14 days during 14 days course).
UNAPPROVED PEDS — Hemophilia A and type 1 von Willebrand's disease: 2 to 4 mcg/kg intranasally or 0.2 to 0.4 mcg/kg IV over 15 to 30 min.
FORMS — Trade only: Stimate nasal spray 150 mcg/0.1 mL (1 spray), 2.5 mL bottle (25 sprays). Generic/Trade (DDAVP nasal spray): 10 mcg/0.1 mL (1 spray), 5 mL bottle (50 sprays). Note difference in concentration of nasal soln. Rhinal Tube: 2.5 mL bottle with 2 flexible plastic tube applicators with graduation marks for dosing. Generic only: Tabs 0.1, 0.2 mg.
NOTES — Monitor serum sodium. Restrict fluid intake 1 h before to 8 h after PO administration. Hold PO treatment for enuresis during acute illnesses that may cause fluid/electrolyte imbalances. Start at lowest dose with Diabetes insipidus. IV/SC doses are approximately 1/10 the intranasal dose. Anaphylaxis reported with both IV and intranasal forms. Do not give if type IIB von Willebrand's disease. Changes in nasal mucosa may impair absorption of nasal spray. Refrigerate nasal spray; stable for 3 weeks at room temperature. 10 mcg = 40 units desmopressin.
MOA — Synthetic vasopressin analogue with a rapid onset that promotes water resorption (antidiuretic effect). Increases Factor VIII and von Willebrand's factor activity.
ADVERSE EFFECTS — Serious: Anaphylaxis, seizures (hyponatremia-associated), hyponatremia, fluid overload, chest pain, thrombotic events (rare). Frequent: Abdominal pain, flushing, headache, nasal congestion, nausea, rhinitis, agitation, balanitis, chills, increased blood pressure, sore throat, local irritation, epistaxis.

DIAZOXIDE (*Hyperstat, Proglycem*) ▶L ♀C ▶– $$$$$
ADULTS — ADULT - Hypoglycemia from hyperinsulinism: Initially 3 mg/kg/day PO divided equally q 8 h, usual maintenance dose 3 to 8 mg/kg/day divided equally q 8 to 12 h, max 10 to 15 mg/kg/day.
PEDS — PEDS - Hypoglycemia from hyperinsulinism: Neonates and infants, initially 10 mg/kg/day divided equally q 8 h, usual maintenance dose 8 to 15 mg/kg/day divided equally q 8 to 12 h; children, same as adult.
FORMS — FORMS - Trade only: Susp 50 mg/mL (30 mL).
NOTES — Close monitoring of blood glucose required. Consider reduced dose in renal impairment. Used for hyperinsulinism associated with islet cell adenoma, carcinoma, or hyperplasia; extrapancreatic malignancy, leucine sensitivity in children, nesidioblastosis. Avoid if hypersensitivity to thiazides or sulfonabmide derivatives. Caution in gout; may increase uric acid. Monitor for edema and heart failure exacerbation during administration; diuretic therapy may be needed.

GALLIUM (*Ganite*) ▶K ♀C ▶? $$$$$
WARNING — Monitor creatinine (contraindicated if > 2.5 mg/dL), urine output, calcium and phosphorous. Avoid concurrent nephrotoxic drugs (eg, aminoglycosides, amphotericin B). Establish urinary output of at least 2 L/day prior to treatment and maintain adequate hydration during therapy.
ADULTS — Hypercalcemia of malignancy: 200 mg/m2/day for 5 days. Shorten course if hypercalcemia is corrected. If mild hypercalcemia with few symptoms, consider 100 mg/m2/day for 5 days. Administer as slow IV infusion over 24 h.
PEDS — Not approved in children.
NOTES — Monitor creatinine (contraindicated if > 2.5 mg/dL), urine output, calcium and phosphorous. Avoid concurrent nephrotoxic drugs (eg, aminoglycosides, amphotericin B). Ensure adequate hydration prior to infusion.
MOA — Inhibits calcium resorption from bone; decreases serum calcium.
ADVERSE EFFECTS — Serious: Hypersensitivity, renal failure, optic neuritis. Frequent: Hypocalcemia, hypophosphatemia, decreased serum bicarbonate, anemia, hypotension.

MECASERMIN (*Increlex*) ▶LK ♀C ▶? $$$$$
ADULTS — Not studied in adults.
PEDS — Growth failure with severe primary insulin-like growth factor-1 deficiency or with neutralizing antibodies to growth hormone in gene deletion: Start 0.04 to 0.08 mg/kg SC bid. As tolerated, increase at weekly intervals by 0.04 mg/kg per dose to maximum of 0.12 mg/kg bid. Administer within 20 min of meal or snack. Omit dose if patient will skip meal.

(cont.)

MECASERMIN (cont.)
FORMS — Trade only: 40 mg multidose vial.
NOTES — Monitor preprandial glucose at initiation and until stable dose. Reduce dose if hypoglycemia occurs despite adequate food intake. Do not use with closed epiphyses or malignancy. Do not give IV. Contains benzyl alcohol.
MOA — Recombinant human IGF-1.
ADVERSE EFFECTS — Serious: Hypoglycemia, intracranial hypertension, hepatomegaly, hypersensitivity, antibody production, slipped capital femoral epiphysis, tonsillar hypertrophy. Frequent: Lipohypertrophy, increased LFTs, snoring, otitis, headache, localized pain, arthralgia, injection site pain.

PEGVISOMANT (*Somavert*) ▶? ♀B ▶? $$$$$
ADULTS — <u>Acromegaly unresponsive to other therapies:</u> Load 40 mg SC on day 1, then maintenance 10 mg SC daily. Max 30 mg/day.
PEDS — Not approved in children.
FORMS — Trade only: 10, 15, 20 mg single-dose vials. Available only from manufacturer.
NOTES — Orphan drug. May cause elevations of growth hormone levels and pituitary tumor growth; periodically image sella turcica. May increase glucose tolerance. May cause IGF-1 deficiency, monitor IGF-1 4 to 6 weeks after initiation or dose change and q 6 months after IGF-1 normalizes. May elevate LFTs; obtain baseline LFTs then check monthly for 6 months, quarterly for the next 6 months and biannually for the next year. Refer to manufacturer's guideline when initiating with abnormal LFTs. Dose adjustment should be every 4 to 6 weeks in 5 mg increment and based on IGF-1. Rotate injection site to prevent lipohypertrophy.
MOA — Growth hormone receptor antagonist.
ADVERSE EFFECTS — Serious: Tumor growth, IGF-1 deficiency. Frequent: Abnormal LFTs, infection, sinusitis, pain, injection site reaction, lipohypertrophy, back pain, dizziness, peripheral edema.

SODIUM POLYSTYRENE SULFONATE (*Kayexalate*)
▶Fecal excretion ♀C ▶? $$$$
ADULTS — <u>Hyperkalemia:</u> 15 g PO daily to qid or 30 to 50 g retention enema (in sorbitol) q 6 h prn. Retain for 30 min to several h. Irrigate with tap water after enema to prevent necrosis.
PEDS — <u>Hyperkalemia:</u> 1 g/kg PO q 6 h.
UNAPPROVED PEDS — <u>Hyperkalemia:</u> 1 g/kg PR q 2 to 6 h.
FORMS — Generic only: Susp 15 g/60 mL. Powdered resin.
NOTES — 1 g binds approximately 1 mEq of potassium. Avoid in bowel obstruction or constipation. Follow aspiration cautions during administration.
MOA — Cation exchange resin that reduces potassium in exchange for sodium.
ADVERSE EFFECTS — Serious: Hypokalemia, hypocalcemia, intestinal obstruction. Frequent: Sodium and water retention, gastric irritation, anorexia, N/V, constipation.

SOMATROPIN (human growth hormone, *Genotropin, Humatrope, Norditropin, Norditropin NordiFlex, Nutropin, Nutropin AQ, Nutropin Depot, Omnitrope, Protropin, Serostim, Serostim LQ, Saizen, Tev-Tropin, Valtropin, Zorbtive*) ▶LK ♀B/C ▶? $$$$$
WARNING — Avoid in patients with Prader-Willi syndrome who are severely obese, have severe respiratory impairment or sleep apnea, or unidentified respiratory infection; fatalities have been reported.
ADULTS — <u>Growth hormone deficiency</u> (Genotropin, Humatrope, Nutropin, Nutropin AQ, Norditropin, Nutropin, Nutropin AQ, Omnitrope, Saizen, Valtropin): Doses vary according to product. <u>AIDS wasting or cachexia</u> (Serostim, Serostim LQ): 0.1 mg/kg SC daily, max 6 mg daily. <u>Short bowel syndrome</u> (Zorbtive): 0.1 mg/kg SC daily, max 8 mg daily.
PEDS — <u>Growth hormone deficiency</u> (Genotropin, Humatrope, Norditropin, Nutropin, Nutropin AQ, Nutropin Depot, Omnitrope, Tev-Tropin, Saizen): Doses vary according to product used. Turner syndrome (Genotropin, Humatrope, Norditropin, Nutropin, Nutropin AQ, Valtropin): Doses vary according to product used. <u>Growth failure in Prader-Willi syndrome</u> (Genotropin, Omnitrope): Individualized dosing. <u>Idiopathic short stature</u> (Genotropin, Humatrope): Individualized dosing. <u>SHOX deficiency</u> (Humatrope): Individualized dosing. <u>Short stature in Noonan syndrome</u> (Norditropin): Individualized dosing. <u>Growth failure in chronic renal insufficiency</u> (Nutropin, Nutropin AQ): Individualized dosing. <u>Short stature in small for gestational age children</u> (Humatrope, Norditropin, Omnitrope): Individualized dosing.
FORMS — Single-dose vials (powder for injection with diluent). Tev-Tropin: 5 mg vial (powder for injection with diluent, stable for 14 days when refrigerated). Genotropin: 1.5, 5.8, 13.8 mg cartridges. Humatrope: 6, 12, 24 mg pen cartridges; 5 mg vial (powder for injection with diluent, stable for 14 days when refrigerated). Nutropin AQ: 10 mg multidose vial, 5, 10, 20 mg/pen cartridges. Norditropin: 5, 10, 15 mg pen cartridges. Norditropin NordiFlex: 5, 10, 15 mg prefilled pens. Omnitrope: 1.5, 5.8 mg vial (powder for injection with diluent). Saizen: Preassembled reconstitution device with autoinjector pen. Serostim: 4, 5, 6 mg single-dose vials; 4, 8.8 mg multidose vials; and 8.8 mg cartridges for autoinjector. Valtropin: 5 mg single-dose vials, 5 mg prefilled syringe. Zorbtive: 8.8 mg vial (powder for injection with diluent, stable for 14 days when refrigerated).
NOTES — Do not use in children with closed epiphyses. Contraindicated in active malignancy or acute critical illness. Monitor glucose for insulin resistance; use with caution if diabetes or risk for diabetes. Transient and dose-dependent fluid retention may occur in adults. May cause hypothyroidism. Monitor thyroid function periodically. Evaluate patients with Prader-Willi syndrome for upper airway obstruction and sleep apnea prior to treatment; control wt and monitor for signs and symptoms of respiratory infection. Avoid if pre-proliferative or proliferative diabetic retinopathy. Perform funduscopic exam initially and then periodically. Monitor other hormonal replacement

(cont.)

SOMATROPIN *(cont.)*
treatments closely in patients with hypopituitarism (multiple pituitary hormone deficiencies).
MOA — Recombinantly derived human growth hormone that stimulates production of IGF-1.
ADVERSE EFFECTS — Serious: Diabetes, antibody production, leukemia, pancreatitis, intracranial hypertension, dyspnea. Frequent: Edema, increased nevi size, gynecomastia, headache, localized pain, weakness, hyperglycemia, injection-site pain, hypothyroidism, hypertension, sleep apnea.

TERIPARATIDE *(Forteo)* ▶LK ♀C ▶– $$$$$
WARNING — Osteosarcoma in animal studies; avoid in those at risk (eg, Paget's disease, prior skeletal radiation).
ADULTS — <u>Treatment of postmenopausal osteoporosis, treatment of men and women with glucocorticoid-induced osteoporosis or to increase bone mass in men with primary or hypogonadal osteoporosis and high risk for fracture:</u> 20 mcg SC daily in thigh or abdomen for no longer than 2 years.
PEDS — Not approved in children.
FORMS — Trade only: 28 dose pen injector (20 mcg/dose).
NOTES — Take with calcium and vitamin D. Pen-like delivery device requires education, and should be discarded 28 days after first injection even if not empty.
MOA — Parathyroid hormone analogue that stimulates trabecular and cortical bone formation.
ADVERSE EFFECTS — Serious: Orthostatic hypotension, HTN, angina, hypercalcemia, hyperuricemia. Frequent: Dizziness, leg cramps/spasms, back spasm, asthenia, arthralgia, depression, insomnia, dyspepsia.

TOLVAPTAN *(Samsca)* ▶K ♀C ▶? $$$$$
WARNING — Start and restart therapy in the hospital setting to closely monitor serum sodium. Avoid rapid correction of serum sodium (> 12 mEq/L/24 h); rapid correction may cause osmotic demyelination causing death or symptoms including dysarthria, dysphagia, lethargy, seizures or coma. Slower correction advised in higher risk patients including malnutrition, alcoholism or advanced liver disease.
ADULTS — <u>Euvolemic or hypervolemic hyponatremia</u> (sodium < 125 mEq/L): Start 15 mg daily. Titrate to desired serum sodium. If needed, increase q 24 h or more slowly to 30 mg daily; max dose 60 mg daily.
PEDS — Not approved in children.
FORMS — Trade only: Tabs 15, 30 mg.
NOTES — Avoid fluid restriction for first 24 h. May use for hyponatremia secondary to heart failure, cirrhosis or SIADH. May use in hyponatremia with sodium > 125 mEq/L if resistant to fluid restriction and symptomatic. Do not use if urgent rise in serum sodium needed or serious neurologic symptoms. Requires frequent monitoring of serum sodium, volume, and neurologic status; monitor potassium if baseline K > 5 mEq/L. Administer through large veins and change infusion site daily to minimize irritation. Avoid concurrent use of strong or moderate CYP3A4 inhibitors or inducers.
MOA — Selective vasopressin V2-receptor antagonist that promotes free water excretion to raise sodium levels.
ADVERSE EFFECTS — Serious: Hypotension, hypovolemia, GI bleed (in cirrhosis). Frequent: Thirst, dry mouth, asthenia, constipation, polyuria, hyperglycemia.

VASOPRESSIN *(Pitressin, ADH, ✦Pressyn AR)* ▶LK ♀C ▶? $$$$$
ADULTS — <u>Diabetes insipidus:</u> 5 to 10 units IM/SC bid to qid prn.
PEDS — Not approved in children.
UNAPPROVED ADULTS — <u>Cardiac arrest:</u> 40 units IV; may repeat if no response after 3 min. <u>Septic shock:</u> 0.01 to 0.1 units/min IV infusion, usual dose less than 0.04 units/min. <u>Bleeding esophageal varices:</u> 0.2 to 0.4 units/min initially (max 0.8 units/min).
UNAPPROVED PEDS — <u>Diabetes insipidus:</u> 2.5 to 10 units IM/SC bid to qid prn. <u>Bleeding esophageal varices:</u> Start 0.002 to 0.005 units/kg/min IV, increase prn to 0.01 units/kg/min. <u>Growth hormone and corticotropin provocative test:</u> 0.3 units/kg IM, max 10 units.
NOTES — Monitor serum sodium. Injectable form may be given intranasally. May cause tissue necrosis with extravasation.
MOA — Promotes water resorption (antidiuretic effect) and smooth muscle contraction; stimulates vasoconstriction of arterioles and capillaries.
ADVERSE EFFECTS — Serious: Angina, arrhythmia, myocardial ischemia, peripheral vasoconstriction, hypersensitivity, anaphylaxis (rare), water intoxication, chronic nephritis, severe vasoconstriction with tissue necrosis (if infusion extravasates). Frequent: Abdominal cramps, dizziness, flatulence, N/V, tremor, sweating, headache.

ENT: Antihistamines—Non-Sedating

NOTE: Antihistamines ineffective when treating the common cold.

DESLORATADINE *(Clarinex, ✦Aerius)* ▶LK ♀C ▶+ $$$
ADULTS — <u>Allergic rhinitis/urticaria:</u> 5 mg PO daily.
PEDS — <u>Allergic rhinitis/urticaria:</u> 2 mL (1 mg) PO daily for age 6 to 11 mo, ½ teaspoonful (1.25 mg) PO daily for age 12 mo to 5 yo, 1 teaspoonful (2.5 mg) PO daily for age 6 to 11 yo, 5 mg PO daily for age older than 12 yo.
FORMS — Trade only: Tabs 5 mg. Fast-dissolve RediTabs 2.5, 5 mg. Syrup 0.5 mg/mL.
NOTES — Increase dosing interval in liver or renal insufficiency to every other day. Use a measured dropper for syrup.
MOA — Antihistamine.
ADVERSE EFFECTS — Serious: None. Frequent: None.

FEXOFENADINE (*Allegra*) ▶LK ♀C ▶+ $$$
ADULTS — Allergic rhinitis, urticaria: 60 mg PO bid or 180 mg PO daily. 60 mg PO daily if decreased renal function.
PEDS — Allergic rhinitis, urticaria: 30 mg PO bid or orally disintegrating tab bid for age 2 to 11 yo. Use adult dose for age older than 12 yo. 30 mg PO daily if decreased renal function. Urticaria: 15 mg (2.5 mL) twice daily for age 6 mo to less than 2 yo. 15 mg PO daily if decreased renal function.
FORMS — Generic/Trade: Tabs 30, 60, 180 mg, Caps 60 mg. Trade only: Susp 30 mg/5 mL, orally disintegrating tab 30 mg.
NOTES — Avoid taking with fruit juice due to a large decrease in bioavailability. Do not remove orally disintegrating tab from its blister package until time of administration.
MOA — Antihistamine.
ADVERSE EFFECTS — Serious: None. Frequent: None.

LORATADINE (*Claritin, Claritin Hives Relief, Claritin ReditTabs, Alavert, Tavist ND*) ▶LK ♀B ▶+ $
ADULTS — Allergic rhinitis/urticaria: 10 mg PO daily.
PEDS — Allergic rhinitis/urticaria: 10 mg PO daily for age older than 6 yo, 5 mg PO daily (syrup) for age 2 to 5 yo.
FORMS — OTC Generic/Trade: Tabs 10 mg. Fast-dissolve tabs (Alavert, Claritin RediTabs) 5, 10 mg. Syrup 1 mg/mL. Rx Trade only (Claritin): Chewable tabs 5 mg, Liqui-gel caps 10 mg.
NOTES — Decrease dose in liver failure or renal insufficiency. Fast-dissolve tabs dissolve on tongue without water. ND indicates nondrowsy (Tavist).
MOA — Antihistamine.
ADVERSE EFFECTS — Serious: None. Frequent: None.

ENT: Antihistamines—Other

NOTE: Antihistamines ineffective when treating the common cold. Contraindicated in narrow-angle glaucoma, BPH, stenosing peptic ulcer disease, and bladder obstruction. Use half the normal dose in the elderly. May cause drowsiness and/or sedation, which may be enhanced with alcohol, sedatives, and other CNS depressants. Deaths have occurred in children younger than 2 yo attributed to toxicity from cough and cold medications; the FDA does not recommend their use in this age group.

CARBINOXAMINE (*Palgic*) ▶L ♀C ▶– $$$
ADULTS — Allergic/vasomotor rhinitis/urticaria: 4 to 8 mg PO tid to qid.
PEDS — Allergic/vasomotor rhinitis/urticaria: Give 2 mg PO tid to qid for age 2 to 3 yo, give 2 to 4 mg PO tid to qid for age 3 to 6 yo, give 4 to 6 mg PO tid to qid for age 6 yo or older.
FORMS — Generic/Trade: Oral soln 4 mg/5 mL. Tab 4 mg.
NOTES — Decrease dose in hepatic impairment.
MOA — Antihistamine.
ADVERSE EFFECTS — Serious: None. Frequent: Sedation, dizziness.

CETIRIZINE (*Zyrtec, ✦Reactine, Aller-Relief*) ▶LK ♀B ▶– $$$
ADULTS — Allergic rhinitis/urticaria: 5 to 10 mg PO daily.
PEDS — Allergic rhinitis/urticaria: 5 to 10 mg PO daily for age older than 6 yo. Peds: Give 2.5 mg PO daily for age 6 to 23 mo, give 2.5 mg PO daily to bid or 5 mg PO daily for age 2 to 5 yo. If age older than 12 mo, may increase to 2.5 mg PO bid.
FORMS — OTC Generic/Trade: Tabs 5, 10 mg. Syrup 5 mg/5 mL. Chewable tabs, grape flavored 5, 10 mg.
NOTES — Decrease dose in renal or hepatic impairment.
MOA — Antihistamine.
ADVERSE EFFECTS — Serious: None. Frequent: Sedation in 14%.

CHLORPHENIRAMINE (*Chlor-Trimeton, Aller-Chlor*) ▶LK ♀B ▶– $
ADULTS — Allergic rhinitis: 4 mg PO q 4 to 6 h. 8 mg PO q 8 to 12 h (timed-release) or 12 mg PO q 12 h (timed-release). Max 24 mg/day.
PEDS — Allergic rhinitis: 2 mg PO q 4 to 6 h (up to 12 mg/day) for age 6 to 11 yo, give adult dose for age 12 yo or older.
UNAPPROVED PEDS — Allergic rhinitis age 2 to 5 yo: 1 mg PO q 4 to 6 h (up to 6 mg/day). Timed release age 6 to 11 yo: 8 mg PO q 12 h prn.
FORMS — OTC Trade only: Tabs extended-release 12 mg. Generic/Trade: Tabs 4 mg. Syrup 2 mg/5 mL. Tabs extended-release 8 mg.
MOA — Antihistamine.
ADVERSE EFFECTS — Serious: None. Frequent: Sedation.

CLEMASTINE (*Tavist-1*) ▶LK ♀B ▶– $
ADULTS — Allergic rhinitis: 1.34 mg PO bid. Max 8.04 mg/day. Urticaria/angioedema: 2.68 mg PO daily-tid. Max 8.04 mg/day.
PEDS — Allergic rhinitis: Give 0.67 mg PO bid. Max 4.02 mg/day for age 6 to 12 yo, give adult dose for age 12 yo or older. Urticaria/angioedema: Give 1.34 mg PO bid (up to 4.02 mg/day) for age 6 to 12 yo, give adult dose for age 6 to 12 yo.
UNAPPROVED PEDS — Allergic rhinitis for age younger than 6 yo: 0.05 mg/kg/day (as clemastine base) PO divided bid to tid. Max dose 1 mg/day.
FORMS — OTC Generic/Trade: Tabs 1.34 mg. Rx: Generic/Trade: Tabs 2.68 mg, Syrup 0.67 mg/5 mL. Rx: Generic only: Syrup 0.5 mg/5 mL.
NOTES — 1.34 mg = 1 mg clemastine base.
MOA — Antihistamine.
ADVERSE EFFECTS — Serious: None. Frequent: Sedation, dry mouth.

CYPROHEPTADINE (*Periactin*) ▶LK ♀B ▶– $
ADULTS — Allergic rhinitis/urticaria: Start 4 mg PO tid, usual effective dose is 12 to 16 mg/day. Max 32 mg/day.

(cont.)

CYPROHEPTADINE (cont.)
PEDS — Allergic rhinitis/urticaria: Start 2 mg PO bid to tid (up to 12 mg/day) for age 2 to 6 yo, Start 4 mg PO bid to tid (up to 16 mg/day) for age 7 to 14 yo.
UNAPPROVED ADULTS — Appetite stimulant: 2 to 4 mg PO tid 1 h before meals. Prevention of cluster headaches: 4 mg PO qid. Treatment of acute serotonin syndrome: 12 mg PO/NG followed by 2 mg q 2 h until symptoms clear, then 8 mg q 6 h maintenance while syndrome remains active.
FORMS — Generic only: Tabs 4 mg. Syrup 2 mg/5 mL.
MOA — Antihistamine/5-HT 2A antagonist.
ADVERSE EFFECTS — Serious: None. Frequent: Sedation.

DEXCHLORPHENIRAMINE (*Polaramine*) ▶LK ♀? ▶– $$
ADULTS — Allergic rhinitis/urticaria: 2 mg PO q 4 to 6 h. Timed-release tabs: 4 or 6 mg PO at bedtime or q 8 to 10 h.
PEDS — Allergic rhinitis/urticaria: Immediate-release tabs and syrup: Give 0.5 mg PO q 4 to 6 h for age 2 to 5 yo, give 1 mg PO q 4 to 6 h for age 6 to 11 yo, give adult dose for age 12 yo or older. Timed Release Tabs age 6 to 12 yo: 4 mg PO daily, preferably at at bedtime.
FORMS — Generic only: Tabs immediate-release 2 mg, timed-release 4, 6 mg. Syrup 2 mg/5 mL.
MOA — Antihistamine.
ADVERSE EFFECTS — Serious: None. Frequent: Sedation.

DIPHENHYDRAMINE (*Benadryl, Banophen, Allermax, Diphen, Diphenhist, Dytan, Siladryl, Sominex, ✦Allerdryl, Nytol*) ▶LK ♀B ▶– $
ADULTS — Allergic rhinitis, urticaria, hypersensitivity reactions: 25 to 50 mg PO/IM/IV q 4 to 6 h. Max 300 to 400 mg/day. Motion sickness: 25 to 50 mg PO pre-exposure and q 4 to 6 h prn. Drug-induced parkinsonism: 10 to 50 mg IV/IM. Antitussive: 25 mg PO q 4 h. Max 100 mg/day. EPS: 25 to 50 mg PO tid to qid or 10 to 50 mg IV/IM tid to qid. Insomnia: 25 to 50 mg PO at bedtime.
PEDS — Hypersensitivity reactions: Give 12.5 to 25 mg PO q 4 to 6 h or 5 mg/kg/day PO/IV/IM divided qid for age 6 to 11 yo, give adult dose for age 12 yo or older. Max 150 mg/day. Antitussive (syrup): Give 6.25 mg PO q 4 h (up to 25 mg/day) for age 2 to 5 yo, give 12.5 mg PO q 4 h (up to 50 mg/day) for age 6 to 12 yo. EPS: 12.5 to 25 mg PO tid to qid or 5 mg/kg/day IV/IM divided qid, max 300 mg/day. Insomnia age 12 yo or older: 25 to 50 mg PO at bedtime.
FORMS — OTC Trade only: Tabs 25, 50 mg, Chewable tabs 12.5 mg. OTC and Rx: Generic only: Caps 25, 50 mg, softgel cap 25 mg. OTC Generic/Trade: Soln 6.25 or 12.5 mg per 5 mL. Rx: Trade only: (Dytan) Susp 25 mg/mL, Chewable tabs 25 mg.
NOTES — Anticholinergic side effects are enhanced in the elderly, and may worsen dementia or delirium. Avoid use with donepezil, rivastigmine, galantamine or tacrine.
MOA — Antihistamine.
ADVERSE EFFECTS — Serious: None. Frequent: Sedation, dry mouth.

HYDROXYZINE (*Atarax, Vistaril*) ▶L ♀C ▶– $$
ADULTS — Pruritus: 25 to 100 mg IM/PO daily to qid or prn.
PEDS — Pruritus: Give 50 mg/day PO divided qid for age younger than 6 yo, give 50 to 100 mg/day PO divided qid for age 6 or older.
FORMS — Generic only: Tabs 10, 25, 50, 100 mg; Caps 100 mg; Syrup 10 mg/5 mL. Generic/Trade: Caps 25, 50 mg, Susp 25 mg/5 mL (Vistaril). (Caps = Vistaril, Tabs = Atarax).
NOTES — Atarax (hydrochloride salt), Vistaril (pamoate salt).
MOA — Antihistamine.
ADVERSE EFFECTS — Serious: None. Frequent: Sedation.

LEVOCETIRIZINE (*Xyzal*) ▶K ♀B ▶– $$$
ADULTS — Allergic rhinitis/urticaria: 5 mg PO daily.
PEDS — Allergic rhinitis/urticaria: Give 2.5 mg PO daily for age 6 to 11 yo, give 5 mg PO daily for age 12 or older.
FORMS — Trade only: Tabs scored 5 mg; Oral soln 2.5 mg/5 mL (148 mL).
NOTES — Decrease dose in renal impairment.
MOA — Antihistamine.
ADVERSE EFFECTS — Serious: None. Frequent: Sedation.

MECLIZINE (*Antivert, Bonine, Medivert, Meclicot, Meni-D, ✦Bonamine*) ▶L ♀B ▶? $
ADULTS — Motion sickness: 25 to 50 mg PO 1 h prior to travel, then 25 to 50 mg PO daily.
PEDS — Not approved in children.
UNAPPROVED ADULTS — Vertigo: 25 mg PO daily to qid prn.
FORMS — Rx/OTC/Generic/Trade: Tabs 12.5, 25 mg; Chewable tabs 25 mg. Rx/Trade only: Tabs 50 mg.
NOTES — FDA classifies meclizine as "possibly effective" for vertigo. May cause dizziness and drowsiness.
MOA — Antihistamine.
ADVERSE EFFECTS — Serious: Tachycardia, confusion. Frequent: Dry mouth, constipation, drowsiness, dizziness, blurred vision, urinary retention, rash.

ENT: Antitussives / Expectorants

BENZONATATE (*Tessalon, Tessalon Perles*) ▶L ♀C ▶? $$
ADULTS — Cough: 100 to 200 mg PO tid. Max 600 mg/day.
PEDS — Cough: give adult dose for age older than 10 yo.
FORMS — Generic/Trade: Softgel caps: 100, 200 mg.
NOTES — Swallow whole. Do not chew. Numbs mouth; possible choking hazard.
MOA — Local anesthetic.
ADVERSE EFFECTS — Serious: None. Frequent: None.

ENT: Combination Products

DEXTROMETHORPHAN (*Benylin, Delsym, Dexalone, Robitussin Cough, Vick's 44 Cough*) ▶L ♀+ ▶+ $
- ADULTS — Cough: 10 to 20 mg PO q 4 h or 30 mg PO q 6 to 8 h. 60 mg PO q 12 h (Delsym).
- PEDS — Cough: Give either 2.5 to 5 mg PO q 4 h or 7.5 mg PO q 6 to 8 h of regular suspension or 15 mg PO q 12 h of sustained action liquid for age 2 to 5 yo, give either 5 to 10 mg PO q 4 h or 15 mg PO q 6 to 8 h of regular suspension, or 30 mg PO q 12 h of sustained action liquid for age 6 to 12 yo, give adult dose for age older than 12 yo.
- FORMS — OTC Trade only: Caps 15 mg (Robitussin), 30 mg (DexAlone), Susp, extended-release 30 mg/5 mL (Delsym). Generic/Trade: Syrup 5, 7.5, 10, 15 mg/5 mL. Generic only: Lozenges 5, 10 mg.
- NOTES — Contraindicated with MAOIs due to potential for serotonin syndrome.
- MOA — Cough suppressant by depressing medullary cough center.
- ADVERSE EFFECTS — Serious: None. Frequent: None.

GUAIFENESIN (*Robitussin, Hytuss, Guiatuss, Mucinex*) ▶L ♀C ▶+ $
- ADULTS — Expectorant: 100 to 400 mg PO q 4 h. 600 to 1200 mg PO q 12 h (extended-release). Max 2.4 g/day.
- PEDS — Expectorant: 50 to 100 mg/dose for age 2 to 5 yo, give 100 to 200 mg/dose for age 6 to 11 yo, give adult dose for age 12 yo or older.
- UNAPPROVED PEDS — Expectorant: Give 25 mg PO q 4 h (up to 150 mg/day) for age 6 to 11 mo, give 50 mg po q 4 h (up to 300 mg/day) for age 12 to 23 mo.
- FORMS — Rx Generic/Trade: Extended-release tabs 600, 1200 mg. OTC Generic/Trade: Liquid, Syrup 100 mg/5 mL. OTC Trade only: Caps 200 mg (Hytuss), Extended-release tabs 600 mg (Mucinex). OTC Generic only: Tabs 100, 200, 400 mg.
- NOTES — Lack of convincing studies to document efficacy.
- MOA — Expectorant.
- ADVERSE EFFECTS — Serious: None. Frequent: None.

ENT: Combination Products—OTC

NOTE: Decongestants in some ENT combination products can increase BP, aggravate anxiety or cause insomnia (use caution). Some contain sedating antihistamines. Sedation can be enhanced by alcohol and other CNS depressants. Some states have restricted or ended OTC sale of pseudoephedrine and pseudoephedrine combination products or reclassified it as a scheduled drug due to the potential for diversion to methamphetamine labs. Deaths have occurred in children younger than 2 yo attributed to toxicity from cough and cold medications; the FDA does not recommend their use in this age group.

ACTIFED COLD AND ALLERGY (phenylephrine + chlorpheniramine) ▶L ♀C ▶+ $
- ADULTS — Allergic rhinitis/nasal congestion: 1 tab PO q 4 to 6 h. Max 4 tabs/day.
- PEDS — Allergic rhinitis/nasal congestion: Give ½ tab PO q 4 to 6 h (up to 2 tabs/day) for age 6 to 12 yo, give adult dose for age older than 12 yo.
- FORMS — OTC Trade only: Tabs 10 mg phenylephrine/4 mg chlorpheniramine.
- MOA — Decongestant/antihistamine combination.
- ADVERSE EFFECTS — Serious: None. Frequent: Insomnia, palpitations, sedation.

ACTIFED COLD AND SINUS (pseudoephedrine + chlorpheniramine + acetaminophen) ▶L ♀C ▶+ $$
- ADULTS — Allergic rhinitis/nasal congestion/headache: 2 caps PO q 6 h. Max 8 caps/day.
- PEDS — Allergic rhinitis/nasal congestion/headache: Age older than 12 yo: Use adult dose.
- FORMS — OTC Trade only: Tabs 30 mg pseudoephedrine/2 mg chlorpheniramine/500 mg acetaminophen.
- MOA — Decongestant/antihistamine/analgesic combination.
- ADVERSE EFFECTS — Serious: None. Frequent: Insomnia, palpitations, sedation.

ALAVERT D-12 (pseudoephedrine + loratadine) ▶LK ♀B ▶– $
- ADULTS — Allergic rhinitis/nasal congestion: 1 tab PO bid.
- PEDS — Not approved in children.
- FORMS — OTC Generic/Trade: Tabs, 12 h extended-release, 120 mg pseudoephedrine/5 mg loratadine.
- NOTES — Decrease dose to 1 tab PO daily with CrCl < 30 mL/min. Avoid in hepatic insufficiency.
- MOA — Decongestant/antihistamine combination.
- ADVERSE EFFECTS — Serious: None. Frequent: Insomnia, palpitations, sedation.

ALEVE COLD AND SINUS (naproxen + pseudoephedrine) ▶L ♀C (D in 3rd trimester) ▶+ $
- ADULTS — Nasal/sinus congestion, fever and pain: 1 caps PO q 12 h.
- PEDS — Nasal/sinus congestion, fever and pain: Age older than 12 yo: Use adult dose.
- FORMS — OTC Generic/Trade: Extended-release caps: 220 mg naproxen sodium/120 mg pseudoephedrine.
- MOA — Decongestant/analgesic/antipyretic.
- ADVERSE EFFECTS — Serious: Hypersensitivity, GI bleeding, nephrotoxicity. Frequent: Insomnia, palpitations.

ALLERFRIM (pseudoephedrine + triprolidine) ▶L ♀C ▶+ $
- ADULTS — Allergic rhinitis/nasal congestion: 1 tab or 10 mL PO q 4 to 6 h. Max 4 tabs/day or 40 mL/day.
- PEDS — Allergic rhinitis/nasal congestion: Give ½ tab or 5 mL PO q 4 to 6 h (up to 2 tabs/day or 20 mL/day) for age 6 to 12 yo, give adult dose for age older than 12 yo.
- FORMS — OTC Trade only: Tabs 60 mg pseudoephedrine/2.5 mg triprolidine. Syrup 30 mg pseudoephedrine/1.25 mg triprolidine/5 mL.

(cont.)

ENT: Combination Products

ALLERFRIM *(cont.)*
MOA — Decongestant/antihistamine combination.
ADVERSE EFFECTS — Serious: None. Frequent: Insomnia, palpitations, sedation.

APRODINE **(pseudoephedrine + triprolidine)** ▶L ♀C ▶+ $
ADULTS — Allergic rhinitis/nasal congestion: 1 tab or 10 mL PO q 4 to 6 h. Max 4 tabs/day or 40 mL/day.
PEDS — Allergic rhinitis/nasal congestion: Age older than 12 yo: Use adult dose. 6 to 12 yo: ½ tab or 5 mL PO q 4 to 6 h. Max 2 tabs/day or 20 mL/day.
FORMS — OTC Trade only: Tabs 60 mg pseudoephedrine/2.5 mg triprolidine. Syrup 30 mg pseudoephedrine/1.25 mg triprolidine/5 mL.
MOA — Decongestant/antihistamine combination.
ADVERSE EFFECTS — Serious: None. Frequent: Insomnia, palpitations, sedation.

BENADRYL ALLERGY AND COLD **(phenylephrine + diphenhydramine + acetaminophen)** ▶L ♀C ▶− $
ADULTS — Allergic rhinitis/nasal congestion/headache: 2 tabs PO q 4 h. Max 12 tabs/day.
PEDS — Allergic rhinitis/nasal congestion/headache: Give 1 tab PO q 4 h (up to 5 tabs/day) for age 6 to 12 yo, give adult dose for age older than 12 yo.
FORMS — OTC Trade only: Tabs 5/12.5/325 mg of phenylephrine/diphenhydramine/acetaminophen.
MOA — Decongestant/antihistamine/analgesic combination.
ADVERSE EFFECTS — Serious: None. Frequent: Insomnia, palpitations, sedation.

BENADRYL-D ALLERGY AND SINUS **(phenylephrine + diphenhydramine)** ▶L ♀C ▶− $
ADULTS — Allergic rhinitis/nasal congestion: 1 tab PO q 4 h. Max 6 tabs/day.
PEDS — Allergic rhinitis/nasal congestion: Age older than 12 yo: Use adult dose.
FORMS — OTC Trade only: Tabs 10/25 mg phenylephrine/diphenhydramine.
MOA — Decongestant/antihistamine combination.
ADVERSE EFFECTS — Serious: None. Frequent: Insomnia, palpitations, sedation.

CHERACOL D COUGH **(guaifenesin + dextromethorphan, ✦*Benylin DME*)** ▶L ♀C ▶? $
ADULTS — Cough: 10 mL PO q 4 h.
PEDS — Cough: Give 2.5 mL PO q 4 h (up to 15 mL/day) for age 2 to 5 yo, give 5 mL PO q 4 h for age 6 to 11 yo, give adult dose for age 12 yo or older.
FORMS — OTC Generic/Trade: Syrup 100 mg guaifenesin/10 mg dextromethorphan/5 mL.
MOA — Expectorant/cough suppressant combination.
ADVERSE EFFECTS — Serious: None. Frequent: None.

CHILDREN'S ADVIL COLD **(ibuprofen + pseudoephedrine)** ▶L ♀C (D in 3rd trimester) ▶+ $
ADULTS — Not approved for use in adults.
PEDS — Nasal congestion/sore throat/fever: Give 5 ml PO q 6 h for age 2 to 5 yo, give 10 mL PO q 6 h for age 6 to 11 yo.
FORMS — OTC Trade only: Susp: 100 mg ibuprofen/15 mg pseudoephedrine/5 mL. Grape flavor, alcohol-free.

NOTES — Shake well before using. Do not use for > 7 days for cold, sinus, and flu symptoms.
MOA — Decongestant/anti-inflammatory/antipyretic combination.
ADVERSE EFFECTS — Serious: Allergic reactions. Frequent: Insomnia, palpitations.

CLARITIN-D 12 HR **(pseudoephedrine + loratadine)** ▶LK ♀B ▶+ $
ADULTS — Allergic rhinitis/nasal congestion: 1 tab PO bid.
PEDS — Not approved in children.
FORMS — OTC Generic/Trade: Tabs, 12 h extended-release: 120 mg pseudoephedrine/5 mg loratadine.
NOTES — Decrease dose to 1 tab PO daily with CrCl < 30 mL/min. Avoid in hepatic insufficiency.
MOA — Decongestant/antihistamine combination.
ADVERSE EFFECTS — Serious: None. Frequent: Insomnia, palpitations, sedation.

CLARITIN-D 24 HR **(pseudoephedrine + loratadine)** ▶LK ♀B ▶+ $
ADULTS — Allergic rhinitis/nasal congestion: 1 tab PO daily.
PEDS — Not approved in children.
FORMS — OTC Generic/Trade: Tabs, 24 h extended-release: 240 mg pseudoephedrine/10 mg loratadine.
NOTES — Decrease dose to 1 tab PO every other day with CrCl < 30 mL/min. Avoid in hepatic insufficiency.
MOA — Decongestant/antihistamine combination.
ADVERSE EFFECTS — Serious: None. Frequent: Insomnia, palpitations, sedation.

CORICIDIN HBP CONGESTION AND COUGH **(guaifenesin + dextromethorphan)** ▶LK ♀B ▶+ $$
ADULTS — Productive cough: 1 to 2 softgels PO q 4 h. Max 12 softgels/day.
PEDS — Productive cough: Give adult dose for 12 yo or older.
FORMS — OTC Trade only: Softgels 200 mg guaifenesin/10 mg dextromethorphan.
MOA — Expectorant/cough suppressant combination.
ADVERSE EFFECTS — Serious: None. Frequent: None.

CORICIDIN HBP COUGH AND COLD **(chlorpheniramine + dextromethorphan)** ▶LK ♀B ▶+ $
ADULTS — Rhinitis/cough: 1 tab q 6 h. Max 4 doses/day.
PEDS — Rhinitis/cough: Give adult dose for 12 yo or older.
FORMS — OTC Trade only: Tabs 4 mg chlorpheniramine/30 mg dextromethorphan.
MOA — Antihistamine/cough suppressant combination.
ADVERSE EFFECTS — Serious: None. Frequent: Sedation.

DIMETAPP COLD AND ALLERGY **(phenylephrine + brompheniramine)** ▶LK ♀C ▶− $
ADULTS — Allergic rhinitis/nasal congestion: 20 mL PO q 4 h. Max 4 doses/day.
PEDS — Allergic rhinitis/nasal congestion: 10 ml PO q 4 h for age 6 to 11 yo, give adult dose for 12 yo or older.
FORMS — OTC Trade only: Liquid, Tabs 2.5 mg phenylephrine/1 mg brompheniramine per tab or 5 mL.

(cont.)

ENT: Combination Products

DIMETAPP COLD AND ALLERGY (cont.)
NOTES — Grape flavor, alcohol-free.
MOA — Decongestant/antihistamine combination.
ADVERSE EFFECTS — Serious: None. Frequent: Insomnia, palpitations, sedation.

DIMETAPP COLD AND COUGH (phenylephrine + brompheniramine + dextromethorphan) ▶LK ♀C ▶– $
ADULTS — Nasal congestion/cough: 20 mL PO q 4 h. Max 6 doses/day.
PEDS — Nasal congestion/cough: Give 10 mL PO q 4 h (up to 6 doses/day) for age 6 to 11 yo, give adult dose for 12 yo or older.
FORMS — OTC Trade only: Liquid 2.5 mg phenylephrine/1 mg brompheniramine/5 mg dextromethorphan/5 mL.
NOTES — Red grape flavor, alcohol-free.
MOA — Decongestant/antihistamine/cough suppressant combination.
ADVERSE EFFECTS — Serious: None. Frequent: Insomnia, palpitations, sedation.

DIMETAPP NIGHTTIME COLD AND CONGESTION (phenylephrine + diphenhydramine) ▶LK ♀C ▶– $
ADULTS — Nasal congestion/runny nose/fever/cough/sore throat: 20 mL PO q 4 h. Max 5 doses/day.
PEDS — Nasal congestion/runny nose/fever/cough/sore throat: Give 10 mL PO q 4 h (up to 5 doses/day) for age 6 to 11 yo, give adult dose for 12 yo or older.
FORMS — OTC Trade only: Syrup 2.5 mg phenylephrine and 6.25 mg diphenhydramine.
NOTES — Bubble gum flavor, alcohol-free.
MOA — Decongestant/antihistamine/cough suppressant/analgesic combination.
ADVERSE EFFECTS — Serious: Hepatotoxicity. Frequent: Insomnia, palpitations, sedation.

DRIXORAL COLD AND ALLERGY (pseudoephedrine + dexbrompheniramine) ▶LK ♀C ▶– $
ADULTS — Allergic rhinitis/nasal congestion: 1 tab PO q 12 h.
PEDS — Allergic rhinitis/nasal congestion give adult dose for 12 yo or older.
FORMS — OTC Trade only: Tabs, sustained-action 120 mg pseudoephedrine/6 mg dexbrompheniramine.
MOA — Decongestant/antihistamine combination.
ADVERSE EFFECTS — Serious: None. Frequent: Insomnia, palpitations, sedation.

GUIATUSS PE (pseudoephedrine + guaifenesin) ▶L ♀C ▶– $
ADULTS — Nasal congestion/cough: 10 mL PO q 4 h. Max 40 mL/day.
PEDS — Nasal congestion/cough: Give 2.5 mL PO q 4 h for age 2 to 5 yo, give 5 mL PO q 4 h for age 6 to 11 yo, give adult dose for 12 yo or older. Max 4 doses/day.
FORMS — OTC Trade only: Syrup 30 mg pseudoephedrine/100 mg guaifenesin/5 mL.
NOTES — PE indicates pseudoephedrine.
MOA — Decongestant/expectorant combination.
ADVERSE EFFECTS — Serious: None. Frequent: Insomnia, palpitations.

MUCINEX D (guaifenesin + pseudoephedrine) ▶L ♀C ▶? $
WARNING — Multiple strengths; write specific product on Rx.
ADULTS — Cough/congestion: 2 tabs (600/60) PO q 12 h; max 4 tabs/24 h. 1 tab (1200/120) PO q 12 h; max 2 tabs/24 h.
PEDS — Cough: Give adult dose for 12 yo or older.
FORMS — OTC Trade only: Tabs, extended-release: 600/60, 1200/120 mg guaifenesin/pseudoephedrine.
NOTES — Do not crush, chew or break the tab. Take with a full glass of water.
MOA — Decongestant/expectorant combination.
ADVERSE EFFECTS — Serious: None. Frequent: Insomnia, palpitations.

MUCINEX DM (guaifenesin + dextromethorphan) ▶L ♀C ▶? $
WARNING — Multiple strengths; write specific product on Rx.
ADULTS — Cough: 1 to 2 tabs (600/30) PO q 12 h; max 4 tabs/24 h. 1 tab (1200/60) PO q 12 h; max 2 tabs/24 h.
PEDS — Cough: Give adult dose for 12 yo or older.
FORMS — OTC Trade only: Tabs, extended-release: 600/30, 1200/60 mg guaifenesin/dextromethorphan.
NOTES — DM indicates dextromethorphan. Do not crush, chew or break the tab. Take with a full glass of water.
MOA — Expectorant/cough suppressant combination.
ADVERSE EFFECTS — Serious: None. Frequent: None.

ROBITUSSIN CF (phenylephrine + guaifenesin + dextromethorphan) ▶L ♀C ▶– $
ADULTS — Nasal congestion/cough: 10 mL PO q 4 h.
PEDS — Nasal congestion/cough: Give 2.5 mL PO q 4 h for age 2 to 5 yo, give 5 mL PO q 4 h for age 6 to 11 yo, give adult dose for 12 yo or older.
FORMS — OTC Generic/Trade: Syrup 5 mg phenylephrine/100 mg guaifenesin/10 mg dextromethorphan/5 mL.
NOTES — CF indicates cough formula.
MOA — Decongestant/expectorant/cough suppressant combination.
ADVERSE EFFECTS — Serious: None. Frequent: Insomnia, palpitations.

ROBITUSSIN DM (guaifenesin + dextromethorphan) ▶L ♀C ▶+ $
ADULTS — Cough: 10 mL PO q 4 h. Max 60 mL/day.
PEDS — Cough: Give 2.5 mL PO q 4 h (up to 15 mL/day) for age 2 to 5 yo, give 5 mL PO q 4 h (up to 30 mL/day) for age 6 to 11 yo, give adult dose for 12 yo or older.
FORMS — OTC Generic/Trade: Syrup 100 mg guaifenesin/10 mg dextromethorphan/5 mL.
NOTES — Alcohol-free. DM indicates dextromethorphan.
MOA — Expectorant/cough suppressant combination.
ADVERSE EFFECTS — Serious: None. Frequent: None.

TRIAMINIC CHEST AND NASAL CONGESTION (phenylephrine + guaifenesin) ▶LK ♀C ▶– $
ADULTS – Child-only preparation.
PEDS – <u>Chest/nasal congestion:</u> Give 5 ml PO q 4 h (up to 6 doses/day) for age 2 to 6 yo, give 10 mL PO q 4 h (up to 6 doses/day) for age 6 to 12 yo.
FORMS – OTC Trade only, yellow label: Syrup 2.5 mg phenylephrine/50 mg guaifenesin/5 mL, tropical flavor.
MOA – Decongestant/expectorant combination.
ADVERSE EFFECTS – Serious: None. Frequent: Insomnia, palpitations.

TRIAMINIC COLD AND ALLERGY (phenylephrine + chlorpheniramine) ▶LK ♀C ▶– $
ADULTS – Child-only preparation.
PEDS – <u>Allergic rhinitis/nasal congestion:</u> 10 mL PO q 4 h to max 6 doses/day for age 6 to 12 yo.
FORMS – OTC Trade only, orange label: Syrup 2.5 mg phenylephrine/1 mg chlorpheniramine/5 mL, orange flavor.
MOA – Decongestant/antihistamine combination.
ADVERSE EFFECTS – Serious: None. Frequent: Insomnia, palpitations, sedation.

TRIAMINIC COUGH AND SORE THROAT (dextromethorphan + acetaminophen) ▶LK ♀C ▶– $
ADULTS – Child-only preparation.
PEDS – <u>Cough/sore throat:</u> Give PO q 4 h to max 5 doses/day: 5 mL or 1 softchew tab per dose for age 2 to 6 yo, give 10 mL or 2 softchew tabs per dose for age 7 to 12 yo.
FORMS – OTC Trade only, purple label: Syrup, Softchew tabs 5 mg dextromethorphan/160 mg acetaminophen/5 mL or tab, grape flavor.
MOA – Cough suppressant/analgesic combination.
ADVERSE EFFECTS – Serious: Hepatotoxicity. Frequent: Insomnia, palpitations.

TRIAMINIC DAY TIME COLD AND COUGH (phenylephrine + dextromethorphan) ▶LK ♀C ▶– $
ADULTS – Child-only preparation.
PEDS – <u>Nasal congestion/cough:</u> Give PO q 4 h to max 6 doses/day: 5 mL or 1 strip per dose for age 2 to 6 yo, give 10 mL or 2 stips per dose for age 7 to 12 yo.
FORMS – OTC Trade only, red label: Syrup, thin strips 2.5 mg phenylephrine/5 mg dextromethorphan/ 5 mL, cherry flavor.
NOTES – Allow strips to dissolve on the tongue.
MOA – Decongestant/cough suppressant combination.
ADVERSE EFFECTS – Serious: None. Frequent: Insomnia, palpitations, sedation.

TRIAMINIC FLU COUGH AND FEVER (acetaminophen + chlorpheniramine + dextromethorphan) ▶LK ♀C ▶– $
ADULTS – Child-only preparation.
PEDS – <u>Fever/cough:</u> 10 mL PO q 6 h to max 4 doses/day for age 6 to 12 yo.
FORMS – OTC Trade only, pink label: Syrup 160 mg acetaminophen/1 mg chlorpheniramine/7.5 mg dextromethorphan/5 mL, bubble gum flavor.
MOA – Analgesic/antihistamine/cough suppressant combination.
ADVERSE EFFECTS – Serious: None. Frequent: Insomnia, palpitations.

TRIAMINIC NIGHT TIME COLD AND COUGH (phenylephrine + diphenhydramine) ▶LK ♀C ▶– $
ADULTS – Child-only preparation.
PEDS – <u>Nasal congestion/cough:</u> 10 mL PO q 4 h to max 6 doses/day for age 6 to 12 yo.
FORMS – OTC Trade only, blue label: Syrup 2.5 mg phenylephrine/6.25 mg diphenhydramine/5 mL, grape flavor.
MOA – Decongestant/antihistamine combination.
ADVERSE EFFECTS – Serious: None. Frequent: Insomnia, palpitations, sedation.

ENT: Combination Products—Rx Only

NOTE: Decongestants in some ENT combination products can increase BP, aggravate anxiety or cause insomnia (use caution). Some contain sedating antihistamines. Sedation can be enhanced by alcohol and other CNS depressants. Deaths have occurred in children younger than 2 yo attributed to toxicity from cough and cold medications; the FDA does not recommend their use in this age group.

ALLEGRA-D 12-HOUR (fexofenadine + pseudoephedrine) ▶LK ♀C ▶+ $$$$
ADULTS – <u>Allergic rhinitis/nasal congestion:</u> 1 tab PO q 12 h.
PEDS – Not approved in children.
FORMS – Trade only: Tabs, extended-release 60/120 mg fexofenadine/pseudoephedrine.
NOTES – Decrease dose to 1 tab PO daily with decreased renal function. Take on an empty stomach. Avoid taking with fruit juice due to a large decrease in bioavailability.
MOA – Decongestant/antihistamine combination.
ADVERSE EFFECTS – Serious: None. Frequent: Insomnia, palpitations.

ALLEGRA-D 24-HOUR (fexofenadine + pseudoephedrine) ▶LK ♀C ▶+ $$$$
ADULTS – <u>Allergic rhinitis/nasal congestion:</u> 1 tab PO daily.
PEDS – Not approved in children.
FORMS – Trade only: Tabs, extended-release 180/240 mg fexofenadine/pseudoephedrine.
NOTES – Decrease dose to 1 tab PO every other days with decreased renal function. Take on an empty stomach. Avoid taking with fruit juice due to a large decrease in bioavailability.
MOA – Decongestant/antihistamine combination.
ADVERSE EFFECTS – Serious: None. Frequent: Insomnia, palpitations.

ENT: Combination Products

ALLERX (pseudoephedrine + methscopolamine + chlorpheniramine) ▶LK ♀C ▶– $$$
- ADULTS – Allergic rhinitis/vasomotor rhinitis/nasal congestion: 1 yellow AM tab qam and 1 blue PM tab qpm.
- PEDS – Allergic rhinitis/vasomotor rhinitis/nasal congestion: Use adult dose for age older than 12 yo.
- FORMS – Trade only: Tabs, AM (yellow): 120 mg pseudoephedrine/2.5 mg methscopolamine. PM (blue): 8 mg chlorpheniramine/2.5 mg methscopolamine.
- NOTES – Contraindicated in severe HTN, CAD, MAOI therapy, narrow angle glaucoma, urinary retention, and peptic ulcer. Caution in elderly, hepatic and renal disease.
- MOA – Decongestant/anticholinergic & antihistamine/anticholinergic combination.
- ADVERSE EFFECTS – Serious: Arrhythmia. Frequent: Insomnia, palpitations, dizziness, dry mouth, blurred vision, urinary retention.

BROMFENEX (pseudoephedrine + brompheniramine) ▶LK ♀C ▶– $
- ADULTS – Allergic rhinitis/nasal congestion: 1 cap PO q 12 h. Max 2 caps/day.
- PEDS – Allergic rhinitis/nasal congestion: Age older than 12 yo: Use adult dose. 6 to 11 yo: 1 cap PO daily.
- FORMS – Generic/Trade: Caps, sustained-release 120 mg pseudoephedrine/12 mg brompheniramine.
- MOA – Decongestant/antihistamine combination.
- ADVERSE EFFECTS – Serious: None. Frequent: Insomnia, palpitations, sedation.

BROMFENEX PD (pseudoephedrine + brompheniramine) ▶LK ♀C ▶– $
- ADULTS – Allergic rhinitis/nasal congestion: 1 to 2 caps PO q 12 h. Max 4 caps/day.
- PEDS – Allergic rhinitis/nasal congestion: Age older than 12 yo: 1 cap PO q 12 h. Max 2 caps/day.
- FORMS – Generic/Trade: Caps, sustained-release 60 mg pseudoephedrine/6 mg brompheniramine.
- NOTES – PD indicates pediatric.
- MOA – Decongestant/antihistamine combination.
- ADVERSE EFFECTS – Serious: None. Frequent: Insomnia, palpitations, sedation.

CARBODEC DM (pseudoephedrine + carbinoxamine + dextromethorphan) ▶L ♀C ▶– $
- ADULTS – Allergic rhinitis/nasal congestion/cough: 5 mL PO qid.
- PEDS – Allergic rhinitis/nasal congestion/cough: Syrup give 2.5 mL PO qid for age 18 mo to 5 yo, give 5 mL PO qid for age older than 6 yo. Infant gtts: Give 0.25 mL PO qid for age 1 to 3 mo, give 0.5 mL PO qid for age 4 to 6 mo, give 0.75 mL PO qid for age 7 to 9 mo, give 1 mL PO qid for age 10 mo to 17 mo.
- FORMS – Generic only: Syrup, 60/4/15 mg pseudoephedrine/carbinoxamine/dextromethorphan/ 5 mL. Gtts, 25/2/4 mg/mL, grape flavor 30 mL with dropper, sugar-free.
- NOTES – Carbinoxamine has potential for sedation similar to diphenhydramine. DM indicates dextromethorphan.
- MOA – Decongestant/antihistamine/cough suppressant combination.
- ADVERSE EFFECTS – Serious: None. Frequent: Insomnia, palpitations, sedation.

CHERATUSSIN AC (guaifenesin + codeine) ▶L ♀C ▶? ©V $
- ADULTS – Cough: 10 mL PO q 4 h. Max 60 mL/day.
- PEDS – Cough: Give 1.25 to 2.5 mL PO q 4 h (up to 15 mL/day) for age 6 to 23 mo, give 2.5 to 5 mL PO q 4 h (up to 30 mL/day) for age 2 to 5 yo, give 5 mL PO q 4 h (up to 30 mL/day) for age 6 to 11 yo, give adult dose for age 12 or older.
- FORMS – Generic/Trade: Syrup 100 mg guaifenesin/10 mg codeine/5 mL. Sugar-free.
- MOA – Expectorant/cough suppressant combination.
- ADVERSE EFFECTS – Serious: Respiratory depression/arrest. Frequent: N/V, constipation, sedation.

CHERATUSSIN DAC (pseudoephedrine + guaifenesin + codeine) ▶L ♀C ▶? ©V $
- ADULTS – Nasal congestion/cough: 10 mL PO q 4 h. Max 40 mL/day.
- PEDS – Nasal congestion/cough: Give 5 mL PO q 4 h (up to 20 mL/day) for age 6 to 11 yo, give adult dose for 12 yo or older.
- FORMS – Generic/Trade: Syrup 30 mg pseudoephedrine/100 mg guaifenesin/10 mg codeine/ 5 mL. Sugar-free.
- NOTES – DAC indicates decongestant and codeine.
- MOA – Decongestant/expectorant/cough suppressant combination.
- ADVERSE EFFECTS – Serious: Respiratory depression/arrest. Frequent: N/V, constipation, sedation, insomnia, palpitations.

CHLORDRINE SR (pseudoephedrine + chlorpheniramine) ▶LK ♀C ▶– $
- ADULTS – Allergic rhinitis/nasal congestion: 1 cap PO q 12 h. Max 2 caps/day.
- PEDS – Allergic rhinitis/nasal congestion: 1 cap PO daily for age 6 to 11 yo, use adult dose for age 12 yo or older.
- FORMS – Generic only: Caps, sustained-release 120 mg pseudoephedrine/8 mg chlorpheniramine.
- MOA – Decongestant/antihistamine combination.
- ADVERSE EFFECTS – Serious: None. Frequent: Insomnia, palpitations, sedation.

CLARINEX-D 12 HOUR (pseudoephedrine + desloratadine) ▶LK ♀C ▶+ $$$$
- ADULTS – Allergic rhinitis: 1 tab PO q 12 h.
- PEDS – Allergic rhinitis age 12 yo or older: Use adult dose.
- FORMS – Trade only: Tabs, extended-release 120 mg pseudoephedrine/2.5 mg desloratadine.
- NOTES – Swallow tabs whole. Avoid with hepatic or renal insufficiency.
- MOA – Decongestant/antihistamine combination.
- ADVERSE EFFECTS – Serious: None. Frequent: Insomnia, palpitations.

CLARINEX-D 24 HOUR (pseudoephedrine + desloratadine) ▶LK ♀C ▶+ $$$$
- ADULTS – Allergic rhinitis: 1 tab PO daily.
- PEDS – Allergic rhinitis age 12 yo or older: Use adult dose.
- FORMS – Trade only: Tabs, extended-release pseudoephedrine + desloratadine, 120/2.5, 240/5 mg.

(cont.)

CLARINEX-D 24 HOUR *(cont.)*
NOTES — Instruct patients to swallow the tab whole. Increase dosing interval in renal insufficiency to every other day. Avoid with hepatic insufficiency.
MOA — Decongestant/antihistamine combination.
ADVERSE EFFECTS — Serious: None. Frequent: Insomnia, palpitations.

DECONAMINE **(pseudoephedrine + chlorpheniramine)** ▶LK ♀C ▶– $$
WARNING — Multiple strengths; write specific product on Rx.
ADULTS — Allergic rhinitis/nasal congestion: 1 tab or 10 mL PO tid to qid. Max 6 tabs or 60 mL/day. Sustained-release: 1 cap PO q 12 h. Max 2 caps/day.
PEDS — Allergic rhinitis/nasal congestion: Age older than 12 yo: Use adult dose. 6 to 11 yo: ½ tab or 5 mL PO tid to qid. Max 3 tabs or 30 mL/day.
FORMS — Trade only: Tabs 60/4 mg pseudoephedrine/chlorpheniramine, scored. Syrup 30/2 mg per 5 mL. Chewable tabs 15/1 mg. Generic/Trade: Caps, sustained-release 120/8 mg (Deconamine SR).
MOA — Decongestant/antihistamine combination.
ADVERSE EFFECTS — Serious: None. Frequent: Insomnia, palpitations, sedation.

DECONSAL II **(phenylephrine + guaifenesin)** ▶L ♀C ▶– $$
ADULTS — Nasal congestion/cough: 1 to 2 tabs PO q 12 h. Max 4 tabs/day.
PEDS — Nasal congestion/cough: Give ½ tab PO q 12 h (up to 1 tab/day) for age 2 to 5 yo, give 1 tab PO q 12 h up to tabs/day for 6 to 12 yo, give adult dose for age older than 12 yo.
FORMS — Trade only: Caps, sustained-release 20 mg phenylephrine/375 mg guaifenesin.
MOA — Decongestant/expectorant combination.
ADVERSE EFFECTS — Serious: None. Frequent: Insomnia, palpitations.

DICEL **(pseudoephedrine + chlorpheniramine)** ▶L ♀C ▶– $$
ADULTS — Allergic rhinitis/nasal congestion: 10 to 20 mL PO q 12 h. Max 40 mL/day.
PEDS — Allergic rhinitis/nasal congestion: Give 2.5 to 5 mL (up to 10 mL/day) PO q 12 h for age 2 to 5 yo, give 5 to 10 mL PO q 12 h (up to 20 mL/day) for age 6 to 11 yo, give adult dose for age 12 yo or older.
FORMS — Generic/Trade: Susp 75 mg pseudoephedrine/4.5 mg chlorpheniramine/5 mL, strawberry-banana flavor.
MOA — Decongestant/antihistamine combination.
ADVERSE EFFECTS — Serious: None. Frequent: Insomnia, palpitations, sedation.

DIMETANE-DX COUGH SYRUP **(pseudoephedrine + brompheniramine + dextromethorphan)** ▶L ♀C ▶– $$$
ADULTS — Nasal congestion/rhinitis/cough: 10 mL PO q 4 h prn.
PEDS — Nasal congestion/rhinitis/cough: Dose by wt: Give 1.25 mL PO qid prn for wt 12 to 22 kg, give 2.5 mL PO qid prn wt 23 to 40 kg. Dose by age: Give 2.5 mL PO q 4 h for age 2 to 5 yo, give 5 mL PO q 4 h for age 6 to 11 yo, give adult dosing for age older than 12 yo.

FORMS — Trade only: Liquid 30 mg pseudoephedrine/2 mg brompheniramine/10 mg dextromethorphan/5 mL, butterscotch flavor. Sugar-free.
MOA — Decongestant/antihistamine/cough suppressant combination.
ADVERSE EFFECTS — Serious: None. Frequent: Insomnia, palpitations, sedation.

DURATUSS **(phenylephrine + guaifenesin)** ▶L ♀C ▶– $
ADULTS — Nasal congestion/cough: 1 tab PO q 12 h.
PEDS — Nasal congestion/cough: Give ½ tab PO q 12 h for age 6 to 12, use adult dosing for age older than 12 yo.
FORMS — Generic/Trade: Tabs, long-acting 25 mg phenylephrine/900 mg guaifenesin.
MOA — Decongestant/expectorant combination.
ADVERSE EFFECTS — Serious: None. Frequent: Insomnia, palpitations.

DURATUSS GP **(phenylephrine + guaifenesin)** ▶L ♀C ▶– $
ADULTS — Nasal congestion/cough: 1 tab PO q 12 h.
PEDS — Not approved in children.
FORMS — Generic/Trade: Tabs, long-acting 25 mg phenylephrine/1200 mg guaifenesin.
MOA — Decongestant/expectorant combination.
ADVERSE EFFECTS — Serious: None. Frequent: Insomnia, palpitations.

DURATUSS HD **(hydrocodone + phenylephrine + guaifenesin)** ▶L ♀C ▶– ©III $$$
ADULTS — Cough/nasal congestion: 10 mL PO q 4 to 6 h.
PEDS — Cough/nasal congestion: Give 5 mL po q 4 to 6 h for age 6 to 12, use adult dosing for age older than 12 yo.
FORMS — Generic/Trade: Elixir 2.5 mg hydrocodone/10 mg phenylephrine/225 mg guaifenesin/5 mL. 5% alcohol.
MOA — Decongestant/expectorant/cough suppressant combination.
ADVERSE EFFECTS — Serious: Respiratory depression/arrest. Frequent: N/V, constipation, sedation, insomnia, palpitations.

ENTEX LA **(phenylephrine + guaifenesin)** ▶L ♀C ▶– $$
ADULTS — Nasal congestion/cough: 1 tab PO q 12 h.
PEDS — Nasal congestion/cough: Give ½ tab PO q 12 h for age 6 to 11 yo, give adult dose for 12 yo or older.
FORMS — Generic/Trade: Tabs, long-acting 30/600 mg phenylephrine/guaifenesin. Caps, long-acting 30/400 mg.
NOTES — Do not crush or chew.
MOA — Decongestant/expectorant combination.
ADVERSE EFFECTS — Serious: None. Frequent: Insomnia, palpitations.

ENTEX LIQUID **(phenylephrine + guaifenesin)** ▶L ♀C ▶– $$$
ADULTS — Nasal congestion/cough: 5 to 10 mL PO q 4 to 6 h. Max 40 mL/day.
PEDS — Nasal congestion/cough: Give 2.5 mL PO q 4 to 6 h (up 10 mL/day) for age 2 to 5 yo, give 5 mL PO q 4 to 6 h (up to 20 mL/day) for age 6 to 11 yo, give adult dose for age 12 or older.

(cont.)

ENT: Combination Products

ENTEX LIQUID *(cont.)*
FORMS – Generic/Trade: Liquid 7.5 mg phenylephrine/100 mg guaifenesin/5 mL. Punch flavor, alcohol-free.
MOA – Decongestant/expectorant combination.
ADVERSE EFFECTS – Serious: None. Frequent: Insomnia, palpitations.

ENTEX PSE (pseudoephedrine + guaifenesin) ▶L ♀C ▶– $
ADULTS – Nasal congestion/cough: 1 tab PO q 12 h.
PEDS – Nasal congestion/cough: Give ½ tab PO q 12 h for age 6 to 12 yo, use adult dosing for age older than 12 yo.
FORMS – Generic/Trade: Tabs, long-acting 120 mg pseudoephedrine/600 mg guaifenesin, scored.
NOTES – PSE indicates pseudoephedrine.
MOA – Decongestant/expectorant combination.
ADVERSE EFFECTS – Serious: None. Frequent: Insomnia, palpitations.

GANI-TUSS NR (guaifenesin + codeine) ▶L ♀C ▶? ©V $
ADULTS – Cough: 10 mL PO q 4 h. Max 60 mL/day.
PEDS – Cough: Give 1.25 to 2.5 mL PO q 4 h (up to 15 mL/day) for age 6 to 23 mo, give 2.5 to 5 mL PO q 4 h (up to 30 mL/day) for age 2 to 5 yo, give 5 mL PO q 4 h (up to 30 mL/day) for age 6 to 11 yo, give adult dosing for age 12 yo or older.
FORMS – Generic/Trade: Syrup 100 mg guaifenesin/10 mg codeine/5 mL. Sugar-free.
MOA – Expectorant/cough suppressant combination.
ADVERSE EFFECTS – Serious: Respiratory depression/arrest. Frequent: N/V, constipation, sedation.

GUAIFENEX DM (guaifenesin + dextromethorphan) ▶L ♀C ▶? $
ADULTS – Cough: 1 to 2 tabs PO q 12 h. Max 4 tabs/day.
PEDS – Cough: Give ½ tab PO q 12 h (up to 1 tab/day) for age 2 to 6 yo, give 1 tab PO q 12 h (up to 2 tabs/day) for age 6 to 12 yo, give adult dose for age 12 yo or older.
FORMS – Generic/Trade: Tabs, sustained-release 600 mg guaifenesin/30 mg dextromethorphan, scored.
NOTES – DM indicates dextromethorphan.
MOA – Expectorant/cough suppressant combination.
ADVERSE EFFECTS – Serious: None. Frequent: None.

GUAIFENEX PSE (pseudoephedrine + guaifenesin) ▶L ♀C ▶– $
WARNING – Multiple strengths; write specific product on Rx.
ADULTS – Nasal congestion/cough: PSE 60: 1 to 2 tabs PO q 12 h. Max 4 tabs/day. PSE 120: 1 tab PO q 12 h.
PEDS – Nasal congestion/cough: PSE 60: Give ½ tab PO q 12 h (up to 1 tab/day) for age 2 to 6 yo, give 1 tab PO q 12 h (up to 2 tabs/day) for age 6 to 12 yo, give adult dose for age 12 yo or older. PSE 120: ½ tab PO q 12 h for age 6 to 12 yo, give adult dose for age older than 12 yo.
FORMS – Generic/Trade: Tabs, extended-release 60/600 mg pseudoephedrine/guaifenesin, scored (Guaifenex PSE 60). Trade only: Tabs, extended-release 120/600 mg (Guaifenex PSE 120).
NOTES – PSE indicates pseudoephedrine.
MOA – Decongestant/expectorant combination.
ADVERSE EFFECTS – Serious: None. Frequent: Insomnia, palpitations.

GUAITEX II SR/PSE (pseudoephedrine + guaifenesin) ▶L ♀C ▶– $
WARNING – Multiple strengths; write specific product on Rx.
ADULTS – Nasal congestion/cough: 1 to 2 tabs PO q 12 h. Max 4 tabs/day (Guaitex II SR). 1 tab PO q 12 h. Max 2 tabs/day (Guaitex PSE).
PEDS – Nasal congestion/cough: (Guaitex II SR) give ½ tab PO q 12 h (up to 1 tab/day) for age 2 to 6 yo, give 1 tab PO q 12 h (up to 2 tabs/day) for age 6 to 12 yo, give adult dose for age 12 yo or older. (Guaitex PSE): Give ½ tab PO q 12 h for age 6 to 12 yo, give adult dose for age older than 12 yo.
FORMS – Generic/Trade: Tabs, sustained-release 60 mg pseudoephedrine/600 mg guaifenesin (Guaitex II SR). Trade only: Tabs, long-acting 120 mg pseudoephedrine/600 mg guaifenesin (Guaitex PSE).
NOTES – PSE indicates pseudoephedrine.
MOA – Decongestant/expectorant combination.
ADVERSE EFFECTS – Serious: None. Frequent: Insomnia, palpitations.

GUIATUSS AC (guaifenesin + codeine) ▶L ♀C ▶? ©V $
ADULTS – Cough: 10 mL PO q 4 h. Max 60 mL/day.
PEDS – Cough: Give 5 mL PO q 4 h (up to 30 mL/day) for age 6 to 11 yo, give adult dose for 12 yo or older.
FORMS – Generic/Trade: Syrup 100 mg guaifenesin/10 mg codeine/5 mL. Sugar-free.
NOTES – AC indicates before meals and codeine.
MOA – Expectorant/cough suppressant combination.
ADVERSE EFFECTS – Serious: Respiratory depression/arrest. Frequent: N/V, constipation, sedation.

GUIATUSSIN DAC (pseudoephedrine + guaifenesin + codeine) ▶L ♀C ▶– ©V $
ADULTS – Nasal congestion/cough: 10 mL PO q 4 h. Max 40 mL/day.
PEDS – Nasal congestion/cough: Give 5 mL PO q 4 h (up to 20 mL/day) for age 6 to 11 yo, give adult dose for 12 yo or older.
FORMS – Generic/Trade: Syrup 30 mg pseudoephedrine/100 mg guaifenesin/10 mg codeine/5 mL. Sugar-free.
NOTES – DAC indicates decongestant and codeine.
MOA – Decongestant/expectorant/cough suppressant combination.
ADVERSE EFFECTS – Serious: Respiratory depression/arrest. Frequent: N/V, constipation, sedation, insomnia, palpitations.

HALOTUSSIN AC (guaifenesin + codeine) ▶L ♀C ▶? ©V $
ADULTS – Cough: 10 mL PO q 4 h. Max 60 mL/day.

(cont.)

HALOTUSSIN AC (*cont.*)
- PEDS – <u>Cough:</u> Give 5 mL PO q 4 h (up to 30 mL/day) for age 6 to 11 yo, give adult dose for 12 yo or older.
- FORMS – Generic/Trade: Syrup 100 mg guaifenesin/10 mg codeine/5 mL. Sugar-free.
- NOTES – AC indicates before meals and codeine.
- MOA – Expectorant/cough suppressant combination.
- ADVERSE EFFECTS – Serious: Respiratory depression/arrest. Frequent: N/V, constipation, sedation.

HALOTUSSIN DAC (**pseudoephedrine + guaifenesin + codeine**) ▶L ♀C ▶– ©V $
- ADULTS – <u>Nasal congestion/cough:</u> 10 mL PO q 4 h. Max 40 mL/day.
- PEDS – <u>Nasal congestion/cough:</u> Give 5 mL PO q 4 h (up to 20 mL/day) for age 6 to 11 yo, give adult dose for 12 yo or older.
- FORMS – Generic/Trade: Syrup 30 mg pseudoephedrine/100 mg guaifenesin/10 mg codeine/5 mL. Sugar-free.
- NOTES – DAC indicates decongestant and codeine.
- MOA – Decongestant/expectorant/cough suppressant combination.
- ADVERSE EFFECTS – Serious: Respiratory depression/arrest. Frequent: N/V, constipation, sedation, insomnia, palpitations.

HISTINEX HC (**phenylephrine + chlorpheniramine + hydrocodone**) ▶L ♀C ▶– ©III $
- ADULTS – <u>Allergic rhinitis/congestion/cough:</u> 10 mL PO q 4 h. Max 40 mL/day.
- PEDS – <u>Allergic rhinitis/congestion/cough:</u> Give 5 mL PO q 4 h (up to 20 mL/day) for age 6 to 11 yo, give adult dose for 12 yo or older.
- FORMS – Generic/Trade: Syrup 5 mg phenylephrine/2 mg chlorpheniramine/2.5 mg hydrocodone/5 mL. Alcohol- and sugar-free.
- MOA – Decongestant/antihistamine/cough suppressant combination.
- ADVERSE EFFECTS – Serious: Respiratory depression/arrest. Frequent: N/V, constipation, sedation, insomnia, palpitations.

HISTUSSIN D (**pseudoephedrine + hydrocodone**) ▶L ♀C ▶– ©III $$
- ADULTS – <u>Nasal congestion/cough:</u> 5 mL PO qid prn.
- PEDS – <u>Nasal congestion/cough:</u> Give 1.25 mL PO qid prn for wt 12 to 22 kg, give 2.5 mL PO qid prn for wt 22 to 40 kg.
- FORMS – Generic/Trade: Liquid 60 mg pseudoephedrine/5 mg hydrocodone/5 mL, cherry/black raspberry flavor.
- MOA – Decongestant/cough suppressant combination.
- ADVERSE EFFECTS – Serious: Respiratory depression/arrest. Frequent: N/V, constipation, sedation, insomnia, palpitations.

HISTUSSIN HC (**phenylephrine + dexbrompheniramine + hydrocodone**) ▶L ♀C ▶– ©III $$
- ADULTS – <u>Allergic rhinitis/congestion/cough:</u> 10 mL PO q 4 h. Max 40 mL/day.
- PEDS – <u>Allergic rhinitis/congestion/cough:</u> Give 5 mL PO q 4 h (up to 20 mL/day) for age 6 to 11 yo, give adult dose for 12 yo or older.
- FORMS – Generic/Trade: Syrup 5 mg phenylephrine/1 mg dexbrompheniramine/2.5 mg hydrocodone/5 mL.
- MOA – Decongestant/antihistamine/cough suppressant combination.
- ADVERSE EFFECTS – Serious: Respiratory depression/arrest. Frequent: N/V, constipation, sedation, insomnia, palpitations.

HUMIBID DM (**guaifenesin + guaiacolsulfonate + dextromethorphan**) ▶L ♀C ▶? $
- ADULTS – <u>Cough:</u> 1 cap PO q 12 h. Max 2 caps/day.
- PEDS – <u>Cough:</u> Give 1 cap PO daily for age 6 to 12 yo, give adult dose for 12 yo or older.
- FORMS – Trade only: Caps, sustained-release 400 mg guaifenesin/200 mg guaiacolsulfonate/50 mg dextromethorphan.
- NOTES – DM indicates dextromethorphan.
- MOA – Expectorant/cough suppressant combination.
- ADVERSE EFFECTS – Serious: None. Frequent: None.

HUMIBID LA (**guaifenesin + guaiacolsulfonate**) ▶L ♀C ▶+ $
- ADULTS – <u>Expectorant:</u> 1 tab PO q 12 h (extended-release). Max 2 tabs/day.
- PEDS – Expectorant age older than 12 yo: Use adult dose.
- FORMS – Trade only: Tabs, extended-release 600 mg guaifenesin/300 mg guaiacolsulfonate.
- MOA – Expectorant combination.
- ADVERSE EFFECTS – Serious: None. Frequent: None.

HYCOCLEAR TUSS (**hydrocodone + guaifenesin**) ▶L ♀C ▶– ©III $
- ADULTS – <u>Cough:</u> 5 mL PO after meals and at bedtime. Max 6 doses/day.
- PEDS – <u>Cough:</u> Give 2.5 mL PO after meals and at bedtime (up to 6 doses/day) for age 6 to 12 yo, give adult dose for age older than 12 yo.
- FORMS – Generic/Trade: Syrup 5 mg hydrocodone/100 mg guaifenesin/5 mL. Generic is alcohol- and sugar-free.
- MOA – Expectorant/cough suppressant combination.
- ADVERSE EFFECTS – Serious: Respiratory depression/arrest. Frequent: N/V, constipation, sedation.

HYCODAN (**hydrocodone + homatropine**) ▶L ♀C ▶– ©III $
- ADULTS – <u>Cough:</u> 1 tab or 5 mL PO q 4 to 6 h. Max 6 doses/day.
- PEDS – <u>Cough:</u> Give 2.5 mg (based on hydrocodone) PO q 4 to 6 h prn (up to 15 mg/day) for age 6 to 12 yo, give adult dose for age older than 12 yo.
- FORMS – Generic/Trade: Syrup 5 mg hydrocodone/1.5 mg homatropine methylbromide/5 mL. Tabs 5/1.5 mg.
- NOTES – May cause drowsiness/sedation. Dosing based on hydrocodone content.
- MOA – Cough suppressant.
- ADVERSE EFFECTS – Serious: Respiratory depression/arrest. Frequent: N/V, constipation, sedation.

ENT: Combination Products

HYCOTUSS (hydrocodone + guaifenesin) ▶L ♀C ▶– ©III $
ADULTS – <u>Cough:</u> 5 mL PO after meals and at bedtime. Max 6 doses/day.
PEDS – <u>Cough:</u> Give 2.5 mL PO after meals and at bedtime (up to 6 doses/day) for age 6 to 12 yo, give adult dose for age older than 12 yo.
FORMS – Generic/Trade: Syrup 5 mg hydrocodone/ 100 mg guaifenesin/5 mL. Generic is alcohol- and sugar-free.
MOA – Expectorant/cough suppressant combination.
ADVERSE EFFECTS – Serious: Respiratory depression/arrest. Frequent: N/V, constipation, sedation.

NOVAFED A (pseudoephedrine + chlorpheniramine) ▶LK ♀C ▶– $
ADULTS – <u>Allergic rhinitis/nasal congestion:</u> 1 cap PO q 12 h. Max 2 caps/day.
PEDS – <u>Allergic rhinitis/nasal congestion:</u> 1 cap PO daily for age 6 to 12 yo, use adult dose for age older than 12 yo.
FORMS – Generic/Trade: Caps, sustained-release 120 mg pseudoephedrine/8 mg chlorpheniramine.
MOA – Decongestant/antihistamine combination.
ADVERSE EFFECTS – Serious: None. Frequent: Insomnia, palpitations, sedation.

PALGIC DS (pseudoephedrine + carbinoxamine) ▶L ♀C ▶– $$
ADULTS – <u>Allergic rhinitis/nasal congestion:</u> 10 mL PO qid.
PEDS – <u>Allergic rhinitis/nasal congestion:</u> Give up to the following PO qid: 1.25 mL for age 1 to 3 mo, 2.5 mL for age 3 to 6 mo, 3.75 mL for age 6 to 9 mo, 3.75 to 5 mL for age 9 to 18 mo, 5 ml for age 18 mo to 6 yo, use adult dose for age older than 6 yo.
FORMS – Generic/Trade: Syrup, 25 mg pseudoephedrine/2 mg carbinoxamine/5 mL. Alcohol- and sugar-free.
NOTES – Carbinoxamine has potential for sedation similar to diphenhydramine.
MOA – Decongestant/antihistamine combination.
ADVERSE EFFECTS – Serious: None. Frequent: Insomnia, palpitations, sedation.

PHENERGAN VC (phenylephrine + promethazine) ▶LK ♀C ▶? $
WARNING – Promethazine contraindicated if age younger than 2 yo due to risk of fatal respiratory depression; caution in older children.
ADULTS – <u>Allergic rhinitis/congestion:</u> 5 mL PO q 4 to 6 h. Max 30 mL/day.
PEDS – <u>Allergic rhinitis/congestion:</u> Give 1.25 to 2.5 mL PO q 4 to 6 h (up to 15 mL/day) for age 2 to 5 yo, give 2.5 to 5 mL PO for age q 4 to 6 h (up to 20 mL/day), give adult dose for age 12 yo or older.
FORMS – Trade unavailable. Generic only: Syrup 6.25 mg promethazine/5 mg phenylephrine/ 5 mL.
NOTES – VC indicates vasoconstrictor.
MOA – Decongestant/antihistamine combination.
ADVERSE EFFECTS – Serious: None. Frequent: Insomnia, palpitations, sedation.

PHENERGAN VC W/CODEINE (phenylephrine + promethazine + codeine) ▶LK ♀C ▶? ©V $
WARNING – Promethazine contraindicated if younger than 2 yo due to risk of fatal respiratory depression; caution in older children.
ADULTS – <u>Allergic rhinitis/congestion/cough:</u> 5 mL PO q 4 to 6 h. Max 30 mL/day.
PEDS – <u>Allergic rhinitis/congestion/cough:</u> Give 1.25 to 2.5 mL PO q 4 to 6 h (up to 10 mL/day) for age 2 to 5 yo, give 2.5 to 5 mL PO for age q 4 to 6 h (up to 20 mL/day), give adult dose for age 12 yo or older.
FORMS – Trade unavailable. Generic only: Syrup 5 mg phenylephrine/6.25 mg promethazine/10 mg codeine/5 mL.
MOA – Decongestant/antihistamine/cough suppressant combination.
ADVERSE EFFECTS – Serious: Respiratory depression/arrest. Frequent: N/V, constipation, sedation, insomnia, palpitations.

PHENERGAN WITH CODEINE (promethazine + codeine) ▶LK ♀C ▶? ©V $
WARNING – Promethazine contraindicated if younger than 2 yo due to risk of fatal respiratory depression; caution in older children.
ADULTS – <u>Allergic rhinitis/cough:</u> 5 mL PO q 4 to 6 h. Max 30 mL/day.
PEDS – <u>Allergic rhinitis/cough:</u> Give 1.25 to 2.5 mL PO q 4 to 6 h (up to 10 mL/day) for age 2 to 5 yo, give 2.5 to 5 mL PO for age q 4 to 6 h (up to 20 mL/day), give adult dose for age 12 yo or older.
FORMS – Trade unavailable. Generic only: Syrup 6.25 mg promethazine/10 mg codeine/5 mL.
MOA – Antihistamine/cough suppressant combination.
ADVERSE EFFECTS – Serious: Respiratory depression/arrest. Frequent: N/V, constipation, sedation.

PHENERGAN/DEXTROMETHORPHAN (promethazine + dextromethorphan) ▶LK ♀C ▶? $
WARNING – Promethazine contraindicated if younger than 2 yo due to risk of fatal respiratory depression; caution in older children.
ADULTS – <u>Allergic rhinitis/cough:</u> 5 mL PO q 4 to 6 h. Max 30 mL/day.
PEDS – <u>Allergic rhinitis/cough:</u> Give 1.25 to 2.5 mL PO q 4 to 6 h (up to 10 mL/day) for age 2 to 5 yo, give 2.5 to 5 mL PO for age q 4 to 6 h (up to 20 mL/day), give adult dose for age 12 yo or older.
FORMS – Trade unavailable. Generic only: Syrup 6.25 mg promethazine/15 mg dextromethorphan/5 mL.
MOA – Decongestant/cough suppressant combination.
ADVERSE EFFECTS – Serious: None. Frequent: Sedation.

PSEUDO-CHLOR (pseudoephedrine + chlorpheniramine) ▶LK ♀C ▶– $
ADULTS – <u>Allergic rhinitis/nasal congestion:</u> 1 cap PO q 12 h. Max 2 caps/day.
PEDS – <u>Allergic rhinitis/nasal congestion:</u> Age older than 12 yo: Use adult dose.

(cont.)

PSEUDO-CHLOR (cont.)
FORMS — Generic/Trade: Caps, sustained-release 120 mg pseudoephedrine/8 mg chlorpheniramine.
MOA — Decongestant/antihistamine combination.
ADVERSE EFFECTS — Serious: None. Frequent: Insomnia, palpitations, sedation.

ROBITUSSIN AC (guaifenesin + codeine) ▶L ♀C ▶? ©V $
ADULTS — The "Robitussin AC" brand is no longer produced; corresponding generics include Cheratussin AC, Gani-Tuss NR, Guiatuss AC, and Halotussin AC.
MOA — Expectorant/cough suppressant combination.
ADVERSE EFFECTS — Serious: Respiratory depression/arrest. Frequent: N/V, constipation, sedation.

ROBITUSSIN DAC (pseudoephedrine + guaifenesin + codeine) ▶L ♀C ▶– ©V $
ADULTS — The "Robitussin DAC" brand is no longer produced; corresponding generics include Cheratussin DAC, Guiatuss DAC, and Halotussin DAC.
MOA — Decongestant/expectorant/cough suppressant combination.
ADVERSE EFFECTS — Serious: Respiratory depression/arrest. Frequent: N/V, constipation, sedation, insomnia, palpitations.

RONDEC (phenylephrine + chlorpheniramine) ▶L ♀C ▶– $$
ADULTS — Allergic rhinitis/nasal congestion: 5 mL syrup PO qid.
PEDS — Allergic rhinitis/nasal congestion: Give 1.25 mL PO qid for age 2 to 5 yo, give 2.5 mL PO qid for age 6 to 12 yo, give adult dose for age older than 12 yo.
FORMS — Trade only: Syrup 12.5 mg phenylephrine/4 mg chlorpheniramine/5 mL, bubble-gum flavor. Alcohol- and sugar-free.
MOA — Decongestant/antihistamine combination.
ADVERSE EFFECTS — Serious: None. Frequent: Insomnia, palpitations, sedation.

RONDEC DM (phenylephrine + chlorpheniramine + dextromethorphan) ▶L ♀C ▶– $$
ADULTS — Allergic rhinitis/nasal congestion/cough: 5 mL syrup PO qid.
PEDS — Allergic rhinitis/nasal congestion/cough: Give 1.25 mL PO qid for age 2 to 5 yo, give 2.5 mL PO qid for age 6 to 12 yo, give adult dose for age older than 12 yo.
FORMS — Trade only: Syrup 12.5 mg phenylephrine/4 mg chlorpheniramine/15 mg dextromethorphan/5 mL, grape flavor. Alcohol- and sugar-free.
NOTES — DM indicates dextromethorphan.
MOA — Decongestant/antihistamine/cough suppressant combination.
ADVERSE EFFECTS — Serious: None. Frequent: Insomnia, palpitations, sedation.

RONDEC INFANT DROPS (phenylephrine + chlorpheniramine) ▶L ♀C ▶– $$
PEDS — Allergic rhinitis/nasal congestion: Give the following dose PO qid: 0.75 ml for age 6 to 12 mo, 1 mL for age 13 to 24 mo.
FORMS — Trade only: Gtts 3.5 mg phenylephrine/1 mg chlorpheniramine/mL, bubble-gum flavor, 30 mL. Alcohol- and sugar-free.
MOA — Decongestant/antihistamine combination.
ADVERSE EFFECTS — Serious: None. Frequent: Insomnia, palpitations, sedation.

RYNA-12 S (phenylephrine + pyrilamine) ▶L ♀C ▶– $$
PEDS — Nasal congestion, allergic rhinitis, sinusitis: Give 2.5 to 5 ML PO q 12 h for age 2 to 6 yo, give 5 to 10 mL PO q 12 h for age older than 6 yo.
FORMS — Generic/Trade: Susp 5 mg phenylephrine/30 mg pyrilamine/5 mL strawberry-currant flavor with graduated oral syringe.
MOA — Decongestant/antihistamine combination.
ADVERSE EFFECTS — Serious: None. Frequent: Insomnia, palpitations, sedation.

RYNATAN (phenylephrine + chlorpheniramine) ▶LK ♀C ▶– $$
ADULTS — Allergic rhinitis/nasal congestion: 1 to 2 tabs PO q 12 h.
PEDS — Allergic rhinitis/nasal congestion age 12 yo or older: 1 tab PO q 12 h.
FORMS — Trade only: Tabs, extended-release: 25/9 mg phenylephrine/chlorpheniramine. Chewable tabs 5/4.5 mg.
MOA — Decongestant/antihistamine combination.
ADVERSE EFFECTS — Serious: None. Frequent: Insomnia, palpitations, sedation.

RYNATAN PEDIATRIC SUSPENSION (phenylephrine + chlorpheniramine) ▶L ♀C ▶– $$$
PEDS — Nasal congestion, allergic rhinitis, sinusitis: Give 2.5 to 5 mL PO q 12 h for age 2 to 6 yo, give 5 to 10 mL PO q 12 h for age older than 6 yo.
FORMS — Trade only: Susp 5 mg phenylephrine/4.5 mg chlorpheniramine/5 mL strawberry-currant flavor.
MOA — Decongestant/antihistamine combination.
ADVERSE EFFECTS — Serious: None. Frequent: Insomnia, palpitations, sedation.

SEMPREX-D (pseudoephedrine + acrivastine) ▶LK ♀C ▶– $$
ADULTS — Allergic rhinitis/nasal congestion: 1 cap PO q 4 to 6 h. Max 4 caps/day.
PEDS — Not approved in children.
FORMS — Trade only: Caps 60 mg pseudoephedrine/8 mg acrivastine.
MOA — Decongestant/antihistamine combination.
ADVERSE EFFECTS — Serious: None. Frequent: Insomnia, palpitations, sedation.

TANAFED DMX (pseudoephedrine + dexchlorpheniramine + dextromethorphan) ▶L ♀C ▶– $$
ADULTS — Allergic rhinitis/nasal congestion: 10 to 20 mL PO q 12 h. Max 40 mL/day.
PEDS — Allergic rhinitis/nasal congestion: Give 2.5 to 5 mL PO q 12 h (up to 10 mL/day) for 2 to 5 yo, give 5 to 10 mL PO q 12 h (up to 20 mL/day) for age 6 to 11 yo, give adult dose for age 12 yo or older.
FORMS — Generic/Trade: Susp 75 mg pseudoephedrine/2.5 mg dexchlorpheniramine/25 mg dextromethorphan/5 mL, strawberry-banana flavor.
MOA — Decongestant/antihistamine/cough suppressant combination.
ADVERSE EFFECTS — Serious: None. Frequent: Insomnia, palpitations, sedation.

TUSS-HC (phenylephrine + chlorpheniramine + hydrocodone) ▶L ♀C ▶− ©III $
ADULTS − Allergic rhinitis/congestion/cough: 10 mL PO q 4 h. Max 40 mL/day.
PEDS − Allergic rhinitis/congestion/cough: Give 5 mL PO q 4 h (up to 20 mL/day) for age 6 to 12 yo, give adult dose for age older than 12 yo.
FORMS − Generic/Trade: Syrup 5 mg phenylephrine/2 mg chlorpheniramine/2.5 mg hydrocodone/5 mL.
MOA − Decongestant/antihistamine/cough suppressant combination.
ADVERSE EFFECTS − Serious: Respiratory depression/arrest. Frequent: N/V, constipation, sedation, insomnia, palpitations.

TUSSICAPS (chlorpheniramine + hydrocodone) ▶L ♀C ▶− ©III $$
ADULTS − Allergic rhinitis/cough: 1 full-strength cap PO q 12 h. Max 2 caps/day.
PEDS − Allergic rhinitis/congestion/cough: Give half strength cap PO q 12 h (up to 2 caps/day) for age 6 to 12 yo, give adult dose for age older than 12 yo.
FORMS − Trade only: Caps, extended-release 4/5 mg (half-strength), 8/10 mg (full strength) chlorpheniramine/hydrocodone.
MOA − Antihistamine/cough suppressant combination.
ADVERSE EFFECTS − Serious: Respiratory depression/arrest. Frequent: N/V, constipation, sedation.

TUSSIONEX (chlorpheniramine + hydrocodone) ▶L ♀C ▶− ©III $$$
ADULTS − Allergic rhinitis/cough: 5 mL PO q 12 h. Max 10 mL/day.
PEDS − Allergic rhinitis/cough: 2.5 mL PO q 12 h (up to 5 mL/day) for age 6 to 12 yo, give adult dose for age older than 12 yo.
FORMS − Generic/Trade: Extended-release susp 8 mg chlorpheniramine/10 mg hydrocodone/5 mL.
MOA − Antihistamine/cough suppressant combination.
ADVERSE EFFECTS − Serious: Respiratory depression/arrest. Frequent: N/V, constipation, sedation.

ZEPHREX-LA (pseudoephedrine + guaifenesin) ▶L ♀C ▶− $
ADULTS − Nasal congestion/cough: 1 tab PO q 12 h.
PEDS − Nasal congestion/cough: Give ½ tab PO q 12 h for age 6 to 12 yo, give adult dosing for age older than 12 yo.
FORMS − Trade only: Tabs, extended-release 120 mg pseudoephedrine/600 mg guaifenesin.
MOA − Decongestant/expectorant combination.
ADVERSE EFFECTS − Serious: None. Frequent: Insomnia, palpitations.

ZYRTEC-D (cetirizine + pseudoephedrine) ▶LK ♀C ▶− $$
ADULTS − Allergic rhinitis/nasal congestion: 1 tab PO q 12 h.
PEDS − Not approved in children.
FORMS − OTC Generic/Trade: Tabs, extended-release 5 mg cetirizine/120 mg pseudoephedrine.
NOTES − Decrease dose to 1 tab PO daily with decreased renal or hepatic function. Take on an empty stomach.
MOA − Decongestant/antihistamine combination.
ADVERSE EFFECTS − Serious: None. Frequent: Insomnia, palpitations, sedation.

ENT: Decongestants

NOTE: See ENT - Nasal Preparations for nasal spray decongestants (oxymetazoline, phenylephrine). Systemic decongestants are sympathomimetic and may aggravate HTN, anxiety, and insomnia. Use cautiously in such patients. Some states have restricted or ended OTC sale of pseudoephedrine or reclassified it as schedule III or V drug due to the potential for diversion to methamphetamine labs. Deaths have occurred in children younger than 2 yo attributed to toxicity from cough and cold medications; the FDA does not recommend their use in this age group.

PHENYLEPHRINE (Sudafed PE) ▶L ♀C ▶+ $
ADULTS − Nasal congestion: 10 mg PO q 4 h prn. Max 6 doses/day.
PEDS − Nasal congestion, age older than 12 yo: Use adult dose.
FORMS − OTC Trade only: Tabs 10 mg.
NOTES − Avoid with MAOIs.
MOA − Decongestant.
ADVERSE EFFECTS − Serious: None. Frequent: Dizziness, anxiety, insomnia.

PSEUDOEPHEDRINE (Sudafed, Sudafed 12 Hour, Efidac/24, Dimetapp Decongestant Infant Drops, PediaCare Infants' Decongestant Drops, Triaminic Oral Infant Drops, ✦Pseudofrin) ▶L ♀C ▶+ $
ADULTS − Nasal congestion: 60 mg PO q 4 to 6 h. 120 mg PO q 12 h (extended-release). 240 mg PO daily (extended-release). Max 240 mg/day.
PEDS − Nasal congestion give 15 mg PO q 4 to 6 h for age 2 to 5 yo, give: 30 mg PO q 4 to 6 h for age 6 to 12 yo, use adult dose for age older than 12 yo.
FORMS − OTC Generic/Trade: Tabs 30, 60 mg, Tabs, extended-release 120 mg (12 h), Soln 15, 30 mg/5 mL. Trade only: Chewable tabs 15 mg, Tabs, extended-release 240 mg (24 h).
NOTES − 12 to 24 h extended-release dosage forms may cause insomnia; use a shorter-acting form if this occurs.
MOA − Decongestant.
ADVERSE EFFECTS − Serious: None. Frequent: Insomnia, palpitations.

ENT: Ear Preparations

AURALGAN **(benzocaine + antipyrine)** ▶Not absorbed ♀C ▶? $
ADULTS — Otitis media, adjunct: Instill 2 to 4 gtts (or enough to fill the ear canal) tid to qid or q 1 to 2 h prn. Cerumen removal: Instill 2 to 4 gtts (or enough to fill the ear canal) tid for 2 to 3 days to detach cerumen, then prn for discomfort. Insert cotton plug moistened with soln after instillation.
PEDS — Otitis media, adjunct: Use adult dose. Cerumen removal: Use adult dose.
FORMS — Generic/Trade: Otic soln 10, 15 mL.
MOA — Local anesthetic/analgesic.
ADVERSE EFFECTS — Serious: None. Frequent: None.

CARBAMIDE PEROXIDE (*Debrox, Murine Ear*) ▶Not absorbed ♀? ▶? $
ADULTS — Cerumen impaction: Instill 5 to 10 gtts into ear bid for 4 days.
PEDS — Not approved in children.
FORMS — OTC Generic/Trade: Otic soln 6.5%, 15, 30 mL.
NOTES — Drops should remain in ear more than 15 min. Do not use for more than 4 days. Remove excess wax by flushing with warm water using a rubber bulb ear syringe.
MOA — Emulsifies/disperses ear wax.
ADVERSE EFFECTS — Serious: None. Frequent: None.

CIPRO HC OTIC **(ciprofloxacin + hydrocortisone)** ▶Not absorbed ♀C ▶− $$$$
ADULTS — Otitis externa: Instill 3 gtts into affected ear(s) bid for 7 days.
PEDS — Otitis externa age 1 yo or older: Use adult dose.
FORMS — Trade only: Otic susp 10 mL.
NOTES — Shake well. Contains benzyl alcohol.
MOA — Fluoroquinolone antibiotic/anti-inflammatory combination.
ADVERSE EFFECTS — Serious: None. Frequent: None.

CIPRODEX OTIC **(ciprofloxacin + dexamethasone)** ▶Not absorbed ♀C ▶− $$$$
ADULTS — Otitis externa: Instill 4 gtts into affected ear(s) bid for 7 days.
PEDS — Otitis externa and otitis media with tympanostomy tubes, age 6 mo or older: Instill 4 gtts into affected ear(s) bid for 7 days.
FORMS — Trade only: Otic susp 5, 7.5 mL.
NOTES — Shake well. Warm susp by holding bottle in hands for 1 to 2 min before instilling.
MOA — Fluoroquinolone antibiotic/anti-inflammatory combination.
ADVERSE EFFECTS — Serious: None. Frequent: None.

CIPROFLOXACIN (*Cetraxal*) ▶Not absorbed ♀C ▶− $$$$
ADULTS — Otitis externa: Instill 1 single-use container into affected ear(s) bid for 7 days.
PEDS — Otitis externa age 1 yo or older: Use adult dose.
FORMS — Trade only: 0.25 mL single-use containers with 0.2% ciprofloxacin soln, #14.
NOTES — Protect from light.
MOA — Fluoroquinolone antibiotic.
ADVERSE EFFECTS — Serious: None. Frequent: None.

CORTISPORIN OTIC **(hydrocortisone + polymyxin + neomycin, Pediotic)** ▶Not absorbed ♀? ▶? $
ADULTS — Otitis externa: Instill 4 gtts in affected ear(s) tid to qid up to 10 days.
PEDS — Otitis externa: Instill 3 gtts in affected ear(s) tid to qid up to 10 days.
FORMS — Generic only: Otic soln or susp 7.5, 10 mL.
NOTES — Caveats with perforated TMs or tympanostomy tubes: (1) Risk of neomycin ototoxicity, especially if use prolonged or repeated; (2) Use susp rather than acidic soln.
MOA — Antibiotic/anti-inflammatory combination.
ADVERSE EFFECTS — Serious: Ototoxicity. Frequent: None.

CORTISPORIN TC OTIC **(hydrocortisone + neomycin + thonzonium + colistin)** ▶Not absorbed ♀? ▶? $$$
ADULTS — Otitis externa: Instill 5 gtts in affected ear(s) tid to qid up to 10 days.
PEDS — Otitis externa: Instill 4 gtts in affected ear(s) tid to qid up to 10 days.
FORMS — Trade only: Otic susp, 10 mL.
MOA — Antibiotic/anti-inflammatory combination.
ADVERSE EFFECTS — Serious: None. Frequent: None.

DOMEBORO OTIC **(acetic acid + aluminum acetate)** ▶Not absorbed ♀? ▶? $
ADULTS — Otitis externa: Instill 4 to 6 gtts in affected ear(s) q 2 to 3 h.
PEDS — Otitis externa: Instill 2 to 3 gtts in affected ear(s) q 3 to 4 h.
FORMS — Generic only: Otic soln 60 mL.
NOTES — Insert a saturated wick. Keep moist for 24 h.
MOA — Antibacterial.
ADVERSE EFFECTS — Serious: None. Frequent: None.

FLUOCINOLONE—OTIC (*DermOtic*) ▶L ♀C ▶? $$
ADULTS — Chronic eczematous external otitis: Instill 5 gtts in affected ear(s) bid for 7 to 14 days.
PEDS — Chronic eczematous external otitis: Age 2 yo or older: Use adult dose.
FORMS — Trade only: Otic oil 0.01% 20 mL.
NOTES — Contains peanut oil.
MOA — Anti-inflammatory.
ADVERSE EFFECTS — Serious: None. Frequent: Burning, itching, irritation.

OFLOXACIN—OTIC (*Floxin Otic*) ▶Not absorbed ♀C ▶− $$$
ADULTS — Otitis externa: Instill 10 gtts in affected ear(s) daily for 7 days. Chronic suppurative otitis

OFLOXACIN—OTIC (cont.)
media: Instill 10 gtts in affected ear(s) bid for 14 days.
PEDS — Otitis externa: Instill 5 gtts in affected ear(s) daily for 7 days for age 1 to 12 yo, use adult dose for age 12 or older. Chronic suppurative otitis media for age older than 12 yo: Use adult dose. Acute otitis media with tympanostomy tubes age 1 to 12 yo: Instill 5 gtts in affected ear(s) bid for 10 days.
FORMS — Generic/Trade: Otic soln 0.3% 5, 10 mL. Trade only: "Singles": Single-dispensing containers 0.25 mL (5 gtts), 2 per foil pouch.
MOA — Fluoroquinolone antibiotic.
ADVERSE EFFECTS — Serious: None. Frequent: None.
SWIM-EAR (isopropyl alcohol + anhydrous glycerins) ▶Not absorbed ♀? ▶? $
ADULTS — Otitis externa, prophylaxis: Instill 4 to 5 gtts in ears after swimming, showering, or bathing.
PEDS — Otitis externa, prophylaxis: Use adult dose.
FORMS — OTC Trade only: Otic soln 30 mL.
MOA — Drying agent.
ADVERSE EFFECTS — Serious: None. Frequent: None.
VOSOL HC (acetic acid + propylene glycol + hydrocortisone) ▶Not absorbed ♀? ▶? $
ADULTS — Otitis externa: Instill 5 gtts in affected ear(s) tid to qid. Insert cotton plug moistened with 3 to 5 gtts q 4 to 6 h for the first 24 h.
PEDS — Otitis externa age older than 3 yo: Instill 3 to 4 gtts in affected ear(s) tid to qid. Insert cotton plug moistened with 3 to 4 gtts q 4 to 6 h for the first 24 h.
FORMS — Generic/Trade: Otic soln 2%/3%/1% 10 mL.
MOA — Antibacterial.
ADVERSE EFFECTS — Serious: None. Frequent: None.

ENT: Mouth and Lip Preparations

AMLEXANOX (*Aphthasol, OraDisc A*) ▶LK ♀B ▶? $
ADULTS — Aphthous ulcers: Apply ¼ inch paste or mucoadhesive patch to ulcer in mouth qid after oral hygiene for up to 10 days.
PEDS — Aphthous ulcers age older than 12 yo: Use adult dose.
FORMS — Trade only: Oral paste 5% (Apthasol), 3, 5 g tube. Mucoadhesive patch (OraDisc) 2 mg, #20.
NOTES — Mucoadhesive patch should be applied ≥80 min before bedtime to ensure its erosion before sleep. Up to 3 patches may be applied at one time. Avoid food or liquid for 1 h after application.
MOA — Anti-inflammatory.
ADVERSE EFFECTS — Serious: None. Frequent: Pain or burning at the site.
CEVIMELINE (*Evoxac*) ▶L ♀C ▶– $$$$$
WARNING — May alter cardiac conduction/heart rate; caution in heart disease. May worsen bronchospasm in asthma/COPD.
ADULTS — Dry mouth due to Sjogren's syndrome: 30 mg PO tid.
PEDS — Not approved in children.
FORMS — Trade only: Caps 30 mg.
NOTES — Contraindicated in narrow-angle glaucoma, acute iritis and severe asthma. May potentiate beta-blockers.
MOA — Cholinergic stimulant.
ADVERSE EFFECTS — Serious: AV block, arrhythmias, brady/tachycardia, pulmonary edema, bronchospasm, blurred vision, cholecystitis. Frequent: Sweating, nausea, rhinitis, flushing.
CHLORHEXIDINE GLUCONATE (*Peridex, Periogard, ✦Denticare*) ▶Fecal excretion ♀B ▶? $
ADULTS — Gingivitis: Bid as an oral rinse, morning and evening after brushing teeth. Rinse with 15 mL of undiluted soln for 30 sec. Do not swallow. Spit after rinsing.
PEDS — Not approved in children.
FORMS — Generic/Trade: Oral rinse 0.12% 473 to 480 mL bottles.
MOA — Antibacterial.
ADVERSE EFFECTS — Serious: Hypersensitivity. Frequent: Staining of teeth, calculus formation, and altered taste.
DEBACTEROL (sulfuric acid + sulfonated phenolics) ▶Not absorbed ♀C ▶+ $$
ADULTS — Aphthous stomatitis, mucositis: Apply to dry ulcer. Rinse with water.
PEDS — Not approved in children younger than 12 yo.
FORMS — Trade only: 1 mL prefilled, single-use applicator.
NOTES — 1 application per ulcer treatment. Dry ulcer area with cotton swab. Apply to ulcer and ring of normal mucosa around it for 5 to 10 sec. Rinse and spit. Return of ulcer pain right after rinsing indicates incomplete application; can be reapplied immediately once. Avoid eye contact. If excess irritation, rinse with dilute bicarbonate soln.
MOA — Topical analgesic + cauterizing agent.
ADVERSE EFFECTS — Serious: None. Frequent: Brief stinging during application.
GELCLAIR (maltodextrin + propylene glycol) ▶Not absorbed ♀+ ▶+ $$$
ADULTS — Aphthous ulcers, mucositis, stomatitis: Rinse mouth with 1 packet tid or prn.
PEDS — Not approved in children.
FORMS — Trade only: 21 packets/box.
NOTES — Mix packet with 3 tablespoons of water. Swish for 1 min, then spit. Do not eat or drink for 1 h after treatment.
MOA — Protective barrier.
ADVERSE EFFECTS — Serious: None. Frequent: None.
LIDOCAINE—VISCOUS (*Xylocaine*) ▶LK ♀B ▶+ $
WARNING — Avoid swallowing during oral or labial use due to GI absorption and toxicity. Measure dose

(cont.)

LIDOCAINE—VISCOUS *(cont.)*
exactly. May apply to small areas in mouth with a cotton-tipped applicator.
ADULTS — Mouth or lip pain: 15 to 20 mL topically or swish and spit q 3 h. Max 8 doses/day.
PEDS — Use with extreme caution, as therapeutic doses approach potentially toxic levels. Use the lowest effective dose. Mouth or lip pain age older than 3 yo: 3.75 to 5 mL topically or swish and spit up to q 3 h.
FORMS — Generic/Trade: Soln 2%, 20 mL unit dose, 100 mL bottle.
NOTES — High risk of adverse effects and overdose in children. Consider benzocaine as a safer alternative. Clearly communicate the amount, frequency, max daily dose, and mode of administration (eg, cotton pledget to individual lesions, ½ dropper to each cheek q 4 h, or 20 min before meals). Do not prescribe on a "prn" basis without specified dosing intervals.
MOA — Local anesthetic.
ADVERSE EFFECTS — Serious: Hypersensitivity. Frequent: Burning, stinging.

MAGIC MOUTHWASH (diphenhydramine + Mylanta + sucralfate) ▶LK ♀B(- in first trimester) ▶- $$$
ADULTS — See components.
PEDS — Not approved in children.
UNAPPROVED ADULTS — Stomatitis: 5 mL PO swish and spit or swish and swallow tid before meals and prn.
UNAPPROVED PEDS — Stomatitis: Apply small amounts to lesions prn.
FORMS — Compounded susp. A standard mixture is 30 mL diphenhydramine liquid (12.5 mg/5 mL)/60 mL Mylanta or Maalox/4 g Carafate.
NOTES — Variations of this formulation are available. The dose and decision to swish and spit or swallow may vary with the indication and/or ingredient. Some preparations may contain: Kaopectate, nystatin, tetracycline, hydrocortisone, 2% lidocaine, cherry syrup (for children). Check local pharmacies for customized formulations. Avoid diphenhydramine formulations that contain alcohol: May cause stinging of mouth sores.
MOA — Antihistamine/antacid/antiulcer combination.
ADVERSE EFFECTS — Serious: None. Frequent: Sedation, constipation, diarrhea.

PILOCARPINE (*Salagen*) ▶L ♀C ▶- $$$$
ADULTS — Dry mouth due to radiation of head and neck: 5 mg PO tid. May increase to 10 mg PO tid. Dry mouth due to Sjogren's syndrome: 5 mg PO qid. Hepatic dysfunction: 5 mg PO bid.
PEDS — Not approved in children.
UNAPPROVED ADULTS — Dry mouth due to Sjogren's syndrome: 2% pilocarpine eye gtts: Swish and swallow 4 gtts diluted in water tid ($).
FORMS — Generic/Trade: Tabs 5, 7.5 mg.
NOTES — Contraindicated in narrow-angle glaucoma, acute iritis and severe asthma. May potentiate beta-blockers.
MOA — Cholinergic stimulant.
ADVERSE EFFECTS — Serious: AV block, arrhythmias, brady/tachycardia, pulmonary edema, bronchospasm, blurred vision. Frequent: Sweating, urinary frequency, nausea, diarrhea, flushing, dizziness.

ENT: Nasal Preparations—Corticosteroids

NOTE: Decrease to the lowest effective dose for maintenance therapy. Tell patients to prime pump before first use and shake well before each subsequent use.

BECLOMETHASONE (*Vancenase, Vancenase AQ Double Strength, Beconase AQ*) ▶L ♀C ▶? $$$$
ADULTS — Allergic rhinitis/nasal polyp prophylaxis: Vancenase: 1 spray in each nostril bid to qid. Beconase AQ: 1 to 2 spray(s) in each nostril bid. Vancenase AQ Double Strength: 1 to 2 spray(s) in each nostril daily.
PEDS — Allergic rhinitis/nasal polyp prophylaxis: 1 spray in each nostril tid for age 6 to 12 yo, give adult dose for age older than 12 yo. Beconase AQ: 1 to 2 spray(s) in each nostril bid for age older than 6 yo. Vancenase AQ Double Strength: 1 to 2 spray(s) in each nostril daily for age older than 6 yo.
FORMS — Trade only: Vancenase 42 mcg/spray, 80 or 200 sprays/bottle. Beconase AQ 42 mcg/spray, 200 sprays/bottle. Vancenase AQ Double Strength 84 mcg/spray, 120 sprays/bottle.
NOTES — AQ (aqueous) formulation may cause less stinging.
MOA — Steroidal anti-inflammatory.
ADVERSE EFFECTS — Serious: Hypersensitivity, anaphylactoid reactions, urticaria, angioedema, bronchospasm, rash. Frequent: Nasal irritation.

BUDESONIDE—NASAL (*Rhinocort Aqua*) ▶L ♀B ▶? $$$$
ADULTS — Allergic rhinitis: 1 to 4 sprays per nostril daily.
PEDS — Allergic rhinitis age 6 yo or older: 1 to 2 sprays per nostril daily.
FORMS — Trade only: Nasal inhaler 120 sprays/bottle.
NOTES — CYP3A4 inhibitors such as ketoconazole, erythromycin, ritonavir, etc significantly increase systemic concentrations, possibly causing adrenal suppression.
MOA — Steroidal anti-inflammatory.
ADVERSE EFFECTS — Serious: Hypersensitivity. Frequent: Nasal irritation.

CICLESONIDE (*Omnaris*) ▶L ♀C ▶? $$$
ADULTS — Allergic rhinitis: 2 sprays per nostril daily.
PEDS — Allergic rhinitis, seasonal give adult dose for age 6 yo or older. Allergic rhinitis perennial give adult dose for age 12 yo or older.

(cont.)

CICLESONIDE (*cont.*)
 FORMS – Trade only: Nasal spray, 50 mcg/spray, 120 sprays/bottle.
 MOA – Steroidal anti-inflammatory.
 ADVERSE EFFECTS – Serious: None. Frequent: Epistaxis, headache.

FLUNISOLIDE (*Nasalide, Nasarel, ♦Rhinalar*) ▶L ♀C ▶? $$$
 ADULTS – Allergic rhinitis: 2 sprays per nostril bid, may increase to tid. Max 8 sprays/nostril/day.
 PEDS – Allergic rhinitis age 6 to 14 yo: 1 spray per nostril tid or 2 sprays per nostril bid. Max 4 sprays/nostril/day.
 FORMS – Generic/Trade: Nasal soln 0.025%, 200 sprays/bottle. Nasalide with pump unit. Nasarel with meter pump and nasal adapter.
 MOA – Steroidal anti-inflammatory.
 ADVERSE EFFECTS – Serious: Hypersensitivity. Frequent: Nasal irritation.

FLUTICASONE—NASAL (*Flonase, Veramyst*) ▶L ♀C ▶? $$$
 ADULTS – Allergic rhinitis: 2 sprays per nostril daily or 1 spray per nostril bid, decrease to 1 spray per nostril daily when appropriate. Seasonal allergic rhinitis alternative: 2 sprays per nostril daily prn.
 PEDS – Allergic rhinitis for age older than 4 yo: 1 to 2 sprays per nostril daily. Max 2 sprays/nostril/day. Seasonal allergic rhinitis alternative for age older than 12 yo: 2 sprays per nostril daily prn.
 FORMS – Generic/Trade: Flonase: Nasal spray 0.05%, 120 sprays/bottle. Trade only: (Veramyst): Nasal spray susp: 27.5 mcg/spray, 120 sprays/bottle.
 NOTES – CYP3A4 inhibitors such as ketoconazole, erythromycin, ritonavir, etc significantly increase systemic concentrations, possibly causing adrenal suppression.
 MOA – Steroidal anti-inflammatory.
 ADVERSE EFFECTS – Serious: Hypersensitivity. Frequent: Nasal irritation.

MOMETASONE—NASAL (*Nasonex*) ▶L ♀C ▶? $$$$
 ADULTS – Allergic rhinitis: 2 sprays per nostril daily.
 PEDS – Allergic rhinitis age 12 yo or older: Use adult dose. 2 to 11 yo: 1 spray per nostril daily.
 FORMS – Trade only: Nasal spray, 120 sprays/bottle.
 MOA – Steroidal anti-inflammatory.
 ADVERSE EFFECTS – Serious: Hypersensitivity. Frequent: Nasal irritation.

TRIAMCINOLONE—NASAL (*Nasacort AQ, Nasacort HFA, Tri-Nasal, AllerNaze*) ▶L ♀C ▶– $$$$
 ADULTS – Allergic rhinitis: Nasacort HFA, Tri-Nasal, AllerNaze: Start 2 sprays per nostril daily, may increase to 2 sprays/nostril bid. Max 4 sprays/nostril/day. Nasacort AQ: 2 sprays per nostril daily.
 PEDS – Allergic rhinitis: Nasacort and Nasacort AQ: 1 to 2 sprays per nostril daily for age 6 to 12 yo, give adult dose for age older than 12 yo. Nasacort AQ: 1 spray in each nostril once daily for age 2 to 5 yo.
 FORMS – Trade only: Nasal inhaler 55 mcg/spray, 100 sprays/bottle (Nasacort HFA). Nasal spray, 55 mcg/spray, 120 sprays/bottle (Nasacort AQ). Nasal spray 50 mcg/spray, 120 sprays/bottle (Tri-Nasal, AllerNaze).
 NOTES – AQ (aqueous) formulation may cause less stinging. Decrease to lowest effective dose after allergy symptom improvement.
 MOA – Steroidal anti-inflammatory.
 ADVERSE EFFECTS – Serious: Hypersensitivity. Frequent: Nasal irritation.

ENT: Nasal Preparations—Other

NOTE: For ALL nasal sprays except saline, oxymetazoline, and phenylephrine, tell patients to prime pump before first use and shake well before each subsequent use.

AZELASTINE—NASAL (*Astelin, Astepro*) ▶L ♀C ▶? $$$$
 ADULTS – Allergic/vasomotor rhinitis: 1 to 2 sprays/nostril bid.
 PEDS – Allergic rhinitis: 1 spray/nostril bid for age 5 to 11 yo, give adult dose for 12 yo or older. Vasomotor rhinitis give adult dose for 12 yo or older.
 FORMS – Generic: Nasal spray, 200 sprays/bottle.
 MOA – Antihistamine.
 ADVERSE EFFECTS – Serious: Atrial fibrillation. Frequent: Bitter taste, sedation.

CROMOLYN—NASAL (*NasalCrom*) ▶LK ♀B ▶+ $
 ADULTS – Allergic rhinitis: 1 spray per nostril tid to qid up to 6 times per day.
 PEDS – Allergic rhinitis for age 2 yo or older: Use adult dose.
 FORMS – OTC Generic/Trade: Nasal inhaler 200 sprays/bottle 13, 26 mL.
 NOTES – Therapeutic effects may not be seen for 1 to 2 weeks.
 MOA – Anti-inflammatory mast-cell stabilizer.
 ADVERSE EFFECTS – Serious: None. Frequent: None.

IPRATROPIUM—NASAL (*Atrovent Nasal Spray*) ▶L ♀B ▶? $$
 ADULTS – Rhinorrhea due to allergic/nonallergic rhinitis: 2 sprays (0.03%) per nostril bid to tid or 2 sprays (0.06%) per nostril qid. Rhinorrhea due to common cold: 2 sprays (0.06%) per nostril tid to qid.
 PEDS – Rhinorrhea due to allergic/nonallergic rhinitis: Give adult dose (0.03% strength) for age 6 yo or older, give adult dose (0.06% strength) for age 5 yo or older. Rhinorrhea due to common cold: 2 sprays (0.06% strength) per nostril tid for age 5 yo or older.
 UNAPPROVED ADULTS – Vasomotor rhinitis: 2 sprays (0.06%) in each nostril tid to qid.
 FORMS – Generic/Trade: Nasal spray 0.03%, 345 sprays/bottle, 0.06%, 165 sprays/bottle.
 MOA – Anticholinergic.
 ADVERSE EFFECTS – Serious: Hypersensitivity. Frequent: Nasal irritation, epistaxis.

LEVOCABASTINE—NASAL (✦Livostin Nasal Spray)
▶L (but minimal absorption) ♀C ▶– $$
ADULTS – Canada only. Allergic rhinitis: 2 sprays per nostril bid; increase prn to 2 sprays per nostril tid to qid.
PEDS – Not approved in children younger than 12 yo.
FORMS – Trade only: Nasal spray 0.5 mg/mL, plastic bottles of 15 mL. 50 mcg/spray.
NOTES – Nasal spray is devoid of CNS effects. Safety/efficacy in patients older than 65 yo has not been established.
MOA – Antihistamine.
ADVERSE EFFECTS – Frequent: Nasal irritation.

OLOPATADINE—NASAL (Patanase) ▶L ♀C ▶? $$$
ADULTS – Allergic rhinitis: 2 sprays/nostril bid.
PEDS – Allergic rhinitis age 12 yo or older: Use adult dose. For age 6-11 yo: 1 spray.nostril bid.
FORMS – Trade only: Nasal spray, 240 sprays/bottle.
MOA – Antihistamine.
ADVERSE EFFECTS – Serious: None. Frequent: Epistaxis, nasal irritation, bitter taste, sedation.

OXYMETAZOLINE (Afrin, Dristan 12 Hr Nasal, Nostrilla, Vicks Sinex 12 Hr) ▶L ♀C ▶? $
ADULTS – Nasal congestion: 2 to 3 sprays or gtts (0.05%) per nostril bid for no more than 3 days.
PEDS – Nasal congestion: Give 2 to 3 gtts (0.025%) per nostril bid no more than 3 days for age 2 to 5 yo, give 2 to 3 sprays or gtts (0.05%) per nostril bid not more than 3 days.
FORMS – OTC Generic/Trade: Nasal spray 0.05% 15, 30 mL; Nose gtts 0.025%, 0.05% 20 mL with dropper.
NOTES – Overuse (more than 3 to 5 days) may lead to rebound congestion. If this occurs, taper to use in 1 nostril only, alternating sides, then discontinue. Substituting an oral decongestant or nasal steroid may also be useful.
MOA – Decongestant.
ADVERSE EFFECTS – Serious: None. Frequent: Stinging, rebound congestion.

PHENYLEPHRINE—NASAL (Neo-Synephrine, Vicks Sinex) ▶L ♀C ▶? $
ADULTS – Nasal congestion: 2 to 3 sprays or gtts (0.25 or 0.5%) per nostril q 4 h prn for 3 days. Use 1% soln for severe congestion.
PEDS – Nasal congestion: Give 1 to 2 gtts (0.125% or 0.16%) per nostril q 4 h prn for 3 days for age 6 to 11 mo, give 2 to 3 gtts (0.125% or 0.16%) per nostril q 4 h prn for 3 days for age 1 to 5 yo, give 2 to 3 gtts or sprays (0.25%) per nostril q 4 h prn for 3 days for age 6 to 12 yo, give adult dose for age older than 12 yo.
FORMS – OTC Generic/Trade: Nasal gtts/spray 0.25, 0.5, 1% (15 mL).
NOTES – Overuse (more 3 to 5 days) may lead to rebound congestion. If this occurs, taper to use in 1 nostril only, alternating sides, then discontinue. Substituting an oral decongestant or nasal steroid may also be useful.
MOA – Decongestant.
ADVERSE EFFECTS – Serious: None. Frequent: Stinging, rebound congestion.

SALINE NASAL SPRAY (SeaMist, Entsol, Pretz, NaSal, Ocean, ✦HydraSense) ▶Not metabolized ♀A ▶+ $
ADULTS – Nasal dryness: 1 to 3 sprays per nostril prn.
PEDS – Nasal dryness: 1 to 3 gtts per nostril prn.
FORMS – Generic/Trade: Nasal spray 0.4, 0.5, 0.65, 0.75%, Nasal gtts 0.4, 0.65%. Trade only: Preservative-free nasal spray 3% (Entsol).
NOTES – May be prepared at home by combining: ¼ teaspoon salt with 8 ounces (1 cup) warm water. Add ¼ teaspoon baking soda (optional) and put in spray bottle, ear syringe, or any container with a small spout. Discard after 1 week.
MOA – Moisturizer.
ADVERSE EFFECTS – Serious: None. Frequent: None.

***CETACAINE* (benzocaine + tetracaine + butamben)** ▶LK ♀C ▶? $$
WARNING – Do not use on the eyes. Hypersensitivity (rare). Methemoglobinemia (rare).
ADULTS – Topical anesthesia of mucous membranes: Spray: Apply for 1 sec or less. Liquid or gel: Apply with cotton applicator directly to site.
PEDS – Use adult dose.
FORMS – Trade only: (14%/2%/2%) Spray 56 mL. Topical liquid 56 mL. Topical gel 5, 29 g.
NOTES – Do not hold cotton applicator in position for extended time due to increased risk of local reactions. Do not use multiple applications. Maximum anesthesia occurs 1 min after application; duration 30 min. May result in potentially dangerous methemoglobinemia; use minimum amount needed.
MOA – Local anesthetic combination.
ADVERSE EFFECTS – Serious: Hypersensitivity, methemoglobinemia. Frequent: Erythema, pruritus.

GASTROENTEROLOGY: Antidiarrheals

BISMUTH SUBSALICYLATE (Pepto-Bismol, Kaopectate) ▶K ♀D ▶? $
WARNING – Avoid in children and teenagers with chickenpox or flu due to possible association with Reye's syndrome.
ADULTS – Diarrhea: 2 tabs or 30 mL (262 mg/15 mL) PO q 30 to 60 min up to 8 doses/day for up to 2 days.
PEDS – Diarrhea: 100 mg/kg/day divided into 5 doses or 1/3 tab or 5 mL (262 mg/15 mL) q 30 to 60 min prn up to 8 doses/day for age 3 to 6 yo, 2/3 tab or 10 mL (262 mg/15 mL) q 30 to 60 min prn up to 8 doses/day for age 7 to 9 yo, 1 tab or 15 mL (262 mg/15 mL) q 30 to 60 min prn up to 8 doses/day for age 10 to 12 yo. Do not take for more than 2 days.
UNAPPROVED ADULTS – Prevention of traveler's diarrhea: 2.1 g/day or 2 tab qid before meals and at bedtime. Has been used as part of a multidrug regimen for Helicobacter pylori.
UNAPPROVED PEDS – Chronic infantile diarrhea: 2.5 mL (262 mg/15 mL) PO q 4 h for age 2 to 24 mo, 5 mL (262 mg/15 mL) PO q 4 h for age 25 to 48 mo, 10 mL (262 mg/15 mL) PO q 4 h for age 49 to 70 mo.

(cont.)

GASTROENTEROLOGY: Antidiarrheals

BISMUTH SUBSALICYLATE (cont.)
FORMS — OTC Generic/Trade: Chewable tabs 262 mg. Susp 262, 525, 750 mg/15 mL. OTC Trade only: Caps 262 mg (Pepto-Bismol). Susp 87 mg/5 mL (Kaopectate Children's Liquid).
NOTES — Use with caution in patients already taking salicylates or warfarin, children recovering from chickenpox or flu. Decreases absorption of tetracycline. May darken stools or tongue.
MOA — Antidiarrheal.
ADVERSE EFFECTS — Frequent: None.

IMODIUM MULTI-SYMPTOM RELIEF (loperamide + simethicone) ▶L ♀C ▶– $
ADULTS — Diarrhea: 2 caps PO initially, then 1 cap PO after each unformed stool to a maximum of 4 caps/day.
PEDS — Diarrhea: 1 cap PO initially, then ½ cap PO after each unformed stool (up to 2 caps/day for age 6 to 8 yo or wt 48 to 59 lbs, up to 3 caps/day for age 9 to 11 yo or wt 60 to 95 lbs).
FORMS — OTC Generic/Trade: Caps, Chewable tabs 2 mg loperamide/125 mg simethicone.
NOTES — Not for C difficile-associated diarrhea, toxigenic bacterial diarrhea, or most childhood diarrhea (difficult to exclude toxigenic).
MOA — Antidiarrheal, inhibits peristalsis of intestinal muscles.
ADVERSE EFFECTS — Frequent: Sedation in children.

LOMOTIL (diphenoxylate + atropine) ▶L ♀C ▶– ©V $
ADULTS — Diarrhea: 2 tabs or 10 mL PO qid.
PEDS — Diarrhea: 0.3 to 0.4 mg diphenoxylate/kg/24 h in 4 divided doses. Max daily dose 20 mg. Not recommended for younger than 2 yo, 1.5 to 3 mL PO qid for age 2 yo or wt 11 to 14 kg; 2 to 3 mL PO qid for age 3 yo or wt 12 to 16 kg; 2 to 4 mL PO qid for age 4 yo or wt 14 to 20 kg; 2.5 to 4.5 mL PO qid for age 5 yo or wt 16 to 23 kg; 2.5 to 5 mL PO qid for age 6 to 8 yo or wt 17 to 32 kg; 3.5 to 5 mL PO qid for 9 to 12 yo or wt 23 to 55 kg.
FORMS — Generic/Trade: Oral soln or tab 2.5 mg/0.025 mg diphenoxylate/atropine per 5 mL or tab.
NOTES — Give with food to decrease GI upset. May cause atropinism in children, especially with Down's syndrome, even at recommended doses. Can cause delayed toxicity. Has been reported to cause severe respiratory depression, coma, brain damage, death after overdose in children. Naltrexone reverses toxicity. Do not use for C difficile-associated diarrhea, toxigenic bacterial diarrhea, or most childhood diarrhea (difficult to exclude toxigenic).
MOA — Antidiarrheal, inhibits peristalsis of intestinal muscles.
ADVERSE EFFECTS — Frequent: Nervousness, dizziness, headache, depression, restlessness.

LOPERAMIDE (Imodium, Imodium AD, ✦Loperacap, Diarr-eze) ▶L ♀C ▶+ $
WARNING — Discontinue if abdominal distention or ileus. Caution in children due to variable response.
ADULTS — Diarrhea: 4 mg PO initially, then 2 mg after each unformed stool to max 16 mg/day.
PEDS — Diarrhea: First dose: 1 mg PO tid for age 2 to 5 yo or wt 13 to 20 kg, 2 mg PO bid for age 6 to 8 yo or wt 21 to 30 kg, 2 mg PO tid for age 9 to 12 yo or wt greater than 30 kg. After first day: give 0.1 mg/kg PO after each loose stool; daily dose not to exceed daily dose of first day.
UNAPPROVED ADULTS — Chronic diarrhea or ileostomy drainage: 4 mg initially then 2 mg after each stool until symptoms are controlled, then reduce dose for maintenance treatment, average adult maintenance dose 4 to 8 mg daily as a single dose or in divided doses.
UNAPPROVED PEDS — Chronic diarrhea: Limited information. Average doses of 0.08 to 0.24 mg/kg/day PO in 2 to 3 divided doses. Max 2 mg/dose. Max 16 mg/day.
FORMS — OTC Generic/Trade: Tabs 2 mg. Oral soln 1 mg/5 mL. OTC Trade only: Oral soln 1 mg/7.5 mL.
NOTES — Not for C difficile-associated diarrhea, toxigenic bacterial diarrhea, or most childhood diarrhea (difficult to exclude toxigenic).
MOA — Antidiarrheal, inhibits peristalsis of intestinal muscles.
ADVERSE EFFECTS — Frequent: Sedation in children.

MOTOFEN (difenoxin + atropine) ▶L ♀C ▶– ©IV $$
ADULTS — Diarrhea: 2 tabs PO initially, then 1 after each loose stool q 3 to 4 h prn (up to 8 tabs/day).
PEDS — Not approved in children. Contraindicated younger than 2 yo.
FORMS — Trade only: Tabs difenoxin 1 mg + atropine 0.025 mg.
NOTES — Do not use for C difficile-associated diarrhea, toxigenic bacterial diarrhea, or most childhood diarrhea (difficult to exclude toxigenic). May cause atropinism in children, especially with Down's syndrome, even at recommended doses. Can cause delayed toxicity. Has been reported to cause severe respiratory depression, coma, brain damage, death after overdose in children. Difenoxin is the primary metabolite of diphenoxylate.
MOA — Antidiarrheal, inhibits peristalsis of intestinal muscles.
ADVERSE EFFECTS — Frequent: Anticholinergic effects, nervousness, dizziness, headache, depression, restlessness.

OPIUM (opium tincture, paregoric) ▶L ♀B (D with long-term use) ▶? ©II (opium tincture), III (paregoric) $$
ADULTS — Diarrhea: 5 to 10 mL paregoric PO daily (up to qid) or 0.3 to 0.6 mL PO opium tincture qid.
PEDS — Diarrhea: 0.25 to 0.5 mL/kg paregoric PO daily (up to qid) or 0.005 to 0.01 mL/kg PO opium tincture q 3 to 4 h (up to 6 doses/day).
FORMS — Trade only: Opium tincture 10% (deodorized opium tincture, 10 mg morphine equivalent/mL). Generic only: Paregoric (camphorated opium tincture, 2 mg morphine equivalent/5 mL).
NOTES — Opium tincture contains 25 times more morphine than paregoric. Do not use for C difficile-associated diarrhea, toxigenic bacterial diarrhea, or most childhood diarrhea.

(cont.)

OPIUM (cont.)
MOA — Antidiarrheal, inhibits peristalsis of intestinal muscles.

ADVERSE EFFECTS — Frequent: Palpitations, hypotension, bradycardia, dizziness, drowsiness, weakness, urinary retention. Severe: Possible biliary tract spasm.

GASTROENTEROLOGY: Antiemetics—5-HT3 Receptor Antagonists

DOLASETRON (*Anzemet*) ▶LK ♀B ▶? $$$
ADULTS — <u>Prevention of N/V with chemo:</u> 1.8 mg/kg (up to 100 mg) IV/PO single dose 30 min (IV) or 60 min (PO) before chemo. <u>Prevention/treatment of post-op N/V:</u> 12.5 mg IV as a single dose 15 min before end of anesthesia or as soon as N/V starts. Alternative for prevention 100 mg PO 2 h before surgery.
PEDS — <u>Prevention of N/V with chemo:</u> 1.8 mg/kg up to 100 mg IV/PO single dose 30 min (IV) or 60 min (PO) before chemo for age 2 to 16 yo. <u>Prevention/treatment of post-op N/V:</u> 0.35 mg/kg IV as single dose 15 minutes before end of anesthesia or as soon as N/V starts for age 2 to 16 yo. Max 12.5 mg. Prevention alternative 1.2 mg/kg PO to max of 100 mg 2 h before surgery. Contraindicated in Canada in children younger than 18 yo.
UNAPPROVED ADULTS — <u>N/V due to radiotherapy:</u> 0.3 mg/kg IV as a single dose.
FORMS — Trade only: Tabs 50, 100 mg.
NOTES — Use caution in patients of any age who have or may develop prolongation of QT interval (ie, hypokalemia, hypomagnesemia, concomitant antiarrhythmic therapy, cumulative high-dose anthracycline therapy). Cimetidine may increase serum concentrations, rifampin may reduce serum concentrations.
MOA — Antiemetic, serotonin antagonist blocking chemoreceptor trigger zone.
ADVERSE EFFECTS — Frequent: None. Severe: Prolongation of cardiac conduction intervals, particularly QTc, ventricular tachycardia, ventricular fibrillation.

GRANISETRON (*Kytril, Sancuso*) ▶L ♀B ▶? $$$$
ADULTS — <u>Prevention of N/V with chemo:</u> 10 mcg/kg over 5 min IV 30 min prior to chemo. Oral: 1 mg PO bid or 2 mg PO every day for 1 day only. <u>Radiation-induced N/V:</u> 2 mg PO 1 h before first irradiation fraction of each day. <u>Prevention/treatment post-op N/V:</u> 1 mg IV.
PEDS — <u>Prevention of N/V with chemo:</u> 10 mcg/kg IV 30 min prior to chemo for age 2 to 16 yo. Max dose 1 mg per dose. Oral form not approved in children.
FORMS — Generic/Trade: Tabs 1 mg. Oral soln 2 mg/10 mL (30 mL). Trade only (Sancuso): Transdermal patch 34.3 mg of granisetron delivering 3.1 mg/24 h.
MOA — Antiemetic, serotonin antagonist blocking chemoreceptor trigger zone.
ADVERSE EFFECTS — Frequent: Headache. Severe: Arrhythmias, QT prolongation.

ONDANSETRON (*Zofran*) ▶L ♀B ▶? $$$$$
ADULTS — <u>Prevention of N/V with chemo:</u> 32 mg IV as a single dose over 15 min, or 0.15 mg/kg IV 30 min prior to chemo and repeated at 4 and 8 h after first dose. Alternatively, 8 mg PO 30 min before moderately emetogenic chemo and 8 h later. Can be given q 12 h for 1 to 2 days after completion of chemo. For <u>single-day highly emetogenic chemo,</u> 24 mg PO 30 min before chemo. <u>Prevention of post-op nausea:</u> 4 mg IV over 2 to 5 min or 4 mg IM or 16 mg PO 1 h before anesthesia. <u>Prevention of N/V associated with radiotherapy:</u> 8 mg PO tid.
PEDS — <u>Prevention of N/V with chemo:</u> IV: 0.15 mg/kg 30 min prior to chemo and repeated at 4 and 8 h after first dose for age greater than 6 mo. PO: Give 4 mg 30 minutes prior to chemo and repeat at 4 and 8 hrs after first dose for age 4 to 11 yo. Can be given q 8 h PO for 1 to 2 days after completion of chemo. Give 8 mg PO 30 min before chemo and 8 h later for age 12 yo or greater. <u>Prevention of post-op N/V:</u> 0.1 mg/kg IV over 2 to 5 min for age 1 mo to 12 yo if wt 40 kg or less; give 4 mg IV over 2 to 5 min if wt greater than 40 kg.
UNAPPROVED ADULTS — Has been used in <u>hyperemesis</u> associated with pregnancy.
UNAPPROVED PEDS — Use with caution if younger than 4 yo. Dosing based on BSA: give 1 mg PO tid for BSA less than 0.3 m2, give 2 mg PO tid for BSA 0.3 to 0.6 m2, give 3 mg PO tid for BSA 0.6 to 1 m2, give 4 mg PO tid for BSA greater than 1 m2. Use caution in infants younger than 6 mo of age.
FORMS — Generic/Trade: Tabs 4, 8, 24 mg. Orally disintegrating tab 4, 8 mg. Oral soln 4 mg/5 mL. Generic only: Tabs 16 mg.
NOTES — Maximum oral dose if severe liver disease is 8 mg/day. Use following abdominal surgery or in those receiving chemotherapy may mask a progressive ileus or gastric distension.
MOA — Antiemetic, serotonin antagonist blocking chemoreceptor trigger zone.
ADVERSE EFFECTS — Frequent: Headache, fever, diarrhea, constipation, transient increases in LFTs. Severe: Transient blindness, especially with IV, arrhythmia, QT prolongation.

PALONOSETRON (*Aloxi*) ▶L ♀B ▶? $$$$$
ADULTS — <u>Prevention of N/V with chemo:</u> 0.25 mg IV over 30 sec, 30 min prior to chemo or 0.5 mg PO 1 h before start of chemotherapy. <u>Prevention of post-op N/V:</u> 0.075 mg IV over 10 sec just prior to anesthesia.
PEDS — Not approved in children.
UNAPPROVED PEDS — Limited information suggests 3 mcg/kg (maximum 0.25 mg) IV is effective and safe in children older than 2 yo.
FORMS — Trade only: Caps 0.5 mg.
MOA — Antiemetic, serotonin antagonist blocking chemoreceptor trigger zone.
ADVERSE EFFECTS — Frequent: Headache, constipation. Severe: Arrhythmia, QT prolongation.

GASTROENTEROLOGY: Antiemetics—Other

APREPITANT (*Emend, fosaprepitant*) ▶L ♀B ▶? $$$$$
ADULTS — Prevention of N/V with moderately to highly emetogenic chemo, in combination with a corticosteroid and a 5-HT3 antagonist: 125 mg PO on day 1 (1 h prior to chemo), then 80 mg PO qam on days 2 and 3. Alternative for first dose only is 115 mg IV (fosaprepitant form) over 15 min given 30 min prior to chemo. Prevention of post-op N/V: 40 mg PO within 3 h prior to anesthesia.
PEDS — Not approved in children.
FORMS — Trade only (aprepitant): Caps 40, 80, 125 mg. IV prodrug form is fosaprepitant.
NOTES — Use caution with other medications metabolized by CYP3A4 hepatic enzyme system and an inducer of the CYP2C9 hepatic enzyme system. Contraindicated with pimozide. May decrease efficacy of oral contraceptives; women should use alternate/back-up method. Monitor INR in patients receiving warfarin. Fosaprepitant is a prodrug of aprepitant.
MOA — Antiemetic, substance P/neurokinin-1 receptor antagonist.
ADVERSE EFFECTS — Frequent: Fatigue, diarrhea, constipation, muscular weakness, hiccups. Severe: Hypersensitivity and anaphylactic reactions.

DICLECTIN (doxylamine + pyridoxine) ▶LK ♀A ▶? $
ADULTS — Canada only. N/V in pregnancy. 2 tabs PO at bedtime. May add 1 tab in am and 1 tab in afternoon, if needed.
PEDS — Not approved in children.
FORMS — Canada Trade only: Delayed-release tabs doxylamine 10 mg + pyridoxine 10 mg.
MOA — Anticholinergic and sedative (doxylamine), coenzyme involved in numerous metabolic transformations of proteins and amino acids (pyridoxine).
ADVERSE EFFECTS — Frequent: Drowsiness, unstable gait, awkwardness of hands, perioral numbness, decreased sensations (touch, temperature, vibrations), paresthesia, photosensitivity, ataxia.

DIMENHYDRINATE (*Dramamine, ✦Gravol*) ▶LK ♀B ▶– $
ADULTS — Nausea: 50 to 100 mg/dose PO/IM/IV q 4 to 6 h prn. Maximum PO dose 400 mg/24 h, maximum IV/IM dose 600 mg/24 h.
PEDS — Nausea: Not recommended for age younger than 2 yo. Give 12.5 to 25 mg PO q 6 to 8 h or 5 mg/kg/day (up to 75 mg/day) PO divided q 6 h for age 2 to 5 yo, give 25 to 50 mg (up to 150 mg/day) PO q 6 to 8 h or for age 6 to 12 yo.
FORMS — OTC Generic/Trade: Tabs 50 mg. Trade only: Chewable tabs 50 mg. Generic only: Oral soln 12.5 mg/5 mL. Canada only: Suppository 25, 50, 100 mg.
NOTES — May cause drowsiness. Use with caution in conditions that may be aggravated by anticholinergic effects (ie, prostatic hypertrophy, asthma, narrow-angle glaucoma). Available as suppositories in Canada.

MOA — Antihistamine.
ADVERSE EFFECTS — Frequent: Blurred vision, dry mouth, dizziness. Severe: Hallucinations, psychosis.

DOMPERIDONE (*✦Motilium*) ▶L ♀? ▶– $$
ADULTS — Canada only. Postprandial dyspepsia: 10 to 20 mg PO tid to qid, 30 min before a meal. N/V: 20 mg PO tid to qid.
PEDS — Not approved in children.
UNAPPROVED ADULTS — Has been used for diabetic gastroparesis, chemotherapy/radiation-induced N/V. Has also been used to increase milk production in lactating mothers although this is not currently recommended due to safety concerns.
UNAPPROVED PEDS — Use in children generally not recommended except for chemotherapy or radiation-induced N/V: 200 to 400 mcg/kg PO q 4 to 8 h.
FORMS — Canada only. Trade/generic: Tabs 10, 20 mg.
NOTES — Similar in efficacy to metoclopramide but less likely to cause EPS.
MOA — Dopamine antagonist at GI muscle receptors and chemoreceptor trigger zone, resulting in improved gastric emptying.
ADVERSE EFFECTS — Serious: Cardiac dysrhythmia. Frequent: galactorrhea, gynecomastia.

DOXYLAMINE (*Unisom Nighttime Sleep Aid, others*) ▶L ♀A ▶? $
PEDS — Not approved in children.
UNAPPROVED ADULTS — Nausea and vomiting associated with pregnancy: 12.5 mg PO bid to qid; often used in combination with pyridoxine.
FORMS — Generic/Trade: Tabs 10 mg.
MOA — Anticholinergic and sedative.
ADVERSE EFFECTS — Frequent: None.

DRONABINOL (*Marinol*) ▶L ♀C ▶– ©III $$$$$
ADULTS — Nausea with chemo: 5 mg/m2 PO 1 to 3 h before chemo then 5 mg/m2/dose q 2 to 4 h after chemo for 4 to 6 doses/day. Dose can be increased to max 15 mg/m2. Anorexia associated with AIDS: Initially 2.5 mg PO bid before lunch and dinner. Maximum 20 mg/day.
PEDS — Nausea with chemo: 5 mg/m2 PO 1 to 3 h before chemo then 5 mg/m2/dose PO q 2 to 4 h after chemo (up to 4 to 6 doses/day). Dose can be increased to max 15 mg/m2. Not approved for anorexia associated with AIDS in children.
UNAPPROVED PEDS — Nausea with chemo: 5 mg/m2 PO 1 to 3 h before chemo then 5 mg/m2/dose PO q 2 to 4 h after chemo (up to 4 to 6 doses/day). Dose can be increased to max 15 mg/m2.
FORMS — Generic/Trade: Caps 2.5, 5, 10 mg.
NOTES — Patient response varies; individualize dosing (start with low doses in elderly). Additive CNS effects with alcohol, sedatives, hypnotics, psychomimetics. Caution if history of seizures.
MOA — Unknown.
ADVERSE EFFECTS — Frequent: Drowsiness, dizziness, anxiety, detachment, mood changes, anorexia. Severe: Syncope.

DROPERIDOL (*Inapsine*) ▶L ♀C ▶? $
WARNING — Cases of fatal QT prolongation and/or torsades de pointes have occurred in patients receiving droperidol at or below recommended doses (some without risk factors for QT prolongation). Reserve for nonresponse to other treatments, and perform 12-lead ECG prior to administration and continue ECG monitoring 2 to 3 h after treatment. Use with extreme caution (if at all) if prolonged baseline QT.
ADULTS — Antiemetic premedication: 0.625 to 2.5 mg IV or 2.5 mg IM then 1.25 mg prn.
PEDS — Pre-op: 0.088 to 0.165 mg/kg IV for age 2 to 12 yo. Children older than 12 yo: 2.5 mg IM/IV, additional doses of 1.25 mg can be given with caution. Post-op antiemetic: 0.01 to 0.03 mg/kg/dose IV q 6 to 8 h prn. Usual dose 0.05 to 0.06 mg/kg/dose (up to 0.1 mg/kg/dose).
UNAPPROVED ADULTS — Chemo-induced nausea: 2.5 to 5 mg IV/IM q 3 to 4 h prn.
UNAPPROVED PEDS — Chemo-induced nausea: 0.05 to 0.06 mg/kg/dose IV/IM q 4 to 6 h prn.
NOTES — Has no analgesic or amnestic effects. Consider lower doses in geriatric, debilitated, or high-risk patients such as those receiving other CNS depressants. May cause hypotension or tachycardia, extrapyramidal reactions, drowsiness.
MOA — Alters action of dopamine to sedate and reduce emesis.
ADVERSE EFFECTS — Frequent: QTc prolongatioon, restlessness, anxiety, dystonic reactions. Severe: Cardiac arrest, sedation, hypotension, seizures, extrapyramidal reactions.

METOCLOPRAMIDE (*Reglan, Metozolv ODT, ✦Maxeran*) ▶K ♀B ▶? $
WARNING — Irreversible tardive dyskinesia with high dose or long-term (greater than 3 months) use.
ADULTS — Gastroesophageal reflux: 10 to 15 mg PO qid 30 min before meals and at bedtime. Diabetic gastroparesis: 10 mg PO/IV/IM 30 min before meals and hs. Prevention of chemo-induced emesis: 1 to 2 mg/kg PO/IV/IM 30 min before chemo and then q 2 h for 2 doses then q 3 h for 3 doses prn. Prevention of post-op nausea: 10 to 20 mg IM/IV near end of surgical procedure, may repeat q 3 to 4 h prn. Intubation of small intestine: 10 mg IV. Radiographic exam of upper GI tract: 10 mg IV.
PEDS — Intubation of small intestine: 0.1 mg/kg IV for age younger than 6 yo, 2.5 to 5 mg IV for age 6 to 14 yo. Radiographic exam of upper GI tract: 0.1 mg/kg IV for age younger than 6 yo: 2.5 to 5 mg IV for age 6 to 14 yo.
UNAPPROVED ADULTS — Prevention/treatment of chemo-induced emesis: 3 mg/kg IV over 1 h followed by continuous IV infusion of 0.5 mg/kg/h for 12 h. Migraine treatment: 10 mg IV. Migraine adjunct: 10 mg PO 5 to 10 min before ergotamine/analgesic/sedative.
UNAPPROVED PEDS — Gastroesophageal reflux: 0.4 to 0.8 mg/kg/day in 4 divided doses. Prevention of chemo-induced emesis: 1 to 2 mg/kg 30 min before chemo and then q 3 h prn (up to 5 doses/day or 5 to 10 mg/kg/day).
FORMS — Generic/Trade: Tabs 5, 10 mg. Trade: Orally disintegrating tabs 5, 10 mg (Metozolv). Generic only: Oral soln 5 mg/5 mL.
NOTES — To reduce incidence and severity of akathisia, consider giving IV doses over 15 min. If extrapyramidal reactions occur (especially with high IV doses) give diphenhydramine IM/IV. Adjust dose in renal dysfunction. Irreversible tardive dyskinesia with high dose or long-term (greater than 3 months) use. May cause drowsiness, agitation, seizures, hallucinations, galactorrhea, hyperprolactinemia, constipation, diarrhea. Increases cyclosporine and ethanol absorption. Do not use if bowel perforation or mechanical obstruction present. Levodopa decreases metoclopramide effects.
MOA — Dopamine blockade; inhibits chemoreceptor trigger zone.
ADVERSE EFFECTS — Frequent: Restlessness, drowsiness, diarrhea, asthenia.

NABILONE (*Cesamet*) ▶L ♀C ▶– ©II $$$$$
ADULTS — N/V in cancer chemotherapy patients with poor response to other agents: 1 to 2 mg PO bid, 1 to 3 h before chemotherapy. Max dose 6 mg/day in 3 divided doses.
PEDS — Not approved in children.
UNAPPROVED PEDS — Children 4 yo or older: wt less than 18 kg: 0.5 mg PO bid, wt 18 to 30 kg: 1 mg PO bid, wt 30 kg or greater: 1 mg PO tid.
FORMS — Trade only: Caps 1 mg.
NOTES — Contraindicated in known sensitivity to marijuana or other cannabinoids. Use with caution with current or past psychiatric reactions. Additive CNS effects with alcohol, sedatives, hypnotics, psychomimetics. Additive cardiac effects with amphetamines, antihistamines, anticholinergic medications.
MOA — Synthetic cannabinoid with antiemetic properties.
ADVERSE EFFECTS — Frequent: Drowsiness, vertigo, dry mouth, euphoria, ataxia, headache, impaired concentration. Serious: Psychotic reactions, seizures, hallucinations.

PHOSPHORATED CARBOHYDRATES (*Emetrol*) ▶L ♀A ▶+ $
ADULTS — Nausea: 15 to 30 mL PO q 15 min until nausea subsides or up to 5 doses.
PEDS — Nausea: 2 to 12 yo: 5 to 10 mL q 15 min until nausea subsides or up to 5 doses.
UNAPPROVED ADULTS — Morning sickness: 15 to 30 mL PO upon rising, repeat q 3 h prn. Motion sickness or nausea due to drug therapy or anesthesia: 15 mL/dose.
UNAPPROVED PEDS — Regurgitation in infants: 5 to 10 mL PO 10 to 15 min prior to each feeding. Motion sickness or nausea due to drug therapy or anesthesia: 5 mL/dose.
FORMS — OTC Generic/Trade: Soln containing dextrose, fructose, and phosphoric acid.

(cont.)

GASTROENTEROLOGY: Antiemetics

PHOSPHORATED CARBOHYDRATES (cont.)
NOTES — Do not dilute. Do not ingest fluids before or for 15 min after dose. Monitor blood glucose in diabetic patients.
MOA — Hyperosmolar effect on GI wall to reduce contraction.
ADVERSE EFFECTS — Frequent: Abdominal pain, diarrhea (in high doses).

PROCHLORPERAZINE (*Compazine,* ✦*Stemetil*) ▶LK ♀C ▶? $
ADULTS — Nausea and vomiting: 5 to 10 mg PO/IM tid to qid (up to 40 mg/day); Sustained release: 10 mg PO q 12 h or 15 mg PO qam; Suppository: 25 mg PR q 12 h; IV/IM: 5 to 10 mg IV over at least 2 min q 3 to 4 h prn (up to 40 mg/day); 5 to 10 mg IM q 3 to 4 h prn (up to 40 mg/day).
PEDS — Nausea and vomiting: Not recommended in age younger than 2 yo or wt less than 10 kg, 0.4 mg/kg/day PO/PR in 3 to 4 divided doses for age older than 2 yo; 0.1 to 0.15 mg/kg/dose IM; IV not recommended in children.
UNAPPROVED ADULTS — Migraine: 10 mg IV/IM or 25 mg PR single dose for acute headache.
UNAPPROVED PEDS — N/V during surgery: 5 to 10 mg IM 1 to 2 h before anesthesia induction, may repeat in 30 min; 5 to 10 mg IV 15 to 30 min before anesthesia induction, may repeat once.
FORMS — Generic only: Tabs 5, 10, 25 mg. Suppository 25 mg.
NOTES — May cause extrapyramidal reactions (especially in elderly), hypotension (with IV), arrhythmias, sedation, seizures, hyperprolactinemia, gynecomastia, dry mouth, constipation, urinary retention, leukopenia, thrombocytopenia. Elderly more prone to adverse effects.
MOA — Blocks post-synaptic dopaminergic receptors.
ADVERSE EFFECTS — Frequent: None. Severe: Cardiac arrest, hypotension, extrapyramidal signs.

PROMETHAZINE (*Phenergan*) ▶LK ♀C ▶– $
WARNING — Contraindicated if age younger than 2 yo due to risk of fatal respiratory depression; caution in older children. Risks of severe tissue injury associated with IV administration including gangrene. Preferred route of administration is deep intramuscular injection, subcutaneous injection is contraindicated.
ADULTS — N/V: 12.5 to 25 mg q 4 to 6 h PO/IM/PR prn. Motion sickness: 25 mg PO/PR 30 to 60 min prior to departure and q 12 h prn. Hypersensitivity reactions: 25 mg IM/IV, may repeat in 2 h. Allergic conditions: 12.5 mg PO/PR/IM/IV qid or 25 mg PO/PR at bedtime.
PEDS — N/V: 0.25 to 1 mg/kg/dose PO/IM/PR q 4 to 6 h prn for age 2 yo or older. Motion sickness: 0.5 mg/kg (up to 25 mg/dose) PO 30 to 60 min prior to departure and q 12 h prn. Hypersensitivity reactions: 6.25 to 12.5 mg PO/PR/IM/IV q 6 h prn for age older than 2 yo.

UNAPPROVED ADULTS — N/V: 12.5 to 25 mg IV q 4 h prn.
UNAPPROVED PEDS — N/V: 0.25 mg/kg/dose IV q 4 h prn for age 2 yo or older.
FORMS — Generic only: Tabs/Suppository 12.5, 25, 50 mg. Syrup 6.25 mg/5 mL.
NOTES — May cause sedation, extrapyramidal reactions (especially with high IV doses), hypotension with rapid IV administration, anticholinergic side effects, eg, dry mouth, blurred vision.
MOA — Antihistamine; blocks post-synaptic dopaminergic receptors.
ADVERSE EFFECTS — Frequent: Sedation, dry mouth. Severe: Cardiac arrest, hypotension, extrapyramidal signs, cholestatic jaundice.

SCOPOLAMINE (*Transderm-Scop, Scopace,* ✦*Transderm-V*) ▶L ♀C ▶+ $$
ADULTS — Motion sickness: 1 disc behind ear at least 4 h before travel and q 3 days prn or 0.4 to 0.8 mg PO 1 h before travel and q 8 h prn. Prevention of post-op N/V: Apply patch behind ear 4 h before surgery, remove 24 h after surgery. Spastic states, postencephalitic parkinsonism: 0.4 to 0.8 mg PO q 8 h prn.
PEDS — Not approved for age younger than 12 yo.
UNAPPROVED PEDS — Pre-op and antiemetic: 6 mcg/kg/dose IM/IV/SC (max dose 0.3 mg/dose). May repeat q 6 to 8 h. Has also been used in severe drooling.
FORMS — Trade only: Topical disc 1.5 mg/72 h, box of 4. Oral tab 0.4 mg.
NOTES — Dry mouth common. Also causes drowsiness, blurred vision.
MOA — Acetylcholine blockage at parasympathetic sites.
ADVERSE EFFECTS — Frequent: Blurred vision, photophobia.

THIETHYLPERAZINE (*Torecan*) ▶L ♀? ▶? $
ADULTS — N/V: 10 mg PO/IM 1 to 3 times/day.
PEDS — Not approved in children.
FORMS — Trade only: Tabs 10 mg.
MOA — Blocks post-synaptic dopaminergic receptors.
ADVERSE EFFECTS — Frequent: Drowsiness, dizziness, xerostomia, dry nose, extrapyramidal symptoms.

TRIMETHOBENZAMIDE (*Tigan*) ▶LK ♀C ▶? $
ADULTS — Nausea and vomiting: 300 mg PO q 6 to 8 h, 200 mg IM q 6 to 8 h.
PEDS — Not approved for use in children.
UNAPPROVED PEDS — 100 to 200 mg PO q 6 to 8 h if wt 13.6 to 40.9 kg.
FORMS — Generic/Trade: Cap 300 mg.
NOTES — Not for IV use. May cause sedation. Reduce starting dose in the elderly or if reduced renal function to minimize risk of adverse effects.
MOA — Inhibits chemoreceptor trigger zone.
ADVERSE EFFECTS — Frequent: Drowsiness. Severe: EPS.

GASTROENTEROLOGY: Antiulcer—Antacids

ALKA-SELTZER (acetylsalicylic acid + citrate + bicarbonate) ▶LK ♀? (- 3rd trimester) ▶? $
- ADULTS — Relief of upset stomach: 2 regular-strength tabs in 4 oz water q 4 h PO prn (up to 8 tabs/day for age younger than 60 yo, up to 4 tabs/day for age 60 yo or older) or 2 extra-strength tabs in 4 oz water q 6 h PO prn (up to 7 tabs/day for age younger than 60 yo, up to 4 tabs/day for age 60 yo or older).
- PEDS — Not approved in children.
- FORMS — OTC Trade only: Regular-strength, original: aspirin 325 mg + citric acid 1000 mg + sodium bicarbonate 1916 mg. Regular-strength lemon lime and cherry: 325 mg + 1000 mg + 1700 mg. Extra-strength: 500 mg + 1000 mg + 1985 mg. Not all forms of Alka Seltzer contain aspirin (eg, Alka Seltzer Heartburn Relief).
- NOTES — Avoid aspirin-containing forms in children and teenagers due to risk of Reye's syndrome.
- MOA — Antacid.
- ADVERSE EFFECTS — Frequent: None. Serious: Sodium content may worsen BP or heart failure; peptic ulcer.

ALUMINUM HYDROXIDE (Alternagel, Amphojel, Alu-Tab, Alu-Cap, ✢Basalgel, Mucaine) ▶K ♀C ▶? $
- ADULTS — Hyperphosphatemia in chronic renal failure (short-term treatment only to avoid aluminum accumulation): 500 to 1,000 mg PO with meals. Upset stomach, indigestion: 5 to 10 mL or 300 to 600 mg PO 6 times per day, between meals and at bedtime and prn.
- PEDS — Not approved in children.
- UNAPPROVED ADULTS — Symptomatic reflux: 15 to 30 mL PO q 30 to 60 min. Long-term management of reflux disease: 15 to 30 mL PO 1 and 3 h after meals and at bedtime prn. Peptic ulcer disease: 15 to 45 mL or 1 to 3 tab PO 1 and 3 h after meals and at bedtime. Prophylaxis against GI bleeding (titrate dose to maintain gastric pH greater than 3.5): 30 to 60 mL or 2 to 4 tab PO q 1 to 2 h.
- UNAPPROVED PEDS — Peptic ulcer disease: 5 to 15 mL PO 1 and 3 h after meals and at bedtime. Prophylaxis against GI bleeding (titrate dose to maintain gastric pH greater than 3.5): Neonates 0.5 to 1 mL/kg/dose PO q 4 h. Infants 2 to 5 mL PO q 1 to 2 h. Child: 5 to 15 mL PO q 1 to 2 h. Child: 5 to 15 mL PO q 1 to 2 h.
- FORMS — OTC Generic/Trade: Susp 320, 600 mg/ 5 mL.
- NOTES — For concentrated suspensions, use ½ the recommended dose. May cause constipation. Avoid administration with tetracyclines, digoxin, iron, isoniazid, buffered/enteric aspirin, diazepam, fluoroquinolones.
- MOA — Antacid.
- ADVERSE EFFECTS — Frequent: Constipation, chalky taste, stomach cramps, fecal impaction.

CITROCARBONATE (bicarbonate + citrate) ▶K ♀? ▶? $
- ADULTS — 1 to 2 teaspoons in cold water PO 15 min to 2 h after meals prn.
- PEDS — give ¼ to ½ teaspoon in cold water PO after meals prn for age 6 to 12 yo.
- FORMS — OTC Trade only: Sodium bicarbonate 0.78 g + sodium citrate anhydrous 1.82 g in each 1 teaspoonful dissolved in water 150, 300 g.
- NOTES — Chronic use may cause metabolic alkalosis. Contains sodium.
- MOA — Antacid.
- ADVERSE EFFECTS — Frequent: None. Serious: Sodium content may worsen blood pressure or heart failure.

GAVISCON (aluminum hydroxide + magnesium carbonate) ▶K ♀? ▶? $
- ADULTS — 2 to 4 tabs or 15 to 30 mL (regular strength) or 10 mL (extra strength) PO qid prn.
- PEDS — Not approved in children.
- UNAPPROVED PEDS — Peptic ulcer disease: 5 to 15 mL PO after meals and at bedtime.
- FORMS — OTC Trade only: Tabs: Regular-strength (Al hydroxide 80 mg + Mg carbonate 20 mg), Extra-strength (Al hydroxide 160 mg + Mg carbonate 105 mg). Liquid: Regular-strength (Al hydroxide 95 mg + Mg carbonate 358 mg per 15 mL), Extra-strength (Al hydroxide 254 mg + Mg carbonate 237.5 mg per 30 mL).
- NOTES — Contains alginic acid or sodium alginate, which is considered an "inactive" ingredient. Alginic acid forms foam barrier which floats in stomach to minimize esophageal contact with acid. Chronic use may cause metabolic alkalosis. Contains sodium.
- MOA — Antacid, "foam barrier" in stomach to minimize esophageal contact with acid (alginic acid).
- ADVERSE EFFECTS — Frequent: Diarrhea, constipation. Serious: Sodium content may worsen BP or heart failure.

MAALOX (aluminum hydroxide + magnesium hydroxide) ▶K ♀C ▶? $
- ADULTS — Heartburn/indigestion: 10 to 20 mL or 1 to 2 tab PO qid, after meals and at bedtime and prn.
- PEDS — Not approved in children.
- UNAPPROVED ADULTS — Peptic ulcer disease: 15 to 45 mL PO 1 and 3 h after meals and at bedtime. Symptomatic reflux: 15 to 30 mL PO q 30 to 60 min prn. Long-term management of reflux disease: 15 to 30 mL PO 1 and 3 h after meals and at bedtime prn. Prophylaxis against GI bleeding (titrate dose to maintain gastric pH greater than 3.5): 30 to 60 mL PO q 1 to 2 h.
- UNAPPROVED PEDS — Peptic ulcer disease: 5 to 15 mL PO 1 and 3 h after meals and at bedtime. Prophylaxis against GI bleeding (titrate dose to maintain gastric pH greater than 3.5): Neonates 1 mL/kg/dose PO q 4 h. Infants 2 to 5 mL PO q 1 to 2 h. Child: 5 to 15 mL PO q 1 to 2 h.
- FORMS — OTC Generic/Trade: Regular-strength chewable tabs (Al hydroxide + Mg hydroxide 200/200 mg), susp (225/200 mg per 5 mL). Other strengths available.

(cont.)

GASTROENTEROLOGY: Antiulcer

MAALOX (cont.)
NOTES — Maalox Extra Strength and Maalox TC are more concentrated than Maalox. Maalox Plus has added simethicone. May cause constipation or diarrhea. Avoid concomitant administration with tetracyclines, digoxin, iron, isoniazid, buffered/enteric aspirin, diazepam, fluoroquinolones. Avoid chronic use in patients with renal dysfunction due to potential for magnesium accumulation.
MOA — Antacid.
ADVERSE EFFECTS — Frequent: None.

MAGALDRATE (Riopan) ▶K ♀C ▶? $
ADULTS — Relief of upset stomach: 5 to 10 mL between meals and at bedtime and prn.
PEDS — Not approved in children.
UNAPPROVED PEDS — Peptic ulcer disease: 5 to 10 mL PO 1 and 3 h after meals and at bedtime.
FORMS — OTC Trade only: Susp 540 mg/5 mL. Riopan Plus (with simethicone) available as susp 540/20 mg/5 mL, chewable tabs 540/20 mg.
NOTES — Riopan Plus has added simethicone. Avoid concomitant administration with tetracyclines, fluoroquinolones, digoxin, iron, isoniazid, buffered/enteric aspirin, diazepam. Avoid chronic use in patients with renal failure.
MOA — Antacid.
ADVERSE EFFECTS — Frequent: None.

MYLANTA (aluminum hydroxide + magnesium hydroxide + simethicone) ▶K ♀C ▶? $
ADULTS — Heartburn/indigestion: 10 to 20 mL or 2 to 4 tab PO qid, after meals and at bedtime and prn.
PEDS — Safe dosing has not been established.
UNAPPROVED ADULTS — Peptic ulcer disease: 15 to 45 mL PO 1 and 3 h after meals and at bedtime. Symptomatic reflux: 15 to 30 mL PO q 30 to 60 min. Long-term management of reflux: 15 to 30 mL PO 1 and 3 h postprandially and at bedtime prn.
UNAPPROVED PEDS — Peptic ulcer disease: 5 to 15 mL PO 1 and 3 h after meals and at bedtime.
FORMS — OTC Generic/Trade: Liquid, Double-strength liquid, Tabs, Double-strength tabs. Trade only: Tabs sodium + sugar + dye-free.
NOTES — Mylanta Gelcaps contain calcium carbonate and magnesium hydroxide. May cause constipation or diarrhea. Avoid concomitant administration with tetracyclines, fluoroquinolones, digoxin, iron, isoniazid, buffered/enteric aspirin, diazepam. Avoid chronic use in renal dysfunction.
MOA — Antacid.
ADVERSE EFFECTS — Frequent: None.

ROLAIDS (calcium carbonate + magnesium hydroxide) ▶K ♀? ▶? $
ADULTS — 2 to 4 tabs PO q 1 h prn, max 12 tabs/day (regular strength) or 10 tabs/day (extra-strength).
PEDS — Not approved in children.
FORMS — OTC Trade only: Tabs regular-strength (Ca carbonate 550 mg, Mg hydroxide 110 mg), extra-strength (Ca carbonate 675 mg, Mg hydroxide 135 mg).
NOTES — Chronic use may cause metabolic alkalosis.
MOA — Antacid.
ADVERSE EFFECTS — Frequent: None. Serious: None.

GASTROENTEROLOGY: Antiulcer—H2 Antagonists

CIMETIDINE (Tagamet, Tagamet HB) ▶LK ♀B ▶+ $
ADULTS — Treatment of duodenal or gastric ulcer: 800 mg PO at bedtime or 300 mg PO qid with meals and at bedtime or 400 mg PO bid. Prevention of duodenal ulcer: 400 mg PO at bedtime. Erosive esophagitis: 800 mg PO bid or 400 mg PO qid. Prevention or treatment of heartburn (OTC product only approved for this indication): 200 mg PO prn max 400 mg/day for up to 14 days. Hypersecretory conditions: 300 mg PO qid with meals and at bedtime. Patients unable to take oral medications: 300 mg IV/IM q 6 to 8 h or 37.5 mg/h continuous IV infusion. Prevention of upper GI bleeding in critically ill patients: 50 mg/h continuous infusion.
PEDS — Not approved in children.
UNAPPROVED ADULTS — Prevention of aspiration pneumonitis during surgery: 300 to 600 mg PO or 200 to 300 mg IV 60 to 90 min prior to anesthesia. Has been used as adjunctive therapy with H1 antagonist for severe allergic reactions.
UNAPPROVED PEDS — Treatment of duodenal or gastric ulcers, erosive esophagitis, Hypersecretory conditions: Neonates: 5 to 10 mg/kg/day PO/IV/IM divided q 8 to 12 h. Infants: 10 to 20 mg/kg/day PO/IV/IM divided q 6 h. Children: 20 to 40 mg/kg/day PO/IV/IM divided q 6 h. Chronic viral warts in children: 25 to 40 mg/kg/day PO in divided doses.
FORMS — Tabs 200, 300, 400, 800 mg. Rx Generic only: Oral soln 300 mg/5 mL. OTC Generic/Trade: Tabs 200 mg.
NOTES — May cause dizziness, drowsiness, headache, diarrhea, nausea. Decreased absorption of ketoconazole, itraconazole. Increased levels of carbamazepine, cyclosporine, diazepam, labetalol, lidocaine, theophylline, phenytoin, procainamide, quinidine, propranolol, TCAs, valproic acid, warfarin. Stagger doses of cimetidine and antacids. Decrease dose with CrCl < 30 mL/min.
MOA — Histamine-2 receptor blocker.
ADVERSE EFFECTS — Frequent: Drowsiness, dizziness, agitation, diarrhea, N/V.

FAMOTIDINE (Pepcid, Pepcid AC, Maximum Strength Pepcid AC) ▶LK ♀B ▶? $
ADULTS — Treatment of duodenal ulcer: 40 mg PO at bedtime or 20 mg PO bid. Maintenance of duodenal ulcer: 20 mg PO at bedtime. Treatment of gastric ulcer: 40 mg PO at bedtime. GERD: 20 mg PO bid. Treatment or prevention of heartburn: (OTC product only approved for this indication) 10 to 20 mg PO prn, up to 2 tabs per day. Hypersecretory conditions: 20 mg PO q 6 h.

(cont.)

HELICOBACTER PYLORI THERAPY

- Quadruple therapy PO for 14 days: bismuth subsalicylate 525 mg (or 30 mL) tid to qid plus metronidazole 500 mg tid to qid plus tetracycline 500 mg tid to qid plus a PPI* or a H2 blocker†
- Quadruple therapy PO for 14 days: bismuth subsalicylate 525 mg (or 30 mL) tid to qid plus metronidazole 500 mg tid to qid plus tetracycline 500 mg tid to qid plus a PPI* or a H2 blocker†
- PPI or H2 blocker may need to be continued past 14 days to heal the ulcer.

*PPIs include esomeprazole 40 mg qd, lansoprazole 30 mg bid, omeprazole 20 mg bid, pantoprazole 40 mg bid, rabeprazole 20 mg bid. †H$_2$ blockers include cimetidine 400 mg bid, famotidine 20 mg bid, nizatidine 150 mg bid, ranitidine 150 mg bid. Adapted from *Medical Letter Treatment Guidelines* 2008:55.

FAMOTIDINE *(cont.)*
Patients unable to take oral medications: 20 mg IV q 12 h.
PEDS — GERD: 0.5 mg/kg/day PO daily for up to 8 weeks for age younger than 3 mo; 0.5 mg/kg PO bid for age 3 to 12 mo; 1 mg/kg/day PO divided bid or 2 mg/kg/day PO daily, max 40 mg PO bid for age 1 to 16 yo. Peptic ulcer: 0.5 mg/kg/day PO at bedtime or divided bid up to 40 mg/day.
UNAPPROVED ADULTS — Prevention of aspiration pneumonitis during surgery: 40 mg PO/IM prior to anesthesia. Upper GI bleeding: 20 mg IV q 12 h. Has been used as adjunctive therapy with H1 antagonist for severe allergic reactions.
UNAPPROVED PEDS — Treatment of Hypersecretory conditions: 0.6 to 0.8 mg/kg/day IV in 2 to 3 divided doses or 1 to 1.2 mg/kg/day PO in 2 to 3 divided doses, maximum 40 mg/day.
FORMS — Generic/Trade: Tabs 10 mg (OTC, Pepcid AC Acid Controller), 20 mg (Rx and OTC, Maximum Strength Pepcid AC), 40 mg. Rx Generic/Trade: Susp 40 mg/5 mL.
NOTES — May cause dizziness, headache, constipation, diarrhea. Decreased absorption of ketoconazole, itraconazole. Adjust dose in patients with CrCl < 50 mL/min.
MOA — Histamine-2 receptor blocker.
ADVERSE EFFECTS — Frequent: Dizziness, headache, nausea. Severe: Convulsion in renal impairment, interstitial pneumonia, Stevens-Johnson syndrome.

NIZATIDINE (*Axid, Axid AR*) ▶K ♀B ▶? $$$$
ADULTS — Treatment of duodenal or gastric ulcer: 300 mg PO at bedtime or 150 mg PO bid. Maintenance of duodenal ulcer: 150 mg PO at bedtime. GERD: 150 mg PO bid. Treatment or prevention of heartburn: (OTC product only approved for this indication) 75 mg PO prn, max 150 mg/day.
PEDS — Esophagitis, GERD: 150 mg PO bid for age 12 yo or older.
UNAPPROVED ADULTS — Has been used as adjunctive therapy with H1 antagonist for severe allergic reactions.
UNAPPROVED PEDS — 6 mo to 11 yo (limited data): 5 to 10 mg/kg/day PO in 2 divided doses.
FORMS — OTC Trade only (Axid AR): Tabs 75 mg. Rx Trade only: Oral soln 15 mg/mL (120, 480 mL). Rx Generic/Trade: Caps 150 mg. Generic: Caps 300 mg.
NOTES — May cause dizziness, headache, constipation, diarrhea. Decrease absorption of ketoconazole, itraconazole. Adjust dose if CrCl < 50 mL/min.
MOA — Histamine-2 receptor blocker.
ADVERSE EFFECTS — Frequent: Dizziness, headache, nausea, constipation.

PEPCID COMPLETE (famotidine + calcium carbonate + magnesium hydroxide) ▶LK ♀B ▶? $
ADULTS — Treatment of heartburn: 1 tab PO prn. Max 2 tabs/day.
PEDS — Not approved in children younger than 12 yo. In children 12 yo or older, use adult dosing for OTC product.
FORMS — OTC trade/generic: Chewable tab, famotidine 10 mg with calcium carbonate 800 mg and magnesium hydroxide 165 mg.
MOA — Histamine-2 receptor blocker, antacid.
ADVERSE EFFECTS — Frequent: Dizziness, headache, nausea.

RANITIDINE (*Zantac, Zantac Efferdose, Zantac 75, Zantac 150, Peptic Relief*) ▶K ♀B ▶? $$$
ADULTS — Treatment of duodenal ulcer: 150 mg PO bid or 300 mg at bedtime. Treatment of gastric ulcer or GERD: 150 mg PO bid. Maintenance of duodenal or gastric ulcer: 150 mg PO at bedtime. Treatment of erosive esophagitis: 150 mg PO qid. Maintenance of erosive esophagitis: 150 mg PO bid. Prevention/treatment of heartburn: (OTC product only approved for this indication) 75 to 150 mg PO prn, max 300 mg/day. Hypersecretory conditions: 150 mg PO bid. Patients unable to take oral meds: 50 mg IV/IM q 6 to 8 h or 6.25 mg/h continuous IV infusion.
PEDS — Treatment of duodenal or gastric ulcers: 2 to 4 mg/kg PO bid (max 300 mg) or 2 to 4 mg/kg/day IV q 6 to 8 h for ages 1 mo to 16 yo. GERD, erosive esophagitis: 2.5 to 5 mg/kg PO bid (max 200 mg/day) or 2 to 4 mg/kg/day IV divided q 6 to 8 h (max 200 mg/day). Maintenance of duodenal or gastric ulcers: 2 to 4 mg/kg/day PO daily (max 150 mg).
UNAPPROVED ADULTS — Prevention of upper GI bleeding in critically ill patients: 6.25 mg/h continuous IV infusion (150 mg/day). Has been used as adjunctive therapy with H1 antagonist for severe allergic reactions.

(cont.)

GASTROENTEROLOGY: Antiulcer

RANITIDINE (cont.)
- UNAPPROVED PEDS – Treatment of duodenal or gastric ulcers, GERD, Hypersecretory conditions: Premature and term infants younger than 2 weeks of age: 1 mg/kg/day PO bid or 1.5 mg/kg IV for one dose then 12 h later 0.75 to 1 mg/kg IV q 12 h. Continuous infusion 1.5 mg/kg for one dose then 0.04 to 0.08 mg/kg/h infusion. Neonates: 1 to 2 mg/kg PO bid or 2 mg/kg/24 h IV divided q 12 h. Infants and children: 2 to 4 mg/kg/24 h IV/IM divided q6 to 12 h or 0.1 to 0.2 mg/kg/h continuous IV infusion.
- FORMS – Generic/Trade: Tabs 75 mg (OTC: Zantac 75), 150 mg (OTC and Rx: Zantac 150), 300 mg. Syrup 75 mg/5 mL. Rx Trade only: Effervescent tabs 25, 150 mg. Rx Generic only: Caps 150, 300 mg.
- NOTES – May cause dizziness, sedation, headache, drowsiness, rash, nausea, constipation, diarrhea. Elevations in SGPT have been observed when H2-antagonists have been administered intravenously greater-than-recommended dosages for 5 days or longer. Bradycardia can occur if the IV form is injected too rapidly. Variable effects on warfarin, decreased absorption of ketoconazole, itraconazole. Dissolve granules and effervescent tabs in water. Stagger doses of ranitidine and antacids. Adjust dose in patients with CrCl < 50 mL/min.
- MOA – Histamine-2 receptor blocker.
- ADVERSE EFFECTS – Frequent: Dizziness, headache, nausea, constipation, taste changes, stool or tongue darkening.

GASTROENTEROLOGY: Antiulcer—Helicobacter pylori Treatment

HELIDAC (bismuth subsalicylate + metronidazole + tetracycline) ▶LK ♀D ▶– $$$$$
- ADULTS – Active duodenal ulcer associated with Helicobacter pylori: 1 dose (2 bismuth subsalicylate chewable tabs, 1 metronidazole tab and 1 tetracycline cap) PO qid, at meals and at bedtime for 2 weeks with an H2 antagonist.
- PEDS – Not approved in children.
- UNAPPROVED ADULTS – Active duodenal ulcer associated with Helicobacter pylori: Same dose as in "adult," but substitute proton pump inhibitor for H2 antagonist.
- FORMS – Trade only: Each dose consists of bismuth subsalicylate 524 mg (2 × 262 mg) chewable tab + metronidazole 250 mg tab + tetracycline 500 mg cap.
- NOTES – See components.

PREVPAC (lansoprazole + amoxicillin + clarithromycin, ✽HP-Pac) ▶LK ♀C ▶? $$$$$
- ADULTS – Active duodenal ulcer associated with Helicobacter pylori: 1 dose PO bid for 10 to 14 days.
- PEDS – Not approved in children.
- FORMS – Trade only: Each does consists of lansoprazole 30 mg cap + amoxicillin 1 g (2 × 500 mg cap), + clarithromycin 500 mg tab.
- NOTES – See components.

- MOA – Antimicrobial treatment for Helicobacter pylori.
- ADVERSE EFFECTS – See components. Frequent: Diarrhea, headache, altered taste. Severe: Colitis, hypersensitivity reactions such as serum-sickness-like reactions, erythema multiforme, Stevens-Johnson syndrome, and exfoliative dermatitis, hepatic dysfunction, hemolytic anemia.

PYLERA (bismuth subcitrate potassium + metronidazole + tetracycline) ▶LK ♀D ▶– $$$$$
- ADULTS – Duodenal ulcer associated with H pylori: 3 caps PO qid (after meals and at bedtime) for 10 days. To be given with omeprazole 20 mg PO bid.
- PEDS – Not approved in children.
- FORMS – Trade only: Each cap contains biskalcitrate 140 mg + metronidazole 125 mg + tetracycline 125 mg.
- NOTES – See components.
- MOA – Antimicrobial treatment for Helicobacter pylori.
- ADVERSE EFFECTS – Frequent: Diarrhea, headache, altered taste. Severe: Colitis, hypersensitivity reactions such as serum-sickness, erythema multiforme, Stevens-Johnson syndrome, and exfoliative dermatitis; hepatic dysfunction, hemolytic anemia.

GASTROENTEROLOGY: Antiulcer—Proton Pump Inhibitors

DEXLANSOPRAZOLE (*Kapidex*) ▶L ♀B ▶? $$$$
- ADULT – Erosive esophagitis: 60 mg PO daily for up to 8 weeks. Maintenance therapy after healing of erosive esophagitis: 30 mg PO daily for up to 6 months. GERD: 30 mg PO daily for up to 4 weeks.
- PEDS – Not approved in children.
- FORMS – Trade only: Cap 30, 60 mg.
- NOTES – May decrease absorption of atazanavir, ketoconazole, itraconazole, ampicillin, digoxin and iron. Monitor INR in patients receiving warfarin. Swallow whole or mix with applesauce and take immediately.

ESOMEPRAZOLE (*Nexium*) ▶L ♀B ▶? $$$$
- ADULTS – Erosive esophagitis: 20 to 40 mg PO daily for 4 to 8 weeks. Maintenance of erosive esophagitis: 20 mg PO daily. Zollinger-Ellison: 40 mg PO bid. GERD: 20 mg PO daily for 4 weeks. GERD with esophagitis: 20 to 40 mg IV daily for 10 days until taking PO. Prevention of NSAID-associated gastric ulcer: 20 to 40 mg PO daily for up to 6 months. H pylori eradication: 40 mg PO daily with amoxicillin 1000 mg PO bid and clarithromycin 500 mg PO bid for 10 days.

(cont.)

ESOMEPRAZOLE (cont.)

PEDS — GERD: wt less than 20 kg: 10 mg PO daily; wt 20 kg or more: 10 to 20 mg daily. Alternatively, 10 to 20 mg PO daily for up to 8 weeks for age 1 to 11 yo, give 20 to 40 mg PO daily for up to 8 weeks for age 12 to 17 yo.
FORMS — Trade only: Cap delayed-release 20, 40 mg. Delayed-release granules for oral susp 10, 20, 40 mg per packet.
NOTES — May decrease absorption of ketoconazole, itraconazole, digoxin, iron, atazanavir, and ampicillin. Concomitant administration with voriconazole, an inhibitor of CYP2C19 and CYP3A4 may lead to a more than doubling of esomeprazole exposure. Conflicting information whether reduces efficacy of clopidogrel.
MOA — H-K ATPase proton pump inhibitor.
ADVERSE EFFECTS — Frequent: Headache, dizziness, rash, diarrhea, N/V, taste perversion. Severe: Anaphylaxis, toxic epidermal necrolysis, Stevens-Johnson syndrome, erythema multiforme, pancreatitis, hepatitis.

LANSOPRAZOLE (*Prevacid*) ▶L ♀B ▶? $$$

ADULTS — Erosive esophagitis: 30 mg PO daily or 30 mg IV daily for 7 days or until taking PO. Maintenance therapy following healing of Erosive esophagitis: 15 mg PO daily. NSAID-induced gastric ulcer: 30 mg PO daily for 8 weeks (treatment), 15 mg PO daily for up to 12 weeks (prevention). GERD: 15 mg PO daily. Duodenal ulcer treatment and maintenance: 15 mg PO daily. Gastric ulcer: 30 mg PO daily. Part of a multidrug regimen for H pylori eradication: 30 mg PO bid with amoxicillin 1000 mg PO bid and clarithromycin 500 mg PO bid for 10 to 14 days (see table) or 30 mg PO tid with amoxicillin 1000 mg PO tid for 14 days. Hypersecretory conditions: 60 mg PO daily.
PEDS — Not effective in patients with symptomatic GERD age 1 mo to younger than 1 year of age. Erosive esophagitis and GERD: give 15 mg PO daily up to 12 weeks for age 1 to 11 yo and wt 30 kg or less, give 30 mg PO daily up to 12 weeks for wt greater than 30 kg. Nonerosive GERD: 15 mg PO daily up to 8 weeks for age 12 to 17 yo. GERD with erosive esophagitis: 30 mg PO daily for up to 8 weeks for age 12 to 17 yo.
FORMS — OTC Trade only: Caps 15 mg. Rx Generic/Trade: 15, 30 mg. Rx Trade only: Susp 15, 30 mg packets. Orally disintegrating tab 15, 30 mg. Prevacid NapraPac: 7 lansoprazole 15 mg caps packaged with 14 naproxen tabs 375 mg or 500 mg.
NOTES — Take before meals. Avoid concomitant administration with sucralfate. May decrease absorption of atazanavir, ketoconazole, itraconazole, ampicillin, digoxin and iron. Potential for PPIs to reduce the response to clopidogrel. Evaluate the need for a PPI in clopidogrel-treated patients and consider H2-blocker/antacid. Orally disintegrating tabs can be dissolved water (15 mg tab in 4 mL, 30 mg tab in 10 mL) and administered via an oral syringe or nasogastric tube at least 8 French within 15 min. Delayed-release orally disintegrating tabs should not be broken or cut.
MOA — H-K ATPase proton pump inhibitor.
ADVERSE EFFECTS — Frequent: fatigue, dizziness, headache, abdominal pain, diarrhea, nausea, increased appetite. Severe: Pancreatitis, severe skin reactions, myositis, interstitial nephritis.

OMEPRAZOLE (*Prilosec, ✦Losec*) ▶L ♀C ▶? OTC $, Rx $$$$

ADULTS — GERD, duodenal ulcer, erosive esophagitis: 20 mg PO daily. Heartburn (OTC): 20 mg PO daily for 14 days. Gastric ulcer: 40 mg PO daily. Hypersecretory conditions: 60 mg PO daily. Part of a multi-drug regimen for H pylori eradication: 20 mg PO bid with amoxicillin 1000 mg PO bid and clarithromycin 500 mg PO bid for 10 day, with additional 18 days of omeprazole 20 mg PO daily if ulcer present (see table). Or 40 mg PO daily with clarithromycin 500 mg PO tid for 14 days, with additional 14 days of omeprazole 20 mg PO daily if ulcer present.
PEDS — GERD, acid-related disorders. maintenance of healing erosive esophagitis: 5 mg PO daily for wt 5 to 9 kg, 10 mg PO daily for wt 10 to 19 kg, give 20 mg PO daily for wt 20 kg or greater.
UNAPPROVED ADULTS — Upper GI bleeding: 80 mg IV, then infusion 8 mg/h until endoscopy.
UNAPPROVED PEDS — Gastric or duodenal ulcers, hypersecretory states: 0.2 to 3.5 mg/kg/dose PO daily. GERD: 1 mg/kg/day PO daily or bid.
FORMS — Rx Generic/Trade: Caps 10, 20, 40 mg. Trade only: Granules for oral susp 2.5 mg, 10 mg. OTC Trade only: Cap 20 mg.
NOTES — Take before meals. Caps contain enteric-coated granules; do not chew. Caps may be opened and administered in acidic liquid (eg, apple juice). May increase levels of diazepam, warfarin, and phenytoin. May decrease absorption of ketoconazole, itraconazole, iron, ampicillin, and digoxin. Reduces plasma levels of atazanavir. Concomitant administration with voriconazole, an inhibitor of CYP2C19 and CYP3A4 may lead to a more than doubling of omeprazole exposure. Avoid administration with sucralfate. Conflicting information whether reduces efficacy of clopidogrel.
MOA — H-K ATPase proton pump inhibitor.
ADVERSE EFFECTS — Frequent: Headache, dizziness, rash, diarrhea, N/V, taste perversion. Severe: Stevens-Johnson syndrome, erythema multiforme, stomatitis, agitation, pancytopenia, agranulocytosis, other blood dyscrasias, pancreatitis, psychiatric disturbances.

PANTOPRAZOLE (*Protonix, ✦Pantoloc*) ▶L ♀B ▶? $$$$

ADULTS — GERD: 40 mg PO daily for 8 to 16 weeks. Maintenance therapy following healing of erosive esophagitis: 40 mg PO daily. Zollinger-Ellison syndrome: 80 mg IV q 8 to 12 h for 7 days until taking PO. GERD associated with a history of erosive esophagitis: 40 mg IV daily for 7 to 10 days until taking PO.

(cont.)

GASTROENTEROLOGY: Antiulcer

PANTOPRAZOLE (cont.)
PEDS – <u>Erosive esophagitis associated with GERD:</u> 15kg to less than 40 kg: 20 mg PO daily for up to 8 weeks. 40 kg or greater: 40 mg PO daily for up to 8 weeks.
UNAPPROVED ADULTS – Has been studied as part of various <u>multi-drug regimens for H pylori eradication.</u> Decreases peptic ulcer re-bleeding after hemostasis: 80 mg IV bolus, then 8 mg/h continuous IV infusion for 3 days, followed by oral therapy (or 40 mg IV q 12 h for 4 to 7 days if unable to tolerate PO).
UNAPPROVED PEDS – <u>GERD associated with a history of erosive esophagitis:</u> 0.5 to 1 mg/kg/day (max 40 mg/day).
FORMS – Generic/Trade: Tabs 20, 40 mg. Trade only: Granules for susp 40 mg/packet.
NOTES – May decrease absorption of ketoconazole, itraconazole, digoxin, iron, and ampicillin. Reduces atazanavir concentrations (avoid together). Can increase INR when used with warfarin.
MOA – H-K ATPase proton pump inhibitor.
ADVERSE EFFECTS – Frequent: Headache. Serious: rhabdomyolysis, anaphylaxis, angioedema, severe dermatologic reactions, hepatocellular damage, interstitial nephritis, pancreatitis, pancytopenia.

RABEPRAZOLE (*AcipHex, ✦Pariet*) ▶L ♀B ▶? $$$$
ADULTS – <u>GERD:</u> 20 mg PO daily for 4 to 16 weeks. <u>Duodenal ulcers:</u> 20 mg PO daily for 4 weeks. <u>Zollinger-Ellison syndrome:</u> 60 mg PO daily, may increase up to 100 mg daily or 60 mg bid. <u>Part of a multidrug regimen for H pylori eradication:</u> 20 mg PO bid, with amoxicillin 1000 mg PO bid and clarithromycin 500 mg PO bid for 7 days.
PEDS – 20 mg PO daily up to 8 weeks for age 12 yo or older.
FORMS – Trade: Tabs 20 mg.
NOTES – May decrease absorption of ketoconazole, itraconazole, digoxin, iron, and ampicillin.
MOA – H-K ATPase proton pump inhibitor.
ADVERSE EFFECTS – Frequent: Headache. Serious: rhabdomyolysis, anaphylaxis, angioedema, severe dermatologic reactions, hepatocellular damage, interstitial nephritis, pancreatitis, pancytopenia.

ZEGERID (omeprazole + bicarbonate) ▶L ♀C ▶? $$$$$
ADULTS – <u>Duodenal ulcer, GERD, erosive esophagitis:</u> 20 mg PO daily for 4 to 8 weeks. <u>Gastric ulcer:</u> 40 mg PO once daily for 4 to 8 weeks. <u>Reduction of risk of upper GI bleed in critically ill</u> (susp only): 40 mg PO, then 40 mg 6 to 8 h later, then 40 mg once daily thereafter for up to 14 days.
PEDS – Not approved in children.
FORMS – OTC Trade only: omerpazole/sodium bicarbonate caps 20 mg/1 g. Rx Trade only: 20 mg/1 g and 40 mg/1 g, powder packets for susp 20 mg/1 g and 40 mg/1 g.
NOTES – Do not combine two 20 mg doses for a 40 mg dose, because the dose of sodium bicarbonate is the same in both dose strengths. May increase levels of diazepam, warfarin, and phenytoin. May decrease absorption of ketoconazole, itraconazole, iron, ampicillin, and digoxin. Reduces plasma levels of atazanavir. Avoid administration with sucralfate.
MOA – H-K ATPase proton pump inhibitor plus antacid combination.
ADVERSE EFFECTS – Frequent: Headache, dizziness, rash, diarrhea, N/V, taste perversion. Severe: Stevens-Johnson syndrome, erythema multiforme, stomatitis, agitation, pancytopenia, agranulocytosis, other blood dyscrasias, pancreatitis, psychiatric disturbances.

GASTROENTEROLOGY: Antiulcer—Other

BELLERGAL-S (phenobarbital + belladonna + ergotamine, ✦*Bellergal Spacetabs*) ▶LK ♀X ▶– $
WARNING – Serious or life-threatening peripheral ischemia has been noted with ergotamine component when used with CYP 3A4 inhibitors such as ritonavir, nelfinavir, indinavir, erythromycin, clarithromycin, ketoconazole, and itraconazole.
ADULTS – <u>Hypermotility/hypersecretion:</u> 1 tab PO bid.
PEDS – Not approved in children.
FORMS – Generic: Tabs phenobarbital 40 mg, ergotamine 0.6 mg, belladonna 0.2 mg.
NOTES – May decrease INR in patients receiving warfarin. Variable effect on phenytoin levels. May cause sedation especially with alcohol, phenothiazines, opioids, or TCAs. Additive anticholinergic effects with TCAs.
MOA – Competitive inhibition of the muscarinic actions of acetylcholine, partial agonist and/or antagonist against tryptaminergic, dopaminergic, and alpha-adrenergic receptors.
ADVERSE EFFECTS – Frequent: xerostomia, blurred vision, urinary retention and hesitancy, N/V, dizziness, tachycardia, bradycardia, claudication, arterial constriction, rebound headache, drowsiness.

DICYCLOMINE (*Bentyl, ✦Bentyol, Formulex, Protylol, Lomine*) ▶LK ♀B ▶– $
ADULTS – <u>Treatment of functional bowel/irritable bowel syndrome (irritable colon, spastic colon, mucous colon):</u> Initiate with 20 mg PO qid and increase to 40 mg PO qid, if tolerated. Patients who are unable to take oral medications: 20 mg IM q 6 h.
PEDS – Not approved in children.
UNAPPROVED PEDS – <u>Treatment of functional/irritable bowel syndrome:</u> 5 to 10 mg PO tid to qid (up to 40 mg/day) for age 6 mo or older.
FORMS – Generic/Trade: Tabs 20 mg. Caps 10 mg. Syrup 10 mg/5 mL. Generic only: Caps 20 mg.
NOTES – Although some use lower doses (ie, 10 to 20 mg PO qid), the only adult oral dose proven to be effective is 160 mg/day.
MOA – Inhibits effect of acetylcholine at parasympathetic receptors.
ADVERSE EFFECTS – Frequent: None specific but generally similar to other anticholinergic drugs.

DONNATAL (phenobarbital + hyoscyamine + atropine + scopolamine) ▶LK ♀C ▶– $$$
ADULTS — Adjunctive therapy of irritable bowel syndrome or adjunctive treatment of duodenal ulcers: 1 to 2 tabs/caps or 5 to 10 mL PO tid to qid or 1 extended-release tab PO q 8 to 12 h.
PEDS — Adjunctive therapy of irritable bowel syndrome, adjunctive treatment of duodenal ulcers: 0.1 mL/kg/dose q 4 h, max 5 mL. Alternative dosing regimen: Give 0.5 mL PO q 4 h or 0.75 mL PO q 6 h for wt 4.5 kg, give 1 mL PO q 4 h or 1.5 mL PO q 6 h for wt 9.1 kg, give 1.5 mL PO q 4 h or 2 mL PO q 6 h for wt 13.6 kg, give 2.5 mL PO q 4 h or 3.75 mL PO q 6 h for wt 22.7 kg, give 3.75 mL PO q 4 h or 5 mL PO q 6 h for wt 34 kg, give 5 mL PO q 4 h or 7.5 mL PO q 6 h for wt 45 kg or greater.
FORMS — Generic/trade: Phenobarbital 16.2 mg + hyoscyamine 0.1 mg + atropine 0.02 mg + scopolamine 6.5 mcg in each tab or 5 mL. Trade only: Extended-release tab 48.6 + 0.3111 + 0.0582 + 0.0195 mg.
NOTES — The FDA has classified Donnatal as "possibly effective" for treatment of irritable bowel syndrome and duodenal ulcer. Heat stroke may occur in hot weather. Can cause anticholinergic side effects; use caution in narrow-angle glaucoma, BPH, etc.
MOA — Anticonvulsant, inhibits effect of acetylcholine at parasympathetic receptors.
ADVERSE EFFECTS — Frequent: xerostomia, blurred vision, urinary retention and hesitancy, N/V, dizziness.

GI COCKTAIL (*green goddess*) ▶LK ♀See individual ▶See individual $
ADULTS — See components.
PEDS — Not approved in children.
UNAPPROVED ADULTS — Acute GI upset: Mixture of Maalox/Mylanta 30 mL + viscous lidocaine (2%) 10 mL + Donnatal 10 mL administered PO in a single dose.
NOTES — Avoid repeat dosing due to risk of lidocaine toxicity.
MOA — Antacid, anesthetic, anti-spasmodic.
ADVERSE EFFECTS — Frequent: None. Severe: Lidocaine toxicity with repeat dosing.

HYOSCINE (✦*Buscopan*) ▶LK ♀C ▶? $$
ADULTS — Canada: GI or bladder spasm: 10 to 20 mg PO/IV up to 60 mg daily (PO) or 100 mg daily (IV).
PEDS — Not approved in children.
FORMS — Canada Trade only: Tabs 10 mg.
NOTES — May cause dizziness, drowsiness, blurred vision, dry mouth, N/V, urinary retention. Contraindicated in glaucoma, obstructive conditions (eg, pyloric, duodenal or other intestinal obstructive lesions, ileus, and obstructive uropathies), and myasthenia gravis.
MOA — Anticholinergic that counteracts urinary and GI smooth muscle contraction.
ADVERSE EFFECTS — Serious: Heat stroke, paralytic ileus, increased ocular pressure, psychosis, anaphylaxis. Frequent: Dry mouth, urinary retention, constipation, headache, dizziness, drowsiness, fever, weakness, impotence, suppressed lactation, confusion, blurred vision, tachycardia, palpitations, anhidrosis, mydriasis, cycloplegia, loss of taste.

HYOSCYAMINE (*Anaspaz, A-spaz, Cystospaz, ED Spaz, Hyosol, Hyospaz, Levbid, Levsin, Levsinex, Medispaz, NuLev, Spacol, Spasdel, Symax*) ▶LK ♀C ▶– $
ADULTS — Bladder spasm, control gastric secretion, GI hypermotility, irritable bowel syndrome: 0.125 to 0.25 mg PO/SL q 4 h or prn. Extended-release 0.375 to 0.75 mg PO q 12 h. Max 1.5 mg/day.
PEDS — Bladder spasm: Use adult dosing in age older than 12 yo. To control gastric secretion, GI hypermotility, irritable bowel syndrome, and others: Initial oral dose by wt for age younger than 2 yo: give 12.5 mcg for 2.3 kg, give 16.7 mcg for 3.4 kg, give 20.8 mcg for 5 kg, give 25 mcg for 7 kg, give 31.3 to 33.3 mcg for 10 kg, give 45.8 mcg for 15 kg. Alternatively, if age younger than 2 yo: 3 gtts for wt 2.3 kg, give 4 gtts for 3.4 kg, give 5 gtts for 5 kg, give 6 gtts for 7 kg, give 8 gtts for 10 kg, give 11 gtts for 15 kg. Doses can be repeated q 4 h prn, but maximum daily dose is six times initial dose. Initial oral dose by wt for age 2 to 12 yo: give 31.3 to 33.3 mcg for 10 kg, give 62.5 mcg for 20 kg, give 93.8 mcg for 40 kg, and give 125 mcg for 50 kg. Doses may be repeated q 4 h, but maximum daily dose should not exceed 750 mcg.
FORMS — Generic/Trade: Tabs 0.125, 0.15 mg. Sublingual tabs 0.125 mg. Chewable tabs 0.125 mg. Extended-release tabs, caps 0.375 mg. Elixir 0.125 mg/5 mL. Gtts 0.125 mg/1 mL.
NOTES — May cause dizziness, drowsiness, blurred vision, dry mouth, N/V, urinary retention. Contraindicated in glaucoma, obstructive conditions (eg, pyloric, duodenal or other intestinal obstructive lesions, ileus, achalasia, GI hemorrhage, and obstructive uropathies), unstable cardiovascular status, and myasthenia gravis.
MOA — Anticholinergic that counteracts urinary and GI smooth muscle contraction.
ADVERSE EFFECTS — Serious: Heat stroke, paralytic ileus, increased ocular pressure, psychosis. Frequent: Dry mouth, urinary retention, constipation, headache, dizziness, drowsiness, fever, weakness, impotence, suppressed lactation, confusion, blurred vision, tachycardia, palpitations, anhidrosis, mydriasis, cycloplegia, loss of taste.

MEPENZOLATE (*Cantil*) ▶K + gut ♀B ▶? $$$$$
ADULTS — Adjunctive therapy in peptic ulcer disease: 25 to 50 mg PO qid, with meals and at bedtime.
PEDS — Not approved in children.
FORMS — Trade only: Tabs 25 mg.
NOTES — Contraindicated in glaucoma, obstructive uropathy, paralytic ileus, toxic megacolon, obstructive diseases of GI tract, intestinal atony in elderly/debilitated, myasthenia gravis, unstable CV status, acute GI bleed.
MOA — Post-ganglionic parasympathetic inhibitor.

(cont.)

MEPENZOLATE (cont.)
ADVERSE EFFECTS — Frequent: Drowsiness, blurred vision, constipation, headache, dry mouth, urinary retention, tachycardia.

METHSCOPOLAMINE (Pamine, Pamine Forte) ▶LK ♀C ▶? $$$$
ADULTS — Adjunctive therapy in peptic ulcer disease: 2.5 mg PO 30 min before meals and 2.5 to 5 mg PO at bedtime, max 12.5 mg/day.
PEDS — Not approved in children.
FORMS — Generic/Trade: Tabs 2.5 mg (Pamine), 5 mg (Pamine Forte).
NOTES — Has not been shown to be effective in treating peptic ulcer disease.
MOA — Anticholinergic.
ADVERSE EFFECTS — Frequent: xerostomia, blurred vision, urinary retention and hesitancy, constipation, N/V, dizziness.

MISOPROSTOL (PGE1, Cytotec) ▶LK ♀X ▶– $$$$
WARNING — Contraindicated in desired early or preterm pregnancy due to its abortifacient property. Pregnant women should avoid contact/exposure to the tabs. Uterine rupture reported with use for labor induction and medical abortion.
ADULTS — Prevention of NSAID-induced gastric ulcers: 200 mcg PO qid. If not tolerated, use 100 mcg PO qid.
PEDS — Not approved in children.
UNAPPROVED ADULTS — Cervical ripening and labor induction: 25 mcg intravaginally q 3 to 6 h (or 50 mcg q 6 h). First trimester pregnancy failure: 800 mcg intravaginally, repeat on day 3 if expulsion incomplete. Medical abortion 63 days gestation or less: With mifepristone, see mifepristone; with methotrexate: 800 mcg intravaginally 5 to 7 days after 50 mg/m2 IM methotrexate. Pre-op cervical ripening: 400 mcg intravaginally 3 to 4 h before mechanical cervical dilation. Postpartum hemorrhage: 800 mcg PR single dose. Oral dosing has been used but is controversial. Treatment of duodenal ulcers: 100 mcg PO qid.
UNAPPROVED PEDS — Improvement in fat absorption in cystic fibrosis in children 8 to 16 yo: 100 mcg PO qid.
FORMS — Generic/Trade: Oral tabs 100, 200 mcg.
NOTES — Contraindicated with prior C-section. Oral tabs can be inserted into the vagina for labor induction/cervical ripening. Monitor for uterine hyperstimulation and abnormal fetal heart rate. Risk factors for uterine rupture: Prior uterine surgery and 5 previous pregnancies or more.
MOA — Prostaglandin E1 analog, uterine stimulant.
ADVERSE EFFECTS — Serious: Uterine hyperstimulation, uterine rupture. Frequent: Diarrhea, abdominal pain.

PROPANTHELINE (Pro-Banthine, *Propanthel) ▶LK ♀C ▶– $$$
ADULTS — Adjunctive therapy in peptic ulcer disease: 7.5 to 15 mg PO 30 min before meals and 30 mg at bedtime.
PEDS — Not approved in children.
UNAPPROVED ADULTS — Irritable bowel, pancreatitis, urinary bladder spasms: 7.5 to 15 mg PO tid and 30 mg at bedtime.
UNAPPROVED PEDS — Antisecretory effects: 1 to 2 mg/kg/day PO in 3 to 4 divided doses. Antispasmodic effects: 2 to 3 mg/kg/day PO divided q 4 to 6 h and at bedtime.
FORMS — Generic only: Tabs 15 mg.
NOTES — For elderly adults and those with small stature use 7.5 mg dose. May cause constipation, dry mucous membranes.
MOA — Antispasmodic.
ADVERSE EFFECTS — Frequent: None

SIMETHICONE (Mylicon, Gas-X, Phazyme, *Ovol) ▶Not absorbed ♀C but + ▶? $
ADULTS — Excessive gas in GI tract: 40 to 250 mg PO after meals and at bedtime prn, max 500 mg/day.
PEDS — Excessive gas in GI tract: 20 mg PO qid prn, max 240 mg/day for age younger than 2 yo, 40 mg PO qid prn for age 2 to 12 yo (max 500 mg/day).
UNAPPROVED PEDS — Although used to treat infant colic (in approved dose for gas), several studies suggest no benefit.
FORMS — OTC Generic/Trade: Chewable tabs 80, 125 mg. Gtts 40 mg/0.6 mL. Trade only: Softgels 166 mg (Gas-X) 180 mg (Phazyme). Strips, oral (Gas-X) 62.5 mg (adults), 40 mg (children).
NOTES — For administration to infants, may mix dose in 30 mL of liquid. Chewable tabs should be chewed thoroughly.
MOA — Theoretically, relieves gas pressure and bloating.
ADVERSE EFFECTS — Frequent: None.

SUCRALFATE (Carafate, *Sulcrate) ▶Not absorbed ♀B ▶? $$
ADULTS — Duodenal ulcer: 1 g PO qid, 1 h before meals and at bedtime. Maintenance therapy of duodenal ulcer: 1 g PO bid.
PEDS — Not approved in children.
UNAPPROVED ADULTS — Gastric ulcer, reflux esophagitis, NSAID-induced GI symptoms, stress ulcer prophylaxis: 1 g PO qid 1 h before meals and at bedtime. Oral and esophageal ulcers due to radiation/chemo/sclerotherapy: (susp only) 5 to 10 mL swish and spit/swallow qid.
UNAPPROVED PEDS — Reflux esophagitis, gastric or duodenal ulcer, stress ulcer prophylaxis: 40 to 80 mg/kg/day PO divided q 6 h. Alternative dosing: 500 mg PO qid for age younger than 6 yo, give 1 g PO qid for age 6 yo or older.
FORMS — Generic/Trade: Tabs 1 g. Susp 1 g/10 mL.
NOTES — May cause constipation. May reduce the absorption of cimetidine, ciprofloxacin, digoxin, ketoconazole, levothyroxine, itraconazole, norfloxacin, phenytoin, ranitidine, tetracycline, theophylline and warfarin; separate doses by at least 2 h. Antacids should be separated by at least 30 min.
MOA — Forms synthetic barrier against peptic acid.
ADVERSE EFFECTS — Frequent: Constipation.

GASTROENTEROLOGY: Laxatives—Bulk-Forming

METHYLCELLULOSE (*Citrucel*) ▶Not absorbed ♀+ ▶? $
ADULTS — Laxative: 1 heaping tablespoon in 8 oz cold water PO daily (up to tid).
PEDS — Laxative: Age 6 to 12 yo: 1½ heaping teaspoons in 4 oz cold water daily (up to tid) PO prn.
FORMS — OTC Trade only: Regular and sugar-free packets and multiple-use canisters, Clear-mix soln, Caps 500 mg.
NOTES — Must be taken with water to avoid esophageal obstruction or choking.
MOA — Osmotic effect in intestinal lumen.
ADVERSE EFFECTS — Frequent: None.

POLYCARBOPHIL (*FiberCon, Konsyl Fiber, Equalactin, Psyllium*) ▶Not absorbed ♀+ ▶? $
ADULTS — Laxative: 1 g PO qid prn.
PEDS — Laxative: Children 3 to 5 yo: 500 mg PO daily (up to bid) prn for age 6 yo or older: 500 mg PO daily (up to qid) prn.
UNAPPROVED ADULTS — Diarrhea: 1 g PO q 30 min prn. Max daily dose 6 g.
UNAPPROVED PEDS — Diarrhea: Give 500 mg PO q 30 min prn (up to 1 g polycarbophil/day for age 3 to 5 yo, and 2 g/day for age older than 6 yo).
FORMS — OTC Generic/Trade: Tabs/Caps 625 mg. OTC Trade only: Chewable tabs 625 mg (Equalactin).
NOTES — When used as a laxative, take dose with at least 8 oz of fluid. Do not administer concomitantly with tetracycline; separate by at least 2 h.
MOA — Bulk-forming laxatives.
ADVERSE EFFECTS — Frequent: None. Severe: Esophageal obstruction, hypersensitivity.

PSYLLIUM (*Metamucil, Fiberall, Konsyl, Hydrocil, ♣Prodium Plain*) ▶Not absorbed ♀+ ▶? $
ADULTS — Laxative: 1 rounded tsp in liquid, 1 packet in liquid or 1 wafer with liquid PO daily (up to tid).
PEDS — Laxative (children 6 to 11 yo): ½ to 1 rounded tsp in liquid, ½ to 1 packet in liquid or 1 wafer with liquid PO daily (up to tid).
UNAPPROVED ADULTS — Reduction in cholesterol: 1 rounded tsp in liquid, 1 packet in liquid or 1 to 2 wafers with liquid PO tid. Prevention of GI side effects with orlistat: 6 g in liquid with each orlistat dose or 12 g in liquid at bedtime.
FORMS — OTC Generic/Trade: Regular and sugar-free powder, Granules, Caps, Wafers, including various flavors and various amounts of psyllium.
NOTES — Powders and granules must be mixed with liquid prior to ingestion. Start with 1 dose/day and gradually increase to minimize gas and bloating. Can bind with warfarin, digoxin, potassium-sparing diuretics, salicylates, tetracycline and nitrofurantoin; space at least 3 h apart.
MOA — Adsorbs water to bulk stool.
ADVERSE EFFECTS — Frequent: None. Severe: Bronchospasm, anaphylaxis.

GASTROENTEROLOGY: Laxatives—Osmotic

GLYCERIN (*Fleet*) ▶Not absorbed ♀C ▶? $
ADULTS — Constipation: 1 adult suppository PR prn.
PEDS — Constipation: Give 0.5 mL/kg/dose as an enema PR prn in neonates, give 1 infant suppository or 2 to 5 mL rectal soln as an enema PR prn for age younger than 6 yo, give 1 adult suppository or 5 to 15 mL of rectal soln as enema PR prn for age 6 yo or older.
FORMS — OTC Generic/Trade: Suppository infant and adult, Soln (Fleet Babylax) 4 mL/applicator.
MOA — Softens and lubricates stool.
ADVERSE EFFECTS — Frequent: None.

LACTULOSE (*Enulose, Kristalose*) ▶Not absorbed ♀B ▶? $$
ADULTS — Constipation: 15 to 30 mL (syrup) or 10 to 20 g (powder for oral soln) PO daily. Evacuation of barium following barium procedures: 15 to 30 mL (syrup) PO daily, may increase to 60 mL. Acute hepatic encephalopathy: 30 to 45 mL syrup/dose PO q 1 h until laxative effect observed or 300 mL in 700 mL water or saline PR as a retention enema q 4 to 6 h. Prevention of encephalopathy: 30 to 45 mL syrup PO tid to qid.
PEDS — Prevention or treatment of encephalopathy: Infants: 2.5 to 10 mL/day (syrup) PO in 3 to 4 divided doses. Children/adolescents: 40 to 90 mL/day (syrup) PO in 3 to 4 divided doses.
UNAPPROVED ADULTS — Restoration of bowel movements in hemorrhoidectomy patients: 15 mL syrup PO bid on days before surgery and for 5 days following surgery.
UNAPPROVED PEDS — Constipation: 7.5 mL syrup PO daily, after breakfast.
FORMS — Generic/Trade: Syrup 10 g/15 mL. Trade only (Kristalose): 10, 20 g packets for oral soln.
NOTES — May be mixed in water, juice, or milk to improve palatability. Packets for oral soln should be mixed in 4 oz of water or juice. Titrate dose to produce 2 to 3 soft stools/day.
MOA — Converts NH3 to NH4+ to prevent rediffusion into plasma.
ADVERSE EFFECTS — Frequent: Flatulence, diarrhea.

MAGNESIUM CITRATE (*♣Citro-Mag*) ▶K ♀B ▶? $
ADULTS — Evacuate bowel prior to procedure: 150 to 300 mL PO once or in divided doses.
PEDS — Evacuate bowel prior to procedure: 2 to 4 mL/kg PO once or in divided doses for age younger than 6 yo. 100 to 150 mL PO once or in divided doses for age 6 to 12 yo.
FORMS — OTC Generic only: Soln 300 mL/bottle. Low-sodium and sugar-free available.
NOTES — Use caution with impaired renal function. May decrease absorption of phenytoin, ciprofloxacin, benzodiazepines, and glyburide. May cause

(cont.)

GASTROENTEROLOGY: Laxatives

MAGNESIUM CITRATE (cont.)
additive CNS depression with CNS depressants. Chill to improve palatability.
MOA — Osmotic effect in intestinal lumen.
ADVERSE EFFECTS — Frequent: None. Severe: Electrolyte disturbances, CNS depression.

MAGNESIUM HYDROXIDE (*Milk of Magnesia*) ▶K ♀+ ▶? $
ADULTS — Laxative: 30 to 60 mL PO as a single dose or divided doses. Antacid: 5 to 15 mL/dose PO qid prn or 622 to 1244 mg PO qid prn.
PEDS — Laxative: Give 0.5 mL/kg PO as a single dose for age younger than 2 yo, give 5 to 15 mL/day PO as a single dose or in divided doses for age 2 to 5 yo, give 15 to 30 mL PO in a single dose or in divided doses for age 6 to 11 yo. Antacid: 2.5 to 5 mL/dose PO qid prn for age older than 12 yo.
FORMS — OTC Generic/Trade: Susp 400 mg/5 mL. Trade only: Chewable tabs 311, 400 mg. Generic only: Susp (concentrated) 1200 mg/5 mL, sugar-free 400 mg/5 mL.
NOTES — Use caution with impaired renal function.
MOA — Osmotic effect in intestinal lumen.
ADVERSE EFFECTS — Frequent: Diarrhea.

POLYETHYLENE GLYCOL (*MiraLax, GlycoLax*) ▶Not absorbed ♀C ▶? $
ADULTS — Constipation: 17 g (1 heaping tablespoon) in 4 to 8 oz water, juice, soda, coffee, or tea PO daily.
PEDS — Not approved in children.
UNAPPROVED PEDS — Children older than 4 yo: 0.1 to 1.5 g/kg/day PO, max 17 g/day.
FORMS — OTC Trade only: Powder for oral soln 17 g/scoop. Rx Generic/Trade: Powder for oral soln 17 g/scoop.
NOTES — Takes 1 to 3 days to produce bowel movement. Indicated for up to 14 days.
MOA — Osmotic and cathartic effect in intestinal lumen.
ADVERSE EFFECTS — Frequent: Nausea, fullness, bloating. Serious: Risk of aspiration in children.

POLYETHYLENE GLYCOL WITH ELECTROLYTES (*GoLytely, Colyte, TriLyte, NuLytely, Moviprep, HalfLytely, and Bisacodyl Tablet Kit, ✦Klean-Prep, Electropeg, Peg-Lyte*) ▶Not absorbed ♀C ▶? $
ADULTS — Bowel cleansing prior to GI examination: 240 mL PO every 10 min or 20 to 30 mL/min NG until 4L are consumed or rectal effluent is clear. Moviprep: 240 mL q 15 min for 4 doses (over 1 h) the night before plus 16 additional ounces of clear liquid and 240 mL q 15 min for 4 doses (over 1 h) plus 16 additional ounces of clear liquid on the morning of the colonoscopy. Alternatively, 240 mL q 15 min for 4 doses (over 1 h) at 6 pm on the evening before the colonoscopy and then 1.5 h later, 240 mL q 15 min for 4 doses (over 1 h) plus 32 additional ounces of clear liquid on the evening before the colonoscopy (Moviprep only).
PEDS — Bowel prep (NuLYTELY, TriLyte): 25 mL/kg/h PO/NG, until rectal effluent is clear, maximum 4L for age greater than 6 mo.
UNAPPROVED ADULTS — Chronic constipation: 125 to 500 mL/day PO daily (up to bid).
UNAPPROVED PEDS — Bowel cleansing prior to GI examination: 25 to 40 mL/kg/h PO/NG for 4 to 10 h or until rectal effluent is clear or 20 to 30 mL/min NG until 4L are consumed or rectal effluent is clear. Whole bowel irrigation in iron overdose: give 0.5 L/h for age younger than 3 yo.
FORMS — Generic/Trade: powder for oral solution in disposable jug 4L or 2L (Moviprep). Also, as a kit of 2L bottle of polyethylene glycol with electrolytes and 2 or 4 bisacodyl tabs 5 mg (HalfLytely and Bisacodyl Tablet Kit). Trade only (GoLytely): packet for oral solution to make 3.785 L.
NOTES — Solid food should not be given within 2 h of soln. Effects should occur within 1 to 2 h. Chilling improves palatability.
MOA — Osmotic and cathartic effect in intestinal lumen.
ADVERSE EFFECTS — Frequent: Nausea, fullness, bloating. Severe: Hypersensitivity reactions.

SODIUM PHOSPHATE (*Fleet enema, Fleet Phospho-Soda, Fleet EZ-Prep, Accu-Prep, Osmoprep, Visicol, ✦Enemol, Phoslax*) ▶Not absorbed ♀C ▶? $
WARNING — Phosphate-containing bowel cleansing regimens have been reported to cause acute phosphate nephropathy. Risk factors include advanced age, kidney disease or decreased intravascular volume, bowel obstruction or active colitis, and medications that affect renal perfusion or function such as diuretics, ACE inhibitors, ARBs, and maybe NSAIDs. Use extreme caution in bowel cleansing.
ADULTS — 1 adult or pediatric enema PR or 20 to 30 mL of oral soln PO prn (max 45 mL/24 h). Visicol: Evening before colonoscopy: 3 tabs with 8 oz clear liquid q 15 min until 20 tabs are consumed. Day of colonoscopy: Starting 3 to 5 h before procedure, 3 tabs with 8 oz clear liquid q 15 min until 20 tabs are consumed.
PEDS — Laxative: 2 to 11 yo: one pediatric enema (67.5 mL) PR prn or 5 to 9 yo: 5 mL of oral soln PO prn. 10 to 12 yo: 10 mL of oral soln PO prn.
UNAPPROVED ADULTS — Visicol: Evening before colonoscopy: 3 tabs with 8 oz clear liquid q 15 min until 20 tabs are consumed. Day of colonoscopy: Starting 3 to 5 h before procedure, 3 tabs with 8 oz clear liquid q 15 min until 8 to 12 tabs are consumed.
FORMS — OTC Generic/Trade: Adult enema, oral soln. OTC Trade only: Pediatric enema, bowel prep. Rx Trade only: Visicol, Osmoprep tab ($$$$) 1.5 g.
NOTES — Taking the last 2 doses of Visicol with ginger ale appears to minimize residue. Excessive doses (more than 45 mL/24 h) of oral products may lead to serious electrolyte disturbances. Use with caution in severe renal impairment.
MOA — Osmotic and cathartic effect in intestinal lumen.
ADVERSE EFFECTS — Frequent: None. Severe: Electrolyte and fluid imbalances.

SORBITOL ▶Not absorbed ♀C ▶? $
ADULTS — Laxative: 30 to 150 mL (of 70% soln) PO or 120 mL (of 25 to 30% soln) PR. Cathartic: 4.3 mL/kg PO.
PEDS — Laxative: Children 2 to 11 yo: 2 mL/kg (of 70% soln) PO or 30 to 60 mL (of 25 to 30% soln) PR.
UNAPPROVED PEDS — Cathartic: 4.3 mL/kg of 35% soln (diluted from 70% soln) PO single dose.
FORMS — Generic only: Soln 70%.
NOTES — When used as a cathartic, can be given with activated charcoal to improve taste and decrease gastric transit time of charcoal. May precipitate electrolyte changes.
MOA — Osmotic and cathartic effect in intestinal lumen.
ADVERSE EFFECTS — Serious: Pulmonary congestion, angina-like pain, acidosis, electrolyte loss, convulsions. Frequent: Hyperglycemia, diarrhea, tachycardia, diuresis, urinary retention, blurred vision, dry mouth, thirst, dehydration, edema, N/V, rhinitis, chills, vertigo, headache, urticaria.

GASTROENTEROLOGY: Laxatives—Stimulant

BISACODYL (*Correctol, Dulcolax, Feen-a-Mint, Fleet*) ▶L ♀C ▶? $
ADULTS — Constipation/colonic evacuation prior to a procedure: 10 to 15 mg PO daily prn, 10 mg PR daily prn.
PEDS — Constipation/colonic evacuation prior to a procedure: 0.3 mg/kg/day PO daily prn. Give 5 mg PR prn for age younger than 2, give 5 to 10 mg PR prn for age 2 to 11 yo, give 10 mg PR prn for 12 yo or older.
FORMS — OTC Generic/Trade: Tabs 5 mg, suppository 10 mg. OTC Trade only (Fleet): Enema, 10 mg/30 mL.
NOTES — Oral tab has onset of 6 to 10 h. Onset of action of suppository is approximately 15 to 60 min. Do not chew tabs, swallow whole. Do not give within 1 h of antacids or dairy products. Chronic use of stimulant laxatives may be habit forming.
MOA — Direct colonic stimulant.
ADVERSE EFFECTS — Frequent: None.
CASCARA ▶L ♀C ▶+ $
ADULTS — Constipation: 325 mg PO at bedtime prn or 5 mL/day of aromatic fluid extract PO at bedtime prn.
PEDS — Constipation: Infants: 1.25 mL/day of aromatic fluid extract PO daily prn. Children 2 to 11 yo: 2.5 mL/day of aromatic fluid extract PO daily prn.
FORMS — OTC Generic only: Tabs 325 mg, liquid aromatic fluid extract.
NOTES — Cascara sagrada fluid extract is 5× more potent than cascara sagrada aromatic fluid extract. Chronic use of stimulant laxatives may be habit forming.
MOA — Direct irritation of intestinal mucosa.
ADVERSE EFFECTS — Frequent: Lightheadedness, fluid/electrolyte imbalance, abdominal cramps, nausea, diarrhea, discoloration of urine.
CASTOR OIL ▶Not absorbed ♀− ▶? $
ADULTS — Constipation: 15 mL PO daily prn. Colonic evacuation prior to procedure: 15 to 30 mL of castor oil or 30 to 60 mL emulsified castor oil PO as a single dose 16 h prior to procedure.
PEDS — Colonic evacuation prior to procedure: Give 1 to 5 mL of castor oil or 5 to 15 mL emulsified castor oil PO as a single dose 16 h prior to procedure for age younger than 2 yo. Give 5 to 15 mL of castor oil or 7.5 to 30 mL of emulsified castor oil PO as a single dose 16 h prior to procedure for age 2 to 11yo.
FORMS — OTC Generic only: Oil 60, 120 mL.
NOTES — Emulsions somewhat mask the bad taste. Onset of action approximately 2 to 6 h. Do not give at bedtime. Chill or administer with juice to improve taste.
MOA — Softens and lubricates stool.
ADVERSE EFFECTS — Frequent: None.
SENNA (*Senokot, SenokotXTRA, Ex-Lax, Fletcher's Castoria, ✦Glysennid*) ▶L ♀C ▶+ $
ADULTS — Laxative or evacuation of the colon for bowel or rectal examinations: 1 tsp granules in water or 10 to 15 mL or 2 tabs PO at bedtime. Max daily dose 4 tsp of granules, 30 mL of syrup, 8 tabs or 2 suppositories.
PEDS — Laxative: 10 to 20 mg/kg/dose PO at bedtime. Alternative regimen: 1 mo to 2 yo: 1.25 to 2.5 mL syrup PO at bedtime, max 5 mL/day; 2 to 5 yo: 2.5 to 3.75 mL syrup PO at bedtime, max 7.5 mL/day; 6 to 12 yo: 5 to 7.5 mL syrup PO at bedtime, max 15 mL/day.
FORMS — OTC Generic/Trade (All dosing is based on sennosides content; 1 mg sennosides = 21.7 mg standardized senna concentrate): Syrup 8.8 mg/5 mL, Liquid 3 mg/mL (Fletcher's Castoria), Tabs 8.6, 15, 17, 25 mg, Chewable tabs 15 mg.
NOTES — Effects occur 6 to 24 h after oral administration. Use caution in renal dysfunction. Chronic use of stimulant laxatives may be habit forming.
MOA — Enhances GI motility.
ADVERSE EFFECTS — Frequent: Potential for severe diaper rash in children wearing diapers.

GASTROENTEROLOGY: Laxatives—Stool Softener

DOCUSATE (*Colace, Surfak, Kaopectate Stool Softener, Enemeez*) ▶L ♀C ▶? $
ADULTS — Constipation. Docusate calcium: 240 mg PO daily. Docusate sodium: 50 to 500 mg/day PO in 1 to 4 divided doses.
PEDS — Constipation. docusate sodium: Give 10 to 40 mg/day for age younger than 3 yo, give 20 to 60 mg/day for age 3 to 6 yo, give 40 to 150 mg/day for age 6 to 12 yo. In all cases doses are divided up to qid.

(cont.)

228　GASTROENTEROLOGY: Ulcerative Colitis

DOCUSATE *(cont.)*
UNAPPROVED ADULTS – Docusate sodium, Constipation. Can be given as a retention enema: Mix 50 to 100 mg docusate liquid with saline or water retention enema for rectal use. Cerumen removal: Instill 1 mL liquid (not syrup) in affected ear; allow to remain for 10 to 15 min, then irrigate with 50 mL lukewarm NS if necessary.
UNAPPROVED PEDS – Docusate sodium: Cerumen removal: Instill 1 mL liquid (not syrup) in affected ear; allow to remain for 10 to 15 min, then irrigate with 50 mL lukewarm NS if necessary.
FORMS – Docusate calcium OTC Generic/Trade: Caps 240 mg. Docusate sodium OTC Generic/Trade: Caps 50, 100, 250 mg. Liquid 50 mg/5 mL. Syrup 20 mg/5 mL. Docusate sodium OTC Trade only (Enemeez): Enema, rectal 283 mg/5 mL.
NOTES – Takes 1 to 3 days to notably soften stools.
MOA – Softens stool, cerumen.
ADVERSE EFFECTS – Frequent: Abdominal cramping.

GASTROENTEROLOGY: Laxatives—Other or Combinations

LUBIPROSTONE *(Amitiza)* ▶Gut ♀C ▶? $$$$$
WARNING – Avoid if symptoms or history of mechanical GI obstruction.
ADULTS – Chronic idiopathic constipation: 24 mcg PO bid with food and water. Irritable bowel syndrome with constipation in age 18 yo or older: 8 mcg PO bid.
PEDS – Not approved in children.
FORMS – Trade only: 8, 24 mcg caps.
MOA – Chloride channel activator which enhances intestinal fluid secretion, thereby increasing intestinal motility.
ADVERSE EFFECTS – Frequent: Nausea, diarrhea, headache, abdominal pain/distension, flatulence.

MINERAL OIL *(Kondremul, Fleet Mineral Oil Enema, Liqui-Doss, ✦Lansoyl)* ▶Not absorbed ♀C ▶? $
ADULTS – Laxative: 15 to 45 mL PO in a single dose or in divided doses, 60 to 150 mL PR.
PEDS – Laxative: Children 6 to 11 yo: 5 to 15 mL PO in a single dose or in divided doses. Children 2 to 11 yo: 30 to 60 mL PR.
FORMS – OTC Generic/Trade: Oil (30, 480 mL), Enema (Fleet). OTC Trade only: Oral liquid (Liqui-Doss) 13.5 mg/15 mL. Oral microemulsion (Kondremul) 2.5 mg/5 mL.
NOTES – Use with caution in children younger than 4 yo and elderly or debilitated patients due to concerns for aspiration pneumonitis. Although usual directions for plain mineral oil are to administer at bedtime, this increases risk of lipid pneumonitis. Mineral oil emulsions may be administered with meals.
MOA – Softens and lubricates stool.
ADVERSE EFFECTS – Frequent: None.

PERI-COLACE (docusate + sennosides) ▶L ♀C ▶? $
ADULTS – Constipation: 2 to 4 tabs PO once daily or in divided doses prn.
PEDS – Constipation 6 to 12 yo: 1 to 2 tabs PO daily prn. 2 to 6 yo: Up to 1 tab PO daily prn.
FORMS – OTC Generic/Trade: Tabs 50 mg docusate + 8.6 mg sennosides.
NOTES – Dilute syrup in 6 to 8 oz. of juice, milk, or infant formula to prevent throat irritation. Chronic use of stimulant laxatives (casanthranol) may be habit forming.
MOA – Softens stool.
ADVERSE EFFECTS – Frequent: Abdominal cramping.

SENOKOT-S (senna + docusate) ▶L ♀C ▶+ $
ADULTS – 2 tabs PO daily, maximum 4 tabs bid.
PEDS – 6 to 12 yo: 1 tab PO daily, max 2 tabs bid. 2 to 6 yo: ½ tab PO daily, max 1 tab bid.
FORMS – OTC Generic/Trade: Tabs 8.6 mg senna concentrate/50 mg docusate.
NOTES – Effects occur 6 to 12 h after oral administration. Use caution in renal dysfunction. Chronic use of stimulant laxatives may be habit forming.
MOA – Natural product; enhances GI motility and softens stool.
ADVERSE EFFECTS – Frequent: None.

GASTROENTEROLOGY: Ulcerative Colitis

BALSALAZIDE *(Colazal)* ▶Minimal absorption ♀B ▶? $$$$$
ADULTS – Ulcerative colitis: 2.25 g PO tid for 8 to 12 weeks.
PEDS – 5 to 17 yo: Mild to moderately active ulcerative colitis: 2.25 g PO tid for 8 weeks. Alternatively, 750 mg PO tid for 8 weeks.
FORMS – Generic/Trade: Caps 750 mg.
NOTES – Contraindicated in salicylate allergy. Caution with renal insufficiency.
MOA – Mesalamine prodrug, inhibits cyclooxygenase pathways.
ADVERSE EFFECTS – Frequent: Headache, abdominal pain, nausea, diarrhea, vomiting, respiratory infection, arthralgias. Severe: Cholestatic jaundice, cirrhosis, liver failure, hypersensitivity, pericarditis.

MESALAMINE *(5-aminosalicylic acid, Apriso, 5-Aspirin, Asacol, Lialda, Pentasa, Canasa, Rowasa, ✦Mesasal, Salofalk)* ▶Gut ♀C ▶? $$$$$
ADULTS – Ulcerative colitis: Asacol: 800 to 1600 mg PO tid. Pentasa: 1 g PO qid. Lialda: 2.4 to 4.8 g PO daily with a meal for 8 weeks. Susp: 4 g (60 mL) PR retained for 8 h at bedtime. Asacol: maintenance of Ulcerative colitis: 1600 mg/day PO in divided doses. Apriso: 1.5 g (4 caps) PO qam. Ulcerative proctitis: Canasa suppository: 500 mg PR bid to tid or 1000 mg PR at bedtime.
PEDS – Not approved in children.

(cont.)

MESALAMINE (cont.)
UNAPPROVED ADULTS – <u>Active Crohn's:</u> 0.4 to 4.8 g/day PO in divided doses. <u>Maintenance of remission of Crohn's:</u> 2.4 g/day in divided doses.
UNAPPROVED PEDS – Tabs: 50 mg/kg/day PO divided q 8 to 12 h. Caps: 50 mg/kg/day PO divided q 6 to 12 h.
FORMS – Trade only: delayed-release tab 400 mg (Asacol), 800 mg (Asacol HD). Controlled-release cap 250, 500 mg (Pentasa). Delayed-release tab 1200 mg (Lialda). Rectal suppository 1000 mg (Canasa). Controlled-release cap 0.375 g (Apriso). Generic/Trade: Rectal susp 4 g/60 mL (Rowasa).
NOTES – Avoid in salicylate sensitivity or hepatic dysfunction. Reports of hepatic failure in patients with pre-existing liver disease. May decrease digoxin levels. May discolor urine yellow-brown. Most common adverse effects include headache, abdominal pain, fever, rash. The coating of Asacol and Asacol HD contain the inactive chemical, dibutyl phthalate (DBP) In animal studies at doses > 190 times the human dose, maternal DBP was associated with external and skeletal malformations and adverse effects on the male reproductive system.
MOA – Unknown.
ADVERSE EFFECTS – Frequent: Headache, malaise, abdominal pain, cramps, flatulence, gas, hair loss. Severe: Cytopenias, myo- and pericarditis, hepatitis, pneumonitis, nephritis.

OLSALAZINE (*Dipentum*) ▶L ♀C ▶– $$$$$
ADULTS – <u>Maintenance of remission of ulcerative colitis in patients intolerant to sulfasalazine:</u> 500 mg PO bid with food.
PEDS – Not approved in children.
UNAPPROVED ADULTS – <u>Crohn's:</u> 1.5 to 3 g/day PO in divided doses with food.
FORMS – Trade only: Caps 250 mg.
NOTES – Diarrhea in up to 17%. Avoid in salicylate sensitivity.
MOA – Unknown.
ADVERSE EFFECTS – Frequent: Diarrhea, cramps, abdominal pain.

SULFASALAZINE (*Azulfidine, Azulfidine EN-tabs, ✦Salazopyrin En-tabs, S.A.S.*) ▶L ♀D ▶– $$
WARNING – Beware of hypersensitivity, marrow suppression, renal and liver damage, irreversible neuromuscular
ADULTS – <u>Colitis:</u> Initially 500 to 1000 mg PO qid. Maintenance: 500 mg PO qid. <u>RA:</u> 500 mg PO bid after meals to start. Increase to 1 g PO bid.
PEDS – <u>JRA:</u> initially 10 mg/kg/day and increase to 30 to 50 mg/kg/day (EN-tabs) PO divided bid to max of 2 g/day for age 6 yo or greater. <u>Colitis:</u> Initially 30 to 60 mg/kg/day PO divided into 3 to 6 doses for age older than 2 yo. Maximum 75 mg/kg/day. Maintenance: 30 to 50 mg/kg/day PO divided q4 to 8 h, max 2 g/day.
UNAPPROVED ADULTS – <u>Ankylosing spondylitis:</u> 1 to 1.5 g PO bid. <u>Psoriasis:</u> 1.5 to 2 g PO bid. <u>Psoriatic arthritis:</u> 1 g PO bid.
FORMS – Generic/Trade: Tabs 500 mg, scored. Enteric-coated, Delayed-release (EN-tabs) 500 mg.
NOTES – Contraindicated in children younger than 2 yo. Avoid with hepatic or renal dysfunction, intestinal or urinary obstruction, porphyria, sulfonamide or salicylate sensitivity. Monitor CBC q 2 to 4 weeks for 3 months then q 3 months. Monitor LFTs and renal function. Oligospermia and infertility, and photosensitivity may occur. May decrease folic acid, digoxin, cyclosporine, and iron levels. May turn body fluids, contact lenses, or skin orange-yellow. Enteric coated (Azulfidine EN, Salazopyrin EN) tabs may cause fewer GI adverse effects. Pregnancy category B, except D at term.
MOA – Immunosuppressant, decreases colonic inflammation.
ADVERSE EFFECTS – Serious: Agranulocytosis, hemolytic anemia, nephro/hepatotoxicity, hepatic failure, drug rash. Frequent: Nausea, dyspepsia, rash.

GASTROENTEROLOGY: Other GI Agents

ALOSETRON (*Lotronex*) ▶L ♀B ▶? $$$$$
WARNING – Can cause severe constipation and ischemic colitis. Concomitant use with fluvoxamine, a potent CYP1A2 inhibitor, is contraindicated. Use caution with moderate CYP1A2 inhibitors such as quinolone antibiotics and cimetidine. Use caution with strong inhibitors of CYP3A4 such as ketoconazole, clarithromycin, protease inhibitors, voriconazole and itraconazole. Can be prescribed only by drug company authorized clinicians using special sticker and written informed consent.
ADULTS – <u>Diarrhea-predominant irritable bowel syndrome in women who have failed conventional therapy:</u> 0.5 mg PO twice a day for 4 weeks; discontinue in patients who become constipated. If well tolerated after 4 weeks, may increase to 1 mg PO bid. Discontinue if symptoms not controlled in 4 weeks on 1 mg PO bid.
PEDS – Not approved in children.
FORMS – Trade only: Tabs 0.5, 1 mg.
NOTES – Specific medication guide must be distributed with prescriptions.
MOA – Selective 5-HT3 receptor antagonist.
ADVERSE EFFECTS – Frequent: Constipation, nausea, abdominal pain. Severe: Severe constipation, ischemic colitis.

ALPHA-GALACTOSIDASE (*Beano*) ▶Minimal absorption ♀? ▶? $
ADULTS – 5 gtts or 1 tab per ½ cup gassy food, 3 tabs PO (chew, swallow or crumble) or 10 to 15 gtts per typical meal.
PEDS – Not approved in age younger than 12 yo.

(cont.)

GASTROENTEROLOGY: Other GI Agents

ALPHA-GALACTOSIDASE (cont.)
FORMS — OTC Trade only: Oral gtts 150 IU/5 gtts, Tabs 150 IU.
NOTES — Beano produces 2 to 6 g of carbohydrates for every 100 g of food treated by Beano; may increase glucose levels.
MOA — Enzyme that breaks down complex sugars in gassy foods making them more digestible.
ADVERSE EFFECTS — Frequent: None. Severe: None.

ALVIMOPAN (*Entereg*) ▶Intestinal flora ♀B ▶? ?
ADULTS — <u>Short-term (up to 15 doses) in hospitalized patients undergoing partial large or small bowel resection surgery with primary anastomosis:</u> 12 mg PO 30 min to 5 h prior to surgery, then 12 mg PO bid starting the day after surgery for up to 7 days.
PEDS — Not approved in children.
FORMS — Trade only: Caps 12 mg.
NOTES — Only available to hospitals who are authorized to use the medication (requires hospital DEA number to be dispensed). Contraindicated in patients who have taken therapeutic doses of opioids for more than 7 consecutive days. Serum concentrations in patients of Japanese descent may be up to 2-fold greater than Caucasian subjects with same dose. Monitor Japanese patients for adverse events.
MOA — Peripherally acting mu-opioid receptor antagonist used for post operative ileus.
ADVERSE EFFECTS — Frequent: Anemia, dyspepsia, hypokalemia, back pain, urinary retention. Severe: Myocardial infarction.

BUDESONIDE (*Entocort EC*) ▶L ♀C ▶? $$$$$
ADULTS — <u>Mild-moderate Crohn's, induction of remission:</u> 9 mg PO daily for up to 8 weeks. May repeat 8 week course for recurring episodes. Maintenance: 6 mg PO daily for 3 months.
PEDS — Not approved in children.
UNAPPROVED PEDS — <u>Mild-moderate Crohn's:</u> 0.45 mg/kg up to 9 mg PO daily for 8 to 12 weeks for age 9 yo or older.
FORMS — Trade only: Caps 3 mg.
NOTES — May taper dose to 6 mg for 2 weeks prior to discontinuation.
MOA — Affects cell motility and protein synthesis; anti-inflammatory.
ADVERSE EFFECTS — Frequent: Palpitations, nervousness, dizziness, headache, pruritus, rash, GI irritation, nausea, bitter taste, hyperglycemia, increased infection rate. Severe: Anaphylaxis.

CERTOLIZUMAB (*Cimzia*) ▶Plasma, K ♀B ▶? $$$$$
WARNING — Increased risk of serious infections leading to hospitalization or death including tuberculosis (TB), bacterial sepsis, invasive fungal infections (such as histoplasmosis), and infections due to other opportunistic pathogens.
ADULTS — <u>Crohn's:</u> 400 mg SQ at 0, 2, and 4 weeks. If response occurs, then 400 mg SQ every 4 weeks. <u>Rheumatoid arthritis:</u> 400 mg SC at 0, 2, and 4 weeks. <u>Maintenance of RA:</u> 200 mg SC every other week or 400 mg SC every 4 weeks.
PEDS — Not approved in children.
FORMS — Trade only: 400 mg kit.
NOTES — Monitor patients for signs and symptoms of TB and other infections.
MOA — TNF blocker.
ADVERSE EFFECTS — Frequent: Arthralgia, UTI, URI. Severe: Cytopenias, arrhythmias, heart failure, pericarditis, seizures, stroke, TB and other serious infections.

CHLORDIAZEPOXIDE-CLIDINIUM (*Librax*) ▶K ♀D ▶– $$$
ADULTS — <u>Irritable bowel syndrome:</u> 1 cap PO tid to qid.
PEDS — Not approved in children.
FORMS — Generic/Trade: Caps, chlordiazepoxide 5 mg + clidinium 2.5 mg.
NOTES — May cause drowsiness. After prolonged use, gradually taper to avoid withdrawal symptoms. Contains ingredients formerly contained in Librax.
MOA — Anticholinergic/benzodiazepine.
ADVERSE EFFECTS — Frequent: Dry mouth, drowsiness, ataxia, memory impairment, rash, decreased libido, xerostomia, changes in appetite, micturation difficulties. Severe: CNS, respiratory depression.

CISAPRIDE (*Propulsid*) ▶LK ♀C ▶? From manufacturer only
WARNING — Available only through limited-access protocol through manufacturer. Can cause potentially fatal cardiac arrhythmias. Many drug and disease interactions.
ADULTS — 10 mg PO qid, at least 15 min before meals and at bedtime. Some patients may require 20 mg PO qid. Max 80 mg/day.
PEDS — Not approved in children.
UNAPPROVED PEDS — <u>GERD:</u> 0.15 mg/kg/dose PO tid to qid. Max 0.8 mg/kg/day for neonates, 10 mg/dose for infants and children.
FORMS — Trade only: Tabs 10, 20 mg, susp 1 mg/1 mL.
MOA — Increases acetylcholine release.
ADVERSE EFFECTS — Frequent: Headache, rash, nausea, cramps, diarrhea, xerostomia. Severe: QT prolongation, torsades de pointes.

GLYCOPYRROLATE (*Robinul, Robinul Forte*) ▶K ♀B ▶? $$$$
ADULTS — <u>Peptic ulcer disease:</u> 1 to 2 mg PO bid to tid. <u>Pre-op/intraoperative respiratory antisecretory:</u> 0.1 mg IV/IM prn.
PEDS — Not approved in age younger than 16 yo.
UNAPPROVED ADULTS — <u>Drooling:</u> 0.1 mg/kg PO bid to tid, max 8 mg/day.
UNAPPROVED PEDS — <u>Drooling:</u> 0.04 to 0.1 mg/kg PO tid to qid, max 8 mg/day. <u>Pre-op/intraoperative respiratory antisecretory:</u> 0.004 to 0.01 mg/kg IV/IM prn, maximum 0.2 mg/dose or 0.8 mg/24h.
FORMS — Generic/Trade: Tabs 1, 2 mg.
NOTES — Contraindicated in glaucoma, obstructive uropathy, paralytic ileus or GI obstruction, myasthenia gravis, severe ulcerative colitis, toxic megacolon and unstable cardiovascular status in acute hemorrhage.

(cont.)

GLYCOPYRROLATE (cont.)
MOA – Inhibits effects of acetylcholine.
ADVERSE EFFECTS – Frequent: Dry skin, dry throat, xerostomia, urinary retention, dry nose, local irritation.

LACTASE (*Lactaid*) ▶Not absorbed ♀+ ▶+ $
ADULTS – Swallow or chew 3 caps (Original strength), 2 caps (Extra strength), 1 caplet (Ultra) with first bite of dairy foods. Adjust dose based on response.
PEDS – Titrate dose based on response.
FORMS – OTC Generic/Trade: Caplets, Chewable tabs.
MOA – Replenish lactase enzymes.
ADVERSE EFFECTS – Frequent: None.

METHYLNALTREXONE (*Relistor*) ▶unchanged ♀B ▶? $$$$$
ADULTS – Opioid-induced constipation in patients with advanced illness who are receiving palliative care, when response to laxative therapy has not been sufficient: Less than 38 kg: 0.15 mg/kg SC every other day; 38 kg to 61 kg: 8 mg SC every other day; 62 kg to 114 kg: 12 mg SC every other day: 115 kg or greater: 0.15 mg/kg SC every other day.
PEDS – Not approved in children.
FORMS – Injectable soln 12 mg/0.6 mL.
NOTES – Do not use with GI obstruction. Usual dose every other day, but no more frequently than once daily.
MOA – Opioid binding at the mu-opioid receptor in periphery.
ADVERSE EFFECTS – Frequent: Abdominal pain, flatulence, nausea, dizziness, diarrhea, hyperhidrosis.

NEOMYCIN—ORAL (*Neo-Fradin*) ▶Minimally absorbed ♀D ▶? $$$
ADULTS – Suppression of intestinal bacteria (given with erythromycin): 1 g PO at 19 h, 18 h and 9 h prior to procedure (ie, 1 pm, 2 pm, 11 pm on prior day). Alternative regimen 1 g PO q 1 h for 4 doses then 1 g PO q 4 h for 5 doses. Hepatic encephalopathy: 4 to 12 g/day PO divided q 4 to 6 h. Diarrhea caused by enteropathogenic E. coli: 3 g/day PO divided q 6 h.
PEDS – Suppression of intestinal bacteria (given with erythromycin): 25 mg/kg PO at 19 h, 18 h and 9 h prior to procedure (ie, 1 pm, 2 pm, 11 pm on prior day). Alternative regimen 90 mg/kg/day PO divided q 4 h for 2 days. Hepatic encephalopathy: 50 to 100 mg/kg/day PO divided q 6 to 8 h. Diarrhea caused by enteropathogenic E. coli: 50 mg/kg/day PO divided q 6 h for 2 to 3 days.
FORMS – Generic only: Tabs 500 mg. Trade only: Soln 125 mg/5 mL.
NOTES – Increased INR with warfarin, decreased levels of digoxin, methotrexate.
MOA – Inhibits bacterial protein synthesis.
ADVERSE EFFECTS – Frequent: None.

OCTREOTIDE (*Sandostatin, Sandostatin LAR*) ▶LK ♀B ▶? $$$$$
ADULTS – Diarrhea associated with carcinoid tumors: 100 to 600 mcg/day SC/IV in 2 to 4 divided doses or 20 mg IM (Sandostatin LAR) q 4 weeks for 2 months. Adjust dose based on response. Diarrhea associated with vasoactive intestinal peptide-secreting tumors: 200 to 300 mcg/day SC/IV in 2 to 4 divided doses or 20 mg IM (Sandostatin LAR) q 4 weeks for 2 months. Adjust dose based on response.
PEDS – Not approved in children.
UNAPPROVED ADULTS – Variceal bleeding: Bolus 25 to 50 mcg IV followed by 25 to 50 mcg/h continuous IV infusion. AIDS diarrhea: 25 to 250mcg SC tid, max 500 mcg SC q8h. Irritable bowel syndrome: 100 mcg as a single dose to 125 mcg SC bid. GI and pancreatic fistulas: 50 to 200 mcg SC/IV q 8 h.
UNAPPROVED PEDS – Diarrhea: Initially 1 to 10 mcg/kg SC/IV q 12 h. Congenital hyperinsulinism 1 to 40 mcg/kg SC daily. Hypothalamic obesity in children 6 to 17 yo: 40 mg IM every 4 weeks (Sandostatin LAR) or 5 to 15 mcg/kg SC daily.
FORMS – Generic/Trade: Injection vials 0.05, 0.1, 0.2, 0.5, 1 mg. Trade only: Long-acting injectable susp (Sandostatin LAR) 10, 20, 30 mg.
NOTES – For the treatment of variceal bleeding, most studies treat for 3 to 5 days. Individualize dose based on response. Dosage reduction often necessary in elderly. May cause hypoglycemia, hyperglycemia; caution especially in diabetes. May cause hypothyroidism, cardiac arrhythmias. Increases bioavailability of bromocriptine. Sandostatin LAR only indicated for patients who are stabilized on Sandostatin.
MOA – Mimics natural somatostatin.
ADVERSE EFFECTS – Frequent: Sinus bradycardia, chest pain, fatigue, headache, malaise, fever, dizziness, pruritis, hyperglycemia, abdominal pain, nausea, diarrhea. Severe: Hepatitis, progressive abdominal distension, severe epigastric pain.

ORLISTAT (*Alli, Xenical*) ▶Gut ♀B ▶? $$$
ADULTS – Weight loss and weight management: 120 mg PO tid with meals or up to 1 h after meals.
PEDS – Children 12 to 16 yo: 120 mg PO tid with meals. Not approved in age younger than 12 yo.
FORMS – OTC Trade only (Alli): Caps 60 mg. Rx Trade only (Xenical): Caps 120 mg.
NOTES – May cause fatty stools, fecal urgency, flatus with discharge and oily spotting in > 20% of patients. GI adverse effects greater when taken with high-fat diet. Can reduce the effect of levothyroxine or increase the effects of warfarin. Administer orlistat and levothyroxine at least 4 h apart.
MOA – Inhibits gastric and pancreatic lipases.
ADVERSE EFFECTS – Frequent: CNS effects, oily stool, fecal incontinence, flatus with discharge Severe: Cholelithiasis, pancreatitis, severe liver injury with hepatocellular necrosis or acute hepatic failure.

PANCREATIN (*Creon, Ku-Zyme, ✦Entozyme*) ▶Gut ♀C ▶? $$$
ADULTS – Enzyme replacement (initial dose): 8000 to 24,000 units lipase (1-2 cap/tab) PO with meals and snacks.
PEDS – Enzyme replacement (initial dose): Give 2000 units lipase PO with meals for age younger

(cont.)

PANCREATIN (*cont.*)
than 1 yo, give 4000 to 8000 units lipase PO with meals or 4000 units lipase with snacks for age 1 to 6 yo, give 4,000 to 12,000 units lipase PO with meals and snacks for age 7 to 12 yo.
FORMS — Tabs, Caps with varying amounts of pancreatin, lipase, amylase, and protease.
NOTES — Titrate dose to stool fat content. Products are not interchangeable. Avoid concomitant calcium carbonate and magnesium hydroxide since these may affect the enteric coating. Do not crush/chew microspheres or tabs. Possible association of colonic strictures and high doses of lipase (> 16,000 units/kg/meal) in pediatric patients.
MOA — Replaces endogenous enzymes.
ADVERSE EFFECTS — Frequent: None.

PANCRELIPASE (*Creon, Pancreaze, Viokase, Pancrease, Pancrecarb, Cotazym, Ku-Zyme HP, Zenpep*) ▶Gut ♀C ▶? $$$
ADULTS — Enzyme replacement (initial dose): 500 lipase units/kg per meal, max 2500 lipase units/kg per meal.
PEDS — Enzyme replacement (initial dose): Infants (up to 12 mos): 2000 to 4000 lipase units per 120 mL of formula or per breastfeeding. 12 mos or older to younger than 4 yo: 1000 lipase units/kg, max 2500 lipase units/kg per meal. 4 yo or older: 500 lipase units/kg per meal, max 2500 lipase units/kg per meal.
FORMS — Tabs, Caps, Powder with varying amounts of lipase, amylase, and protease.
NOTES — Titrate dose to stool fat content. Products are not interchangeable. Avoid concomitant calcium carbonate and magnesium hydroxide since these may affect the enteric coating. Do not crush/chew microspheres or tabs. Possible association of colonic strictures and high doses of lipase (> 16,000 units/kg/meal) in pediatric patients. Not all products FDA approved. Creon, Zenpep, Pancreaze FDA-approved products.
MOA — Replaces endogenous enzymes.
ADVERSE EFFECTS — Frequent: None.

PINAVERIUM (*✦Dicetel*) ▶? ♀C ▶– $$$
ADULTS — Canada only. Irritable bowel syndrome: 50 mg PO tid, may increase to maximum of 100 mg tid.
PEDS — Not for children.
FORMS — Trade only: tabs 50, 100 mg.
NOTES — Take with a full glass of water during meal or snack.
MOA — Calcium antagonist; blocks voltage-dependent calcium channels at the smooth muscle cell level; highly selective for intestinal smooth muscle.
ADVERSE EFFECTS — Frequent: Epigastric pain, nausea, constipation.

SECRETIN (*SecreFlo, ChiRhoStim*) ▶Serum ♀C ▶? $$$$$
ADULTS — Stimulation of pancreatic secretions, to aid in diagnosis of exocrine pancreas dysfunction: Test dose 0.2 mcg IV. If tolerated, 0.2 mcg/kg IV over 1 min. Stimulation of gastrin to aid in diagnosis of gastrinoma: Test dose 0.2 mcg IV. If tolerated, 0.4 mcg/kg IV over 1 min. Identification of ampulla of Vater and accessory papilla during ERCP: 0.2 mcg/kg IV over 1 min.
PEDS — Not approved in children.
UNAPPROVED PEDS — Has been used in autism.
NOTES — Previously known as SecreFlo. Contraindicated in acute pancreatitis.
MOA — Increases volume and bicarbonate content of secreted pancreatic juices.
ADVERSE EFFECTS — Frequent: Abdominal discomfort, hypotension, diaphoresis, flushing, nausea.

TEGASEROD (*Zelnorm*) ▶stomach/L ♀B ▶? Free (investigational)
WARNING — Restricted (investigational) use; contact manufacturer to obtain. Severe diarrhea leading to hypovolemia, hypotension, and syncope has been reported, as has ischemic colitis and other forms of intestinal ischemia; discontinue immediately if symptoms occur.
ADULTS — Constipation-predominant irritable bowel syndrome in women younger than the age of 55 yo: 6 mg PO bid before meals for 4 to 6 weeks. May repeat for an additional 4 to 6 weeks.
PEDS — Not approved in children.
FORMS — Restricted use only. Trade only: Tabs 2, 6 mg.
MOA — 5-HT4 receptor agonist.
ADVERSE EFFECTS — Frequent: Abdominal pain, diarrhea, nausea, flatulence, headache. Severe: Severe diarrhea, hypovolemia, hypotension, syncope; ischemic colitis, other forms of intestinal ischemia.

URSODIOL (*Actigall, URSO, URSO Forte*) ▶Bile ♀B ▶? $$$$
ADULTS — Radiolucent gallstone dissolution (Actigall): 8 to 10 mg/kg/day PO divided in 2 to 3 doses. Prevention of gallstones associated with rapid wt loss (Actigall): 300 mg PO bid. Primary biliary cirrhosis (URSO): 13 to 15 mg/kg/day PO divided in 2 to 4 doses.
PEDS — Not approved in children.
UNAPPROVED ADULTS — Cholestasis of pregnancy: 300 to 600 mg PO bid.
UNAPPROVED PEDS — Biliary atresia: 10 to 15 mg/kg/day PO once daily. Cystic fibrosis with liver disease: 30 mg/kg/day PO divided bid. TPN-induced cholestasis: 30 mg/kg/day PO divided tid.
FORMS — Generic/Trade: Caps 300 mg, Tabs 250, 500 mg.
NOTES — Gallstone dissolution requires month of therapy. Complete dissolution does not occur in all patients and 5-year recurrence up to 50%. Does not dissolve calcified cholesterol stones, radiopaque stones, or radiolucent bile pigment stones. Avoid concomitant antacids, cholestyramine, colestipol, estrogen, oral contraceptives.
MOA — Decreases cholesterol content of bile and bile stones.
ADVERSE EFFECTS — Frequent: Diarrhea, constipation, nausea, vomiting, dizziness. Serious: Thrombocytopenia, hypersensitivity reactions.

HEMATOLOGY: Anticoagulants—LMW Heparins, and Fondaparinux

NOTE: See cardiovascular section for antiplatelet drugs and thrombolytics. Contraindicated in active major bleeding. High risk of spinal/epidural hematoma if spinal puncture or neuraxial anesthesia before/during treatment (see http://journals.lww.com/rapm/Fulltext/2010/01000/Regional_Anesthesia_in_the_Patient_Receiving.13.aspx). Risk of bleeding increased by oral anticoagulants, aspirin, dipyridamole, dextran, glycoprotein IIb/IIIa inhibitors, NSAIDs (including ketorolac), ticlopidine, clopidogrel, and thrombolytics. Monitor platelets, Hb, stool for occult blood.

DALTEPARIN (*Fragmin*) ▶KL ♀B ▶+ $$$$$
ADULTS — DVT prophylaxis, acute medical illness with restricted mobility: 5000 units SC daily for 12 to 14 days. DVT prophylaxis, abdominal surgery: 2500 units SC 1 to 2 h preop and daily postop for 5 to 10 days. DVT prophylaxis, abdominal surgery in patients with malignancy: 5000 units SC evening before surgery and daily postop for 5 to 10 days. Alternatively, 2500 units SC 1 to 2 h preop and 12 h later, then 5000 units SC daily for 5 to 10 days. DVT prophylaxis, hip replacement: Give SC for up to 14 days. Preop start (day of surgery): 2500 units 2 h preop and 4 to 8 h postop, then 5000 units daily starting at least 6 h after second dose. Preop start (evening before surgery): 5000 units SC given evening before surgery then 5000 units daily starting at least 4 to 8 h postop (approximately 24 h between doses). Postop start regimen: 2500 units 4 to 8 h postop, then 5000 units daily starting at least 6 h after first dose. Treatment of DVT/PE in cancer: 200 units/kg SC daily for 1 month, then 150 units/kg SC daily for 5 months. Max 18,000 units/day, round to nearest commercially available syringe dose (if CrCl < 30 mL/min then target therapeutic anti-Xa level of anti-Xa of 0.5 to 1.5 units/mL; recheck 4 to 6 h after dose following at least 3 to 4 doses.). Unstable angina or non-Q-wave MI: 120 units/kg up to 10,000 units SC q 12 h with aspirin (75 to 165 mg/day PO) until clinically stable.
PEDS — Not approved in children.
UNAPPROVED ADULTS — Therapeutic anticoagulation: 200 units/kg SC daily or 100 to 120 units/kg SC bid. Venous thromboembolism in pregnancy. Prevention: 5000 units SC daily. Treatment: 100 units/kg SC q 12 h or 200 units/kg SC daily. To avoid unwanted anticoagulation during delivery, stop LMWH 24 h before elective induction of labor.
FORMS — Trade only: Single-dose syringes 2500, 5000 anti-Xa units/0.2 mL, 7500 anti-Xa/0.3 mL, 10,000 anti-Xa units/1 mL, 12,500 anti-Xa units/0.5 mL, 15,000 anti-Xa units/0.6 mL, 18,000 anti-Xa units/0.72 mL; multidose vial 10,000 units/mL, 9.5 mL and 25,000 units/mL, 3.8 mL.
NOTES — Longer prophylaxis may be warranted based on individual thromboembolic risk. ACCP recommendations suggest that patients with total hip or knee replacement or hip fracture surgery receive prophylaxis for at least 10 days; consider extended prophylaxis (28 to 35 days) in hip replacement or hip fracture surgery. Contraindicated in heparin or pork allergy, history of heparin-induced thrombocytopenia. Use caution and consider monitoring anti-Xa levels if morbidly obese, underweight, pregnant, or renal/liver failure. Drug effect can be reversed with protamine.
MOA — Low molecular weight heparin, antithrombin activator that preferentially inhibits factor Xa and inhibits factor IIa.
ADVERSE EFFECTS — Serious: Major bleeding, HIT (rare), spinal/epidural hematomas associated with neuraxial anesthesia/spinal punctures before/during treatment. Frequent: Asymptomatic increase in hepatic transaminases, injection site pain.

ENOXAPARIN (*Lovenox*) ▶KL ♀B ▶+ $$$$$
ADULTS — DVT prophylaxis, acute medical illness with restricted mobility: 40 mg SC daily for no more than 14 days (CrCl < 30 mL/min): 30 mg SC daily. DVT prophylaxis, hip/knee replacement: 30 mg SC q 12 h starting 12 to 24 h postop for no more than 14 days (CrCl < 30 mL/min: 30 mg SC daily). Alternative for hip replacement: 40 mg SC daily starting 12 h preop. After hip replacement may continue 40 mg SC daily for 3 weeks. DVT prophylaxis, abdominal surgery: 40 mg SC daily starting 2 h preop for no more than 12 days (CrCl < 30 mL/min: 30 mg SC daily). Outpatient treatment of DVT without pulmonary embolus: 1 mg/kg SC q 12 h. Inpatient treatment of DVT with/without pulmonary embolus: 1 mg/kg SC q 12 h or 1.5 mg/kg SC q 24 h (CrCl < 30 mL/min: 1 mg/kg SC daily). Give at the same time each day. Continue enoxaparin for at least 5 days and until therapeutic oral anticoagulation established. Unstable angina or non-Q-wave MI (NSTEMI): 1 mg/kg SC q 12 h with aspirin (100 to 325 mg PO daily) for at least 2 days and until clinically stable (CrCl < 30 mL/min: 1 mg/kg SC daily). Acute ST-elevation MI: If age 75 yo or younger: 30 mg IV bolus followed 15 min later by 1 mg/kg SC dose then 1 mg/kg (max 100 mg/dose for the 1st two doses) SC q 12 h (CrCl < 30 mL/min: 30 mg IV bolus followed 15 min later by 1 mg/kg SC dose then 1 mg/kg SC daily); if age older than 75 yo: 0.75 mg/kg (max 75 mg/dose for the 1st two doses, no bolus) SC q 12 h (CrCl < 30 mL/min: 1 mg/kg SC daily, no bolus). Given with aspirin (75 to 325 mg PO daily) until hospital discharge or for at least 8 days.
PEDS — Not approved in children.
UNAPPROVED ADULTS — Prevention of venous thromboembolism. After major trauma: 30 mg SC q 12 h starting 12 to 36 h postinjury if hemostasis achieved. Acute spinal cord injury: 30 mg SC q 12 h. Venous thromboembolism in pregnancy: Prevention: 40 mg SC daily. Treatment: 1 mg/kg SC q 12 h. To avoid unwanted anticoagulation during delivery, stop LMWH 24 h before elective induction of labor.
UNAPPROVED PEDS — Therapeutic anticoagulation: Age younger than 2 mo: 1.5 mg/kg/dose SC q 12 h titrated to anti-Xa level of 0.5 to 1 units/mL. Age

(cont.)

ENOXAPARIN (cont.)

2 mo or older: 1 mg/kg/dose SC q 12 h titrated to anti-Xa level of 0.5 to 1 units/mL. <u>DVT prophylaxis:</u> Age younger than 2 mo: 0.75 mg/kg/dose q 12 h. Age 2 mo or older: 0.5 mg/kg/dose q 12 h.
FORMS — Trade only: Multidose vial 300 mg; Syringes 30, 40 mg; graduated syringes 60, 80, 100, 120, 150 mg. Concentration is 100 mg/mL except for 120, 150 mg, which are 150 mg/mL.
NOTES — Longer prophylaxis may be warranted based on individual thromboembolic risk. ACCP recommendations suggest that patients with total hip or knee replacement or hip fracture surgery receive prophylaxis for at least 10 days; consider extended prophylaxis (28 to 35 days) in hip replacement or hip fracture surgery. Dosage adjustments for CrCl < 30 mL/min. Use caution and consider monitoring anti-Xa levels if renal dysfunction, pregnancy, morbidly obese, underweight, or abnormal coagulation/bleeding. In unstable angina or NSTEMI, can give 30 mg IV bolus 15 min before first SC dose. In acute ST-elevation MI, if administered with thrombolytic give between 15 min before or 30 min after start of thrombolytic therapy. In PCI, if last enoxaparin administration was more than 8 h before balloon inflation, give 0.3 mg/kg IV bolus. Contraindicated in patients with heparin or pork allergy, history of heparin-induced thrombocytopenia. Use caution in mechanical heart valves, especially in pregnancy; reports of valve thrombosis (maternal and fetal deaths reported). Congenital anomalies linked to enoxaparin use during pregnancy; causality unclear. Multidose formulation contains benzyl alcohol, which can cause hypersensitivity and cross placenta in pregnancy. Drug effect can be reversed with protamine.
MOA — Low molecular weight heparin, antithrombin activator that preferentially inhibits factor Xa and inhibits factor IIa.
ADVERSE EFFECTS — Serious: Major bleeding, thrombocytopenia (rare), spinal/epidural hematomas associated with neuraxial anesthesia/spinal punctures before/during treatment. Reports of valve thrombosis when used for thromboprophylaxis in patients with prosthetic heart valves, especially pregnant women (maternal and fetal deaths reported). Frequent: Asymptomatic increase in hepatic transaminases, injection site reactions, peripheral edema.

FONDAPARINUX (*Arixtra*) ▶K ♀B ▶? $$$$$
ADULTS — <u>DVT prophylaxis, hip/knee replacement or hip fracture surgery, abdominal surgery:</u> 2.5 mg SC daily starting 6 to 8 h postop (giving earlier increases risk of bleeding). Usual duration is 5 to 9 days; extend prophylaxis up to 24 additional days (max 32 days) in hip fracture surgery. <u>DVT/PE treatment based on wt:</u> 5 mg (if wt less than 50 kg), 7.5 mg (if 50 to 100 kg), 10 mg (if wt greater than 100 kg) SC daily for at least 5 days and therapeutic oral anticoagulation.
PEDS — Not approved in children. Since risk for bleeding is increased if weight less than 50 kg, bleeding may be a particular concern in pediatrics.
UNAPPROVED ADULTS — <u>Unstable angina or non-ST-elevation MI:</u> 2.5 mg SC daily until hospital discharge or for up to 8 days. <u>ST-elevation MI and creatinine < 3 mg/dL:</u> 2.5 mg IV loading dose, then 2.5 mg SC daily until hospital discharge or for up to 8 days.
FORMS — Trade only: Prefilled syringes 2.5 mg/0.5 mL, 5 mg/0.4 mL, 7.5 mg/0.6 mL, 10 mg/0.8 mL.
NOTES — May cause thrombocytopenia; however, lacks in vitro cross-reactivity with heparin-induced thrombocytopenia antibodies. Risk of major bleeding increased in elderly. Contraindicated if CrCl < 30 mL/min due to increased bleeding risk. Caution advised if CrCl 30 to 50 mL/min. Monitor renal function in all patients; discontinue if severely impaired or labile. In DVT prophylaxis, contraindicated if body wt less than 50 kg. Protamine ineffective for reversing anticoagulant effect. Factor VIIa partially reverses anticoagulant effect in small studies. Risk of catheter thrombosis in PCI; use in conjunction with anticoagulant with anti-IIa activity. Store at room temperature.
MOA — Synthetic pentasaccharide sequence of heparin that binds with antithrombin III to inactivate factor Xa.
ADVERSE EFFECTS — Serious: Major bleeding (especially in elderly, low body weight, or renal dysfunction), thrombocytopenia (rare), spinal/epidural hematomas associated with neuraxial anesthesia/spinal punctures before/during treatment. Frequent: None.

TINZAPARIN (*Innohep*) ▶K ♀B ▶+ $$$$$
ADULTS — <u>DVT with/without pulmonary embolus:</u> 175 units/kg SC daily for at least 6 days and until adequate anticoagulation with warfarin.
PEDS — Not approved in children.
UNAPPROVED ADULTS — <u>Treatment of venous thromboembolism in pregnancy:</u> 175 units/kg SC daily.
FORMS — Trade only: 20,000 anti-Xa units/mL, 2 mL multidose vial.
NOTES — Contraindicated if history of heparin-induced thrombocytopenia, or allergy to heparin, pork, sulfites, or benzyl alcohol. Can cause thrombocytopenia, priapism (rare), increased AST/ALT. Tinzaparin may slightly prolong PT; draw blood for INR just before giving tinzaparin. Use caution and consider monitoring anti-Xa levels if morbidly obese, underweight, pregnant, or renal dysfunction. Drug effect can be reversed with protamine. Consider alternatives in patients age 70 or older with renal impairment and DVT/PE due to increased all-cause mortality in one trial.
MOA — Low molecular weight heparin, antithrombin activator that preferentially inhibits factor Xa and inhibits factor IIa.
ADVERSE EFFECTS — Serious: Major bleeding, HIT (rare), priapism (rare), spinal/epidural hematomas associated with neuraxial anesthesia/spinal punctures before/during treatment. Frequent: Asymptomatic increase in hepatic transaminases.

HEMATOLOGY: Anticoagulants—Other

ARGATROBAN ▶L ♀B ▶– $$$$$
ADULTS — <u>Prevention/treatment of thrombosis in heparin-induced thrombocytopenia:</u> Start 2 mcg/kg/min IV infusion. Get PTT at baseline and 2 h after starting infusion. Adjust dose (up to 10 mcg/kg/min) until PTT is 1.5 to 3× baseline (but not > 100 sec). <u>Percutaneous coronary intervention in those with or at risk for heparin-induced thrombocytopenia:</u> Bolus 350 mcg/kg IV over 3 to 5 min then 25 mcg/kg/min infusion. Target activated clotting time (ACT): 300 to 450 sec. If ACT < 300 sec, give 150 mcg/kg bolus and increase infusion rate to 30 mcg/kg/min. If ACT > 450 sec, reduce infusion rate to 15 mcg/kg/min. Maintain ACT 300 to 450 sec for the duration of the procedure.
PEDS — Not approved in children.
NOTES — ACCP recommends starting at lower doses of 0.5 to 1.2 mcg/kg/min in patients with heart failure, multiorgan failure, anasarca or postcardiac surgery. Argatroban prolongs INR with warfarin; discontinue when INR > 4 on combined therapy, recheck INR in 4 to 6 h and restart argatroban if INR subtherapeutic. Dosage reduction recommended in liver dysfunction.
MOA — Direct thrombin inhibitor, synthetic derivative of L-arginine.
ADVERSE EFFECTS — Serious: Major bleeding, hypotension. Frequent: Fever, diarrhea.

BIVALIRUDIN (Angiomax) ▶proteolysis/K ♀B ▶? $$$$$
ADULTS — <u>Anticoagulation in patients undergoing PCI (including patients with or at risk of heparin-induced thrombocytopenia or heparin-induced thrombocytopenia and thrombosis syndrome):</u> 0.75 mg/kg IV bolus prior to intervention, then 1.75 mg/kg/h for duration of procedure (with provisional Gp IIb/IIIa inhibition) and optionally up to 4 h postprocedure. For CrCl < 30 mL/min, reduce infusion dose to 1 mg/kg/h after bolus. For patients on dialysis, reduce infusion dose to 0.25 mg/kg/h. Use with aspirin 300 to 325 mg PO daily. Additional bolus of 0.3 mg/kg if activated clotting time < 225 sec. Can additionally infuse 0.2 mg/kg/h for up to 20 h more.
PEDS — Not approved in children.
UNAPPROVED ADULTS — <u>Acute coronary syndrome (with or without Gp IIb/IIIa inhibition):</u> 0.1 mg/kg bolus followed by 0.25 mg/kg/h. If PCI, then additional bolus 0.5 mg/kg then 1.75 mg/kg/h. Use with aspirin.
NOTES — Contraindicated in active major bleeding. Monitor activated clotting time. Former trade name Hirulog.
MOA — Direct thrombin inhibitor (reversible).
ADVERSE EFFECTS — Serious: Major bleeding. Frequent: Back pain, nausea.

DESIRUDIN (Iprivask) ▶K ♀C ▶?
WARNING — Contraindicated in active major bleeding. High risk of spinal/epidural hematoma if spinal puncture or neuraxial anesthesia before/during treatment. Risk increased by drugs that affect hemostasis including NSAIDs, antiplatelets and other anticoagulants. Risk also increased by use of indwelling catheters, history of trauma or repeated epidural punctures, spinal deformity or spinal surgery.
ADULTS — <u>DVT prophylaxis (hip replacement surgery):</u> 15 mg SC q12 hours (if CrCl ≤ 31-60 ml/min give 5 mg SC q12 h, if CrCl < 31 ml/min give 1.7 mg SC q12 h)
PEDS — Not approved in children.
NOTES — ACCP guidelines recommend against use if CrCl < 30 ml/min and against repeated use due to risk of anaphylaxis. Severe anaphylactic reactions resulting in death have been reported upon initial or re-exposure.
MOA — Direct thrombin inhibitor.
ADVERSE EFFECTS — Serious: Anaphylaxis, major hemorrhage (including fatal, intracranial, intraspinal, intraocular), hypotension. Frequent: Injection site reactions, hematoma, minor bleeding, nausea.

HEPARIN (✦Hepalean) ▶Reticuloendothelial system ♀C but + ▶+ $$
ADULTS — <u>Venous thrombosis/pulmonary embolus treatment:</u> Load 80 units/kg IV, then initiate infusion at 18 units/kg/h. Adjust based on coagulation testing (PTT). <u>DVT prophylaxis:</u> 5000 units SC q 8 to 12 h. <u>Low-dose for prevention of thromboembolism in pregnancy:</u> 5000 to 10,000 units SC q 12 h. <u>Treatment of thromboembolism in pregnancy:</u> 80 units/kg IV load, then infuse 18 units/kg/h with dose titrated to achieve full anticoagulation for at least 5 days. Then continue via SC route with at least 10,000 units SC q 8 to 12 h adjusted to achieve PTT of 1.5 to 2.5× control. To avoid unwanted anticoagulation during delivery, stop SC heparin 24 h before elective induction of labor.
PEDS — <u>Venous thrombosis/pulmonary embolus treatment:</u> Load 50 units/kg IV, then 25 units/kg/h infusion.
UNAPPROVED ADULTS — <u>Venous thrombosis/pulmonary embolus treatment:</u> Load 333 units/kg SC, then 250 units/kg SC q 12 h based on max 100 kg wt. Adjust to achieve goal PTT 1.5 to 2× control (~50–70 sec). <u>Anticoagulation for acute MI not treated with thrombolytics:</u> 75 units/kg IV load, then initiate infusion at 1000 to 1200 units/h adjusted to achieve PTT of 1.5 to 2.5× control. <u>Unstable angina/non-ST-elevation MI:</u> 60 to 70 units/kg IV load (max 5000 units), then initiate infusion at 12 to 15 units/kg/h (max 1000 units) and adjust to achieve goal PTT 1.5 to 2.5× control. <u>Adjunct to thrombolytics for acute MI.</u> For use with alteplase, reteplase, or tenecteplase: 60 units/kg IV load (max 4000 units), then initial infusion 12 units/kg/h (max 1000 units/h) adjusted to achieve goal PTT 1.5 to 2× control (~50–70 sec). Maintain for at least 48 h, duration based on concomitant therapy and patient thromboembolic risk.

(cont.)

HEMATOLOGY: Anticoagulants

WEIGHT-BASED HEPARIN DOSING FOR DVT/PE*

Initial dose: 80 units/kg IV bolus, then 18 units/kg/h. Check PTT in 6 h.

PTT less than 35 sec (less than 1.2 × control): 80 units/kg IV bolus, then increase infusion rate by 4 units/kg/h.

PTT 35–45 sec (1.2–1.5 × control): 40 units/kg IV bolus, then increase infusion by 2 units/kg/h.

PTT 46–70 sec (1.5–2.3 × control): No change.

PTT 71–90 sec (2.3–3 × control): decrease infusion rate by 2 units/kg/h.

PTT greater than 90 sec (greater than 3 × control): Hold infusion for 1 h, then decrease infusion rate by 3 units/kg/h.

*PTT = Activated partial thromboplastin time. Reagent-specific target PTT may differ; use institutional nomogram when available. Consider establishing a max bolus dose/max initial infusion rate or use an adjusted body wt in obesity. Monitor PTT 6 h after heparin initiation and 6 h after each dosage adjustment. When PTT is stable within therapeutic range, monitor every morning. Therapeutic PTT range corresponds to anti-factor Xa activity of 0.3–0.7 units/mL. Check platelets between days 3 and 5. Can begin warfarin on first day of heparin; continue heparin for ≥4 to 5 days of combined therapy. Adapted from *Ann Intern Med* 1993;119:874; *Chest* 2008:133:463S–464S, *Circulation* 2001; 103:2994.

HEPARIN (*cont.*)

UNAPPROVED PEDS – <u>Venous thrombosis/pulmonary embolus treatment:</u> Load 75 units/kg IV over 10 min, then 28 units/kg/h if age younger than 1 yo, 20 units/kg/h if age 1 yo or older.

FORMS – Generic only: 1000, 5000, 10,000, 20,000 units/mL in various vial and syringe sizes.

NOTES – Beware of heparin-induced thrombocytopenia, elevated LFTs, hyperkalemia/hypoaldosteronism. Heparin-induced thrombocytopenia can occur up to several weeks after heparin discontinued. Osteoporosis with long-term use. Bleeding risk increased by high dose; concomitant thrombolytic or platelet GPIIb/IIIa receptor inhibitor; recent surgery, trauma, or invasive procedure; concomitant hemostatic defect. Monitor platelets, Hb, stool for occult blood. Anti-Xa is an alternative to PTT for monitoring. Drug effect can be reversed with protamine. Do not administer heparin preserved with benzyl alcohol (porcine) to neonates, infants or pregnant or lactating women.

MOA – Antithrombin activator that inhibits factors Xa and IIa.

ADVERSE EFFECTS – Serious: Major bleeding, HIT, elevated LFTs, hyperkalemia/hypoaldosteronism, osteoporosis (with long-term use). Frequent: None.

LEPIRUDIN (*Refludan*) ▶K ♀B ▶? $$$$$

ADULTS – <u>Anticoagulation in heparin-induced thrombocytopenia (HIT) and associated thromboembolic disease:</u> Bolus 0.4 mg/kg up to 44 mg IV over 15 to 20 sec, then infuse 0.15 mg/kg/h up to 16.5 mg/h for 2 to 10 days. Adjust dose to maintain APTT ratio of 1.5 to 2.5. <u>Adjunct to thrombolytic therapy:</u> Bolus 0.2 mg/kg IV over 15 to 20 sec, then infuse 0.1 mg/kg/h.

PEDS – Not approved in children.

UNAPPROVED ADULTS – <u>Anticoagulation in HIT:</u> Bolus 0.2 mg/kg IV then infuse 0.05-0.1 mg/kg/h. Adjust dose to maintain aPTT ratio of 1.5 to 2.5.

NOTES – Dosing for HIT recommended by ACCP guidelines is lower than FDA-approved dosing due to higher rates of bleeding with FDA-approved dosing. Dosage adjustment for renal impairment per ACCP guidelines: Bolus 0.2 mg/kg IV (bolus only if life or limb threatening thrombosis) followed by 0.05 mg/kg/h for Cr 1.0 to 1.6 mg/dL, 0.01 mg/kg/h for Cr 1.7 to 4.5 mg/dL, 0.005 mg/kg/h for Cr > 4.5 to 6.0 mg/dL. Avoid or stop infusion if Cr> 6.0. May increase INR. Severe anaphylactic reactions resulting in death have been reported upon initial or re-exposure.

MOA – Direct thrombin inhibitor (irreversible).

ADVERSE EFFECTS – Serious: Severe anaphylactic reactions resulting in death have been reported upon initial or re-exposure. May have higher risk of bleeding than reversible thrombin inhibitors. Post-marketing reports of intracranial bleeding in absence of thrombolytics. Frequent: Abnormal LFTs.

WARFARIN (*Coumadin, Jantoven*) ▶L ♀X ▶+ $

WARNING – Major or fatal bleeding possible. Higher risk during initiation and when INR elevated. Additional risk factors include: High intensity of anticoagulation (INR > 4.0), age ≤ 65, highly variable INRs, history of GI bleed, hypertension, cerebrovascular disease, heart disease, anemia, malignancy, trauma, renal insufficiency and long duration of therapy. Regular monitoring of INR needed; monitor those at higher risk more frequently. Educate patients about signs and symptoms of bleeding, measures to reduce risk and how to manage/seek treatment if bleeding occurs. Many important drug interactions that increase/decrease INR, see table.

ADULTS – <u>Oral anticoagulation for prophylaxis/ treatment of DVT/PE, thromboembolic complications associated with A-fib, mechanical and bioprosthetic heart valves:</u> Start 2 to 5 mg PO daily for 1 to 2 days, then adjust dose to maintain

(cont.)

HEMATOLOGY: Antihemophilic Agents

THERAPEUTIC GOALS FOR ANTICOAGULATION

INR Range*	Indication
2.0–3.0	Atrial fibrillation, deep venous thrombosis†, pulmonary embolism†, bioprosthetic heart valve, mechanical prosthetic heart valve (aortic position, bileaflet or tilting disk with normal sinus rhythm and normal left atrium)
2.5–3.5	Mechanical prosthetic heart valve: (1) mitral position, (2) aortic position with atrial fibrillation, (3) caged ball or caged disk

*Aim for an INR in the middle of the INR range (eg, 2.5 for range of 2 to 3 and 3.0 for range of 2.5 to 3.5). Adapted from: Chest 2008; 133: 456-7S, 459S, 547S, 594-5S; see this manuscript for additional information and other indications. †For first-event unprovoked DVT/PE, after 3 months of therapy at goal INR 2 to 3, may consider low-intensity therapy (INR range 1.5 to 2.0) in patients with strong preference for less frequent INR testing.

WARFARIN (cont.)
therapeutic PT/INR. Consider using an initial dose of less than 5 mg/day if elderly, malnourished, liver disease, or high bleeding risk. Target INR of 2 to 3 for most indications, 2.5 to 3.5 for mechanical heart valves. See table for specific target INR.
PEDS — Not approved in children.
UNAPPROVED ADULTS — <u>Oral anticoagulation treatment of acute DVT/PE:</u> Start 5 to 10 mg PO daily (with at least 5 days of LMWH/heparin) until target INR (2.0 to 3.0) reached. See table for target INR.
FORMS — Generic/Trade: Tabs 1, 2, 2.5, 3, 4, 5, 6, 7.5, 10 mg.
NOTES — Loading doses not recommended. ACCP guidelines suggest initial dose of 2 to 10 mg, with lower doses if high risk of bleeding, elderly, malnourished or congestive heart failure. Consider lower initial dose if genetic variation in CYP2C9 and VKORC1 enzymes. Clinical factors that may affect maintenance dose needed to achieve target PT/INR include age, race, weight, sex, medications and comorbidities. Many important drug interactions that increase/decrease INR, see table for significant drug interactions. Warfarin onset of action is within 24 h, peak effect delayed by 3 to 4 days. Most patients can begin warfarin at the same time as heparin/LMWH. Continue heparin/LMWH treatment for thrombosis until the INR has been in the therapeutic range for at least 2 days. Tissue necrosis in protein C or S deficiency. See phytonadione (vitamin K) entry for management of abnormally high INR.
MOA — Inhibits vitamin K-dependent coagulation factors II, VII, IX, X. Also inhibits biologic anticoagulant proteins C&S.
ADVERSE EFFECTS — Serious: Major bleeding, tissue necrosis in protein C or S deficiency (rare), systemic cholesterol microembolization, purple toe syndrome. Frequent: Bruising.

HEMATOLOGY: Antihemophilic Agents

ANTI-INHIBITOR COAGULANT COMPLEX (*Feiba VH, Feiba NF, ✦Feiba VH Immuno*) ▶L ♀C ▶? $$$$$
ADULTS — <u>Hemophilia A or B with factor VIII inhibitors, XI and XII (if surgery or active bleeding):</u> 50 to 100 units/kg IV; specific dose and frequency based on site of bleeding, max 200 units/kg/day.
PEDS — Not approved in children.
FORMS — Trade only: Single-dose vials 500, 1000, 2500 units/vial.
NOTES — Contraindicated if normal coagulation. Human plasma product, thus risk of infectious agent transmission. Avoid in active or impending disseminated intravascular coagulation (DIC).
MOA — Coagulation factors II, IX, X and activated factor VII with factor VIII inhibitor bypassing activity that shortens the APTT of plasma containing factor VIII inhibitor.
ADVERSE EFFECTS — Serious: DIC, thromboembolic events, myocardial infarction, anaphylaxis, infectious agent transmission. Frequent: Hypersensitivity (rash, urticaria), anamnestic response (increase in factor VIII inhibitor titer).

FACTOR IX (*AlphaNine SD, Benefix, Mononine, ✦Immunine VH*) ▶L ♀C ▶? $$$$$
ADULTS — <u>Hemophilia B:</u> Individualize factor IX dose.
PEDS — <u>Hemophilia B:</u> Individualize factor IX dose.
FORMS — Specific formulation usually chosen by specialist in Hemophilia Treatment Center.
NOTES — Risk of HIV/hepatitis transmission varies by product. Products that contain factors II, VII, and X may cause thrombosis in at-risk patients. Stop infusion if signs of DIC.
MOA — Coagulation factor in the intrinsic coagulation pathway. Activated factor IXa in combination with Factor VIII:C activates Factor X to Xa.
ADVERSE EFFECTS — Serious: HIV/hepatitis transmission (risk varies by product). Products that contain factors II, VII, & X may cause thrombosis in at-risk patients. Frequent: Infusion-related fever, chills, flushing, nausea, IV-site discomfort.

FACTOR VIIA (*NovoSeven, NovoSeven RT, ✦Niastase*) ▶L ♀C ▶? $$$$$
WARNING — Serious thrombotic events reported when used outside of labeled indications, including

(cont.)

HEMATOLOGY: Antihemophilic Agents

WARFARIN—SELECTED DRUG INTERACTIONS

Assume possible interactions with any new medication. When starting/stopping a medication, the INR should be checked at least weekly for ≥2 to 3 weeks and dose adjusted accordingly. For further information regarding mechanism or management, refer to the Tarascon Pocket Pharmacopoeia drug interactions database (mobile or web edition). Similarly monitor if significant change in diet (including supplements) or illness resulting in decreased oral intake.

Increased anticoagulant effect of warfarin / Increased risk of bleeding

Monitor INR when agents below started, stopped, or dosage changed. Consider alternative agent.
acetaminophen ≥2 g/day for ≥3 to 4 days, allopurinol, amiodarone*, amprenavir, **anabolic steroids**, ASA¶, cefixime, cefoperazone, cefotetan, celecoxib, chloramphenicol, cimetidine†, **corticosteroids**, danazol, danshen, disulfiram, dong quai, erlotinib, etravirine, **fibrates**, fish oil, fluconazole, **fluoroquinolones**, fluorouracil, fluvoxamine, fosphenytoin (acute), garlic supplements, gemcitabine, gemfibrozil, glucosamine-chondroitin, ginkgo, ifosfamide, imatinib, isoniazid, itraconazole, ketoconazole, leflunomide, lepirudin, levothyroxine#, **macrolides**‡, metronidazole, miconazole (intravaginal), neomycin (PO for >1 to 2 days), **NSAIDs**¶, olsalazine, omeprazole, paroxetine, penicillin (high-dose IV), pentoxifylline, phenytoin (acute), propafenone, propoxyphene, quinidine, quinine, **statins**§, sulfinpyrazone (with later inhibition), **sulfonamides**, tamoxifen, **testosterones**, **tetracyclines**, tramadol, tigecycline, tipranavir, **TCAs**, valproate, voriconazole, vorinostat, vitamin A (high-dose), vitamin E, zafirlukast, zileuton

Decreased anticoagulant effect of warfarin / Increased risk of thrombosis

Monitor INR when agents below started, stopped, or dosage changed. Consider alternative agent.
A cefotetan, prepitant, azathioprine, barbiturates, bosentan, carbamazepine, coenzyme Q-10, dicloxacillin, fosphenytoin (chronic), ginseng (American), griseofulvin, mercaptopurine, mesalamine, methimazole#, mitotane, nafcillin, oral contraceptives**, phenytoin (chronic), primidone, propylthiouracil#, raloxifene, ribavirin, rifabutin, rifampin, rifapentine, ritonavir, St John's wort, vitamin C (high-dose).
Use alternative to agents below. Or give at different times of day and monitor INR when agent started, stopped, or dose/dosing schedule changed
cholestyramine, colestipol††, sucralfate

*Interaction may be delayed; monitor INR for several weeks after starting & several months after stopping amiodarone. May need to decrease warfarin dose by 33% to 50%.
† Famotidine, nizatidine or ranitidine are alternatives.
‡ Azithromycin appears to have lower risk of interaction than clarithromycin or erythromycin.
§ Pravastatin appears to have lower risk of interaction.
# Hyperthyroidism/thyroid replacement increases metabolism of clotting factors, increasing response to warfarin therapy and increased bleed risk (typically requires lowering warfarin dose).
¶ Does not necessarily increase INR, but increases bleeding risk. Check INR frequently and monitor for GI bleeding.
**Do not necessarily ↓ INR, but may induce hypercoagulability.
†† Likely lower risk than cholestyramine
Table Adapted from: Coumadin® product information; *Am Fam Phys* 1999;59:635; *Chest* 2004;126:204S; Hansten and Horn's Drug Interactions Analysis and Management; *Ann Intern Med* 2004;141:23; *Arch Intern Med* 2005;165:1095. Tarascon Pocket Pharmacopoeia drug interactions database (Mobile or web edition).

FACTOR VIIA (*cont.*)
fatal arterial and venous events. Thrombotic events also reported when used for labeled uses. Monitor all patients for thrombosis. Patients with DIC, advanced atherosclerotic disease, crush injury or septicemia may be at increase thrombotic risk. Use with caution in those with thromboembolic risk factors. If DIC or thrombosis confirmed, reduce dose or stop treatment depending on symptoms.
ADULTS — <u>Hemophilia A or B:</u> Individualize factor VIIa dose.
PEDS — <u>Hemophilia A or B:</u> Individualize factor VIIa dose.
UNAPPROVED ADULTS — <u>Reversal of excessive warfarin anticoagulation (INR > 10):</u> 15 to 20 mcg/kg IV over 3 to 5 min. <u>Intracerebral hemorrhage (within 4 h of symptom onset):</u> 40 to 160 mcg/kg IV over 1 to 2 min. <u>Perioperative blood loss in retropubic prostatectomy:</u> 20 or 40 mcg/kg IV bolus.
FORMS — Trade only: 1200, 2400, 4800 mcg/vial.
NOTES — Contraindicated with hypersensitivity to mouse, hamster or bovine proteins.
MOA — Coagulation factor that acts as a cofactor in extrinsic pathway of coagulation by conversion of Factor IX to IXa and X to Xa.
ADVERSE EFFECTS — Serious: DIC, hemorrhage, hemarthrosis, arterial and venous thromboembolic events. Frequent: Fever, plasma fibrinogen decrease, hyper/hypotension, allergic reactions, infusion site reactions.
FACTOR VIII (*Advate, Alphanate, Helixate, Hemofil M, Humate P, Koate, Kogenate, Monoclate P, Monarc-M, Recombinate, ReFacto, Xyntha*) ▶L ♀C ▶? $$$$$

(cont.)

FACTOR VIII *(cont.)*
ADULTS — Hemophilia A: Individualize factor VIII dose. Surgical procedures in patients with von Willebrand disease (Alphanate, Humate P): Individualized dosing. Bleeding in patients with von Willebrand disease (Humate P): Individualized dosing.
PEDS — Hemophilia A: Individualize factor VIII dose.
FORMS — Specific formulation usually chosen by specialist in Hemophilia Treatment Center. Recombinant formulations: Advate, Helixate, Kogenate, Recombinate, ReFacto, Xyntha. Human plasma-derived formulations: Alphanate, Hemofil M, Humate P, Koate, Monoclate P, Monarc-M.
NOTES — Risk of HIV/hepatitis transmission varies by product; no such risk with recombinant product. Reduced response with development of factor VIII inhibitors. Hemolysis with large/repeated doses in patients with A, B, AB blood type.
MOA — Coagulation factor in the intrinsic coagulation pathway, activated factor VIII acts as a cofactor for conversion of Factor X to Xa.
ADVERSE EFFECTS — Serious: HIV/hepatitis transmission (risk varies by product; no such risk if recombinant). Reduced response with development of factor VIII inhibitors (antibodies). Hemolysis with large/repeated doses in patients with A, B, AB blood type. Frequent: Allergic reactions, infusion site reactions.

HEMATOLOGY: Colony Stimulating Factors

DARBEPOETIN (*Aranesp, NESP*) ▶cellular sialidases, L ♀C ▶? $$$$$
WARNING — Increased risk of death and serious cardiovascular events, including arterial and venous thrombotic events; may shorten time to tumor progression in in cancer patients. To minimize risks in cancer patients, use lowest effective dose to avoid blood transfusion. To minimize risks in chronic renal failure, individualize dosing to maintain Hb 10 to 12 g/dL; risks have not been excluded with targeted Hb < 12 g/dL. Consider antithrombotic DVT prophylaxis, especially in peri-operative period. Not approved for use in cancer patients unless anemia is caused by concurrent myelosuppressive chemotherapy; discontinue when chemotherapy completed. Not for patients receiving myelosuppressive chemotherapy in whom anticipated outcome is cure.
ADULTS — Anemia of chronic renal failure: 0.45 mcg/kg IV/SC q week, or 0.75 mcg/kg SC q 2 weeks for some nondialysis patients. Maintenance dose may be lower in predialysis patients than dialysis patients. Adjust dose based on Hb to maintain Hg 10 to 12 g/dL. Anemia in cancer chemo patients: Initially 2.25 mcg/kg SC q week, or 500 mcg SC every 3 weeks. For weekly administration, max 4.5 mcg/kg/dose. Adjust dose based on Hb to maintain lowest level to avoid transfusion. Weekly dose conversion to darbepoetin (D) from erythropoietin (E): 6.25 mcg D for less than 2500 units E; 12.5 mcg D for 2500 to 4999 units E; 25 mcg D for 5000 to 10,999 units E; 40 mcg D for 11,000 to 17,999 units E; 60 mcg D for 18,000 to 33,999 units E; 100 mcg D for 34,000 to 89,999 units E; 200 mcg D for 90,000 units E or greater. Give D once a week for patients taking E 2 to 3 times per week; give D once every 2 weeks for patients taking E once a week. Monitor Hb weekly until stable, then at least monthly.
PEDS — Not approved in children.
UNAPPROVED ADULTS — Chemotherapy-induced anemia: 3 mcg/kg or 200 mcg SC q 2 weeks.
FORMS — Trade only: All forms are available with or without albumin. Single-dose vials: 25, 40, 60, 100, 200, 300, 500 mcg/1 mL, and 150 mcg/0.75 mL. Single-dose prefilled syringes or autoinjectors: 25 mcg/0.42 mL, 40 mcg/0.4 mL, 60 mcg/0.3 mL, 100 mcg/0.5 mL, 150 mcg/0.3 mL, 200 mcg/0.4 mL, 300 mcg/0.6 mL, 500 mcg/1 mL.
NOTES — May exacerbate HTN; contraindicated if uncontrolled HTN. Not for immediate correction of anemia. Evaluate iron stores before and during treatment; most patients eventually require iron supplements. Consider other causes of anemia if no response. Use only 1 dose per vial/syringe; discard any unused portion. Do not shake. Protect from light.
MOA — Long-acting form of erythropoietin that gains its increased serum half-life and biologic activity from increased sialic acid content; stimulates erythroid progenitor cells to increase RBC production.
ADVERSE EFFECTS — Serious: Hypertension, seizures, pure red cell aplasia, thrombotic events, severe anemia secondary to antibodies. Frequent: Iatrogenic iron deficiency, myalgia/arthralgia, headache, edema, GI complaints.

EPOETIN ALFA (*Epogen, Procrit,* erythropoietin alpha, ✦*Eprex*) ▶L ♀C ▶? $$$$$
WARNING — Increased risk of death and serious cardiovascular events, including arterial and venous thrombotic events; may shorten time to tumor progression in cancer patients. To minimize risks in cancer patients, use lowest dose to minimum level to avoid blood transfusion. To minimize risks in chronic renal failure, individualize dosing to maintain Hb 10 to 12 g/dL; risks have not been excluded with targeted Hb < 12 g/dL. Consider antithrombotic DVT prophylaxis, especially in the peri-operative period. Not approved for use in cancer patients unless anemia is caused by concurrent myelosuppressive chemotherapy; discontinue when chemotherapy completed. Not for patients receiving myelosuppressive chemotherapy in whom anticipated outcome is cure.
ADULTS — Anemia of chronic renal failure: Initial dose 50 to 100 units/kg IV/SC 3 times per week.

(cont.)

HEMATOLOGY: Colony Stimulating Factors

EPOETIN ALFA *(cont.)*
Adjust dose based on Hb to maintain Hg 10 to 12 g/dL. Adjust dose based on Hb to maintain lowest level to avoid transfusion. <u>Zidovudine-induced anemia in HIV-infected patients:</u> 100 to 300 units/kg IV/SC 3 times per week. <u>Anemia in cancer chemo patients:</u> 150 to 300 units/kg SC 3 times per week or 40,000 units SC once a week. Monitor Hb weekly until stable, then at least monthly. <u>Reduction of allogeneic blood transfusion in surgical patients:</u> 300 units/kg/day SC for 10 days preop, on the days of surgery, and 4 days postop. Or 600 units/kg SC once a week starting 21 days preop and ending on days of surgery (4 doses).
PEDS — Not approved in children.
UNAPPROVED PEDS — <u>Anemia of chronic renal failure:</u> Initial dose 50 to 100 units/kg IV/SC 3 times per week. <u>Zidovudine-induced anemia in HIV-infected patients:</u> 100 units/kg SC 3 times per week; max of 300 units/kg/dose.
FORMS — Trade only: Single-dose 1 mL vials 2000, 3000, 4000, 10,000, 40,000 units/mL. Multidose vials 10,000 units/mL 2 mL, 20,000 units/mL 1 mL.
NOTES — May exacerbate HTN; contraindicated if uncontrolled HTN. Not for immediate correction of anemia. Evaluate iron stores before and during treatment; most patients eventually require iron supplements. Consider other causes of anemia if no response. Single-dose vials contain no preservatives. Use 1 dose per vial; do not re-enter vial. Discard unused portion.
MOA — Stimulates erythroid progenitor cells to increase red blood cell production.
ADVERSE EFFECTS — Serious: Hypertension in patients with chronic renal failure, seizures, pure red cell aplasia, thrombotic events, severe anemia secondary to antibodies. Frequent: Iatrogenic iron deficiency, headache, arthralgia, fever.

FILGRASTIM (*G-CSF, Neupogen*) ▶L ♀C ▶? $$$$$
ADULTS — <u>Neutropenia from myelosuppressive chemotherapy:</u> 5 mcg/kg/day SC/IV until postnadir ANC is at least 10,000/mm3 for no more than 2 weeks. Can increase by 5 mcg/kg/day with each cycle prn. <u>Bone Marrow Transplant:</u> 10 mcg/kg/day IV infusion over 4 to 24 hours or 24-hour SC infusion. Administer first dose at least 24 hours after cytotoxic chemotherapy and at least 24 hours after bone marrow. Adjust to neutrophil response (see product information). <u>Peripheral blood progenitor cell collection:</u> 10 mcg/kg/day in donors for at least 4 days (usually 6 to 7 days) before the first leukapheresis and continued until the final leukapheresis. Consider decreased dose if WBC greater than 100,000/mm3. <u>Severe chronic neutropenia</u> (congenital): Start 6 mcg/kg SC bid. <u>Severe chronic neutropenia</u> (idiopathic or cyclic): Start 5 mcg/kg SC daily.
PEDS — <u>Neutropenia from myelosuppressive chemotherapy:</u> 5 mcg/kg/day SC/IV for no more than 2 weeks until postnadir ANC is at least 10,000/mm3. 10,000/mm3 for no more than 2 weeks. Can increase by 5 mcg/kg/day with each cycle prn. <u>Bone Marrow Transplant:</u> 10 mcg/kg/day IV infusion over 4 to 24 hours or 24-hour SC infusion. Administer first dose at least 24 hours after cytotoxic chemotherapy and at least 24 hours after bone marrow. Adjust to neutrophil response (see product information). <u>Peripheral blood progenitor cell collection:</u> 10 mcg/kg/day in donors for at least 4 days (usually 6 to 7 days) before the first leukapheresis and continued until the final leukapheresis. Consider decreased dose if WBC greater than 100,000/mm3. <u>Severe chronic neutropenia (congenital):</u> Start 6 mcg/kg SC bid. <u>Severe chronic neutropenia (idiopathic or cyclic):</u> Start 5 mcg/kg SC daily.
UNAPPROVED ADULTS — <u>AIDS:</u> 0.3 to 3.6 mcg/kg/day.
FORMS — Trade only: Single-dose vials: 300 mcg/1 mL, 480 mcg/1.6 mL. Single-dose syringes: 300 mcg/0.5 mL, 480 mcg/0.8 mL.
NOTES — Allergic-type reactions, bone pain, cutaneous vasculitis. Do not give within 24 h before/after cytotoxic chemotherapy. Store in refrigerator; use within 24 h when kept at room temperature.
MOA — Granulocyte colony-stimulating factor, a colony-stimulating factor that stimulates neutrophil production.
ADVERSE EFFECTS — Serious: Allergic-type reactions, cutaneous vasculitis. Frequent: Bone pain, increased levels of LDH and alkaline phosphatase.

OPRELVEKIN (*Neumega*) ▶K ♀C ▶? $$$$$
WARNING — Risk of allergic reactions and anaphylaxis.
ADULTS — <u>Prevention of severe thrombocytopenia after chemo for nonmyeloid malignancies:</u> 50 mcg/kg SC daily starting 6 to 24 h after chemo and continuing until postnadir platelet count is at least 50,000 cells/mcL (usual duration 10-21 days).
PEDS — Not approved in children. Safe and effective dose not established. Papilledema with 100 mcg/kg; 50 mcg/kg ineffective.
FORMS — Trade only: 5 mg single-dose vials with diluent.
NOTES — Fluid retention: Monitor fluid and electrolyte balance. Transient atrial arrhythmias, visual blurring, papilledema.
MOA — Interleukin-11, thrombopoietic growth factor that increases platelet production.
ADVERSE EFFECTS — Serious: Anaphylaxis, allergy, papilledema. Frequent: Edema, dyspnea, pleural effusions, transient atrial arrhythmias, transient visual blurring, conjunctival injection, thrush, asthenia.

PEGFILGRASTIM (*Neulasta*) ▶Plasma ♀C ▶? $$$$$
WARNING — Do not use if wt less than 45 kg.
ADULTS — <u>To reduce febrile neutropenia after chemo for nonmyeloid malignancies:</u> 6 mg SC once each chemo cycle.
PEDS — Not approved in children.
FORMS — Trade only: Single-dose syringes 6 mg/0.6 mL.
NOTES — Bone pain common. Do not give in the time period between 14 days prior to and 24 h after

(cont.)

PEGFILGRASTIM *(cont.)*
cytotoxic chemo. Store in refrigerator. Stable at room temperature for no more than 48 h. Protect from light.
MOA — Long-acting form of filgrastim that is conjugated to polyethylene glycol (pegylated).
ADVERSE EFFECTS — Similar to filgrastim. Serious: None. Frequent: Bone pain, reversible increases in LDH, alkaline phosphatase, uric acid.
SARGRAMOSTIM (*GM-CSF, Leukine*) ▶L ♀C ▶? $$$$$

ADULTS — Specialized dosing for leukemia, bone marrow transplantation.
PEDS — Not approved in children.
MOA — Granulocyte-macrophage colony-stimulating factor, a colony-stimulating factor that stimulates the production of neutrophils, monocytes, and eosinophils.
ADVERSE EFFECTS — Serious: Capillary leak syndrome, dyspnea due to sequestration of WBCs in lungs (rare). Frequent: Fluid retention, fever, asthenia, headache, bone pain, chills, myalgia.

HEMATOLOGY: Other Hematological Agents

AMINOCAPROIC ACID (*Amicar*) ▶K ♀D ▶? $ IV $$$$$ Oral
ADULTS — <u>To improve hemostasis when fibrinolysis contributes to bleeding:</u> 4 to 5 g IV/PO over 1 h, then 1 g/h for 8 h or until bleeding controlled.
PEDS — Not approved in children.
UNAPPROVED ADULTS — <u>Prevention of recurrent subarachnoid hemorrhage:</u> 6 g IV/PO q 4 h (6 doses/day). <u>Reduction of postop bleeding after cardiopulmonary bypass:</u> 5 g IV, then 1 g/h for 6 to 8 h.
UNAPPROVED PEDS — <u>To improve hemostasis when fibrinolysis contributes to bleeding:</u> 100 mg/kg or 3 g/m2 IV infusion during 1st h, then continuous infusion of 33.3 mg/kg/h or 1 g/m2/h. Max dose of 18 g/m2/day. IV prep contains benzyl alcohol; do not use in newborns.
FORMS — Generic/Trade: Syrup 250 mg/mL, Tabs 500 mg. Trade only: Tabs 1000 mg.
NOTES — Contraindicated in active intravascular clotting. Do not use in DIC without heparin. Can cause intrarenal thrombosis, hyperkalemia. Skeletal muscle weakness, necrosis with prolonged use; monitor CPK. Use with estrogen/oral contraceptives can cause hypercoagulability. Rapid IV administration can cause hypotension, bradycardia, arrhythmia.
MOA — Inhibits fibrinolysis.
ADVERSE EFFECTS — Serious: Skeletal muscle weakness and necrosis with prolonged use. Rapid IV administration can cause hypotension, bradycardia, arrhythmia. Frequent: None.
ANAGRELIDE (*Agrylin*) ▶LK ♀C ▶? $$$$$
ADULTS — <u>Thrombocythemia due to myeloproliferative disorders (including essential thrombocythemia):</u> Start 0.5 mg PO qid or 1 mg PO bid, then after 1 week adjust to lowest effective dose that maintains platelet count < 600,000/mcL. Max 10 mg/day or 2.5 mg as a single dose. Usual dose 1.5 to 3 mg/day.
PEDS — Limited data. <u>Thrombocythemia due to myeloproliferative disorders (including essential thrombocythemia):</u> Start 0.5 mg PO daily, then after 1 week adjust to lowest effective dose that maintains platelet count < 600,000/mcL. Max 10 mg/day or 2.5 mg as a single dose. Usual dose 1.5 to 3 mg/day.
FORMS — Generic/Trade: Caps 0.5 mg. Generic only: Caps 1 mg.

NOTES — Caution with heart disease, may cause vasodilation, tachycardia, palpitations, heart failure. Contraindicated in severe hepatic impairment, use with caution in mild to moderate hepatic impairment. Monitor LFTs baseline and during therapy. Caution in lung disease and renal insufficiency. Dosage should be increased by not more than 0.5 mg/day in any 1 week.
MOA — Unknown; a decrease in megakaryocyte hypermaturation may decrease platelet production.
ADVERSE EFFECTS — Serious: May cause cardiovascular events including vasodilation, tachycardia, palpitations, and heart failure, renal failure, pulmonary disorders, hepatotoxicity. Frequent: Headache, diarrhea, edema, palpitation, abdominal pain.
DABIGATRAN (*Pradaxa*) ▶K ♀C ▶– $$$$$
ADULTS — <u>Stroke prevention in atrial fibrillation:</u> 150 mg PO BID (if CrCl 15-30 ml/min: 75 mg PO BID).
PEDS — Not approved in children.
FORMS — Trade only: caps 75, 150 mg.
NOTES — Do not break, open or chew capsules. May cause gastritis. Avoid interruptions in therapy as this may increase risk of stroke. Avoid use with rifampin.
DEFERASIROX (*Exjade*) ▶L ♀B ▶? $$$$$
WARNING — Monitor renal and hepatic function closesly. Renal impairment, including failure, has been reported; assess serum creatinine and creatnine clearance before therapy and monthly thereafter. Fatal hepatic failure has been reported; monitor LFTs and bilirubin baseline, q 2 weeks for 1 month, then monthly. Gastrointestinal bleeding reported.
ADULTS — <u>Chronic iron overload:</u> 20 mg/kg PO daily; adjust dose q 3 to 6 months based on ferritin trends. Max 40 mg/kg/day.
PEDS — <u>Chronic iron overload,</u> age 2 yo or older: 20 mg/kg PO daily; adjust dose q 3 to 6 months based on ferritin trends. Max 40 mg/kg/day.
FORMS — Trade only: Tabs for dissolving into oral susp 125, 250, 500 mg.
NOTES — Do not use if CrCl < 40 ml/min, serum creatnine greater than twice upper limit of normal. Contraindicated if high-risk fmyelodysplastic syndrome, advanced malignancy or poor performance status. Give on an empty stomach, 30 min or more before food. Reports of fatal cytopenias, monitor CBC regularly. Perform auditory and ophthalmic

(cont.)

DEFERASIROX (cont.)
testing before initiation of therapy and yearly thereafter. Do not take with aluminum-containing antacids. May decrease serum ferritin and liver iron concentrations.
MOA — Chelates free serum iron.
ADVERSE EFFECTS — Serious: Renal failure, hepatic failure, hearing disturbance/loss, ocular disturbances, optic neuritis, neutropenia, thrombocytopenia, GI hemorrhage/ulcer, erythema multiforme. Frequent: Fever, headache, abdominal pain, cough, diarrhea, creatinine increase, N/V, rash, arthralgia, fatigue.

HYDROXYUREA (Hydrea, Droxia) ▶LK ♀D ▶− $ varies by therapy
WARNING — Mutagenic and clastogenic; may cause secondary leukemia. Instruct patients to report promptly fever, sore throat, signs of local infection, bleeding from any site, or symptoms suggestive of anemia. Cutaneous vasculitic toxicities, including vasculitic ulcerations and gangrene, have been reported most often in patients on interferon therapy.
ADULTS — Sickle cell anemia.(Droxia): Start 15 mg/kg PO daily while monitoring CBC q 2 weeks. If WBC is 2500/mm3 or greater, platelet count is 95,000/mm3 or greater, and Hb is above 5.3 g/dL, then increase dose q 12 weeks by 5 mg/kg/day (max 35 mg/kg/day). Give concomitant folic acid 1 mg/day. Chemotherapy: Doses vary by indication, eg, melanoma, CML, recurrent, metastatic or inoperable carcinoma of the ovary, squamous cell carcinoma of the head and neck, acute leukemia.
PEDS — Not approved in children.
UNAPPROVED ADULTS — Essential thrombocythemia at high risk for thrombosis: 0.5 to 1 g PO daily adjusted to keep platelets < 400/mm3. Also has been used for HIV, psoriasis, polycythemia vera.
UNAPPROVED PEDS — Sickle cell anemia.
FORMS — Generic/Trade: Caps 500 mg. Trade only: (Droxia) Caps 200, 300, 400 mg.
NOTES — Reliable contraception is recommended. Monitor CBC and renal function. Elderly may need lower doses. Minimize exposure to the drug by wearing gloves during handling.
MOA — Antimetabolite.
ADVERSE EFFECTS — Serious: Bone marrow suppression, nephrotoxicity. Frequent: Bone marrow suppression, erythropoiesis, mucositis, rash.

PLERIXAFOR (Mozobil) ▶K ♀D ▶? $$$$$
ADULTS — Hematopoietic stem cell mobilization with G-CSF for autologous transplantation in non-Hodgkin's lymphoma and multiple myeloma: 0.24 mg/kg (actual body wt) SC once daily for up to 4 days, max 40 mg/day.
PEDS — Not approved in children.
FORMS — Trade only: Single-dose vials 20 mg/mL, 1.2 mL vial.
NOTES — Use with G-CSF; initiate after patient has received G-CSF daily for 4 days. Administer 11 h prior to apheresis. If CrCl < 50 mL/min, decrease dose to 0.16 mg/kg. Do not use in leukemia. Monitor CBC, may increase WBC and decrease platelets. May mobilize tumor cells from marrow. Evaluate for splenic rupture if left upper abdominal, scapular or shoulder pain.
MOA — CXCR4 chemokine antagonist.
ADVERSE EFFECTS — Serious: Leukocytosis, thrombocytopenia, splenic rupture. Frequent: Diarrhea, nausea, fatigue, injection site reactions, headache, arthralgia, dizziness, vomiting.

PROTAMINE ▶Plasma ♀C ▶? $
WARNING — Hypotension, cardiovascular collapse, pulmonary edema/vasoconstriction/hypertension may occur. May be more common with higher doses, overdose or repeated doses, including previous exposure to protamine or protamine-containing drugs (including insulin). Other risk factors include fish allergy, vasectomy, LV dysfunction and pulmonary hemodynamic instability.
ADULTS — Heparin overdose: 1 mg antagonizes about 100 units heparin. Give IV over 10 min in doses of no greater than 50 mg.
PEDS — Not approved in children.
UNAPPROVED ADULTS — Reversal of low-molecular-weight heparin: 1 mg protamine per 100 anti-Xa units of dalteparin or tinzaparin. Give additional 0.5 mg protamine per 100 anti-Xa units of tinzaparin if PTT remains prolonged 2 to 4 h after first infusion of protamine. 1 mg protamine per 1 mg enoxaparin.
UNAPPROVED PEDS — Heparin overdose: Within 30 min of last heparin dose, give 1 mg protamine per 100 units of heparin received; between 30 to 60 min since last heparin dose, give 0.5 to 0.75 mg protamine per 100 units of heparin received; between 60 to 120 min since last heparin dose, give 0.375 to 0.5 mg protamine per 100 units of heparin; more than 120 min since last heparin dose, give 0.25 to 0.375 mg protamine per 100 units of heparin.
NOTES — Severe hypotension/anaphylactoid reaction possible with too rapid administration. Additional doses of protamine may be required in some situations (neutralization of SC heparin, heparin rebound after cardiac surgery). Monitor APTT to confirm heparin neutralization.
MOA — Binds with and neutralizes heparin and some LMWHs.
ADVERSE EFFECTS — Serious: Severe hypotension/anaphylactoid reaction with too rapid administration, allergic reactions in patients with fish allergy, previous exposure to protamine (including insulin), pulmonary edema, circulatory collapse. Frequent: Back pain, transient flushing.

ROMIPLOSTIN (Nplate) ▶L ♀C ▶? $$$$$
ADULTS — Chronic immune idiopathic thrombocytopenic purpura: 1 mcg/kg SC weekly. Adjust by 1 mcg/kg weekly to achieve and maintain platelet count at least 50,000 cells/mcL; max 10 mcg/kg weekly. Hold dose if platelet count is 400,000 cells/mcL or greater.
PEDS — Not approved in children.
NOTES — Use only for chronic ITP; do not use if low platelets from other causes. Use only if increased

(cont.)

ROMIPLOSTIN (cont.)

risk of bleeding and insufficient response to corticosteroids, immunoglobulins or splenectomy. Do not use to normalize platelet counts; excessive therapy may increase risk of thrombosis. May increase risk for fibrous deposits in bone marrow. Monitor CBC (platelets and peripheral blood smears) weekly until stable dose; then monthly. Platelet counts may drop below baseline following discontinuation; monitor CBC for 2 weeks following cessation of therapy. May increase risk of hematologic malignancies, especially if myelodysplastic syndrome. Available only through restricted distribution program.
MOA — Throbopoietin receptor agonist.
ADVERSE EFFECTS — Serious: Thrombosis, bone marrow fibrosis. Frequent: Headache, arthralgia, dizziness, insomnia, myalgia, pain in extremity, shoulder pain, dyspepsia, paresthesia.

THROMBIN—TOPICAL (*Evithrom, Recothrom, Thrombin-JMI*) ▶? ♀C ▶? $$$
WARNING — The bovine form (Thrombin-JMI) has been associated with rare but potentially fatal abnormalities in hemostasis ranging from asymptomatic alterations in PT and/or aPTT to severe bleeding or thrombosis. Hemostatic abnormalities are likely due to antibody formation, may cause factor V deficiency, and are more likely with repeated applications. Consult hematologist if abnormal coagulation, bleeding or thrombosis after topical thrombin use.
ADULTS — <u>Hemostatic aid for minor bleeding:</u> Apply topically to site of bleeding; dose depends on area to be treated.
PEDS — <u>Hemostatic aid for minor bleeding</u> (Evithrom): Apply topically to site of bleeding; dose depends on area to be treated. Recothrom/Thrombin-JMI not approved in children.
NOTES — Do not inject; for topical use only. Do not use for severe or brisk arterial bleeding. Thaw Evithrom prior to use. Reconstitute Recothrom and Thrombin-JMI prior to use. Evithrom is human-derived and carries risk of viral transmission. Recothrom is a recombinant product; risk of allergic reaction in known hypersensitivity to snake proteins; contraindicated in hypersensitivity to hamster proteins. Thrombin-JMI is a bovine origin product; contraindicated in hypersensitivity to products of bovine origin.
MOA — Promotes clot formation by activating platelets and catalyzing the conversion of fibrinogen to fibrin.
ADVERSE EFFECTS — Serious: Anaphylaxis, antibody development, hemostatic abnormalities, thrombosis, severe bleeding. Frequent: Pruritus, incision/procedure site complications.

TRANEXAMIC ACID (*Cyklokapron, Lysteda*) ▶K ♀B ▶– $$$
ADULTS — <u>Prophylaxis/reduction of bleeding during tooth extraction in hemophilia patients:</u> 10 mg/kg IV immediately before surgery, then 25 mg/kg PO 3 to 4 times per day for 2 to 8 days following surgery. Additional regimens include: 10 mg/kg IV 3 to 4 times per day if intolerant of oral therapies or 25 mg/kg PO 3 to 4 times per day beginning 1 day before surgery. <u>Heavy menstrual bleeding (Lysteda):</u> 1300 mg PO TID for up to 5 days during menstruation.
PEDS — Not approved in children.
FORMS — Oral: Trade only, tab: 650 mg.
NOTES — Dose adjust in renal impairment.
MOA — Competitively inhibits plasminogen activator and noncompetitively plasmin (at higher doses).
ADVERSE EFFECTS — Hypotension (infusion rate limiting), DVT, PE, vision abnormalities, giddiness, N/V, diarrhea.

HERBAL & ALTERNATIVE THERAPIES

NOTE: In the United States, herbal and alternative therapy products are regulated as dietary supplements, not drugs. Premarketing evaluation and FDA approval are not required unless specific therapeutic claims are made. Because these products are not required to demonstrate efficacy, it is unclear whether many of them have health benefits. In addition, there may be considerable variability in content from lot to lot or between products. See www.tarascon.com/herbals for the evidence-based efficacy ratings used by Tarascon editorial staff.

ALOE VERA (*acemannan, burn plant*) ▶LK ♀oral– topical+? ▶oral- topical+? $
UNAPPROVED ADULTS — Topical: Efficacy unclear for seborrheic dermatitis, psoriasis, genital herpes, partial-thickness skin burns. Does not prevent radiation-induced skin injury. Do not apply to surgical incisions; impaired healing reported. Oral: Efficacy unclear for active ulcerative colitis or type 2 diabetes.
UNAPPROVED PEDS — Not for use in children.
FORMS — Not by prescription.
NOTES — OTC laxatives containing aloe were removed from the US market due to concerns about increased risk of colon cancer. International Aloe Science Council seal may help ensure aloe content. Cases of Henoch-Schonlein purpura and hepatotoxicity reported with oral administration.
MOA — Topical: Constituents of gel from within leaves have skin-moisturizing, immunomodulatory, anti-inflammatory, and antiviral activity in vitro. Oral: Aloe latex contains anthraquinone glycosides (stimulant laxative). Pancreatic beta cell stimulation in vitro.
ADVERSE EFFECTS — Topical: Contact dermatitis, pruritus. Oral: Abdominal cramping, diarrhea. Potassium depletion or electrolyte imbalance possible with chronic administration. Hepatotoxicity (hypersensitivity probable mechanism). Henoch-Schonlein purpura (several case reports).

ANDROSTENEDIONE (*andro*) ▶L, peripheral conversion to estrogens and androgens ♀− ▶− $
UNAPPROVED ADULTS − Was marketed as anabolic steroid to enhance athletic performance. Advise patients against use because of potential for androgenic (primarily in women) and estrogenic (primarily in men) side effects.
UNAPPROVED PEDS − Not for use in children.
FORMS − Not by prescription.
NOTES − Banned as dietary supplement by FDA. Also banned by many athletic organizations. In theory, chronic use may increase risk of hormone-related cancers (prostate, breast, endometrial, ovarian). Increase in androgen levels could exacerbate hyperlipidemia.
MOA − Anabolic steroid precursor; converted to estrogen and testosterone.
ADVERSE EFFECTS − Potential long-term effects include: Testicular atrophy, impotence, and gynecomastia in men; acne, male pattern baldness, deep voice, hirsutism, clitoral enlargement, abnormal menstrual cycles, and thromboembolism in women; premature puberty and short stature in children/adolescents. May exacerbate hyperlipidemia.

ARISTOLOCHIC ACID (*Aristolochia, Asarum, Bragantia, Mu Tong, Fangchi*) ▶? ♀− ▶− $
UNAPPROVED ADULTS − Do not use due to well-documented risk of nephrotoxicity. Was promoted for wt loss.
UNAPPROVED PEDS − Do not use.
FORMS − Not by prescription.
NOTES − Banned by FDA due to risk of nephrotoxicity and cancer. Possible adulterant in other Chinese herbal products like Akebia, Clematis, Stephania, and others. Rule out aristolochic acid nephrotoxicity in cases of unexplained renal failure.
MOA − Nephrotoxic (causes interstitial renal fibrosis). Also caused lymphoma and kidney, bladder, stomach, and lung cancer in animal studies.
ADVERSE EFFECTS − Serious: End-stage renal disease and urothelial carcinoma reported in humans.

ARNICA (*Arnica montana, leopard's bane, wolf's bane*) ▶? ♀− ▶− $
UNAPPROVED ADULTS − Toxic if taken by mouth. Topical preparations promoted for treatment of bruises, aches, and sprains; but insufficient data to assess efficacy. Do not use on open wounds.
UNAPPROVED PEDS − Not for use in children.
FORMS − Not by prescription.
NOTES − Repeated topical application can cause skin reactions.
MOA − Contains derivatives of thymol. Thymol is a subcutanuos vasodilator, may have anti-inflammatory and analgesic effects. Helenalin in the product is a GI toxin.
ADVERSE EFFECTS − Repeated topical application can cause skin reactions. Contact dermatitis; cross-hypersensitivity possible with other plants in Compositae family, including chamomile, chrysanthemum, echinacea, feverfew, ragweed, Artemisia. If ingested, may cause gastroenteritis and GI bleeding.

ARTICHOKE LEAF EXTRACT (*Cynara scolymus*) ▶? ♀? ▶? $
UNAPPROVED ADULTS − May reduce total cholesterol, but clinical significance is unclear. Possibly effective for functional dyspepsia. Does not appear to prevent alcohol-induced hangover.
UNAPPROVED PEDS − Not for use in children.
FORMS − Not by prescription.
NOTES − Advise against use by patients with bile duct obstruction or gallstones.
MOA − Contains cynarine, a choleretic that increases bile secretion.
ADVERSE EFFECTS − Contact dermatitis (rare).

ASTRAGALUS (*Astragalus membranaceus, huang qi, Jin Fu Kang, vetch*) ▶? ♀? ▶? $
UNAPPROVED ADULTS − Used in combination with other herbs in traditional Chinese medicine for CHD, CHF, chronic kidney disease, viral infections, upper respiratory tract infections. Early studies suggested that astragalus might improve efficacy of platinum-based chemotherapy for non-small-cell lung cancer. However, an astragalus-based herbal formula (Jinfukang) did not affect survival in phase II study of non-small cell lung cancer.
UNAPPROVED PEDS − Not for use in children.
FORMS − Not by prescription.
NOTES − Not used for more than 3 weeks without close follow-up in traditional Chinese medicine. In theory, may enhance activity of drugs for diabetes, HTN, and anticoagulation.
MOA − Has immunostimulant properties. Contains saponins, astragalosides, high-weight polysaccharides, amino acids, and trace minerals.
ADVERSE EFFECTS − None found.

BILBERRY (*Vaccinium myrtillus, huckleberry, Tegens, VMA extract*) ▶Bile, K ♀− ▶− $
UNAPPROVED ADULTS − Insufficient data to evaluate efficacy for macular degeneration or cataracts. Does not appear to improve night vision.
UNAPPROVED PEDS − Supplements not for use in children.
FORMS − Not by prescription.
NOTES − High doses may impair platelet aggregation, affect clotting time, and cause GI distress.
MOA − Contains bioflavonoids (antioxidants) and anthocyanosides (stabilize collagen).
ADVERSE EFFECTS − GI distress, rash. High doses may impair platelet aggregation and affect clotting time.

BITTER MELON (*Momordica charantia, ampalaya, karela*) ▶? ♀− ▶− $$
UNAPPROVED ADULTS − Efficacy unclear for type 2 diabetes. Dose unclear; juice may be more potent than dried fruit powder.
UNAPPROVED PEDS − Not for use in children. Two cases of hypoglycemic coma in children ingesting bitter melon tea.
FORMS − Not by prescription.
MOA − Mechanism of hypoglycemic action unknown but contains insulin-like peptide. MAP30 protein in seeds has in vitro antiviral and antineoplastic activity.

(cont.)

BITTER MELON (cont.)

ADVERSE EFFECTS – Two cases of hypoglycemic coma in children ingesting bitter melon tea. Seeds can cause hemolytic anemia in G6PD deficiency.

BITTER ORANGE (Citrus aurantium, Seville orange, Acutrim Natural AM, Dexatrim Natural Ephedrine Free) ▶K ♀– ▶– $

UNAPPROVED ADULTS – Marketed as substitute for ephedra in weight-loss dietary supplements; safety and efficacy not established.

UNAPPROVED PEDS – Not for use in children.

FORMS – Not by prescription.

NOTES – Contains sympathomimetics including synephrine and octopamine. Synephrine banned by some sports organizations. Do not use within 14 days of an MAOI. Juice may inhibit intestinal CYP3A4.

MOA – Contains sympathomimetics, including synephrine (similar to phenylephrine) and octopamine. May increase blood pressure and heart rate. Juice contains furocoumarin which inhibits CYP3A4.

ADVERSE EFFECTS – Treatment-resistant hypertension. Supplements containing synephrine linked to reports of rhabdomyolysis, MI, stroke, ischemic colitis, and ventricular tachycardia. Ephedra, a related compound, was banned from US market due to similar adverse effects. Bitter orange peel oil may be phototoxic.

BLACK COHOSH (Cimicifuga racemosa, Remifemin, Menofem) ▶Bile + Feces ♀– ▶– $

UNAPPROVED ADULTS – Ineffective for relief of menopausal symptoms.

UNAPPROVED PEDS – Not for use in children.

FORMS – Not by prescription.

NOTES – US Pharmacopoeia concluded black cohosh is possible cause of hepatotoxicity in 30 case reports. Does not alter vaginal epithelium, endometrium, or estradiol levels in postmenopausal women.

MOA – Contains triterpene glycosides. Mechanism of action unknown, but does not appear to interact directly with estrogen receptors.

ADVERSE EFFECTS – GI distress, rash. United States Pharmacopoeia determined black cohosh to be possible cause of hepatotoxicity in 30 case reports.

BUTTERBUR (Petasites hybridus, Petadolex, Petaforce, Tesalin, ZE 339) ▶? ♀– ▶– $

UNAPPROVED ADULTS – <u>Migraine prophylaxis</u> (possibly effective): Petadolex 50 to 75 mg PO bid. <u>Allergic rhinitis prophylaxis</u> (possibly effective): Petadolex 50 mg PO bid or Tesalin (ZE 339; 8 mg petasin/tab) 1 tab PO qid or 2 tabs tid. Efficacy unclear for asthma.

UNAPPROVED PEDS – Not for children.

FORMS – Not by prescription. Standardized pyrrolizidine-free extracts: Petadolex (7.5 mg of petasin and isopetasin/50 mg tab). Tesalin (ZE 339; 8 mg petasin/tab).

NOTES – Do not use raw butterbur; it may contain hepatotoxic pyrrolizidine alkaloids which are removed by processing. Butterbur is related to Asteraceae and Compositae; consider the potential for cross-allergenicity between plants in these families.

MOA – Cerebrovascular smooth muscle relaxant and inhibitor of leukotriene synthesis.

ADVERSE EFFECTS – Serious: None reported. Frequent: Nausea, burping, stomach pain. No long-term safety data.

CESIUM CHLORIDE (none) ▶K ♀– ▶–

UNAPPROVED ADULTS – Health Canada and FDA are taking action against Internet sellers promoting cesium chloride as alternative treatment of late-stage cancer. Evidence for benefit as cancer treatment is lacking.

FORMS – Not by prescription.

NOTES – Can prolong QT interval and cause torsades. Toxicity can be prolonged due to extremely long-half life (approximately 200 days to reach steady-state). Prussian blue has been used to speed cesium chloride elimination.

MOA – Claims that cesium (a group 1a element) kills tumor cells by increasing intracellular pH are unproven. Cesium prolongs QT interval by blocking potassium channels; effect is so reproducible that it is used in animal model of long-QT syndrome.

ADVERSE EFFECTS – Syncope, QT interval prolongation, torsades de pointes, hypokalemia, diarrhea, paresthesias.

CHAMOMILE (Matricaria recutita - German chamomile, Anthemis nobilis - Roman chamomile) ▶? ♀– ▶– $

UNAPPROVED ADULTS – Promoted as a sedative or anxiolytic, to relieve GI distress, for skin infections or inflammation, many other indications. Efficacy unclear for any indication. Does not appear to reduce mucositis caused by 5-fluorouracil or radiation.

UNAPPROVED PEDS – Supplements not for use in children. Efficacy and safety unclear for treatment of infant colic with multi-ingredient teas/extracts of chamomile, fennel, and lemon balm.

FORMS – Not by prescription.

NOTES – Theoretical concern (no clinical evidence) for interactions due to increased sedation, increased risk of bleeding (contains coumarin derivatives), delayed GI absorption of other drugs (due to antispasmodic effect). Increased INR with warfarin attributed to chamomile in single case report.

MOA – Contains compounds with antispasmodic, antiinflammatory, antimicrobial, and mild sedative effects in animal and in vitro studies.

ADVERSE EFFECTS – Rare allergic reactions including anaphylaxis, contact dermatitis. Cross-hypersensitivity with other plants in Compositae family, including arnica, chrysanthemum, echinacea, feverfew, ragweed, Artemisia. Topical application to the eye can cause conjunctivitis.

CHASTEBERRY (Vitex agnus castus fruit extract, Femaprin) ▶? ♀– ▶– $

UNAPPROVED ADULTS – <u>Premenstrual syndrome</u> (possibly effective): 20 mg PO daily of extract ZE 440 (ratio 6–12:1; standardized for casticin).

UNAPPROVED PEDS – Not for use in children.

FORMS – Not by prescription.

(cont.)

CHASTEBERRY (cont.)

NOTES − Liquid formulations may contain alcohol. Avoid concomitant dopamine antagonists such as haloperidol or metoclopramide.
MOA − Higher doses may reduce prolactin levels by binding to dopamine D2 receptors in the pituitary. Low doses may increase serum prolactin levels.
ADVERSE EFFECTS − Rash, acne, GI upset, intermenstrual bleeding.

CHONDROITIN ▶K ♀? ▶? $

UNAPPROVED ADULTS − Does not appear effective for relief of OA pain overall. Glucosamine/Chondroitin Arthritis Intervention Trial (GAIT) did not find improvement in pain of knee OA with chondroitin 400 mg PO tid ± glucosamine. Glucosamine + chondroitin improved pain in subgroup of patients with moderate to severe knee OA.
UNAPPROVED PEDS − Not for use in children.
FORMS − Not by prescription.
NOTES − Chondroitin content not standardized and known to vary. Cosamin DS contains 3 mg manganese/cap; tolerable upper limit of manganese is 11 mg/day. Some products made from bovine cartilage. Case reports of increased INR/bleeding with warfarin in patient taking chondroitin + glucosamine.
MOA − Glycosaminoglycan that may stimulate production of cartilage matrix.
ADVERSE EFFECTS − GI distress, allergic reactions. Adverse effects appear minor and infrequent.

CINNAMON (*Cinnamomum Cassia, Aromaticum*) ▶? ♀+ in food, - in supplements ▶+ in food, - in supplements $

UNAPPROVED ADULTS − Doses of 1 to 6 g/day do not appear to reduce HgA1c, fasting glucose, or lipids in type 2 diabetes.
UNAPPROVED PEDS − Does not appear to improve glycemic control in adolescents with type 1 diabetes.
FORMS − Not by prescription.
NOTES − A ½ teaspoon of powdered cinnamon from grocery store is approximately 1 g.

COENZYME Q10 (*CoQ-10, ubiquinone*) ▶Bile ♀− ▶− $

UNAPPROVED ADULTS − Heart failure: 100 mg/day PO divided bid to tid (conflicting clinical trials; may reduce hospitalization, dyspnea, edema, but AHA does not recommend). Statin-induced myalgia: 100 to 200 mg PO daily (efficacy unclear; conflicting clinical trials). Parkinson's disease: 1200 mg/day PO divided qid at meals and hs ($$$$; efficacy unclear; might slow progression slightly, but American Academy of Neurology does not recommend). Study for progression of Huntington's disease was inconclusive. Prevention of migraine: 100 mg PO tid (possibly effective). Efficacy unclear for hypertension, and improving athletic performance. Appears ineffective for diabetes, amyotrophic lateral sclerosis.
UNAPPROVED PEDS − Not for use in children.
FORMS − Not by prescription.
NOTES − Case reports of increased INR with warfarin; but a crossover study did not find an interaction.
MOA − Coenzyme in mitochondrial metabolism; also an antioxidant.
ADVERSE EFFECTS − Mild insomnia, increased LFTs, rash, GI distress.

CRANBERRY (*Cranactin, Vaccinium macrocarpon*) ▶? ♀+ in food, - in supplements ▶ + in food, - in supplements $

UNAPPROVED ADULTS − Prevention of UTI (possibly effective): 300 mL/day PO cranberry juice cocktail. Usual dose of cranberry juice extract caps/tabs is 300 to 400 mg PO bid. Insufficient data to assess efficacy for treatment of UTI. Does not appear to prevent UTI in spinal cord injury; IDSA advises against routine use to reduce bacteriuria/UTI in neurogenic bladder managed with intermittent/indwelling catheter.
UNAPPROVED PEDS − Insufficient data to assess efficacy for prevention/treatment of UTI in children. Does not appear to prevent UTI in spinal cord injury; IDSA advises against routine use to reduce bacteriuria/UTI in neurogenic bladder managed with intermittent/indwelling catheter.
FORMS − Not by prescription.
NOTES − Warfarin product labeling advises patients to avoid ingestion of cranberry products based on case reports of increased INRs and bleeding. However, most clinical trials did not find an increase in the INR with cranberry. Approximately 100 calories/6 oz of cranberry juice cocktail. Advise diabetics that some products have high sugar content. Increases urinary oxalate excretion; may increase risk of oxalate kidney stones.
MOA − Proanthocyanidin or fructose appears to block adhesion of bacteria to uroepithelial cells. Although cranberry juice is acidic, it does not appear to significantly change urine pH.
ADVERSE EFFECTS − GI distress and diarrhea with more than 3 L/day.

CREATINE ▶LK ♀− ▶− $

UNAPPROVED ADULTS − Promoted to enhance athletic performance. No benefit for endurance exercise, but modest benefit for intense anaerobic tasks lasting less than 30 sec. Usually taken as loading dose of 20 g/day PO for 5 days, then 2 to 5 g/day. A 5-year phase III NIH trial is evaluating for neuroprotection in Parkinson's disease (http://www.parkinsontrial.ninds.nih.gov). Possibly effective for increasing muscle strength in Duchenne muscular dystrophy, polymyositis/dermatomyositis. Does not appear effective for myotonic dystrophy Type 1, amyotrophic lateral sclerosis. Research ongoing in Huntington's disease.
UNAPPROVED PEDS − Not usually for use in children. The AAP strongly discourages performance-enhancing substances by athletes. Possibly effective for increasing muscle strength in Duchenne muscular dystrophy.
FORMS − Not by prescription.
NOTES − Caffeine may antagonize the ergogenic effects of creatine. Creatine is metabolized to creatinine. In young healthy adults, large doses can increase serum creatinine slightly without affecting CrCl. The effect in elderly is unknown.

(cont.)

CREATINE (cont.)
MOA — Endogenous product converted in muscle to creatine phosphate which may increase ATP levels and increase the force of muscle contraction. Improved mitochondrial function and antioxidant activity are proposed mechanism in Parkinson's disease.
ADVERSE EFFECTS — Single case of lone atrial fibrillation (causality unclear). Manic switch reported in two patients in pilot study of bipolar depression. Anecdotal reports of GI distress and myalgia. Diarrhea with doses at least 10 g. Creatine is metabolized to creatinine. Supplements slightly increase serum creatinine in young healthy adults; effect in elderly is unknown. Infrequent reports of renal impairment are unconfirmed. Creatine, especially when taken with protein supplements, has led to misdiagnosis of chronic kidney disease.

DANSHEN (*Salvia miltiorrhiza*) ▶? ♀? ▶? $
UNAPPROVED ADULTS — Used for treatment of cardiovascular diseases in traditional Chinese medicine.
UNAPPROVED PEDS — Not for use in children.
FORMS — Not by prescription.
NOTES — Case reports of increased INR with warfarin.
MOA — Tanoshionones may cause coronary artery vasodilation. Fatty acids in danshen may inhibit thromboxane formation and platelet aggregation/adhesion.
ADVERSE EFFECTS — May increase INR with warfarin.

DEHYDROEPIANDROSTERONE (*DHEA, Aslera, Fidelin, Prasterone*) ▶Peripheral conversion to estrogens and androgens ♀– ▶– $
UNAPPROVED ADULTS — Does not improve cognition, quality of life, or sexual function in elderly. Not recommended as androgen replacement in late-onset male hypogonadism. To improve well-being in women with adrenal insufficiency: 50 mg PO daily (possibly effective; conflicting clinical trials). Used by athletes as a substitute for anabolic steroids; but no convincing evidence of enhanced athletic performance or increased muscle mass. Banned by many sports organizations.
UNAPPROVED PEDS — Not for use in children.
FORMS — Not by prescription.
NOTES — In theory, chronic use may increase risk of hormone-related cancers (prostate, breast, ovarian). But epidemiologic studies found no link between sex hormone serum levels and prostate cancer.
MOA — Adrenal steroid precursor for estrogen and testosterone. Physiologic doses increase androgen and estrogen levels in women, and estrogen levels in men. May increase insulin sensitivity.
ADVERSE EFFECTS — Acne, hirsutism, and decreased HDL with 100-200 mg/day in women. Case reports of mania induction.

DEVIL'S CLAW (*Harpagophytum procumbens, Phyto Joint, Doloteffin, Harpadol*) ▶? ♀– ▶– $
UNAPPROVED ADULTS — OA, acute exacerbation of chronic low-back pain (possibly effective): 2400 mg extract/day (50 to 100 mg harpagoside/day) PO divided bid to tid.
UNAPPROVED PEDS — Not for children.
FORMS — Not by prescription. Extracts standardized to harpagoside (iridoid glycoside) content.
MOA — Contains harpagoside and other iridoid glycosides with antiinflammatory and analgesic effects. Appears to inhibit COX-2 (but not COX-1), and nitric oxide synthetase. May increase gastric acid secretion. May decrease heart rate and contractility.
ADVERSE EFFECTS — Serious: Bradycardia. Frequent: Dyspepsia, diarrhea. No long-term safety data.

DONG QUAI (*Angelica sinensis*) ▶? ♀– ▶– $
UNAPPROVED ADULTS — Appears ineffective for postmenopausal symptoms; North American Menopause Society recommends against use. Used with other herbs for treatment and prevention of dysmenorrhea, TIA, CVA, PAD, and cardiovascular conditions in traditional Chinese medicine.
UNAPPROVED PEDS — Not for use in children.
FORMS — Not by prescription.
NOTES — Increased risk of bleeding with warfarin with/without increase in INR; avoid concurrent use.
MOA — Unknown. In vitro evidence of platelet antagonism; contains natural coumarins.
ADVERSE EFFECTS — Photosensitivity possible. A case of subarachnoid hemorrhage attributed to supplement containing Siberian ginseng, dong quai, red clover.

ECHINACEA (*E. purpurea, E. angustifolia, E. pallida, cone flower, EchinaGuard, Echinacin Madaus*) ▶ L ♀– ▶– $
UNAPPROVED ADULTS — Promoted as immune stimulant. Conflicting clinical trials for prevention or treatment of upper respiratory infections.
UNAPPROVED PEDS — Not for use in children. Appears ineffective for treatment of upper respiratory tract infections in children.
FORMS — Not by prescription.
NOTES — Single case reports of precipitation of thrombotic thrombocytopenic purpura and exacerbation of pemphigus vulgaris; causality unclear. Rare allergic reactions including anaphylaxis. Cross-hypersensitivity possible with other plants in Compositae family. Photosensitivity possible. Could interact with immunosuppressants due to immunomodulating effects. Some experts limit use to no more than 8 weeks and recommend against use in patients with autoimmune disorders. May inhibit CYP1A2.
MOA — May have immunomodulating and/or antiviral effects.
ADVERSE EFFECTS — Serious: Rare allergic reactions including anaphylaxis (may be more common in atopic individuals), photosensitivity possible. Single case reports of precipitation of thrombotic thrombocytopenic purpura and exacerbation of pemphigus vulgaris; causality unclear. Other: GI complaints. Frequent: Rash in children.

ELDERBERRY (*Sambucus nigra, Rubini, Sambucol, Sinupret*) ▶? ♀– ▶– $
UNAPPROVED ADULTS — Efficacy unclear for influenza, sinusitis, and bronchitis.
UNAPPROVED PEDS — Not for use in children.

(cont.)

ELDERBERRY (cont.)
FORMS — Not by prescription.
NOTES — Sinupret and Sambucol also contain other ingredients. Eating uncooked elderberries may cause nausea or cyanide toxicity.
MOA — Stimulates cytokine production and inhibits influenza virus replication in vitro. Flowers and berries contain flavonoids and antioxidant with immunomodulating activity. Also reported to have diuretic and hypoglycemic effects.
ADVERSE EFFECTS — Eating uncooked elderberries may cause nausea or cyanide toxicity.

EPHEDRA (*Ephedra sinica, ma huang*) ▶K ♀− ▶− $
UNAPPROVED ADULTS — Little evidence of efficacy for obesity, other than modest short-term wt loss. Traditional use as a bronchodilator. FDA banned ephedra supplements in 2004.
UNAPPROVED PEDS — Not for use in children.
FORMS — Not by prescription.
NOTES — FDA banned ephedra supplements because of link to CVA, MI, sudden death, HTN, palpitations, tachycardia, seizures. Risk of serious reactions may increase with dose, strenuous exercise, or concomitant use of other stimulants like caffeine. Country mallow (Sida cordifolia) contains ephedrine.
MOA — Contains sympathomimetics, ephedrine and pseudoephedrine, which cause CNS stimulation, bronchodilation, hypertension, and chronotropic and inotropic effects.
ADVERSE EFFECTS — Serious: Linked to stroke, myocardial infarction, sudden death, HTN, tachycardia, seizures, psychiatric symptoms. Case reports of ephedra kidney stones. Frequent: N/V, palpitations, tremor, insomnia.

EVENING PRIMROSE OIL (*Oenothera biennis*) ▶? ♀? ▶? $
UNAPPROVED ADULTS — Appears ineffective for premenstrual syndrome, postmenopausal symptoms, atopic dermatitis. Inadequate data to evaluate efficacy for cervical ripening.
UNAPPROVED PEDS — Not for use in children.
FORMS — Not by prescription.
MOA — Contains gamma linolenic acid and linoleic acid, precursors of arachidonic acid and other eicosanoids. Promoted to have anti-inflammatory properties.
ADVERSE EFFECTS — No significant health hazards identified other than mild nausea, diarrhea, headache.

FENUGREEK (*Trigonelle foenum-graecum*) ▶? ♀− ▶? $$
UNAPPROVED ADULTS — Efficacy unclear for diabetes or hyperlipidemia. Insufficient data to evaluate efficacy as galactagogue.
UNAPPROVED PEDS — Not for use in children.
FORMS — Not by prescription.
NOTES — Case report of increased INR with warfarin possibly related to fenugreek. Can cause maple syrup-like body odor. Fiber content could decrease GI absorption of some drugs.
MOA — A legume that is a good source of fiber. Hydroxyisoleucine may increase glucose-mediated insulin release. Sapogenins may increase biliary cholesterol excretion.
ADVERSE EFFECTS — Abdominal pain, flatulence, diarrhea. Generally regarded as safe as food by FDA.

FEVERFEW (*Chrysanthemum parthenium, MIG-99, Migra-Lief, MigraSpray, Tanacetum parthenium L.*) ▶? ♀− ▶− $
UNAPPROVED ADULTS — Prevention of migraine (possibly effective): 50 to 100 mg extract PO daily; 2 to 3 fresh leaves PO daily; 50 to 125 mg freeze-dried leaf PO daily. Take either leaf form with or after meals. Benefit of alcoholic extract questioned. May take 1 to 2 months to be effective. Inadequate data to evaluate efficacy for acute migraine.
UNAPPROVED PEDS — Not for use in children.
FORMS — Not by prescription.
NOTES — May cause uterine contractions; avoid in pregnancy. Migra-Lief contains feverfew, riboflavin and magnesium. MigraSpray and Gelstat are homeopathic products that are unlikely to be beneficial.
MOA — Parthenolide may inhibit prostaglandin synthesis or act as serotonin antagonist. Inhibition of platelet aggregation in vitro, but not in humans. Leaves contain tiny amount of melatonin.
ADVERSE EFFECTS — Mouth and lip irritation after chewing fresh leaves. Mild GI complaints. Rebound headache reported after chronic use. Cross-hypersensitivity possible with other composite flowers (arnica, chamomile, echinacea, ragweed, marigolds, chrysanthemums, daisies).

FLAVOCOXID (*Limbrel, UP446*) ▶L ♀− ▶− $$$
UNAPPROVED ADULTS — OA (efficacy unclear): 250 to 500 mg PO bid. Max 2000 mg/day short-term. Taking 1 h before or after meals may increase absorption.
UNAPPROVED PEDS — Not for use in children.
FORMS — Caps 250, 500 mg. Marketed as medical food by prescription only (not all medical foods require a prescription). Medical foods are intended to be given under physician supervision to meet distinctive nutritional needs of a disease, but they do not undergo an approval process to establish safety and efficacy.
NOTES — Be alert for confusion between the brand names, Limbrel and Enbrel, as well as misidentification of flavocoxid as a COX-2 inhibitor. Baicalin, a component of Limbrel, may reduce exposure to rosuvastatin in some patients. Each cap contains 10 mg elemental zinc.
MOA — Contains flavonoids (baicalin, catechin) from Scutellaria baicalensis and Acacia catechu that may inhibit the production of inflammatory prostaglandins and leukotrienes in the arachidonic acid pathway. Flavonoids may also act as antioxidants. Flavocoxid is not a COX-2 inhibitor.
ADVERSE EFFECTS — Rash, synovitis, hypersensitivity, pneumonitis, increased LFTs, possible reports of hepatotoxicity. Frequent: Nausea, diarrhea, flatulence.

GARCINIA (*Garcinia cambogia, Citri Lean*) ▶? ♀− ▶− $
UNAPPROVED ADULTS − Appears ineffective for wt loss.
UNAPPROVED PEDS − Not for use in children.
FORMS − Not by prescription.
MOA − Contains hydroxycitric acid which may inhibit lipogenesis.
ADVERSE EFFECTS − Case reports of hepatotoxicity and rhabdomyolysis with multi-ingredient wt loss supplements containing Garcinia.

GARLIC SUPPLEMENTS (*Allium sativum, Kwai, Kyolic*) ▶LK ♀− ▶− $
UNAPPROVED ADULTS − Ineffective for hyperlipidemia; Am College of Cardiology does not recommend for this indication. Small reduction in BP, but efficacy in HTN unclear. Does not appear effective for diabetes.
UNAPPROVED PEDS − Not for use in children.
FORMS − Not by prescription.
NOTES − Topical application of garlic can cause burn/rash. Significantly decreases saquinavir levels; may also interact with other protease inhibitors. May increase bleeding risk with warfarin with/without increase in INR. However, Kyolic (aged garlic extract) and enteric-coated garlic did not affect the INR in clinical studies.
MOA − May inhibit HMG-CoA reductase; may inhibit platelet aggregation and enhances fibrinolytic activity; may have antioxidant activity; may cause vasodilation.
ADVERSE EFFECTS − GI irritation, bad breath.

GINGER (*Zingiber officinale*) ▶bile ♀? ▶? $
UNAPPROVED ADULTS − <u>Prevention of motion sickness (efficacy unclear):</u> 500 to 1000 mg powdered rhizome PO single dose 1 h before exposure. American College of Obstetrics and Gynecology considers ginger 250 mg PO qid a nonpharmacologic option for N/V of pregnancy. Some experts advise pregnant women to limit dose to usual dietary amount (no more than 1 g/day). <u>Acute chemotherapy-induced nausea (possibly effective adjunct to standard antiemetics):</u> 250 to 500 mg PO bid for 6 days, starting 3 days before chemo. No benefit for chemo-induced acute vomiting, or delayed nausea/vomiting. Does not appear effective for postoperative N/V. Efficacy unclear for relief of OA pain.
UNAPPROVED PEDS − Not for use in children.
FORMS − Not by prescription.
NOTES − Increased INR more than 10 attributed to ginger in a phenprocoumon-treated patient, but study in healthy volunteers found no effect of ginger on INR or pharmacokinetics of warfarin. Some European countries advise pregnant women to avoid ginger in supplements because it is cytotoxic in vitro. A ½ teaspoon of ground ginger is about 1 g of ginger.
MOA − Gingerols and shogaols may increase rate of gastric emptying. Ginger is cytotoxic in vitro, raising concern about use by pregnant women.
ADVERSE EFFECTS − GI irritation possible at high doses.

GINKGO BILOBA (*EGb 761, Ginkgold, Ginkoba*) ▶K ♀− ▶− $
UNAPPROVED ADULTS − <u>Dementia</u> (efficacy unclear): 40 mg PO tid of standardized extract containing 24% ginkgo flavone glycosides and 6% terpene lactones. Am Psychiatric Assn and others find evidence too weak to recommend for Alzheimer's or other dementias. Does not prevent dementia in elderly with normal or mildly impaired cognitive function. Does not improve cognition in healthy younger people. Does not appear effective for intermittent claudication or prevention of acute altitude sickness.
UNAPPROVED PEDS − Not for use in children.
FORMS − Not by prescription.
NOTES − Possible increased risk of stroke. Case reports of intracerebral, subdural, and ocular bleeding; but no increase in major bleeding in large clinical trial. Does not appear to increase INR with warfarin, but monitoring for bleeding is advised. May reduce efficacy of efavirenz. Ginkgo seeds contain a neurotoxin. A few reports attributing exacerbation or precipitation of seizures to ginkgo supplements have raised concern about possible contamination with the neurotoxin. Some experts advise caution or avoidance of ginkgo by those with seizures or taking drugs that lower the seizure threshold.
MOA − May decrease capillary fragility or blood viscosity, cause vasodilation, increase peripheral blood flow, affect neurotransmitters, and act as antioxidant.
ADVERSE EFFECTS − Serious: Seizures possible (rare), intracerebral, subdural, ocular bleeding (rare). Higher risk of stroke in clinical trial of ginkgo for prevention of cognitive decline in elderly. Other: GI complaints, headache, allergy, anxiety/restlessness, sleep disturbances.

GINSENG—AMERICAN (*Panax quinquefolius L., Cold-fX*) ▶K ♀− ▶− $
UNAPPROVED ADULTS − <u>Reduction of postprandial glucose in type 2 diabetes</u> (possibly effective): 3 g PO taken with or up to 2 h before meal. Cold-fX (1 cap PO bid) may modestly reduce the frequency of colds/flu; approved in Canada to strengthen immune system. <u>Cancer-related fatigue</u> (possibly effective): 500-1000 mg PO bid in am and midafternoon with food.
UNAPPROVED PEDS − Usually not for use in children. Cold-fX (1 cap PO bid) may modestly reduce the frequency of colds/flu; approved in Canada for children 12 yo and older to strengthen immune system.
FORMS − Not by prescription.
NOTES − Ginseng content varies widely and some products are mislabeled or adulterated with caffeine. American, Asian, and Siberian ginseng are often misidentified. Decreased INR with warfarin.
MOA − Ginsenosides may increase insulin sensitivity or secretion. Polysaccharides in Cold-fX may have immunomodulating effect; it does not contain ginsenosides.
ADVERSE EFFECTS − None found.

GINSENG—ASIAN (*Panax ginseng, Ginsana, G115, Korean red ginseng*) ▶? ♀– ▶– $
UNAPPROVED ADULTS – <u>Promoted to improve vitality and well-being:</u> 200 mg PO daily. Ginsana: 2 caps PO daily or 1 cap PO bid. Ginsana Sport: 1 cap PO daily. Preliminary evidence of efficacy for erectile dysfunction. Efficacy unclear for improving physical or psychomotor performance, diabetes, herpes simplex infections, cognitive or immune function. American College of Obstetrics and Gynecology and North American Menopause Society recommend against use for postmenopausal hot flashes.
UNAPPROVED PEDS – Not for use in children.
FORMS – Not by prescription.
NOTES – Some formulations may contain up to 34% alcohol. Ginsana Gold also contains vitamins and minerals. Reports of an interaction with the MAOI, phenelzine. May decrease INR with warfarin. Ginseng content varies widely and some products are mislabeled or adulterated with caffeine. American, Asian, and Siberian ginseng are often misidentified. May interfere with some digoxin assays.
MOA – Unknown. Considered an adaptogen.
ADVERSE EFFECTS – Hypertension, headache, restlessness, estrogenic effects (swollen breasts, menstrual bleeding), a case report of mania, and a case report of hypertensive crisis and TIA.

GINSENG—SIBERIAN (*Eleutherococcus senticosus, Ci-wu-jia*) ▶? ♀– ▶– $
UNAPPROVED ADULTS – Does not appear to improve athletic endurance. Did not appear effective in single clinical trial for chronic fatigue syndrome.
UNAPPROVED PEDS – Not for use in children.
FORMS – Not by prescription.
NOTES – May interfere with some digoxin assays. A case report of thalamic CVA attributed to Siberian ginseng plus caffeine.
MOA – Considered an adaptogen. Vasodilatory and antiviral activity reported. Not related to Asian or American ginseng (Panax ginseng or quinquefolius).
ADVERSE EFFECTS – A case of thalamic stroke attributed to Siberian ginseng plus caffeine. A case of subarachnoid hemorrhage attributed to supplement containing Siberian ginseng, dong quai, red clover. Hypertension and dysrhythmia also reported.

GLUCOSAMINE (*Cosamin DS, Dona*) ▶L ♀– ▶– $
UNAPPROVED ADULTS – <u>OA:</u> Glucosamine HCl 500 mg PO tid or glucosamine sulfate (Dona $$) 1500 mg PO once daily. Appears ineffective overall for OA pain, but glucosamine plus chondroitin may improve pain in moderate to severe knee OA.
UNAPPROVED PEDS – Not for use in children.
FORMS – Not by prescription.
NOTES – Use cautiously or avoid in patients with shellfish allergy. Case reports of increased INR/bleeding with warfarin in patient taking chondroitin + glucosamine. Cosamin DS contains 3 mg manganese/cap; tolerable upper limit of manganese is 11 mg/day.
MOA – May stimulate production of cartilage matrix.
ADVERSE EFFECTS – GI complaints, allergic skin reactions (rare). Well-tolerated in the GAIT study.

GOLDENSEAL (*Hydrastis canadensis*) ▶? ♀– ▶– $
UNAPPROVED ADULTS – Often used in attempts to achieve false-negative urine test for illicit drug use (efficacy unclear). Often combined with echinacea in cold remedies; but insufficient data to assess efficacy of goldenseal for the common cold or URIs.
UNAPPROVED PEDS – Not for use in children.
FORMS – Not by prescription.
NOTES – Alkaloids in goldenseal with antibacterial activity not well-absorbed orally. Oral use contraindicated in pregnancy (may cause uterine contractions), newborns (may cause kernicterus), and HTN (high doses may cause peripheral vasoconstriction). Adding goldenseal directly to urine turns it brown. May inhibit CYP2D6 and 3A4. Berberine, a component of goldenseal, may increase cyclosporine levels.
MOA – Contains isoquinoline alkaloids (berberine and others) with antimicrobial activity.
ADVERSE EFFECTS – Oral use contraindicated in pregnancy (may cause uterine contractions), newborns (may cause kernicterus), and hypertension (high doses may cause peripheral vasoconstriction). Berberine doses more than 500 mg may be toxic; may cause ventricular arrhythmias in patients with heart failure. Possible exacerbation of severe hypernatremia reported in child with type I diabetes.

GRAPE SEED EXTRACT (*Vitis vinifera L., procyanidolic oligomers, PCO*) ▶? ♀? ▶? $
UNAPPROVED ADULTS – Small clinical trials suggest benefit in chronic venous insufficiency. No benefit in single study of seasonal allergic rhinitis.
UNAPPROVED PEDS – Not for use in children.
FORMS – Not by prescription.
NOTES – Pine bark (pycnogenol) and grape seed extract are often confused; they both contain oligomeric proanthocyanidins.
MOA – Contains oligomeric proanthocyanidins (OPC/PCO) with antioxidant properties. May inhibit platelet aggregation or reactivity.
ADVERSE EFFECTS – None.

GREEN TEA (*Camellia sinensis, Polyphenon E*) ▶LK
♀+ in moderate amount in food, – in supplements
▶+ in moderate amount in food, - in supplements $
UNAPPROVED ADULTS – Some population studies suggest a reduction in adenomatous polyps and chronic atrophic gastritis in green tea drinkers. Efficacy unclear for cancer prevention, wt loss, hypercholesterolemia. Green tea catechins (Polyphenon E) under evaluation for chronic lymphocytic leukemia and prevention of prostate cancer in men with high-grade prostate intraepithelial neoplasia.
UNAPPROVED PEDS – Not for children.
FORMS – Not by prescription. Green tea extract available in caps standardized to polyphenol content.
NOTES – Case report of decreased INR with warfarin attributed to drinking large amounts of green tea

(cont.)

GREEN TEA (cont.)
(due to vitamin K content). The vitamin K content of green tea is low with usual consumption.
MOA − Contains caffeine (approximately 50 mg/cup of tea), catechins, polyphenols including (-)-epigallocatechin-3-gallate (ECGC; primary catechin in Polyphenon E), trace elements, vitamins. Has antioxidant activity.
ADVERSE EFFECTS − Case reports of hepatotoxicity with supplements (not tea). N/V, insomnia, fatigue, diarrhea, abdominal pain, and confusion reported in clinical trials.

GUARANA (*Paullinia cupana*) ▶? ♀+ in food, − in supplements ▶+ in food, - in supplements $
UNAPPROVED ADULTS − Marketed as a source of caffeine in weight-loss dietary supplements. Guarana in weight-loss dietary supplements may provide high doses of caffeine.
UNAPPROVED PEDS − Not for children.
FORMS − Not by prescription.
MOA − Stimulant effects. Contains caffeine.
ADVERSE EFFECTS − Sympathomimetic effect may increase the risk of serious cardiovascular adverse effects. Case reports of rhabdomyolysis and seizures possibly related to caffeine intoxication from sports drinks containing caffeine, guarana, garcinia, and other ingredients.

GUGGULIPID (*Commiphora mukul extract, guggul*) ▶? ♀− ▶− $$
UNAPPROVED ADULTS − Does not appear effective for hyperlipidemia with doses up to 2000 mg PO tid.
UNAPPROVED PEDS − Not for use in children.
FORMS − Not by prescription.
NOTES − May decrease levels of propranolol and diltiazem. A randomized controlled trial conducted in the United States with 1000 mg or 2000 mg PO tid reported no change in total cholesterol, triglycerides, or HDL, and a small increase in LDL. Earlier studies of weaker design reported reductions in total cholesterol of up to 27%.
MOA − Resin from the mukul mirth tree traditionally used in Ayurvedic medicine. Contains E and Z guggalsterones which may facilitate cholesterol catabolism via FXR receptor. May reduce C-reactive protein and improve insulin sensitivity at high doses.
ADVERSE EFFECTS − GI distress, headache, and rash. Allergic contact dermatitis reported with guggulipid anticellulite cream.

HAWTHORN (*Crataegus laevigata, monogyna, oxyacantha, standardized extract WS 1442 - Crataegutt novo, HeartCare*) ▶? ♀− ▶− $
UNAPPROVED ADULTS − Symptomatic improvement of mild CHF (NYHA I–II; possibly effective): 80 mg PO bid to 160 mg PO tid of standardized extract (19% oligomeric procyanidins; WS 1442; HeartCare 80 mg tabs); doses as high as 900 to 1800 mg/day have been studied. Initial presentation of SPICE study found no benefit for primary outcome (composite of cardiac death/hospitalization) but possible reduction of sudden cardiac death for LVEF 25 to 35%. Am College of Cardiology found evidence insufficient to recommend for mild heart failure. Does not appear effective for HTN.
UNAPPROVED PEDS − Not for use in children.
FORMS − Not by prescription.
NOTES − Unclear whether hawthorn and digoxin should be used together; mechanisms of action may be similar.
MOA − Contains oligomeric procyanidins and flavonoids with positive inotropic and vasodilatory properties, and possible antioxidant activity. May have anti-ischemic activity.
ADVERSE EFFECTS − GI distress, dizziness, palpitations (rare). Some inotropic agents increase mortality in heart failure. Initial presentation of SPICE study did not report increased mortality; hawthorn was safe in combo with other heart failure meds.

HONEY (*Medihoney*) ▶? ♀+ ▶+ $ for oral $$$ for Medihoney
UNAPPROVED ADULTS − Topical for burn/wound care (including pressure ulcers, 1st and 2nd degree partial thickness burns, donor sites, surgical/traumatic wounds): Apply Medihoney to wound for 12 to 24 h/day. Efficacy of topical honey unclear for prevention of dialysis catheter infections. Oral. Constipation (efficacy unclear): 1 to 2 tbsp (30 to 60 g) in glass of water.
UNAPPROVED PEDS − Topical for burn/wound care (including pressure ulcers, 1st and 2nd degree partial thickness burns, donor sites, surgical/traumatic wounds): Apply Medihoney to wound for 12 to 24 h/day. Do not feed honey to children younger than 1 yo due to risk of infant botulism. Nocturnal cough due to upper RTI in children (efficacy unclear): Give PO within 30 min before sleep. Give ½ tsp for 2 to 5 yo, 1 tsp for 6 to 11 yo, 2 tsp for 12 to 18 yo. WHO considers honey a cheap, popular, and safe demulcent for children.
FORMS − Mostly not by prescription. Medihoney is FDA-approved.
NOTES − Honey may contain trace amounts of antimicrobials used to treat infection in honeybee hives. Medihoney sterile dressings contain Leptospermum (Manuka) honey that is irradiated to inactivate C botulinum spores.
MOA − Topical: Antimicrobial due to hygroscopic property, low pH, generation of hydrogen peroxide. May also have anti-inflammatory activity. Leptospermum honey may have unique antimicrobial properties. Oral: May act as a demulcent. Laxative effect due to unabsorbed fructose.
ADVERSE EFFECTS − Serious: Botulism from ingestion of honey by infants younger than 1 yo; anaphylaxis reported after honey ingestion in patient with history of Compositae pollen allergy. Topical: Stinging sensation after application in ~5% of patients; local atopic reaction in atopic patients. Oral: Well-tolerated, diarrhea.

HORSE CHESTNUT SEED EXTRACT (*Aesculus hippocastanum, buckeye, HCE50, Venastat*) ▶? ♀− ▶− $
UNAPPROVED ADULTS − Chronic venous insufficiency (effective): 1 cap Venastat PO bid with water

(cont.)

HORSE CHESTNUT SEED EXTRACT (cont.)
before meals. Response within 1 month. Venastat is 16% escin in standardized extract. Am College of Cardiology found evidence insufficient to recommend for peripheral arterial disease.
UNAPPROVED PEDS — Not for use in children.
FORMS — Not by prescription.
NOTES — Venastat does not contain aesculin, a toxin in horse chestnuts.
MOA — Escin increases venous pressure; may prevent leukocyte activation or inhibit elastase and hyaluronidase.
ADVERSE EFFECTS — Mild and infrequent GI distress, dizziness, headache.

KAVA (*Piper methysticum*) ▶K ♀− ▶− $
UNAPPROVED ADULTS — Promoted as anxiolytic (possibly effective) or sedative; recommend against use due to hepatotoxicity.
UNAPPROVED PEDS — Not for use in children.
FORMS — Not by prescription.
NOTES — Reports of severe hepatotoxicity leading to liver transplantation. May potentiate CNS effects of benzodiazepines and other sedatives, including alcohol. Reversible yellow skin discoloration with long-term use.
MOA — Anxiolytic and sedative effects.
ADVERSE EFFECTS — Serious: Reports of severe hepatotoxicity leading to death or liver transplantation. Most cases used kava products prepared by ethanol or acetone extraction methods. Reversible yellow skin discoloration with long-term use.

KOMBUCHA TEA (*Manchurian or Kargasok tea*) ▶? ♀− ▶− $
UNAPPROVED ADULTS — Promoted for many indications, but no scientific evidence to support benefit for any condition. FDA advises caution due to a case of fatal acidosis.
UNAPPROVED PEDS — Not for use in children.
FORMS — Not by prescription.
NOTES — Acidic fermented drink made from addition of bacterial and yeast culture to sweetened black or green tea. It may contain alcohol, ethyl acetate, acetic acid, and lactate.
MOA — Culture of bacteria and yeast that is very acidic after preparation.
ADVERSE EFFECTS — Serious: Fatal acidosis, hepatic dysfunction.

LICORICE (*Cankermelt, Glycyrrhiza glabra, Glycyrrhiza uralensis*) ▶Bile ♀− ▶− $
UNAPPROVED ADULTS — Insufficient data to assess efficacy for postmenopausal vasomotor symptoms. Cankermelt (dissolving oral patch): Efficacy unclear for pain relief and healing of aphthous stomatitis. Apply patch to ulcer for 16 h/day until ulcer is healed.
UNAPPROVED PEDS — Not for use in children.
FORMS — Not by prescription.
NOTES — Chronic high doses can cause pseudo-primary aldosteronism (with hypertension, edema, hypokalemia). Case reports of myopathy. Diuretics or stimulant laxatives could potentiate licorice-induced hypokalemia. In the United States, "licorice" candy usually does not contain licorice. Deglycyrrhizinated licorice does not have mineralocorticoid effects.
MOA — Has in vitro antioxidant, antimicrobial, antiviral, and anti-inflammatory activity. Glycyrrhizin has mineralocorticoid activity (not present in deglycyrrhizinated licorice).
ADVERSE EFFECTS — Pseudo-primary aldosteronism (with hypertension, edema, hypokalemia) possible with chronic high doses. Case reports of myopathy. Transient visual loss.

MELATONIN (*N-acetyl-5-methoxytryptamine*) ▶L ♀− ▶− $
UNAPPROVED ADULTS — To reduce jet lag after flights across more than 5 time zones (effective; especially traveling East; may also help for 2 to 4 time zones): 0.5 to 5 mg PO at bedtime (10 pm to midnight) for 3 to 6 nights starting on day of arrival. Faster onset and better sleep quality with 5 mg. No benefit with use before departure or slow-release formulations. Do not take earlier in day (may cause drowsiness and delay adaptation to local time). To promote daytime sleep in night shift workers: 1.8 to 3 mg PO prior to daytime sleep. Delayed sleep phase disorder: 0.3 to 5 mg PO 1.5 to 6 h before habitual bedtime. Orphan drug for treatment of circadian rhythm-related sleep disorders in blind patients with no light perception. Possibly effective for difficulty falling asleep but not for staying asleep. Am Academy of Sleep Medicine does not recommend for chronic insomnia but does recommend for jet lag.
UNAPPROVED PEDS — Not usually used in children. Sleep-onset insomnia in ADHD, age 6 yo or older (possibly effective): 3 to 6 mg PO at bedtime. Orphan drug treatment of circadian rhythm-related sleep disorders in blind patients with no light perception.
FORMS — Not by prescription.
NOTES — High melatonin levels linked to nocturnal asthma; some experts advise patients with nocturnal asthma to avoid melatonin supplements until more data available.
MOA — Pineal hormone related to 5-hydroxytryptamine. Synthesis is controlled by environmental factors including light. Melatonin helps to regulate circadian rhythms, induces pigment lightening of skin cells, and suppresses ovarian function at high doses. May reset endogenous circadian pacemaker.
ADVERSE EFFECTS — Occasional short-term use appears safe. May cause drowsiness for 4-5 h after the dose; warn against hazardous tasks. May increase withdrawn behavior in elderly patients with dementia.

METHYLSULFONYLMETHANE (*MSM, dimethyl sulfone, crystalline DMSO2*) ▶? ♀− ▶− $
UNAPPROVED ADULTS — Insufficient data to assess efficacy of oral and topical MSM for arthritis pain.
UNAPPROVED PEDS — Not for use in children.
FORMS — Not by prescription.

(cont.)

HERBAL & ALTERNATIVE THERAPIES

METHYLSULFONYLMETHANE *(cont.)*
NOTES — Can cause nausea, diarrhea, headache. DMSO metabolite promoted as a source of sulfur without odor.
MOA — DMSO metabolite promoted as a source of sulfur without odor.
ADVERSE EFFECTS — Nausea, diarrhea, headache.

MILK THISTLE (*Silybum marianum, Legalon, silymarin, Thisylin*) ▶LK ♀– ▶– $
UNAPPROVED ADULTS — Hepatic cirrhosis (efficacy unclear): 100 to 200 mg PO tid of standardized extract with 70 to 80% silymarin. Guidelines for management of alcoholic liver disease recommend against use. Hepatitis C: May decrease serum transaminases, but does not appear to improve viral load or liver histology; the American Gastroenterological Association recommends against use. Used in Europe to treat Amanita mushroom poisoning.
UNAPPROVED PEDS — Not for use in children.
FORMS — Not by prescription.
NOTES — May inhibit CYP2C9. May decrease blood glucose in patients with cirrhosis and diabetes.
MOA — Hepatoprotectant with antioxidant, membrane-stabilizing, liver cell regeneration properties.
ADVERSE EFFECTS — Serious: Anaphylaxis. Other: GI distress, headache, skin reactions, arthralgias.

NETTLE ROOT (*stinging nettle, Urtica dioica radix*) ▶? ♀– ▶– $
UNAPPROVED ADULTS — Efficacy unclear for treatment of BPH or osteoarthritis.
UNAPPROVED PEDS — Not for use in children.
FORMS — Not by prescription.
NOTES — Can cause allergic skin reactions, mild GI upset, sweating. Case reports of gynecomastia in a man and galactorrea in a woman.
MOA — May have anti-inflammatory effects. Contains phytosterols.
ADVERSE EFFECTS — Allergic skin reactions, mild GI upset, sweating. Case reports of gynecomastia in a man and galactorrhea in a woman.

NONI (*Morinda citrifolia*) ▶? ♀– ▶– $$$
UNAPPROVED ADULTS — Promoted for many medical disorders; but insufficient data to assess efficacy.
UNAPPROVED PEDS — Not for use in children.
FORMS — Not by prescription.
NOTES — Potassium concentration comparable to orange juice. Hyperkalemia reported in a patient with chronic renal failure. Case reports of hepatotoxicity.
MOA — Antineoplastic, anthelmintic, and immunostimulant activity in vitro and in animal studies.
ADVERSE EFFECTS — Hyperkalemia reported in a patient with chronic renal failure. Three case reports of hepatotoxicity.

PEPPERMINT OIL (*Mentha x piperita oil*) ▶LK ♀+ in food, ? in supplements ▶+ in food, ? in supplements $
UNAPPROVED ADULTS — Irritable bowel syndrome (possibly effective): 0.2 to 0.4 mL enteric-coated caps PO tid before meals. Efficacy of peppermint oil plus caraway seed is unclear for dyspepsia.
UNAPPROVED PEDS — Irritable bowel syndrome, age 8 yo or older (possibly effective): 0.1 to 0.2 mL enteric-coated capsules PO tid before meals.
FORMS — Not by prescription.
NOTES — Generally regarded as safe as food by FDA. May exacerbate GERD. For irritable bowel syndrome, use enteric-coated caps that deliver peppermint oil to lower GI tract. Drugs that increase gastric pH (antacids, H2 blockers, proton pump inhibitors) may dissolve enteric-coated capsules too soon, causing heart burn and reducing benefit. Separate peppermint oil and antacid doses by at least 2 hours.
ADVERSE EFFECTS — Perianal burning, nausea.

POLICOSANOL (*CholeRx, Cholestin*) ▶? ♀– ▶– $
UNAPPROVED ADULTS — Ineffective for hyperlipidemia. A Cuban formulation (unavailable in the United States) 5 mg bid reduced LDL cholesterol in studies by a single group of researchers, but studies by other groups found no benefit. Clinical study of a US formulation also found no benefit.
UNAPPROVED PEDS — Not for use in children.
FORMS — Not by prescription.
NOTES — An old formulation of Cholestin contained red yeast rice; the current formulation contains policosanol.
MOA — Mixture of aliphatic alcohols extracted from sugar cane wax (octacosanol); may inhibit platelet aggregation and anitoxidants. Mechanism of action in hyperlipidemia unknown.
ADVERSE EFFECTS — Serious: None reported.

PROBIOTICS (*Acidophilus, Align, Bifantis, Bifidobacteria, Lactobacillus, Bacid, Culturelle, Florastor, IntestiFlora, Lactinex, LiveBac, Power-Dophilus, Primadophilus, Probiotica, Saccharomyces boulardii, VSL#3*) ▶? ♀+ ▶+ $
ADULTS — VSL#3 approved as medical food. Ulcerative colitis (possibly effective); 1 to 2 packets or 4 to 8 caps/day. Active ulcerative colitis: 4 to 8 packets or 16 to 32 caps/day. Pouchitis (effective): 2 to 4 packets or 6 to 18 caps/day. Irritable bowel syndrome (may relieve gas and bloating): ½ to 1 packet PO daily or 2 to 4 caps daily. Mix powder from packets with at least 4 oz of cold water before taking.
PEDS — VSL#3 approved as medical food for ulcerative colitis (possibly effective) or pouchitis (effective), for age 3 mo or older: Dose based on wt and number of bowel movements/day. See http://www.vsl3.com/. Use adult dose for age 15 yo or older. Mix powder with at least 4 oz of cold water before taking.
UNAPPROVED ADULTS — Antibiotic-associated diarrhea (effective): Saccharomyces boulardii 500 mg PO bid (Florastor 2 caps PO bid). Give 2 h before/after antibiotic so culture isn't killed. IDSA recommends against probiotics to prevent C difficile associated diarrhea; safety and efficacy is unclear. Probiotics may reduce GI side effects of H pylori eradication regimens. Bifido bacterium and some combo products improve abdominal pain and

(cont.)

PROBIOTICS (cont.)

bloating in <u>Irritable bowel syndrome</u> (eg, Align 1 cap PO once daily), but Lactobacillus alone did not improve symptoms. Efficacy of probiotics unclear for travelers' diarrhea (conflicting evidence), Crohn's disease, H pylori, radiation enteritis. Lactobacillus GG appears ineffective for prevention of post-antibiotic vulvovaginitis.

UNAPPROVED PEDS — <u>Prevention of antibiotic-associated diarrhea</u> (effective): Lactobacillus GG 10 to 20 billion cells/day PO (Culturelle 1 cap PO once daily or bid) or S boulardii 250 mg PO bid (Floraster 1 cap PO bid). IDSA recommends against probiotics to prevent C difficile associated diarrhea; safety and efficacy is unclear. <u>Rotavirus gastroenteritis:</u> Lactobacillus GG at least 10 billion cells/day PO started early in illness. Efficacy of probiotics unclear for travelers' diarrhea (conflicting evidence), radiation enteritis. Lactobacillus GG does not appear effective for Crohn's disease in children. Research ongoing for prevention and treatment of atopic dermatitis.

FORMS — Not by prescription. Culturelle contains Lactobacillus GG 10 billion cells/cap. Florastor contains Saccharomyces boulardii 5 billion cells/250 mg cap. Probiotica contains Lactobacillus reuteri 100 million cells/chewable tab. VSL#3 contains 450 billion cells/packet, 225 billion cells/2 caps (Bifidobacterium breve, longum, infantis; Lactobacillus acidophilus, plantarum, casei, bulgaricus; Streptococcus thermophilus). Align contains Bifidobacterium infantis 35624, 1 billion cells/cap. VSL#3 is marketed as nonprescription medical food. Medical foods are intended to be given under physician supervision to meet distinctive nutritional needs of a disease, but they do not undergo an approval process to establish safety and efficacy.

NOTES — Do not use probiotics in patients with acute pancreatitis; increased mortality and bowel ischemia reported in clinical trial. Acquired infection possible, especially in immunocompromised or critically ill patients; bacteremia, endocarditis, abscess reported, with possible contamination of central venous access port in some cases. Microbial type and content varies by product. Pick yogurt products labeled "Live and active cultures." Refrigerate packets of VSL#3; can store at room temp for 1 week.

MOA — Lactobacillus bacteria and Saccharomyces boulardii, a nonpathogenic yeast, are part of gut normal flora. They inhibit pathogen attachment in colon, modulate intestinal inflammation, reduce colonic permeability, and may enhance barrier function. Bifidobacterium infantis may reduce gut transit time.

ADVERSE EFFECTS — Serious: Acquired infection possible, especially in immunocompromised or critically ill patients; bacteremia, endocarditis, abscess reported, with possible contamination of central venous access port in some cases. Increased risk of bowel ischemia and death in clinical trial evaluting probiotics for acute pancreatitis.

PYCNOGENOL (French maritime pine tree bark) ▶L ♀? ▶? $

UNAPPROVED ADULTS — Promoted for many medical disorders, but efficacy unclear for chronic venous insufficiency, sperm dysfunction, melasma, OA, HTN, type 2 diabetes, diabetic retinopathy, and ADHD.

UNAPPROVED PEDS — Not for use in children.

FORMS — Not by prescription.

NOTES — Pine bark (pycnogenol) and grape seed extract are often confused; they both contain oligomeric proanthocyanidins.

MOA — Antioxidant. Contains oligomeric proanthocyanidins and bioflavonoids.

ADVERSE EFFECTS — GI distress.

PYGEUM AFRICANUM (African plum tree) ▶? ♀— ▶— $

UNAPPROVED ADULTS — <u>Benign prostatic hypertrophy</u> (may have modest efficacy): 50 to 100 mg PO bid or 100 mg PO daily of standardized extract containing 14% triterpenes.

UNAPPROVED PEDS — Not for use in children.

FORMS — Not by prescription.

NOTES — Appears well-tolerated. Self-treatment could delay diagnosis of prostate cancer.

MOA — Unknown, but may inhibit 5-alpha reductase.

ADVERSE EFFECTS — Well-tolerated, GI distress.

RED CLOVER (red clover isoflavone extract, Trifolium pratense, trefoil, Promensil, Rimostil, Trinovin) ▶Gut, L, K ♀— $$

UNAPPROVED ADULTS — Promensil (1 tab PO daily to bid with meals) marketed for menopausal symptoms; Rimostil (1 tab PO daily) for bone and cholesterol health, and to promote health and well-being after menopause; Trinovin (1 tab PO daily) for maintaining prostate health and urinary function in men. Conflicting evidence of efficacy for postmenopausal vasomotor symptoms. Does not appear effective overall, but may have modest benefit for severe symptoms. Efficacy unclear for prevention of osteoporosis and treatment of hyperlipidemia in postmenopausal women, and for BPH symptoms in men.

UNAPPROVED PEDS — Not for use in children.

FORMS — Not by prescription. Isoflavone content (genistein, daidzein, biochanin, formononetin) is 40 mg/tab in Promensil and Trinovin, 57 mg/tab in Rimostil.

NOTES — Does not appear to stimulate endometrium. Effect on breast cancer risk is unclear; some experts recommend against use of isoflavone supplements by women with breast cancer. No effect on breast density in women with Wolfe P2 or DY mammographic breast density patterns. H2 blockers, proton pump inhibitors, and antibiotics may decrease metabolic activation of isoflavones in GI tract. Ingesting large amounts of red clover can cause bleeding in cattle; bleeding risk of supplements in humans is theoretical.

MOA — Contains isoflavone phytoestrogens (biochanin, formononetin, genistein, daidzein), which may act as selective estrogen receptor modulators. Biochanin and formononetin metabolized to genistein and daidzein.

ADVERSE EFFECTS — Appears well tolerated. May increase hepatic transaminases. Safety of isoflavone

(cont.)

RED CLOVER (cont.)
supplements unclear in women with breast cancer. A case of subarachnoid hemorrhage attributed to supplement containing Siberian ginseng, dong quai, red clover.

RED YEAST RICE (*Monascus purpureus, Xuezhikang, Zhibituo, Hypocol, Lipolysar*) ▶L ♀− ▶− $$
UNAPPROVED ADULTS − Hyperlipidemia: Usual dose is 1200 mg PO bid. Efficacy for hyperlipidemia depends on whether formulation contains lovastatin or other statins. In the US, red yeast rice should not contain more than trace amounts of statins, but some products contain up to 10 mg lovastatin per cap. Some clinicians consider red yeast rice an alternative for patients who develop myalgia with prescription statins. In China, red yeast rice was effective for secondary prevention of CHD events.
UNAPPROVED PEDS − Not for use in children.
FORMS − Not by prescription. Xuezhikang marketed in Asia, Norway (HypoCol), Italy (Lipolysar).
NOTES − In 1997, a red yeast rice product called Cholestin was marketed in the United States as a cholesterol-lowering supplement. It was removed from the market in 2001 after a judge ruled it an unapproved drug because it contained lovastatin. Cholestin later returned to the market; it now contains policosanol (ineffective for hyperlipidemia). Current red yeast rice products should not contain more than trace amounts of statins, but tests show they may contain up to 10 mg lovastatin per capsule. Can cause myopathy. Case reports of hepatotoxicity. Consider the potential for lovastatin drug interactions.
MOA − Fermentation product of red yeast (Monascus purpureus) grown on rice; it contains some statins (monacolins) and sterols, including lovastatin (Monocolin K).
ADVERSE EFFECTS − Case reports of myopathy, including rhabdomyolysis in a transplant patient treated with cyclosporine. Case reports of hepatotoxicity. A potential nephrotoxin, citrinin, can be produced with improper fermentation of red yeast rice and has been found in some products in the United States. Usual adverse effects of Xuezhikang/Zibituo: Dizziness, stomach ache, abdominal distension, nausea, diarrhea.

S-ADENOSYLMETHIONINE (*SAM-e, sammy*) ▶L ♀? ▶? $$$
UNAPPROVED ADULTS − Mild to moderate Depression (effective): 800 to 1600 mg/day PO in divided doses with meals. Efficacy unclear for OA and alcoholic liver disease.
UNAPPROVED PEDS − Not for use in children.
FORMS − Not by prescription.
NOTES − Serotonin syndrome possible when co-administered with SSRIs. Do not use within 2 weeks of an MAOI or in bipolar disorder.
MOA − Acts as a methyl group donor in methylation reactions. Mechanism of action in depression and osteoarthritis unknown.
ADVERSE EFFECTS − Anxiety, headache, insomnia, nausea, induction of mania in bipolar disorder.

SAINT JOHN'S WORT (*Hypericum perforatum, Kira, Movana, LI-160*) ▶L ♀− ▶− $

UNAPPROVED ADULTS − Mild to moderate depression (effective): 300 mg PO tid of standardized extract (0.3% hypericin).
UNAPPROVED PEDS − Not for use in children. Does not appear effective for ADHD.
FORMS − Not by prescription.
NOTES − Photosensitivity possible with more than 1800 mg/day. Inducer of hepatic CYP3A4, CYP2C9, CYP2C19, and P-glycoprotein. May decrease efficacy of drugs with hepatic metabolism including alprazolam, cyclosporine, methadone, non-nucleoside reverse transcriptase inhibitors, omeprazole, oral contraceptives, oxycodone, protease inhibitors, statins, voriconazole. May need increased dose of digoxin, theophylline, TCAs. Decreased INR with warfarin. Administration with SSRIs, SNRIs, triptans may cause serotonin syndrome. Do not use within 14 days of a MAOI.
MOA − May inhibit uptake of serotonin, dopamine, norepinephrine, GABA, or L-glutamate.
ADVERSE EFFECTS − Serious: Induction of mania/hypomania, serotonin syndrome. Other: Photosensitivity possible with more than 1800 mg/day, dry mouth, dizziness, GI symptoms, fatigue, headache. Better tolerated than paroxetine in short-term trial for depression.

SAW PALMETTO (*Serenoa repens*) ▶? ♀− ▶− $
UNAPPROVED ADULTS − BPH (does not appear effective): 160 mg PO bid or 320 mg PO daily of standardized liposterolic extract. Take with food.
UNAPPROVED PEDS − Not for use in children.
FORMS − Not by prescription.
NOTES − Not for use by women of childbearing potential. Does not interfere with PSA test. Self-treatment could delay diagnosis of prostate cancer.
MOA − May have anti-androgenic anti-estrogenic, and estrogenic effects.
ADVERSE EFFECTS − Adverse reactions are mild and infrequent. May cause nausea, diarrhea, abdominal pain. Less erectile dysfunction than finasteride. Single case reports of intraoperative hemorrhage and acute pancreatitis.

SHARK CARTILAGE (*BeneFin, Cartilade*) ▶? ♀− ▶− $$$$$
UNAPPROVED ADULTS − Appears ineffective for palliative care of advanced cancer. A derivative of shark cartilage was ineffective in a phase III clinical trial for non-small cell lung cancer.
UNAPPROVED PEDS − Not for use in children.
FORMS − Not by prescription.
NOTES − Case reports of hypercalcemia linked to high calcium content (up to 600 to 780 mg/day elemental calcium in BeneFin or Cartilade). Contamination with salmonella was reported in some shark cartilage caps.
MOA − Contains proteins, glycoproteins, and glycosaminoglycans (chondroitin). Inhibits tumor angiogenesis in animal models.
ADVERSE EFFECTS − Hypercalcemia (has high calcium content; up to 600-780 mg/day elemental calcium with BeneFin or Cartilade), hyperglycemia, GI distress, constipation, hypotension.

SILVER—COLLOIDAL (*mild and strong silver protein, silver ion*) ▶ tissues ♀− ▶− $
UNAPPROVED ADULTS − The FDA does not recognize OTC colloidal silver products as safe or effective for any use.
UNAPPROVED PEDS − Not for use in children.
FORMS − Not by prescription. May come as silver chloride, cyanide, iodide, oxide, or phosphate.
NOTES − Silver accumulates in skin (leads to permanent grey tint), conjunctiva, and internal organs with chronic use.
MOA − Suspension of silver particles in a colloidal (gelatinous) base. Silver has antimicrobial effects.
ADVERSE EFFECTS − Serious: Silver accumulates in skin (leads to gray tint), conjunctiva, and internal organs with chronic use.

SOY (*Genisoy, Healthy Woman, Novasoy, Phytosoya, Supro*) ▶Gut, L, K ♀+ for food, ? for supplements ▶+ for food, ? for supplements $
UNAPPROVED ADULTS − Cardiovascular risk reduction: At least 25 g/day soy protein (50 mg/day isoflavones) PO. Hypercholesterolemia: About 50 g/day soy protein PO reduces LDL cholesterol by approximately 3%; effects on HDL, triglycerides, BP appear insignificant. No apparent benefit for isoflavone supplements. Postmenopausal vasomotor symptoms (modest benefit if any): 20 to 60 g/day soy protein PO (40 to 80 mg/day isoflavones). Conflicting clinical trials for reducing postmenopausal bone loss. AHA recommends against isoflavone supplements for treatment or prevention of hyperlipidemia, or breast, endometrial, or prostate cancer.
UNAPPROVED PEDS − Soy foods are regarded as safe for children.
FORMS − Not by prescription.
NOTES − Effect of soy supplements on breast cancer risk is unclear; some experts recommend against use of isoflavone or phytoestrogen supplements by women with endometrial or breast cancer (esp. estrogen receptor-positive tumor or receiving tamoxifen). Case report of decreased INR with ingestion of soy milk by patient taking warfarin. Report of decreased levothyroxine absorption with soy protein.
MOA − Contains isoflavone phytoestrogens (genistein, daidzein), which may act as estrogen receptor agonists or antagonists. In 30-50% of the population, gut microbes convert daidzein to equol, a nonsteroidal estrogen. Benefit for postmenopausal symptoms may be limited to equol producers. Soy foods are low in saturated fat and high in fiber, vitamins, and minerals.
ADVERSE EFFECTS − Soy is generally regarded as safe as a food. Protein powder may cause GI complaints. High doses (150 mg/day isoflavones) may cause endometrial hyperplasia.

STEVIA (*Stevia rebaudiana*) ▶L ♀− ▶? $
ADULTS − Rebaudioside A (a component of stevia) is FDA approved as a general purpose sweetener.
PEDS − Rebaudioside A (a component of stevia) is FDA approved as a general purpose sweetener.
UNAPPROVED ADULTS − Leaves traditionally used as a sweetener but not enough safety data for FDA approval as such. WHO acceptable daily intake of up to 4 mg/kg/day of steviol glycosides. Health Canada advises a max of 280 mg/day of stevia leaf powder in adults.
UNAPPROVED PEDS − Stevia leaves not for use in children.
FORMS − Not by prescription. Rebaudioside A available as Rebiana, Truvia, PureVia.
NOTES − Unrefined stevia is available as a dietary supplement in US, but is not FDA approved as a food sweetener. In December 2008, FDA approved rebaudioside A (a component of stevia) as a general purpose sweetener. Rebaudioside A lacks bitter aftertaste of unrefined stevia. Canadian labeling advises against use by pregnant women, children, or those with low BP.
MOA − Leaves of stevia plant contain glycosides (stevioside and rebaudioside). Stevioside is 100-fold sweeter than sucrose; rebaudioside A is even sweeter. Stevia may stimulate insulin secretion by pancreatic beta cells at high glucose levels.
ADVERSE EFFECTS − No effect of rebaudioside A on blood pressure or glycemic control in type 2 diabetes.

TEA TREE OIL (*melaleuca oil, Melaleuca alternifolia*) ▶? ♀− ▶− $
UNAPPROVED ADULTS − Not for oral use; CNS toxicity reported. Efficacy unclear for topical treatment of onychomycosis, tinea pedis, acne vulgaris, dandruff, pediculosis.
UNAPPROVED PEDS − Not for use in children.
FORMS − Not by prescription.
NOTES − Can cause allergic contact dermatitis, especially with concentration of 2% or greater.
MOA − Antimicrobial, scabicidal, and antifungal effects in vitro. Weak estrogenic and antiandrogenic activity in vitro. Oil is distilled from leaves of Melaleuca alternifolia.
ADVERSE EFFECTS − Allergic contact dermatitis; products with concentration of 2% or greater linked to skin reactions. Single case reports of immediate hypersensitivity reaction, and gynecomastia in prepubertal boy.

VALERIAN (*Valeriana officinalis, Alluna*) ▶? ♀− ▶− $
UNAPPROVED ADULTS − Insomnia (possibly modestly effective; conflicting clinical trials): 400 to 900 mg of standardized extract PO 30 min before bedtime. Response reported in 2 to 4 weeks. Alluna (valerian + hops): 2 tabs PO 1 h before bedtime. Am Academy of Sleep Medicine does not recommend for chronic insomnia due to inadequate safety and efficacy data.
UNAPPROVED PEDS − Not for use in children.
FORMS − Not by prescription.
NOTES − Do not combine with CNS depressants. Withdrawal symptoms reported after long-term use. Some products have unpleasant smell.
MOA − Valerenic acid inhibits breakdown of GABA in CNS.
ADVERSE EFFECTS − Headache. Some products have unpleasant smell. Withdrawal symptoms

(cont.)

VALERIAN (cont.)
reported after long-term use. Serious: Case reports of possible hepatotoxicity.

WILD YAM (*Dioscorea villosa*) ▶L ♀? ▶? $
UNAPPROVED ADULTS — Ineffective as topical "natural progestin."
UNAPPROVED PEDS — Not for use in children.
FORMS — Not by prescription.
MOA — Contains diosgenin which is structurally similar to cholesterol. Was used historically to synthesize progestins, cortisone, and androgens; it is not converted to them or DHEA in the body.
ADVERSE EFFECTS — None known.

WILLOW BARK EXTRACT (*Salix alba, Salicis cortex, Assalix, salicin*) ▶K ♀– ▶– $
UNAPPROVED ADULTS — OA, low-back pain (possibly effective): 60 to 240 mg/day salicin PO divided bid to tid. Onset of pain relief is approximately 2 h. Often included in multi-ingredient weight-loss supplements based on preliminary research suggesting that aspirin increases thermogenesis.
UNAPPROVED PEDS — Not for use in children.
FORMS — Not by prescription. Some products standardized to 15% salicin content.
NOTES — Contraindicated in 3rd trimester of pregnancy and in patients with intolerance or allergy to aspirin or other NSAIDs. Consider contraindications and precautions that apply to other salicylates. Avoid concomitant use of NSAIDs.
MOA — Antipyretic, anti-inflammatory, and analgesic activity. Inhibits prostaglandin synthesis. Salicin, the primary component, is a prodrug that is metabolized to salicylic acid. Salicin does not irreversibly inhibit platelet aggregation like aspirin. The pharmacologic activity of willow is not due solely to salicin.
ADVERSE EFFECTS — Serious: Anaphylactic reactions possible in patients with a history of aspirin hypersensitivity; risk of gastrointestinal bleeding unclear. Frequent: Dose-related tinnitus; GI complaints.

YOHIMBE (*Corynanthe yohimbe, Pausinystalia yohimbe*) ▶L ♀– ▶– $
UNAPPROVED ADULTS — Nonprescription yohimbe promoted for impotence and as aphrodisiac, but some products contain little yohimbine (active constituent). FDA considers yohimbe bark in herbal remedies an unsafe herb. Yohimbine HCl is available in the United States as a prescription drug, but Am Urological Assoc does not recommend for erectile dysfunction.
UNAPPROVED PEDS — Not for use in children.
FORMS — Yohimbine is the primary alkaloid in the bark of the yohimbe tree. Yohimbine HCl is a prescription drug in the United States; yohimbe bark is available without prescription. Yohimbe bark (not by prescription) and prescription yohimbine HCl are not interchangeable.
NOTES — Can cause CNS stimulation. High doses of yohimbine have MAOI activity and can increase BP. Avoid in patients with hypotension, diabetes, heart, liver or kidney disease. Reports of renal failure, seizures, death in patients taking products containing yohimbe.
MOA — Yohimbine is the primary alkaloid in the bark of the yohimbe tree. Yohimbine is an alpha 2-adrenergic receptor blocker.
ADVERSE EFFECTS — High doses can increase blood pressure. Can also cause tachycardia, GI distress, and anxiety/agitation. Case report of priapism.

IMMUNOLOGY: Immunizations

NOTE: For vaccine info see CDC website (www.cdc.gov).

AVIAN INFLUENZA VACCINE H5N1—INACTIVATED INJECTION ▶Immune system ♀C ▶? ?
ADULTS — 18 to 64 yo: 1 mL IM for 2 doses, separated by 21 to 35 days.
PEDS — Not approved for use in children.
NOTES — Caution if hypersensitivity to chicken or egg proteins. The immunocompromised may have a blunted immune response.
MOA — Active immunity, stimulates antibody production.
ADVERSE EFFECTS — Frequent: Fever, malaise, pain, tenderness and erythema at injection site. Severe: Allergic reactions/anaphylaxis, Guillain-Barré syndrome, angioedema.

BCG VACCINE (*Tice BCG, ✱Oncotice, Immucyst*) ▶Immune system ♀C ▶? $$$$
WARNING — BCG infections reported in health care workers following exposure from accidental needle sticks or skin lacerations. Nosocomial infections reported in patients receiving parenteral drugs that were prepared in areas in which BCG was reconstituted. Serious infections, including fatal infections, have been reported in patients receiving intravesical BCG.
ADULTS — 0.2 to 0.3 mL percutaneously (using 1 mL sterile water for reconstitution).
PEDS — Decrease concentration by 50% using 2 mL sterile water for reconstitution, then 0.2 to 0.3 mL percutaneously for age younger than 1 mo. May revaccinate with full dose (adult dose) after 1 yo if necessary. Use adult dose for age older than 1 mo.
MOA — Active immunity, stimulates antibody production.
ADVERSE EFFECTS — Frequent: None.

COMVAX (haemophilus B vaccine + hepatitis B vaccine) ▶Immune system ♀C ▶? $$$
ADULTS — Do not use in adults.
PEDS — Infants born of HBsAg (–) mothers: 0.5 mL IM for 3 doses at 2, 4, and 12 to 15 mo.
NOTES — Combination is made of PedvaxHIB (haemophilus b vaccine) + Recombivax HB (hepatitis B vaccine). For infants 8 weeks of age or older.
MOA — Active immunity, stimulates antibody production.
ADVERSE EFFECTS — Frequent: Acute febrile reaction.

IMMUNOLOGY: Immunizations

TETANUS WOUND CARE (www.cdc.gov)		
	Unknown or less than 3 prior tetanus immunizations	3 or more prior tetanus immunizations
Non-tetanus prone wound (e.g., clean and minor)	Td (DT age younger than 7 yo)	Td if more than 10 years since last dose
Tetanus prone wound (eg, dirt, contamination, punctures, crush components)	Td (DT age younger than 7 yo), tetanus immune globulin 250 units IM at site other than Td	Td if more than 5 years since last dose

If patient age 10 yo or older has never received a pertussis booster consider DTaP (*Boostrix* if 10–18 yo, *Adacel* if 11–64 yo).

DIPHTHERIA TETANUS AND ACELLULAR PERTUSSIS VACCINE (*DTaP, Tdap, Tripedia, Infanrix, Daptacel, Boostrix, Adacel, ✦Tripacel*) ▶Immune system ♀C ▶– $$
ADULTS – 0.5 mL IM in deltoid as a single dose, 2 to 5 years since last tetanus dose (Adacel, only) one time only.
PEDS – Check immunization history: DTaP is preferred for all DTP doses. Give first dose of 0.5 mL IM at approximately 2 mo, 2nd dose at 4 mo, 3rd dose at 6 mo, 4th dose at 15 to 18 mo, and 5th dose (booster) at 4 to 6 yo. Use Boostrix only if adolescents age 10 to 18 yo, and at least 2 to 5 years after the last childhood dose of DTaP. Use Adacel only in adolescents 11 yo or older and at least 2 to 5 years after last childhood dose of DTaP or Td.
NOTES – When feasible, use same brand for first 3 doses. Do not give if prior DTaP vaccination caused anaphylaxis or encephalopathy within 7 days. Avoid Tripedia in thimerosal allergic patients. Do not use Boostrix or Adacel for primary childhood vaccination series, if prior DTaP vaccination caused anaphylaxis or encephalopathy, or if progressive neurologic disorders (eg, encephalopathy) or uncontrolled epilepsy. Adacel is only DTaP vaccine approved for use in adults up to age 64 yo. For adolescents and adults, only 1 dose should be given, at least 2 to 5 years after last tetanus dose. Specify Adacel/Boostrix vaccine for adolescent and adult booster as pediatric formulations have increased pertussis concentrations and may increase local reaction. No information available on repeat doses in adolescents or adults.
MOA – Active immunity, stimulates antibody production.
ADVERSE EFFECTS – Frequent: Agitation, drowsiness, pain, redness and swelling at injection site, headache, fatigue.

DIPHTHERIA-TETANUS TOXOID (*Td, DT, ✦D2T5*) ▶Immune system ♀C ▶? $
ADULTS – 0.5 mL IM, 2nd dose 4 to 8 weeks later, and 3rd dose 6 to 12 months later. Give 0.5 mL booster dose at 10 year intervals. Use adult formulation (Td) for adults and children at least 7 yo.
PEDS – 0.5 mL IM for age 6 weeks to 6 yo, 2nd dose 4 to 8 weeks later, and 3rd dose 6 to 12 months later using DT for pediatric use. If immunization of infants begins in the first year of life using DT rather than DTP (ie, pertussis is contraindicated), give three 0.5 mL doses 4 to 8 weeks apart, followed by a fourth dose 6 to 12 months later.
FORMS – Injection DT (pediatric: 6 weeks to 6 yo). Td (adult and children at least 7 yo).
NOTES – DTaP is preferred for most children age less than 7 yo. Td is preferred for adults and children at least 7 yo. Avoid in thimerosal allergy.
MOA – Active immunity, stimulates antibody production.
ADVERSE EFFECTS – Frequent: Agitation, drowsiness.

HAEMOPHILUS B VACCINE (*ActHIB, HibTITER, PedvaxHIB*) ▶Immune system ♀C ▶? $$
PEDS – Doses vary depending on formulation used and age at first dose. ActHIB/OmniHIB/HibTITER: Give 0.5 mL IM for 3 doses at 2 month intervals for age 2 to 6 mo, give 0.5 mL IM for 2 doses at 2 month intervals for age 7 to 11 mo, give 0.5 mL IM for 1 dose for age 12 to 14 mo. A single 0.5 mL IM booster dose is given to previously immunized children at least 15 mo, and at least 2 months after the previous injection. For children age 15 mo to 5 yo at age of first dose, give 0.5 mL IM for 1 dose (no booster). PedvaxHIB: 0.5 mL IM for 2 doses at 2 month intervals for age 2 to 14 mo. If the 2 doses are given before 12 mo of age, a third 0.5 mL IM (booster) dose is given at least 2 months after the second dose. 0.5 mL IM for 1 dose (no booster) for age 15 mo to 5 yo.
UNAPPROVED ADULTS – <u>Asplenia, at least 14 days prior to elective splenectomy, or immunodeficiency:</u> 0.5 mL IM for 1 dose of any Hib conjugate vaccine.
UNAPPROVED PEDS – <u>Asplenia, at least 14 days prior to elective splenectomy, or immunodeficiency</u> age 5 yo or older: 0.5 mL IM for 1 dose of any Hib vaccine.
NOTES – Not for IV use. No data on interchangeability between brands; AAP and ACIP recommend use of any product in children age 12 to 15 mo.
MOA – Active immunity, stimulates antibody production.
ADVERSE EFFECTS – Frequent: Acute febrile reaction, soreness and redness at injection site.

HEPATITIS A VACCINE (*Havrix, Vaqta, ✦Avaxim, Epaxal*) ▶ ♀C ▶+ $$$
ADULTS – Havrix: 1 mL (1440 ELU) IM, then 1 mL (1440 ELU) IM booster dose 6 to 12 months later.

(cont.)

CHILDHOOD IMMUNIZATION SCHEDULE*

Age	Birth	1	2	4	6	12 (Months)	15	18	2 (Years)	4–6	11–12
Hepatitis B	HB	HB				HB					
Rotavirus			Rota	Rota	Rota@						
DTP			DTaP	DTaP	DTaP		DTaP			DTaP	DTaP***
H influenza b			Hib	Hib	Hib	Hib					
Pneumococci**			PCV	PCV	PCV	PCV					
Polio			IPV	IPV		IPV				IPV#	
Influenza†						Influenza (yearly)†					
MMR						MMR				MMR	
Varicella						Varicella				Vari	
Hepatitis A¶						Hep A × 2¶					
Papillomavirus§											HPV × 3§
Meningococcal^											MCV^

*2010 schedule from the CDC, ACIP, AAP, & AAFP, see CDC website (www.cdc.gov/vaccines/recs/schedules/default.htm).
**Administer 1 dose to all healthy children 24–59 months having an incomplete schedule.
***When immunizing adolescents 10 yo or older, consider DTaP if patient has never received a pertussis booster (*Boostrix* if 10–18 yo, *Adacel* if 11–64 yo).
@If using *Rotarix* at 2 and 4 months, dose at 6 months is not indicated.
Last IPV on or after 4th birthday, and at least 6 months since last dose. If 4 doses given before 4th birthday, give 5th dose at ages 4 to 6 yo.
†For healthy patients age 2 yo or greater can use intranasal form. If age less than 9 yo and receiving for first time, administer 2 doses 4 or more weeks apart for injected form and 6 or more weeks apart for intranasal form.
¶Two doses at least 6 months apart. §Second and third doses 2 and 6 months after first dose. Also approved for males 9–18 yo to reduce risk of genital warts. ^For children 2–10 yo at high risk for meningococcal disease, vaccinate with meningococcal polysaccharide vaccine (*Menactra*). Revaccinate after 3 years (if first dose was at 2–6 yo) for children who remain at high risk or after 5 years (if first dose was a 7 yo or older).

HEPATITIS A VACCINE (*cont.*)

Vaqta: 1 mL (50 units) IM, then 1 mL (50 units) IM booster 6 months later for age 18 yo or older.
PEDS — Havrix: 0.5 mL (720 ELU) IM for 1 dose, then 0.5 mL (720 ELU) IM booster 6 to 12 months after first dose for age 1 to 18 yo. Vaqta: 0.5 mL (25 units) IM for 1 dose, then 0.5 mL (25 units) IM booster 6 to 18 months later for age 1 to 18 yo.
FORMS — Single-dose vial (specify pediatric or adult).
NOTES — Do not inject IV, SC, or ID. Brands may be used interchangeably. Need for boosters is unclear. Postexposure prophylaxis with hepatitis A vaccine alone is not recommended. Should be given 4 weeks prior to travel to endemic area. May be given at the same time as immune globulin, but preferably at different site.
MOA — Active immunity, stimulates antibody production.
ADVERSE EFFECTS — Frequent: Headache, pain, tenderness, warmth, soreness and redness at injection site.

HEPATITIS B VACCINE (*Engerix-B, Recombivax HB*)
▶ ♀C ▶+ $$$
ADULTS — Engerix-B: 1 mL (20 mcg) IM, repeat in 1 and 6 months for age 20 yo or older.
Hemodialysis: Give 2 mL (40 mcg) IM, repeat in 1, 2, and 6 months. Give 2 mL (40 mcg) IM booster when antibody levels decline to less than 10 mIU/mL. Recombivax HB: 1 mL (10 mcg) IM, repeat in 1 and 6 months. Hemodialysis: 1 mL (40 mcg) IM, repeat in 1 and 6 months. Give 1 mL (40 mcg) IM booster when antibody levels decline to less than 10 mIU/mL.
PEDS — Specialized dosing based on age and maternal HBsAg status. Engerix-B 10 mcg (0.5 mL) IM 0, 1, 6 months for infants of hepatitis B negative and positive mothers and children age 15 to 20 yo. Recombivax 5 mcg (0.5 mL) IM 0, 1, 6 months for infants of hepatitis B negative and positive mothers and children age 15 to 20 yo. A 2-dose schedule can be used (Recombivax HB 10 mcg (1 mL) IM at 0 and 4 to 6 months for age 11 to 15 yo.
NOTES — Infants born to hepatitis B positive mothers should also receive hepatitis B immune globulin and hepatitis B vaccine within 12 h of birth. Not for IV or ID use. May interchange products. Recombivax HB Dialysis Formulation is intended for adults only. Avoid if yeast allergy.
MOA — Active immunity, stimulates antibody production.
ADVERSE EFFECTS — Frequent: Dizziness, malaise, pain and tenderness at injection site.

IMMUNOLOGY: Immunizations

HUMAN PAPILLOMAVIRUS RECOMBINANT VACCINE (*Gardasil*) ▶ ♀B ▶? $$$$$
ADULTS — <u>Prevention of cervical cancer, vulvar and vaginal cancer:</u> Females up to age 26 yo: 0.5 mL IM at time 0, 2 and 6 months.
PEDS — <u>Prevention of cervical cancer, vulvar and vaginal cancer:</u> Females for age 9 yo or older: 0.5 mL IM at time 0, 2 and 6 months.
NOTES — Includes types 6, 11, 16, 18. Patients must be counseled to continue to use condoms. Immunosuppression may reduce response. Fainting and falling may occur after vaccination; observe patient for 15 min after vaccination.
MOA — Active immunity, stimulates antibody production.
ADVERSE EFFECTS — Frequent: Pain, tenderness, pruritus and erythema at injection site, fainting.

INFLUENZA VACCINE—INACTIVATED INJECTION (*Afluria, Fluarix, FluLaval, Fluzone, Fluvirin, ✽Fluviral, Vaxigrip*) ▶Immune system ♀C ▶+ $
ADULTS — 0.5 mL IM single dose once a year.
PEDS — Fluarix and FluLaval are not indicated for age younger than 18 yo, Fluvirin not indicated for age younger than 4 yo. Give 0.25 mL IM for age 6 to 35 mo, repeat dose after 4 weeks if previously unvaccinated. Give 0.5 mL IM for age 3 to 8 yo, repeat dose after 4 weeks if previously unvaccinated. Give 0.5 mL IM once a year for age 9 to 12 yo.
NOTES — Avoid in Guillain-Barré syndrome, chicken egg allergy, aspirin therapy in children (Reye's risk), thimerosal allergy (Fluzone is thimerosal-free). Optimal administration October to November.
MOA — Active immunity, stimulates antibody production.
ADVERSE EFFECTS — Frequent: Fever, malaise, pain, tenderness and erythema at injection site. Severe: Allergic or anaphylactoid reactions in egg-allergic persons, Guillain-Barré syndrome, angioedema.

INFLUENZA VACCINE—LIVE INTRANASAL (*FluMist*) ▶Immune system ♀C ▶+ $
ADULTS — 1 dose (0.2 mL) intranasally once a year for health adults age 18 to 49 yo.
PEDS — 1 dose (0.2 mL) intranasally for healthy children age 2 to 17 yo, repeat dose after 4 weeks if previously unvaccinated and age 2 to 8 yo.
NOTES — Avoid in Guillain-Barré syndrome, chicken egg allergy, aspirin therapy in children (Reye's risk), pregnancy, chronic illness that could increase vulnerability to influenza complications (CHF, asthma, diabetes, renal failure), recurrent wheezing and in children younger than 2 yo. Optimal administration October to November. Since FluMist is a live vaccine, do not use with immune deficiencies (eg, HIV, malignancy, etc.) or altered immune status (eg, taking systemic corticosteroids, chemotherapy, radiation, etc.).
MOA — Active immunity, stimulates antibody production.
ADVERSE EFFECTS — Frequent: Fever, malaise. Severe: Allergic or anaphylactoid reactions in egg-allergic persons, Guillain-Barré syndrome, angioedema.

JAPANESE ENCEPHALITIS VACCINE (*JE-Vax*) ▶ ♀C ▶? $$$$
ADULTS — 1 mL SC for 3 doses on day 0, 7, and 30.
PEDS — 0.5 mL SC for 3 doses on day 0, 7, and 30 for age 1 to 3 yo. Give 1 mL SC for 3 doses on day 0, 7, and 30. for age 3 yo or older.
NOTES — Give at least 10 days before travel to endemic areas. An abbreviated schedule on day 0, 7, and 14 can be given if time limits. A booster dose may be given after 2 years. Avoid in thimerosal allergy.
MOA — Active immunity, stimulates antibody production.
ADVERSE EFFECTS — Frequent: Tenderness, redness and swelling at injection site. Severe: Anaphylactic reaction, angioedema, dyspnea, encephalitis, encephalopathy, erythema nodosum, erythema multiforme, peripheral neuropathy, seizures.

MEASLES MUMPS & RUBELLA VACCINE (*M-M-R II, ✽Priorix*) ▶Immune system ♀C ▶+ $$$
ADULTS — 0.5 mL (1 vial) SC.
PEDS — 0.5 mL (1 vial) SC for age 12 to 15 mo. Revaccinate prior to elementary and/or middle school according to local health guidelines. If measles outbreak, may immunize infants 6 to 12 mo with 0.5 mL SC; then start 2-dose regimen between 12 to 15 mo.
NOTES — Do not inject IV. Contraindicated in pregnancy. Advise women to avoid pregnancy for 4 weeks following vaccination. Live virus, contraindicated in immunocompromised patients. Avoid if allergic to neomycin or gelatin; caution in egg allergy.
MOA — Active immunity, stimulates antibody production.
ADVERSE EFFECTS — Frequent: Fever, burning, induration, rash. Severe: Allergic reactions, encephalitis, convulsions, erythema multiforme, prolonged high fever, Guillain-Barré syndrome, thrombocytopenia.

MENINGOCOCCAL VACCINE (*Menomune-A/C/Y/W-135, Menactra, ✽Menjugate*) ▶ ♀C ▶? $$$$
WARNING — Reports of associated Guillain-Barré syndrome; avoid if prior history of this condition.
ADULTS — 0.5 mL SC (Menomune) or IM (Menactra).
PEDS — 0.5 mL SC for age 2 yo or older.
UNAPPROVED PEDS — 0.5 mL SC for 2 doses separated by 3 mo for age 3 to 18 mo.
NOTES — Give 2 weeks before elective splenectomy or travel to endemic areas. May consider revaccination q 3 to 5 year in high-risk patients. Do not inject IV. Contraindicated in pregnancy. Consider vaccinating 11 to 12 yo and first year college students living in dormitories. Avoid in thimerosal allergy (except Menactra which is thimerosal-free).
MOA — Active immunity, stimulates antibody production.
ADVERSE EFFECTS — Frequent: Pain, erythema, induration, tenderness. Severe: Guillain-Barré syndrome.

PEDIARIX (**diphtheria tetanus and acellular pertussis vaccine + hepatitis B vaccine + polio vaccine**) ▶Immune system ♀C ▶? $$$
PEDS — 0.5 mL at 2, 4, 6 mo IM.
NOTES — Do not administer before 6 weeks of age.
MOA — Active immunity, stimulates antibody production.
ADVERSE EFFECTS — Frequent: Local injection site reactions (pain, swelling, redness), fever, fussiness. Severe: Convulsions, encephalopathy.

PLAGUE VACCINE ▶Immune system ♀C ▶+ $
ADULTS — 1 mL IM for 1 dose, then 0.2 mL IM 1 to 3 months after the first injection, then 0.2 mL IM 5 to 6 months after the second injection for age 18 to 61 yo.
PEDS — Not approved in children.
NOTES — Up to 3 booster doses (0.2 mL) may be administered at 6 month intervals in high-risk patients. Jet injector gun may be used for IM administration.
MOA — Active immunity, stimulates antibody production.
ADVERSE EFFECTS — Frequent: Malaise, fever, headache, tenderness, nausea.

PNEUMOCOCCAL 23-VALENT VACCINE (*Pneumovax, ✢Pneumo 23*) ▶Immune system ♀C ▶+ $$
ADULTS — All adults 65 yo or older: 0.5 mL IM/SC for 1 dose. Vaccination also recommended for high-risk individuals younger than age 65 yo. Routine revaccination in immunocompetent patients is not recommended. Consider revaccination once in patients age 65 yo or greater who were vaccinated before the age of 65 or patients at high risk of developing serious pneumococcal infection if more than 5 years from initial vaccine.
PEDS — 0.5 mL IM/SC for age 2 yo or older. Consider revaccination once in patients at high risk of developing serious pneumococcal infection after 3 to 5 yo from initial vaccine in patients who would be 10 yo or younger at time of revaccination.
NOTES — Do not give IV or ID. May be given in conjunction with influenza virus vaccine at different site. OK for high-risk children at least 2 yo who received Prevnar series already to provide additional serotype coverage.
MOA — Active immunity, stimulates antibody production.
ADVERSE EFFECTS — Frequent: Induration and soreness at the injection site. Severe: Anaphylaxis, Guillain-Barré syndrome,

PNEUMOCOCCAL 7-VALENT CONJUGATE VACCINE (*Prevnar*) ▶ ♀C ▶? $$$
ADULTS — Not approved in adults.
PEDS — 0.5 mL IM for 3 doses 6 to 8 weeks apart starting at 2 to 6 mo of age, followed by a fourth dose of 0.5 mL IM at 12 to 15 mo. For previously unvaccinated older infants and children age 7 to 11 mo: 0.5 mL for 2 doses 6 to 8 weeks apart, followed by a third dose of 0.5 mL at 12 to 15 mo. Give 0.5 mL for 2 doses 6 to 8 weeks apart for age 12 to 23 mo. Give 0.5 mL for 1 dose; give second dose 4 weeks later in immunocompromised or chronically ill children for age 2 to 9 yo.
NOTES — For IM use only; do not inject IV. Shake susp vigorously prior to administration.
MOA — Active immunity, stimulates antibody production.
ADVERSE EFFECTS — Frequent: Erythema, induration, tenderness. Severe: Component hypersensitivity.

POLIO VACCINE (*IPOL*) ▶ ♀C ▶ $$
ADULTS — Previously unvaccinated adults at increased risk of exposure should receive a complete primary immunization series of 3 doses (2 doses at intervals of 4 to 8 weeks; a third dose at 6 to 12 months after the second dose). Accelerated schedules are available. Travelers to endemic areas who have received primary immunization should receive a single booster in adulthood.
PEDS — 0.5 mL IM or SC at age 2 mo, with second dose at 4 mo, third dose at 6 to 18 mo, and fourth dose at 4 to 6 yo.
NOTES — Oral polio vaccine no longer available.
MOA — Active immunity, stimulates antibody production.
ADVERSE EFFECTS — Frequent; Fever, erythema, induration, pain, irritability, sleepiness, fussiness, crying.

PROQUAD (measles mumps & rubella vaccine + varicella vaccine, MMRV) ▶Immune system ♀C ▶? $$$$
ADULTS — Not indicated in adults.
PEDS — 0.5 mL (1 vial) SC for age 12 mo to 12 yo.
NOTES — Give at least 1 month after a MMR-containing vaccine and at least 3 months after a varicella-containing vaccine. Do not inject IV. Contraindicated in pregnancy. Following vaccination avoid pregnancy for 3 months and aspirin/salicylates for 6 weeks. Live virus, contraindicated in immunocompromise or untreated TB. Avoid if allergic to neomycin; caution with egg allergies.
MOA — Active immunity, stimulates antibody production.
ADVERSE EFFECTS — Frequent: Fever, pain, tenderness, soreness, swelling, rash. Severe: Allergic reactions, encephalitis, convulsions, erythema multiforme, prolonged high fever, Guillain-Barré syndrome, thrombocytopenia.

RABIES VACCINE (*RabAvert, Imovax Rabies, BioRab, Rabies Vaccine Adsorbed*) ▶ ♀C ▶? $$$$$
ADULTS — Postexposure prophylaxis: Give rabies immune globulin (20 international units/kg) immediately after exposure, then give rabies vaccine 1 mL IM in deltoid region on day 0, 3, 7, 14, and 28. If patients have received pre-exposure immunization, give 1 mL IM rabies vaccine on day 0 and 3 only, without rabies immune globulin. Pre-exposure immunization: 1 mL IM rabies vaccine on day 0, 7, and between days 21 and 28. Or 0.1 mL ID on day 0, 7, and between days 21 and 28. (Imovax Rabies I.D. vaccine formula only). Repeat q 2 to 5 y based on antibody titer.
PEDS — Same as adults.
NOTES — Do not use ID preparation for postexposure prophylaxis.
MOA — Active immunity, stimulates antibody production.
ADVERSE EFFECTS — Frequent: Pain, swelling, erythema, pruritus. Severe: Immune-complex like reactions, Guillain-Barré syndrome.

ROTAVIRUS VACCINE (*RotaTeq, Rotarix*) ▶▶? $$$$$
ADULTS — Not recommended.
PEDS — RotaTeq: Give the first dose (2 mL PO) between 6 to 12 weeks of age, and then the second

(cont.)

ROTAVIRUS VACCINE (cont.)
and third doses at 4 to 10 weeks intervals thereafter (last dose no later than 32 weeks). Rotarix: Give first dose (1 mL) at 6 weeks of age, and second dose (1 mL) at least 4 weeks later, and prior to 24 weeks of age.
FORMS — Trade only: Oral susp 2 mL (RotaTeq), 1 mL (Rotarix).
NOTES — Live vaccine so potential for transmission, especially to immunodeficient close contacts. Safety unclear in immunocompromised infants.
MOA — Active immunity, stimulates antibody production.
ADVERSE EFFECTS — Frequent: Diarrhea, vomiting.

SMALLPOX VACCINE (*ACAM 2000, vaccinia vaccine*) ▶Immune system ♀C ▶— Not available to civilians.
ADULTS — Prevention of smallpox or monkeypox: Specialized administration using bifurcated needle SC for 1 dose.
PEDS — Specialized administration using bifurcated needle SC for 1 dose for children older than 1 yo.
NOTES — Caution in polymyxin, neomycin, tetracycline, or streptomycin allergy. Avoid in those (or household contacts of those) with eczema or a history of eczema, those with a rash due to other causes (eg, burns, zoster, impetigo, psoriasis), immunocompromised, or pregnancy. Persons with known cardiac disease or at least 3 risk factors for cardiac disease should not be vaccinated.
MOA — Active immunity, stimulates antibody production.
ADVERSE EFFECTS — Frequent: Fever, malaise, swelling/tenderness of regional lymph nodes. Severe: Generalized vaccinia, encephalitis, encephalopathy, eczema vaccinatum, myopericarditis, myocardial infarction, angina, death.

TETANUS TOXOID ▶Immune system ♀C ▶+ $$
WARNING — Td is preferred in adults and children age 7 yo or older. DTaP is preferred in children younger than 7 yo. Use fluid tetanus toxoid in assessing cell-mediated immunity only.
ADULTS — 0.5 mL IM (adsorbed) for 2 doses 4 to 8 weeks apart. Give third dose 6 to 12 months after second injection. Give booster q 10 years. Assess cell-mediated immunity: 0.1 mL of 1:100 diluted skin-test reagent or 0.02 mL of 1:10 diluted skin-test reagent injected intradermally.
PEDS — 0.5 mL IM (adsorbed) for 2 doses 4 to 8 weeks apart. Give third dose 6 to 12 months after second injection. Give booster q 10 years.
NOTES — May use tetanus toxoid fluid for active immunization in patients hypersensitive to the aluminum adjuvant of the adsorbed formulation: 0.5 mL IM or SC for 3 doses at 4 to 8 week intervals. Give fourth dose 6 to 12 months after third injection. Give booster dose q 10 years. Avoid in thimerosal allergy.
MOA — Active immunity, stimulates antibody production.
ADVERSE EFFECTS — Frequent: Local induration at the injection site, chills, fever. Severe: Hypersensitivity reactions, fever (>103 F), neurological disturbances.

TRIHIBIT (haemophilus B vaccine + diphtheria tetanus and acellular pertussis vaccine) ▶Immune system ♀C ▶— $$$
PEDS — For fourth dose only, 15 to 18 mo: 0.5 mL IM.
NOTES — Tripedia (DTaP) is used to reconstitute ActHIB (Haemophilus b) to make TriHIBit and will appear whitish in color. Use within 30 min. Avoid in thimerosal allergy.
MOA — Active immunity, stimulates antibody production.
ADVERSE EFFECTS — Frequent: Acute febrile reactions, edema, erythema, focal neurologic signs, arthralgias, induration, urticaria. Severe: Convulsions, collapse, screaming episodes.

TWINRIX (hepatitis A vaccine + hepatitis B vaccine) ▶Immune system ♀C ▶? $$$$
ADULTS — 1 mL IM in deltoid only for age 18 yo or older, repeat at 1 and 6 months. Accelerated dosing schedule: 0, 7, 21 to 30 days and booster dose at 12 months.
PEDS — Not approved in children.
NOTES — Not for IV or ID use. 1 mL is equivalent to 720 ELU inactivated hepatitis A + 20 mcg hepatitis B surface antigen.
MOA — Active immunity, stimulates antibody production.
ADVERSE EFFECTS — Frequent: Headache, local pain, tenderness, warmth, dizziness, malaise, urticaria, rash, erythema. Severe: Angioedema, anaphylaxis.

TYPHOID VACCINE—INACTIVATED INJECTION (*Typhim Vi, ✦Typherix*) ▶Immune system ♀C ▶? $$
ADULTS — 0.5 mL IM for 1 dose given at least 2 weeks prior to potential exposure. May consider revaccination q 2 y in high-risk patients.
PEDS — Same as adult dose for age 2 years or older.
NOTES — Recommended for travel to endemic areas.
MOA — Active immunity, stimulates antibody production.
ADVERSE EFFECTS — Frequent: Headache, fever, local tenderness at site, erythema, induration, myalgia.

TYPHOID VACCINE—LIVE ORAL (*Vivotif Berna*) ▶Immune system ♀C ▶? $$
ADULTS — 1 cap 1 h before a meal with cold or lukewarm drink every other day for 4 doses to be completed at least 1 week prior to potential exposure. May consider revaccination q 5 years in high-risk patients.
PEDS — Give adult dose for age 6 yo or older.
FORMS — Trade only: Caps.
NOTES — Recommended for travel to endemic areas. Oral vaccine may be inactivated by antibiotics, including antimalarials.
MOA — Active immunity, stimulates antibody production.
ADVERSE EFFECTS — Frequent (oral): Rash, abdominal pain, diarrhea, N/V.

VARICELLA VACCINE (*Varivax,* ✦*Varilrix*) ▶ ♀C ▶+ $$$$
ADULTS — 0.5 mL SC. Repeat 4 to 8 weeks later.
PEDS — 0.5 mL SC for 1 dose for age 1 to 12 yo. Repeat at ages 4 yo, 6 yo. Use adult dose for age 13 yo or older. Not recommended for infants less than 1 yo.
UNAPPROVED PEDS — Postexposure prophylaxis: 0.5 mL SC within 3 to 5 days of exposure.
NOTES — Do not inject IV. Following vaccination avoid pregnancy for 3 months and aspirin/salicylates for 6 weeks. This live vaccine is contraindicated in immunocompromised. Vaccine is stored in freezer; thawed vaccine must be used within 30 min.
MOA — Active immunity, stimulates antibody production.
ADVERSE EFFECTS — Frequent: Fever, inflammation at the injection site.

YELLOW FEVER VACCINE (*YF-Vax*) ▶ ♀C ▶+ $$$
ADULTS — 0.5 mL SC.
PEDS — 0.5 mL SC into thigh (6 mo to 3 yo) or deltoid region for age 3 yo or older.
NOTES — Must be accredited site to administer vaccination. International Certificate of Vaccination obligatory for some travel destinations. Consult CDC traveler's health website for accredited sites or to apply for accreditation. A booster dose (0.5 mL) may be administered q 10 years.
MOA — Active immunity, stimulates antibody production.
ADVERSE EFFECTS — Frequent: Fever, malaise, headache, myalgia.

ZOSTER VACCINE—LIVE (*Zostavax*) ▶Immune system ♀C ▶? $$$$
ADULTS — 0.65 mL SC for 1 dose for age 60 yo or older.
PEDS — Not approved in children.
NOTES — Avoid if history of anaphylactic/anaphylactoid reaction to gelatin or neomycin, if primary or acquired immunodeficiency states, or if taking immunosuppressives. Do not administer if active untreated TB or in possible pregnancy. Theoretically possible to transmit to pregnant household contact who has not had varicella infection or immunocompromised contact. Do not substitute for Varivax in children.
MOA — Active immunity, boosts pre-existing immunity on individuals who have a history of varicella disease.
ADVERSE EFFECTS — Frequent: Pain, tenderness, pruritus and erythema at injection site.

IMMUNOLOGY: Immunoglobulins

NOTE: Adult IM injections should be given in the deltoid region; injection in the gluteal region may result in suboptimal response.

ANTIVENIN—CROTALIDAE IMMUNE FAB OVINE POLYVALENT (*CroFab*) ▶? ♀C ▶? $$$$$
ADULTS — Rattlesnake envenomation: Give 4 to 6 vials IV infusion over 60 min, within 6 h of bite if possible. Administer 4 to 6 additional vials if no initial control of envenomation syndrome, then 2 vials q 6 h for up to 18 h (3 doses) after initial control has been established.
PEDS — Same as adults, although specific studies in children have not been conducted.
NOTES — Contraindicated in allergy to papaya or papain. Start IV infusion slowly over the first 10 min at 25 to 50 mL/h and observe for allergic reaction, then increase to full rate of 250 mL/h.
MOA — Antivenom.
ADVERSE EFFECTS — Frequent: None,

ANTIVENIN—CROTALIDAE POLYVALENT ▶L ♀C ▶? $$$$$
ADULTS — Pit viper envenomation: 20 to 40 mL (2 to 4 vials) IV infusion for minimal envenomation, 50 to 90 mL (5 to 9 vials) IV infusion for moderate envenomation; give at least 100 to 150 mL (10–15 vials) IV infusion for severe envenomation. Administer within 4 h of bite, less effective after 8 h, and of questionable value after 12 h. May give additional 10 to 50 mL (1 to 5 vials) IV infusion based on clinical assessment and response to initial dose.
PEDS — Larger relative doses of antivenin are needed in children and small adults because of small volume of body fluid to dilute the venom. The dose is not based on wt.
NOTES — Test first for sensitivity to horse serum. Serum sickness may occur 5 to 24 days after dose. IV route is preferred. May give IM.
MOA — Antivenom.
ADVERSE EFFECTS — Frequent: None.

ANTIVENIN—LATRODECTUS MACTANS ▶L ♀C ▶? $$
ADULTS — Specialized dosing for black widow spider toxicity; consult poison center.
PEDS — Specialized dosing for black widow spider toxicity; consult poison center.
NOTES — Test first for horse serum sensitivity. Serum sickness may occur 5 to 24 days after dose.
MOA — Antivenom.
ADVERSE EFFECTS — Frequent: None.

BOTULISM IMMUNE GLOBULIN (*BabyBIG*) ▶L ♀? ▶? $$$$$
ADULTS — Not approved in age 1 yo or older.
PEDS — Infant botulism: 1 mL (50 mg)/kg IV for age younger than 1 yo.
MOA — Passive immunity.
ADVERSE EFFECTS — Frequent: Mild, transient erythematous rash of face or trunk. Severe: Anaphylaxis, angioedema, urticaria, renal dysfunction/failure.

ADULT IMMUNIZATION SCHEDULE*

Tetanus, diphtheria (Td): For all ages, 1 dose booster every 10 years. *Pertussis*: Consider single dose of pertussis in adults younger than 65 yo (as part of Tdap), at least 10 years since last tetanus dose. If patient has never received a pertussis booster use Boostrix if 10 to 18 yo, Adacel if 11 to 64 yo, *Influenza*: 1 yearly dose if age 50 yo or older. If younger than 50 yo, then 1 yearly dose if healthcare worker, pregnant, chronic underlying illness, household contact of person with chronic underlying illness or household contact with children younger than 5 yo, or those who request vaccination. Intranasal vaccine indicated for healthy adults younger than 50 yo. *Pneumococcal* (polysaccharide): 1 dose if age 65 yo or older. If younger than 65 yo, consider immunizing if chronic underlying illness, nursing home resident. Consider revaccination 5 years later if high risk or if age 65 yo or older and received primary dose before age 65 yo. *Hepatitis A*: For all ages with clotting factor disorders, chronic liver disease, or exposure risk (travel to endemic areas, illegal drug use, men having sex with men), 2 doses (0, 6-12 months). *Hepatitis B*: For all ages with medical (hemodialysis, clotting factor recipients, chronic liver disease), occupational (healthcare or public safety workers with blood exposure), behavioral (illegal drug use, multiple sex partners, those seeking evaluation or treatment of sexually transmitted disease, men having sex with men) or other (household/sex contacts of those with chronic HBV or HIV infections, clients/staff of developmentally disabled, >6 month travel to high risk areas, inmates of correctional facilities) indications, 3 doses (0, 1-2, 4-6 months). Hemodialysis patients require 4 doses and higher dose (40 mcg). *Measles, mumps, rubella (MMR)*: If born during or after 1957 and immunity in doubt, see cdc.gov. *Varicella*: For all ages if immunity in doubt, age 13 yo or older, 2 doses separated by 4 to 8 weeks. *Meningococcal* (conjugate vaccine is preferred for age 55 or less): For all ages with medical indications (complement deficiency, anatomic or functional asplenia) or other indications (travel to endemic regions, college dormitory residents, military recruits), administer 1 dose. Consider revaccination in 3 to 5 years if high-risk. *Human papillomavirus*: Consider HPV vaccine in women 9 to 26 yo at 0, 2 and 6 months. Can be used in males 9 to 26 yo to decrease risk of genital warts. *Herpes zoster*: Consider single dose of HZ vaccine in individuals for age 60 or older. Haemophilus influenzae type b (Hib): 1 dose in high risk adults (sickle cell, leukemia, HIV, splenectomy), if not previously immunized.

*2010 schedule from the CDC, ACIP, & AAFP, see: ww.cdc.gov/vaccines/recs/schedules/default.htm

CYTOMEGALOVIRUS IMMUNE GLOBULIN HUMAN (*Cytogam*) ▶L ♀C ▶? $$$$$
ADULTS — Specialized dosing based on indication and time since transplant.
PEDS — Specialized dosing based on indication and time since transplant.
MOA — Passive immunity.
ADVERSE EFFECTS — Frequent: Flushing, fever, pain, N/V. Severe: Anaphylaxis.

HEPATITIS B IMMUNE GLOBULIN (*H-BIG, HyperHep B, HepaGam B, NABI-HB*) ▶L ♀C ▶? $$$
ADULTS — Postexposure prophylaxis for needlestick, ocular, mucosal exposure: 0.06 mL/kg IM (usual dose 3 to 5 mL) within 24 h of exposure. Initiate hepatitis B vaccine series within 7 days. Consider a second dose of hepatitis B immune globulin (HBIG) 1 month later if patient refuses hepatitis B vaccine series. Postexposure prophylaxis for sexual exposure: 0.06 mL/kg IM within 14 days of sexual contact. Initiate hepatitis B vaccine series. Prevention of hepatitis B recurrence following liver transplantation in HBsAg-positive (HepaGam B): first dose given during transplantation surgery. Subsequent doses daily for 7 days, then biweekly up to 3 months and monthly thereafter. Doses adjusted based on regular monitoring of HBsAg, HBV-DNA, HBeAg, and anti-HBs antibody levels.
PEDS — Prophylaxis of infants born to HBsAg (+) mothers: 0.5 mL IM within 12 h of birth. Initiate hepatitis B vaccine series within 7 days. If hepatitis B vaccine series is refused, repeat HBIG dose at 3 and 6 mo. Household exposure age younger than 12 mo: give 0.5 mL IM within 14 days of exposure. Initiate hepatitis B vaccine series.
NOTES — HBIG may be administered at the same time or up to 1 month prior to hepatitis B vaccine without impairing the active immune response from hepatitis B vaccine.
MOA — Passive immunity.
ADVERSE EFFECTS — Frequent: Pain at injection site. Severe: Anaphylaxis, angioedema, urticaria.

IMMUNE GLOBULIN—INTRAMUSCULAR (*Baygam, ◆Gamastan*) ▶L ♀C ▶? $$$$
ADULTS — Hepatitis A postexposure prophylaxis for household or institutional contacts: 0.02 mL/kg IM within 2 weeks of exposure. Hepatitis A pre-exposure prophylaxis (ie, travel to endemic area): give 0.02 mL/kg IM for length of stay less than 3 months, give 0.06 mL/kg IM and repeat q 4 to 6 months for length of stay greater than 3 months. Measles: 0.2 to 0.25 mL/kg IM within 6 days of exposure, max 15 mL. Varicella zoster (if VariZIG unavailable): 0.6 to 1.2 mL/kg IM. Rubella exposure in pregnant, susceptible women: 0.55 mL/kg IM. Immunoglobulin deficiency: 0.66 mL/kg IM every 3 to 4 weeks.
PEDS — Not approved in children.
UNAPPROVED PEDS — Measles: 0.2 to 0.25 mL/kg IM within 6 days of exposure. In susceptible immunocompromised children use 0.5 mL/kg IM (max 15 mL) immediately after exposure. Varicella zoster (if VariZIG unavailable): 0.6 to 1.2 mL/kg IM.

(cont.)

IMMUNE GLOBULIN—INTRAMUSCULAR (cont.)
NOTES – Human derived product, increased infection risk. Hepatitis A vaccine preferred over immune globulin for age 2 yo or older who plan to travel to high-risk areas repeatedly or for long periods of time.
MOA – Passive immunity.
ADVERSE EFFECTS – Frequent: Pain at injection site, tenderness, muscle stiffness, HA. Severe: Anaphylaxis, angioedema, urticaria, nephrotic syndrome.

IMMUNE GLOBULIN—INTRAVENOUS (*Carimune, Flebogamma, Gammagard, Gammaplex, Gamunex, Octagam, Privigen*) ▶L ♀C ▶? $$$$$
WARNING – Renal dysfunction, acute renal failure, osmotic nephrosis, and death may be associated with IV immune globulins, especially those containing sucrose. Administer at the minimum concentration available and the minimum practical infusion rate.
ADULTS – Idiopathic thrombocytopenic purpura (induction): 400 mg/kg IV daily for 5 days (or 1 g/kg IV daily for 1 to 2 days). Bone marrow transplant: 500 mg/kg IV daily, given 7 and 2 days before transplant, and then weekly until 90 days post transplant for age older than 20 yo. Primary humoral immunodeficiency: 200 to 300 mg/kg IV each month; increase as needed to max 400 to 800 mg/kg/month. B-cell chronic lymphocytic leukemia: Specialized dosing. Chronic inflammatory demyelinating polyneuropathy (CIDP): (Gamunex) 2 g/kg IV loading dose followed by 1 g/kg IV every 3 weeks.
PEDS – Pediatric HIV: 400 mg/kg IV q 28 days. Idiopathic thrombocytopenic purpura (induction): 400 mg/kg IV daily for 5 days (or 1 g/kg IV daily for 1 to 2 days). Kawasaki syndrome (acute): 400 mg/kg IV daily for 4 days (or 2 g/kg IV for 1 dose over 10 h). Primary humoral immunodeficiency: 200 to 300 mg/kg IV each month; increase as needed to max 400 to 800 mg/kg/month.
UNAPPROVED ADULTS – First line therapy in severe Guillain-Barré syndrome, chronic inflammatory demyelinating polyneuropathy, multifocal motor neuropathy, severe posttransfusion purpura, inclusion body myositis, fetomaternal alloimmune thrombocytopenia; 2nd line therapy in stiff-person syndrome, dermatomyositis, myasthenia gravis, and Lambert-Eaton myasthenic syndrome. Various dosing regimens have been used; a common one is myasthenia gravis (induction): 400 mg/kg IV daily for 5 days (total 2 g/kg). Has been used in multiple sclerosis and inflammatory myositis (polymyositis and dermatomyositis), renal transplant rejection, systemic lupus erythematosus, toxic epidermal necrolysis and Stevens-Johnson syndrome, Clostridium difficile colitis, Graves' ophthalmopathy, pemphigus, Wegener's granulomatosis, Churg-Strauss syndrome, and Duchenne muscular dystrophy.
UNAPPROVED PEDS – Myasthenia gravis (induction): 400 mg/kg IV daily for 5 days. Other dosing regimens have been used.
NOTES – Indications and doses vary by product. Follow LFTs, renal function, vital signs, and urine output closely. Contraindicated in IgA deficiency. Use caution (and lower infusion rates) if risk factors for thrombosis, heart failure, or renal insufficiency. Use slower infusion rates for initial doses. Consider pretreatment with acetaminophen and/or diphenhydramine to minimize some infusion-related adverse effects. Human-derived product; although donors are carefully screened there is risk of transmission of infectious agents.
MOA – Immunomodulatory effects through exogenous immunoglobulins.
ADVERSE EFFECTS – Serious: Acute renal failure, non-cardiogenic pulmonary edema, hemolysis, heart failure, stroke, MI, DVT, aseptic meningitis, anaphylaxis. Frequent: Infusion reactions, HA, vomiting, fever, chills, hypotension, rash, back pain, reversible neutropenia, pain at injection site.

IMMUNE GLOBULIN—SUBCUTANEOUS (*Vivaglobulin, Hizentra*) ▶L ♀C ▶? $$$$$
ADULTS – Primary immune deficiency: 100 to 200 mg/kg SC weekly. In patients already receiving IV immune globulin: SC dose is equivalent to (previous IV dose × 1.37) divided by frequency of IV regimen in week.
PEDS – Limited information. Dosing appears to be same as in adults.
NOTES – Do not administer IV. Contraindicated in IgA deficiency. Human-derived product, increased infection risk.
MOA – Passive immunity.
ADVERSE EFFECTS – Serious: Acute hypersensitivity reactions, anaphylaxis. Frequent: Injection site reactions, HA, nausea/vomiting, fever, rash, pain, diarrhea, sore throat.

LYMPHOCYTE IMMUNE GLOBULIN (*Atgam*) ▶L ♀C ▶? $$$$$
ADULTS – Renal allograft recipients: 10 to 30 mg/kg IV daily. Delaying onset of allograft rejection: 15 mg/kg IV daily for 14 days, then every other day for 14 days. Treatment of renal transplant rejection: 10 to 15 mg/kg IV for 14 days. Aplastic anemia: 10 to 20 mg/kg IV daily for 8 to 14 days, then every other day, as needed, up to 21 total doses.
PEDS – Limited experience. Has been safely administered to a limited number of children with renal transplant and aplastic anemia at doses comparable to adults.
NOTES – Equine product. Doses should be administered over at least 4 h.
MOA – Lymphocyte-specific immunosuppressant.
ADVERSE EFFECTS – Frequent: Fever, chills, skin reactions, systemic infections, abnormal renal function, serum-sickness-like reactions, dyspnea, arthralgia, chest, back, flank pain, diarrhea, N/V. Severe: Anaphylaxis, hemolysis, thrombocytopenia, leukopenia.

RABIES IMMUNE GLOBULIN HUMAN (*Imogam Rabies-HT, HyperRAB S/D*) ▶L ♀C ▶? $$$$$
ADULTS — <u>Postexposure prophylaxis:</u> 20 units/kg (0.133 mL/kg), with as much as possible infiltrated around the bite and the rest given IM. Give as soon as possible after exposure. Administer with the first dose of vaccine, but in a different extremity.
PEDS — Not approved in children.
UNAPPROVED PEDS — Use adult dosing.
NOTES — Do not repeat dose once rabies vaccine series begins. Do not give to patients who have been completely immunized with rabies vaccine. Do not administer IV.
MOA — Passive immunity.
ADVERSE EFFECTS — Frequent: Pain at injection site, sensitization. Severe: Anaphylaxis, angioedema, skin rash, nephrotic syndrome.

RSV IMMUNE GLOBULIN (*RespiGam*) ▶Plasma ♀C ▶? $$$$$
PEDS — <u>RSV prophylaxis:</u> 1.5 mL/kg/h for 15 min for age younger than 24 mo. Increase rate as clinical condition permits to 3 mL/kg/h for 15 min, then to a maximum rate of 6 mL/kg/h. Max total dose/month is 750 mg/kg.
NOTES — May cause fluid overload; monitor vital signs frequently during IV infusion. RSV season is typically November-April.
MOA — Passive immunity.
ADVERSE EFFECTS — Frequent: Rash, fever, tachycardia, hypotension, hypertension, vomiting, diarrhea, gastroenteritis.

TETANUS IMMUNE GLOBULIN (*BayTet, ✦Hypertet*) ▶L ♀C ▶? $$$$
ADULTS — See tetanus wound management table. <u>Postexposure prophylaxis in tetanus prone wounds for age 7 yo or greater:</u> if less than 3 doses of tetanus vaccine have been administered or if history is uncertain, give 250 units IM for 1 dose along with dT. If at least 3 doses of tetanus vaccine have been administered in the past, do not give tetanus immune globulin. <u>Tetanus treatment:</u> 3000 to 6000 units IM in combination with other therapies.
PEDS — 4 units/kg IM or 250 units IM for age younger than 7 yo. Initiate tetanus toxoid vaccine (DTP or DT).
NOTES — Do not give tetanus immune globulin for clean, minor wounds. May be given at the same time as tetanus toxoid active immunization. Do not inject IV.
MOA — Passive immunity.
ADVERSE EFFECTS — Frequent: Pain at injection site, sensitization. Severe: Anaphylaxis, angioedema, skin rash, nephrotic syndrome.

VARICELLA-ZOSTER IMMUNE GLOBULIN (*VariZIG, VZIG*) ▶L ♀C ▶? $$$$$
ADULTS — Specialized dosing for postexposure prophylaxis.
PEDS — Specialized dosing for postexposure prophylaxis.
MOA — Passive immunity.
ADVERSE EFFECTS — Frequent: Pain at injection site, sensitization. Severe: Anaphylaxis, angioedema, skin rash, nephrotic syndrome.

IMMUNOLOGY: Immunosuppression

BASILIXIMAB (*Simulect*) ▶Plasma ♀B ▶? $$$$$
WARNING — To be used only by trained physicians. To be given only in facility with adequate laboratory and supportive medical resources.
ADULTS — Specialized dosing for <u>organ transplantation.</u>
PEDS — Specialized dosing for <u>organ transplantation.</u>
MOA — Immunosuppressant, prophylaxis of acute organ rejection.
ADVERSE EFFECTS — Frequent: Administration did not increase the incidence or severity of adverse events over placebo in immunosuppressed patients.

CYCLOSPORINE (*Sandimmune, Neoral, Gengraf*) ▶L ♀C ▶– $$$$$
WARNING — Should only be prescribed by physicians who are knowledgeable about the drug. Serious adverse effects can occur.
ADULTS — Specialized dosing <u>for organ transplantation, RA, and psoriasis.</u>
PEDS — Not approved in children.
UNAPPROVED ADULTS — Specialized dosing for <u>autoimmune eye disorders, vasculitis, inflammatory myopathies, Behcet's disease, psoriatic arthritis, chronic refractory idiopathic thrombocytopenia.</u>
UNAPPROVED PEDS — Specialized dosing for <u>organ transplantation, chronic refractory idiopathic thrombocytopenia.</u>
FORMS — Generic/Trade: Microemulsion Caps 25, 100 mg. Generic/Trade: Caps (Sandimmune) 25, 100 mg. Soln (Sandimmune) 100 mg/mL. Microemulsion soln (Neoral, Gengraf) 100 mg/mL.
NOTES — Monitor cyclosporine blood concentrations closely. Many drug interactions including atorvastatin, azithromycin, lovastatin, oral contraceptives, rosuvastatin, simvastatin, sirolimus, terbinafine, voriconazole. Use caution when combining with methotrexate or potassium sparing drugs such as ACE inhibitors. Reduce dose in renal dysfunction. Monitor BP and renal function closely. Avoid excess UV light exposure. Monitor patients closely when switching from Sandimmune to microemulsion formulations.
MOA — Immunosuppressant, prophylaxis of acute organ rejection.
ADVERSE EFFECTS — Frequent: Hypertension, hirsutism, hypomagnesemia, hypokalemia, gingival hypertrophy, tremor, nephrotoxicity. Severe: Anaphylaxis, infection and increased risk of lymphoma and other malignancies, especially those of the skin, risk, optic disc edema, benign intracranial hypertension, papilledema, visual impairment.

IMMUNOLOGY: Immunosuppression

DACLIZUMAB (*Zenapax*) ▶L ♀C ▶? $$$$$
WARNING — Should only be prescribed by physicians who are knowledgeable about the drug. Serious adverse effects have been reported.
ADULTS — Specialized dosing for organ transplantation.
PEDS — Not approved in children.
UNAPPROVED PEDS — Specialized dosing for organ transplantation.
MOA — Immunosuppressant, prophylaxis of acute organ rejection.
ADVERSE EFFECTS — Frequent: Hyperglycemia.

MYCOPHENOLATE MOFETIL (*Cellcept, Myfortic*) ▶? ♀D ▶? $$$$$
WARNING — Has been associated with lymphoma, malignancy, increased risk of infection, and progressive multifocal leukoencephalopathy (PML).
ADULTS — Specialized dosing for organ transplantation.
PEDS — Not approved in children.
UNAPPROVED ADULTS — Lupus nephritis: 1000 mg PO bid. Has been used in pemphigus, bullous pemphigoid, and refractory uveitis.
UNAPPROVED PEDS — Specialized dosing for organ transplantation.
FORMS — Generic/Trade: Caps 250 mg. Tabs 500 mg. Trade only (CellCept): Susp 200 mg/mL. Trade only (Myfortic): Tabs Extended-release: 180, 360 mg.
NOTES — Increased risk of 1st trimester pregnancy loss and increased risk of congenital malformations, especially external ear and facial abnormalities.
MOA — Immunosuppressant, prophylaxis of acute organ rejection.
ADVERSE EFFECTS — Frequent: GI upset, thrombophlebitis, thrombosis (with IV administration). Severe: Infection, GI bleeding, nephrotic syndrome, bone marrow suppression, leukopenia, lymphoma, malignancy, progressive multifocal leukoencephalopathy, pure red cell aplasia.

SIROLIMUS (*Rapamune*) ▶L ♀C ▶– $$$$$
WARNING — Increased risk of infection and lymphoma. Combination of sirolimus plus cyclosporine or tacrolimus is associated with hepatic artery thrombosis in liver transplant patients. Combination with tacrolimus and corticosteroids in lung transplant patients may cause bronchial anastomotic dehiscence. Possible increased mortality in stable liver transplant patients after conversion from a calcineurin inhibitor (CNI)-based immunosuppressive regimen to sirolimus. Can cause hypersensitivity reactions including anaphylactic and/or anaphylactoid reactions, angioedema, vasculitis. Avoid with strong inhibitors of CYP3A4 and/or P-glycoprotein (ketoconazole, voriconazole, itraconazole, erythromycin, clarithromycin) or strong inducers CYP3A4 and/or P-glycoprotein (rifampin, rifabutin). Monitor level if cyclosporine is discontinued or has dose markedly changed.
ADULTS — Specialized dosing for organ transplantation.
PEDS — Not approved in children.
UNAPPROVED PEDS — Specialized dosing for organ transplantation.
FORMS — Trade only: Soln 1 mg/mL (60 mL). Tabs 1, 2 mg.
NOTES — Wear protective clothing and sunscreen when exposed to sunlight to reduce the risk of skin cancer. Be aware of site-specific assay method, as this may affect reported serum concentrations. Adjust dose by 1/3 to 1/2 in liver dysfunction. Monitor trough levels, particularly in patients likely to have altered drug metabolism, age 13 yo or older with wt less than 40 kg, hepatic impairment, when changing doses or with interacting medications. Do not adjust dose more frequently than q 1 to 2 weeks. Oral soln and tabs are clinically equivalent from a dosing standpoint at the 2 mg level; however, this is unknown at higher doses.
MOA — Immunosuppressant, prophylaxis of acute organ rejection in solid organ transplant.
ADVERSE EFFECTS — Frequent: Hypertension, edema, chest pain, fever, headache, pain, insomnia, rash, hypercholesterolemia, increased triglycerides, abdominal pain, renal dysfunction, nausea, diarrhea, anemia, thrombocytopenia, arthralgia, dyspnea. Severe: Hepatic artery thrombosis in liver transplant patients, hypersensitivity reactions, nephrotic syndrome, exfoliative dermatitis, impaired wound healing, angioedema, vasculitis, interstitial lung disease, hemolytic uremic syndrome/thrombotic thrombocytopenic purpura/thrombotic microangiopathy, increased risk of infections such as tuberculosis, especially when used with calcineurin inhibitor.

TACROLIMUS (*Prograf, FK 506*) ▶L ♀C ▶– $$$$$
ADULTS — Specialized dosing for organ transplantation.
PEDS — Specialized dosing for organ transplantation.
UNAPPROVED ADULTS — RA (approved in Canada), active vasculitis, systemic lupus erythematosus nephritis, and vasculitis.
FORMS — Generic/Trade: Caps 0.5, 1, 5 mg.
NOTES — Reduce dose in renal dysfunction. Monitor BP and renal function closely. Neurotoxic, especially in high doses. Many drug interactions. Increased risk of infections.
MOA — Immunosuppressant, prophylaxis of acute organ rejection.
ADVERSE EFFECTS — Frequent: Hypertension, peripheral edema, headache, insomnia, pain, fever, pruritus, N/V, diarrhea, abdominal pain, tremors, paresthesias. Severe: Anaphylaxis, edema, hypertrophic cardiomyopathy, myocardial hypertrophy, ECG abnormalities and arrhythmias, paralysis, stroke, hemolytic uremic syndrome, nephrotoxicity, secondary malignancy.

IMMUNOLOGY: Other

HYMENOPTERA VENOM ▶Serum ♀C ▶? $$$$
ADULTS — Specialized desensitization dosing protocol.
PEDS — Specialized desensitization dosing protocol.
NOTES — Venom products available: Honey bee (Apis mellifera) and yellow jacket (Vespula sp.), yellow hornet (Dolichovespula arenaria), white-faced hornet (D maculata) and wasp (Polistes sp.). Mixed vespid venom protein (yellow jacket, yellow hornet and white-faced hornet) is also available.
MOA — Desensitization protein.
ADVERSE EFFECTS — Frequent: Erythema, swelling, pruritus, burning. Severe: Systemic reactions, anaphylaxis, death.

TUBERCULIN PPD (*Aplisol, Tubersol, Mantoux, PPD*) ▶L ♀C ▶+ $
ADULTS — 5 TU (0.1 mL) intradermally.
PEDS — Same as adult dose. AAP recommends screening at 12 mo, 4 to 6 yo, and 14 to 16 yo.
NOTES — Avoid SC injection. Read 48 to 72 h after intradermal injection. Repeat testing in patients with known prior positive PPD may cause scarring at injection site.
MOA — Skin test for diagnosis of tuberculosis.
ADVERSE EFFECTS — Frequent: Ulceration, necrosis, vesiculation.

NEUROLOGY: Alzheimer's Disease—Cholinesterase Inhibitors

NOTE: Avoid concurrent use of anticholinergic agents. Use caution in asthma/COPD. May be coadministered with memantine.

DONEPEZIL (*Aricept*) ▶LK ♀C ▶? $$$$
ADULTS — <u>Alzheimer's disease:</u> Start 5 mg PO at bedtime. May increase to 10 mg PO at bedtime in 4 to 6 weeks for mild to moderate disease. For moderate to severe disease (MMSE 10 or less), may increase after 3 months to 23 mg/day.
PEDS — Not approved in children.
UNAPPROVED ADULTS — <u>Dementia in Parkinson's disease:</u> 5 to 10 mg/day.
FORMS — Generic/Trade: Tabs 5, 10 mg. Trade only: Tab 23 mg. Orally disintegrating tabs 5, 10 mg.
NOTES — Some clinicians start with 5 mg PO every other day to minimize GI side effects.
MOA — Reversible acetylcholinesterase inhibitor.
ADVERSE EFFECTS — Serious: Cholinergic crisis, seizures, bradycardia, syncope, hypotension, respiratory depression. Frequent: N/V, diarrhea, anorexia, insomnia, muscle cramps, fatigue, ecchymosis.

GALANTAMINE (*Razadyne, Razadyne ER, ✦Reminyl*) ▶LK ♀B ▶? $$$$
ADULTS — <u>Alzheimer's disease:</u> Extended-release: Start 8 mg PO qam with food; increase to 16 mg qam after 4 weeks. May increase to 24 mg qam after another 4 weeks. Immediate-release: Start 4 mg PO bid with food; increase to 8 mg bid after 4 weeks. May increase to 12 mg PO bid after another 4 weeks.
PEDS — Not approved in children.
UNAPPROVED ADULTS — <u>Dementia in Parkinson's disease:</u> 4 to 8 mg PO bid (immediate-release).
FORMS — Generic/Trade: Tabs 4, 8, 12 mg. Extended-release caps 8, 16, 24 mg. Oral soln 4 mg/mL. Prior to April 2005 was called Reminyl.
NOTES — Do not exceed 16 mg/day with renal or hepatic impairment. Use caution with CYP3A4 and CYP2D6 inhibitors. Avoid abrupt discontinuation. If therapy has been interrupted for several days or more, then restart at the lowest dose.
MOA — Reversible acetylcholinesterase inhibitor.
ADVERSE EFFECTS — Serious: Cholinergic crisis, seizures, bradycardia, syncope, hypotension. Frequent: N/V, diarrhea, anorexia, weight loss, muscle cramps.

RIVASTIGMINE (*Exelon, Exelon Patch*) ▶K ♀B ▶? $$$$$
ADULTS — <u>Alzheimer's disease:</u> Start 1.5 mg PO bid with food. Increase to 3 mg bid after 2 weeks. Usual effective dose is 6 to 12 mg/day. Max 12 mg/day. Patch: Start 4.6 mg/24 h once daily; may increase after 1 month or more to max 9.5 mg/24 h. <u>Dementia associated with Parkinson's disease:</u> Start 1.5 mg PO bid with food. Increase by 3 mg/day at intervals more than 4 weeks to max 12 mg/day. Patch: Start 4.6 mg/24 h once daily; may increase after 1 month or more to max 9.5 mg/24 h.
PEDS — Not approved in children.
FORMS — Trade only: Caps 1.5, 3, 4.5, 6 mg. Oral soln 2 mg/mL (120 mL). Transdermal patch: 4.6 mg/24 h (9 mg/patch), 9.5 mg/24 h (18 mg/patch).
NOTES — Restart treatment with the lowest daily dose (ie, 1.5 mg PO bid) if discontinued for several days to reduce the risk of severe vomiting. Use soln if difficulty swallowing. When changing from PO to patch, patients taking less than 6 mg/day can be placed on 4.6 mg/24 h patch. For those taking 6 to 12 mg/day, may start with 9.5 mg/24 h patch. Have patient start the day after stopping oral dosing. Rotate application sites and do not apply to same spot for 14 days.
MOA — Reversible acetylcholinesterase inhibitor.
ADVERSE EFFECTS — Serious: Cholinergic crisis, seizures, bradycardia, syncope, hypotension, respiratory depression. Frequent: N/V, diarrhea, dyspepsia, anorexia, weight loss, muscle cramps, headache, dizziness, asthenia.

NEUROLOGY: Alzheimer's Disease—NMDA Receptor Antagonists

MEMANTINE (*Namenda, Namenda XR, ♣Ebixa*) ▶KL ♀B ▶? $$$$
ADULTS — Alzheimer's disease (moderate to severe): Start 5 mg PO daily. Increase by 5 mg/day at weekly intervals to max 20 mg/day. Doses greater than 5 mg/day should be divided bid. Extended-release: Start 7 mg once daily. Increase at weekly intervals to target dose of 28 mg/day. Reduce to 14 mg/day with renal impairment.
PEDS — Not approved in children.
FORMS — Trade only: Tabs 5, 10 mg. Oral soln 2 mg/mL. Extended-release caps 7, 14, 21, 28 mg.
NOTES — May be used in combination with acetylcholinesterase inhibitors. Reduce target dose to 5 mg PO bid in severe renal impairment (CrCl 5 to 29 mL/min). No dosage adjustment needed for mild–moderate renal impairment. When switching to extended-release caps patients taking 10 mg bid can be changed to 28 mg/day of ER after last regular dose. Patients switched from 5 mg bid can be changed to 14 mg/day of ER.
MOA — N-methyl-D-aspartate (NMDA) receptor antagonist.
ADVERSE EFFECTS — Serious: None. Frequent: Hypertension, dizziness, headache, constipation, confusion.

NEUROLOGY: Anticonvulsants

NOTE: Avoid rapid discontinuation of anticonvulsants, since this can precipitate seizures or other withdrawal symptoms. Recent data suggest an increased risk of suicidal ideation or behaviors with antiepileptic drugs. Monitor closely for signs of depression, anxiety, hostility, hypomania/mania, or suicidality. Symptoms may develop within 1 week of initiation, and risk continues for at least 24 weeks.

CARBAMAZEPINE (*Tegretol, Tegretol XR, Carbatrol, Epitol, Equetro*) ▶LK ♀D ▶+ $$
WARNING — Risk of aplastic anemia and agranulocytosis; contraindicated if prior marrow depression. Monitor CBC at baseline and periodically.
ADULTS — Epilepsy: Start 200 mg PO bid. Increase by 200 mg/day at weekly intervals, divided tid to qid (regular-release), bid (extended-release), or qid (susp) to max 1600 mg/day. Trigeminal neuralgia: Start 100 mg PO bid or 50 mg PO qid (susp); increase by 200 mg/day until pain relief. Max 1200 mg/day. Bipolar disorder, acute manic/mixed episodes (Equetro): Start 200 mg PO bid; increase by 200 mg/day to max 1600 mg/day. See "unapproved adult" section for alternative bipolar dosing.
PEDS — Epilepsy, age younger than 6 yo: Start 10 to 20 mg/kg/day PO divided bid to tid or qid (suspension). Increase weekly prn. Max 35 mg/kg/day. Epilepsy, age 6 to 12 yo: Start 100 mg PO bid or 50 mg PO qid (susp); increase by 100 mg/day at weekly intervals divided tid to qid (regular-release), bid (extended-release), or qid (susp) to max 1000 mg/day. Epilepsy, age 13 yo or older: Start 200 mg PO bid or 100 mg PO qid (suspension); increase by 200 mg/day at weekly intervals, divided tid to qid (regular release), bid (extended-release), or qid (suspension) to max 1000 mg/day (age 13 to 15 yo) or 1200 mg/day (age older than 15 yo).
UNAPPROVED ADULTS — Neuropathic pain: Start 100 mg PO bid; usual effective dose is 200 mg PO bid to qid. Max 1200 mg/day. Mania (American Psychiatric Association guidelines): Start 200 to 600 mg/day divided tid to qid (standard-release) or bid (extended-release), then increase by 200 mg/day q 2 to 4 days. Mean effective dose is 1000 mg/day. Max 1600 mg/day.
UNAPPROVED PEDS — Bipolar disorder (manic or mixed phase): Start 100 to 200 mg PO daily or bid; titrate to usual effective dose of 200 to 600 mg/day for children and up to 1200 mg/day for adolescents.
FORMS — Generic/Trade: Tabs 200 mg, Chewable tabs 100 mg, Susp 100 mg/5 mL. Extended-release tabs (Tegretol XR) 100, 200, 400 mg. Generic only: Tabs 100, 300, 400 mg, Chewable tabs 200 mg. Trade only: Extended-release caps (Carbatrol and Equetro): 100, 200, 300 mg.
NOTES — Usual therapeutic level is 4 to 12 mcg/mL. Stevens-Johnson syndrome, hepatitis, aplastic anemia, and hyponatremia may occur. Monitor CBC and LFTs. Many drug interactions. Should not be used for absence or atypical absence seizures. Dangerous and possibly fatal skin reactions are more common with the HLA-B*1502 allele most common in people of Asian and Indian ancestry; screen new patients for this allele prior to starting therapy.
MOA — Anticonvulsant, sodium channel blocker.
ADVERSE EFFECTS — Serious: Aplastic anemia and other blood dyscrasias, hepatotoxicity, SIADH/hyponatremia, rash, Stevens-Johnson syndrome, toxic epidermal necrolysis, hypersensitivity reactions, suicidality. Frequent: Drowsiness, ataxia, dizziness, confusion, N/V, blurred vision, nystagmus.

CLOBAZAM (*♣Frisium*) ▶L ♀X (first trimester) D (second/third trimesters) ▶– $
WARNING — Caution in the elderly; may accumulate and cause side effects such as psychomotor impairment.
ADULTS — Canada only. Epilepsy, adjunctive: Start 5 to 15 mg PO daily. Gradually increase prn to max 80 mg/day.
PEDS — Canada only. Epilepsy, adjunctive: Start 0.5 to 1 mg/kg PO daily for age younger than 2 yo, start 5 mg daily for age 2 to 16 yo: Then may increase prn to max 40 mg/day.
FORMS — Generic/Trade: Tabs 10 mg.

(cont.)

NEUROLOGY: Anticonvulsants

DERMATOMES MOTOR FUNCTION BY NERVE ROOTS	
Level	Motor Function
C3/C4/C5	Diaphragm
C5/C6	Deltoid/biceps
C7/C8	Triceps
C8/T1	Finger flexion/intrinsics
T1–T12	Intercostal/abd muscles
L2/L3	Hip flexion
L2/L3/L4	Hip adduction/quads
L4/L5	Ankle dorsiflexion
S1/S2	Ankle plantarflexion
S2/S3/S4	Rectal tone

	Root	Motor	Sensory	Reflex
LUMBOSACRAL	L4	quadriceps	medial foot	knee-jerk
NERVE ROOT	L5	dorsiflexors	dorsum of foot	medial hamstring
COMPRESSION	S1	plantarflexors	lateral foot	ankle-jerk

GLASGOW COMA SCALE

	Verbal Activity	Motor Activity
Eye Opening	5. Oriented	6. Obeys commands
4. Spontaneous	4. Confused	5. Localizes pain
3. To command	3. Inappropriate	4. Withdraws to pain
2. To pain	2. Incomprehensible	3. Flexion to pain
1. None	1. None	2. Extension to pain
		1. None

CLOBAZAM *(cont.)*
 NOTES — Reduce dose in hepatic or renal dysfunction. Drug interactions with enzyme-inducing anticonvulsants such as carbamazepine and phenytoin; may need to adjust dose.
 MOA — Benzodiazepine; potentiates GABA-ergic transmission.
 ADVERSE EFFECTS — Serious: Respiratory and CNS depression, tolerance, dependence, suicidality. Frequent: Drowsiness, dizziness, fatigue, orthostatic hypotension.

ETHOSUXIMIDE (*Zarontin*) ▶LK ♀C ▶+ $$$$
 ADULTS — Absence seizures: Start 500 mg PO given once daily or divided bid. Increase by 250 mg/day q 4 to 7 d prn. Max 1.5 g/day.
 PEDS — Absence seizures: Start 250 mg PO daily or divided bid. (up to 500 mg/day) for age 3 to 6 yo. Use adult dosing for age older than 6 yo.
 UNAPPROVED PEDS — Absence seizures, age younger than 3 yo: Start 15 mg/kg/day PO divided bid. Increase q 4 to 7 d prn. Usual effective dose is 15 to 40 mg/kg/day divided bid. Max 500 mg/day.
 FORMS — Generic/Trade: Caps 250 mg. Syrup 250 mg/5 mL.
 NOTES — Usual therapeutic level is 40 to 100 mcg/mL. Monitor CBC for blood dyscrasias. Use caution in hepatic and renal impairment. May increase the risk of grand mal seizures in some patients.
 MOA — Increases seizure threshold by reducing current in T-type calcium channels.
 ADVERSE EFFECTS — Serious: Blood dyscrasias, hepatotoxicity, Stevens-Johnson syndrome, drug-induced lupus, suicidality. Frequent: N/V, anorexia, weight loss, abdominal pain, rash, drowsiness, irritability, headache, fatigue, ataxia, euphoria.

FELBAMATE (*Felbatol*) ▶KL ♀C ▶– $$$$$
 WARNING — Aplastic anemia and fatal hepatic failure have occurred.
 ADULTS — Severe, refractory epilepsy: Start 400 mg PO tid. Increase by 600 mg/day q 2 weeks to max 3600 mg/day.
 PEDS — Lennox-Gastaut syndrome, adjunctive therapy, age 2 to 14 yo: Start 15 mg/kg/day PO in 3 to 4 divided doses. Increase by 15 mg/kg/day at weekly intervals to max 45 mg/kg/day.
 FORMS — Trade only: Tabs 400, 600 mg. Susp 600 mg/5 mL.
 NOTES — Use only after discussing the risks and obtaining written informed consent. Many drug interactions.
 MOA — Increases seizure threshold by blocking glycine binding to NMDA receptors.
 ADVERSE EFFECTS — Serious: Aplastic anemia, hepatotoxicity, liver failure, purpura, maculopapular rash, suicidality. Frequent: Insomnia, headache, anxiety, N/V, diarrhea, constipation, rhinitis.

NEUROLOGY: Anticonvulsants

FOSPHENYTOIN (*Cerebyx*) ▶L ♀D ▶+ $$$$$
ADULTS — Status epilepticus: Load 15 to 20 mg "phenytoin equivalents" (PE) per kg IV no faster than 100 to 150 mg PE/min. Nonemergent loading dose: 10 to 20 mg PE/kg IM/IV at rate no greater than 150 mg/min. Maintenance: 4 to 6 mg PE/kg/day.
PEDS — Not approved in children.
UNAPPROVED PEDS — Status epilepticus: 15 to 20 mg PE/kg IV at a rate less than 2 mg PE/kg/min. Nonemergent use age older than 7 yo: 4 to 6 mg PE/kg/24 h IV/IM no faster than 100 to 150 mg PE/min.
NOTES — Fosphenytoin is dosed in "phenytoin equivalents" (PE). Use beyond 5 days has not been systematically studied. Monitor ECG and vital signs continuously during and after infusion. Contraindicated in cardiac conduction block. Many drug interactions. Usual therapeutic level is 10 to 20 mcg/mL in normal hepatorenal function. Renal/hepatic disease may change protein binding and levels. Low albumin levels may increase free fraction.
MOA — Prodrug for phenytoin. Increases seizure threshold by modulating sodium and calcium channels.
ADVERSE EFFECTS — Serious: Cardiovascular collapse, CNS depression, hypotension, arrhythmias, hypersensitivity reactions, Stevens-Johnson syndrome, blood dyscrasias, hepatotoxicity, suicidality. Frequent: Nystagmus, dizziness, pruritus, paresthesia, headache, drowsiness, ataxia.

GABAPENTIN (*Neurontin*) ▶K ♀C ▶? $$$$
ADULTS — Partial seizures, adjunctive therapy: Start 300 mg PO at bedtime. Increase gradually to usual effective dose of 300 to 600 mg PO tid. Max 3600 mg/day. Postherpetic neuralgia: Start 300 mg PO on day 1. Increase to 300 mg bid on day 2, and to 300 mg tid on day 3. Max 1800 mg/day divided tid.
PEDS — Partial seizures, adjunctive therapy: Start 10 to 15 mg/kg/day PO divided tid for age 3 to 12 yo. Titrate over 3 days to usual effective dose of 25 to 40 mg/kg/day divided tid. Max 50 mg/kg/day. Use adult dosing for age older than 12 yo.
UNAPPROVED ADULTS — Partial seizures, initial monotherapy: Titrate as above. Usual effective dose is 900 to 1800 mg/day. Neuropathic pain: 300 mg PO tid, max 3600 mg/day in 3 to 4 divided doses. Migraine prophylaxis: Start 300 mg PO daily, then gradually increase to 1200 to 2400 mg/day in 3 to 4 divided doses. Restless legs syndrome: Start 300 mg PO at bedtime. Max 3600 mg/day divided tid. Hot flashes: 300 mg PO tid.
UNAPPROVED PEDS — Neuropathic pain: Start 5 mg/kg PO at bedtime. Increase to 5 mg/kg bid on day 2 and 5 mg/kg tid on day 3. Titrate to usual effective level of 8 to 35 mg/kg/24 h.
FORMS — Generic only: Tabs 100, 300, 400 mg. Generic/Trade: Caps 100, 300, 400 mg. Tabs scored 600, 800 mg. Soln 50 mg/mL.
NOTES — Decrease dose in renal impairment (CrCl < 60 mL/min); table in package insert. Discontinue gradually over ≥1 week.
MOA — Unknown. Does not appear to be a GABA analog.
ADVERSE EFFECTS — Serious: Leukopenia. Frequent: Fatigue, drowsiness, dizziness, ataxia, nystagmus, tremor, peripheral edema, weight gain, suicidality. Peds only: Emotional lability, hostility, hyperactivity.

LACOSAMIDE (*Vimpat*) ▶KL ♀C ▶? $$$$$
ADULTS — Partial onset seizures, adjunctive (17 yo and older): Start 50 mg PO/IV bid. Increase by 50 mg bid to recommended dose of 100 to 200 mg bid. Max 600 mg/day or 300 mg/day in mild/mod hepatic failure or severe renal impairment (CrCl < 30 mL/min).
PEDS — Not approved in children.
FORMS — Trade only: Tabs 50, 100, 150, 200 mg.
NOTES — Use caution in patients with cardiac conduction problems or on drugs that increase the PR interval.
MOA — Enhances slow inactivation of voltage-gated sodium channels.
ADVERSE EFFECTS — Severe: Increased PR interval, AV block, suicidality, syncope. Frequent: Dizziness, ataxia, nausea/vomiting, diplopia, vertigo, blurred vision, headache.

LAMOTRIGINE (*Lamictal, Lamictal CD, Lamictal ODT*) ▶LK ♀C (see notes) ▶− $$$$
WARNING — Potentially life-threatening rashes (eg, Stevens-Johnson Syndrome) have been reported in 0.3% of adults and 0.8% of children, usually within 2 to 8 weeks of initiation; discontinue at first sign of rash. Drug interaction with valproate; see adjusted dosing guidelines.
ADULTS — Partial seizures, Lennox-Gastaut syndrome, or generalized tonic-clonic seizures, adjunctive therapy with an enzyme-inducing anticonvulsant (age older than 12 yo): Start 50 mg PO daily for 2 weeks, then 50 mg PO bid for 2 weeks. Increase by 100 mg/day q 1 to 2 weeks to usual maintenance dose of 150 to 250 mg PO bid. Partial seizures, conversion to monotherapy from adjunctive therapy with a single enzyme-inducing anticonvulsant (age 16 yo): Use above guidelines to gradually increase the dose to 250 mg PO bid; then taper the enzyme-inducing anticonvulsant by 20% per week over 4 weeks. Partial seizures, Lennox-Gastaut syndrome, or generalized tonic-clonic seizures, adjunctive therapy with valproate (age > 12 yo): Start 25 mg PO every other day for 2 weeks, then 25 mg PO daily for 2 weeks. Increase by 25 to 50 mg/day q 1 to 2 weeks to usual maintenance dose of 100 to 400 mg/day (when used with valproate + other anticonvulsants) or 100 to 200 mg/day (when used with valproate alone) given once daily or divided bid. Partial seizures, conversion to monotherapy from adjunctive therapy with valproate (age 16 yo): Use above guidelines to gradually increase the dose to 200 mg/day PO given daily or divided bid; then decrease valproate weekly in increments less than or equal to 500 mg/day to an initial goal of 500 mg/day. After 1 week at these doses, increase lamotrigine to 300 mg/day and decrease

(cont.)

LAMOTRIGINE (cont.)

valproate to 250 mg/day divided bid. A week later, discontinue valproate; then increase lamotrigine weekly by 100 mg/day to usual maintenance dose of 500 mg/day. Partial seizures, Lennox-Gastaut syndrome, or generalized tonic-clonic seizures, adjunctive therapy with other anticonvulsants (not valproate or enzyme inducers) (age older than 12 yo): Start 25 mg PO daily for 2 weeks, then 50 mg PO daily for 2 weeks. Increase by 50 mg/day every 1 to 2 weeks to usual maintenance dose of 225 to 375 mg/day divided bid. See psychiatry section for bipolar disorder dosing.

PEDS — Partial seizures, Lennox-Gastaut syndrome or generalized tonic-clonic seizures, adjunctive therapy with an enzyme-inducing anticonvulsant, age 2 to 12 yo: Start 0.6 mg/kg/day PO divided bid for 2 weeks, then 1.2 mg/kg/day PO divided bid for 2 weeks. Increase every 1 to 2 weeks by 1.2 mg/kg/day (rounded down to the nearest whole tab) to usual maintenance dose of 5 to 15 mg/kg/day. Max 400 mg/day. Partial seizures, Lennox-Gastaut syndrome, or generalized tonic-clonic seizures, adjunctive therapy with valproate, age 2 to 12 yo: Start 0.15 mg/kg/day PO (given daily or divided bid) for 2 weeks, then 0.3 mg/kg/day PO (given daily or divided bid) for 2 weeks. Increase every 1 to 2 weeks by 0.3 mg/kg/day (rounded down to nearest whole tab) to usual maintenance dose of 1 to 5 mg/kg/day (lamotrigine + valproate and other anticonvulsants) or 1 to 3 mg/kg/day if used with valproate alone. Max 200 mg/day. Partial seizures, Lennox-Gastaut syndrome, or generalized tonic-clonic seizures, adjunctive therapy with other anticonvulsants (not valproate or enzyme inducers), age 2 to 12 yo: Start 0.3 mg/kg/day (given daily or divided bid) for 2 weeks, then 0.6 mg/kg/day for 2 weeks. Increase every 1 to 2 weeks by 0.6 mg/kg/day (rounded down to nearest whole tab) to usual maintenance dose of 4.5 to 7.5 mg/kg/day. Max 300 mg/day. Age older than 12 yo: Use adult dosing for all of the above indications.

UNAPPROVED ADULTS — Initial monotherapy for partial seizures: Start 25 mg PO daily. Usual maintenance dose is 100 to 300 mg/day divided bid. Max 500 mg/day.

UNAPPROVED PEDS — Initial monotherapy for partial seizures: Start 0.5 mg/kg/day given daily or divided bid. Max 10 mg/kg/day. Newly-diagnosed absence seizures: Titrate as above. Usual effective dose is 2 to 15 mg/kg/day.

FORMS — Generic/Trade: Chewable dispersible tabs (Lamictal CD) 2, 5, 25 mg. Tabs, 25, 100, 150, 200 mg. Trade only: Orally disintegrating tabs (Lamictal ODT) 25, 50, 100, 200 mg. Chewable dispersible tabs (Lamictal CD) 2 mg may not be available in all pharmacies; obtain through manufacturer representative, or by calling 888-825-5249.

NOTES — Drug interactions with valproate and enzyme-inducing antiepileptic drugs (ie, carbamazepine, phenobarbital, phenytoin, primidone); may need to adjust dose. May increase carbamazepine toxicity. Women taking estrogen-containing oral contraceptives without an enzyme-inducing anticonvulsant will generally require an increase of the lamotrigine maintenance dose by up to 2-fold. Consider increasing the lamotrigine dose when the contraceptive is started. Taper lamotrigine by 25% or less of daily dose q week over a 2 week period if the contraceptive is stopped. Preliminary evidence suggests that exposure during the first trimester of pregnancy is associated with a risk of cleft palate and/or cleft lip. Please report all fetal exposure to the Lamotrigine Pregnancy Registry (800-336-2176) and the North American Antiepileptic Drug Pregnancy Registry (888-233-2334).

MOA — Blocks sodium channels and inhibits the release of glutamate.

ADVERSE EFFECTS — Serious: Stevens-Johnson syndrome, toxic epidermal necrolysis, hypersensitivity reactions, blood dyscrasias, multiorgan failure, suicidality. Frequent: Rash, dizziness, diplopia, ataxia, drowsiness, headache, blurred vision, N/V, somnolence, insomnia.

LEVETIRACETAM (Keppra, Keppra XR) ▶K ♀C ▶? $$$$$

ADULTS — Partial seizures, juvenile myoclonic epilepsy (JME), or primary generalized tonic-clonic seizures (GTC), adjunctive therapy: Start 500 mg PO/IV bid (IV route not approved for GTC) or 1000 mg PO daily (Keppra XR, partial seizures only); increase by 1000 mg/day q 2 weeks prn to max 3000 mg/day (partial seizures) or to target dose of 3000 mg/day (JME or GTC).

PEDS — Partial seizures, adjunctive therapy for age older than 4 yo: Start 20 mg/kg/day PO (or IV if 16 yo or older) divided bid. Increase q 2 weeks as tolerated to target dose of 60 mg/kg/day. Juvenile myoclonic epilepsy, adjunctive therapy, age 12 yo or older: See adult dosing (IV approved for 16 yo or older only). Primary generalized tonic-clonic seizures (GTC), adjunctive therapy, age 6 to 15 yo: Start 20 mg/kg/day PO (or IV if 16 yo or older) divided bid. Increase by 20 mg/kg/day q 2 weeks to target dose of 60 mg/kg/day.

UNAPPROVED ADULTS — Myoclonus: Start 500 to 1000 mg/day in divided doses. May increase to max 1500 to 3000 mg/day or 50 mg/kg/day.

FORMS — Generic/Trade: Tabs 250, 500, 750, 1000 mg, Oral soln 100 mg/mL. Trade only: Tabs extended-release 500, 750 mg.

NOTES — Drug interactions unlikely. Decrease dose in renal dysfunction (CrCl < 80 mL/min). Emotional lability, hostility, and depression may occur. Use same dose when switching between IV and PO forms.

MOA — Unknown but may involve opposition of negative modulators of GABA and glycine-gated currents and inhibition of N-type calcium currents.

ADVERSE EFFECTS — Serious: Pancytopenia, pancreatitis, psychosis, depression, suicidality. Frequent: Drowsiness, dizziness, fatigue, asthenia, nervousness, emotional lability, hostility, ataxia.

NEUROLOGY: Anticonvulsants

OXCARBAZEPINE (*Trileptal*) ▶LK ♀C ▶– $$$$$
WARNING – Serious multiorgan hypersensitivity reactions and life-threatening rashes (eg, Stevens-Johnson syndrome, toxic epidermal necrolysis) have occurred, with some fatalities. Consider discontinuation if skin reactions occur.
ADULTS – <u>Partial seizures, monotherapy:</u> Start 300 mg PO bid. Increase by 300 mg/day q 3 day to usual effective dose of 1200 mg/day. Max 2400 mg/day. <u>Partial seizures, adjunctive:</u> Start 300 mg PO bid. Increase by no more than 600 mg/day at weekly intervals to usual effective dose of 1200 mg/day. Max 2400 mg/day.
PEDS – <u>Partial seizures, adjunctive,</u> age 2 to 16 yo: Start 8 to 10 mg/kg/day PO divided bid (max starting dose 600 mg/day). Titrate to max 60 mg/kg/day for age 2 to less than 4 yo, titrate to max 900 mg/day for wt 20 to 29 kg, titrate to max 1200 mg/day for wt 29.1 to 39 kg, titrate to max 1800 mg/day for wt greater than 39 kg. Consider using a starting dose of 16 to 20 mg/kg for children aged 2 to less than 4 yo who weigh less than 20 kg to account for higher clearance. <u>Partial seizures, initial monotherapy,</u> age 4 to 16 yo: Start 8 to 10 mg/kg/day divided bid. Increase by 5 mg/kg/day q 3 days to recommended dose (in mg/day based on wt rounded to nearest 5 kg) as follows: 600 to 900 for wt 20 kg, 900 to 1200 for wt 25 and 30 kg, 900 to 1500 for wt 35 and 40 kg, 1200 to 1500 for wt 45 kg, 1200 to 1800 for wt 50 and 55 kg, 1200 to 2100 for wt 60 and 65 kg, 1500 to 2100 for wt 70 kg. <u>Partial seizures, conversion to monotherapy,</u> age 4 to 16 yo: Start 8 to 10 mg/kg/day divided bid. Increase at weekly intervals by no more than 10 mg/kg/day to target dose listed for initial monotherapy.
FORMS – Generic/Trade: Tabs (scored) 150, 300, 600 mg. Trade only: Oral susp 300 mg/5 mL.
NOTES – Monitor serum sodium. Decrease initial dose by ½ in renal dysfunction (CrCl < 30 mL/min). Inhibits CYP2C19 and induces CYP3A4/5. Interactions with other antiepileptic drugs, oral contraceptives, and dihydropyridine calcium channel blockers.
MOA – Unknown. May inhibit sodium channels, increase potassium conductance, and modulate calcium channels.
ADVERSE EFFECTS – Serious: Stevens-Johnson syndrome, toxic epidermal necrolysis, hyponatremia / SIADH, leukopenia, angioedema, suicidality. Frequent: Dizziness, drowsiness, fatigue, headache, ataxia, diplopia, nystagmus, gait disturbance, tremor, N/V, abdominal pain.

PHENOBARBITAL (*Luminal*) ▶L ♀D ▶– ©IV $
ADULTS – <u>Epilepsy:</u> 100 to 300 mg/day PO divided daily to tid. <u>Status epilepticus:</u> 20 mg/kg IV at rate no faster than 60 mg/min.
PEDS – <u>Epilepsy:</u> 3 to 5 mg/kg/day PO divided bid to tid. <u>Status epilepticus:</u> 20 mg/kg IV at rate no faster than 60 mg/min.
UNAPPROVED ADULTS – <u>Status epilepticus:</u> May give up to a total dose of 30 mg/kg IV.
UNAPPROVED PEDS – <u>Status epilepticus:</u> 15 to 20 mg/kg IV load; may give additional 5 mg/kg doses q 15 to 30 mins to max total dose of 30 mg/kg. <u>Epilepsy:</u> Give 3 to 5 mg/kg/day given once daily or divided bid for neonates, give 5 to 6 mg/kg/day once daily or divided bid for infants, give 6 to 8 mg/kg/day given once daily or divided bid for age 1 to 5 yo, give 4 to 6 mg/kg/day once daily or divided bid for age 6 to 12 yo, give 1 to 3 mg/kg/day once daily or divided bid for age older than 12 yo.
FORMS – Generic only: Tabs 15, 16.2, 30, 32.4, 60, 100 mg. Elixir 20 mg/5 mL.
NOTES – Usual therapeutic level is 15 to 40 mcg/mL. Monitor cardiopulmonary function closely when administering IV. Decrease dose in renal or hepatic dysfunction. Many drug interactions.
MOA – Nonselective CNS depressant.
ADVERSE EFFECTS – Serious: Respiratory and CNS depression, blood dyscrasias, anemia, thrombocytopenia, Stevens-Johnson syndrome, angioedema, suicidality. Frequent: Drowsiness, fatigue, N/V, bradycardia, ataxia, nystagmus, dizziness, cognitive symptoms, paradoxical CNS excitation.

PHENYTOIN (*Dilantin, Phenytek*) ▶L ♀D ▶+ $$
ADULTS – <u>Status epilepticus:</u> 15-20 mg/kg IV at rate no faster than 50 mg/min, then 100 mg IV/PO q 6 to 8 h. <u>Epilepsy,</u> oral loading dose: 400 mg PO initially, then 300 mg in 2 h and 4 h. <u>Epilepsy,</u> maintenance dose: 300 mg/day PO given once daily (extended release) or divided tid (standard release) and titrated to a therapeutic level.
PEDS – <u>Epilepsy,</u> age older than 6 yo: 5 mg/kg/day PO divided bid to tid, to max 300 mg/day. <u>Status epilepticus:</u> 15 to 20 mg/kg IV at a rate no faster than 1 mg/kg/min.
FORMS – Generic/Trade: Extended-release caps 30, 100 mg (Dilantin). Susp 125 mg/5 mL. Trade only: Extended-release caps 200, 300 mg (Phenytek). Chewable tabs 50 mg (Dilantin Infatabs). Generic only: Extended-release caps 200, 300 mg.
NOTES – Usual therapeutic level is 10 to 20 mcg/mL. Monitor ECG and vital signs when administering IV. Many drug interactions. Monitor serum levels closely when switching between forms (free acid vs. sodium salt). The free fraction may be increased in patients with low albumin levels. IV loading doses of 15 to 20 mg/kg have also been recommended. May need to reduce loading dose if patient is already on phenytoin. Avoid in patients known to be positive for HLA-B*1502 due to possible increased risk of Stevens-Johnson syndrome as with carbamazepine.
MOA – Increases seizure threshold through modulation of sodium and calcium channels.
ADVERSE EFFECTS – Serious: Arrhythmias, blood dyscrasias, Stevens-Johnson syndrome, toxic epidermal necrolysis, hypotension, cardiovascular collapse, thrombocytopenia, anemia, hypersensitivity, local skin necrosis (IV only), suicidality. Frequent: Rash, nystagmus, tremor, ataxia, dizziness, sedation, lymphadenopathy. Frequent (chronic use): gingival hyperplasia, osteomalacia, coarse facies.

NEUROLOGY: Anticonvulsants

PREGABALIN (Lyrica) ▶K ♀C ▶? ©V $$$$$
ADULTS — Painful diabetic peripheral neuropathy: Start 50 mg PO tid; may increase within 1 week to max 100 mg PO tid. Postherpetic neuralgia: Start 150 mg/day PO divided bid to tid; may increase within 1 week to 300 mg/day divided bid to tid; max 600 mg/day. Partial seizures (adjunctive): Start 150 mg/day PO divided bid to tid; may increase prn to max 600 mg/day divided bid to tid. Fibromyalgia: Start 75 mg PO bid; may increase to 150 mg bid within 1 week; max 225 mg bid.
PEDS — Not approved in children.
FORMS — Trade only: Caps 25, 50, 75, 100, 150, 200, 225, 300 mg. Oral solution 20 mg/mL (480 mL).
NOTES — Adjust dose if CrCl < 60 mL/min; refer to package insert. Warn patients to report changes in visual acuity and muscle pain. May increase creatine kinase. Must taper if discontinuing to avoid withdrawal symptoms. Increased risk of peripheral edema when used in conjunction with thiazolidinedione antidiabetic agents.
MOA — Unknown. Binds to alpha-2-delta subunit of voltage-gated calcium channels and reduces neurotransmitter release.
ADVERSE EFFECTS — Serious: Visual field changes, reduced visual acuity, thrombocytopenia, suicidality. Frequent: Dizziness, somnolence, dry mouth, decreased concentration/attention, blurred vision, peripheral edema, weight gain, ataxia, withdrawal reactions.

PRIMIDONE (Mysoline) ▶LK ♀D ▶– $$$$
ADULTS — Epilepsy: Start 100 to 125 mg PO at bedtime. Increase over 10 days to usual maintenance dose of 250 mg PO tid to qid. Max 2 g/day.
PEDS — Epilepsy age younger than 8 yo: Start 50 mg PO at bedtime. Increase over 10 days to usual maintenance dose of 125 to 250 mg PO tid or 10 to 25 mg/kg/day.
UNAPPROVED ADULTS — Essential tremor: Start 12.5 to 25 mg PO at bedtime. May increase weekly prn by 50 mg/day to 250 mg/day given once daily or in divided doses. Max 750 mg/day.
FORMS — Generic/Trade: Tabs 50, 250 mg.
NOTES — Usual therapeutic level is 5 to 12 mcg/mL. Metabolized to phenobarbital.
MOA — Converted to phenobarbital and PEMA. Nonselective CNS depressant.
ADVERSE EFFECTS — Serious: Respiratory and CNS depression, anemia, thrombocytopenia, suicidality. Frequent: Drowsiness, ataxia, vertigo, lethargy, irritability, emotional lability, nystagmus, rash, N/V, paradoxical CNS excitation.

RUFINAMIDE (Banzel) ▶K ♀C ▶? $$$$$
ADULTS — Epilepsy, Lennox-Gastaut syndrome (adjunctive): Start 400 to 800 mg/day PO divided bid. Increase by 400 to 800 mg/day q 2 d to max 3200 mg/day divided bid.
PEDS — Epilepsy, Lennox-Gastaut syndrome (adjunctive) age 4 yo or older: Start 10 mg/kg/day PO given bid. Increase by 10 mg/kg every other day to target of 45 mg/kg/day divided bid.
FORMS — Trade only: Tabs 200, 400 mg.
NOTES — Give with food.
MOA — Modulates activity of sodium channels.
ADVERSE EFFECTS — Serious: Suicidality, multiorgan hypersensitivity. Frequent: Headache, dizziness, fatigue, somnolence, nausea.

TIAGABINE (Gabitril) ▶L ♀C ▶? $$$$$
WARNING — New onset-seizures and status epilepticus may occur when used in patients without epilepsy, particularly when combined with other medications that lower the seizure threshold. Avoid off-label use.
ADULTS — Partial seizures, adjunctive therapy with an enzyme-inducing anticonvulsant: Start 4 mg PO daily. Increase by 4 to 8 mg/day prn at weekly intervals to max 56 mg/day divided bid to qid.
PEDS — Partial seizures, adjunctive therapy with an enzyme-inducing anticonvulsant for age 12 to 18 yo: Start 4 mg PO daily. Increase by 4 mg/day prn q 1 to 2 weeks to max 32 mg/day divided bid to qid.
FORMS — Trade only: Tabs 2, 4, 12, 16 mg.
NOTES — Take with food. Dosing is for patients on enzyme-inducing anticonvulsants such as carbamazepine, phenobarbital, phenytoin, or primidone. Reduce dosage in patients who are not taking enzyme-inducing medications, and in those with liver dysfunction.
MOA — Inhibits presynaptic reuptake of GABA.
ADVERSE EFFECTS — Serious: Stevens-Johnson syndrome, generalized weakness, status epilepticus (with overdose); new onset seizures or status epilepticus (with off-label use), suicidality. Frequent: Dizziness, lightheadedness, asthenia, sedation, tremor, confusion, ataxia, nervousness, depression, decreased concentration, N/V, diarrhea.

TOPIRAMATE (Topamax) ▶K ♀C ▶? $$$$$
ADULTS — Partial seizures or primary generalized tonic-clonic seizures, monotherapy: Start 25 mg PO bid (week 1), 50 mg bid (week 2), 75 mg bid (week 3), 100 mg bid (week 4), 150 mg bid (week 5), then 200 mg bid as tolerated. Partial seizures, primary generalized tonic-clonic seizures, or Lennox-Gastaut syndrome, adjunctive therapy: Start 25 to 50 mg PO at bedtime. Increase weekly by 25 to 50 mg/day to usual effective dose of 200 mg PO bid. Doses greater than 400 mg/day not shown to be more effective. Migraine prophylaxis: Start 25 mg PO at bedtime (week 1), then 25 mg bid (week 2), 25 mg qam and 50 mg qpm (week 3), then 50 mg bid (week 4 and thereafter).
PEDS — Partial seizures or primary generalized tonic-clonic seizures, monotherapy age older than 10 yo: Use adult dosing. Partial seizures, primary generalized tonic-clonic seizures, or Lennox-Gastaut syndrome, adjunctive therapy age 2 to 16 yo: Start 1 to 3 mg/kg (max 25 mg) PO at bedtime. Increase by 1 to 3 mg/kg/day q 1 to 2 weeks to usual effective dose of 5 to 9 mg/kg/day divided bid.
UNAPPROVED ADULTS — Essential tremor: Start 25 mg PO daily. Increase by 25 mg/day at weekly intervals to 100 mg/day; max 400 mg/day. Bipolar

(cont.)

TOPIRAMATE (cont.)

disorder: Start 25 to 50 mg PO daily. Titrate prn to max 400 mg/day. Alcohol dependence: Start 25 mg PO every day; increase by 25 mg/day at weekly intervals as tolerated to 300 mg/day for up to 14 weeks total.

FORMS — Trade: Tabs 25, 50, 100, 200 mg. Sprinkle Caps 15, 25 mg.

NOTES — Give ½ usual adult dose in renal impairment (CrCl < 70 mL/min). Confusion, nephrolithiasis, glaucoma, and wt loss may occur. Risk of oligohidrosis and hyperthermia, particularly in children; use caution in warm ambient temperatures and/or with vigorous physical activity. Hyperchloremic, nonanion gap metabolic acidosis may occur; monitor serum bicarbonate and either reduce dose or taper off entirely if this occurs. Max dose tested was 1600 mg/day.

MOA — Unknown. May modulate sodium channels and enhance GABA action.

ADVERSE EFFECTS — Serious: Acute angle-closure glaucoma, nephrolithiasis, oligohidrosis, hyperthermia, metabolic acidosis, suicidality. Frequent: Somnolence, fatigue, ataxia, psychomotor slowing, cognitive symptoms, confusion, diplopia, nystagmus, dizziness, depression, nervousness, weight loss, paresthesia.

VALPROIC ACID (*Depakene, Depakote, Depakote ER, Depacon, Stavzor, divalproex, sodium valproate, ♣Epival, Deproic*) ▶L ♀D ▶+ $$$$

WARNING — Fatal hepatic failure has occurred; monitor LFTs during first 6 month of treatment. Life-threatening pancreatitis has been reported after initial or prolonged use. Evaluate for abdominal pain, N/V, and/or anorexia. Discontinue if pancreatitis occurs. May be more teratogenic than other anticonvulsants (eg, carbamazepine, lamotrigine, and phenytoin). Hepatic failure and clotting disorders have occurred when used during pregnancy.

ADULTS — Epilepsy: 10 to 15 mg/kg/day (absence start 15 mg/kg/day) PO or IV infusion over 60 min (rate no faster than 20 mg/min) divided bid to qid (standard-release, delayed-release, or IV) or given once daily (Depakote ER). Increase dose by 5 to 10 mg/kg/day at weekly intervals to max 60 mg/kg/day. Migraine prophylaxis: Start 250 mg PO bid (Depakote or Stavzor) or 500 mg PO daily (Depakote ER) for 1 week, then increase to max 1000 mg/day PO divided bid (Depakote or Stavzor) or given once daily (Depakote ER).

PEDS — Seizures age older than 2 yo: 10 to 15 mg/kg/day PO or IV infusion over 60 min (rate no faster than 20 mg/min). Increase dose by 5 to 10 mg/kg/day at weekly intervals to max 60 mg/kg/day. Divide doses which are greater than 250 mg/day into bid to qid; may give once daily (Depakote ER) if age older than 10 yo. For complex partial seizures: Stavzor used for ages 10 yo older.

UNAPPROVED ADULTS — Status epilepticus (not first line): Load 20 to 40 mg/kg IV (rate no faster than 6 mg/kg/min), then continue 4 to 8 mg/kg IV tid to achieve therapeutic level. May use lower loading dose if already on valproate.

UNAPPROVED PEDS — Status epilepticus, age older than 2 yo (not first line): Load 20 to 40 mg/kg IV over 1 to 5 min, then 5 mg/kg/h adjusted to achieve therapeutic level. May use lower loading dose if already on valproate.

FORMS — Generic/Trade: Immediate-release caps 250 mg (Depakene), syrup (Depakene, valproic acid) 250 mg/5 mL. Delayed-release tabs (Depakote) 125, 250, 500 mg, Extended-release tabs (Depakote ER) 250, 500 mg, Delayed-release sprinkle caps (Depakote) 125 mg. Trade only (Stavzor): Delayed-release caps 125, 250, 500 mg.

NOTES — Contraindicated in urea cycle disorders or hepatic dysfunction. Usual therapeutic trough level is 50 to 100 mcg/mL. Depakote and Depakote ER are not interchangeable. Depakote ER is approximately 10% less bioavailable than Depakote. Depakote-releases divalproex sodium over 8 to 12 h (daily to qid dosing); Depakote ER-releases divalproex sodium over 18 to 24 h (daily dosing). Many drug interactions. Patients receiving other anticonvulsants may require higher doses of valproic acid. Reduce dose in the elderly. Hyperammonemia, GI irritation, or thrombocytopenia may occur.

MOA — May increase GABA levels and modulate sodium channels.

ADVERSE EFFECTS — Serious: Hepatotoxicity, anaphylaxis, polycystic ovarian syndrome, bone marrow suppression, thrombocytopenia, pancreatitis, SIADH, Stevens-Johnson syndrome, hyperammonemia, suicidality. Frequent: N/V, diarrhea, weight gain, CNS depression, drowsiness, tremor, alopecia, rash, nystagmus, asthenia.

VIGABATRIN (*♣Sabril*) ▶K ♀C ▶– $$$$

WARNING — Ophthalmologic abnormalities have been reported. Visual field testing should be performed prior to treatment and q 3 months thereafter. Given the limitations of visual field testing in children younger than 9 yo, vigabatrin should be used in this age group only if clearly indicated. Do not use with other retinotoxic drugs.

ADULTS — Canada only. Epilepsy (adjunct treatment): Start: 1 g/day in divided doses. Maintenance: 2 to 3 g/day in divided doses.

PEDS — Canada only. Epilepsy (adjunct treatment) or infantile spasms (monotherapy): Start: 40 mg/kg/day, maintenance: 50 to 100 mg/kg/day in divided doses.

FORMS — Trade only: Tabs 500 mg. Oral powder 500 mg/sachet.

MOA — Irreversible inhibitor of GABA-transaminase; increases CNS levels of GABA.

ADVERSE EFFECTS — Serious: Ophthalmologic abnormalities: Retinal atrophy, optic neuritis, optic atrophy, suicidality. Frequent: Drowsiness, dizziness, headache.

ZONISAMIDE (*Zonegran*) ▶LK ♀C ▶? $$$$
ADULTS — <u>Partial seizures, adjunctive:</u> Start 100 mg PO daily for 2 weeks, then increase to 200 mg PO daily. May increase prn q 2 weeks to 300 to 400 mg/day, given once daily or divided bid. Max 600 mg/day.
PEDS — Not approved in children.
FORMS — Generic/Trade: Caps 25, 50, 100 mg.
NOTES — This is a sulfonamide; contraindicated in sulfa allergy. Fatalities and severe reactions including Stevens-Johnson syndrome, toxic epidermal necrolysis, fulminant hepatic necrosis, and blood dyscrasias have occurred with sulfonamides. Clearance is affected by CYP3A4 inhibitors or inducers such as phenytoin, carbamazepine, phenobarbital, and valproic acid. Nephrolithiasis may occur. Oligohidrosis and hyperthermia may occur, and are more common in children. Patients with renal disease may require slower titration.
MOA — Unknown. May involve inhibition of sodium and calcium channels.
ADVERSE EFFECTS — Serious: Toxic epidermal necrolysis, Stevens-Johnson syndrome, hepatic necrosis, agranulocytosis, aplastic anemia, hypersensitivity, nephrolithiasis, psychosis, suicidality, oligohidrosis, hyperthermia. Frequent: Abdominal pain, headache, somnolence, fatigue, N/V, anorexia, dizziness, drowsiness, cognitive symptoms, ataxia, diplopia, confusion, depression, irritability, agitation, insomnia, weight loss.

NEUROLOGY: Migraine Therapy—Triptans (5-HT1 Receptor Agonists)

NOTE: May cause vasospasm. Avoid in ischemic or vasospastic heart disease, cerebrovascular syndromes, peripheral arterial disease, uncontrolled HTN, and hemiplegic or basilar migraine. Do not use within 24 h of ergots or other triptans. Risk of serotonin syndrome if used with SSRIs or MAOIs.

ALMOTRIPTAN (*Axert*) ▶LK ♀C ▶? $$
ADULTS — <u>Migraine treatment:</u> 6.25 to 12.5 mg PO. May repeat in 2 h prn. Max 25 mg/day.
PEDS — <u>Migraine treatment</u> for age 12 to 17 yo: 6.25 to 12.5 mg PO. May repeat in 2 h prn. Max 25 mg/day.
FORMS — Trade only: Tabs 6.25, 12.5 mg.
NOTES — MAOIs inhibit almotriptan metabolism; use together only with extreme caution. Use lower doses (6.25 mg) in renal and/or hepatic dysfunction. Use with caution in patients with known hypersensitivity to sulfonamides.
MOA — Serotonin 5-HT1B/D agonist.
ADVERSE EFFECTS — Serious: Chest pain/tightness, coronary vasospasm, acute MI, arrhythmias, peripheral ischemia, stroke. Frequent: N/V, headache, paresthesias, sedation, dry mouth.
ELETRIPTAN (*Relpax*) ▶LK ♀C ▶? $$$
ADULTS — <u>Migraine treatment:</u> 20 to 40 mg PO at onset. May repeat after 2 h prn. Max 40 mg/dose or 80 mg/day.
PEDS — Not approved in children.
FORMS — Trade only: Tabs 20, 40 mg.
NOTES — Do not use within 72 h of potent CYP3A4 inhibitors such as ketoconazole, itraconazole, nefazodone, troleandomycin, clarithromycin, ritonavir, or nelfinavir.
MOA — Serotonin 5-HT1B/D agonist.
ADVERSE EFFECTS — Serious: Chest pain/tightness, coronary vasospasm, acute MI, arrhythmias, peripheral ischemia, stroke, HTN, seizures. Frequent: Dizziness, somnolence, nausea, asthenia, chest tightness.
FROVATRIPTAN (*Frova*) ▶LK ♀C ▶? $
ADULTS — <u>Migraine treatment:</u> 2.5 mg PO. May repeat in 2 h prn. Max 7.5 mg/24 h.
PEDS — Not approved in children.
FORMS — Trade only: Tabs 2.5 mg.
MOA — Serotonin 5-HT1B/D agonist.
ADVERSE EFFECTS — Serious: Chest pain/tightness, coronary vasospasm, acute MI, arrhythmias, peripheral ischemia, stroke, HTN. Frequent: N/V, headache, paresthesias, sedation, dizziness, fatigue, dry mouth.
NARATRIPTAN (*Amerge*) ▶KL ♀C ▶? $$$
ADULTS — <u>Migraine treatment:</u> 1 to 2.5 mg PO. May repeat in 4 h prn. Max 5 mg/24 h.
PEDS — Not approved in children.
FORMS — Generic/Trade: Tabs 1, 2.5 mg.
NOTES — Contraindicated in severe renal or hepatic impairment.
MOA — Serotonin 5-HT1B/D agonist.
ADVERSE EFFECTS — Serious: Chest pain/tightness, coronary vasospasm, acute MI, arrhythmias, peripheral ischemia, stroke, HTN. Frequent: Paresthesia, dizziness, drowsiness, malaise, fatigue.
RIZATRIPTAN (*Maxalt, Maxalt MLT*) ▶LK ♀C ▶? $$
ADULTS — <u>Migraine treatment:</u> 5 to 10 mg PO; May repeat in 2 h prn. Max 30 mg/24 h.
PEDS — Not approved in children.
FORMS — Trade only: Tabs 5, 10 mg. Orally disintegrating tabs (MLT) 5, 10 mg.
NOTES — Should not be combined with MAOIs. MLT form dissolves on tongue without liquids.
MOA — Serotonin 5-HT1B/D agonist.
ADVERSE EFFECTS — Serious: Chest pain/tightness, coronary vasospasm, acute MI, arrhythmias, peripheral ischemia, stroke, HTN. Frequent: Asthenia, fatigue, drowsiness, pain/pressure sensation, dizziness, paresthesia.
SUMATRIPTAN (*Imitrex, Alsuma*) ▶LK ♀C ▶+ $$$
ADULTS — <u>Migraine treatment:</u> 4 to 6 mg SC. May repeat in 1 h prn. Max 12 mg/24 h. Tabs: 25 to 100 mg PO (50 mg most common). May repeat q 2 h prn with 25 to 100 mg doses. Max 200 mg/24 h. Intranasal spray: 5 to 20 mg. May repeat q 2 h prn. Max 40 mg/24 h. <u>Cluster headache treatment:</u> 6 mg SC. May repeat in > 1 h

(cont.)

SUMATRIPTAN (cont.)
prn. Max 12 mg/24 h. Initial oral dose of 50 mg appears to be more effective than 25 mg. If HA returns after initial SC injection, then tabs may be used q 2 h prn, max 100 mg/24 h.
PEDS — Not approved in children.
UNAPPROVED PEDS — Acute migraine, intranasal spray, for age 8 to 17 yo: Give 20 mg for wt 40 kg or greater or 10 mg for wt 20 to 39 kg intranasally at headache onset. May repeat after 2 h prn.
FORMS — Injection (STATdose System) 4, 6 mg prefilled cartridges.
NOTES — Should not be combined with MAOIs. Avoid IM/IV route.
MOA — Serotonin 5-HT1B/D agonist.
ADVERSE EFFECTS — Serious: Chest pain/tightness, coronary vasospasm, acute MI, arrhythmias, peripheral ischemia, stroke, seizures, HTN. Frequent: Dizziness, lightheadedness, weakness, myalgias, muscle cramps, N/V, fatigue, drowsiness, flushing, pain/pressure sensation.

TREXIMET (sumatriptan + naproxen) ▶LK ♀C ▶– $$
WARNING — May cause vasospasm. Avoid in ischemic or vasospastic heart disease, cerebrovascular syndromes, peripheral arterial disease, uncontrolled HTN, and hemiplegic or basilar migraine. Do not use within 24 h of ergots or other triptans. There is a risk of GI bleeding and perforation. Do not use ergots within 24 h of Treximet.
ADULTS — Migraine treatment: 1 tab PO at onset; may repeat after 2 h. Max 2 tabs/24 h.
PEDS — Not approved in children.
FORMS — Trade only: Tabs 85 mg sumatriptan + 500 mg naproxen sodium.

NOTES — Avoid if CrCl < 30 mL/min, hepatic impairment, cerebrovascular, cardiovascular, or peripheral vascular disease, uncontrolled HTN. Contraindicated with MAOIs.
MOA — Combination of serotonin 5-HT1B/D agonist and anti-inflammatory/analgesic.
ADVERSE EFFECTS — Serious: Serotonin syndrome, renal toxicity, anaphylactic reactions, chest pain/tightness, coronary vasospasm, acute MI, arrhythmias, peripheral ischemia, stroke, seizures, HTN. Frequent: Dizziness, lightheadedness, weakness, myalgias, muscle cramps, N/V, fatigue, drowsiness, flushing, pain/pressure sensation.

ZOLMITRIPTAN (*Zomig, Zomig ZMT*) ▶L ♀C ▶? $$
ADULTS — Migraine treatment: Tabs: 1.25 to 2.5 mg PO q 2 h. Max 10 mg/24 h. Orally disintegrating tabs (ZMT): 2.5 mg PO. May repeat in 2 h prn. Max 10 mg/24 h. Nasal spray: 5 mg (1 spray) in 1 nostril. May repeat in 2 h prn. Max 10 mg/24 h.
PEDS — Not approved in children.
FORMS — Trade only: Tabs 2.5, 5 mg. Orally disintegrating tabs (ZMT) 2.5, 5 mg. Nasal spray 5 mg/spray.
NOTES — Risk of vasospastic complications. Should not be combined with MAOIs. Use lower doses (< 2.5 mg) in hepatic dysfunction. May break 2.5 mg tabs in half.
MOA — Serotonin 5-HT1B/D agonist.
ADVERSE EFFECTS — Serious: Chest pain/tightness, coronary vasospasm, acute MI, arrhythmia, peripheral and splenic ischemia, stroke, HTN. Frequent: Asthenia, pain/pressure, diaphoresis, dizziness, drowsiness, dyspepsia, flushing, paresthesia, dysgeusia (nasal spray only).

NEUROLOGY: Migraine Therapy—Other

CAFERGOT (ergotamine + caffeine) ▶L ♀X ▶– $
WARNING — Contraindicated with concomitant use of potent CYP3A4 inhibitors (eg, macrolides, protease inhibitors) due to risk of serious/life-threatening peripheral ischemia. Ergots have been associated with potentially life-threatening fibrotic complications.
ADULTS — Migraine and cluster headache treatment: 2 tabs PO at onset, then 1 tab q 30 min prn to max 6 tabs/attack or 10 tabs/week.
PEDS — Not approved in children.
UNAPPROVED PEDS — Migraine treatment: 1 tab PO at onset, then 1 tab q 30 min prn to max 3 tabs/attack.
FORMS — Trade only: Tabs 1/100 mg ergotamine/caffeine.
NOTES — Contraindicated in sepsis, CAD, peripheral arterial disease, HTN, impaired hepatic or renal function, malnutrition, or severe pruritus.
MOA — Vasoconstrictor. Partial agonist/antagonist at alpha-adrenergic and serotonin receptors (ergotamine).
ADVERSE EFFECTS — Serious: Coronary vasospasm, coronary or peripheral ischemia, arrhythmias, HTN; retroperitoneal, pleural, pericardial, or cardiac valvular fibrosis. Frequent: N/V, dry mouth, abdominal pain, localized edema and pruritus, myalgias, leg weakness, peripheral ischemia, paresthesias, asthenia

DIHYDROERGOTAMINE (*D.H.E. 45, Migranal*) ▶L ♀X ▶– $$
WARNING — Contraindicated with concomitant use of potent CYP3A4 inhibitors (eg, macrolides, protease inhibitors) due to risk of serious/life-threatening peripheral ischemia. Ergots have been associated with potentially life-threatening fibrotic complications.
ADULTS — Migraine treatment: Soln (DHE 45): 1 mg IV/IM/SC; may repeat q 1 h prn to max 2 mg (IV) or 3 mg (IM/SC) per 24 h. Nasal spray (Migranal): 1 spray (0.5 mg) in each nostril; may repeat in 15 min prn to max 6 sprays (3 mg)/24 h or 8 sprays (4 mg)/week.
PEDS — Not approved in children.
FORMS — Trade only: Nasal spray 0.5 mg/spray (Migranal). Self-injecting soln (D.H.E 45): 1 mg/mL.
NOTES — Contraindicated in basilar or hemiplegic migraine, sepsis, ischemic or vasospastic

(cont.)

NEUROLOGY: Multiple sclerosis

DIHYDROERGOTAMINE (cont.)
cardiac disease, peripheral vascular disease, vascular surgery, impaired hepatic or renal function, or uncontrolled HTN. Avoid concurrent ergotamine, methysergide, or triptan use.
MOA – Serotonin 5-HT1D receptor agonist.
ADVERSE EFFECTS – Serious: Coronary vasoconstriction, MI, ventricular arrhythmias, stroke, HTN, peripheral ischemia; retroperitoneal, pleural, pericardial, or cardiac valvular fibrosis. Frequent: N/V, diarrhea, paresthesia, chest pain. Rhinitis and dysgeusia (nasal spray only).

FLUNARIZINE (✦*Sibelium*) ▶L ♀C ▶– $$
ADULTS – Canada only. Migraine prophylaxis: 10 mg PO at bedtime; if side effects occur, then reduce dose to 5 mg at bedtime. Safety of long-term use (more than 4 months) has not been established.
PEDS – Not approved in children.
FORMS – Generic/Trade: Caps 5 mg.
NOTES – Gradual onset of benefit, over 6 to 8 weeks. Not for acute therapy. Contraindicated if history of depression or extrapyramidal disorders.
MOA – Selective calcium channel blocker.

ADVERSE EFFECTS – Serious: Depression, extrapyramidal symptoms, tardive syndromes. Frequent: Drowsiness, weight gain.

MIDRIN (isometheptene + dichloralphenazone + acetaminophen, Amidrine, Durdrin, Migquin, Migratine, Migrazone, Va-Zone) ▶L ♀? ▶? ©IV $
ADULTS – Tension and vascular headache treatment: 1 to 2 caps PO q 4 h, to max of 8 caps/day. Migraine treatment: 2 caps PO single dose, then 1 cap q 1 h prn to max 5 caps within 12 h.
PEDS – Not approved in children.
FORMS – Generic only: Caps (isometheptene/dichloralphenazone/acetaminophen) 65/100/325 mg.
NOTES – Midrin brand no longer available; generics only. FDA has classified as possibly effective for migraine treatment. Contraindicated in glaucoma, severe renal disease, heart disease, hepatic disease, or concurrent MAOI use. Use caution in HTN, peripheral arterial disease, or recent MI.
MOA – Combination sympathomimetic (vasoconstrictor), CNS depressant, and analgesic.
ADVERSE EFFECTS – Serious: Hepatotoxicity, renal tubular necrosis, chronic analgesic nephropathy. Frequent: Rash, dizziness.

NEUROLOGY: Multiple sclerosis

DALFAMPRIDINE (*Ampyra*) ▶K - ♀C ▶?
ADULTS – Multiple sclerosis: 10 mg PO bid
PEDS – Not approved for use in children or adolescents
FORMS – Trade: Extended-release tabs 10 mg.
NOTES – Contraindicated with moderate to severe renal impairment and history of seizures.
MOA – Broad spectrum potassium channel blocker.
ADVERSE EFFECTS – Serious: Seizures. Frequent: Urinary tract infection, insomnia, dizziness, headache, nausea, asthenia, back pain, balance disorder, multiple sclerosis relapse, paresthesia, nasopharyngitis, constipation, dyspepsia, pharyngolaryngeal pain.

GLATIRAMER (*Copaxone*) ▶Serum ♀B ▶? $$$$$
ADULTS – Multiple sclerosis (relapsing-remitting): 20 mg SC daily.
PEDS – Not approved in children.
FORMS – Trade only: Injection 20 mg single-dose vial.
NOTES – Do not inject IV.
MOA – Immunomodulator.
ADVERSE EFFECTS – Serious: Anaphylaxis. Frequent: Injection site reactions, flu-like symptoms, flushing, dyspnea, chest pain, anxiety, palpitations, asthenia, pain, N/V, arthralgia.

INTERFERON BETA-1A (*Avonex, Rebif*) ▶L ♀C ▶? $$$$$
WARNING – Risk of severe hepatic injury and failure, possibly greater when used with other hepatotoxic drugs. Monitor LFTs. Suicidality risk; use caution in depression.
ADULTS – Multiple sclerosis (relapsing forms): Avonex 30 mcg (6 million units) IM q week. Rebif start 8.8 mcg SC 3 times weekly; titrate over 4 weeks to maintenance dose of 44 mcg 3 times weekly.
PEDS – Not approved in children.
FORMS – Trade only (Avonex): Injection 30 mcg single-dose vial with or without albumin. Prefilled syringe 30 mcg. Trade only (Rebif): Starter kit 20 mcg prefilled syringe. Prefilled syringe 22, 44 mcg.
NOTES – Use caution in patients with depression, seizure disorders, or cardiac disease. Follow LFTs and CBC. Avonex: Indicated for the first attack of MS. Rebif: Give same dose 3 days each week, with at least 48 h between doses.
MOA – Immunomodulator.
ADVERSE EFFECTS – Serious: Depression, suicidal ideation, psychosis, hepatotoxicity, anaphylaxis, autoimmune disorders (idiopathic thrombocytopenia, hyper- and hypothyroidism, hepatitis), cytopenias, seizures, cardiomyopathy, cardiac failure. Frequent: Injection site reactions, headache, fever, chills, N/V, diarrhea, flu-like symptoms, fatigue, muscle pain.

INTERFERON BETA-1B (*Betaseron*) ▶L ♀C ▶? $$$$$
ADULTS – Multiple sclerosis (relapsing-remitting): Start 0.0625 mg SC every other day; titrate over 6 weeks to 0.25 mg (8 million units) SC every other day.
PEDS – Not approved in children.
FORMS – Trade only: Injection 0.3 mg (9.6 million units) single-dose vial.
NOTES – Suicidality risk; use caution in depression. Check LFTs after 1, 3, and 6 months and then periodically. Product can be stored at room temp until reconstituted; then refrigerate and use within 3 h.
MOA – Immunomodulator.

(cont.)

INTERFERON BETA-1B (cont.)

ADVERSE EFFECTS — Serious: Depression, suicidality, autoimmune hepatitis, hepatic failure, hypersensitivity, leukopenia, injection site necrosis, hypertension. Frequent: Injection site reactions, headache, fever, chills, N/V, diarrhea, constipation, abdominal pain, edema, flu-like symptoms, myalgia, palpitations, dizziness, somnolence, increased LFTs, abnormal menses.

NATALIZUMAB (*Tysabri*) ▶Serum ♀C ▶? $$$$$
WARNING — May cause progressive multifocal leukoencephalopathy; avoid concomitant use of other immunomodulators. Risk of severe hepatotoxicity; discontinue if jaundice or evidence of liver injury. Risk of anaphylaxis or other hypersensitivity reactions; permanently discontinue if they occur.
ADULTS — Refractory, relapsing multiple sclerosis (monotherapy) and Crohn's disease: 300 mg IV infusion over 1 h q 4 weeks.
PEDS — Not approved in children.
NOTES — Not first line; recommended only when there has been an inadequate response or failure to tolerate other therapies. Available only through the MS-TOUCH or CD-TOUCH prescribing programs at 800-456-2255. Observe closely for infusion reactions. Avoid other immunosuppressants when using for Crohn's disease; discontinue if no response by 12 weeks. For patients on steroids, taper them as soon as a benefit is noted and discontinue natalizumab if steroids cannot be tapered off within 6 months. Consider stopping natalizumab in patients who require steroids more than 3 months/year. Severe hepatotoxicity has been reported; discontinue if jaundice or evidence of liver injury.
MOA — Specific mechanism unknown. Monoclonal antibody that blocks interaction of alpha-4-beta 1-integrin expressed inflammatory cells to vascular endothelium and parenchymal cells in the brain.
ADVERSE EFFECTS — Serious: Progressive multifocal leukoencephalopathy, cholelithiasis, hepatotoxicity, depression, suicidality, anaphylaxis, hypersensitivity reactions, infection. Frequent: Infusion reactions, headache, fatigue, arthralgia, urinary urgency/frequency, abdominal discomfort, diarrhea, rash, irregular menstruation/dysmenorrhea.

NEUROLOGY: Myasthenia Gravis

EDROPHONIUM (*Tensilon, Enlon*) ▶Plasma ♀C ▶? $
ADULTS — Evaluation for myasthenia gravis: 2 mg IV over 15 to 30 sec (test dose) while on cardiac monitor, then 8 mg IV after 45 sec. Reversal of neuromuscular blockade: 10 mg IV over 30 to 45 sec; repeat prn to max 40 mg.
PEDS — Evaluation for myasthenia gravis: Give 1 mg IV (test dose), then 1 mg IV q 30 to 45 sec to max 5 mg for wt 34 kg or less, give 2 mg IV (test dose), then 2 mg IV q 30 to 45 sec to max 10 mg for wt greater than 34 kg.
UNAPPROVED ADULTS — Reversal of nondepolarizing neuromuscular blocking agents: 0.5 to 1 mg/kg IV together with atropine 0.007 to 0.014 mg/kg.
FORMS — 10 mg/mL MDV vial.
NOTES — Not for maintenance therapy of myasthenia gravis because of short duration of action (5 to 10 min). May give IM. Monitor cardiac function. Atropine should be readily available in case of cholinergic reaction. Contraindicated in mechanical urinary or intestinal obstruction.
MOA — Reversible cholinesterase inhibitor.
ADVERSE EFFECTS — Serious: Arrhythmias, bradycardia, respiratory paralysis, cholinergic toxicity, dysphagia, seizures. Frequent: N/V, abdominal cramping, diarrhea, miosis, lacrimation, diplopia, fasciculations.

NEOSTIGMINE (*Prostigmin*) ▶L ♀C ▶? $$$$
ADULTS — Myasthenia gravis: 15 to 375 mg/day PO in divided doses, or 0.5 mg IM/SC when oral therapy is not possible. Reversal of nondepolarizing neuromuscular blocking agents: 0.5 to 2 mg slow IV (preceded by atropine 0.6 to 1.2 mg or glycopyrrolate 0.2 to 0.6 mg); repeat prn to max 5 mg.
PEDS — Not approved in children.
UNAPPROVED PEDS — Myasthenia gravis: 7.5 to 15 mg PO tid to qid; or 0.03 mg/kg IM q 2 to 4 h. Reversal of nondepolarizing neuromuscular blocking agents: 0.025 to 0.08 mg/kg/dose slow IV, preceded by either atropine (0.4 mg for each mg of neostigmine) or glycopyrrolate (0.2 mg for each mg of neostigmine).
FORMS — Trade only: Tabs 15 mg.
NOTES — Oral route preferred when possible.
MOA — Reversible cholinesterase inhibitor.
ADVERSE EFFECTS — Serious: Cholinergic toxicity, respiratory paralysis, bronchospasm, arrhythmias, cardiac arrest, seizures. Frequent: N/V, diarrhea, abdominal cramping, dizziness, headache, muscle cramps/weakness, fasciculations, hypersalivation, increased bronchial secretions, miosis.

PYRIDOSTIGMINE (*Mestinon, Mestinon Timespan, Regonal*) ▶Plasma, K ♀C ▶+ $$
ADULTS — Myasthenia gravis, standard-release tabs: Start 60 mg PO tid; gradually increase to usual therapeutic dose of 200 mg PO tid. Extended-release tabs: Start 180 mg PO daily or divided bid. Max 1500 mg/day. May give 2 mg IM or slow IV injection q 2 to 3 h.
PEDS — Not approved in children.
UNAPPROVED PEDS — Myasthenia gravis, neonates: 5 mg PO q 4 to 6 h or 0.05 to 0.15 mg/kg IM/IV q 4 to 6 h. Myasthenia gravis, children: 7 mg/kg/day PO in 5 to 6 divided doses, or 0.05 to 0.15 mg/kg/dose IM/IV q 4 to 6 h. Max 10 mg IM/IV single dose.
FORMS — Generic/Trade: Tabs 60 mg. Trade only: Extended-release tabs 180 mg. Syrup 60 mg/ 5 mL.
NOTES — Give injection at 1/30th of oral dose when oral therapy is not possible.

(cont.)

PYRIDOSTIGMINE (cont.)
MOA — Reversible cholinesterase inhibitor.
ADVERSE EFFECTS — Serious: Cholinergic toxicity, bronchospasm, respiratory paralysis, bradycardia, arrhythmias, cardiac arrest. Frequent: N/V, diarrhea, abdominal cramps/pain, muscle cramps/weakness, fasciculation, miosis, hypersalivation, increased bronchial secretions.

NEUROLOGY: Parkinsonian Agents—Anticholinergics

NOTE: Anticholinergic medications may cause memory loss, delirium, or psychosis, particularly in elderly patients or those with baseline cognitive impairment.

BENZTROPINE MESYLATE (*Cogentin*) ▶LK ♀C ▶? $
ADULTS — Parkinsonism: Start 0.5 to 2 mg/day PO/IM/IV. Increase in 0.5 mg increments at weekly intervals to max 6 mg/day. May divide doses daily to qid. Drug-induced extrapyramidal disorders: 1 to 4 mg PO/IM/IV given once daily or divided bid.
PEDS — Not approved in children.
UNAPPROVED PEDS — Parkinsonism in age older than 3 yo: 0.02 to 0.05 mg/kg/dose given once daily or divided bid. Use caution; potential for undesired anticholinergic effects.
FORMS — Generic only: Tabs 0.5, 1, 2 mg.
NOTES — Contraindicated in narrow-angle glaucoma. Avoid concomitant use of donepezil, rivastigmine, galantamine, or tacrine.
MOA — Anticholinergic.
ADVERSE EFFECTS — Serious: Tachycardia, anticholinergic toxicity, psychosis, delirium. Frequent: Dry mouth, constipation, urinary retention, blurred vision, drowsiness, dizziness, headache, rash, N/V, memory problems.

BIPERIDEN (*Akineton*) ▶LK ♀C ▶? $$$
ADULTS — Parkinsonism: 2 mg PO tid to qid. Titrate to max 16 mg/day. Drug-induced extrapyramidal disorders: 2 mg PO daily to tid to max 8 mg/24 h.
PEDS — Not approved in children.
FORMS — Trade only: Tabs 2 mg.
NOTES — Contraindicated in narrow-angle glaucoma, bowel obstruction, and megacolon.
MOA — Anticholinergic.
ADVERSE EFFECTS — Serious: Tachycardia, anticholinergic toxicity, psychosis, delirium. Frequent: Dry mouth, constipation, urinary retention, blurred vision, drowsiness, dizziness, headache, rash, N/V, memory problems, delirium.

TRIHEXYPHENIDYL (*Artane*) ▶LK ♀C ▶? $
ADULTS — Parkinsonism: 1 mg PO daily. Increase by 2 mg/day at 3- to 5-day intervals to usual therapeutic dose of 6 to 10 mg/day divided tid with meals. Max 15 mg/day.
PEDS — Not approved in children.
FORMS — Generic only: Tabs 2, 5 mg. Elixir 2 mg/5 mL.
MOA — Anticholinergic.
ADVERSE EFFECTS — Serious: Tachycardia, anticholinergic toxicity, psychosis, delirium. Frequent: Dry mouth, constipation, urinary retention, blurred vision, drowsiness, dizziness, headache, rash, N/V, memory problems.

NEUROLOGY: Parkinsonian Agents—COMT Inhibitors

ENTACAPONE (*Comtan*) ▶L ♀C ▶? $$$$$
ADULTS — Parkinson's disease, adjunctive: Start 200 mg PO with each dose of carbidopa/levodopa. Max 8 tabs (1600 mg)/day.
PEDS — Not approved in children.
FORMS — Trade only: Tabs 200 mg.
NOTES — Adjunct to carbidopa/levodopa in patients who have end-of-dose "wearing off." Has no antiparkinsonian effect on its own. Avoid concomitant use of nonselective MAOIs. Use caution in hepatobiliary dysfunction. Avoid rapid withdrawal, which may precipitate neuroleptic malignant syndrome.
MOA — Blocks dopamine breakdown by inhibiting catechol-o-methyltransferase.
ADVERSE EFFECTS — Serious: Orthostatic hypotension, rhabdomyolysis, hallucinations, delirium, severe diarrhea, impulse control disorders. Frequent: Dyskinesia, hyperkinesia, N/V, abdominal pain, diarrhea, urine discoloration.

NEUROLOGY: Parkinsonian Agents—Dopaminergic Agents and Combinations

NOTE: Dopaminergic medications may cause hallucinations, particularly when used in combination. They have also been associated with sudden-onset episodes of sleep without warning ("sleep attacks"), and with the development of impulse control disorders such as compulsive gambling, hypersexuality, and hyperphagia. This is more common with dopamine agonists than L-dopa. Avoid rapid discontinuation, which may precipitate neuroleptic malignant syndrome.

APOMORPHINE (*Apokyn*) ▶L ♀C ▶? $$$$$
WARNING — Never administer IV due to risk of severe adverse effects including pulmonary embolism.
ADULTS — Acute, intermittent treatment of hypomobility ("off episodes") in Parkinson's disease: Start 0.2 mL SC test dose in the presence of medical personnel. May increase dose by 0.1 mL every few days as tolerated. Max 0.6 mL/dose or 2 mL/day. Monitor for orthostatic hypotension after initial dose and with dose escalation. Potent emetic; pretreat with

(cont.)

APOMORPHINE (cont.)
trimethobenzamide 300 mg PO tid (or domperidone 20 mg PO tid) starting 3 days prior to use, and continue for ≥2 months before weaning.
PEDS — Not approved in children.
FORMS — Trade only: Cartridges (for injector pen, 10 mg/mL) 3 mL. Ampules (10 mg/mL) 2 mL.
NOTES — Write doses exclusively in mL rather than mg to avoid errors. Most effective when administered at (or just prior to) the onset of an "off" episode. Avoid concomitant use of 5HT3 antagonists (eg, ondansetron, granisetron, dolasetron, palonosetron, alosetron), which can precipitate severe hypotension and loss of consciousness. Inform patients that the dosing pen is labeled in mL (not mg), and that it is possible to dial in a dose of medication even if the cartridge does not contain sufficient drug. Rotate injection sites. Restart at 0.2 mL/day if treatment is interrupted for 1 week or more. Use cautiously with hepatic impairment. Reduce starting dose to 0.1 mL in patients with mild or moderate renal failure. Contains sulfites.
MOA — Dopamine agonist (non-ergot).
ADVERSE EFFECTS — Serious: Syncope, orthostatic hypotension, QT prolongation, arrhythmias, myocardial infarction, anaphylaxis, sleep attacks, priapism, inappropriate sexual behavior, impulse control disorders. Frequent: N/V, yawning, chest pain, confusion, hallucinations, sedation, drowsiness, dyskinesia, dizziness, rhinorrhea, peripheral edema, injection site reactions.

CARBIDOPA (*Lodosyn*) ▶LK ♀C ▶? $$$
ADULTS — Parkinson's disease, adjunct to carbidopa/levodopa: Start 25 mg PO daily with first daily dose of carbidopa/levodopa. May give an additional 12.5 to 25 mg with each dose of carbidopa/levodopa as needed. Max 200 mg/day.
PEDS — Not approved in children.
FORMS — Trade only: Tabs 25 mg.
NOTES — Adjunct to carbidopa/levodopa to reduce peripheral side-effects such as nausea. Also increases the CNS availability of levodopa. Monitor for CNS side-effects such as dyskinesias and hallucinations when initiating therapy, and reduce the dose of levodopa as necessary.
MOA — Blocks the peripheral conversion of levodopa to dopamine.
ADVERSE EFFECTS — Serious: None. Frequent: None. The adverse effects of carbidopa/levodopa are due to the levodopa component.

CARBIDOPA-LEVODOPA (*Sinemet, Sinemet CR, Parcopa*) ▶L ♀C ▶– $$$$
ADULTS — Parkinsonism: Standard-release and orally disintegrating tab: Start 1 tab (25/100 mg) PO tid. Increase by 1 tab/day q 1 to 2 days prn. Use 1 tab (25/250 mg) PO tid to qid when higher levodopa doses are needed. Sustained-release: Start 1 tab (50/200 mg) PO bid; separate doses by at least 4 h. Increase as needed at intervals of 3 days or more. Typical max dose is 1600 to 2000 mg/day of levodopa, but higher doses have been used.
PEDS — Not approved in children.
UNAPPROVED ADULTS — Restless legs syndrome: Start ½ tab (25/100 mg) PO at bedtime; increase q 3 to 4 days to max 50/200 mg (two 25/100 tabs) at bedtime. If symptoms recur during the night, then a combination of standard-release (25/100 mg, 1 to 2 tabs at bedtime) and sustained-release (25/100 or 50/200 mg at bedtime) tabs may be used. Dopa-responsive dystonia: Start 1 tab (25/100) PO daily and titrate to max 1000 mg of levodopa daily.
FORMS — Generic/Trade: Tabs (carbidopa/levodopa) 10/100, 25/100, 25/250 mg. Tabs, sustained-release (Sinemet CR, carbidopa-levodopa ER) 25/100, 50/200 mg. Trade only: Orally disintegrating tab (Parcopa) 10/100, 25/100, 25/250.
NOTES — Motor fluctuations and dyskinesias may occur. The 25/100 mg tabs are preferred as initial therapy, since most patients require at least 70 to 100 mg/day of carbidopa to reduce the risk of N/V. The 10/100 mg tabs have limited clinical utility. Extended-release formulations have a lower bioavailability than conventional preparations. Do not use within 2 weeks of a nonselective MAOI. When used for restless legs syndrome, may precipitate rebound (recurrence of symptoms during the night) or augmentation (earlier daily onset of symptoms). Orally disintegrating tab is placed on top of the tongue and does not require water or swallowing, but is absorbed through the GI tract (not sublingually). Use caution in patients with undiagnosed skin lesions or a history of melanoma. Intense urges (gambling and sexual for example) have been reported. Consider discontinuing the medication or reducing the dose if these occur.
MOA — Levodopa is a dopamine precursor. Carbidopa blocks the peripheral conversion of levodopa to dopamine.
ADVERSE EFFECTS — Serious: Orthostatic hypotension, psychosis, agranulocytosis, leukopenia, hepatotoxicity, thrombocytopenia, pathologic gambling. Frequent: Dyskinesia, dystonia, orthostatic hypotension, N/V, abdominal cramps, confusion, hallucinations.

PRAMIPEXOLE (*Mirapex, Mirapex ER*) ▶K ♀C ▶? $$$$$
ADULTS — Parkinson's disease: Start 0.125 mg PO tid for 1 week, then 0.25 mg for 1 week; after that, increase by 0.75 mg/week divided tid. Usual effective dose is 0.5 to 1.5 mg PO tid. Extended release: Start 0.375 mg daily. May increase q 5-7 days first to 0.75 mg/day then by 0.75 mg/day increments to max 4.5 mg/day. Restless legs syndrome: Start 0.125 mg PO 2 to 3 h prior to bedtime. May increase q 4 to 7 d to 0.25 mg then 0.5 mg if needed.
PEDS — Not approved in children.
FORMS — Generic/Trade: Tabs 0.125, 0.25, 0.5, 1, 1.5 mg. Trade only: Tabs 0.75 mg, Tabs extended release 0.375, 0.75, 1.5, 3, 4.5 mg.
NOTES — Decrease dose in renal impairment. Sleep attacks, syncope, and/or orthostatic hypotension may occur. Titrate slowly. Intense urges (gambling

(cont.)

NEUROLOGY: Parkinsonian Agents

PRAMIPEXOLE (cont.)
and sexual for example) have been reported. Consider discontinuing the medication or reducing the dose if these occur. May change to extended-release tabs at same daily dose as regular tabs overnight.
MOA — Dopamine agonist (non-ergot).
ADVERSE EFFECTS — Serious: Sleep attacks, orthostatic hypotension, psychosis, impulse control disorders. Frequent: Edema, N/V, dizziness, drowsiness, insomnia, constipation, dry mouth, orthostatic hypotension, dyskinesia, dystonia, hallucinations.

ROPINIROLE (*Requip, Requip XL*) ▶L ♀C ▶? $$$$$
ADULTS — <u>Parkinson's disease:</u> Start 0.25 mg PO tid. Increase by 0.25 mg/dose at weekly intervals to 1 mg PO tid. Extended-release: Start 2 mg PO daily, then gradually titrate dose at weekly intervals or longer. Max 24 mg/day. <u>Restless legs syndrome:</u> Start 0.25 mg PO 1 to 3 h before sleep for 2 days, then increase to 0.5 mg/day on day 3 to 7. Increase by 0.5 mg/day at weekly intervals prn to max 4 mg/day given 1 to 3 h before sleep.
PEDS — Not approved in children.
FORMS — Generic/Trade: Tabs, immediate-release 0.25, 0.5, 1, 2, 3, 4, 5 mg. Trade only: Tabs extended-release 2, 3, 4, 6, 8 mg.
NOTES — Sleep attacks, impulse control disorders, syncope, and/or orthostatic hypotension may occur. Titrate slowly. Retitrate if significant interruption of therapy occurs. Intense urges (gambling and sexual for example) have been reported. Consider discontinuing the medication or reducing the dose if these occur.
MOA — Dopamine agonist (non-ergot).
ADVERSE EFFECTS — Serious: Sleep attacks, atrial fibrillation, syncope, orthostatic hypotension, HTN, psychosis, impulse control disorders. Frequent: N/V, dizziness, syncope, drowsiness, fatigue, asthenia, headache, dyspepsia, constipation, abdominal pain, dyskinesia, dystonia, pain, edema, diaphoresis, dry mouth, confusion, hallucinations, visual changes.

ROTIGOTINE (*Neupro*) ▶L ♀C ▶? $$$$
ADULTS — Product being discontinued altogether spring 2008. <u>Parkinson's disease:</u> Start 2 mg/24 h patch daily for 1 week, then increase to lowest effective dose of 4 mg/24 h. May increase prn after 1 week to max 6 mg/24 h.
PEDS — Not approved in children.
FORMS — Trade only: Transdermal patch 2, 4, 6 mg/24 h.
NOTES — Contains sulfites. Remove prior to MRI or cardioversion to avoid burns. Apply to clean, dry, intact skin of the abdomen, thigh, flank, shoulder, or upper arm, and hold in place for 20 to 30 sec. Rotate application sites daily, and wash skin after removal. Taper by 2 mg/24 h every other day when discontinuing.
MOA — Dopamine agonist (non-ergot).
ADVERSE EFFECTS — Serious: Sleep attacks, orthostatic hypotension, psychosis, syncope, HTN, impulse control disorders. Frequent: N/V, application site reactions, weight gain, fluid retention, dyskinesia, somnolence, dizziness, headache, insomnia, constipation.

STALEVO (carbidopa + levodopa + entacapone) ▶L ♀C ▶– $$$$$
ADULTS — <u>Parkinson's disease</u> (converting from prior treatment using carbidopa-levodopa with or without entacapone): Start Stalevo tab that contains the same amount of carbidopa-levodopa as the patient was previously taking, and titrate to desired response. May need to lower the dose of levodopa in patients not already taking entacapone. Max 1600 mg/day of entacapone or 1600 to 2000 mg/day of levodopa.
PEDS — Not approved in children.
FORMS — Trade only: Tabs (carbidopa/levodopa/entacapone): Stalevo 50 (12.5/50/200 mg), Stalevo 75 (18.75/75/200), Stalevo 100 (25/100/200 mg), Stalevo 125 (31.25/125/200), Stalevo 150 (37.5/150/200 mg), Stalevo 200 (50/200/200 mg).
NOTES — Patients who are not currently taking entacapone may benefit from titration of the individual components of this medication before conversion to this fixed-dose preparation. Avoid concomitant use of nonselective MAOIs. Use caution in hepatobiliary dysfunction. Motor fluctuations and dyskinesias may occur. Should not be used in patients with undiagnosed skin lesions or a history of melanoma.
MOA — Levodopa is a dopamine precursor. Carbidopa blocks the peripheral conversion of levodopa to dopamine. Entacapone blocks the peripheral metabolism of dopamine by inhibiting catechol-o-methyltransferase.
ADVERSE EFFECTS — Serious: Orthostatic hypotension, psychosis, agranulocytosis, leukopenia, hepatotoxicity, thrombocytopenia, rhabdomyolysis, severe diarrhea. Frequent: Dyskinesia, hyperkinesia, dystonia, orthostatic hypotension, N/V, abdominal cramps, diarrhea, confusion, hallucinations, urine discoloration.

NEUROLOGY: Parkinsonian Agents—Monoamine Oxidase Inhibitors (MAOIs)

RASAGILINE (*Azilect*) ▶L ♀C ▶? $$$$$
ADULTS — <u>Parkinson's disease, monotherapy:</u> 1 mg PO qam. <u>Parkinson's disease, adjunctive:</u> 0.5 mg PO qam. Max 1 mg/day.
PEDS — Not approved in children.
FORMS — Trade only: Tabs 0.5, 1 mg.
NOTES — Requires an MAOI diet. Contraindicated (risk of hypertensive crisis) with meperidine, methadone, tramadol, propoxyphene, dextromethorphan, sympathomimetic amines (eg, pseudoephedrine, phenylephrine, ephedrine), antidepressants, other MAOIs, cyclobenzaprine, and general anesthesia.

(cont.)

RASAGILINE *(cont.)*
Discontinue at least 14 days before liberalizing diet, starting one of these medications, or proceeding with elective surgery that requires general anesthesia. May need to reduce levodopa dose when used in combination. Reduce dose to 0.5 mg when used with CYP1A2 inhibitors (eg, ciprofloxacin) and in mild hepatic impairment. Do not use in moderate or severe liver disease. Consider periodic skin exams for melanoma.
MOA — Irreversible MAO inhibitor.
ADVERSE EFFECTS — Serious: Hypertensive crisis with food/drug interactions, psychosis, orthostatic hypotension, injury/falls, melanoma. Frequent: Worsening of levodopa-induced dyskinesias, anorexia, N/V, constipation, abdominal pain, weight loss, hallucinations, arthralgia, dry mouth, rash, ecchymosis, somnolence, paresthesia.

SELEGILINE (*Eldepryl, Zelapar*) ▶LK ♀C ▶? $$$$
ADULTS — Parkinsonism (adjunct to levodopa): 5 mg PO q am and q noon; max 10 mg/day. Zelapar ODT: Start 1.25 mg sublingual qam for at least 6 weeks, then increase prn to max 2.5 mg qam.
PEDS — Not approved in children.
UNAPPROVED ADULTS — Parkinsonism (monotherapy): 5 mg PO q am and q noon; max 10 mg/day.
FORMS — Generic/Trade: Caps 5 mg. Tabs 5 mg. Trade only: Oral disintegrating tabs (Zelapar ODT) 1.25 mg.
NOTES — Should not be combined with meperidine or other opioids. Do not exceed max recommended dose; risk of nonselective MAO inhibition. Zelapar should be taken in the morning before food and without water. Intense urges (gambling and sexual for example) have been reported. Consider discontinuing the medication or reducing the dose if these occur.
MOA — Selective MAO-B inhibitor.
ADVERSE EFFECTS — Serious: Angina, syncope, mood lability, psychosis, orthostatic hypotension, impulse control disorders. Frequent: N/V, confusion, depression, ataxia, insomnia, orthostatic hypotension, hallucinations.

NEUROLOGY: Other Agents

BETAHISTINE (✦*Serc*) ▶LK ♀? ▶? $
ADULTS — Canada only. Vertigo of Meniere's disease: 8 to 16 mg PO tid.
PEDS — Not approved in children.
FORMS — Trade only: Tabs 8, 16 mg.
NOTES — Contraindicated in peptic ulcer disease and pheochromocytoma; use caution in asthmatics.
MOA — Histamine H1-receptor agonist.
ADVERSE EFFECTS — Frequent: Urticaria, pruritus, gastrointestinal upset, nausea, headache.

BOTULINUM TOXIN TYPE A (*Botox, Botox Cosmetic*) ▶Not absorbed ♀C ▶? $$$$$
WARNING — Symptoms of systemic botulism have been reported, particularly in children treated for spasticity due to cerebral palsy.
ADULTS — Moderate to severe glabellar lines in patients no older than age 65 yo: Inject 0.1 mL into each of 5 sites. Blepharospasm: 1.25 to 5 units IM into each of several sites in the orbicularis oculi of upper and lower lids q 3 months; use lower doses at initial visit. Strabismus: 1.25 to 5 units depending on diagnosis, injected into extraocular muscles. Cervical dystonia: 15 to 100 units IM (with or without EMG guidance) into affected muscles q 3 months (eg, splenius capitis/cervicis, sternocleidomastoid, levator scapulae, trapezius, semispinalis, scalene, longissimus); usual total dose is 200 to 300 units/treatment. Primary axillary hyperhidrosis: 50 units/axilla intradermally, divided over 10 to 15 sites. Upper limb spasticity: Biceps brachii, 100-200 units IM divided into 4 sites; flexor carpi radialis, 12.5-50 units IM in 1 site; flexor carpi ulnaris, 12.5-50 units IM in 1 site; flexor digitorum profundus, 30-50 units IM in 1 site; flexor digitorum sublimis, 30-50 units IM in 1 site.
PEDS — Not approved in children younger than 12 yo for blepharospasm, younger than 16 yo for cervical dystonia, or younger than 18 yo for hyperhidrosis.
UNAPPROVED ADULTS — Hemifacial spasm: 1.25 to 2.5 units IM into affected muscles q 3 to 4 months (eg, corrugator, orbicularis oculi, zygomaticus major, buccinator, depressor anguli oris, platysma); usual total dose is 10 to 34 units/treatment.
FORMS — Trade only: 100 unit single-use vials.
NOTES — Clinical benefit occurs within 2 weeks (2 to 3 days for facial injections), peaks at 1 to 6 weeks, and wears off in approximately 3 months. Contraindicated in peripheral motor neuropathic disease (eg, ALS, motor neuropathy) or neuromuscular junction disease (eg, myasthenia gravis, Lambert-Eaton syndrome). The use of lower doses and longer dosing intervals may decrease the risk of producing neutralizing antibodies. Increased risk of dysphagia when more than 100 units are injected into the sternocleidomastoid or with bilateral sternocleidomastoid injections. When used for upper limb spasticity, the dose may be repeated when effect diminishes, but no sooner than 12 weeks. Potency units of Botox cannot be interchanged with other products.
MOA — Neuromuscular transmission blockade; inhibits presynaptic acetylcholine release.
ADVERSE EFFECTS — Severe: Anaphylaxis, dysphagia, arrhythmias, myocardial infarction, systemic botulism, death. Frequent: Rash, urticaria, pruritus, flu-like symptoms, excessive weakness, upper respiratory tract infection, neck pain, headache. Periorbital injections may cause ptosis, dry eyes, superficial keratosis, or lacrimation; injections of facial muscles may cause facial asymmetry.

BOTULINUM TOXIN TYPE B (*Myobloc*) ▶Not significantly absorbed ♀+ ▶? $$$$$
WARNING — Symptoms of systemic botulism have been reported, particularly in children treated for spasticity due to cerebral palsy.
ADULTS — <u>Cervical dystonia:</u> Start 2500 to 5000 units IM in affected muscles. Use lower initial dose if no prior history of botulinum toxin therapy. Benefits usually last for 12 to 16 weeks when a total dose of 5000 to 10,000 units has been administered. Titrate to effective dose. Give treatments at least 3 months apart to decrease the risk of producing neutralizing antibodies.
PEDS — Not approved in children.
NOTES — Low systemic concentrations are expected with IM injection; monitor closely for dysphagia. Use caution in peripheral motor neuropathic disease (eg, ALS, motor neuropathy) or neuromuscular junction disease (eg, myasthenia gravis, Lambert-Eaton syndrome due to an increased risk of systemic effects) and with other drugs that block neuromuscular function (eg, aminoglycosides, curare-like compounds).
MOA — Neuromuscular transmission blockade; inhibits presynaptic acetylcholine release.
ADVERSE EFFECTS — Serious: Systemic botulism, dysphagia, respiratory compromise, hypersensitivity. Frequent: Dry mouth, dyspepsia/nausea, injection site pain, flu-like syndrome, arthralgia, back pain, cough, myasthenia, asthenia, dizziness.

MANNITOL (*Osmitrol, Resectisol*) ▶K ♀C ▶? $$
ADULTS — <u>Intracranial HTN:</u> 0.25 to 2 g/kg IV over 30 to 60 min as a 15, 20, or 25% soln.
PEDS — Not approved in children.
UNAPPROVED ADULTS — <u>Increased ICP or Head trauma:</u> 0.25 to 1 g/kg IV push over 20 min. Repeat q 4 to 6 h prn.
UNAPPROVED PEDS — <u>Increased ICP/Cerebral edema:</u> 0.25 to 1 g/kg/dose IV push over 20 to 30 min, then 0.25 to 0.5 g/kg/dose IV q 4 to 6 h prn.
NOTES — Monitor fluid and electrolyte balance and cardiac function. Filter IV solns with concentrations ≥20%; crystals may be present.
MOA — Osmotic diuretic.
ADVERSE EFFECTS — Serious: Congestive heart failure, pulmonary edema, seizures, electrolyte changes, CNS depression, acute renal failure. Frequent: Headache, dizziness, N/V, polydipsia.

MILNACIPRAN (*Savella*) ▶KL ♀C ▶? $$$$
ADULTS — <u>Fibromyalgia:</u> Start day 1: 12.5 mg PO once, then days 2 to 3: 12.5 mg bid, days 4 to 7: 25 mg bid, then 50 mg bid. Max 200 mg/day.
PEDS — Not approved for use in children.
FORMS — Trade only: Tabs 12.5, 25, 50, 100 mg.
NOTES — Reduce dose by 50% for severe renal impairment with CrCl < 30 mL/min. Taper if discontinued.
MOA — Selective serotonin/norepinephrine reuptake inhibitor.
ADVERSE EFFECTS — Severe: Worsening of depression, suicidality, serotonin syndrome, hypertension, tachycardia, seizures, hepatotoxicity, abnormal bleeding, hyponatremia. Frequent: Nausea/vomiting, headache, dizziness, insomnia, hot flushes, hyperhidrosis, palpitations, dry mouth.

NIMODIPINE (*Nimotop*) ▶L ♀C ▶− $$$$$
ADULTS — <u>Subarachnoid hemorrhage:</u> 60 mg PO q 4 h for 21 days.
PEDS — Not approved in children.
FORMS — Generic only: Caps 30 mg.
NOTES — Begin therapy within 96 h. Give 1 h before or 2 h after meals. May give cap contents SL or via NG tube. Reduce dose in hepatic dysfunction.
MOA — Calcium channel blocker.
ADVERSE EFFECTS — Serious: Heart failure, disseminated intravascular coagulation, deep vein thrombosis, neurological deterioration. Frequent: Hypotension, N/V, diarrhea, flushing, edema, headache.

OXYBATE (*Xyrem, GHB, gamma hydroxybutyrate*) ▶L ♀B ▶? ©III $$$$$
WARNING — CNS depressant with abuse potential; avoid concurrent alcohol or sedative use.
ADULTS — <u>Narcolepsy-associated cataplexy or excessive daytime sleepiness:</u> 2.25 g PO at bedtime. Repeat in 2.5 to 4 h. May increase by 1.5 g/day at 2-week intervals to max 9 g/day. Dilute each dose in 60 mL water.
PEDS — Not approved in children.
FORMS — Trade only: Soln 180 mL (500 mg/mL) supplied with measuring device and child-proof dosing cups.
NOTES — Available only through the Xyrem Success Program centralized pharmacy (866-997-3688). Adjust dose in hepatic dysfunction. Prepare doses just prior to bedtime, and use within 24 h. May need an alarm to signal 2nd dose.
MOA — Unknown.
ADVERSE EFFECTS — Serious: Abuse and dependence, depression, syncope, seizures, CNS and respiratory depression, coma. Frequent: Headache, nausea, dizziness, pain, somnolence, pharyngitis, infection, flu-like symptoms, accidental injury, diarrhea, urinary incontinence, confusion, sleepwalking.

RILUZOLE (*Rilutek*) ▶LK ♀C ▶− $$$$$
ADULTS — <u>Amyotrophic lateral sclerosis:</u> 50 mg PO q 12 h.
PEDS — Not approved in children.
FORMS — Trade only: Tabs 50 mg.
NOTES — Take 1 h before or 2 h after meals. Monitor LFTs.
MOA — Glutamate antagonist.
ADVERSE EFFECTS — Serious: Tachycardia, hypertension, hepatotoxicity, neutropenia, interstitial lung disease. Frequent: Asthenia, N/V, diarrhea, abdominal pain, pneumonia, dizziness, paresthesia, drowsiness.

TETRABENAZINE (*Xenazine, ✦Nitoman*) ▶L ♀C ▶? ? $$$$$
WARNING — Contraindicated with untreated or inadequately responding depression or suicidality; monitor closely and discontinue at the first signs thereof.

(cont.)

TETRABENAZINE *(cont.)*
- ADULTS — <u>Chorea associated with Huntington's disease:</u> Start 12.5 mg PO qam. Increase after 1 week to 12.5 mg PO bid. May increase by 12.5 mg/day weekly. For doses greater than 37.5 to 50 mg/day divide doses tid. For doses greater than 50 mg/day genotype the patient for CYP2D6 activity and titrate by 12.5 mg/day weekly and divide tid to max 100 mg/day and 37.5 mg/dose (extensive/intermediate metabolizers) or 50 mg/day and 25 mg/dose (poor metabolizers).
- PEDS — Not approved in children.
- UNAPPROVED ADULTS — <u>Hyperkinetic movement disorders such as hemiballismus, senile chorea, tic disorders including Tourette's syndrome</u> (approved dosing in Canada): Start 12.5 mg PO bid to tid. May increase by 12.5 mg/day q 3 to 5 days to usual dose of 25 mg PO tid. Max 200 mg/day, but most patients do not tolerate more than 75 mg/day. Discontinue if there is no benefit after 7 days of treatment at max tolerated dose.
- UNAPPROVED PEDS — Limited data suggest that ½ of the adult dose may be used and titrated as tolerated.
- FORMS — Trade only: Tabs 12.5, 25 mg.
- NOTES — Contraindicated in hepatic impairment, suicidality, untreated/inadequately responding depression, and with MAOIs. Reduce dose by 50% if used with potent CYP2D6 inhibitors. Monitor patient for depression, akathisia, sedation/somnolence, and parkinsonism, which may respond to lowering the dose. Retitrate dose if interrupted > 5 days. Use caution when combined with antipsychotics and other dopamine receptor blocking agents. May attenuate the effects of levodopa and antidepressants. Increases QTc by approximately 8 msec.
- MOA — Depletes monoamines from storage sites.
- ADVERSE EFFECTS — Serious: Parkinsonism, cognitive decline, orthostatic hypotension, depression, suicidality, neuroleptic malignant syndrome. Frequent: Drowsiness, fatigue, weakness, anxiety, insomnia, akathisia, sialorrhea, irritability, agitation, N/V, epigastric pain, confusion, disorientation, dizziness.

OB/GYN: Contraceptives—Oral Biphasic

NOTE: Not recommended in women greater than 35 yo who smoke or have complex migraine headaches. Increased risk of thromboembolism, CVA, MI, hepatic neoplasia, and gallbladder disease. Nausea, breast tenderness, and breakthrough bleeding are common transient side effects. Nighttime dosing may minimize nausea. Effectiveness is reduced by hepatic enzyme-inducing drugs such as certain anticonvulsants and barbiturates, rifampin, rifabutin, griseofulvin and protease inhibitors. Additionally, products that contain St. John's wort may decrease efficacy. Vomiting or diarrhea may also increase the risk of contraceptive failure. An additional form of birth control may be advisable. Advise patients to take at the same time every days. See PI for instructions on missing doses. Most available in 21 and 28 day packs. Although not approved by the FDA, combined OCPs are used for dysfunctional uterine bleeding, dysmenorrhea, pelvic pain, and hirsutism (with spironolactone): 1 tab PO daily. Wait 6 weeks postpartum to initiate combination OCPs to decrease the risk of thromboembolism and to support lactation.

NECON 10/11 (ethinyl estradiol + norethindrone) ▶L ♀X ▶– $$
- ADULTS — <u>Contraception:</u> 1 tab PO daily.
- PEDS — Not approved in children.
- FORMS — Trade only: Tabs 35 mcg ethinyl estradiol/0.5 mg norethindrone (10), 35 mcg ethinyl estradiol/1 mg norethindrone (11).
- NOTES — Same as Ortho-Novum 10/11.
- MOA — Contraceptive steroid combination.
- ADVERSE EFFECTS — Serious: DVT/PE, stroke, MI, hepatic neoplasia, and gallbladder disease. Frequent: Nausea, breast tenderness, and breakthrough bleeding.

ORTHO NOVUM 10/11 (ethinyl estradiol + norethindrone) ▶L ♀X ▶– $$$
- ADULTS — <u>Contraception:</u> 1 tab PO daily.
- PEDS — Not approved in children.
- FORMS — Trade only: Tabs 35 mcg ethinyl estradiol/0.5 mg norethindrone (10), 35 mcg ethinyl estradiol/1 mg norethindrone (11).
- MOA — Contraceptive steroid combination.
- ADVERSE EFFECTS — Serious: DVT/PE, stroke, MI, hepatic neoplasia, and gallbladder disease. Frequent: Nausea, breast tenderness, and breakthrough bleeding.

OB/GYN: Contraceptives—Oral Monophasic

NOTE: Not recommended in women greater than 35 yo who smoke or have complex migraine headaches. Increased risk of thromboembolism, CVA, MI, hepatic neoplasia and gallbladder disease. Nausea, breast tenderness, and breakthrough bleeding are common transient side effects. Nighttime dosing may minimize nausea. Effectiveness is reduced by hepatic enzyme-inducing drugs such as certain anticonvulsants and barbiturates, rifampin, rifabutin, griseofulvin, and protease inhibitors. Additionally, products that contain St John's wort may decrease efficacy. Vomiting or diarrhea may also increase the risk of contraceptive failure. An additional form of birth control may be advisable. Advise patients to take at the same time every days. See PI for instructions on missing doses. Most available in 21 and 28 day packs. Although not approved by the FDA, combined OCPs are used for dysfunctional uterine bleeding, emergency contraception, dysmenorrhea, pelvic pain, and hirsutism (with spironolactone): 1 tab PO daily. Wait 6 weeks postpartum to initiate combination OCPs to decrease the risk of thromboembolism and to support lactation.

OB/GYN: Contraceptives

ALESSE (ethinyl estradiol + levonorgestrel) ▶L ♀X ▶– $$
ADULTS – Contraception: 1 tab PO daily.
PEDS – Not approved in children.
UNAPPROVED ADULTS – Postcoital contraception: See table.
FORMS – Trade only: Tabs 20 mcg ethinyl estradiol/0.1 mg levonorgestrel.
NOTES – May cause less nausea and breast tenderness and may increase breakthrough bleeding due to lower estrogen content.
MOA – Contraceptive steroid combination.
ADVERSE EFFECTS – Serious: DVT/PE, stroke, MI, hepatic neoplasia, and gallbladder disease. Frequent: Nausea, breast tenderness, and breakthrough bleeding.

APRI (ethinyl estradiol + desogestrel, ✢Marvelon) ▶L ♀X ▶– $$
ADULTS – Contraception: 1 tab PO daily.
PEDS – Not approved in children.
FORMS – Trade only: Tabs 30 mcg ethinyl estradiol/0.15 mg desogestrel.
NOTES – Same as Desogen.
MOA – Contraceptive steroid combination.
ADVERSE EFFECTS – Serious: DVT/PE, stroke, MI, hepatic neoplasia, and gallbladder disease. Frequent: Nausea, breast tenderness, and breakthrough bleeding.

AVIANE (ethinyl estradiol + levonorgestrel) ▶L ♀X ▶– $$
ADULTS – Contraception: 1 tab PO daily.
PEDS – Not approved in children.
UNAPPROVED ADULTS – Postcoital contraception: See table.
FORMS – Trade only: Tabs 20 mcg ethinyl estradiol/0.1 mg levonorgestrel.
NOTES – May cause less nausea and breast tenderness and may increase breakthrough bleeding due to lower estrogen content. Same as Alesse.
MOA – Contraceptive steroid combination.
ADVERSE EFFECTS – Serious: DVT/PE, stroke, MI, hepatic neoplasia, and gallbladder disease. Frequent: Nausea, breast tenderness, and breakthrough bleeding.

BALZIVA (ethinyl estradiol + norethindrone) ▶L ♀X ▶– $$
ADULTS – Contraception: 1 tab PO daily.
PEDS – Not approved in children.
FORMS – Trade only: Tabs 35 mcg ethinyl estradiol/0.4 mg norethindrone.
NOTES – Same as Ovcon-35.
MOA – Contraceptive steroid combination.
ADVERSE EFFECTS – Serious: DVT/PE, stroke, MI, hepatic neoplasia, and gallbladder disease. Frequent: Nausea, breast tenderness, and breakthrough bleeding.

BREVICON (ethinyl estradiol + norethindrone) ▶L ♀X ▶– $$$
ADULTS – Contraception: 1 tab PO daily.
PEDS – Not approved in children.
FORMS – Trade only: Tabs 35 mcg ethinyl estradiol/0.5 mg norethindrone.

MOA – Contraceptive steroid combination.
ADVERSE EFFECTS – Serious: DVT/PE, stroke, MI, hepatic neoplasia, and gallbladder disease. Frequent: Nausea, breast tenderness, and breakthrough bleeding.

CRYSELLE (ethinyl estradiol + norgestrel) ▶L ♀X ▶– $$
ADULTS – Contraception: 1 tab PO daily.
PEDS – Not approved in children.
UNAPPROVED ADULTS – Postcoital contraception: See table.
FORMS – Trade only: Tabs: 30 mcg ethinyl estradiol/0.3 mg norgestrel.
NOTES – Same as Lo/Ovral.
MOA – Contraceptive steroid combination.
ADVERSE EFFECTS – Serious: DVT/PE, stroke, MI, hepatic neoplasia, and gallbladder disease. Frequent: Nausea, breast tenderness, and breakthrough bleeding.

DEMULEN (ethinyl estradiol + ethynodiol) ▶L ♀X ▶– $$
WARNING – Multiple strengths; see FORMS and write specific product on Rx.
ADULTS – Contraception: 1 tab PO daily.
PEDS – Not approved in children.
FORMS – Trade only: Tabs 35 mcg ethinyl estradiol/1 mg ethynodiol (Demulen 1/35); 50 mcg ethinyl estradiol/1 mg ethynodiol (Demulen 1/50).
NOTES – 50 mcg estrogen component rarely necessary.
MOA – Contraceptive steroid combination.
ADVERSE EFFECTS – Serious: DVT/PE, stroke, MI, hepatic neoplasia, and gallbladder disease. Frequent: Nausea, breast tenderness, and breakthrough bleeding.

DESOGEN (ethinyl estradiol + desogestrel, ✢Marvelon) ▶L ♀X ▶– $$
ADULTS – Contraception: 1 tab PO daily.
PEDS – Not approved in children.
FORMS – Trade only: Tabs 30 mcg ethinyl estradiol/0.15 mg desogestrel.
MOA – Contraceptive steroid combination.
ADVERSE EFFECTS – Serious: DVT/PE, stroke, MI, hepatic neoplasia, and gallbladder disease. Frequent: Nausea, breast tenderness, and breakthrough bleeding.

FEMCON FE (ethinyl estradiol + norethindrone) ▶L ♀X ▶– $$$
ADULTS – Contraception: 1 tab PO daily.
PEDS – Not approved in children.
FORMS – Trade only: Chewable tabs 35 mcg ethinyl estradiol/0.4 mg norethindrone. Placebo tabs are ferrous fumarate 75 mg.
NOTES – Chewable formulation may be swallowed whole or chewed. If chewed, follow with 8 ounces liquid.
MOA – Contraceptive steroid combination.
ADVERSE EFFECTS – Serious: DVT/PE, stroke, MI, hepatic neoplasia, and gallbladder disease. Frequent: Nausea, breast tenderness, and breakthrough bleeding.

JUNEL (ethinyl estradiol + norethindrone) ▶L ♀X ▶– $$
WARNING – Multiple strengths; see FORMS and write specific product on Rx.
ADULTS – Contraception: 1 tab PO daily.
PEDS – Not approved in children.
FORMS – Trade only: Tabs 1 mg norethindrone/20 mcg ethinyl estradiol (Junel 1/20). 1.5 mg norethindrone/30 mcg ethinyl estradiol (Junel 1.5/30).
NOTES – Junel 1/20 may cause less nausea and breast tenderness and may increase breakthrough bleeding due to lower estrogen content. Same as Loestrin.
MOA – Contraceptive steroid combination.
ADVERSE EFFECTS – Serious: DVT/PE, stroke, MI, hepatic neoplasia, and gallbladder disease. Frequent: Nausea, breast tenderness, and breakthrough bleeding.

JUNEL FE (ethinyl estradiol + norethindrone + ferrous fumarate) ▶L ♀X ▶– $$
WARNING – Multiple strengths; see FORMS and write specific product on Rx.
ADULTS – Contraception: 1 tab PO daily.
PEDS – Not approved in children.
FORMS – Trade only: Tabs 1 mg norethindrone/20 mcg ethinyl estradiol with 7 days 75 mg ferrous fumarate (Junel Fe 1/20). 1.5 mg norethindrone/30 mcg ethinyl estradiol with 7 days 75 mg ferrous fumarate (1.5/30).
NOTES – Junel Fe 1/20 may cause less nausea and breast tenderness and may increase breakthrough bleeding due to lower estrogen content. Same as Loestrin Fe.
MOA – Contraceptive steroid combination.
ADVERSE EFFECTS – Serious: DVT/PE, stroke, MI, hepatic neoplasia, and gallbladder disease. Frequent: Nausea, breast tenderness, and breakthrough bleeding.

KARIVA (ethinyl estradiol + desogestrel) ▶L ♀X ▶– $$$
ADULTS – Contraception: 1 tab PO daily.
PEDS – Not approved in children.
FORMS – Trade only: Tabs 20 mcg ethinyl estradiol/0.15 mg desogestrel (21), 10 mcg ethinyl estradiol (5).
NOTES – May have less breakthrough bleeding. All 28 tabs must be taken. Same as Mircette.
MOA – Contraceptive steroid combination.
ADVERSE EFFECTS – Serious: DVT/PE, stroke, MI, hepatic neoplasia, and gallbladder disease. Frequent: Nausea, breast tenderness, and breakthrough bleeding.

KELNOR (ethinyl estradiol + ethynodiol) ▶L ♀X ▶– $$
ADULTS – Contraception: 1 tab PO daily.
PEDS – Not approved in children.
FORMS – Generic/Trade: Tabs 35 mcg ethinyl estradiol/1 mg ethynodiol.
NOTES – Same as Demulen.
MOA – Contraceptive steroid combination.
ADVERSE EFFECTS – Serious: DVT/PE, stroke, MI, hepatic neoplasia, and gallbladder disease. Frequent: Nausea, breast tenderness, and breakthrough bleeding.

LESSINA (ethinyl estradiol + levonorgestrel) ▶L ♀X ▶– $$
ADULTS – Contraception: 1 tab PO daily.
PEDS – Not approved in children.
UNAPPROVED ADULTS – Postcoital contraception: See table.
FORMS – Generic/Trade: Tabs 20 mcg ethinyl estradiol/0.1 mg levonorgestrel.
NOTES – May cause less nausea and breast tenderness and may increase breakthrough bleeding due to lower estrogen content. Same as Levlite.
MOA – Contraceptive steroid combination.
ADVERSE EFFECTS – Serious: DVT/PE, stroke, MI, hepatic neoplasia, and gallbladder disease. Frequent: Nausea, breast tenderness, and breakthrough bleeding.

LEVLEN (ethinyl estradiol + levonorgestrel, ✽Min-Ovral) ▶L ♀X ▶– $$
ADULTS – Contraception: 1 tab PO daily.
PEDS – Not approved in children.
UNAPPROVED ADULTS – Postcoital contraception: See table.
FORMS – Trade only: Tabs 30 mcg ethinyl estradiol/0.15 mg levonorgestrel.
NOTES – Same as Nordette.
MOA – Contraceptive steroid combination.
ADVERSE EFFECTS – Serious: DVT/PE, stroke, MI, hepatic neoplasia, and gallbladder disease. Frequent: Nausea, breast tenderness, and breakthrough bleeding.

LEVLITE (ethinyl estradiol + levonorgestrel) ▶L ♀X ▶– $$
ADULTS – Contraception: 1 tab PO daily.
PEDS – Not approved in children.
UNAPPROVED ADULTS – Postcoital contraception: See table.
FORMS – Generic/Trade: Tabs 20 mcg ethinyl estradiol/0.1 mg levonorgestrel.
NOTES – May cause less nausea and breast tenderness and may increase breakthrough bleeding due to lower estrogen content. Same as Alesse.
MOA – Contraceptive steroid combination.
ADVERSE EFFECTS – Serious: DVT/PE, stroke, MI, hepatic neoplasia, and gallbladder disease. Frequent: Nausea, breast tenderness, and breakthrough bleeding.

LEVORA (ethinyl estradiol + levonorgestrel, ✽Min-Ovral) ▶L ♀X ▶– $$
ADULTS – Contraception: 1 tab PO daily.
PEDS – Not approved in children.
UNAPPROVED ADULTS – Postcoital contraception: See table.
FORMS – Trade only: Tabs 30 mcg ethinyl estradiol/0.15 mg levonorgestrel.
NOTES – Same as Levlen.
MOA – Contraceptive steroid combination.
ADVERSE EFFECTS – Serious: DVT/PE, stroke, MI, hepatic neoplasia, and gallbladder disease. Frequent: Nausea, breast tenderness, and breakthrough bleeding.

OB/GYN: Contraceptives

LO/OVRAL (ethinyl estradiol + norgestrel) ▶L ♀X ▶– $$
ADULTS – <u>Contraception:</u> 1 tab PO daily.
PEDS – Not approved in children.
UNAPPROVED ADULTS – <u>Postcoital contraception:</u> See table.
FORMS – Trade only: Tabs: 30 mcg ethinyl estradiol/0.3 mg norgestrel.
MOA – Contraceptive steroid combination.
ADVERSE EFFECTS – Serious: DVT/PE, stroke, MI, hepatic neoplasia, and gallbladder disease. Frequent: Nausea, breast tenderness, and breakthrough bleeding.

LOESTRIN (ethinyl estradiol + norethindrone, ✦Minestrin 1/20) ▶L ♀X ▶– $$$
WARNING – Multiple strengths; see FORMS and write specific product on Rx.
ADULTS – <u>Contraception:</u> 1 tab PO daily.
PEDS – Not approved in children.
FORMS – Trade only: Tabs 1 mg norethindrone/20 mcg ethinyl estradiol (Loestrin 1/20). 1.5 mg norethindrone/30 mcg ethinyl estradiol (Loestrin 1.5/30).
NOTES – Loestrin 1/20 may cause less nausea and breast tenderness and may increase breakthrough bleeding due to lower estrogen content.
MOA – Contraceptive steroid combination.
ADVERSE EFFECTS – Serious: DVT/PE, stroke, MI, hepatic neoplasia, and gallbladder disease. Frequent: Nausea, breast tenderness, and breakthrough bleeding.

LOESTRIN 24 FE (ethinyl estradiol + norethindrone + ferrous fumarate) ▶L ♀X ▶– $$$
ADULTS – <u>Contraception:</u> 1 tab PO daily.
PEDS – Not approved in children.
FORMS – Trade only: Tabs 1 mg norethindrone/20 mcg ethinyl estradiol (24 days) with 4 days 75 mg ferrous fumarate.
NOTES – Loestrin 24 Fe 1/20 may cause less nausea and breast tenderness and may increase breakthrough bleeding due to lower estrogen content.
MOA – Contraceptive steroid combination.
ADVERSE EFFECTS – Serious: DVT/PE, stroke, MI, hepatic neoplasia, and gallbladder disease. Frequent: Nausea, breast tenderness, and breakthrough bleeding.

LOESTRIN FE (ethinyl estradiol + norethindrone + ferrous fumarate) ▶L ♀X ▶– $$$
WARNING – Multiple strengths; see FORMS and write specific product on Rx.
ADULTS – <u>Contraception:</u> 1 tab PO daily.
PEDS – Not approved in children.
FORMS – Trade only: Tabs 1 mg norethindrone/20 mcg ethinyl estradiol with 7 days 75 mg ferrous fumarate (Loestrin Fe 1/20); 1.5 mg norethindrone/30 mcg ethinyl estradiol with 7 days 75 mg ferrous fumarate (1.5/30).
NOTES – Loestrin Fe 1/20 may cause less nausea and breast tenderness and may increase breakthrough bleeding due to lower estrogen content. All 28 tabs must be taken.
MOA – Contraceptive steroid combination.
ADVERSE EFFECTS – Serious: DVT/PE, stroke, MI, hepatic neoplasia, and gallbladder disease. Frequent: Nausea, breast tenderness, and breakthrough bleeding.

LOSEASONIQUE (ethinyl estradiol + levonorgestrel) ▶L ♀X ▶– $$$
ADULTS – <u>Contraception:</u> 1 tab PO daily.
PEDS – Not approved in children.
FORMS – Trade only: Tabs 20 mcg ethinyl estradiol/0.1 mg levonorgestrel. 84 orange active pills followed by 7 yellow pills with 10 mcg ethinyl estradiol.
NOTES – Decreases menstrual periods from q month to q 3 months; however, intermenstrual bleeding and spotting is more frequent than with 28-day regimens. All 91 tabs must be taken.
MOA – Contraceptive steroid combination.
ADVERSE EFFECTS – Serious: DVT/PE, stroke, MI, hepatic neoplasia, and gallbladder disease. Frequent: Nausea, breast tenderness, and breakthrough bleeding.

LOW-OGESTREL (ethinyl estradiol + norgestrel) ▶L ♀X ▶– $$
ADULTS – <u>Contraception:</u> 1 tab PO daily.
PEDS – Not approved in children.
UNAPPROVED ADULTS – <u>Postcoital contraception:</u> See table.
FORMS – Trade only: Tabs: 30 mcg ethinyl estradiol/0.3 mg norgestrel.
NOTES – Same as Lo/Ovral.
MOA – Contraceptive steroid combination.
ADVERSE EFFECTS – Serious: DVT/PE, stroke, MI, hepatic neoplasia, and gallbladder disease. Frequent: Nausea, breast tenderness, and breakthrough bleeding.

LUTERA (ethinyl estradiol + levonorgestrel) ▶L ♀X ▶– $$
ADULTS – <u>Contraception:</u> 1 tab PO daily.
PEDS – Not approved in children.
UNAPPROVED ADULTS – <u>Postcoital contraception:</u> See table.
FORMS – Trade only: Tabs 20 mcg ethinyl estradiol/0.1 mg levonorgestrel.
NOTES – May cause less nausea and breast tenderness and may increase breakthrough bleeding due to lower estrogen content. Same as Alesse.
MOA – Contraceptive steroid combination.
ADVERSE EFFECTS – Serious: DVT/PE, stroke, MI, hepatic neoplasia, and gallbladder disease. Frequent: Nausea, breast tenderness, and breakthrough bleeding.

LYBREL (ethinyl estradiol + levonorgestrel) ▶L ♀X ▶– $$$
ADULTS – <u>Contraception:</u> 1 tab PO daily.
PEDS – Not approved in children.
FORMS – Trade only: Tabs 20 mcg ethinyl estradiol/90 mcg levonorgestrel.
NOTES – Approved for continuous use without a "pill-free" period. May cause breakthrough bleeding.
MOA – Contraceptive steroid combination.

(cont.)

LYBREL (cont.)
ADVERSE EFFECTS – Serious: DVT/PE, stroke, MI, hepatic neoplasia, and gallbladder disease. Frequent: Nausea, breast tenderness, and breakthrough bleeding.

MICROGESTIN FE (ethinyl estradiol + norethindrone + ferrous fumarate) ▶L ♀X ▶– $$
WARNING – Multiple strengths; see FORMS and write specific product on Rx.
ADULTS – <u>Contraception</u>: 1 tab PO daily.
PEDS – Not approved in children.
FORMS – Trade only: Tabs 1 mg norethindrone/20 mcg ethinyl estradiol with 7 days 75 mg ferrous fumarate (Microgestin Fe 1/20). 1.5 mg norethindrone/30 mcg ethinyl estradiol with 7 days 75 mg ferrous fumarate (1.5/30).
NOTES – Microgestin Fe 1/20 may cause less nausea and breast tenderness and may increase breakthrough bleeding due to lower estrogen content. Same as Loestrin Fe. All 28 tabs must be taken.
MOA – Contraceptive steroid combination.
ADVERSE EFFECTS – Serious: DVT/PE, stroke, MI, hepatic neoplasia, and gallbladder disease. Frequent: Nausea, breast tenderness, and breakthrough bleeding.

MIRCETTE (ethinyl estradiol + desogestrel) ▶L ♀X ▶– $$$
ADULTS – <u>Contraception</u>: 1 tab PO daily.
PEDS – Not approved in children.
FORMS – Trade only: Tabs 20 mcg ethinyl estradiol/0.15 mg desogestrel (21), 10 mcg ethinyl estradiol (5).
NOTES – May have less breakthrough bleeding. All 28 tabs must be taken.
MOA – Contraceptive steroid combination.
ADVERSE EFFECTS – Serious: DVT/PE, stroke, MI, hepatic neoplasia, and gallbladder disease. Frequent: Nausea, breast tenderness, and breakthrough bleeding.

MODICON (ethinyl estradiol + norethindrone) ▶L ♀X ▶– $$$
ADULTS – <u>Contraception</u>: 1 tab PO daily.
PEDS – Not approved in children.
FORMS – Trade only: Tabs 35 mcg ethinyl estradiol/0.5 mg norethindrone.
NOTES – Same as Brevicon.
MOA – Contraceptive steroid combination.
ADVERSE EFFECTS – Serious: DVT/PE, stroke, MI, hepatic neoplasia, and gallbladder disease. Frequent: Nausea, breast tenderness, and breakthrough bleeding.

MONONESSA (ethinyl estradiol + norgestimate) ▶L ♀X ▶– $$
ADULTS – <u>Contraception</u>: 1 tab PO daily.
PEDS – Not approved in children.
FORMS – Trade only: Tabs: 35 mcg ethinyl estradiol/0.25 mg norgestimate.
NOTES – Same as Ortho-Cyclen.
MOA – Contraceptive steroid combination.
ADVERSE EFFECTS – Serious: DVT/PE, stroke, MI, hepatic neoplasia, and gallbladder disease. Frequent: Nausea, breast tenderness, and breakthrough bleeding.

NECON (ethinyl estradiol + norethindrone, ✜Select 1/35, Brevicon 1/35) ▶L ♀X ▶– $$
WARNING – Multiple strengths; see FORMS and write specific product on Rx.
ADULTS – <u>Contraception</u>: 1 tab PO daily.
PEDS – Not approved in children.
FORMS – Trade only: Tabs 0.5 mg norethindrone/35 mcg ethinyl estradiol (Necon 0.5/35). 1 mg norethindrone/35 mcg ethinyl estradiol (Necon 1/35).
NOTES – Same as Brevicon (0.5/35), Ortho-Novum 1/35 (1/35).
MOA – Contraceptive steroid combination.
ADVERSE EFFECTS – Serious: DVT/PE, stroke, MI, hepatic neoplasia, and gallbladder disease. Frequent: Nausea, breast tenderness, and breakthrough bleeding.

NECON 1/50 (mestranol + norethindrone) ▶L ♀X ▶– $$
ADULTS – <u>Contraception</u>: 1 tab PO daily.
PEDS – Not approved in children.
FORMS – Trade only: Tabs: 1 mg norethindrone/50 mcg mestranol.
NOTES – 50 mcg estrogen component rarely necessary. Same as Ortho-Novum 1/50.
MOA – Contraceptive steroid combination.
ADVERSE EFFECTS – Serious: DVT/PE, stroke, MI, hepatic neoplasia, and gallbladder disease. Frequent: Nausea, breast tenderness, and breakthrough bleeding.

NORDETTE (ethinyl estradiol + levonorgestrel, ✜Min-Ovral) ▶L ♀X ▶– $$$
ADULTS – <u>Contraception</u>: 1 tab PO daily.
PEDS – Not approved in children.
UNAPPROVED ADULTS – <u>Postcoital contraception</u>: See table.
FORMS – Trade only: Tabs 30 mcg ethinyl estradiol/0.15 mg levonorgestrel.
NOTES – Same as Levlen.
MOA – Contraceptive steroid combination.
ADVERSE EFFECTS – Serious: DVT/PE, stroke, MI, hepatic neoplasia, and gallbladder disease. Frequent: Nausea, breast tenderness, and breakthrough bleeding.

NORINYL 1+35 (ethinyl estradiol + norethindrone, ✜Select 1/35, Brevicon 1/35) ▶L ♀X ▶– $$
ADULTS – <u>Contraception</u>: 1 tab PO daily.
PEDS – Not approved in children.
FORMS – Trade only: Tabs 1 mg norethindrone/35 mcg ethinyl estradiol.
NOTES – Same as Ortho-Novum 1/35.
MOA – Contraceptive steroid combination.
ADVERSE EFFECTS – Serious: DVT/PE, stroke, MI, hepatic neoplasia, and gallbladder disease. Frequent: Nausea, breast tenderness, and breakthrough bleeding.

NORINYL 1+50 (mestranol + norethindrone) ▶L ♀X ▶– $$
ADULTS – <u>Contraception</u>: 1 tab PO daily.
PEDS – Not approved in children.

(cont.)

NORINYL 1+50 (cont.)
FORMS — Trade only: Tabs: 1 mg norethindrone/50 mcg mestranol.
NOTES — 50 mcg estrogen component rarely necessary. Same as Ortho-Novum 1/50.
MOA — Contraceptive steroid combination.
ADVERSE EFFECTS — Serious: DVT/PE, stroke, MI, hepatic neoplasia, and gallbladder disease. Frequent: Nausea, breast tenderness, and breakthrough bleeding.

NORTREL (ethinyl estradiol + norethindrone) ▶L ♀X ▶– $$
WARNING — Multiple strengths; see FORMS and write specific product on Rx.
ADULTS — Contraception: 1 tab PO daily.
PEDS — Not approved in children.
FORMS — Trade only: Tabs 35 mcg ethinyl estradiol/1 mg norethindrone (Nortrel 1/35). 35 mcg ethinyl estradiol/0.5 mg norethindrone (Nortrel 0.5/35).
NOTES — Same as Brevicon (0.5/35), Ortho-Novum 1/35 (1/35).
MOA — Contraceptive steroid combination.
ADVERSE EFFECTS — Serious: DVT/PE, stroke, MI, hepatic neoplasia, and gallbladder disease. Frequent: Nausea, breast tenderness, and breakthrough bleeding.

OGESTREL (ethinyl estradiol + norgestrel) ▶L ♀X ▶– $$
ADULTS — Contraception: 1 tab PO daily.
PEDS — Not approved in children.
UNAPPROVED ADULTS — Postcoital contraception: See table.
FORMS — Trade only: Tabs: 50 mcg ethinyl estradiol/0.5 mg norgestrel.
NOTES — 50 mcg estrogen component rarely necessary. Same as Ovral.
MOA — Contraceptive steroid combination.
ADVERSE EFFECTS — Serious: DVT/PE, stroke, MI, hepatic neoplasia, and gallbladder disease. Frequent: Nausea, breast tenderness, and breakthrough bleeding.

ORTHO-CEPT (ethinyl estradiol + desogestrel, ♣Marvelon) ▶L ♀X ▶– $$$
ADULTS — Contraception: 1 tab PO daily.
PEDS — Not approved in children.
FORMS — Trade only: Tabs 30 mcg ethinyl estradiol/0.15 mg desogestrel.
NOTES — Same as Desogen.
MOA — Contraceptive steroid combination.
ADVERSE EFFECTS — Serious: DVT/PE, stroke, MI, hepatic neoplasia, and gallbladder disease. Frequent: Nausea, breast tenderness, and breakthrough bleeding.

ORTHO-CYCLEN (ethinyl estradiol + norgestimate, ♣Cyclen) ▶L ♀X ▶– $$
ADULTS — Contraception: 1 tab PO daily.
PEDS — Not approved in children.
FORMS — Generic/Trade: Tabs: 35 mcg ethinyl estradiol/0.25 mg norgestimate.
MOA — Contraceptive steroid combination.
ADVERSE EFFECTS — Serious: DVT/PE, stroke, MI, hepatic neoplasia, and gallbladder disease. Frequent: Nausea, breast tenderness, and breakthrough bleeding.

ORTHO-NOVUM 1/35 (ethinyl estradiol + norethindrone) ▶L ♀X ▶– $$$
ADULTS — Contraception: 1 tab PO daily.
PEDS — Not approved in children.
FORMS — Trade only: Tabs 1 mg norethindrone/ 35 mcg ethinyl estradiol.
MOA — Contraceptive steroid combination.
ADVERSE EFFECTS — Serious: DVT/PE, stroke, MI, hepatic neoplasia, and gallbladder disease. Frequent: Nausea, breast tenderness, and breakthrough bleeding.

ORTHO-NOVUM 1/50 (mestranol + norethindrone) ▶L ♀X ▶– $$$
ADULTS — Contraception: 1 tab PO daily.
PEDS — Not approved in children.
FORMS — Trade only: Tabs: 1 mg norethindrone/ 50 mcg mestranol.
NOTES — 50 mcg estrogen component rarely necessary.
MOA — Contraceptive steroid combination.
ADVERSE EFFECTS — Serious: DVT/PE, stroke, MI, hepatic neoplasia, and gallbladder disease. Frequent: Nausea, breast tenderness, and breakthrough bleeding.

OVCON-35 (ethinyl estradiol + norethindrone) ▶L ♀X ▶– $$$
ADULTS — Contraception: 1 tab PO daily.
PEDS — Not approved in children.
FORMS — Trade only: Tabs 35 mcg ethinyl estradiol/0.4 mg norethindrone.
MOA — Contraceptive steroid combination.
ADVERSE EFFECTS — Serious: DVT/PE, stroke, MI, hepatic neoplasia, and gallbladder disease. Frequent: Nausea, breast tenderness, and breakthrough bleeding.

OVCON-50 (ethinyl estradiol + norethindrone) ▶L ♀X ▶– $$$
ADULTS — Contraception: 1 tab PO daily.
PEDS — Not approved in children.
FORMS — Trade only: Tabs 50 mcg ethinyl estradiol/0.4 mg norethindrone.
NOTES — 50 mcg estrogen component rarely necessary.
MOA — Contraceptive steroid combination.
ADVERSE EFFECTS — Serious: DVT/PE, stroke, MI, hepatic neoplasia, and gallbladder disease. Frequent: Nausea, breast tenderness, and breakthrough bleeding.

OVRAL (ethinyl estradiol + norgestrel) ▶L ♀X ▶– $$$
ADULTS — Contraception: 1 tab PO daily.
PEDS — Not approved in children.
UNAPPROVED ADULTS — Postcoital contraception: See table.
FORMS — Trade only: Tabs: 50 mcg ethinyl estradiol/0.5 mg norgestrel.
NOTES — 50 mcg estrogen component rarely necessary.

(cont.)

OVRAL (*cont.*)
MOA — Contraceptive steroid combination.
ADVERSE EFFECTS — Serious: DVT/PE, stroke, MI, hepatic neoplasia, and gallbladder disease. Frequent: Nausea, breast tenderness, and breakthrough bleeding.

PORTIA (ethinyl estradiol + levonorgestrel) ▶L ♀X ▶– $$
ADULTS — <u>Contraception:</u> 1 tab PO daily.
PEDS — Not approved in children.
UNAPPROVED ADULTS — <u>Postcoital contraception:</u> See table.
FORMS — Trade only: Tabs 30 mcg ethinyl estradiol/0.15 mg levonorgestrel.
NOTES — Same as Nordette.
MOA — Contraceptive steroid combination.
ADVERSE EFFECTS — Serious: DVT/PE, stroke, MI, hepatic neoplasia, and gallbladder disease. Frequent: Nausea, breast tenderness, and breakthrough bleeding.

PREVIFEM (ethinyl estradiol + norgestimate) ▶L ♀X ▶– $$
ADULTS — <u>Contraception:</u> 1 tab PO daily.
PEDS — Not approved in children.
FORMS — Trade only: Tabs: 35 mcg ethinyl estradiol/0.25 mg norgestimate.
MOA — Contraceptive steroid combination.
ADVERSE EFFECTS — Serious: DVT/PE, stroke, MI, hepatic neoplasia, and gallbladder disease. Frequent: Nausea, breast tenderness, and breakthrough bleeding.

QUASENSE (ethinyl estradiol + levonorgestrel) ▶L ♀X ▶– $$$
ADULTS — <u>Contraception:</u> 1 tab PO daily.
PEDS — Not approved in children.
FORMS — Generic/Trade: Tabs 30 mcg ethinyl estradiol/0.15 mg levonorgestrel. 84 white active pills followed by 7 peach placebo pills.
NOTES — Decreases menstrual periods from q month to q 3 months; however, intermenstrual bleeding and spotting is more frequent than with 28-day regimens. Same as Seasonale.
MOA — Contraceptive steroid combination.
ADVERSE EFFECTS — Serious: DVT/PE, stroke, MI, hepatic neoplasia, and gallbladder disease. Frequent: Nausea, breast tenderness, and breakthrough bleeding.

RECLIPSEN (ethinyl estradiol + desogestrel) ▶L ♀X ▶– $$
ADULTS — <u>Contraception:</u> 1 tab PO daily.
PEDS — Not approved in children.
FORMS — Trade only: Tabs 30 mcg ethinyl estradiol/0.15 mg desogestrel.
NOTES — Same as Desogen.
MOA — Contraceptive steroid combination.
ADVERSE EFFECTS — Serious: DVT/PE, stroke, MI, hepatic neoplasia, and gallbladder disease. Frequent: Nausea, breast tenderness, and breakthrough bleeding.

SEASONALE (ethinyl estradiol + levonorgestrel) ▶L ♀X ▶– $$$
ADULTS — <u>Contraception:</u> 1 tab PO daily.
PEDS — Not approved in children.
FORMS — Generic/Trade: Tabs 30 mcg ethinyl estradiol/0.15 mg levonorgestrel. 84 pink active pills followed by 7 white placebo pills.
NOTES — Decreases menstrual periods from q month to q 3 months; however, intermenstrual bleeding and spotting is more frequent than with 28-day regimens.
MOA — Contraceptive steroid combination.
ADVERSE EFFECTS — Serious: DVT/PE, stroke, MI, hepatic neoplasia, and gallbladder disease. Frequent: Nausea, breast tenderness, and breakthrough bleeding.

SEASONIQUE (ethinyl estradiol + levonorgestrel) ▶L ♀X ▶– $$$
ADULTS — <u>Contraception:</u> 1 tab PO daily.
PEDS — Not approved in children.
FORMS — Trade only: Tabs 30 mcg ethinyl estradiol/0.15 mg levonorgestrel. 84 light blue-green active pills followed by 7 yellow pills with 10 mcg ethinyl estradiol.
NOTES — Decreases menstrual periods from q month to q 3 months; however, intermenstrual bleeding and spotting is more frequent than with 28-day regimens. All 91 tabs must be taken.
MOA — Contraceptive steroid combination.
ADVERSE EFFECTS — Serious: DVT/PE, stroke, MI, hepatic neoplasia, and gallbladder disease. Frequent: Nausea, breast tenderness, and breakthrough bleeding.

SPRINTEC (ethinyl estradiol + norgestimate) ▶L ♀X ▶– $$
ADULTS — <u>Contraception:</u> 1 tab PO daily.
PEDS — Not approved in children.
FORMS — Trade only: Tabs: 35 mcg ethinyl estradiol/0.25 mg norgestimate.
NOTES — Same as Ortho-Cyclen.
MOA — Contraceptive steroid combination.
ADVERSE EFFECTS — Serious: DVT/PE, stroke, MI, hepatic neoplasia, and gallbladder disease. Frequent: Nausea, breast tenderness, and breakthrough bleeding.

YASMIN (ethinyl estradiol + drospirenone) ▶L ♀X ▶– $$$
ADULTS — <u>Contraception:</u> 1 tab PO daily.
PEDS — Not approved in children.
FORMS — Trade only: Tabs: 30 mcg ethinyl estradiol/3 mg drospirenone.
NOTES — May cause hyperkalemia due to antimineralocorticoid activity of drospirenone (equal to 25 mg spironolactone). Monitor potassium in patients on ACE inhibitors, ARBs, potassium-sparing diuretics, heparin, aldosterone antagonists, and NSAIDs.
MOA — Contraceptive steroid combination.
ADVERSE EFFECTS — Serious: DVT/PE, stroke, MI, hepatic neoplasia, and gallbladder disease. Frequent: Nausea, breast tenderness, and breakthrough bleeding.

YAZ (ethinyl estradiol + drospirenone) ▶L ♀X ▶– $$$
ADULTS — <u>Contraception, premenstrual dysphoric disorder, acne:</u> 1 tab PO daily.

(cont.)

OB/GYN: Contraceptives

YAZ (cont.)
PEDS — Not approved in children.
FORMS — Trade only: Tabs: 20 mcg ethinyl estradiol/3 mg drospirenone. 24 active pills are followed by 4 inert pills.
NOTES — May cause hyperkalemia due to antimineralocorticoid activity of drospirenone (equal to 25 mg spironolactone). Monitor potassium in patients on ACE inhibitors, ARBs, potassium-sparing diuretics, heparin, aldosterone antagonists, and NSAIDs.
MOA — Contraceptive steroid combination.
ADVERSE EFFECTS — Serious: DVT/PE, stroke, MI, hepatic neoplasia, and gallbladder disease. Frequent: Nausea, breast tenderness, and breakthrough bleeding.

ZOVIA (ethinyl estradiol + ethynodiol) ▶L ♀X ▶– $$
WARNING — Multiple strengths; see FORMS and write specific product on Rx.
ADULTS — Contraception: 1 tab PO daily.
PEDS — Not approved in children.
FORMS — Trade only: Tabs 1 mg ethynodiol/35 mcg ethinyl estradiol (Zovia 1/35E). 1 mg ethynodiol/50 mcg ethinyl estradiol (Zovia 1/50E).
NOTES — 50 mcg estrogen component rarely necessary. Same as Demulen.
MOA — Contraceptive steroid combination.
ADVERSE EFFECTS — Serious: DVT/PE, stroke, MI, hepatic neoplasia, and gallbladder disease. Frequent: Nausea, breast tenderness, and breakthrough bleeding.

OB/GYN: Contraceptives—Oral Triphasic

NOTE: Not recommended in women greater than 35 yo who smoke. Increased risk of thromboembolism, CVA, MI, hepatic neoplasia, and gallbladder disease. Nausea, breast tenderness, and breakthrough bleeding are common transient side effects. Nighttime dosing may minimize nausea. Effectiveness is reduced by hepatic enzyme-inducing drugs such as certain anticonvulsants and barbiturates, rifampin, rifabutin, griseofulvin, and protease inhibitors. Additionally, products that contain St John's wort may decrease efficacy. Vomiting or diarrhea may also increase the risk of contraceptive failure. An additional form of birth control may be advisable. Advise patients to take at the same time every day. See PI for instructions on missing doses. Most available in 21- and 28-day packs. Although not approved by the FDA, combined OCPs are used for dysfunctional uterine bleeding, emergency contraception, dysmenorrhea, pelvic pain, and hirsutism (with spironolactone): 1 tab PO daily. Wait 6 weeks postpartum to initiate combination OCPs to decrease the risk of thromboembolism and to support lactation.

ARANELLE (ethinyl estradiol + norethindrone) ▶L ♀X ▶– $$
ADULTS — Contraception: 1 tab PO daily.
PEDS — Not approved in children.
FORMS — Trade only: Tabs 35 mcg ethinyl estradiol/0.5, 1, 0.5 mg norethindrone.
NOTES — Same as Tri-Norinyl.
MOA — Contraceptive steroid combination.
ADVERSE EFFECTS — Serious: DVT/PE, stroke, MI, hepatic neoplasia, and gallbladder disease. Frequent: Nausea, breast tenderness, and breakthrough bleeding.

CYCLESSA (ethinyl estradiol + desogestrel) ▶L ♀X ▶– $$
ADULTS — Contraception: 1 tab PO daily.
PEDS — Not approved in children.
FORMS — Generic/Trade: Tabs 25 mcg ethinyl estradiol/0.100, 0.125, 0.150 mg desogestrel.
MOA — Contraceptive steroid combination.
ADVERSE EFFECTS — Serious: DVT/PE, stroke, MI, hepatic neoplasia, and gallbladder disease. Frequent: Nausea, breast tenderness, and breakthrough bleeding.

ENPRESSE (ethinyl estradiol + levonorgestrel, ✣Triquilar) ▶L ♀X ▶– $$
ADULTS — Contraception: 1 tab PO daily.
PEDS — Not approved in children.
UNAPPROVED ADULTS — Postcoital contraception: See table.
FORMS — Trade only: Tabs 30, 40, 30 mcg ethinyl estradiol/0.05, 0.075, 0.125 mg levonorgestrel.

NOTES — Same as Triphasil.
MOA — Contraceptive steroid combination.
ADVERSE EFFECTS — Serious: DVT/PE, stroke, MI, hepatic neoplasia, and gallbladder disease. Frequent: Nausea, breast tenderness, and breakthrough bleeding.

ESTROSTEP FE (ethinyl estradiol + norethindrone + ferrous fumarate) ▶L ♀X ▶– $$$
ADULTS — Contraception: 1 tab PO daily.
PEDS — Not approved in children.
FORMS — Generic/Trade: Tabs 20, 30, 35 mcg ethinyl estradiol/1 mg norethindrone + "placebo" tabs with 75 mg ferrous fumarate. Packs of 28 only.
NOTES — All 28 tabs must be taken.
MOA — Contraceptive steroid combination.
ADVERSE EFFECTS — Serious: DVT/PE, stroke, MI, hepatic neoplasia, and gallbladder disease. Frequent: Nausea, breast tenderness, and breakthrough bleeding.

LEENA (ethinyl estradiol + norethindrone) ▶L ♀X ▶– $$
ADULTS — Contraception: 1 tab PO daily.
PEDS — Not approved in children.
FORMS — Trade only: Tabs 35 mcg ethinyl estradiol/0.5, 1, 0.5 mg norethindrone.
NOTES — Same as Tri-Norinyl.
MOA — Contraceptive steroid combination.
ADVERSE EFFECTS — Serious: DVT/PE, stroke, MI, hepatic neoplasia, and gallbladder disease. Frequent: Nausea, breast tenderness, and breakthrough bleeding.

NECON 7/7/7 (ethinyl estradiol + norethindrone) ▶L ♀X ▶– $$
ADULTS – Contraception: 1 tab PO daily.
PEDS – Not approved in children.
FORMS – Trade only: Tabs 35 mcg ethinyl estradiol/0.5, 0.75, 1 mg norethindrone.
NOTES – Same as Ortho-Novum 7/7/7.
MOA – Contraceptive steroid combination.
ADVERSE EFFECTS – Serious: DVT/PE, stroke, MI, hepatic neoplasia, and gallbladder disease. Frequent: Nausea, breast tenderness, and breakthrough bleeding.

NORTREL 7/7/7 (ethinyl estradiol + norethindrone) ▶L ♀X ▶– $$
ADULTS – Contraception: 1 tab PO daily.
PEDS – Not approved in children.
FORMS – Trade only: Tabs 35 mcg ethinyl estradiol/0.5, 0.75, 1 mg norethindrone.
NOTES – Same as Ortho-Novum 7/7/7.
MOA – Contraceptive steroid combination.
ADVERSE EFFECTS – Serious: DVT/PE, stroke, MI, hepatic neoplasia, and gallbladder disease. Frequent: Nausea, breast tenderness, and breakthrough bleeding.

ORTHO TRI-CYCLEN (ethinyl estradiol + norgestimate, ✢Tri-Cyclen) ▶L ♀X ▶– $$
ADULTS – Contraception, adult acne: 1 tab PO daily.
PEDS – Not approved in children.
FORMS – Generic/Trade: Tabs 35 mcg ethinyl estradiol/0.18, 0.215, 0.25 mg norgestimate.
MOA – Contraceptive steroid combination.
ADVERSE EFFECTS – Serious: DVT/PE, stroke, MI, hepatic neoplasia, and gallbladder disease. Frequent: Nausea, breast tenderness, and breakthrough bleeding.

ORTHO TRI-CYCLEN LO (ethinyl estradiol + norgestimate) ▶L ♀X ▶– $$$
ADULTS – Contraception: 1 tab PO daily.
PEDS – Not approved in children.
FORMS – Trade only: Tabs 25 mcg ethinyl estradiol/0.18, 0.215, 0.25 mg norgestimate.
MOA – Contraceptive steroid combination.
ADVERSE EFFECTS – Serious: DVT/PE, stroke, MI, hepatic neoplasia, and gallbladder disease. Frequent: Nausea, breast tenderness, and breakthrough bleeding.

ORTHO-NOVUM 7/7/7 (ethinyl estradiol + norethindrone) ▶L ♀X ▶– $$
ADULTS – Contraception: 1 tab PO daily.
PEDS – Not approved in children.
FORMS – Trade only: Tabs 35 mcg ethinyl estradiol/0.5, 0.75, 1 mg norethindrone.
MOA – Contraceptive steroid combination.
ADVERSE EFFECTS – Serious: DVT/PE, stroke, MI, hepatic neoplasia, and gallbladder disease. Frequent: Nausea, breast tenderness, and breakthrough bleeding.

TRI-LEGEST (ethinyl estradiol + norethindrone) ▶L ♀X ▶– $$$
ADULTS – Contraception: 1 tab PO daily.
PEDS – Not approved in children.
FORMS – Trade only: Tabs 20, 30, 35 mcg ethinyl estradiol/1 mg norethindrone.
MOA – Contraceptive steroid combination.
ADVERSE EFFECTS – Serious: DVT/PE, stroke, MI, hepatic neoplasia, and gallbladder disease. Frequent: Nausea, breast tenderness, and breakthrough bleeding.

TRI-LEGEST FE (ethinyl estradiol + norethindrone + ferrous fumarate) ▶L ♀X ▶– $$$
ADULTS – Contraception: 1 tab PO daily.
PEDS – Not approved in children.
FORMS – Trade only: Tabs 20, 30, 35 mcg ethinyl estradiol/1 mg norethindrone + "placebo" tabs with 75 mg ferrous fumarate.
NOTES – Same as Estrostep Fe. All 28 tabs must be taken.
MOA – Contraceptive steroid combination.
ADVERSE EFFECTS – Serious: DVT/PE, stroke, MI, hepatic neoplasia, and gallbladder disease. Frequent: Nausea, breast tenderness, and breakthrough bleeding.

TRI-LEVLEN (ethinyl estradiol + levonorgestrel) ▶L ♀X ▶– $$
ADULTS – Contraception: 1 tab PO daily.
PEDS – Not approved in children.
UNAPPROVED ADULTS – Postcoital contraception: See table.
FORMS – Trade only: Tabs 30, 40, 30 mcg ethinyl estradiol/0.05, 0.075, 0.125 mg levonorgestrel.
NOTES – Same as Triphasil.
MOA – Contraceptive steroid combination.
ADVERSE EFFECTS – Serious: DVT/PE, stroke, MI, hepatic neoplasia, and gallbladder disease. Frequent: Nausea, breast tenderness, and breakthrough bleeding.

TRINESSA (ethinyl estradiol + norgestimate) ▶L ♀X ▶– $$
ADULTS – Contraception, adult acne: 1 tab PO daily.
PEDS – Not approved in children.
FORMS – Trade only: Tabs 35 mcg ethinyl estradiol/0.18, 0.215, 0.25 mg norgestimate.
NOTES – Same as Ortho Tri-Cyclen.
MOA – Contraceptive steroid combination.
ADVERSE EFFECTS – Serious: DVT/PE, stroke, MI, hepatic neoplasia, and gallbladder disease. Frequent: Nausea, breast tenderness, and breakthrough bleeding.

TRI-NORINYL (ethinyl estradiol + norethindrone, ✢Synphasic) ▶L ♀X ▶– $$
ADULTS – Contraception: 1 tab PO daily.
PEDS – Not approved in children.
FORMS – Trade only: Tabs 35 mcg ethinyl estradiol/0.5, 1, 0.5 mg norethindrone.
MOA – Contraceptive steroid combination.
ADVERSE EFFECTS – Serious: DVT/PE, stroke, MI, hepatic neoplasia, and gallbladder disease. Frequent: Nausea, breast tenderness, and breakthrough bleeding.

TRIPHASIL (ethinyl estradiol + levonorgestrel) ▶L ♀X ▶– $$
ADULTS – Contraception: 1 tab PO daily.

(cont.)

OB/GYN: Contraceptives

TRIPHASIL (cont.)
PEDS — Not approved in children.
UNAPPROVED ADULTS — Postcoital contraception: See table.
FORMS — Trade only: Tabs 30, 40, 30 mcg ethinyl estradiol/0.05, 0.075, 0.125 mg levonorgestrel.
MOA — Contraceptive steroid combination.
ADVERSE EFFECTS — Serious: DVT/PE, stroke, MI, hepatic neoplasia, and gallbladder disease. Frequent: Nausea, breast tenderness, and breakthrough bleeding.

TRI-PREVIFEM (ethinyl estradiol + norgestimate) ▶L ♀X ▶– $$
ADULTS — Contraception, adult acne: 1 tab PO daily.
PEDS — Not approved in children.
FORMS — Trade only: Tabs 35 mcg ethinyl estradiol/0.18, 0.215, 0.25 mg norgestimate.
NOTES — Same as Ortho Tri-Cyclen.
MOA — Contraceptive steroid combination.
ADVERSE EFFECTS — Serious: DVT/PE, stroke, MI, hepatic neoplasia, and gallbladder disease. Frequent: Nausea, breast tenderness, and breakthrough bleeding.

TRI-SPRINTEC (ethinyl estradiol + norgestimate) ▶L ♀X ▶– $$
ADULTS — Contraception, adult acne: 1 tab PO daily.
PEDS — Not approved in children.
FORMS — Trade only: Tabs 35 mcg ethinyl estradiol/0.18, 0.215, 0.25 mg norgestimate.
NOTES — Same as Ortho Tri-Cyclen.

MOA — Contraceptive steroid combination.
ADVERSE EFFECTS — Serious: DVT/PE, stroke, MI, hepatic neoplasia, and gallbladder disease. Frequent: Nausea, breast tenderness, and breakthrough bleeding.

TRIVORA-28 (ethinyl estradiol + levonorgestrel) ▶L ♀X ▶– $$
ADULTS — Contraception: 1 tab PO daily.
PEDS — Not approved in children.
UNAPPROVED ADULTS — Postcoital contraception: See table.
FORMS — Trade only: Tabs 30, 40, 30 mcg ethinyl estradiol/0.05, 0.075, 0.125 mg levonorgestrel.
NOTES — Same as Triphasil.
MOA — Contraceptive steroid combination.
ADVERSE EFFECTS — Serious: DVT/PE, stroke, MI, hepatic neoplasia, and gallbladder disease. Frequent: Nausea, breast tenderness, and breakthrough bleeding.

VELIVET (ethinyl estradiol + desogestrel) ▶L ♀X ▶– $$
ADULTS — Contraception: 1 tab PO daily.
PEDS — Not approved in children.
FORMS — Generic/Trade: Tabs 25 mcg ethinyl estradiol/0.100, 0.125, 0.150 mg desogestrel.
NOTES — Same as Cyclessa.
MOA — Contraceptive steroid combination.
ADVERSE EFFECTS — Serious: DVT/PE, stroke, MI, hepatic neoplasia, and gallbladder disease. Frequent: Nausea, breast tenderness, and breakthrough bleeding.

OB/GYN: Contraceptives—Other

ETONOGESTREL (Implanon) ▶L ♀X ▶+ $$$$$
WARNING — Increased risk of thromboembolism and CVA. Effectiveness may be reduced by hepatic enzyme-inducing drugs such as certain anticonvulsants, barbiturates, griseofulvin, rifampin. Additionally, products that contain St John's wort may decrease efficacy; an additional form of birth control may be advisable.
ADULTS — Contraception: 1 subdermal implant every 3 years.
PEDS — Not approved in children.
FORMS — Trade only: Single rod implant, 68 mg etonogestrel.
NOTES — Not studied in women greater than 130% of ideal body wt; may be less effective if overweight. Implant should be palpable immediately after insertion.
MOA — Contraceptive steroid combination.
ADVERSE EFFECTS — Serious: DVT/PE, stroke. Frequent: Weight gain & bleeding irregularities.

LEVONORGESTREL (Plan B) ▶L ♀X ▶– $$
ADULTS — Emergency contraception: 1 tab PO ASAP but within 72 h of intercourse. 2nd tab 12 h later.
PEDS — Not approved in children.
UNAPPROVED ADULTS — 2 tabs (1.5 mg) PO ASAP but within 72 h of intercourse (lesser efficacy at up to 120 h).
FORMS — OTC Trade only: Kit contains 2 tabs 0.75 mg.
NOTES — OTC if at least 18 yo; Rx if younger. Nausea uncommon; however, if vomiting occurs within 1 h, initial dose must be given again. Consider adding an antiemetic. Patients should be instructed to then contact their healthcare providers. Can be used at any time during the menstrual cycle.
MOA — Gonadal steroid.
ADVERSE EFFECTS — Serious: None. Frequent: None.

LEVONORGESTREL 1S (Plan B One-Step) ▶L ♀X ▶– $$
ADULTS — Emergency contraception: 1 tab PO ASAP but within 72 h of intercourse.
PEDS — Not approved in children.
FORMS — OTC Trade only: Tabs 1.5 mg.
NOTES — OTC if at least 17 yo; Rx if younger. Nausea uncommon; however, if vomiting occurs within 1 h, initial dose must be given again. Consider adding an antiemetic. Patients should be instructed to then contact their healthcare providers. Can be used at any time during the menstrual cycle. Lesser efficacy at up to 120 h.
MOA — Gonadal steroid.
ADVERSE EFFECTS — Serious: None. Frequent: None.

OB/GYN: Contraceptives

ORAL CONTRACEPTIVES* ▶L ♀X *Monophasic*	Estrogen (mcg)	Progestin (mg)
Norinyl 1+50, Ortho-Novum 1/50, Necon 1/50	50 mestranol	1 norethindrone
Ovcon-50	50 ethinyl estradiol	
Demulen 1/50, Zovia 1/50E		1 ethynodiol
Ovral, Ogestrel		0.5 norgestrel
Norinyl 1+35, Ortho-Novum 1/35, Necon 1/35, Nortrel 1/35	35 ethinyl estradiol	1 norethindrone
Brevicon, Modicon, Necon 0.5/35, Nortrel 0.5/35		0.5 norethindrone
Ovcon-35, Femcon Fe, Balziva		0.4 norethindrone
Previfem		0.18 norgestimate
Ortho-Cyclen, MonoNessa, Sprintec-28		0.25 norgestimate
Demulen 1/35, Zovia 1/35E, Kelnor 1/35		1 ethynodiol
Loestrin 21 1.5/30, Loestrin Fe 1.5/30, Junel 1.5/30, Junel 1.5/30 Fe, Microgestin Fe 1.5/30	30 ethinyl estradiol	1.5 norethindrone
Cryselle, Lo/Ovral, Low-Ogestrel		0.3 norgestrel
Apri, Desogen, Ortho-Cept, Reclipsen		0.15 desogestrel
Levlen, Levora, Nordette, Portia, Solia		0.15 levonorgestrel
Yasmin, Ocella		3 drospirenone
Loestrin 21 1/20, Loestrin Fe 1/20, Loestin 24 Fe, Junel 1/20, Junel Fe 1/20, Microgestin Fe 1/20	20 ethinyl estradiol	1 norethindrone
Alesse, Aviane, Lessina, Levlite, Lutera, Sronyx		0.1 levonorgestrel
Lybrel†		0.09 levonorgestrel
Yaz		3 drospirenone
Kariva, Mircette	20/10 eth estrad	0.15 desogestrel
Progestin-only		
Micronor, Nor-Q.D., Camila, Errin, Jolivette, Nora-BE	none	0.35 norethindrone
Biphasic (estrogen & progestin contents vary)		
Ortho Novum 10/11, Necon 10/11	35 eth estradiol	0.5/1 norethindrone
Triphasic (estrogen & progestin contents vary)		
Cyclessa, Velivet, Cesia	25 ethinyl estradiol	0.100/0.125/0.150 desogestrel
Ortho-Novum 7/7/7, Necon 7/7/7, Nortrel 7/7/7	35 ethinyl estradiol	0.5/0.75/1 norethindr
Tri-Norinyl, Leena, Aranelle		0.5/1/0.5 norethindr
Enpresse, Tri-Levlen, Triphasil, Trivora-28	30/40/30 ethinyl estradiol	0.5/0.75/0.125 levonorgestrel
Ortho Tri-Cyclen, Trinessa, Tri-Sprintec, Tri-Previfem	35 eth estradiol	00.18/0.215/0.25 norgestimate
Ortho Tri-Cyclen Lo	25 eth estradiol	
Estrostep Fe, Tri-Legest, Tri-Legest Fe, Tilia Fe	20/30/35 eth estr	1 norethindrone
Extended Cycle††		
Seasonale, Quasense, Jolessa	30 ethinyl estradiol	0.15 levonorgestrel
Seasonique	30/10 eth estrad	0.15 levonorgestrel
LoSeasonique	20 ethinyl estradiol	0.1 levonorgestrel

***All**: Not recommended in smokers. Increase risk of thromboembolism, CVA, MI, hepatic neoplasia, & gallbladder disease. Nausea, breast tenderness, & breakthrough bleeding are common transient side effects. Effectiveness reduced by hepatic enzyme-inducing drugs such as certain anticonvulsants and barbiturates, rifampin, rifabutin, griseofulvin, & protease inhibitors. Coadministration with St. John's wort may decrease efficacy. Vomiting or diarrhea may also increase the risk of contraceptive failure. Consider an additional form of birth control in above circumstances. See product insert for instructions on missing doses. Most available in 21 and 28 day packs. **Progestin only**: Must be taken at the same time every day. Because much of the literature regarding OC adverse effects pertains mainly to estrogen/progestin combinations, the extent to which progestin-only contraceptives cause these effects is unclear. No significant interaction has been found with broad-spectrum antibiotics. The effect of St. John's wort is unclear. No placebo days, start new pack immediately after finishing current one. Available in 28 day packs. Readers may find the following website useful: www.managingcontraception.com. † Approved for continuous use without a "pill-free" period. †† 84 active pills and 7 placebo pills.

EMERGENCY CONTRACEPTION Emergency contraception within 72 h of unprotected sex. Progestin-only methods (causes less nausea & may be more effective): *Plan B One-Step* (levonorgestrel 1.5 mg tab, OTC for age at least 17 yo): take one pill. *Plan B* (levonorgestrel 0.75 mg, OTC for age at least 18 yo): take one tab ASAP and 2nd dose 12 h later. Progestin and estrogen method: Dose is defined as 2 pills of *Ovral or Ogestrel*, 4 pills of *Cryselle, Levlen, Levora, Lo/Ovral, Nordette, Tri-Levlen*, Triphasil*, Trivora*, or Low Ogestrel*, or 5 pills of *Alesse, Aviane, Lessina, or Levlit*: Take first dose ASAP and 2nd dose 12 h later. If vomiting occurs within 1 h of taking dose, consider repeating that dose with an antiemetic 1 h prior. More info at: www.not-2-late.com.

*Use 0.125 mg levonorgestrel/30 mcg ethinyl estradiol tabs.

NUVARING (ethinyl estradiol vaginal ring + etonogestrel) ▶L ♀X ▶– $$$
WARNING – Not recommended in women greater than 35 yo who smoke. Increased risk of thromboembolism, CVA, MI, hepatic neoplasia and gallbladder disease. Vaginitis, headache, nausea and wt gain are common side effects. Effectiveness is reduced by hepatic enzyme-inducing drugs, such as certain anticonvulsants and barbiturates, rifampin, rifabutin, griseofulvin and protease inhibitors. Additionally, products that contain St John's wort may decrease efficacy. An additional form of birth control may be advisable.
ADULTS – Contraception: 1 ring intravaginally for 3 weeks each month.
PEDS – Not approved in children.
FORMS – Trade only: Flexible intravaginal ring, 15 mcg ethinyl estradiol/0.120 mg etonogestrel/day in 1, 3 rings/box.
NOTES – Insert on day 5 of cycle or within 7 days of the last oral contraceptive pill. The ring must remain in place continuously for 3 weeks, including during intercourse. Remove for 1 week, then insert a new ring. May be used continuously for 4 weeks and replaced immediately to skip a withdrawal week. Store at room temperature. In case of accidental removal, reinsert ASAP after rinsing with cool to lukewarm water. If removal is greater than 3 h, use back up method until ring in place for at least 7 days. Rare reports of urinary bladder insertion; assess if persistent urinary symptoms and unable to locate the ring.
MOA – Contraceptive steroid combination.
ADVERSE EFFECTS – Serious: DVT/PE, stroke, MI, hepatic neoplasia, and gallbladder disease. Frequent: Nausea, breast tenderness, breakthrough bleeding, asymptomatic vaginal discharge.

ORTHO EVRA (norelgestromin + ethinyl estradiol transdermal, *◆Evra*) ▶L ♀X ▶– $$$
WARNING – Average estrogen concentration 60% higher than common oral contraceptives (ie, 35 mcg ethinyl estradiol), which may further increase the risk of thromboembolism. Not recommended in women greater than 35 yo who smoke. Increased risk of thromboembolism, CVA, MI, hepatic neoplasia and gallbladder disease. Nausea, breast tenderness, and breakthrough bleeding are common, transient side effects. Effectiveness is reduced by hepatic enzyme-inducing drugs, such as certain anticonvulsants and barbiturates, rifampin, rifabutin, griseofulvin and protease inhibitors. Additionally, products that contain St John's wort may decrease efficacy. An additional form of birth control may be advisable.
ADULTS – Contraception: 1 patch q week for 3 weeks, then 1 week patch-free.
PEDS – Not approved in children.
FORMS – Trade only: Transdermal patch: 150 mcg norelgestromin/20 mcg ethinyl estradiol/day in 1, 3 patches/box.
NOTES – May be less effective in women 90 kg or greater (198 lbs). Apply new patch on the same days each week. Do not exceed 7 days between patches. Rotate application sites, avoid the waistline. Do not use earlier than 4 weeks postpartum if not breastfeeding.
MOA – Contraceptive steroid combination.
ADVERSE EFFECTS – Serious: DVT/PE, stroke, MI, hepatic neoplasia, and gallbladder disease. Frequent: Nausea, breast tenderness, breakthrough bleeding.

OB/GYN: Estrogens

NOTE: See also Hormone Combinations. Unopposed estrogens increase the risk of endometrial cancer in postmenopausal women. Malignancy should be ruled out in cases of persistent or recurrent abnormal vaginal bleeding. In women with an intact uterus, a progestin should be administered daily throughout the month or for the last 10–12 days of the month. Do not use during pregnancy. May increase the risk of DVT/PE, gallbladder disease. Interactions with oral anticoagulants, certain anticonvulsants, rifampin, barbiturates, corticosteroids, and St. John's wort. Estrogens should not be used in the prevention of cardiovascular disease. In the Women's Health Initiative, the use of conjugated estrogens (Premarin) caused an increase in the risk of CVA and PE. Additionally, the combination with medroxyprogesterone increased the risk of breast cancer and MI. Women greater than 65 yo with 4 years of therapy had an increased risk of dementia. Estrogens should be prescribed at the lowest effective doses and for the shortest durations. Patients should be counseled regarding the risks/benefits of HRT.

ESTERIFIED ESTROGENS (*Menest*) ▶L ♀X ▶– $$
ADULTS – <u>Moderate to severe menopausal vasomotor symptoms:</u> 1.25 mg PO daily. <u>Atrophic vaginitis:</u> 0.3 to 1.25 mg PO daily. <u>Female hypogonadism:</u> 2.5 to 7.5 mg PO daily in divided doses for 20 days followed by a 10-day rest period. Repeat until bleeding occurs. <u>Bilateral oophorectomy and ovarian failure:</u> 1.25 mg PO daily. <u>Prevention of postmenopausal osteoporosis:</u> 0.3 to 1.25 mg PO daily.
PEDS – Not approved in children.
FORMS – Trade only: Tabs 0.3, 0.625, 1.25, 2.5 mg.
NOTES – Typical hormone replacement regimen consists of a daily estrogen dose with a progestin added either daily or for the last 10 to 12 days of the cycle.
MOA – Gonadal steroid.
ADVERSE EFFECTS – Serious: Endometrial cancer, DVT/PE, gallbladder disease, breast cancer, MI, CVA. Frequent: Nausea, breast tenderness.

ESTRADIOL (*Estrace, Gynodiol*) ▶L ♀X ▶– $
ADULTS – <u>Moderate to severe menopausal vasomotor symptoms and atrophic vaginitis, female hypogonadism, bilateral oophorectomy and ovarian failure:</u> 1 to 2 mg PO daily. <u>Prevention of postmenopausal osteoporosis:</u> 0.5 mg PO daily.
PEDS – Not approved in children.
FORMS – Generic/Trade: Tabs, micronized 0.5, 1, 2 mg, scored. Trade only: 1.5 mg (Gynodiol).
NOTES – Typical hormone replacement regimen consists of a daily estrogen dose with a progestin added either daily or for the last 10 to 12 days of the cycle.
MOA – Gonadal steroid.
ADVERSE EFFECTS – Serious: Endometrial cancer, DVT/PE, gallbladder disease, breast cancer, MI, CVA. Frequent: Nausea, breast tenderness.

ESTRADIOL ACETATE (*Femtrace*) ▶L ♀X ▶– $$
ADULTS – <u>Moderate to severe menopausal vasomotor symptoms:</u> 0.45 to 1.8 mg PO daily.
PEDS – Not approved in children.
FORMS – Trade only: Tabs, 0.45, 0.9, 1.8 mg.
NOTES – Typical hormone replacement regimen consists of a daily estrogen dose with a progestin added either daily or for the last 10 to 12 days of the cycle.
MOA – Gonadal steroid.
ADVERSE EFFECTS – Serious: Endometrial cancer, DVT/PE, gallbladder disease, breast cancer, MI, CVA. Frequent: Nausea, breast tenderness.

ESTRADIOL ACETATE VAGINAL RING (*Femring*) ▶L ♀X ▶– $$$
WARNING – A few cases of toxic shock syndrome have been reported. Bowel obstruction.
ADULTS – <u>Menopausal atrophic vaginitis or vasomotor symptoms:</u> Insert ring into the vagina and replace after 90 days.
PEDS – Not approved in children.
FORMS – Trade only: 0.05 mg/day and 0.1 mg/day.
NOTES – Should the ring fall out or be removed during the 90-day period, rinse in lukewarm water and re-insert. Ring adhesion to vaginal wall has been reported, making removal difficult.
MOA – Gonadal steroid.
ADVERSE EFFECTS – Serious: Toxic shock, bowel obstruction. Frequent: Breast tenderness, breakthrough bleeding.

ESTRADIOL CYPIONATE (*Depo-Estradiol*) ▶L ♀X ▶– $
ADULTS – <u>Moderate to severe menopausal vasomotor symptoms:</u> 1 to 5 mg IM q 3 to 4 weeks. Female hypogonadism: 1.5 to 2 mg IM q month.
PEDS – Not approved in children.
MOA – Gonadal steroid.
ADVERSE EFFECTS – Serious: Endometrial cancer, DVT/PE, gallbladder disease, breast cancer, MI, CVA. Frequent: Nausea, breast tenderness.

ESTRADIOL GEL (*Divigel, Estrogel, Elestrin*) ▶L ♀X ▶– $$$
ADULTS – <u>Moderate to severe menopausal vasomotor symptoms and atrophic vaginitis:</u> Thinly apply contents of 1 complete pump depression to one entire arm, from wrist to shoulder (Estrogel) or upper arm (Elestrin) or contents of 1 foil packet to left or right upper thigh on alternating days. Allow to dry completely before dressing. Wash both hands thoroughly after application.
PEDS – Not approved in children.
FORMS – Trade only: Gel 0.06% in nonaerosol, metered-dose pump with #64 or #32 1.25 g doses (Estrogel), #100 0.87 g doses (Elestrin). Gel 0.1% in single-dose foil packets of 0.25, 0.5, 1.0 g, carton of 30 (Divigel).
NOTES – Depress the pump 2 times to prime. Concomitant sunscreen may increase absorption. Typical hormone replacement regimen consists of a daily estrogen dose with a progestin added either daily or for the last 10 to 12 days of the cycle.
MOA – Gonadal steroid.
ADVERSE EFFECTS – Serious: Endometrial cancer, DVT/PE, gallbladder disease, breast cancer, MI, CVA. Frequent: Nausea, breast tenderness, rash.

ESTRADIOL TOPICAL EMULSION (*Estrasorb*) ▶L ♀X ▶– $$
ADULTS – <u>Moderate to severe menopausal vasomotor symptoms:</u> Apply entire contents of 1 pouch each to left and right legs (spread over thighs and calves) qam. Rub for 3 min until entirely absorbed. Allow to dry completely before dressing. Wash both hands thoroughly after application. Daily dose is two 1.74 g pouches.
PEDS – Not approved in children.
FORMS – Trade only: Topical emulsion, 56 pouches/carton.
NOTES – Typical hormone replacement regimen consists of a daily estrogen dose with a progestin added either daily or for the last 10 to 12 days of the cycle. Concomitant sunscreen may increase absorption.
MOA – Gonadal steroid.
ADVERSE EFFECTS – Serious: Endometrial cancer, DVT/PE, gallbladder disease, breast cancer, MI, CVA. Frequent: Nausea, breast tenderness.

ESTRADIOL TRANSDERMAL PATCH (*Alora, Climara, Esclim, Estraderm, FemPatch, Menostar, Vivelle, Vivelle Dot, ♦Estradot, Oesclim*) ▶L ♀X ▶– $$
ADULTS – Moderate to severe menopausal vasomotor symptoms and atrophic vaginitis, female hypogonadism, bilateral oophorectomy and ovarian failure: Initiate with 0.025 to 0.05 mg/day patch once or twice per week, depending on the product (see FORMS). Prevention of postmenopausal osteoporosis: 0.025 to 0.1 mg/day patch.
PEDS – Not approved in children.
FORMS – Generic/Trade: Transdermal patches doses in mg/day: Climara (once a week) 0.025, 0.0375, 0.05, 0.06, 0.075, 0.1. Trade only: FemPatch (once a week) 0.025. Esclim (twice per week) 0.025, 0.0375, 0.05, 0.075, 0.1. Vivelle, Vivelle Dot (twice per week) 0.025, 0.0375, 0.05, 0.075, 0.1. Estraderm (twice per week) 0.05, 0.1. Alora (twice per week) 0.025, 0.05, 0.075, 0.1.
NOTES – Rotate application sites, avoid the waistline. Transdermal may be preferable for women with high triglycerides and chronic liver disease.
MOA – Gonadal steroid.
ADVERSE EFFECTS – Serious: Endometrial cancer, DVT/PE, gallbladder disease, breast cancer, MI, CVA. Frequent: Nausea, breast tenderness.

ESTRADIOL TRANSDERMAL SPRAY (*Evamist*) ▶L ♀X ▶– $$$
ADULTS – Moderate to severe menopausal vasomotor symptoms: Initial: 1 spray daily to adjacent non-overlapping inner surface of the forearm. Allow to dry for 2 min and do not wash for 30 min. Adjust up to 3 sprays daily based on clinical response.
PEDS – Not approved in children.
FORMS – Trade only: Spray: 1.53 mg estradiol per 90 mcL spray, 56 sprays per metered-dose pump.
NOTES – Depress the pump 3 times with the cover on to prime each new applicator. Hold upright and vertical for spraying; rest the plastic cone against the skin. Typical hormone replacement regimen consists of a daily estrogen dose with a progestin added either daily or for the last 10 to 12 days of the cycle.
MOA – Gonadal steroid.
ADVERSE EFFECTS – Serious: Endometrial cancer, DVT/PE, gallbladder disease, breast cancer, MI, CVA. Frequent: Nausea, breast tenderness, rash.

ESTRADIOL VAGINAL RING (*Estring*) ▶L ♀X ▶– $$$
WARNING – Do not use during pregnancy. Toxic shock syndrome has been reported.
ADULTS – Menopausal atrophic vaginitis: Insert ring into upper 1/3 of the vaginal vault and replace after 90 days.
PEDS – Not approved in children.
FORMS – Trade only: 2 mg ring single pack.
NOTES – Should the ring fall out or be removed during the 90-day period, rinse in lukewarm water and re-insert. Reports of ring adhesion to the vaginal wall making ring removal difficult. Minimal systemic absorption, probable lower risk of adverse effects than systemic estrogens.
MOA – Gonadal steroid.
ADVERSE EFFECTS – Serious: Toxic shock, bowel obstruction, vaginal wall adhesion. Frequent: None.

ESTRADIOL VAGINAL TAB (*Vagifem*) ▶L ♀X ▶– $$$
WARNING – Do not use during pregnancy.
ADULTS – Menopausal atrophic vaginitis: Begin with 1 tab vaginally daily for 2 weeks, maintenance 1 tab vaginally twice per week.
PEDS – Not approved in children.
FORMS – Trade only: Vaginal tab: 25 mcg in disposable single-use applicators, 8, 18/pack.
MOA – Gonadal steroid.
ADVERSE EFFECTS – Serious: None. Frequent: None.

ESTRADIOL VALERATE (*Delestrogen*) ▶L ♀X ▶– $$
ADULTS – Moderate to severe menopausal vasomotor symptoms and atrophic vaginitis, female hypogonadism, bilateral oophorectomy and ovarian failure: 10 to 20 mg IM q 4 weeks.
PEDS – Not approved in children.
MOA – Gonadal steroid.
ADVERSE EFFECTS – Serious: Endometrial cancer, DVT/PE, gallbladder disease, breast cancer, MI, CVA. Frequent: Nausea, breast tenderness.

ESTROGEN VAGINAL CREAM (*Premarin, Estrace*) ▶L ♀X ▶? $$$$
ADULTS – Menopausal atrophic vaginitis: Premarin: 0.5 to 2 g intravaginally daily. Estrace: 2 to 4 g intravaginally daily for 1 to 2 weeks. Gradually reduce to a maintenance dose of 1 g 1 to 3 times per week. Moderate to severe menopausal dyspareunia: Premarin: 0.5 g daily; reduce to twice per week.
PEDS – Not approved in children.
FORMS – Trade only: Vaginal cream (Premarin) 0.625 mg conjugated estrogens/g in 42.5 g with or without calibrated applicator. Estrace: 0.1 mg estradiol/g in 42.5 g with calibrated applicator. Generic only: Cream 0.625 mg synthetic conjugated estrogens/g in 30 g with calibrated applicator.
NOTES – Possibility of absorption through the vaginal mucosa. Uterine bleeding might be provoked by excessive use in menopausal women. Breast tenderness and vaginal discharge due to mucus hypersecretion may result from excessive estrogenic stimulation. Endometrial withdrawal bleeding may occur if use is discontinued.
MOA – Gonadal steroid.
ADVERSE EFFECTS – Serious: Endometrial cancer, DVT/PE, gallbladder disease. Frequent: Nausea, breast tenderness.

ESTROGENS CONJUGATED (*Premarin, C.E.S., Congest*) ▶L ♀X ▶– $$$
ADULTS – Moderate to severe menopausal vasomotor symptoms, atrophic vaginitis, and urethritis: 0.3 to 1.25 mg PO daily. Female hypogonadism: 0.3 to 0.625 mg PO daily for 3 weeks with 1 week off every month. Bilateral oophorectomy and ovarian failure: 1.25 mg PO daily for 3 weeks with 1 week off every month. Prevention of

(cont.)

ESTROGENS CONJUGATED (cont.)
postmenopausal osteoporosis: 0.625 mg PO daily. Abnormal uterine bleeding: 25 mg IV/IM. Repeat in 6 to 12 h if needed.
PEDS — Not approved in children.
UNAPPROVED ADULTS — Prevention of postmenopausal osteoporosis: 0.3 mg PO daily. Normalizing bleeding time in patients with AV malformations or underlying renal impairment: 30 to 70 mg IV/PO daily until bleeding time normalized.
FORMS — Trade only: Tabs 0.3, 0.45, 0.625, 0.9, 1.25 mg.
MOA — Gonadal steroid.
ADVERSE EFFECTS — Serious: Endometrial cancer, DVT/PE, gallbladder disease, breast cancer, MI, CVA. Frequent: Nausea, breast tenderness.

ESTROGENS SYNTHETIC CONJUGATED A (*Cenestin*) ▶L ♀X ▶– $$$
ADULTS — Moderate to severe menopausal vasomotor symptoms: 0.3 to 1.25 mg PO daily.
PEDS — Not approved in children.
FORMS — Trade only: Tabs 0.3, 0.45, 0.625, 0.9, 1.25 mg.
NOTES — The difference between synthetic conjugated estrogens A and B is the additional component of delta-8,9-dehydroestrone sulfate in the B preparation. The clinical significance of this is unknown.
MOA — Gonadal steroid.
ADVERSE EFFECTS — Serious: Endometrial cancer, DVT/PE, gallbladder disease, breast cancer, MI, CVA. Frequent: Nausea, breast tenderness.

ESTROGENS SYNTHETIC CONJUGATED B (*Enjuvia*) ▶L ♀X ▶– $$
ADULTS — Moderate to severe menopausal vasomotor symptoms: 0.3 to 1.25 mg PO daily.
PEDS — Not approved in children.
FORMS — Trade only: Tabs 0.3, 0.45, 0.625, 0.9, 1.25 mg.
NOTES — Typical hormone replacement regimen consists of a daily estrogen dose with a progestin either daily or for the last 10 to 12 days of the cycle. The difference between synthetic conjugated estrogens A and B is the additional component of delta-8,9-dehydroestrone sulfate in the B preparation. The clinical significance of this is unknown.
MOA — Gonadal steroid.
ADVERSE EFFECTS — Serious: Endometrial cancer, DVT/PE, gallbladder disease, breast cancer, MI, CVA. Frequent: Nausea, breast tenderness.

ESTROPIPATE (*Ogen, Ortho-Est*) ▶L ♀X ▶– $
ADULTS — Moderate to severe menopausal vasomotor symptoms, vulvar and vaginal atrophy: 0.75 to 6 mg PO daily. Female hypogonadism, bilateral oophorectomy, or ovarian failure: 1.5 to 9 mg PO daily. Prevention of osteoporosis: 0.75 mg PO daily.
PEDS — Not approved in children.
FORMS — Generic/Trade: Tabs 0.75, 1.5, 3, 6 mg of estropipate.
NOTES — 6 mg estropipate is 5 mg sodium estrone sulfate.
MOA — Gonadal steroid.
ADVERSE EFFECTS — Serious: Endometrial cancer, DVT/PE, gallbladder disease, breast cancer, MI, CVA. Frequent: Nausea, breast tenderness.

OB/GYN: GnRH Agents

NOTE: Anaphylaxis has occurred with synthetic GnRH agents.

CETRORELIX ACETATE (*Cetrotide*) ▶Plasma ♀X ▶– $$$$$
ADULTS — Infertility: Multiple dose regimen: 0.25 mg SC daily during the early to mid follicular phase. Continue treatment daily until the days of hCG administration. Single-dose regimen: 3 mg SC for 1 usually on stimulation day 7.
PEDS — Not approved in children.
FORMS — Trade only: Injection 0.25 mg and 3 mg vials.
NOTES — Best sites for SC self-injection are on the abdomen around the navel. Storage in original carton: 0.25 mg refrigerated (36–46F); 3 mg room temperature (77F). Contraindicated with severe renal impairment.
MOA — GnRH analog.
ADVERSE EFFECTS — Serious: Anaphylaxis, ovarian hyperstimulation syndrome. Frequent: Injection site reaction.

GANIRELIX (*Follistim-Antagon Kit, ✦Orgalutran*) ▶Plasma ♀X ▶? $$$$$
ADULTS — Infertility: 250 mcg SC daily during the early to mid follicular phase. Continue treatment daily until the days of hCG administration.
PEDS — Not approved in children.
FORMS — Trade only: Injection 250 mcg/0.5 mL in prefilled, disposable syringes with 3 vials follitropin beta.
NOTES — Best sites for SC self-injection are on the abdomen around the navel or upper thigh. Store at room temperature (77F) for up to 3 months. Protect from light. Packaging contains natural rubber latex which may cause allergic reactions.
MOA — GnRH analog.
ADVERSE EFFECTS — Serious: Anaphylaxis, ovarian hyperstimulation syndrome. Frequent: Injection site reaction.

NAFARELIN (*Synarel*) ▶L ♀X ▶– $$$$$
ADULTS — Endometriosis: 200 mcg spray into 1 nostril qam and the other nostril qpm. May be increased to one 200 mcg spray into each nostril bid. Duration of treatment: 6 months.
PEDS — Central precocious puberty: 2 sprays into each nostril bid for a total of 1600 mcg/day. May be increased to 1800 mcg/day. Allow 30 sec to elapse between sprays.
FORMS — Trade only: Nasal soln 2 mg/mL in 8 mL bottle (200 mcg per spray) approximately 80 sprays/bottle.

(cont.)

NAFARELIN (cont.)
NOTES — Ovarian cysts have occurred in the first 2 months of therapy. Symptoms of hypoestrogenism may occur. Elevations of phosphorus and eosinophil counts, and decreases in serum calcium and WBC counts have been documented. Consider norethindrone as "add back" therapy to decrease bone loss (see norethindrone).
MOA — GnRH analog.
ADVERSE EFFECTS — Serious: Anaphylaxis. Frequent: Hot flashes, nasal irritation.

OB/GYN: Hormone Combinations

NOTE: See also Estrogens. Unopposed estrogens increase the risk of endometrial cancer in postmenopausal women. Malignancy should be ruled out in cases of persistent or recurrent abnormal vaginal bleeding. Do not use during pregnancy. May increase the risk of DVT/PE, gallbladder disease. Interactions with oral anticoagulants, phenytoin, rifampin, barbiturates, corticosteroids, and St. John's wort. For preparations containing testosterone derivatives, observe women for signs of virilization, and lipid abnormalities. In the Women's Health Initiative, the combination of conjugated estrogens and medroxyprogesterone (PremPro) caused an increase in the risk of breast cancer, MI, CVA, and DVT/PE and did not improve overall quality of life. Women greater than 65 yo with 4 years of therapy had an increased risk of dementia. Estrogen/progestin combinations should be prescribed at the lowest effective doses and for the shortest durations. Patients should be counseled regarding the risks/benefits of hormone replacement.

ACTIVELLA (estradiol + norethindrone) ▶L ♀X ▶– $$$
ADULTS — Moderate to severe menopausal vasomotor symptoms, vulvar and vaginal atrophy, prevention of postmenopausal osteoporosis: 1 tab PO daily.
PEDS — Not approved in children.
FORMS — Trade only: Tabs 1/0.5 mg and 0.5/0.1 mg estradiol/norethindrone acetate in calendar dial pack dispenser.
MOA — Gonadal steroid combination.
ADVERSE EFFECTS — Serious: DVT/PE, gallbladder disease, breast cancer, MI, CVA. Frequent: Nausea, breast tenderness.

ANGELIQ (estradiol + drospirenone) ▶L ♀X ▶– $$$
ADULTS — Moderate to severe menopausal vasomotor symptoms, vulvar and vaginal atrophy: 1 tab PO daily.
PEDS — Not approved in children.
FORMS — Trade only: Tabs 1 mg estradiol/0.5 mg drospirenone.
NOTES — May cause hyperkalemia in high-risk patients due to antimineralocorticoid activity of drospirenone. Monitor potassium in patients on ACE inhibitors, ARBs, potassium-sparing diuretics, heparin, aldosterone antagonists, and NSAIDs. Should not be used if renal insufficiency, hepatic dysfunction or adrenal insufficiency.
MOA — Gonadal steroid combination.
ADVERSE EFFECTS — Serious: DVT/PE, gallbladder disease, breast cancer, MI, CVA. Frequent: Nausea, breast tenderness.

CLIMARA PRO (estradiol + levonorgestrel) ▶L ♀X ▶– $$$
ADULTS — Moderate to severe menopausal vasomotor symptoms, prevention of postmenopausal osteoporosis: 1 patch weekly.
PEDS — Not approved in children.
FORMS — Trade only: Transdermal 0.045/0.015 estradiol/levonorgestrel in mg/day, 4 patches/box.
NOTES — Rotate application sites; avoid the waistline.
MOA — Gonadal steroid combination.
ADVERSE EFFECTS — Serious: DVT/PE, gallbladder disease, breast cancer, MI, CVA. Frequent: Nausea, breast tenderness.

COMBIPATCH (estradiol + norethindrone, ✦Estalis) ▶L ♀X ▶– $$$
ADULTS — Moderate to severe menopausal vasomotor symptoms, vulvar and vaginal atrophy, female hypogonadism, bilateral oophorectomy, and ovarian failure, prevention of postmenopausal osteoporosis: 1 patch twice per week.
PEDS — Not approved in children.
FORMS — Trade only: Transdermal patch 0.05 estradiol/0.14 norethindrone and 0.05 estradiol/0.25 norethindrone in mg/day, 8 patches/box.
NOTES — Rotate application sites, avoid the waistline.
MOA — Gonadal steroid combination.
ADVERSE EFFECTS — Serious: DVT/PE, gallbladder disease, breast cancer, MI, CVA. Frequent: Nausea, breast tenderness.

ESTRATEST (esterified estrogens + methyltestosterone) ▶L ♀X ▶– $$$$
ADULTS — Moderate to severe menopausal vasomotor symptoms: 1 tab PO daily.
PEDS — Not approved in children.
UNAPPROVED ADULTS — Menopause-associated decrease in libido: 1 tab PO daily.
FORMS — Trade only: Tabs 1.25 mg esterified estrogens/2.5 mg methyltestosterone.
NOTES — Monitor LFTs and lipids.
MOA — Gonadal steroid combination.
ADVERSE EFFECTS — Serious: DVT/PE, gallbladder disease, breast cancer, MI, CVA, virilization. Frequent: Nausea, breast tenderness.

ESTRATEST H.S. (esterified estrogens + methyltestosterone) ▶L ♀X ▶– $$$
ADULTS — Moderate to severe menopausal vasomotor symptoms: 1 tab PO daily.
PEDS — Not approved in children.
UNAPPROVED ADULTS — Menopause-associated decrease in libido: 1 tab PO daily.
FORMS — Trade only: Tabs 0.625 mg esterified estrogens/1.25 mg methyltestosterone.
NOTES — HS indicates half-strength. Monitor LFTs and lipids.
MOA — Gonadal steroid combination.

(cont.)

DRUGS GENERALLY ACCEPTED AS SAFE IN PREGNANCY (selected)

<u>Analgesics:</u> acetaminophen, codeine*, meperidine*, methadone*. <u>Antimicrobials:</u> penicillins, cephalosporins, erythromycins (not estolate), azithromycin, nystatin, clotrimazole, metronidazole, nitrofurantoin***, Nix. <u>Antivirals:</u> acyclovir, valacyclovir, famciclovir. <u>CV:</u> labetalol, methyldopa, hydralazine, nifedipine. <u>Derm:</u> erythromycin, clindamycin, benzoyl peroxide. <u>Endo:</u> insulin, liothyronine, levothyroxine. <u>ENT:</u> chlorpheniramine, diphenhydramine, dimenhydrinate, dextromethorphan, guaifenesin, nasal steroids, nasal cromolyn. <u>GI:</u> trimethobenzamide, antacids*, simethicone, cimetidine, famotidine, ranitidine, nizatidine, psyllium, metoclopramide, bisacodyl, docusate, doxylamine, meclizine. <u>Heme:</u> Heparin, low molecular wt heparins. <u>Psych:</u> desipramine, doxepin. <u>Pulmonary:</u> short-acting inhaled beta-2 agonists, cromolyn, nedocromil, beclomethasone, budesonide, theophylline, prednisone**. *Except if used long-term or in high dose at term. **Except 1st trimester.   ***Contraindicated at term and during labor and delivery.

ESTRATEST H.S. (cont.)
ADVERSE EFFECTS — Serious: DVT/PE, gallbladder disease, breast cancer, MI, CVA, virilization. Frequent: Nausea, breast tenderness.

FEMHRT (ethinyl estradiol + norethindrone) ▶L ♀X ▶– $$$
WARNING — Multiple strengths; see FORMS and write specific product on Rx.
ADULTS — <u>Moderate to severe menopausal vasomotor symptoms, prevention of postmenopausal osteoporosis:</u> 1 tab PO daily.
PEDS — Not approved in children.
FORMS — Trade only: Tabs 5/1, 2.5/0.5 mcg ethinyl estradiol/mg norethindrone, 28/blister card.
MOA — Gonadal steroid combination.
ADVERSE EFFECTS — Serious: DVT/PE, gallbladder disease, breast cancer, MI, CVA. Frequent: Nausea, breast tenderness.

PREFEST (estradiol + norgestimate) ▶L ♀X ▶– $$$
ADULTS — <u>Moderate to severe menopausal vasomotor symptoms, vulvar atrophy, atrophic vaginitis, prevention of postmenopausal osteoporosis:</u> 1 pink tab PO daily for 3 days followed by 1 white tab PO daily for 3 days, sequentially throughout the month.
PEDS — Not approved in children.
FORMS — Trade only: Tabs in 30 days blister packs 1 mg estradiol (15 pink), 1 mg estradiol/0.09 mg norgestimate (15 white).
MOA — Gonadal steroid combination.
ADVERSE EFFECTS — Serious: DVT/PE, gallbladder disease, breast cancer, MI, CVA. Frequent: Nausea, breast tenderness.

PREMPHASE (estrogens conjugated + medroxyprogesterone) ▶L ♀X ▶– $$$
ADULTS — <u>Moderate to severe menopausal vasomotor symptoms, vulvar/vaginal atrophy, and prevention of postmenopausal osteoporosis:</u> 0.625 mg conjugated estrogens PO daily on days 1 to 14 and 0.625 mg conjugated estrogens/5 mg medroxyprogesterone PO daily on days 15 to 28.
PEDS — Not approved in children.
FORMS — Trade only: Tabs in 28 days EZ-Dial dispensers: 0.625 mg conjugated estrogens (14), 0.625 mg/5 mg conjugated estrogens/medroxyprogesterone (14).
MOA — Gonadal steroid combination.
ADVERSE EFFECTS — Serious: DVT/PE, gallbladder disease, breast cancer, MI, CVA. Frequent: Nausea, breast tenderness.

PREMPRO (estrogens conjugated + medroxyprogesterone, ✦*Premplus*) ▶L ♀X ▶– $$$
WARNING — Multiple strengths; see FORMS and write specific product on Rx.
ADULTS — <u>Moderate to severe menopausal vasomotor symptoms, vulvar/vaginal atrophy, and prevention of postmenopausal osteoporosis:</u> 1 PO daily.
PEDS — Not approved in children.
FORMS — Trade only: Tabs in 28-day EZ-Dial dispensers: 0.625 mg/5 mg, 0.625 mg/2.5 mg, 0.45 mg/1.5 mg (Prempro low dose), or 0.3 mg/1.5 mg conjugated estrogens/medroxyprogesterone.
MOA — Gonadal steroid combination.
ADVERSE EFFECTS — Serious: DVT/PE, gallbladder disease, breast cancer, MI, CVA. Frequent: Nausea, breast tenderness.

SYNTEST D.S. (esterified estrogens + methyltestosterone) ▶L ♀X ▶– $$$
ADULTS — <u>Moderate to severe menopausal vasomotor symptoms:</u> 1 tab PO daily.
PEDS — Not approved in children.
UNAPPROVED ADULTS — <u>Menopause-associated decrease in libido:</u> 1 tab PO daily.
FORMS — Generic only: Tabs 1.25 mg esterified estrogens/2.5 mg methyltestosterone.
NOTES — Monitor LFTs and lipids. Same as Estratest.
MOA — Gonadal steroid combination.
ADVERSE EFFECTS — Serious: DVT/PE, gallbladder disease, breast cancer, MI, CVA, virilization. Frequent: Nausea, breast tenderness.

SYNTEST H.S. (esterified estrogens + methyltestosterone) ▶L ♀X ▶– $$$
ADULTS — <u>Moderate to severe menopausal vasomotor symptoms:</u> 1 tab PO daily.
PEDS — Not approved in children.
UNAPPROVED ADULTS — <u>Menopause-associated decrease in libido:</u> 1 tab PO daily.
FORMS — Generic only: Tabs 0.625 mg esterified estrogens/1.25 mg methyltestosterone.
NOTES — HS indicates half-strength. Monitor LFTs and lipids. Same as Estratest-HS.
MOA — Gonadal steroid combination.
ADVERSE EFFECTS — Serious: DVT/PE, gallbladder disease, breast cancer, MI, CVA, virilization. Frequent: Nausea, breast tenderness.

OB/GYN: Labor Induction / Cervical Ripening

NOTE: Fetal well-being should be documented prior to use.

DINOPROSTONE (*PGE2, Prepidil, Cervidil, Prostin E2*) ▶Lung ♀C ▶? $$$$$
ADULTS — <u>Cervical ripening:</u> Gel: 1 syringe via catheter placed into cervical canal below the internal os. May be repeated q 6 h to a max of 3 doses. Vaginal insert: Place in posterior fornix. Evacuation of uterine contents after fetal death up to 28 weeks or termination of pregnancy 12 to 20th gestational week: 20 mg intravaginal suppository; repeat at 3 to 5 h intervals until abortion occurs. Do not use for more than 2 days.
PEDS — Not approved in children.
FORMS — Trade only: Gel (Prepidil) 0.5 mg/3 g syringe. Vaginal insert (Cervidil) 10 mg. Vaginal supps (Prostin E2) 20 mg.
NOTES — Patient should remain supine for 15 to 30 min after gel and 2 h after vaginal insert. For hospital use only. Monitor for uterine hyperstimulation and abnormal fetal heart rate. Caution with asthma or glaucoma. Contraindicated in prior C-section or major uterine surgery due to potential for uterine rupture.
MOA — Uterine stimulant.
ADVERSE EFFECTS — Serious: Uterine hyperstimulation, uterine rupture. Frequent: N/V, diarrhea.

MISOPROSTOL- OB (*PGE1, Cytotec*) ▶LK ♀X ▶− $$$$
WARNING — Contraindicated in desired early or preterm pregnancy due to its abortifacient property. Pregnant women should avoid contact/exposure to the tabs. Uterine rupture reported with use for labor induction and medical abortion.
UNAPPROVED ADULTS — <u>Cervical ripening and labor induction:</u> 25 mcg intravaginally q 3 to 6 h (or 50 mcg q 6 h). <u>First trimester pregnancy failure:</u> 800 mcg intravaginally, repeat on day 3 if expulsion incomplete. <u>Medical abortion less than 50 days gestation:</u> With mifepristone, see mifepristone; with methotrexate: 800 mcg intravaginally 5 to 7 days after 50 mg/m2 PO or IM methotrexate. <u>Preop cervical ripening:</u> 400 mcg intravaginally 3 to 4 h before mechanical cervical dilation. <u>Postpartum hemorrhage:</u> 800 mcg PR for 1 dose. Oral dosing has been used but is controversial. Treatment of duodenal ulcers: 100 mcg PO qid.
FORMS — Generic/Trade: Oral tabs 100, 200 mcg.
NOTES — Contraindicated with prior C-section. Oral tabs can be inserted into the vagina for labor induction/cervical ripening. Monitor for uterine hyperstimulation and abnormal fetal heart rate. Risk factors for uterine rupture: Prior uterine surgery and 5 or more previous pregnancies.
MOA — Prostaglandin E1 analog, uterine stimulant.
ADVERSE EFFECTS — Serious: Uterine hyperstimulation, uterine rupture. Frequent: diarrhea, abdominal pain.

OXYTOCIN (*Pitocin*) ▶LK ♀? ▶− $
WARNING — Not approved for elective labor induction, although widely used.
ADULTS — <u>Induction/stimulation of labor:</u> 10 units in 1000 mL NS, 1 to 2 milliunits/min IV as a continuous infusion (6 to 12 mL/h). Increase in increments of 1 to 2 milliunits/min q 30 min until a contraction pattern is established, up to a max of 20 milliunits/min. <u>Postpartum bleeding:</u> 10 units IM after delivery of the placenta. 10 to 40 units in 1000 mL NS IV infusion, infuse 20 to 40 milliunits/min.
PEDS — Not approved in children.
UNAPPROVED ADULTS — <u>Augmentation of labor:</u> 0.5 to 2 milliunits/min IV as a continuous infusion, increase by 1 to 2 milliunits/min q 30 min until adequate pattern of labor to a max of 40 milliunits/min.
NOTES — Use a pump to accurately control the infusion while patient is under continuous observation. Continuous fetal monitoring is required. Concurrent sympathomimetics may result in postpartum HTN. Anaphylaxis and severe water intoxication have occurred. Caution in patients undergoing a trial of labor after c-section.
MOA — Uterine stimulant.
ADVERSE EFFECTS — Serious: Anaphylaxis, water intoxication. Frequent: N/V.

OB/GYN: Ovulation Stimulants

NOTE: Potentially serious adverse effects include DVT/PE, ovarian hyperstimulation syndrome, adnexal torsion, ovarian enlargement and cysts, and febrile reactions.

CHORIOGONADOTROPIN ALFA (*hCG, Ovidrel*) ▶L ♀X ▶? $$$
ADULTS — <u>Specialized dosing for ovulation induction.</u>
PEDS — Not approved in children.
FORMS — Trade only: Powder for injection or, prefilled syringe 250 mcg.
NOTES — Best site for SC self-injection is on the abdomen below the navel. Beware of multiple pregnancy and multiple adverse effects. Store in original package and protect from light. Use immediately after reconstitution.
MOA — Ovulation induction.
ADVERSE EFFECTS — Serious: Arterial thromboembolism, PE, ovarian hyperstimulation syndrome, adnexal torsion, ovarian enlargement & cysts, & febrile reactions. Frequent: Injection site reactions.

CHORIONIC GONADOTROPIN (*hCG, Pregnyl, Novarel*) ▶L ♀X ▶? $$$
ADULTS — <u>Specialized dosing for ovulation induction.</u>
PEDS — Not approved in children.
NOTES — Beware of multiple pregnancy and multiple adverse effects. For IM use only.

(cont.)

CHORIONIC GONADOTROPIN (cont.)
MOA — Ovulation induction.
ADVERSE EFFECTS — Serious: Arterial thromboembolism, PE, ovarian hyperstimulation syndrome, ovarian cysts, & ascites. Frequent: Injection site reactions.

CLOMIPHENE (*Clomid, Serophene*) ▶L ♀D ▶? $$$$$
ADULTS — Specialized dosing for infertility.
PEDS — Not approved in children.
FORMS — Generic/Trade: Tabs 50 mg, scored.
NOTES — Beware of multiple pregnancy and multiple adverse effects.
MOA — Ovulation induction.
ADVERSE EFFECTS — Serious: Blurred vision, ovarian hyperstimulation syndrome, ovarian enlargement & cysts. Frequent: hot flashes, abdominal discomfort.

FOLLITROPIN ALFA (*FSH, Gonal-F, Gonal-F RFF Pen*) ▶L ♀X ▶? $$$$$
ADULTS — Specialized dosing for infertility.
PEDS — Not approved in children.
FORMS — Trade only: Powder for injection, 75 international units FSH activity, multidose vial 450, 1050 international units FSH activity. Prefilled, multiple-dose pen, 300 international units, 450 international units, 900 international units FSH activity with single-use disposable needles.
NOTES — Best site for SC self-injection is on the abdomen below the navel. Beware of multiple gestation pregnancy and multiple adverse effects. Store in original package and protect from light. Use immediately after reconstitution. Pen may be stored at room temperature for up to 1 month or expiration, whichever is first.
MOA — Ovulation induction.
ADVERSE EFFECTS — Serious: Arterial thromboembolism, DVT/PE, ovarian hyperstimulation syndrome, adnexal torsion, ovarian cysts, & febrile reactions. Frequent: Injection site reactions.

FOLLITROPIN BETA (*FSH, Follistim AQ, ✦Puregon*) ▶L ♀X ▶? $$$$$
ADULTS — Specialized dosing for infertility.
PEDS — Not approved in children.
FORMS — Trade only: Cartridge, for use with the Follistim Pen, 150, 300, 600, 900 international units. Aqueous soln 75, 150 international units FSH activity.
NOTES — Best site for SC self-injection is on the abdomen below the navel. Beware of multiple pregnancy and multiple adverse effects. Store in original package and protect from light. Use powder for injection immediately after reconstitution. Cartridge may be stored for up to 28 days. Store aqueous soln in refrigerator.
MOA — Ovulation induction.
ADVERSE EFFECTS — Serious: Arterial thromboembolism, DVT/PE, ovarian hyperstimulation syndrome, adnexal torsion, ovarian cysts, & febrile reactions. Frequent: Injection site reactions.

GONADOTROPINS (*menotropins, FSH and LH, Menopur, Pergonal, Repronex, ✦Propasi HP*) ▶L ♀X ▶? $$$$$
ADULTS — Specialized dosing for infertility.
PEDS — Not approved in children.
FORMS — Trade only: Powder for injection, 75 international units FSH/LH activity.
NOTES — Best site for SC self-injection is on the abdomen below the navel. Beware of multiple pregnancy and numerous adverse effects. Use immediately after reconstitution.
MOA — Ovulation induction.
ADVERSE EFFECTS — Serious: Anaphylaxis, arterial thromboembolism, DVT/PE, ovarian hyperstimulation syndrome, adnexal torsion, ovarian cysts, & febrile reactions. Frequent: Injection site reactions.

LUTROPIN ALFA (*Luveris*) ▶L ♀X ▶— $$$$$
ADULTS — Specialized dosing for infertility.
PEDS — Not approved in children.
FORMS — Trade only: Powder for injection, 75 international units LH activity.
NOTES — For use with follitropin alfa. Best site for SC self-injection is on the abdomen below the navel. Protect from light. Use immediately after reconstitution.
MOA — Ovulation induction.
ADVERSE EFFECTS — Serious: Anaphylaxis, ovarian hyperstimulation syndrome, ovarian cysts, arterial thromboembolism, DVT/PE. Frequent: Headache, abdominal pain, breast pain.

UROFOLLITROPIN (*Bravelle, FSH, Fertinex*) ▶L ♀X ▶? $$$$$
ADULTS — Specialized dosing for infertility and polycystic ovary syndrome.
PEDS — Not approved in children.
FORMS — Trade only: Powder for injection, 75 international units FSH activity.
NOTES — Best site for SC self-injection is on the abdomen below the navel. Beware of multiple pregnancy and numerous adverse effects. Use immediately after reconstitution.
MOA — Ovulation induction.
ADVERSE EFFECTS — Serious: Arterial thromboembolism, DVT/PE, ovarian hyperstimulation syndrome, adnexal torsion, ovarian cysts, & febrile reactions. Frequent: Injection site reactions.

OB/GYN: Progestins

NOTE: Do not use in pregnancy. DVT, PE, cerebrovascular disorders, and retinal thrombosis may occur. Effectiveness may be reduced by hepatic enzyme-inducing drugs such as certain anticonvulsants and barbiturates, rifampin, rifabutin, griseofulvin, and protease inhibitors. The effects of St. John's wort-containing products on progestin-only pills is currently unknown. In the Women's Health Initiative, the combination of conjugated estrogens and medroxyprogesterone (PremPro) caused a statistically significant increase in the risk of breast cancer, MI, CVA, and DVT/PE. Additionally, women greater than 65 yo with 4 years of therapy had an increased risk of dementia. Estrogen/progestin combinations should be prescribed at the lowest effective doses and for the shortest durations. Patients should be counseled regarding the risks/benefits of hormone replacement.

HYDROXYPROGESTERONE CAPROATE ▶L ♀X ▶? $
ADULTS — <u>Amenorrhea, dysfunctional uterine bleeding, metrorrhagia:</u> 375 mg IM. <u>Production of secretory endometrium and desquamation:</u> 125 to 250 mg IM on 10th days of the cycle, repeat q 7 d until suppression no longer desired.
PEDS — Not approved in children.
UNAPPROVED ADULTS — <u>Endometrial hyperplasia:</u> 500 mg IM weekly. <u>Prevention of preterm delivery in patients with a history of preterm birth:</u> 250 mg IM weekly starting at 16 to 20 weeks gestation until 36 weeks or delivery.
MOA — Gonadal steroid.
ADVERSE EFFECTS Serious: Thrombophlebitis, cerebrovascular disorders, retinal thrombosis, DVT/PE. Frequent: Injection site reactions, breakthrough bleeding.

MEDROXYPROGESTERONE (Provera) ▶L ♀X ▶+ $
ADULTS — <u>Secondary amenorrhea:</u> 5 to 10 mg PO daily for 5 to 10 days. <u>Abnormal uterine bleeding:</u> 5 to 10 mg PO daily for 5 to 10 days beginning on the 16th or 21st day of the cycle (after estrogen priming). Withdrawal bleeding usually occurs 3 to 7 days after therapy ends.
PEDS — Not approved in children.
UNAPPROVED ADULTS — <u>Add to estrogen replacement therapy to prevent endometrial hyperplasia:</u> 10 mg PO daily for 10 to 12 days each month, or 2.5 to 5 mg PO daily. <u>Endometrial hyperplasia:</u> 10 to 30 mg PO daily (long-term); 40 to 100 mg PO daily (short-term) or 500 mg IM twice per week.
FORMS — Generic/Trade: Tabs 2.5, 5, 10 mg, scored.
NOTES — Breakthrough bleeding/spotting may occur. Amenorrhea usually after 6 months of continuous dosing.
MOA — Gonadal steroid.
ADVERSE EFFECTS — Serious: Thrombophlebitis, cerebrovascular disorders, retinal thrombosis, DVT/PE. Frequent: Breakthrough bleeding.

MEDROXYPROGESTERONE—INJECTABLE (Depo-Provera, depo-subQ provera 104) ▶L ♀X ▶+ $
WARNING — Risk of significant bone loss, possibly irreversible, increases with duration of use. Long-term use (greater than 2 years) only recommended if other methods of birth control are inadequate or symptoms of endometriosis return after discontinuation.
ADULTS — <u>Contraception/Endometriosis:</u> 150 mg IM in deltoid or gluteus maximus or 104 mg SC in anterior thigh or abdomen q 13 weeks. Also used for adjunctive therapy in endometrial and renal carcinoma.
PEDS — Not approved in children.
UNAPPROVED ADULTS — <u>Dysfunctional uterine bleeding:</u> 150 mg IM in deltoid or gluteus maximus q 13 weeks.

NOTES — Breakthrough bleeding/spotting may occur. Amenorrhea usually after 6 months. Wt gain is common. To be sure that the patient is not pregnant give this injection only during the first 5 days after the onset of a normal menstrual period or after a negative pregnancy test. May be given immediately post-pregnancy termination as well as postpartum, including breastfeeding women. May be given as often as 11 weeks apart. If the time between injections is greater than 14 weeks, exclude pregnancy before administering. Return to fertility can be variably delayed after last injection, with the median time to pregnancy being 10 months. Bone loss may occur with prolonged administration. Evaluate bone mineral density if considering retreatment for endometriosis.
MOA — Progestational agent that inhibits release of LH.
ADVERSE EFFECTS — Serious: Thrombophlebitis, cerebrovascular disorders, retinal thrombosis, DVT/PE, bone loss. Frequent: Injection site reactions, breakthrough bleeding, weight gain.

MEGESTROL (Megace, Megace ES) ▶L ♀D ▶? $$$$$
ADULTS — <u>AIDS anorexia:</u> 800 mg (20 mL) susp PO daily or 625 mg (5 mL) ES daily. <u>Palliative treatment for advanced breast carcinoma:</u> 40 mg (tabs) PO qid. <u>Endometrial carcinoma:</u> 40 to 320 mg/day (tabs) in divided doses.
PEDS — Not approved in children.
UNAPPROVED ADULTS — <u>Endometrial hyperplasia:</u> 40 to 160 mg PO daily for 3 to 4 months. <u>Cancer-associated anorexia/cachexia:</u> 80 to 160 mg PO qid.
FORMS — Generic/Trade: Tabs 20, 40 mg. Susp 40 mg/mL in 240 mL. Trade only: Megace ES susp 125 mg/mL (150 mL).
NOTES — In HIV-infected women, breakthrough bleeding/spotting may occur.
MOA — Gonadal steroid.
ADVERSE EFFECTS — Serious: Thrombophlebitis, cerebrovascular disorders, retinal thrombosis, DVT/PE. Frequent: Breakthrough bleeding, weight gain.

NORETHINDRONE (Aygestin, Micronor, Nor-Q.D., Camila, Errin, Jolivette, Nora-BE) ▶L ♀D/X ▶See notes $
ADULTS — <u>Contraception:</u> 0.35 mg PO daily. <u>Amenorrhea, abnormal uterine bleeding:</u> 2.5 to 10 mg PO daily for 5 to 10 days during the second half of the menstrual cycle. <u>Endometriosis:</u> 5 mg PO daily for 2 weeks. Increase by 2.5 mg q 2 weeks to 15 mg/day.
PEDS — Not approved in children.
UNAPPROVED ADULTS — <u>"Add back" therapy with GnRH agonists (eg, leuprolide) to decrease bone loss:</u> 5 mg PO daily.
FORMS — Generic/Trade: Tabs scored 5 mg. Trade only: 0.35 mg tabs.

(cont.)

NORETHINDRONE (cont.)
NOTES — Contraceptive doses felt compatible with breast feeding, but not higher doses.
MOA — Gonadal steroid.
ADVERSE EFFECTS — Serious: Thrombophlebitis, cerebrovascular disorders, retinal thrombosis, DVT/PE. Frequent: Nausea, breast tenderness, breakthrough bleeding.

PROGESTERONE GEL (*Crinone, Prochieve*) ▶Plasma ♀–▶? $$$
ADULTS — Secondary amenorrhea: 45 mg (4%) intravaginally every other day up to 6 doses. If no response, use 90 mg (8%) intravaginally every other day up to 6 doses. Specialized dosing for infertility.
PEDS — Not approved in children.
FORMS — Trade only: 4%, 8% single-use, prefilled applicators.
NOTES — An increase in dose from the 4% gel can only be accomplished using the 8% gel; doubling the volume of 4% does not increase absorption.
MOA — Gonadal steroid.
ADVERSE EFFECTS — Serious: Thrombophlebitis, cerebrovascular disorders, retinal thrombosis, DVT/PE. Frequent: Vaginal discharge.

PROGESTERONE IN OIL ▶L ♀X ▶? $$
WARNING — Contraindicated in peanut allergy since some products contain peanut oil.
ADULTS — Amenorrhea, uterine bleeding: 5 to 10 mg IM daily for 6 to 8 days.
PEDS — Not approved in children.
NOTES — Discontinue with thrombotic disorders, sudden or partial loss of vision, proptosis, diplopia or migraine.

MOA — Gonadal steroid.
ADVERSE EFFECTS — Serious: Thrombophlebitis, cerebrovascular disorders, retinal thrombosis, DVT/PE. Frequent: Breakthrough bleeding.

PROGESTERONE MICRONIZED (*Prometrium*) ▶L ♀B ▶+ $$
WARNING — Contraindicated in patients allergic to peanuts since caps contain peanut oil.
ADULTS — Hormone therapy to prevent endometrial hyperplasia: 200 mg PO at bedtime 10 to 12 days/month. Secondary amenorrhea: 400 mg PO at bedtime for 10 days.
PEDS — Not approved in children.
UNAPPROVED ADULTS — Hormone therapy to prevent endometrial hyperplasia: 100 mg at bedtime daily.
FORMS — Trade only: Caps 100, 200 mg.
NOTES — Breast tenderness, dizziness, headache and abdominal cramping may occur.
MOA — Gonadal steroid.
ADVERSE EFFECTS — Serious: Thrombophlebitis, cerebrovascular disorders, retinal thrombosis, DVT/PE. Frequent: Breakthrough bleeding.

PROGESTERONE VAGINAL INSERT (*Endometrin*) ▶Plasma ♀–▶? $$$$
ADULTS — Specialized dosing for infertility.
PEDS — Not approved in children.
FORMS — Trade only: 100 mg vaginal insert.
NOTES — Do not use concomitantly with other vaginal products, such as antifungals, as this may alter absorption.
MOA — Gonadal steroid.
ADVERSE EFFECTS — Serious: Thrombophlebitis, cerebrovascular disorders, retinal thrombosis, DVT/PE. Frequent: Vaginal discharge.

OB/GYN: Selective Estrogen Receptor Modulators

RALOXIFENE (*Evista*) ▶L ♀X ▶– $$$$
WARNING — Increases the risk of venous thromboembolism and CVA. Do not use during pregnancy.
ADULTS — Postmenopausal osteoporosis prevention/treatment, breast cancer prevention: 60 mg PO daily.
PEDS — Not approved in children.
FORMS — Trade only: Tabs 60 mg.
NOTES — Contraindicated with history of venous thromboembolism. Interactions with oral anticoagulants and cholestyramine. May increase risk of DVT/PE. Discontinue use 72 h prior to and during prolonged immobilization because of DVT risk. Does not decrease (and may increase) hot flashes. Leg cramps. Triglyceride levels may increase in women with prior estrogen-associated hypertriglyceridemia (> 500 mg/dL).
MOA — Selective Estrogen Receptor Modulator.
ADVERSE EFFECTS — Serious: DVT/PE, hypertriglyceridemia, stroke. Frequent: Hot flashes, leg cramps.

TAMOXIFEN (*Nolvadex, Soltamox, Tamone, ✦Tamofen*) ▶L ♀D ▶– $$
WARNING — Uterine malignancies, CVA and pulmonary embolism, sometimes fatal. Visual disturbances, cataracts, hypercalcemia, increased LFTs, bone pain, fertility impairment, hot flashes, menstrual irregularities, endometrial hyperplasia and cancer, alopecia. Do not use during pregnancy.
ADULTS — Breast cancer prevention in high-risk women: 20 mg PO daily for 5 years. Breast cancer: 10 to 20 mg PO bid for 5 years.
PEDS — Not approved in children.
UNAPPROVED ADULTS — Mastalgia: 10 mg PO daily for 4 months. Anovulation: 5 to 40 mg PO bid for 4 days.
FORMS — Generic/Trade: Tabs 10, 20 mg. Trade only (Soltamox): Sugar-free soln 10 mg/5 mL (150 mL).
NOTES — Reliable contraception is recommended. Monitor CBCs, LFTs. Regular gynecologic and ophthalmologic examinations. Interacts with oral anticoagulants. Does not decrease hot flashes.
MOA — Selective Estrogen Receptor Modulator.
ADVERSE EFFECTS — Serious: DVT/PE, retinal thrombosis, hepatotoxicity, endometrial cancer,. Frequent: Hot flashes, leg cramps, vaginal discharge.

OB/GYN: Uterotonics

CARBOPROST (*Hemabate, 15-methyl-prostaglandin F2 alpha*) ▶LK ♀C ▶? $$$
ADULTS – <u>Refractory postpartum uterine bleeding:</u> 250 mcg deep IM. If necessary, may repeat at 15 to 90 min intervals up to a total dose of 2 mg (8 doses).
PEDS – Not approved in children.
NOTES – Caution with asthma. Transient fever, HTN, nausea, bronchoconstriction and flushing. May augment oxytocics.
MOA – Uterotonic.
ADVERSE EFFECTS – Serious: Pulmonary edema. Frequent: Fever, flushing, nausea, diarrhea.

METHYLERGONOVINE (*Methergine*) ▶LK ♀C ▶? $$
ADULTS – <u>To increase uterine contractions and decrease postpartum bleeding:</u> 0.2 mg IM after delivery of the placenta, delivery of the anterior shoulder, or during the puerperium. Repeat q 2 to 4 h prn. 0.2 mg PO tid to qid in the puerperium for a max of 1 week.
PEDS – Not approved in children.
FORMS – Trade only: Tabs 0.2 mg.
NOTES – Contraindicated in pregnancy-induced HTN/preeclampsia. Avoid IV route due to risk of sudden HTN and CVA. If IV absolutely necessary, give slowly over no less than 1 min, monitor BP.
MOA – Uterotonic.
ADVERSE EFFECTS – Serious: CVA, seizure. Frequent: Hypertension, headache, nausea.

OB/GYN: Vaginitis Preparations

NOTE: See also STD/vaginitis table in antimicrobial section. Many experts recommend 7 days antifungal therapy for pregnant women with candida vaginitis. Many of these creams and supps are oil-based and may weaken latex condoms and diaphragms. Do not use latex products for 72 h after last dose.

BORIC ACID ▶Not absorbed ♀? ▶– $
PEDS – Not approved in children.
UNAPPROVED ADULTS – <u>Resistant vulvovaginal candidiasis:</u> 600 mg suppository intravaginally at bedtime for 2 weeks.
FORMS – No commercial preparation; must be compounded by pharmacist. Vaginal supps 600 mg in gelatin caps.
NOTES – Reported use for azole-resistant nonalbicans (C glabrata) or recurrent albicans failing azole therapy. Do not use if abdominal pain, fever or foul-smelling vaginal discharge is present. Avoid vaginal intercourse during treatment.
MOA – Antifungal.
ADVERSE EFFECTS – Serious: None. Frequent: Vulvovaginal irritation, erythema, & erosions.

BUTOCONAZOLE (*Gynazole, Mycelex-3*) ▶LK ♀C ▶? $(OTC), $$$(Rx)
ADULTS – <u>Local treatment of vulvovaginal candidiasis,</u> nonpregnant patients: Mycelex 3: 1 applicatorful (~5 g) intravaginally at bedtime for 3 days, up to 6 days, if necessary. Pregnant patients: (second and third trimesters only) 1 applicatorful (~5 g) intravaginally at bedtime for 6 days. Gynazole-1: 1 applicatorful (~5 g) intravaginally once daily.
PEDS – Not approved in children.
FORMS – OTC Trade only (Mycelex 3): 2% vaginal cream in 5 g prefilled applicators (3s), 20 g tube with applicators. Rx: Trade only (Gynazole-1): 2% vaginal cream in 5 g prefilled applicator.
NOTES – Do not use if abdominal pain, fever or foul-smelling vaginal discharge is present. Since small amount may be absorbed from the vagina, use during the first trimester only when essential. During pregnancy, use of a vaginal applicator may be contraindicated and manual insertion may be preferred. Vulvar/vaginal burning may occur. Avoid vaginal intercourse during treatment.
MOA – Antifungal.
ADVERSE EFFECTS – Serious: None. Frequent: Vulvovaginal irritation.

CLINDAMYCIN—VAGINAL (*Cleocin, Clindesse, ✦Dalacin*) ▶L ♀– ▶+ $$
ADULTS – <u>Bacterial vaginosis:</u> Cleocin: 1 applicatorful (~100 mg clindamycin phosphate in 5 g cream) intravaginally at bedtime for 7 days, or 1 suppository at bedtime for 3 days. Clindesse: 1 applicatorful cream × 1.
PEDS – Not approved in children.
FORMS – Generic/Trade: 2% vaginal cream in 40 g tube with 7 disposable applicators (Cleocin). Vag suppository (Cleocin Ovules) 100 mg (3) with applicator. 2% vaginal cream in a single-dose prefilled applicator (Clindesse).
NOTES – Clindesse may degrade latex/rubber condoms and diaphragms for 5 days after the last dose (Cleocin for up to 3 days). Not recommended during pregnancy despite B rating, as it does not prevent the adverse effects of bacterial vaginosis (eg, preterm birth, neonatal infection). Cervicitis, vaginitis, and vulvar irritation may occur. Avoid vaginal intercourse during treatment.
MOA – Antibiotic.
ADVERSE EFFECTS – Serious: None. Frequent: Cervicitis, vaginitis, & vulvar irritation.

CLOTRIMAZOLE—VAGINAL (*Mycelex 7, Gyne-Lotrimin, ✦Canesten, Clotrimaderm*) ▶LK ♀B ▶? $
ADULTS – <u>Local treatment of vulvovaginal candidiasis:</u> 1 applicatorful 1% cream at bedtime for 7 days. 1 applicatorful 2% cream at bedtime for 3 days. 100 mg suppository intravaginally at bedtime for 7 days. 200 mg suppository at bedtime for 3 days. Topical cream for external symptoms bid for 7 days.
PEDS – Not approved in children.
FORMS – OTC Generic/Trade: 1% vaginal cream with applicator (some prefilled). 2% vaginal cream

(cont.)

OB/GYN: Vaginitis Preparations

CLOTRIMAZOLE—VAGINAL (cont.)
with applicator and 1% topical cream in some combination packs. OTC Trade only (Gyne-Lotrimin): Vaginal suppository 100 mg (7), 200 mg (3) with applicators.
NOTES — Do not use if abdominal pain, fever or foul-smelling vaginal discharge is present. Since small amounts of these drugs may be absorbed from the vagina, use during the 1st trimester only when essential. During pregnancy, use of a vaginal applicator may be contraindicated; manual insertion of tabs may be preferred. Skin rash, lower abdominal cramps, bloating, vulvar irritation may occur. Avoid vaginal intercourse during treatment.
MOA — Antifungal.
ADVERSE EFFECTS — Serious: None. Frequent: Vulvovaginal irritation.

METRONIDAZOLE—VAGINAL (*MetroGel-Vaginal, Vandazole*) ▶LK ♀B ▶? $$
ADULTS — Bacterial vaginosis: 1 applicatorful (approximately 5 g containing approximately 37.5 mg metronidazole) intravaginally at bedtime or bid for 5 days.
PEDS — Not approved in children.
FORMS — Generic/Trade: 0.75% gel in 70 g tube with applicator.
NOTES — Cure rate same with at bedtime and bid dosing. Vaginally applied metronidazole could be absorbed in sufficient amounts to produce systemic effects. Caution in patients with CNS diseases due to rare reports of seizures, neuropathy, and numbness. Do not administer to patients who have taken disulfiram within the last 2 weeks. Interaction with ethanol. Caution with warfarin. Candida cervicitis and vaginitis, and vaginal, perineal, or vulvar itching may occur. Avoid vaginal intercourse during treatment.
MOA — Antibiotic.
ADVERSE EFFECTS — Serious: Seizures. Frequent: Cervicitis, vaginitis, & vulvar irritation.

MICONAZOLE (*Monistat, Femizol-M, M-Zole, Micozole, Monazole*) ▶LK ♀+ ▶? $
ADULTS — Local treatment of vulvovaginal candidiasis: 1 applicatorful 2% cream intravaginally at bedtime for 7 days or 4% cream at bedtime for 3 days. 100 mg suppository intravaginally at bedtime for 7 days, 400 mg at bedtime for 3 days, or 1200 mg for 1 dose. Topical cream for external symptoms bid for 7 days.
PEDS — Not approved in children.
FORMS — OTC Generic/Trade: 2% vaginal cream in 45 g with 1 applicator or 7 disposable applicators. Vaginal suppository 100 mg (7) OTC Trade only: 400 mg (3), 1200 mg (1) with applicator. Generic/Trade: 4% vaginal cream in 25 g tubes or 3 prefilled applicators. Some in combination packs with 2% miconazole cream for external use.
NOTES — Do not use if abdominal pain, fever or foul-smelling vaginal discharge is present. Since small amounts of these drugs may be absorbed from the vagina, use during the 1st trimester only when essential. During pregnancy, use of a vaginal applicator may be contraindicated; manual insertion of suppositories may be preferred. Vulvovaginal burning, itching, irritation and pelvic cramps may occur. Avoid vaginal intercourse during treatment. May increase warfarin effect.
MOA — Antifungal.
ADVERSE EFFECTS — Serious: None. Frequent: Vulvovaginal irritation.

NYSTATIN—VAGINAL (*Mycostatin, ✦Nilstat, Nyaderm*) ▶Not metabolized ♀A ▶? $$
ADULTS — Local treatment of vulvovaginal candidiasis: 100,000 units tab intravaginally at bedtime for 2 weeks.
PEDS — Not approved in children.
FORMS — Generic only: Vaginal tabs 100,000 units in 15s with applicator.
NOTES — Topical azole products more effective. Do not use if abdominal pain, fever, or foul-smelling vaginal discharge is present. During pregnancy use of a vaginal applicator may be contraindicated, manual insertion of tabs may be preferred. Avoid vaginal intercourse during treatment.
MOA — Antifungal.
ADVERSE EFFECTS — Serious: None. Frequent: Vulvovaginal irritation.

TERCONAZOLE (*Terazol*) ▶LK ♀C ▶− $$
ADULTS — Local treatment of vulvovaginal candidiasis: 1 applicatorful 0.4% cream intravaginally at bedtime for 7 days. 1 applicatorful 0.8% cream intravaginally at bedtime for 3 days. 80 mg suppository intravaginally at bedtime for 3 days.
PEDS — Not approved in children.
FORMS — All forms supplied with applicators: Generic/Trade: Vaginal cream 0.4% (Terazol 7) in 45 g tube, 0.8% (Terazol 3) in 20 g tube. Vaginal suppository (Terazol 3) 80 mg (#3).
NOTES — Do not use if abdominal pain, fever, or foul-smelling vaginal discharge is present. Since small amounts of these drugs may be absorbed from the vagina, use during the 1st trimester only when essential. During pregnancy, use of a vaginal applicator may be contraindicated; manual insertion of supps may be preferred. Avoid vaginal intercourse during treatment. Vulvovaginal irritation, burning, and pruritus may occur.
MOA — Antifungal.
ADVERSE EFFECTS — Serious: None. Frequent: Vulvovaginal irritation.

TIOCONAZOLE (*Monistat 1-Day, Vagistat-1*) ▶Not absorbed ♀C ▶− $
ADULTS — Local treatment of vulvovaginal candidiasis: 1 applicatorful (~ 4.6 g) intravaginally at bedtime for 1 dose.
PEDS — Not approved in children.
FORMS — OTC Trade only: Vaginal ointment: 6.5% (300 mg) in 4.6 g prefilled single-dose applicator.
NOTES — Do not use if abdominal pain, fever or foul-smelling vaginal discharge is present. Since small amounts of these drugs may be absorbed

(cont.)

TIOCONAZOLE (cont.)
from the vagina, use during the first trimester only when essential. During pregnancy, use of a vaginal applicator may be contraindicated. Avoid vaginal intercourse during treatment. Vulvovaginal burning and itching may occur.
MOA — Antifungal.
ADVERSE EFFECTS — Serious: None. Frequent: Vulvovaginal irritation.

OB/GYN: Other OB/GYN Agents

DANAZOL (*Danocrine*, ✦*Cyclomen*) ▶L ♀X ▶– $$$$$
ADULTS — <u>Endometriosis:</u> Start 400 mg PO bid, then titrate downward to a dose sufficient to maintain amenorrhea for 3 to 6 months, up to 9 months. <u>Fibrocystic breast disease:</u> 100 to 200 mg PO bid for 4 to 6 months.
PEDS — Not approved in children.
UNAPPROVED ADULTS — <u>Menorrhagia:</u> 100 to 400 mg PO daily for 3 months. <u>Cyclical mastalgia:</u> 100 to 200 mg PO bid for 4 to 6 months.
FORMS — Generic only: Caps 50, 100, 200 mg.
NOTES — Contraindications: Impaired hepatic, renal or cardiac function. Androgenic effects may not be reversible even after the drug is discontinued. May alter voice. Hepatic dysfunction has occurred. Insulin requirements may increase in diabetics. Prolongation of PT/INR has been reported with concomitant warfarin.
MOA — Androgen.
ADVERSE EFFECTS — Serious: Stroke, intracranial hypertension, hepatic adenoma. Frequent: Acne, edema, hirsutism, deepening voice, emotional lability, depression.

MIFEPRISTONE (*Mifeprex, RU-486*) ▶L ♀X ▶? $$$$$
WARNING — Rare cases of sepsis and death have occurred. Surgical intervention may be necessary with incomplete abortions. Patients need to be given info on where such services are available and what do in case of an emergency.
ADULTS — <u>Termination of pregnancy, up to 49 days:</u> Day 1: 600 mg PO. Day 3: 400 mcg misoprostol (unless abortion confirmed). Day 14: Confirmation of pregnancy termination.
PEDS — Not approved in children.
UNAPPROVED ADULTS — <u>Termination of pregnancy, up to 63 days:</u> 200 mg PO followed by 800 mcg misoprostol intravaginally 24 to 72 h later.
FORMS — Trade only: Tabs 200 mg.
NOTES — Bleeding/spotting and cramping most common side effects. Prolonged heavy bleeding may be a sign of incomplete abortion. Contraindications: Ectopic pregnancy, IUD use, adrenal insufficiency and long-term steroid use, use of anticoagulants, hemorrhagic disorders and porphyrias. CYP3A4 inducers may increase metabolism and lower levels. Available through physician offices only.
MOA — Anti-progestational/abortifacient.
ADVERSE EFFECTS — Serious: Sepsis, incomplete abortion. Frequent: Bleeding, spotting, cramping, N/V.

PREMESIS-RX (pyridoxine + folic acid + cyanocobalamin + calcium carbonate) ▶L ♀A ▶+ $$
ADULTS — <u>Treatment of pregnancy-induced nausea:</u> 1 tab PO daily.
PEDS — Unapproved in children.
FORMS — Trade only: Tabs 75 mg vitamin B6 (pyridoxine), sustained-release, 12 mcg vitamin B12 (cyanocobalamin), 1 mg folic acid, and 200 mg calcium carbonate.
NOTES — May be taken in conjunction with prenatal vitamins.
MOA — Vitamin combination.
ADVERSE EFFECTS — Serious: None. Frequent: None.

RHO IMMUNE GLOBULIN (*HyperRHO S/D, MICRhoGAM, RhoGAM, Rhophylac, WinRho SDF*) ▶L ♀C ▶? $$$$$
ADULTS — <u>Prevention of hemolytic disease of the newborn if mother Rh– and baby is or might be Rh+:</u> 300 mcg vial IM to mother at 28 weeks gestation followed by a second dose < 72 h of delivery. Doses more than 1 vial may be needed if large fetal-maternal hemorrhage occurs during delivery (see complete prescribing information to determine dose). <u>Following amniocentesis, miscarriage, abortion, or ectopic pregnancy at least 13 weeks gestation:</u> 1 vial (300 mcg) IM. < 12 weeks gestation: 1 vial (50 mcg) microdose IM. <u>Immune thrombocytopenic purpura (ITP), nonsplenectomized</u> (WinRho): 250 units/kg/dose (50 mcg/kg/dose) IV for 1 dose if hemoglobin > 10 g/dL or 125 to 200 units/kg/dose (25 to 40 mcg/kg/dose) IV for 1 dose if hemoglobin < 10 g/dL. Additional doses of 125 to 300 units/kg/dose (25 to 60 mcg/kg/dose) IV may be given as determined by patient's response.
PEDS — <u>Immune thrombocytopenic purpura (ITP), nonsplenectomized</u> (WinRho): 250 units/kg/dose (50 mcg/kg/dose) IV for 1 dose if hemoglobin > 10 g/dL or 125 to 200 units/kg/dose (25 to 40 mcg/kg/dose) IV for 1 dose if hemoglobin < 10 g/dL. Additional doses of 125 to 300 units/kg/dose (25 to 60 mcg/kg/dose) IV may be given as determined by patient's response.
UNAPPROVED ADULTS — <u>Rh-incompatible transfusion:</u> Specialized dosing.
NOTES — One 300 mcg vial prevents maternal sensitization to the Rh factor if the fetomaternal hemorrhage is less than 15 mL fetal RBCs (30 mL of whole blood). When the fetomaternal hemorrhage exceeds this (as estimated by Kleihauer-Betke testing), administer more than one 300 mcg vial.
MOA — Immune globulin.
ADVERSE EFFECTS — Serious: None. Frequent: Injection site reactions.

ONCOLOGY: Alkylating agents

ALTRETAMINE (*Hexalen*) ▶L ♀D ▶– $ varies by therapy
WARNING – Peripheral neuropathy, bone marrow suppression, fertility impairment, N/V, alopecia. Instruct patients to report promptly fever, sore throat, signs of local infection, bleeding from any site, or symptoms suggestive of anemia.
ADULTS – Chemotherapy doses vary by indication. Ovarian cancer.
PEDS – Not approved in children.
UNAPPROVED ADULTS – Lung, breast, cervical cancer, non-Hodgkin's lymphoma.
FORMS – Trade only: Caps 50 mg.
NOTES – Reliable contraception is recommended. Monitor CBCs. Cimetidine increases toxicity. MAOIs may cause severe orthostatic hypotension.
MOA – Alkylating agent.
ADVERSE EFFECTS – Serious: Bone marrow suppression, peripheral neuropathy. Frequent: Bone marrow suppression, N/V, peripheral neuropathy, bone marrow suppression, adverse CNS symptoms.

BENDAMUSTINE (*Treanda*) ▶Plasma ♀D ▶– $ varies by therapy
WARNING – Anaphylaxis, bone marrow suppression, nephrotoxicity, Stevens-Johnson syndrome, toxic epidermal necrolysis. Instruct patients to report promptly fever, sore throat, signs of local infection, bleeding from any site, or symptoms suggestive of anemia. Take precautions to avoid extravasation, including monitoring intravenous infusion site during and after administration.
ADULTS – Chemotherapy doses vary by indication. CLL, non-Hodgkin's lymphoma.
PEDS – Not approved in children.
NOTES – Reliable contraception is recommended. Monitor CBCs and renal function.
MOA – Alkylating agent.
ADVERSE EFFECTS – Serious: Anaphylaxis, bone marrow suppression, nephrotoxicity, Stevens-Johnson syndrome, toxic epidermal necrolysis. Frequent: Bone marrow suppression, N/V.

BUSULFAN (*Myleran, Busulfex*) ▶LK ♀D ▶– $ varies by therapy
WARNING – Secondary malignancies, bone marrow suppression, adrenal insufficiency, hyperuricemia, pulmonary fibrosis, seizures (must initiate prophylactic anticonvulsant therapy prior to use of busulfan), cellular dysplasia, hepatic veno-occlusive disease, fertility impairment, alopecia. Instruct patients to report promptly fever, sore throat, signs of local infection, bleeding from any site, symptoms suggestive of anemia, or yellow discoloration of the skin or eyes.
ADULTS – Chemotherapy doses vary by indication. Tabs: CML. Injection: Conditioning regimen prior to allogeneic hematopoietic progenitor cell transplantation for CML. in combination with cyclophosphamide.
PEDS – Chemotherapy doses vary by indication. Tabs: CML. Safety of the injection has not been established.
UNAPPROVED ADULTS – High dose in conjunction with stem cell transplant for leukemia and lymphoma.
FORMS – Trade only (Myleran) Tabs 2 mg. Busulfex injection for hospital/oncology clinic use; not intended for outpatient prescribing.
NOTES – Reliable contraception is recommended. Monitor CBCs and LFTs. Hydration and allopurinol to decrease adverse effects of uric acid. Acetaminophen and itraconazole decrease busulfan clearance. Phenytoin increases clearance.
MOA – Alkylating agent.
ADVERSE EFFECTS – Serious: Bone marrow suppression, adrenal insufficiency, seizures, pulmonary fibrosis, hepatic veno-occlusive disease. Frequent: Bone marrow suppression, hyperpigmentation.

CARMUSTINE (*BCNU, BiCNU, Gliadel*) ▶Plasma ♀D ▶– $ varies by therapy
WARNING – Secondary malignancies, bone marrow suppression, pulmonary fibrosis, nephrotoxicity, hepatotoxicity, ocular nerve fiber-layer infarcts and retinal hemorrhages, fertility impairment, alopecia. Wafer: Seizures, brain edema and herniation, intracranial infection. Instruct patients to report promptly fever, sore throat, signs of local infection, bleeding from any site, symptoms suggestive of anemia, or yellow discoloration of the skin or eyes.
ADULTS – Chemotherapy doses vary by indication. Injection: Glioblastoma, brainstem glioma, medulloblastoma, astrocytoma, ependymoma and metastatic brain tumors, multiple myeloma with prednisone; Hodgkin's disease and non-Hodgkin's lymphomas, in combination regimens. Wafer: Glioblastoma multiforme, adjunct to surgery. High-grade malignant glioma, adjunct to surgery and radiation.
PEDS – Not approved in children.
UNAPPROVED ADULTS – Mycosis fungoides, topical soln.
NOTES – Reliable contraception is recommended. Monitor CBCs, PFTs, LFTs and renal function. May decrease phenytoin and digoxin levels. Cimetidine may increase myelosuppression.
MOA – Alkylating agent.
ADVERSE EFFECTS – Serious: Bone marrow suppression, pulmonary fibrosis, nephrotoxicity, hepatotoxicity, ocular nerve fiber-layer infarcts and retinal hemorrhages. Wafer: Seizures, brain edema and herniation, intracranial infection. Frequent: Bone marrow suppression, N/V.

CHLORAMBUCIL (*Leukeran*) ▶L ♀D ▶– $ varies by therapy
WARNING – Secondary malignancies, bone marrow suppression, seizures, fertility impairment, alopecia. Instruct patients to report promptly fever, sore

(cont.)

ONCOLOGY: Alkylating agents

CHLORAMBUCIL (*cont.*)
throat, signs of local infection, bleeding from any site, or symptoms suggestive of anemia.
ADULTS — Chemotherapy doses vary by indication. CLL. Lymphomas including indolent lymphoma and Hodgkin's disease.
PEDS — Not approved in children.
UNAPPROVED ADULTS — Uveitis and meningoencephalitis associated with Behcet's disease. Idiopathic membranous nephropathy. Ovarian carcinoma.
FORMS — Trade only: Tabs 2 mg.
NOTES — Reliable contraception is recommended. Monitor CBCs. Avoid live vaccines.
MOA — Alkylating agent.
ADVERSE EFFECTS — The most common side effect is bone marrow suppression, anemia, leukopenia, neutropenia, thrombocytopenia, or pancytopenia. Seizures.

CYCLOPHOSPHAMIDE (*Cytoxan, Neosar*) ▶L ♀D ▶− $ varies by therapy
WARNING — Secondary malignancies, leukopenia, cardiac toxicity, acute hemorrhagic cystitis, hypersensitivity, fertility impairment, alopecia. Instruct patients to report promptly fever, sore throat, signs of local infection, bleeding from any site, symptoms suggestive of anemia, or yellow discoloration of the skin or eyes.
ADULTS — Chemotherapy doses vary by indication. Non-Hodgkin's lymphomas, Hodgkin's disease. Multiple myeloma. Disseminated neuroblastoma. Adenocarcinoma of the ovary. Retinoblastoma. Carcinoma of the breast. CLL. CML. AML. Mycosis fungoides.
PEDS — Chemotherapy doses vary by indication. ALL. "Minimal change" nephrotic syndrome.
UNAPPROVED ADULTS — Wegener's granulomatosis, other steroid-resistant vasculitides. Severe progressive RA. Systemic lupus erythematosus. Multiple sclerosis. Polyarteritis nodosa. Lung, testicular and bladder cancer, sarcoma.
FORMS — Generic only: Tabs 25, 50 mg. Injection for hospital/oncology clinic use; not intended for outpatient prescribing.
NOTES — Reliable contraception is recommended. Monitor CBCs, urine for red cells. Allopurinol may increase myelosuppression. Thiazides may prolong leukopenia. May reduce digoxin levels, reduce fluoroquinolone activity. May increase anticoagulant effects. Coadministration with mesna reduces hemorrhagic cystitis when used in high doses.
MOA — Alkylating agent.
ADVERSE EFFECTS — Serious: Leukopenia, cardiac toxicity, acute hemorrhagic cystitis, hypersensitivity. Frequent: Alopecia, leukopenia.

DACARBAZINE (*DTIC-Dome*) ▶LK ♀C ▶− $ varies by therapy
WARNING — Extravasation associated with severe necrosis. Secondary malignancies, bone marrow suppression, hepatotoxicity, anorexia, N/V, anaphylaxis, alopecia. Instruct patients to report promptly fever, sore throat, signs of local infection, bleeding from any site, symptoms suggestive of anemia, or yellow discoloration of the skin or eyes.
ADULTS — Chemotherapy doses vary by indication. Metastatic melanoma. Hodgkin's disease, in combination regimens.
PEDS — Not approved in children.
UNAPPROVED ADULTS — Malignant pheochromocytoma, in combination regimens. Sarcoma.
NOTES — Monitor CBCs and LFTs.
MOA — Alkylating agent.
ADVERSE EFFECTS — Serious: Bone marrow suppression, hepatotoxicity, anaphylaxis. Frequent: Bone marrow suppression, N/V, anorexia.

IFOSFAMIDE (*Ifex*) ▶L ♀D ▶− $ varies by therapy
WARNING — Secondary malignancies, hemorrhagic cystitis, confusion, coma, bone marrow suppression, hematuria, nephrotoxicity, alopecia. Instruct patients to report promptly fever, sore throat, signs of local infection, bleeding from any site, symptoms suggestive of anemia, or yellow discoloration of the skin or eyes.
ADULTS — Chemotherapy doses vary by indication. Germ cell testicular cancer, in combination regimens.
PEDS — Not approved in children.
UNAPPROVED ADULTS — Lung, breast, ovarian, pancreatic and gastric cancer; sarcomas, acute leukemias (except AML), lymphomas.
NOTES — Reliable contraception is recommended. Monitor CBCs, renal function and urine for red cells. Coadministration with mesna reduces hemorrhagic cystitis.
MOA — Alkylating agent.
ADVERSE EFFECTS — Serious: Hemorrhagic cystitis, coma, bone marrow suppression, hematuria, nephrotoxicity. Frequent: Bone marrow suppression, CNS, N/V, hematuria, alopecia.

LOMUSTINE (*CeeNu, CCNU*) ▶L ♀D ▶− $ varies by therapy
WARNING — Secondary malignancies, bone marrow suppression, hepatotoxicity, nephrotoxicity, pulmonary fibrosis, fertility impairment, alopecia. Instruct patients to report promptly fever, sore throat, signs of local infection, bleeding from any site, symptoms suggestive of anemia, or yellow discoloration of the skin or eyes.
ADULTS — Chemotherapy doses vary by indication. Brain tumors. Hodgkin's disease, in combination regimens.
PEDS — Chemotherapy doses vary by indication. Brain tumors. Hodgkin's disease, in combination regimens.
FORMS — Trade only: Caps 10, 40, 100 mg.
NOTES — Reliable contraception is recommended. Monitor CBCs, LFTs, PFTs and renal function. Avoid alcohol.
MOA — Alkylating agent.
ADVERSE EFFECTS — Serious: Bone marrow suppression, hepatotoxicity, nephrotoxicity, pulmonary fibrosis. Frequent: Bone marrow suppression, N/V.

ONCOLOGY: Alkylating agents

MECHLORETHAMINE (*Mustargen*) ▶Plasma ♀D ▶– $ varies by therapy
WARNING – Extravasation associated with severe necrosis. Secondary malignancies, bone marrow suppression, amyloidosis, herpes zoster, anaphylaxis, fertility impairment, alopecia. Instruct patients to report promptly fever, sore throat, signs of local infection, bleeding from any site, or symptoms suggestive of anemia.
ADULTS – Chemotherapy doses vary by indication. Intravenous: Hodgkin's disease (Stages III and IV). Lymphosarcoma. Chronic myelocytic or chronic lymphocytic leukemia. Polycythemia vera. Mycosis fungoides. Bronchogenic carcinoma. Intrapleurally, intraperitoneally or intrapericardially: Metastatic carcinoma resulting in effusion.
PEDS – Not approved in children.
UNAPPROVED ADULTS – Cutaneous mycosis fungoides: Topical soln or ointment.
UNAPPROVED PEDS – Hodgkin's disease (Stages III and IV), in combination regimens.
NOTES – Reliable contraception is recommended. Monitor CBCs.
MOA – Alkylating agent.
ADVERSE EFFECTS – Serious: Bone marrow suppression, amyloidosis, herpes zoster, anaphylaxis. Frequent: Bone marrow suppression, N/V.

MELPHALAN (*Alkeran*) ▶Plasma ♀D ▶– $ varies by therapy
WARNING – Secondary malignancies, bone marrow suppression, anaphylaxis, fertility impairment, alopecia. Instruct patients to report promptly fever, sore throat, signs of local infection, bleeding from any site, or symptoms suggestive of anemia.
ADULTS – Chemotherapy doses vary by indication. Multiple myeloma and nonresectable epithelial ovarian carcinoma.
PEDS – Not approved in children.
UNAPPROVED ADULTS – Non-Hodgkin's lymphoma in high doses for stem cell transplant, testicular cancer.
FORMS – Trade only: Tabs 2 mg. Injection for hospital/clinic use; not intended for outpatient prescribing.
NOTES – Reliable contraception is recommended. Monitor CBCs. Avoid live vaccines.
MOA – Alkylating agent.
ADVERSE EFFECTS – Serious: Bone marrow suppression, anaphylaxis. Frequent: Bone marrow suppression, N/V.

PROCARBAZINE (*Matulane*) ▶LK ♀D ▶– $ varies by therapy
WARNING – Secondary malignancies, bone marrow suppression, hemolysis and Heinz-Ehrlich inclusion bodies in erythrocytes, hypersensitivity, fertility impairment, alopecia. Peds: Tremors, convulsions and coma have occurred. Instruct patients to report promptly fever, sore throat, signs of local infection, bleeding from any site, symptoms suggestive of anemia, black tarry stools or vomiting of blood.
ADULTS – Chemotherapy doses vary by indication. Hodgkin's disease (Stages III and IV), in combination regimens.
PEDS – Chemotherapy doses vary by indication. Hodgkin's disease (Stages III and IV), in combination regimens.
FORMS – Trade only: Caps 50 mg.
NOTES – Reliable contraception is recommended. Monitor CBCs. Renal/hepatic function impairment may predispose toxicity. UA, LFTs, and BUN weekly. May decrease digoxin levels. May increase effects of opioids, sympathomimetics, TCAs. Ingestion of foods with high tyramine content may result in a potentially fatal hypertensive crisis. Alcohol may cause a disulfiram-like reaction.
MOA – Alkylating agent.
ADVERSE EFFECTS – Serious: Bone marrow suppression, hemolysis and Heinz-Ehrlich inclusion bodies in erythrocytes, hypersensitivity. Frequent: Bone marrow suppression, N/V.

STREPTOZOCIN (*Zanosar*) ▶Plasma ♀C ▶– $ varies by therapy
WARNING – Extravasation associated with severe necrosis. Secondary malignancies, nephrotoxicity, N/V, hepatotoxicity, decrease in hematocrit, hypoglycemia, fertility impairment, alopecia.
ADULTS – Chemotherapy doses vary by indication. Metastatic islet cell carcinoma of the pancreas.
PEDS – Not approved in children.
NOTES – Hydration important. Monitor renal function, CBCs and LFTs.
MOA – Alkylating agent.
ADVERSE EFFECTS – Serious: Nephrotoxicity, N/V, hepatotoxicity. Frequent: N/V, hepatotoxicity.

TEMOZOLOMIDE (*Temodar*, ♣*Temodal*) ▶Plasma ♀D ▶– $ varies by therapy
WARNING – Secondary malignancies, bone marrow suppression, fertility impairment, alopecia. Instruct patients to report promptly fever, sore throat, signs of local infection, bleeding from any site, or symptoms suggestive of anemia. Cases of interstitial pneumonitis, alveolitis, and pulmonary fibrosis have been reported.
ADULTS – Chemotherapy doses vary by indication. Anaplastic astrocytoma, glioblastoma multiforme.
PEDS – Not approved in children.
UNAPPROVED ADULTS – Metastatic melanoma, renal cell carcinoma. Cutaneous T-cell lymphomas.
FORMS – Trade only: Caps 5, 20, 100, 140, 180, 250 mg.
NOTES – Reliable contraception is recommended. Monitor CBCs. Valproic acid decreases clearance.
MOA – Alkylating agent.
ADVERSE EFFECTS – Serious: Bone marrow suppression, erythema multiforme. Frequent: N/V, fatigue, headache.

THIOTEPA (*Thioplex*) ▶L ♀D ▶– $ varies by therapy
WARNING – Secondary malignancies, bone marrow suppression, hypersensitivity, fertility impairment, alopecia. Instruct patients to report promptly fever, sore throat, signs of local infection, bleeding from

(cont.)

THIOTEPA (cont.)
any site, symptoms suggestive of anemia, black tarry stools or vomiting of blood.
ADULTS — Chemotherapy doses vary by indication. Adenocarcinoma of the breast or ovary. Control of intracavitary malignant effusions. Superficial papillary carcinoma of the urinary bladder. Hodgkin's disease. Lymphosarcoma.
PEDS — Not approved in children.
NOTES — Reliable contraception is recommended. Monitor CBCs.
MOA — Alkylating agent.
ADVERSE EFFECTS — Serious: Bone marrow suppression, hypersensitivity. Frequent: Bone marrow suppression.

ONCOLOGY: Antibiotics

BLEOMYCIN (*Blenoxane*) ▶K ♀D ▶– $ varies by therapy
WARNING — Pulmonary fibrosis, skin toxicity, nephro/hepatotoxicity, alopecia, and severe idiosyncratic reaction consisting of hypotension, mental confusion, fever, chills, and wheezing. Because of the possibility of an anaphylactoid reaction, lymphoma patients should be treated with 2 units or less for the first 2 doses. If no acute reaction occurs, then the regular dosage schedule may be followed.
ADULTS — Chemotherapy doses vary by indication. Squamous cell carcinoma of the head and neck. Carcinoma of the skin, penis, cervix, and vulva. Hodgkin's and non-Hodgkin's lymphoma. Testicular carcinoma. Malignant pleural effusion: Sclerosing agent.
PEDS — Not approved in children.
UNAPPROVED ADULTS — Treatment of ovarian germ cell tumors.
NOTES — Reliable contraception is recommended. Frequent chest x-rays. May decrease digoxin and phenytoin levels. Risk of pulmonary toxicity increases with lifetime cumulative dose > 400 units.
MOA — Antibiotic.
ADVERSE EFFECTS — Serious: Pulmonary fibrosis, skin toxicity, nephro/hepatotoxicity, severe idiosyncratic reaction: hypotension, mental confusion, fever, chills, and wheezing. Frequent: Pulmonary fibrosis, stomatitis, vomiting, weight loss, alopecia.

DACTINOMYCIN (*Cosmegen*) ▶Not metabolized ♀C ▶– $ varies by therapy
WARNING — Extravasation associated with severe necrosis. Contraindicated with active chicken pox or herpes zoster. Erythema and vesiculation (with radiation), bone marrow suppression, alopecia. Instruct patients to report promptly fever, sore throat, signs of local infection, bleeding from any site, or symptoms suggestive of anemia.
ADULTS — Chemotherapy doses vary by indication. Wilms' tumor. Rhabdomyosarcoma. Metastatic and nonmetastatic choriocarcinoma. Nonseminomatous testicular carcinoma. Ewing's sarcoma. Sarcoma botryoides. Most in combination regimens.
PEDS — Chemotherapy doses vary by indication. See adult. Contraindicated in infants less than 6 mo.
NOTES — Monitor CBCs.
MOA — Antibiotic.
ADVERSE EFFECTS — Serious: Erythema and vesiculation (with radiation), bone marrow suppression. Frequent: Bone marrow suppression, N/V, alopecia.

DAUNORUBICIN (*DaunoXome, Cerubidine*) ▶L ♀D ▶– $ varies by therapy
WARNING — Extravasation associated with severe necrosis. Cardiac toxicity, more frequent in children. Bone marrow suppression, infusion-related reactions. Instruct patients to report promptly fever, sore throat, signs of local infection, bleeding from any site, or symptoms suggestive of anemia.
ADULTS — Chemotherapy doses vary by indication. First-line treatment of Advanced HIV-associated Kaposi's sarcoma (DaunoXome). AML, in combination regimens. ALL (Cerubidine).
PEDS — Chemotherapy doses vary by indication. ALL (Cerubidine). DaunoXome not approved in children.
NOTES — Reliable contraception is recommended. Monitor CBCs, cardiac, renal and hepatic function (toxicity increased with impaired function). Transient urine discoloration (red).
MOA — Antibiotic.
ADVERSE EFFECTS — Serious: Cardiac toxicity, bone marrow suppression, secondary malignancies, infusion-related reactions, anaphylaxis. Frequent: Cardiac toxicity, bone marrow suppression, urine discoloration.

DOXORUBICIN LIPOSOMAL (*Doxil, ✦Caelyx, Myocet*) ▶L ♀D ▶– $ varies by therapy
WARNING — Extravasation associated with severe necrosis. Cardiac toxicity, more frequent in children. Bone marrow suppression, infusion-associated reactions, necrotizing colitis, mucositis, hyperuricemia, palmar-plantar erythrodysesthesia. Secondary malignancies. Instruct patients to report promptly fever, sore throat, signs of local infection, bleeding from any site, or symptoms suggestive of anemia.
ADULTS — Chemotherapy doses vary by indication. Advanced HIV-associated Kaposi's sarcoma, multiple myeloma, ovarian carcinoma.
PEDS — Not approved in children.
UNAPPROVED ADULTS — Breast cancer, Hodgkin's Lymphoma, non-Hodgkin's lymphoma, soft tissue sarcomas.
NOTES — Heart failure with cumulative doses. Monitor ejection fraction, CBCs, LFTs, uric acid levels, and renal function (toxicity increased with impaired function). Reliable contraception is recommended. Transient urine discoloration (red).
MOA — Antibiotic.

(cont.)

DOXORUBICIN LIPOSOMAL (cont.)
ADVERSE EFFECTS − Serious: Cardiac toxicity, bone marrow suppression, infusion-associated reactions, necrotizing colitis, palmar-plantar erythrodysesthesia, secondary malignancies. Frequent: Cardiac toxicity, bone marrow suppression, hyperuricemia, fatigue, fever, anorexia, N/V, stomatitis, diarrhea, urine discoloration.

DOXORUBICIN NON-LIPOSOMAL (*Adriamycin, Rubex*) ▶L ♀D ▶− $ varies by therapy
WARNING − Extravasation associated with severe necrosis. Cardiac toxicity, more frequent in children. Bone marrow suppression, infusion-associated reactions, necrotizing colitis, mucositis, hyperuricemia, alopecia. Secondary malignancies. Instruct patients to report promptly fever, sore throat, signs of local infection, bleeding from any site, or symptoms suggestive of anemia.
ADULTS − Chemotherapy doses vary by indication. ALL. AML. Wilms' tumor. Neuroblastoma. Soft tissue and bone sarcomas. Breast carcinoma. Ovarian carcinoma. Transitional cell bladder carcinoma. Thyroid carcinoma. Hodgkin's and non-Hodgkin's lymphomas. Bronchogenic carcinoma. Gastric carcinoma.
PEDS − Chemotherapy doses vary by indication: See adult.
UNAPPROVED ADULTS − Sarcoma, small cell lung cancer.
NOTES − Heart failure with cumulative doses. Monitor ejection fraction, CBCs, LFTs, uric acid levels, and renal function (toxicity increased with impaired function). Reliable contraception is recommended. Transient urine discoloration (red).
MOA − Antibiotic.
ADVERSE EFFECTS − Serious: Cardiac toxicity, bone marrow suppression, secondary malignancies, infusion-associated reactions, necrotizing colitis. Frequent: Cardiac toxicity, bone marrow suppression, secondary malignancies, hyperuricemia, alopecia, urine discoloration.

EPIRUBICIN (*Ellence, ✦Pharmorubicin*) ▶L ♀D ▶− $ varies by therapy
WARNING − Extravasation associated with severe necrosis. Cardiac toxicity, bone marrow suppression, secondary malignancy (AML), hyperuricemia, fertility impairment, alopecia. Instruct patients to report promptly fever, sore throat, signs of local infection, bleeding from any site, or symptoms suggestive of anemia.
ADULTS − Chemotherapy doses vary by indication. Adjuvant therapy for breast cancer, axillary-node positive.
PEDS − Not approved in children.
UNAPPROVED ADULTS − Neoadjuvant and metastatic breast cancer. Cervical cancer, esophageal cancer, gastric cancer, soft tissue sarcomas, uterine sarcoma.
NOTES − Reliable contraception is recommended. Monitor CBCs, cardiac, hepatic and renal function (toxicity increased with impaired function). Cimetidine increase levels. Transient urine discoloration (red).
MOA − Antibiotic.
ADVERSE EFFECTS − Serious: Cardiac toxicity, bone marrow suppression, secondary malignancies. Frequent: Cardiac toxicity, bone marrow suppression, N/V, mucositis, hyperuricemia, alopecia.

IDARUBICIN (*Idamycin*) ▶? ♀D ▶− $ varies by therapy
WARNING − Extravasation associated with severe necrosis. Cardiac toxicity, bone marrow suppression, hyperuricemia, alopecia. Instruct patients to report promptly fever, sore throat, signs of local infection, bleeding from any site, or symptoms suggestive of anemia.
ADULTS − Chemotherapy doses vary by indication. AML, in combination regimens.
PEDS − Not approved in children.
UNAPPROVED ADULTS − ALL, CML.
NOTES − Reliable contraception is recommended. Monitor CBCs, LFTs, cardiac and renal function (toxicity increased with impaired function).
MOA − Antibiotic.
ADVERSE EFFECTS − Serious: Cardiac toxicity, bone marrow suppression, secondary malignancies. Frequent: Cardiac toxicity, bone marrow suppression, N/V, hyperuricemia, alopecia.

MITOMYCIN (*Mutamycin, Mitomycin-C*) ▶L ♀D ▶− $ varies by therapy
WARNING − Extravasation associated with severe necrosis. Bone marrow suppression, hemolytic uremic syndrome, nephrotoxicity, adult respiratory distress syndrome, alopecia. Instruct patients to report promptly fever, sore throat, signs of local infection, bleeding from any site, or symptoms suggestive of anemia.
ADULTS − Chemotherapy doses vary by indication. Disseminated adenocarcinoma of stomach, pancreas, or colorectum, in combination regimens.
PEDS − Not approved in children.
UNAPPROVED ADULTS − Superficial bladder cancer, intravesical route; pterygia, adjunct to surgical excision: Ophthalmic soln.
NOTES − Reliable contraception is recommended. Monitor CBCs and renal function.
MOA − Antibiotic.
ADVERSE EFFECTS − Serious: Bone marrow suppression, hemolytic uremic syndrome, nephrotoxicity, adult respiratory distress syndrome. Frequent: Bone marrow suppression, N/V, anorexia.

MITOXANTRONE (*Novantrone*) ▶LK ♀D ▶− $ varies by therapy
WARNING − Secondary malignancies (AML), bone marrow suppression, cardiac toxicity/heart failure, hyperuricemia, increased LFTs. Instruct patients to report promptly fever, sore throat, signs of local infection, bleeding from any site, or symptoms suggestive of anemia.
ADULTS − Chemotherapy doses vary by indication. AML, in combination regimens. Symptomatic patients with hormone refractory prostate cancer.

(cont.)

ONCOLOGY: Antimetabolites

MITOXANTRONE (cont.)
Multiple sclerosis (secondary progressive, progressive relapsing, or worsening relapsing-remitting): 12 mg/m2 of BSA IV q 3 months.
PEDS — Not approved in children.
UNAPPROVED ADULTS — Breast cancer. Non-Hodgkin's lymphoma. ALL, CML, Ovarian carcinoma. Sclerosing agent for malignant pleural effusions.
NOTES — Reliable contraception is recommended. Monitor CBCs and LFTs. Baseline echocardiogram and repeat echoes prior to each dose are recommended. Transient urine and sclera discoloration (blue-green).
MOA — Antibiotic.
ADVERSE EFFECTS — Serious: Bone marrow suppression, cardiac toxicity, secondary malignancies. Frequent: Bone marrow suppression, N/V, menstrual disorders, stomatitis, urine and sclera discoloration, alopecia.

VALRUBICIN (Valstar, ✦Valtaxin) ▶K ♀C ▶— $ varies by therapy
WARNING — Induces complete responses in only 1 in 5 patients. Delaying cystectomy could lead to development of lethal metastatic bladder cancer. Irritable bladder symptoms, alopecia.
ADULTS — Chemotherapy doses vary by indication. Bladder cancer, intravesical therapy of BCG-refractory carcinoma in situ.
PEDS — Not approved in children.
NOTES — Reliable contraception is recommended. Transient urine discoloration (red).
MOA — Antibiotic.
ADVERSE EFFECTS — Serious: None. Frequent: Irritable bladder symptoms.

ONCOLOGY: Antimetabolites

AZACITIDINE (Vidaza) ▶K ♀D ▶— $ varies by therapy
WARNING — Contraindicated with malignant hepatic tumors. Bone marrow suppression. Fertility impairment. Instruct patients to report promptly fever, sore throat, or signs of local infection or bleeding from any site.
ADULTS — Chemotherapy doses vary by indication. Myelodysplastic syndrome subtypes.
PEDS — Not approved in children.
NOTES — Reliable contraception is recommended. Men should not father children while on this drug. Monitor CBC, renal and hepatic function.
MOA — Antimetabolite.
ADVERSE EFFECTS — Serious: Bone marrow suppression, hepatotoxicity, renal failure. Frequent: N/V, bone marrow suppression, fever, diarrhea, fatigue, constipation.

CAPECITABINE (Xeloda) ▶L ♀D ▶— $ varies by therapy
WARNING — Increased INR and bleeding with warfarin. Contraindicated in severe renal dysfunction (CrCl < 30 mL/min). Severe diarrhea, fertility impairment, palmar-plantar erythrodysesthesia or chemotherapy-induced acral erythema, cardiac toxicity, hyperbilirubinemia, neutropenia, alopecia. Instruct patients to report promptly fever, sore throat, or signs of local infection or bleeding from any site.
ADULTS — Chemotherapy doses vary by indication. Metastatic breast and colorectal cancer.
PEDS — Not approved in children.
UNAPPROVED ADULTS — Gastric cancer, esophageal cancer, pancreatic cancer, hepatocellular carcinoma, ovarian cancer, metastatic renal cell cancer, neuroendocrine tumors, metastatic CNS lesions.
FORMS — Trade only: Tabs 150, 500 mg.
NOTES — Reliable contraception is recommended. Antacids containing aluminum hydroxide and magnesium hydroxide increase levels. May increase phenytoin levels.
MOA — Antimetabolite.
ADVERSE EFFECTS — Serious: Bleeding with warfarin, severe diarrhea, palmar-plantar erythrodysesthesia, cardiac toxicity, neutropenia. Frequent: Palmar-plantar erythrodysesthesia, N/V, diarrhea, stomatitis, hyperbilirubinemia.

CLADRIBINE (Leustatin, chlorodeoxyadenosine)
▶intracellular ♀D ▶— $ varies by therapy
WARNING — Bone marrow suppression, nephrotoxicity, neurotoxicity, fever, fertility impairment, alopecia. Instruct patients to report promptly fever, sore throat, or signs of local infection, bleeding from any site, or symptoms suggestive of anemia.
ADULTS — Chemotherapy doses vary by indication. Hairy cell leukemia.
PEDS — Not approved in children.
UNAPPROVED ADULTS — Advanced cutaneous T-cell lymphomas. Chronic lymphocytic leukemia, non-Hodgkin's lymphomas. AML. Autoimmune hemolytic anemia. Mycosis fungoides. Sezary syndrome. Progressive multiple sclerosis.
NOTES — Reliable contraception is recommended. Monitor CBCs and renal function.
MOA — Antimetabolite.
ADVERSE EFFECTS — Serious: Bone marrow suppression, nephrotoxicity, neurotoxicity, fever. Frequent: Bone marrow suppression, fever, N/V, diarrhea, rash.

CLOFARABINE (Clolar) ▶K ♀D ▶— $ varies by therapy
WARNING — Myelodysplastic syndrome, bone marrow suppression, tumor lysis syndrome, hepatotoxicity. Instruct patients to report promptly fever, sore throat, or signs of local infection, bleeding from any site, or symptoms suggestive of anemia.
ADULTS — Not approved in adults.
PEDS — 1 to 21 yo: Chemotherapy doses vary by indication. Relapsed or refractory acute lymphoblastic leukemia.
NOTES — Reliable contraception is recommended. Monitor CBCs, LFTs and renal function.
MOA — Antimetabolite.

(cont.)

ONCOLOGY: Antimetabolites

CLOFARABINE (cont.)
ADVERSE EFFECTS − Serious: Myelodysplastic syndrome, bone marrow suppression, tumor lysis syndrome, hepatotoxicity. Frequent: Bone marrow suppression, N/V, diarrhea.

CYTARABINE (*Cytosar-U, Tarabine, Depo-Cyt, AraC*) ▶LK ♀D ▶− $ varies by therapy
WARNING − Bone marrow suppression, hepatotoxicity, N/V/D, hyperuricemia, pancreatitis, peripheral neuropathy, "cytarabine syndrome" (fever, myalgia, bone pain, occasional chest pain, maculopapular rash, conjunctivitis, and malaise), alopecia. Neurotoxicity. Chemical arachnoiditis (N/V, headache, and fever) with Depo-Cyt. Instruct patients to report promptly fever, sore throat, or signs of local infection, bleeding from any site, symptoms suggestive of anemia, or yellow discoloration of the skin or eyes.
ADULTS − Chemotherapy doses vary by indication. AML. ALL. CML. Prophylaxis and treatment of meningeal leukemia, intrathecal (Cytosar-U, Tarabine). Lymphomatous meningitis, intrathecal (Depo-Cyt).
PEDS − Chemotherapy doses vary by indication. AML. ALL. Chronic myelocytic leukemia. Prophylaxis and treatment of meningeal leukemia, intrathecal (Cytosar-U, Tarabine). Depo-Cyt not approved in children.
NOTES − Reliable contraception is recommended. Monitor CBCs, LFTs and renal function. Decreases digoxin levels. Chemical arachnoiditis can be reduced by coadministration of dexamethasone. Use dexamethasone eye drops with high doses.
MOA − Antimetabolite.
ADVERSE EFFECTS − Serious: Bone marrow suppression, hepatotoxicity, pancreatitis, peripheral neuropathy, "cytarabine syndrome" (fever, myalgia, bone pain, occasional chest pain, maculopapular rash, conjunctivitis, and malaise). Neurotoxicity. Chemical arachnoiditis (N/V, headache, and fever) with Depo-Cyt. Frequent: Bone marrow suppression, N/V, diarrhea, rash.

DECITABINE (*Dacogen*) ▶L ♀D ▶− $ varies by therapy
WARNING − Bone marrow suppression, pulmonary edema. Instruct patients to report promptly fever, sore throat, or signs of local infection, bleeding from any site, or symptoms suggestive of anemia.
ADULTS − Myelodysplastic syndromes. Treatment Regimen: Option 1 - Administer at a dose of 15 mg/m2 by continuous intravenous infusion over 3 hours repeated every 8 hours for 3 days. Repeat cycle every 6 weeks. Option 2 - Administer at a dose of 20 mg/m2 by continuous intravenous infusion over 1 hour repeated daily for 5 days. Repeat cycle every 4 weeks.
PEDS − Not approved in children.
NOTES − Reliable contraception is recommended. Men should not father children during and 2 months after therapy. Monitor CBCs, baseline LFTs.
MOA − Antimetabolite.
ADVERSE EFFECTS − Serious: Bone marrow suppression, pulmonary edema. Frequent: Bone marrow suppression, N/V, fatigue, fever, diarrhea, constipation, hyperglycemia, stomatitis.

FLOXURIDINE (*FUDR*) ▶L ♀D ▶− $ varies by therapy
WARNING − Bone marrow suppression, nephrotoxicity, increased LFTs, alopecia. Instruct patients to report promptly fever, sore throat, or signs of local infection, bleeding from any site, or symptoms suggestive of anemia.
ADULTS − Chemotherapy doses vary by indication. GI adenocarcinoma metastatic to the liver given by intrahepatic arterial pump.
PEDS − Not approved in children.
NOTES − Reliable contraception is recommended. Monitor CBCs, LFTs and renal function.
MOA − Antimetabolite.
ADVERSE EFFECTS − Serious: Bone marrow suppression. Frequent: Bone marrow suppression, N/V, stomatitis, alopecia.

FLUDARABINE (*Fludara*) ▶Serum ♀D ▶− $ varies by therapy
WARNING − Neurotoxicity (agitation, blindness, and coma), progressive multifocal leukoencephalopathy and death, bone marrow suppression, hemolytic anemia, thrombocytopenia, ITP, Evan's syndrome, acquired hemophilia, pulmonary toxicity, fertility impairment, hyperuricemia, alopecia. Instruct patients to report promptly fever, sore throat, or signs of local infection, bleeding from any site, or symptoms suggestive of anemia.
ADULTS − Chemotherapy doses vary by indication. Chronic lymphocytic leukemia.
PEDS − Not approved in children.
UNAPPROVED ADULTS − Non-Hodgkin's lymphoma. Mycosis fungoides. Hairy-cell leukemia. Hodgkin's disease.
NOTES − Reliable contraception is recommended. Monitor CBCs and renal function; watch for hemolysis.
MOA − Antimetabolite.
ADVERSE EFFECTS − Serious: Neurotoxicity (agitation, blindness, coma), progressive multifocal leukoencephalopathy and death, bone marrow suppression, hemolytic anemia, pulmonary toxicity. Frequent: Bone marrow suppression, edema, N/V, fever, diarrhea, rash, alopecia.

FLUOROURACIL (*Adrucil, 5-FU*) ▶L ♀D ▶− $ varies by therapy
WARNING − Increased INR and bleeding with warfarin. Bone marrow suppression, angina, fertility impairment, alopecia, diarrhea, mucositis, hand and foot syndrome (palmar plantar erythrodysesthesia). Instruct patients to report promptly fever, sore throat, signs of local infection, bleeding from any site, or symptoms suggestive of anemia.
ADULTS − Chemotherapy doses vary by indication. Colon, rectum, breast, stomach, and pancreatic carcinoma. Dukes' stage C colon cancer with irinotecan or leucovorin after surgical resection.
PEDS − Not approved in children.

(cont.)

ONCOLOGY: Antimetabolites

FLUOROURACIL (cont.)
UNAPPROVED ADULTS — <u>Head and neck, renal cell, prostate, ovarian, esophageal, anal and topical to skin for basal and squamous cell carcinoma.</u>
NOTES — Reliable contraception is recommended. Monitor CBCs.
MOA — Antimetabolite.
ADVERSE EFFECTS — Serious: Bone marrow suppression, bleeding with warfarin, palmar-plantar erythrodysesthesia, angina. Frequent: Bone marrow suppression, N/V, diarrhea, stomatitis, alopecia.

GEMCITABINE (*Gemzar*) ▶intracellular ♀D ▶– $ varies by therapy
WARNING — Bone marrow suppression, fever, rash, increased LFTs, proteinuria, hematuria, alopecia. Instruct patients to report promptly fever, sore throat, signs of local infection, bleeding from any site, or symptoms suggestive of anemia.
ADULTS — Chemotherapy doses vary by indication. <u>Adenocarcinoma of the pancreas. Non-small-cell lung cancer, in combination regimens. Metastatic breast cancer, in combination regimens. Advanced ovarian cancer.</u>
PEDS — Not approved in children.
NOTES — Reliable contraception is recommended. Monitor CBCs, LFTs and renal function.
MOA — Antimetabolite.
ADVERSE EFFECTS — Serious: Bone marrow suppression. Frequent: Bone marrow suppression, fever, rash, proteinuria, hematuria, increased LFTs.

MERCAPTOPURINE (*6-MP, Purinethol*) ▶L ♀D ▶– $ varies by therapy
WARNING — Bone marrow suppression, hepatotoxicity, hyperuricemia, alopecia. Instruct patients to report promptly fever, sore throat, signs of local infection, bleeding from any site, symptoms suggestive of anemia, or yellow discoloration of the skin or eyes.
ADULTS — Chemotherapy doses vary by indication. <u>ALL. AML. CML.</u>
PEDS — Chemotherapy doses vary by indication. <u>ALL. AML.</u>
UNAPPROVED ADULTS — <u>Inflammatory bowel disease:</u> Start at 50 mg PO daily, titrate to response. Typical dose range 0.5 to 1.5 mg/kg PO daily.
UNAPPROVED PEDS — <u>Inflammatory bowel disease:</u> 1.5 mg/kg PO daily.
FORMS — Generic/Trade: Tabs 50 mg.
NOTES — Reliable contraception is recommended. Monitor CBCs, LFTs and renal function. Consider folate supplementation. Allopurinol and trimethoprim/sulfamethoxazole increase toxicity.
MOA — Antimetabolite.
ADVERSE EFFECTS — Serious: Bone marrow suppression, hepatotoxicity, oligospermia. Frequent: Bone marrow suppression, alopecia, rash, diarrhea.

NELARABINE (*Arranon*) ▶LK ♀D ▶– $ varies by therapy
WARNING — Peripheral neuropathy, paralysis, demyelination, severe somnolence, convulsions. Bone marrow suppression.
ADULTS — Chemotherapy doses vary by indication. <u>ALL, T-cell lymphoblastic lymphoma.</u>
PEDS — Chemotherapy doses vary by indication. <u>ALL, T-cell lymphoblastic lymphoma.</u>
NOTES — Reliable contraception is recommended. Monitor renal function.
MOA — Antimetabolite.
ADVERSE EFFECTS — Serious: Bone marrow suppression, peripheral neuropathy, paralysis, demyelination, convulsions. Frequent: Bone marrow suppression, fatigue, somnolence, N/V/D.

PEMETREXED (*Alimta*) ▶K ♀D ▶– $ varies by therapy
WARNING — Bone marrow suppression, rash. Instruct patients to report promptly fever, sore throat, signs of local infection, bleeding from any site, symptoms suggestive of anemia.
ADULTS — Chemotherapy doses vary by indication. <u>Malignant pleural mesothelioma, in combination with cisplatin. Nonsquamous non-small cell lung cancer. Supplement with folic acid and B12.</u>
PEDS — Not approved in children.
UNAPPROVED ADULTS — <u>Metastatic bladder cancer, cervical cancer, thymic malignancies.</u>
NOTES — Reliable contraception is recommended. Monitor CBCs and renal function. Do not use in patients with CrCl < 45 mL/min. Avoid NSAIDs around the time of administration.
MOA — Antimetabolite.
ADVERSE EFFECTS — Serious: Bone marrow suppression, severe rash. Frequent: Bone marrow suppression, fatigue, fever, N/V, stomatitis, dyspnea, rash.

PENTOSTATIN (*Nipent*) ▶K ♀D ▶– $ varies by therapy
WARNING — Bone marrow suppression, nephrotoxicity, hepatotoxicity, CNS toxicity, pulmonary toxicity, severe rash, fertility impairment, alopecia. Instruct patients to report promptly fever, sore throat, signs of local infection, bleeding from any site, symptoms suggestive of anemia, or yellow discoloration of the skin or eyes.
ADULTS — Chemotherapy doses vary by indication. <u>Hairy cell leukemia, refractory to alpha-interferon.</u>
PEDS — Not approved in children.
UNAPPROVED ADULTS — <u>ALL, CLL, non-Hodgkin's lymphoma, Mycosis fungoides.</u>
NOTES — Reliable contraception is recommended. Monitor CBCs and renal function.
MOA — Antimetabolite.
ADVERSE EFFECTS — Serious: Bone marrow suppression, nephrotoxicity, hepatotoxicity, CNS toxicity, pulmonary toxicity, severe rash. Frequent: N/V, fever.

PRALATREXATE (*Folotyn*) ▶ + intracellular ♀D ▶–WARNING — Bone marrow suppression, mucositis and hepatotoxicity may require dosage modification. Concomitant administration of drugs that are subject to substantial renal clearance (eg, NSAIDs, trimethoprim/sulfamethoxazole) may result in delayed clearance of pralatrexate.
ADULTS — 30mg/m2 IV once weekly for 6 out of 7 weeks. <u>Treatment of relapsed/refractory peripheral T-cell lymphoma.</u> (PTCL)

(cont.)

PRALATREXATE (cont.)
- PEDS — Not approved in pediatrics
- NOTES — Folic Acid and Vitamin B12 supplementation needed to reduce hematologic toxicity and treatment related mucositis. Folic Acid 1-1.25mg p.o. daily should be started within 10 days prior to starting pralatrexate, and continued for 30 days post last pralatrexate dose. Vitamin B12 1000mcg I.M. should be administered within 10 weeks prior to starting pralatrexate, and every 8 to 10 weeks thereafter. B12 may be given same day as pralatrexate after the initial dose.
- MOA — Antifolate analog. Inhibits DNA, RNA and protein synthesis by entering cells expressing reduced folate carrier. After polyglutamylation by FPGS (folylpolyglutamate synthetase), competes for DHFR-folate binding site to inhibit DHFR (dihydrofolate reductase).
- ADVERSE EFFECTS — Significant: Edema, fatigue, fever, rash, mucositis, nausea, vomiting, diarrhea, constipation, bone marrow suppression, increased LFTs, back and limb pain, cough, epistaxis, night sweats.

THIOGUANINE (*Tabloid*, ✦*Lanvis*) ▶L ♀D ▶– $ varies by therapy
- WARNING — Bone marrow suppression, hepatotoxicity, hyperuricemia, alopecia. Instruct patients to report promptly fever, sore throat, signs of local infection, bleeding from any site, symptoms suggestive of anemia, or yellow discoloration of the skin or eyes.
- ADULTS — Chemotherapy doses vary by indication. Acute nonlymphocytic leukemias.
- PEDS — Chemotherapy doses vary by indication. Acute nonlymphocytic leukemias.
- FORMS — Generic only: Tabs 40 mg, scored.
- NOTES — Reliable contraception is recommended. Monitor CBCs and LFTs.
- MOA — Antimetabolite.
- ADVERSE EFFECTS — Serious: Bone marrow suppression, hepatotoxicity. Frequent: Bone marrow suppression, diarrhea.

ONCOLOGY: Cytoprotective Agents

AMIFOSTINE (*Ethyol*) ▶plasma ♀C ▶– $ varies by therapy
- WARNING — Hypotension, hypocalcemia, N/V, hypersensitivity.
- ADULTS — Doses vary by indication. Reduction of renal toxicity with cisplatin. Reduction of xerostomia and mucositis with radiation.
- PEDS — Not approved in children.
- NOTES — Monitor calcium and BP.
- MOA — Cytoprotective.
- ADVERSE EFFECTS — Serious: Hypotension, hypocalcemia. Frequent: N/V.

DEXRAZOXANE (*Totect, Zinecard*) ▶plasma ♀C ▶– $ varies by therapy
- WARNING — Additive bone marrow suppression, secondary malignancies, fertility impairment, N/V.
- ADULTS — Doses vary by indication. Reduction of cardiac toxicity with doxorubicin. Treatment of anthracycline extravasation; give ASAP within 6 h of extravasation.
- PEDS — Not approved in children.
- NOTES — Monitor CBCs.
- MOA — Cytoprotective.
- ADVERSE EFFECTS — Serious: Additive bone marrow suppression, secondary malignancies. Frequent: N/V.

MESNA (*Mesnex*, ✦*Uromitexan*) ▶plasma ♀B ▶– $ varies by therapy
- WARNING — Hypersensitivity, bad taste in the mouth.
- ADULTS — Doses vary by indication. Reduction of hemorrhagic cystis with ifosfamide.
- PEDS — Not approved in children.
- UNAPPROVED ADULTS — Doses vary by indication. Reduction of hemorrhagic cystis with high-dose cyclophosphamide.
- UNAPPROVED PEDS — Doses vary by indication.
- FORMS — Trade only: Tabs 400 mg, scored.
- NOTES — False positive test urine ketones.
- MOA — Cytoprotective.
- ADVERSE EFFECTS — Serious: Hypersensitivity. Frequent: Bad taste in mouth.

PALIFERMIN (*Kepivance*) ▶plasma ♀C ▶? $ varies by therapy
- ADULTS — Doses vary by indication. Decreases incidence, duration, and severity of severe oral mucositis in patients receiving therapy for hematologic malignancies.
- PEDS — Not approved in children.
- MOA — Cytoprotective — human keratinocyte growth factor.
- ADVERSE EFFECTS — Serious: Fever. Frequent: Rash, erythema, edema, pruritus, oral/perioral dysesthesia, tongue discoloration or thickening, alteration of taste.

ONCOLOGY: Hormones

ANASTROZOLE (*Arimidex*) ▶L ♀X ▶– $ varies by therapy
- WARNING — Patients with estrogen receptor-negative disease and patients who do not respond to tamoxifen therapy rarely respond to anastrozole. Fertility impairment, vaginal bleeding, hot flashes, alopecia, decrease in bone mineral density. Increase in cardiovascular ischemia in women with preexisting ischemic heart disease.
- ADULTS — Chemotherapy doses vary by indication. Locally advanced or metastatic breast cancer. Adjuvant early breast cancer.
- PEDS — Not approved in children.
- FORMS — Generic/Trade: Tabs 1 mg.

(cont.)

ONCOLOGY: Hormones

ANASTROZOLE (*cont.*)
NOTES — Reliable contraception is recommended. Monitor CBCs. Contraindicated in premenopausal women.
MOA — Aromatase inhibitor.
ADVERSE EFFECTS — Serious: Cardiovascular ischemia. None. Frequent: Hot flashes, nausea.

BICALUTAMIDE (*Casodex*) ▶L ♀X ▶– $ varies by therapy
WARNING — Hypersensitivity, hepatotoxicity, interstitial lung disease, gynecomastia/breast pain, fertility impairment, hot flashes, diarrhea, alopecia.
ADULTS — <u>Prostate cancer:</u> 50 mg PO daily in combination with a LHRH analog (eg, goserelin or leuprolide). Not indicated in women.
PEDS — Not approved in children.
UNAPPROVED ADULTS — <u>Adjuvant prostate cancer.</u>
FORMS — Generic/Trade: Tabs 50 mg.
NOTES — Monitor PSA levels and LFTs. Displaces warfarin, possibly increasing anticoagulant effects. Gynecomastia and breast pain occur.
MOA — Anti-androgen.
ADVERSE EFFECTS — Serious: Hypersensitivity, hepatotoxicity, angioedema, urticaria, interstitial lung disease. Frequent: Gynecomastia, breast pain, hot flashes, general pain, impotence.

CYPROTERONE (*✦Androcur, Androcur Depot*) ▶L ♀X ▶– $ varies by therapy
ADULTS — <u>Prostate cancer.</u>
PEDS — Not approved in children.
FORMS — Generic/Trade: Tabs 50 mg.
NOTES — Dose-related hepatotoxicity has occurred, monitor LFTs at initiation and during treatment. Monitor adrenocortical function periodically. May impair carbohydrate metabolism; monitor blood glucose, especially in diabetics.
MOA — Antiandrogen.
ADVERSE EFFECTS — Serious: Hepatotoxicity, thromboembolism, depression. Frequent: Decreased libido, gynecomastia, impotence, abnormal spermatozoa.

DEGARELIX ▶LK ♀X ▶– $ varies by therapy
WARNING — QT prolongation.
ADULTS — <u>Advanced prostate cancer:</u> Initial dose: 240 mg SC; maintenance: 80 mg SC q 28 days.
PEDS — Not approved in children.
NOTES — Monitor LFTs and PSA. May prolong QT interval. May decrease bone mineral density.
MOA — Gonadotropin-releasing hormone antagonist that suppresses LH and FSH secretion thus lowering serum testosterone.
ADVERSE EFFECTS — Serious: Allergic reactions, hepatotoxicity, QT prolongation. Frequent: Hot flashes, weight gain, increased LFTs, night sweats.

ESTRAMUSTINE (*Emcyt*) ▶L ♀X ▶– $ varies by therapy
WARNING — Thrombosis, including MI, glucose intolerance, HTN, fluid retention, increased LFTs, alopecia.
ADULTS — Chemotherapy doses vary by indication. <u>Hormone refractory prostate cancer.</u>
PEDS — Not approved in children.
FORMS — Trade only: Caps 140 mg.
NOTES — Reliable contraception is recommended. Monitor LFTs, glucose and BP. Milk, milk products and calcium-rich foods or drugs may impair absorption.
MOA — Alkylating agent.
ADVERSE EFFECTS — Serious: Thrombosis, MI, glucose intolerance, HTN, fluid retention. Frequent: None.

EXEMESTANE (*Aromasin*) ▶L ♀D ▶– $ varies by therapy
WARNING — Lymphocytopenia, alopecia.
ADULTS — Chemotherapy doses vary by indication. <u>Breast cancer.</u>
PEDS — Not approved in children.
UNAPPROVED ADULTS — Chemotherapy doses vary by indication. <u>Prevention of prostate cancer.</u>
FORMS — Trade only: Tabs 25 mg.
NOTES — Contraindicated in premenopausal women. Reliable contraception is recommended. Monitor CBCs.
MOA — Aromatase inhibitor.
ADVERSE EFFECTS — Serious: Lymphocytopenia. Frequent: Lymphocytopenia, nausea, hot flashes

FLUTAMIDE (*Eulexin,* ✦*Euflex*) ▶L ♀D ▶– $ varies by therapy
WARNING — Hepatic failure, methemoglobinemia, hemolytic anemia, breast neoplasms, gynecomastia, fertility impairment, photosensitivity, alopecia.
ADULTS — <u>Prostate cancer:</u> 250 mg PO q 8 h in combination with a LHRH analog (eg, goserelin or leuprolide). Not indicated in women.
PEDS — Not approved in children.
UNAPPROVED ADULTS — <u>Hirsutism in women.</u>
FORMS — Generic only: Caps 125 mg.
NOTES — Monitor LFTs, PSA, methemoglobin levels. Transient urine discoloration (amber or yellow-green). Avoid exposure to sunlight/use sunscreen. Increased INR with warfarin. Gynecomastia and breast pain occur.
MOA — Anti-androgen.
ADVERSE EFFECTS — Serious: Hepatic failure, methemoglobinemia, hemolytic anemia. Frequent: Gynecomastia, urine discoloration, hot flashes, diarrhea, photosensitivity, impotence.

FULVESTRANT (*Faslodex*) ▶L ♀D ▶– $ varies by therapy
WARNING — Contraindicated in pregnancy. Hypersensitivity, N/V/D, constipation, abdominal pain, hot flashes.
ADULTS — Chemotherapy doses vary by indication. <u>Breast cancer.</u>
PEDS — Not approved in children.
NOTES — Reliable contraception is recommended.
MOA — Estrogen receptor antagonist.
ADVERSE EFFECTS — Serious: Hypersensitivity. Frequent: N/V, diarrhea, abdominal pain, hot flashes.

GOSERELIN (*Zoladex*) ▶LK ♀D/X ▶– $ varies by therapy
WARNING — Transient increases in sex hormones, increases in lipids, hypercalcemia, decreases in

(cont.)

ONCOLOGY: Hormones

GOSERELIN *(cont.)*
bone mineral density, vaginal bleeding, fertility impairment, hot flashes, decreased libido, alopecia.
ADULTS — Prostate cancer: 3.6 mg implant SC into upper abdominal wall every 28 days, or 10.8 mg implant SC q 12 weeks. Endometriosis: 3.6 mg implant SC q 28 days or 10.8 mg implant q 12 weeks for 6 months. Specialized dosing for breast cancer.
PEDS — Not approved in children.
UNAPPROVED ADULTS — Adjuvant prostate cancer. Palliative treatment of breast cancer. 3.6 mg implant SC q 28 days indefinitely. Endometrial thinning prior to ablation for dysfunctional uterine bleeding: 3.6 mg SC 4 weeks prior to surgery or 3.6 mg SC q 4 weeks for 2 doses with surgery 2 to 4 weeks after last dose.
FORMS — Trade only: Implants 3.6, 10.8 mg.
NOTES — Transient increases in testosterone and estrogen occur. Hypercalcemia may occur in patients with bone metastases. Vaginal bleeding may occur during the first 2 months of treatment and should stop spontaneously. Reliable contraception is recommended. Consider norethindrone as "add back" therapy to decrease bone loss (see norethindrone).
MOA — Gonadotropin inhibitor.
ADVERSE EFFECTS — Serious: Hypersensitivity, anaphylaxis, antibody formation, pituitary apoplexy, osteoporosis, decreased bone mineral density, angina, thromboembolism, heart failure, hypercalcemia. Frequent: Decrease in bone mineral density, vaginal bleeding, hot flashes, gynecomastia, transient worsening of pain.

HISTRELIN (*Vantas, Supprelin LA*) ▶Not metabolized ♀X ▶– $ varies by therapy
WARNING — Worsening of symptoms, especially during the first weeks of therapy: Increase in bone pain, difficulty urinating. Decreases in bone mineral density.
ADULTS — Palliative treatment of advanced prostate cancer: Insert 1 implant SC in the inner upper arm q 12 mo. May repeat if appropriate after 12 months.
PEDS — Central precocious puberty (Supprelin LA), in age greater than 2 yo: Insert 1 implant SC in the inner upper arm. May repeat if appropriate after 12 months.
FORMS — Trade only: 50 mg implant.
NOTES — Causes transient increase of testosterone level during the first weeks of treatment which may create or exacerbate symptoms. Patients with metastatic vertebral lesions and/or urinary tract obstruction should be closely observed during the first few weeks of therapy. Avoid wetting arm for 24 h after implant insertion and from heavy lifting or strenuous exertion of the involved arm for 7 days after insertion. Measure testosterone levels and PSA periodically. May decrease bone density. Monitor LH, FSH, estradiol or testosterone, height and bone age in children with central precocious puberty at 1 month post implantation and q 6 mo thereafter.
MOA — Gonadotropin inhibitor.
ADVERSE EFFECTS — Serious: Bladder outlet obstruction, hematuria, bone pain, neuropathy, spinal cord compression. Frequent: Implant site reaction, erectile dysfunction, gynecomastia, hot flashes, testicular atrophy, transient worsening of pain.

LETROZOLE (*Femara*) ▶LK ♀D ▶– $$$$$
WARNING — Fertility impairment, decreases in lymphocytes, increased LFTs, alopecia.
ADULTS — 2.5 mg PO daily. Adjuvant treatment of postmenopausal, hormone receptor positive, early breast cancer. Extended adjuvant treatment of early breast cancer after 5 years of tamoxifen therapy. Advanced breast cancer with disease progression after antiestrogen therapy, hormone receptor positive or hormone receptor unknown, locally advanced or metastatic breast cancer.
PEDS — Not approved in children.
UNAPPROVED ADULTS — Ovarian (epithelial) cancer. Endometrial cancer.
FORMS — Trade only: Tabs 2.5 mg.
NOTES — Reliable contraception is recommended. Monitor CBCs, LFTs, and lipids.
MOA — Aromatase inhibitor.
ADVERSE EFFECTS — Serious: Lymphocytopenia, angioedema, anaphylaxis, toxic epidermal necrolysis, erythema multiforme, and hepatitis. Frequent: Lymphocytopenia, nausea, hot flashes, bone pain, fatigue, dizziness, increased cholesterol, decreased bone mineral density.

LEUPROLIDE (*Eligard, Lupron, Lupron Depot, Lupron Depot-Ped*) ▶L ♀X ▶– $ varies by therapy
WARNING — Possible increase of diabetes and cardiovascular disease in men receiving leuprolide for prostate cancer. Worsening of symptoms: Increase in bone pain, difficulty urinating. Decreases in bone mineral density. Anaphylaxis, alopecia.
ADULTS — Advanced prostate cancer: Lupron: 1 mg SC daily. Eligard: 7.5 mg SC q month, 22.5 mg SC q 3 months, 30 mg SC q 4 months, or 45 mg SC q 6 months. Lupron depot: 7.5 mg IM q month, 22.5 mg IM q 3 months or 30 mg IM q 4 months. Viadur: 65 mg SC implant q 12 months. Endometriosis or uterine leiomyomata (fibroids): 3.75 mg IM q month or 11.25 mg IM q 3 months for total therapy of 6 months (endometriosis) or 3 months (fibroids). Administer concurrent iron for fibroid-associated anemia.
PEDS — Central precocious puberty: Injection: 50 mcg/kg/day SC. Increase by 10 mcg/kg/day until total down regulation. Depot-Ped: 0.3 mg/kg q 4 weeks IM (minimum dose 7.5 mg). Increase by 3.75 mg q 4 weeks until adequate down regulation.
UNAPPROVED ADULTS — Treatment of breast cancer, infertility, menses cessation in patients receiving high dose chemotherapy, prostatic hyperplasia.
NOTES — For prostate cancer, monitor testosterone, prostatic acid phosphatase and PSA levels. Transient increases in testosterone and estrogen occur. For endometriosis, a fractional dose of the

(cont.)

ONCOLOGY: Immunomodulators

LEUPROLIDE (cont.)
3 month depot preparation is not equivalent to the same dose of the monthly formulation. Rotate the injection site periodically. Consider norethindrone as "add back" therapy to decrease bone loss (see norethindrone).
MOA – Gonadotropin inhibitor.
ADVERSE EFFECTS – Serious: Anaphylaxis, urinary obstruction, erythema multiforme, pituitary apoplexy. Frequent: Decrease in bone mineral density, vaginal bleeding, hot flashes, gynecomastia, transient worsening of pain.

NILUTAMIDE (*Nilandron*) ▶L ♀C ▶– $ varies by therapy
WARNING – Interstitial pneumonitis, hepatitis, aplastic anemia (isolated cases), delay in adaptation to the dark, hot flashes, alcohol intolerance, alopecia.
ADULTS – Prostate cancer: 300 mg PO daily for 30 days, then 150 mg PO daily. Begin therapy on same day as surgical castration.
PEDS – Not approved in children.
FORMS – Trade only: Tabs 150 mg.
NOTES – Monitor CBCs, LFTs and chest X-rays. Caution patients who experience delayed adaptation to the dark about driving at night or through tunnels; suggest wearing tinted glasses. May increase phenytoin and theophylline levels. Avoid alcohol.
MOA – Anti-androgen.
ADVERSE EFFECTS – Serious: Interstitial pneumonitis, hepatitis, aplastic anemia. Frequent: Delay in adaptation to the dark, hot flashes, gynecomastia, alcohol intolerance, alopecia.

TOREMIFENE (*Fareston*) ▶L ♀D ▶– $ varies by therapy
WARNING – Hypercalcemia and tumor flare, endometrial hyperplasia, thromboembolism, hot flashes, vaginal bleeding, fertility impairment, alopecia.
ADULTS – Chemotherapy doses vary by indication. Breast cancer.
PEDS – Not approved in children.
FORMS – Trade only: Tabs 60 mg.
NOTES – Reliable contraception is recommended. Monitor CBCs, calcium levels and LFTs. May increase effects of anticoagulants.
MOA – Selective estrogen receptor modulator.
ADVERSE EFFECTS – Serious: DVT/PE, endometrial cancer, visual disturbances, cataracts, hypercalcemia, tumor flare, hepatotoxicity. Frequent: Hot flashes, vaginal bleeding.

TRIPTORELIN (*Trelstar Depot*) ▶LK ♀X ▶– $ varies by therapy
WARNING – Transient increases in sex hormones, bone pain, neuropathy, hematuria, urethral/bladder outlet obstruction, spinal cord compression, anaphylaxis, hot flashes, impotence, alopecia.
ADULTS – Chemotherapy doses vary by indication. Prostate cancer.
PEDS – Not approved in children.
MOA – Gonadotropin inhibitor.
ADVERSE EFFECTS – Serious: Bone pain, neuropathy, hematuria, urethral/bladder outlet obstruction, spinal cord compression, anaphylaxis. Frequent: Transient worsening of symptoms, hot flashes, impotence.

ONCOLOGY: Immunomodulators

ALDESLEUKIN (*Proleukin, interleukin-2*) ▶K ♀C ▶– $ varies by therapy
WARNING – Capillary leak syndrome, resulting in hypotension and reduced organ perfusion. Exacerbation of autoimmune diseases and symptoms of CNS metastases, impaired neutrophil function, hepato/nephrotoxicity, mental status changes, decreased thyroid function, anemia, thrombocytopenia, fertility impairment, alopecia.
ADULTS – Chemotherapy doses vary by indication. Renal-cell carcinoma.
PEDS – Not approved in children.
UNAPPROVED ADULTS – Kaposi's sarcoma. Metastatic melanoma. Colorectal cancer. Non-Hodgkin's lymphoma.
NOTES – Monitor CBCs, electrolytes, LFTs, renal function and chest X-rays. Baseline PFTs. Avoid iodinated contrast media. Antihypertensives potentiate hypotension.
MOA – Aldesleukin stimulates a cytokine cascade involving various interferons, interleukins, and tumor necrosis factors, which induces the proliferation and differentiation of B and T-cells, monocytes, macrophages, natural killer cells, and other cytotoxic cells.
ADVERSE EFFECTS – Serious: Capillary leak syndrome, resulting in hypotension and reduced organ perfusion. Exacerbation of autoimmune diseases and of symptoms of CNS metastases, immunosuppression, hepato/nephrotoxicity, decreased thyroid function, anemia, thrombocytopenia. Frequent: Hypotension, tachycardia, mental status changes, anemia, thrombocytopenia, N/V, fever, chills, rigors, pruritus.

ALEMTUZUMAB (*Campath, ✦MabCampath*) ▶? ♀C ▶– $ varies by therapy
WARNING – Idiopathic thrombocytopenic purpura, bone marrow suppression, hemolytic anemia, hypersensitivity, and immunosuppression.
ADULTS – Chemotherapy doses vary by indication. B-cell chronic lymphocytic leukemia.
PEDS – Not approved in children.
NOTES – Monitor CBC.
MOA – The exact mechanism of alemtuzumab is unknown; however, the proposed mechanism involves the binding of alemtuzumab to CD52, a nonmodulating antigen that is present on the surface of essentially all B and T lymphocytes, a majority of monocytes, macrophages, NK cells, and a subpopulation of granulocytes, causing an antibody-dependent lysis of leukemic cells.

(cont.)

ALEMTUZUMAB (cont.)
ADVERSE EFFECTS — Serious: Idiopathic thrombocytopenic purpura, bone marrow suppression, hemolytic anemia, hypersensitivity, and immunosuppression. Frequent: Hypotension, rigors, fever, shortness of breath, bronchospasm, chills, rash, N/V.

BCG (*Bacillus of Calmette and Guerin, Pacis, TheraCys, Tice BCG, ✦Oncotice, Immucyst*) ▶Not metabolized ♀C ▶? $ varies by therapy
WARNING — Hypersensitivity, hematuria, urinary frequency, dysuria, bacterial UTI, flu-like syndrome, alopecia.
ADULTS — Chemotherapy doses vary by indication. Carcinoma in situ of the urinary bladder, intravesical.
PEDS — Not approved in children.
NOTES — Bone marrow depressants, immunosuppressants and antimicrobial therapy may impair response. Increase fluid intake after treatments.
MOA — BCG is an immunostimulant used to stimulate the immune system to produce immunity against tuberculosis or to mount a local inflammation and immune reaction against superficial cancers from the activation of T-lymphocytes, B-lymphocytes, and natural killer cells.
ADVERSE EFFECTS — Serious: Hypersensitivity, hematuria, urinary frequency, dysuria, bacterial urinary tract infection. Frequent: Flu-like syndrome.

BEVACIZUMAB (*Avastin*) ▶? ♀C ▶− $ varies by therapy
WARNING — CVA, MI, TIA, angina, GI perforation, wound dehiscence, serious hemorrhage, HTN, heart failure, nephrotic syndrome, reversible posterior leukoencephalopathy syndrome (brain capillary leak syndrome), nasal septum perforation. Tracheoesophageal fistula has been reported. Microangiopathic hemolytic anemia (MAHA) in patients on concomitant sunitinib malate.
ADULTS — Chemotherapy doses vary by indication. Metastatic colorectal carcinoma, non-small-cell lung cancer, glioblastoma, metastatic HER-2 negative breast cancer, metastatic renal cell cancer.
PEDS — Not approved in children.
UNAPPROVED ADULTS — Recurrent ovarian cancer, age-related macular degeneration.
NOTES — Monitor BP, and UA for protein. Do not use in combination with sunitinib.
MOA — Bevacizumab is a humanized monoclonal antibody which binds the vascular endothelial growth factor (VEGF) preventing the interaction of VEGF to its receptors. In human cancers, VEGF expression is associated with increased microvascular density, tumor growth, metastasis, and poor prognosis.
ADVERSE EFFECTS — Serious: CVA, MI, TIA, angina, GI perforation, wound dehiscence, serious hemorrhage, HTN, heart failure, nephrotic syndrome, reversible posterior leukoencephalopathy syndrome (brain capillary leak syndrome), microangiopathic hemolytic anemia, nasal septum perforation. Frequent: Headache, HTN, stomatitis, constipation, diarrhea, abdominal pain, N/V, epistaxis, dyspnea, proteinuria.

CETUXIMAB (*Erbitux*) ▶? ♀C ▶− $ varies by therapy
WARNING — Anaphylaxis, cardiopulmonary arrest/sudden death, pulmonary toxicity, rash, sepsis, renal failure, pulmonary embolus, hypomagnesemia.
ADULTS — Chemotherapy doses vary by indication. Metastatic colorectal carcinoma, head and neck squamous cell carcinoma.
PEDS — Not approved in children.
UNAPPROVED ADULTS — EGFR-expressing advanced nonsmall cell lung cancer.
NOTES — Monitor renal function and electrolytes including magnesium. Caution with known CAD, heart failure, or arrhythmias. Premedication with a H1 antagonist and a 1-hour observation period after infusion is recommended due to potential for anaphylaxis. Use is not recommended in patients with codon 12 or 13 KRAS mutations.
MOA — Cetuximab is a recombinant chimeric monoclonal antibody that binds to and blocks the binding of ligands (eg, epidermal growth factor and tissue growth factor) to the epidermal growth factor receptor (EGFR, HER1, c-ErbB-1) on the surface of normal and tumor cells, resulting in inhibition of cell growth, induction of apoptosis, and decreased vascular endothelial growth factor (VEGF) production.
ADVERSE EFFECTS — Serious: Anaphylaxis, cardiopulmonary arrest/sudden death, pulmonary toxicity, rash, sepsis, renal failure, pulmonary embolus, hypomagnesemia. Frequent: Rash, pruritus, nail changes, malaise, diarrhea, abdominal pain, N/V, hypomagnesemia.

DENILEUKIN (*Ontak*) ▶Plasma ♀C ▶− $ varies by therapy
WARNING — Hypersensitivity, vascular leak syndrome (hypotension, edema, hypoalbuminemia), visual loss, thrombosis, rash, diarrhea, alopecia.
ADULTS — Chemotherapy doses vary by indication. Cutaneous T-cell lymphoma.
PEDS — Not approved in children.
UNAPPROVED ADULTS — Mycosis fungoides, Sezary syndrome. second line treatment for peripheral T-cell lymphoma.
NOTES — Monitor CBCs, LFTs and renal function. Visual loss is usually persistent.
MOA — Denileukin diftitox is a recombinant DNA-derived cytotoxic protein composed of the amino acid sequences for diphtheria toxin fragments A and B, followed by the sequences for interleukin-2, designed to be cytotoxic to cells that express certain high-affinity interleukin (IL)-2 receptors.
ADVERSE EFFECTS — Serious: Hypersensitivity, vascular leak syndrome (hypotension, edema, hypoalbuminemia), visual loss, infection, DVT/PE. Frequent: Hypersensitivity, vascular leak syndrome (hypotension, edema, hypoalbuminemia), fever, rash, N/V, diarrhea.

ONCOLOGY: Immunomodulators

EVEROLIMUS (*Afinitor*) ▶L ♀D ▶– $ varies by therapy
WARNING – Noninfectious pneumonitis, hyperglycemia, bone marrow suppression. Avoid live vaccines.
ADULTS – Chemotherapy doses vary by indication. Advanced renal cell carcinoma.
PEDS – Not approved in children.
UNAPPROVED ADULTS – Treatment of pancreatic neuroendocrine tumors.
NOTES – Reliable contraception is recommended. Drugs that induce the CYP450 3A4 system such as phenytoin, phenobarbital, rifampin may decrease concentrations. Inhibitors such as clarithromycin, itraconazole, ketoconazole and ritonavir may increase concentrations. Avoid live vaccines. Monitor CBC, hepatic and renal function, glucose and lipid profile. Increased risk of proteinuria when used in combination with cyclosporine.
MOA – Protein kinase inhibitor that inhibits phosphorylation in ribosomal protein and cell division in renal cell lines.
ADVERSE EFFECTS – Serious: Immunosuppressant properties leading to serious infection, and development of malignancy including lymphoma and skin cancer. Noninfectious pneumonitis, bone marrow suppression. Frequent: Hyperglycemia, hypertriglyceridemia, rash, mucositis, stomatitis, N/V.

IBRITUMOMAB (*Zevalin*) ▶L ♀D ▶– $ varies by therapy
WARNING – Contraindicated in patients with allergy to murine proteins. Fatal infusion reactions, severe cutaneous and mucocutaneous reactions, bone marrow suppression, hypersensitivity.
ADULTS – Chemotherapy doses vary by indication. Non-Hodgkin's lymphoma.
PEDS – Not approved in children.
NOTES – Reliable contraception is recommended. Monitor CBCs.
MOA – Ibritumomab tiuxetan contains a monoclonal antibody linked to an active chelator that accounts for its cytotoxic activity. The antibody moiety contains a murine IgG1 kappa monoclonal antibody directed against the CD20 antigen, once bound, the beta emission from the tiuxetan portion induces cellular damage through the formation of free radicals in the target and neighboring cells.
ADVERSE EFFECTS – Serious: Fatal infusion reactions, erythema multiforme, Stevens-Johnson syndrome, toxic epidermal necrolysis, bullous and exfoliative dermatitis, bone marrow suppression, hypersensitivity. Frequent: Bone marrow suppression, N/V, diarrhea.

INTERFERON ALFA-2A (*Roferon-A*) ▶Plasma ♀C ▶– $ varies by therapy
WARNING – GI hemorrhage, CNS reactions, leukopenia, increased LFTs, anemia, neutralizing antibodies, depression/suicidal behavior, alopecia.
ADULTS – Discontinued by manufacturer February 2008. Chemotherapy doses vary by indication. Hairy cell leukemia. AIDS-related Kaposi's sarcoma. CML.
PEDS – Not approved in children.
UNAPPROVED ADULTS – Superficial bladder tumors. Carcinoid tumor. Cutaneous T-cell lymphoma. Essential thrombocythemia. Non-Hodgkin's lymphoma.
NOTES – Reliable contraception is recommended. Monitor CBCs and LFTs. Hydration important. Decreases clearance of theophylline.
MOA – Interferons exert their cellular activities by binding to specific membrane receptors on the cell surface. Once bound to the cell membrane, interferons initiate a complex sequence of intracellular events. In vitro studies demonstrated that these include the induction of certain enzymes, suppression of cell proliferation, immunomodulating activities such as enhancement of the phagocytic activity of macrophages and augmentation of the specific cytotoxicity of lymphocytes for target cells, and inhibition of virus replication in virus-infected cells.
ADVERSE EFFECTS – Serious: Depression/suicidal behavior, GI hemorrhage, CNS reactions, leukopenia, increased LFTs, anemia. Frequent: Rash, N/V, diarrhea, flu-like syndrome.

LENALIDOMIDE (*Revlimid*) ▶K ♀X ▶– $ varies by therapy
WARNING – Potential for human birth defects, bone marrow suppression, DVT and PE. Instruct patients to report promptly fever, sore throat, signs of local infection, bleeding from any site, or symptoms suggestive of anemia.
ADULTS – Chemotherapy doses vary by indication. Transfusion-dependent anemia due to myelodysplastic syndromes. Multiple myeloma.
PEDS – Not approved in children.
FORMS – Trade only: Caps 5, 10, 15, 25 mg.
NOTES – Analog of thalidomide; can cause birth defects or fetal death. Available only through a restricted distribution program. Reliable contraception is mandated; males must use a latex condom. Monitor CBCs. Do not break, chew or open the caps. Adjust dose for CrCl < 60 mL/min.
MOA – Immunomodulator and angiogenesis inhibitor.
ADVERSE EFFECTS – Serious: Potential for birth defects, neutropenia and thrombocytopenia, DVT/PE. Frequent: Bone marrow suppression, diarrhea, pruritus, rash, fatigue.

OFATUMUMAB (*ARZERRA*) ▶immune system - ♀C ▶?
WARNING – May cause cause serious infusion reactions. Premedicate with acetaminophen, an antihistamine, and a corticosteroid. May cause prolonged cytopenias. Progressive multifocal leukoencephalopathy (PML) can occur. Hepatitis B reactivation may occur. Intestinal obstruction may occur.
ADULTS – 300 mg IV initial dose (Dose 1), followed 1 week later by 2,000 mg IV weekly for 7 doses (Doses 2 through 8), followed 4 weeks later by 2,000 mg IV every 4 weeks for 4 doses (Doses 9 through 12). Treatment of patients with chronic lymphocytic leukemia (CLL) refractory to fludarabine and alemtuzumab.
PEDS – Not approved for pediatric use.

(cont.)

OFATUMUMAB (cont.)
NOTES — Premedicate 30 min. to 2 hours prior to ofatumumab infusion with acetaminopen, antihistamine, and corticosteroid. See product labeling for dose reduction guidelines of corticosteroids.
MOA — Binds specifically to both the small and large extracellular loops of the CD20 molecule on B-lymphocytes resulting in complement dependent cell lysis and antibody-dependent cell mediated toxicity.
ADVERSE EFFECTS — Neutropenia, pneumonia, pyrexia, cough, diarrhea, anemia, fatigue, dyspnea, rash, nausea, bronchitis, and upper respiratory tract infections.

PANITUMUMAB (*Vectibix*) ▶Not metabolized ♀C ▶— $ varies by therapy
WARNING — Skin exfoliation, severe dermatologic reactions complicated by sepsis and death. Anaphylaxis.
ADULTS — Chemotherapy doses vary by indication. Metastatic colorectal carcinoma.
PEDS — Not approved in children.
NOTES — Reliable contraception is recommended. Monitor potassium and magnesium.
MOA — Panitumumab is a monoclonal antibody that binds to epidermal growth factor receptor (EGFR) on tumor cells preventing autophosphorylation and activation of receptor-associated kinases, resulting in inhibition of cell growth, induction of apoptosis, decreased proinflammatory cytokine and vascular growth factor production.
ADVERSE EFFECTS — Serious: Infusion-related reactions, anaphylaxis, sepsis, pulmonary fibrosis. Frequent: Hypomagnesemia, acne, pruritus, erythema, rash, skin exfoliation, paronychia, stomatitis, mucositis, diarrhea, photosensitivity.

RITUXIMAB (*Rituxan*) ▶Not metabolized ♀C ▶— $ varies by therapy
WARNING — Contraindicated if allergy to murine proteins. Fatal infusion reactions, tumor lysis syndrome, severe mucocutaneous reactions, cardiac arrhythmias, nephrotoxicity, bowel obstruction/perforation, hypersensitivity, neutropenia, thrombocytopenia, anemia, serious viral infections with death. Hepatitis B virus reactivation with fulminant hepatitis, liver failure and death in patients with hematologic malignancies have been reported; monitor hepatitis B carriers closely. Cases of fatal progressive multifocal leukoencephalopathy have been reported.
ADULTS — RA: 1000 mg IV infusion weekly for 2 doses in combination with methotrexate and methylprednisolone 100 mg IV pretreatment. Chemotherapy doses vary by indication. Non-Hodgkin's lymphoma, rheumatoid arthritis with methotrexate. Treatment of patients previously treated for CD20-positive chronic lymphocytic leukemia (CLL) in combination with fludarabine and cyclophosphamide (FC).
PEDS — Not approved in children.
UNAPPROVED ADULTS — Immune thrombocytopenic purpura (ITP), thrombotic thrombocytopenic purpura (TTP), multiple sclerosis, Hodgkin's lymphoma, treatment of systemic autoimmune diseases other than RA, treatment of steroid-refractory chronic graft-versus-host disease.
UNAPPROVED PEDS — Autoimmune hemolytic anemia in children.
NOTES — Monitor CBCs.
MOA — Rituximab is a chimeric monoclonal antibody that binds to the antigen CD20, a hydrophobic transmembrane protein found on the surface of B-cell precursors and mature B-lymphocytes, which mediates cell lysis.
ADVERSE EFFECTS — Serious: Fatal infusion reactions, hepatitis, hepatic failure, tumor lysis syndrome, severe mucocutaneous reactions, cardiac arrhythmias, nephrotoxicity, bowel obstruction and perforation, hypersensitivity, bone marrow suppression, infection. Frequent: Bone marrow suppression, infection.

TEMSIROLIMUS (*Torisel*) ▶L ♀C ▶— $ varies by therapy
WARNING — Hypersensitivity, interstitial lung disease, bowel perforation, renal failure, hyperglycemia, bone marrow suppression. Avoid live vaccines.
ADULTS — Chemotherapy doses vary by indication. Advanced renal cell carcinoma.
PEDS — Not approved in children.
UNAPPROVED ADULTS — Relapsed or refractory mantle cell lymphoma.
NOTES — Reliable contraception is recommended. Drugs that induce the CYP4503A4 system such as phenytoin, phenobarbital, rifampin may decrease concentrations. Inhibitors such as clarithromycin, itraconazole, ketoconazole and ritonavir may increase concentrations. Avoid live vaccines. Monitor CBC, hepatic and renal function, glucose and lipid profile. Premedicate with an H1 antagonist 30 minutes prior to infusion to prevent infusion reactions,
MOA — Targeted inhibitor of mTOR (mammalian target of rapamycin) kinase activity, halting the cell cycle at the G1 phase in tumor cells. Also reduces levels of HIF-1 (hypoxia inducible factor) and HIF-2 alpha, and VEGF (vascular endothelial growth factor) thus exhibiting angiogenic activity in renal cell carcinoma.
ADVERSE EFFECTS — Serious: Hypersensitivity, interstitial lung disease, bowel perforation, renal failure, bone marrow suppression. Frequent: Hyperglycemia, hypertriglyceridemia, rash, mucositis, anorexia, N/V.

THALIDOMIDE (*Thalomid*) ▶Plasma ♀X ▶? $$$$$
WARNING — Pregnancy category X. Has caused severe, life-threatening human birth defects. Available only through special restricted distribution program. Prescribers and pharmacists must be registered in this program in order to prescribe or dispense.
ADULTS — Chemotherapy doses vary by indication. Multiple myeloma, with dexamethasone. Erythema nodosum leprosum: 100 to 400 mg PO at bedtime.

(cont.)

THALIDOMIDE (cont.)
Use low end of dose range for initial episodes and if wt less than 50 kg.
PEDS — Not approved in children.
UNAPPROVED ADULTS — Graft vs. Host reactions after bone marrow transplant, Crohn's disease, Waldenstrom's macroglobinemia. Langerhans cell histiocytosis, AIDs related aphthous stomatitis.
UNAPPROVED PEDS — Clinical trials show beneficial effects when combined with dexamethasone in multiple myeloma.
FORMS — Trade only: Caps 50, 100, 150, 200 mg.
MOA — Immunomodulatory agent. Exact mechanism unknown.
ADVERSE EFFECTS — Serious: Birth defects, permanent peripheral neuropathy, bradycardia, Stevens-Johnson syndrome, toxic epidermal necrolysis. Frequent: Somnolence, drowsiness, dizziness, orthostatic hypotension, rash, leukopenia.

TOSITUMOMAB (*Bexxar*) ▶Not metabolized ♀X ▶– $ varies by therapy
WARNING — Contraindicated in patients with allergy to murine proteins. Hypersensitivity, anaphylaxis, infusion reactions, neutropenia, thrombocytopenia, anemia. Hypothyroidism.
ADULTS — Chemotherapy doses vary by indication. Follicular, non-Hodgkin's lymphoma unresponsive to rituximab.
PEDS — Not approved in children.
NOTES — This product is a combination of tositumomab + iodine I 131 tositumomab. Reliable contraception is recommended. Monitor CBC, TSH.
MOA — Tositumomab induces cytotoxicity by combining the immunological effects of antibody binding with the preferential targeting of radiation therapy. Tositumomab, an anti-CD20 monoclonal antibody, targets B-lymphocytes and induces complement-mediated cytolysis, antibody-dependent cellular cytotoxicity, apoptosis, and cell death caused by ionizing radiation from the radioisotope.
ADVERSE EFFECTS — Serious: Infusion reactions, hypersensitivity, bone marrow suppression, hypothyroidism. Frequent: Bone marrow suppression, N/V.

TRASTUZUMAB (*Herceptin*) ▶Not metabolized ♀B ▶– $ varies by therapy
WARNING — Hypersensitivity, including fatal anaphylaxis, fatal infusion-related reactions, pulmonary events including ARDS and death, ventricular dysfunction and heart failure. Anemia, leukopenia, diarrhea, alopecia.
ADULTS — Chemotherapy doses vary by indication. Breast cancer with tumors overexpressing the HER2 NEU protein.
PEDS — Not approved in children.
NOTES — Monitor with ECG, echocardiogram, or MUGA scan. CBCs.
MOA — Trastuzumab is a recombinant DNA-derived humanized monoclonal antibody that selectively binds to the extracellular domain of the human epidermal growth factor receptor 2 protein (HER2) expressed in breast, ovarian, and colon cancers, leading to cell cycle arrest.
ADVERSE EFFECTS — Serious: Anaphylaxis, fatal infusion-related reactions, ARDS, heart failure, bone marrow suppression. Frequent: Fever, chills, N/V, diarrhea, rash.

ONCOLOGY: Mitotic Inhibitors

DOCETAXEL (*Taxotere*) ▶L ♀D ▶– $ varies by therapy
WARNING — Severe hypersensitivity with anaphylaxis, bone marrow suppression, fluid retention, neutropenia, rash, erythema of the extremities, nail hypo- or hyperpigmentation, hepatotoxicity, treatment related mortality, paresthesia/dysesthesia, asthenia, fertility impairment, alopecia. Instruct patients to report promptly fever, sore throat, or signs of local infection.
ADULTS — Chemotherapy doses vary by indication. Breast cancer. Non-small-cell lung cancer. Prostate cancer, in combination with prednisone. Advanced gastric adenocarcinoma with cisplatin and fluorouracil. Squamous cell carcinoma of the head and neck.
PEDS — Not approved in children.
UNAPPROVED ADULTS — Gastric cancer. Melanoma. Non-Hodgkin's lymphoma. Ovarian cancer. Pancreatic cancer. Prostate cancer. Small-cell lung cancer. Soft-tissue sarcoma. Urothelial cancer. Adjuvant and neo-adjuvant breast cancer.
NOTES — Reliable contraception is recommended. Monitor CBCs and LFTs. CYP3A4 inhibitors or substrates may lead to significant increases in blood concentrations.
MOA — Mitotic Inhibitor.
ADVERSE EFFECTS — Serious: Hypersensitivity/anaphylaxis, edema, neutropenia, rash, erythema of the extremities, nail hypo- or hyperpigmentation, hepatotoxicity, paresthesia/dysesthesia. Frequent: Rash, N/V, diarrhea, bone marrow suppression.

IXABEPILONE (*Ixempra*) ▶L ♀D ▶– $ varies by therapy
WARNING — Contraindicated in patients with AST or ALT > 2.5 ULN or bilirubin > 1 times ULN upper limit of normal or higher. Contraindicated in patients with hypersensitivity reactions to products containing Cremophor EL (polyoxyethylated castor oil). Neutropenia. Instruct patients to report promptly fever, sore throat, signs of local infection or anemia. Peripheral neuropathy (sensory and motor) occurs commonly. Dose reductions, delays or discontinuations may be necessary. Usually occurs during the first 3 cycles of treatment.
ADULTS — Chemotherapy doses vary by indication. Metastatic or locally advanced breast cancer.
PEDS — Not approved in children.
FORMS — 15mg and 45mg powder for injection.

(cont.)

IXABEPILONE (cont.)
NOTES — CYP450 inhibitors such as ketoconazole may increase concentration; inducers such as rifampin, phenytoin or carbamazepine may reduce levels Patients should receive an H1 and H2 blocker one hour prior to ixabepilone infusion to minimize hypersensitivity reactions. If patients experience such a reaction, they should also receive a corticosteroid prior to the next dose.
MOA — Mitotic Inhibitor.
ADVERSE EFFECTS — Serious: Anaphylaxis, bone marrow suppression, peripheral neuropathy, MI, ventricular dysfunction. Frequent: Bone marrow suppression, peripheral neuropathy, N/V/D, palmar-plantar erythrodysesthesia syndrome, myalgias.

PACLITAXEL (*Taxol, Abraxane, Onxol*) ▶L ♀D ▶– $ varies by therapy
WARNING — Anaphylaxis, bone marrow suppression, cardiac conduction abnormalities, peripheral neuropathy, fertility impairment, alopecia. Contraindicated in patients with hypersensitivity reactions to products containing Cremophor EL (polyoxyethylated castor oil). Instruct patients to report promptly fever, sore throat, signs of local infection or anemia.
ADULTS — Chemotherapy doses vary by indication. Ovarian cancer. Metastatic breast cancer. Non-small cell lung cancer, in combination regimens. AIDS-related Kaposi's sarcoma.
PEDS — Not approved in children.
UNAPPROVED ADULTS — Advanced head and neck cancer. Small-cell lung cancer. Adenocarcinoma of the upper GI tract. Gastric, esophageal and colon adenocarcinoma. Hormone-refractory prostate cancer. Non-Hodgkin's lymphoma. Transitional cell carcinoma of the urothelium. Adenocarcinoma or unknown primary, adjuvant and neoadjuvant breast cancer, uterine cancer. Pancreatic cancer. Polycystic kidney disease.
NOTES — Abraxane is a form of paclitaxel bound to albumin. Reliable contraception is recommended. Monitor CBCs. Ketoconazole, felodipine, diazepam, and estradiol may increase paclitaxel.
MOA — Mitotic Inhibitor.
ADVERSE EFFECTS — Serious: Anaphylaxis, bone marrow suppression, cardiac conduction abnormalities, peripheral neuropathy. Frequent: Bone marrow suppression, peripheral neuropathy, hypotension, mucositis, N/V.

VINBLASTINE (*Velban, VLB*) ▶L ♀D ▶– $ varies by therapy
WARNING — Extravasation associated with severe necrosis. Leukopenia, fertility impairment, bronchospasm, alopecia. Instruct patients to report promptly fever, sore throat, or signs of local infection.
ADULTS — Chemotherapy doses vary by indication. Hodgkin's disease. Non-Hodgkin's lymphoma. Histiocytic lymphoma. Mycosis fungoides. Advanced testicular carcinoma. Kaposi's sarcoma. Letterer-Siwe disease (histiocytosis X). Choriocarcinoma. Breast cancer.
PEDS — Not approved in children.
UNAPPROVED ADULTS — Non-small-cell lung cancer, renal cancer, CML.
NOTES — Reliable contraception is recommended. May decrease phenytoin levels. Erythromycin/drugs that inhibit CYP450 enzymes may increase toxicity.
MOA — Mitotic Inhibitor.
ADVERSE EFFECTS — Serious: Leukopenia, fertility impairment, bronchospasm. Frequent: Leukopenia, alopecia.

VINCRISTINE (*Oncovin, Vincasar, VCR*) ▶L ♀D ▶– $ varies by therapy
WARNING — Extravasation associated with severe necrosis. CNS toxicity, hypersensitivity, bone marrow suppression, hyperuricemia, bronchospasm, fertility impairment, alopecia. Instruct patients to report promptly fever, sore throat, signs of local infection or anemia.
ADULTS — Chemotherapy doses vary by indication. ALL. Hodgkin's disease. Non-Hodgkin's lymphomas. Rhabdomyosarcoma. Neuroblastoma. Wilms' tumor. All in combination regimens.
PEDS — Chemotherapy doses vary by indication. Acute leukemia. Sarcoma, multiple myeloma.
UNAPPROVED ADULTS — Idiopathic thrombocytopenic purpura. Kaposi's sarcoma. Breast cancer. Bladder cancer.
NOTES — Reliable contraception is recommended. Monitor CBCs. May decrease phenytoin and digoxin levels.
MOA — Mitotic Inhibitor.
ADVERSE EFFECTS — Serious: CNS toxicity, hypersensitivity, bone marrow suppression, uric acid nephropathy, bronchospasm. Frequent: Paresthesias, alopecia.

VINORELBINE (*Navelbine*) ▶L ♀D ▶– $ varies by therapy
WARNING — Extravasation associated with severe necrosis. Granulocytopenia, pulmonary toxicity, bronchospasm, peripheral neuropathy, increased LFTs, alopecia. Instruct patients to report promptly fever, sore throat, or signs of local infection.
ADULTS — Chemotherapy doses vary by indication. Non-small-cell lung cancer, alone or in combination regimens.
PEDS — Not approved in children.
UNAPPROVED ADULTS — Breast cancer. Cervical carcinoma. Desmoid tumors. Kaposi's sarcoma. Ovarian, Hodgkin's disease, head and neck cancer.
NOTES — Reliable contraception is recommended. Monitor CBCs. Drugs that inhibit CYP450 enzymes may increase toxicity.
MOA — Mitotic Inhibitor.
ADVERSE EFFECTS — Serious: Granulocytopenia, pulmonary toxicity, bronchospasm, peripheral neuropathy, ileus. Frequent: Granulocytopenia, alopecia, peripheral neuropathy, N/V.

ONCOLOGY: Platinum-Containing Agents

CARBOPLATIN (*Paraplatin*) ▶K ♀D ▶– $ varies by therapy
WARNING – Secondary malignancies, bone marrow suppression, increased in patients with renal insufficiency; emesis, anaphylaxis, nephrotoxicity, peripheral neuropathy, increased LFTs, alopecia. Instruct patients to report promptly fever, sore throat, signs of local infection, bleeding from any site, symptoms suggestive of anemia, or yellow discoloration of the skin or eyes.
ADULTS – Chemotherapy doses vary by indication. Ovarian carcinoma.
PEDS – Not approved in children.
UNAPPROVED ADULTS – Small cell lung cancer, in combination regimens. Squamous cell carcinoma of the head and neck. Advanced endometrial cancer. Acute leukemia. Seminoma of testicular cancer. Non-small-cell lung cancer. Adenocarcinoma of unknown primary. Cervical cancer. Bladder carcinoma.
NOTES – Reliable contraception is recommended. Monitor CBCs, LFTs and renal function. May decrease phenytoin levels.
MOA – Alkylating agent.
ADVERSE EFFECTS – Serious: Bone marrow suppression, peripheral neuropathy, anaphylaxis, nephrotoxicity. Frequent: Bone marrow suppression, N/V, increased LFTs, alopecia.

CISPLATIN (*Platinol-AQ*) ▶K ♀D ▶– $ varies by therapy
WARNING – Secondary malignancies, nephrotoxicity, bone marrow suppression, N/V, very highly emetogenic, ototoxicity, anaphylaxis, hepatotoxicity, vascular toxicity, hyperuricemia, electrolyte disturbances, optic neuritis, papilledema and cerebral blindness, neuropathies, muscle cramps, alopecia. Amifostine can be used to reduce renal toxicity in patients with advanced ovarian cancer. Instruct patients to report promptly fever, sore throat, signs of local infection, bleeding from any site, symptoms suggestive of anemia, or yellow discoloration of the skin or eyes.
ADULTS – Chemotherapy doses vary by indication. Metastatic testicular and ovarian tumors, bladder cancer.
PEDS – Not approved in children.
UNAPPROVED ADULTS – Esophageal cancer, gastric cancer, non-small-cell lung cancer and small cell lung cancer, head and neck cancer, endometrial cancer, cervical cancer, neoadjuvant bladder sparing chemotherapy, sarcoma.
NOTES – Reliable contraception is recommended. Monitor CBCs, LFTs, renal function and electrolytes. Audiometry. Aminoglycosides potentiate renal toxicity. Decreases phenytoin levels. Patients older than 65 yo may be more susceptible to nephrotoxicity, bone marrow suppression and peripheral neuropathy.
MOA – Alkylating agent.
ADVERSE EFFECTS – Serious: Bone marrow suppression, nephrotoxicity, ototoxicity, anaphylaxis, optic neuritis, papilledema and cerebral blindness, peripheral neuropathy. Frequent: Bone marrow suppression, N/V, nephrotoxicity, ototoxicity, hyperuricemia, muscle cramps.

OXALIPLATIN (*Eloxatin*) ▶LK ♀D ▶– $ varies by therapy
WARNING – Anaphylaxis, neuropathy, pulmonary fibrosis, bone marrow suppression, transient vision loss, N/V/D, fertility impairment. Instruct patients to report promptly fever, sore throat, signs of local infection, bleeding from any site, or symptoms suggestive of anemia.
ADULTS – Chemotherapy doses vary by indication. Colorectal cancer with 5-FU + leucovorin.
PEDS – Not approved in children.
UNAPPROVED ADULTS – Esophageal cancer, gastric cancer, non-Hodgkin's Lymphoma, ovarian cancer, testicular cancer, hepatobiliary cancer, pancreatic cancer.
NOTES – Reliable contraception is recommended. Monitor CBCs and renal function.
MOA – Alkylating agent.
ADVERSE EFFECTS – Serious: Bone marrow suppression, anaphylaxis, neuropathy, pulmonary fibrosis. Frequent: N/V, diarrhea.

ONCOLOGY: Radiopharmaceuticals

SAMARIUM 153 (*Quadramet*) ▶Not metabolized ♀C ▶– $ varies by therapy
WARNING – Bone marrow suppression, flare reactions. Instruct patients to report promptly fever, sore throat, signs of local infection or anemia.
ADULTS – Chemotherapy doses vary by indication. Osteoblastic metastatic bone lesions, relief of pain.
PEDS – Not approved in children.
UNAPPROVED ADULTS – Ankylosing spondylitis. Paget's disease. RA.
NOTES – Reliable contraception is recommended. Monitor CBCs. Radioactivity in excreted urine for 12 h after dose.
MOA – Radiopharmaceutical.
ADVERSE EFFECTS – Serious: Bone marrow suppression, flare reactions. Frequent: Bone marrow suppression, N/V.

STRONTIUM-89 (*Metastron*) ▶K ♀D ▶– $ varies by therapy
WARNING – Bone marrow suppression, flare reactions, flushing sensation. Instruct patients to report promptly fever, sore throat, signs of local infection or anemia.
ADULTS – Chemotherapy doses vary by indication. Painful skeletal metastases, relief of bone pain.
PEDS – Not approved in children.

(cont.)

STRONTIUM-89 (cont.)
NOTES — Reliable contraception is recommended. Monitor CBCs. Radioactivity in excreted urine for 12 h after dose.

MOA — Radiopharmaceutical.
ADVERSE EFFECTS — Serious: Bone marrow suppression, flare reactions, flushing sensation. Frequent: Bone marrow suppression.

ONCOLOGY: Miscellaneous

ARSENIC TRIOXIDE (*Trisenox*) ▶L ♀D ▶– $ varies by therapy
WARNING — APL differentiation syndrome: Fever, dyspnea, wt gain, pulmonary infiltrates and pleural/pericardial effusions, occasionally with impaired myocardial contractility and episodic hypotension, with or without leukocytosis. QT prolongation, AV block, torsade de pointes, N/V/D, hyperglycemia, alopecia.
ADULTS — Chemotherapy doses vary by indication. Acute promyelocytic leukemia, refractory.
PEDS — Not approved in children less than 5 yo. Chemotherapy doses vary by indication. Acute promyelocytic leukemia, refractory.
UNAPPROVED ADULTS — Chemotherapy doses vary by indication. Chronic myeloid leukemia. ALL.
NOTES — Reliable contraception is recommended. Monitor ECG, electrolytes, renal function, CBCs and PT.
MOA — Unknown.
ADVERSE EFFECTS — Serious: APL differentiation syndrome: fever, dyspnea, weight gain, pulmonary infiltrates and pleural/pericardial effusions, with or w/o leukocytosis. QT prolongation, tachycardia, AV block, torsade de pointes, hyperleukocytosis. Frequent: Hypotension, N/V, diarrhea, hyperglycemia, fever, fatigue, dermatitis, nausea, electrolyte abnormalities.

ASPARAGINASE (*Elspar, ✦Kidrolase*) ▶? ♀C ▶– $ varies by therapy
WARNING — Contraindicated with previous/current pancreatitis. Anaphylaxis, bone marrow suppression, bleeding, hyperglycemia, pancreatitis, hepato/nephrotoxicity, alopecia. Instruct patients to report promptly fever, sore throat, signs of local infection, bleeding from any site, or symptoms suggestive of anemia.
ADULTS — Chemotherapy doses vary by indication. ALL, in combination regimens.
PEDS — Chemotherapy doses vary by indication. ALL, in combination regimens.
NOTES — Toxicity greater in children. Monitor CBCs, LFTs, renal function, PT, glucose and amylase. May interfere with interpretation of thyroid function tests.
MOA — Unknown.
ADVERSE EFFECTS — Serious: Anaphylaxis, bone marrow suppression, bleeding, hyperglycemia, pancreatitis, hepato/nephrotoxicity. Frequent: Hepatotoxicity, hypersensitivity, N/V.

BEXAROTENE (*Targretin*) ▶L ♀X ▶– $ varies by therapy
WARNING — Gel: Rash, pruritus, contact dermatitis. Caps: Lipid abnormalities, increased LFTs, pancreatitis, hypothyroidism, leukopenia, cataracts, photosensitivity, alopecia.
ADULTS — Chemotherapy doses vary by indication. Cutaneous T-cell lymphoma.
PEDS — Not approved in children.
FORMS — Trade only: 1% gel (60 g). Caps 75 mg.
NOTES — Gel: Do not use with DEET (insect repellant) or occlusive dressings. Caps: Monitor lipids, LFTs, thyroid function tests, CBCs. Multiple drug interactions; consult product insert for info. Reliable contraception is recommended.
MOA — Unknown.
ADVERSE EFFECTS — Gel- Serious: None. Frequent: Rash, pruritus, contact dermatitis. Caps- Serious: Hyperlipidemia, increased LFTs, pancreatitis, hypothyroidism, leukopenia, cataracts, pseudotumor cerebri. Frequent: Nausea, photosensitivity.

BORTEZOMIB (*Velcade*) ▶L ♀D ▶– $ varies by therapy
WARNING — Peripheral neuropathy, orthostatic hypotension, heart failure, pneumonia, acute respiratory distress syndrome, thrombocytopenia, neutropenia, N/V/D. Instruct patients to report promptly acute onset of dyspnea, cough and low-grade fever and bleeding from any site.
ADULTS — Chemotherapy doses vary by indication. Multiple myeloma, mantle cell lymphoma.
PEDS — Not approved in children.
NOTES — Reliable contraception is recommended. Monitor CBCs.
MOA — Inhibits 26S proteasome.
ADVERSE EFFECTS — Serious: Peripheral neuropathy, thrombocytopenia, neutropenia, orthostatic hypotension, heart failure, pneumonia, acute respiratory distress syndrome. Frequent: Peripheral neuropathy, thrombocytopenia, fatigue, nausea, diarrhea, anorexia, constipation, anemia, rash.

DASATINIB (*Sprycel*) ▶L ♀D ▶– $ varies by therapy
WARNING — Bone marrow suppression, hemorrhage, prolonged QT interval, pleural effusion.
ADULTS — Chemotherapy doses vary by indication. CML. ALL.
PEDS — Not approved in children.
UNAPPROVED ADULTS — Post allogeneic stem cell transplant treatment of CML.
FORMS — Trade only: Tabs 20, 50, 70, 100 mg.
NOTES — Reliable contraception is recommended. Monitor LFTs, CBCs, and wt. Monitor for signs and symptoms of fluid retention. Increased by ketoconazole, erythromycin, itraconazole, clarithromycin, ritonavir, atazanavir, indinavir, nelfinavir, saquinavir and telithromycin. Decreased by rifampin, phenytoin, carbamazepine, phenobarbital and dexamethasone. Increases simvastatin. Antacids

(cont.)

ONCOLOGY: Miscellaneous

DASATINIB (cont.)
should be taken at least 2 h pre or post dose. Avoid H2 blockers and PPIs.
MOA — Protein-tyrosine kinase inhibitor that inhibits the Bcr-Abl tyrosine kinase, the constitutive abnormal tyrosine kinase created by the Philadelphia chromosome abnormality in chronic myeloid leukemia, and the SRC family kinases.
ADVERSE EFFECTS — Serious: Bone marrow suppression, hemorrhage, pleural effusion. Frequent: Bone marrow suppression, N/V, diarrhea, edema.

ERLOTINIB (*Tarceva*) ▶L ♀D ▶– $ varies by therapy
WARNING — Interstitial lung disease, acute renal failure, hepatic failure, GI perforations, exfoliative skin disorders, MI, CVA, microangiopathic hemolytic anemia, corneal perforation.
ADULTS — Chemotherapy doses vary by indication. Non-small-cell lung cancer, pancreatic cancer. Monotherapy for the maintenance treatment of patients with locally advanced or metastatic non-small-cell lung cancer whose disease has not progressed after four cycles of platinum-based first-line chemotherapy.
PEDS — Not approved in children.
FORMS — Trade only: Tabs 25, 100, 150 mg.
NOTES — Reliable contraception is recommended. Hepato-renal syndrome has been reported; monitor LFTs and SCr. CYP3A4 inhibitors such as ketoconazole increase concentrations. CYP3A4 inducers such as rifampin decrease concentrations. Increases INR in patients on warfarin. Monitor LFTs. Avoid concomitant use of erlotinib with H2 blockers and PPIs.
MOA — Inhibits the intracellular phosphorylation of tyrosine kinase associated with epidermal growth factor receptor, which is expressed on the surface of normal cells and cancer cells.
ADVERSE EFFECTS — Serious: Pulmonary toxicity, GI bleeding, acute renal failure due to dehydration, hepatic failure, GI perforations, exfoliative skin disorders, MI, CVA, microangiopathic hemolytic anemia, corneal perforation. Frequent: Diarrhea, anorexia, fatigue, stomatitis, rash, infection, pruritus.

ETOPOSIDE (*VP-16, Etopophos, Toposar, VePesid*) ▶K ♀D ▶– $ varies by therapy
WARNING — Bone marrow suppression, anaphylaxis, hypotension, CNS depression, alopecia. Instruct patients to report promptly fever, sore throat, or signs of local infection.
ADULTS — Chemotherapy doses vary by indication. Testicular cancer. Small cell lung cancer, in combination regimens.
PEDS — Not approved in children.
UNAPPROVED ADULTS — AML. Hodgkin's disease. Non-Hodgkin's lymphomas. Kaposi's sarcoma. Neuroblastoma. Choriocarcinoma. Rhabdomyosarcoma. Hepatocellular carcinoma. Epithelial ovarian, non-small- and small-cell lung, testicular, gastric, endometrial and breast cancers. ALL. Soft tissue sarcoma.
FORMS — Generic/Trade: Caps 50 mg. Injection for hospital/clinic use; not intended for outpatient prescribing.
NOTES — Reliable contraception is recommended. Monitor CBCs, LFTs and renal function. May increase INR with warfarin.
MOA — Mitotic Inhibitor.
ADVERSE EFFECTS — Serious: Bone marrow suppression, anaphylaxis, hypotension, CNS depression. Frequent: Alopecia, bone marrow suppression, N/V, diarrhea.

GEFITINIB (*Iressa*) ▶L ♀D ▶– $ varies by therapy
WARNING — Pulmonary toxicity, corneal erosion, N/V. Instruct patients to report promptly acute onset of dyspnea, cough and low-grade fever.
ADULTS — Chemotherapy doses vary by indication. Non-small-cell lung cancer.
PEDS — Not approved in children.
FORMS — Trade only: Tabs 250 mg.
NOTES — Reliable contraception is recommended. Monitor LFTs. Potent inducers of CYP3A4 (eg, rifampin, phenytoin) decrease concentration; use 500 mg. May increase warfarin effect; monitor INR. Potent inhibitors of CYP3A4 (eg, ketoconazole, itraconazole) increase toxicity. Ranitidine increases concentrations.
MOA — Inhibits phosphorylation of tyrosine kinases.
ADVERSE EFFECTS — Serious: Pulmonary toxicity, corneal erosion. Frequent: Increased LFTs, diarrhea, rash, acne, dry skin, N/V.

IMATINIB (*Gleevec*) ▶L ♀D ▶– $ varies by therapy
WARNING — Bone marrow suppression, increased LFTs, hemorrhage, erythema multiforme, Stevens-Johnson syndrome, N/V, pulmonary edema, CHF, muscle cramps.
ADULTS — Chemotherapy doses vary by indication. CML. GI stromal tumors (GISTs), Ph+ ALL, agressive systemic mastocytosis, dermatofibrosarcoma protuberans, hypereosinophillic syndrome, myelodysplastic/myeloproliferative disease associated with platelet-derived growth factor recptor mutations.
PEDS — Chemotherapy doses vary by indication. CML.
UNAPPROVED ADULTS — Treatment of desmoid tumors, poststem cell transplant follow-up treatment in CML.
FORMS — Trade only: Tabs 100, 400 mg.
NOTES — Reliable contraception is recommended. Monitor LFTs, CBCs, and wt. Monitor for signs and symptoms of fluid retention. Increased by ketoconazole, erythromycin, itraconazole, clarithromycin. Decreased by phenytoin, carbamazepine, rifampin, phenobarbital, St. John's wort. Increases acetaminophen levels and warfarin effects. Monitor INR. Reduce dose with renal insufficiency.
MOA — Imatinib mesylate is a protein-tyrosine kinase inhibitor that inhibits the Bcr-Abl tyrosine kinase, the constitutive abnormal tyrosine kinase created by the Philadelphia chromosome abnormality in chronic myeloid leukemia.

(cont.)

ONCOLOGY: Miscellaneous

IMATINIB (cont.)
ADVERSE EFFECTS — Serious: Bone marrow suppression, hepatotoxicity, hemorrhage, erythema multiforme, Stevens-Johnson syndrome, pulmonary edema, cardiac tamponade, CHF, increased intracranial pressure and papilledema. Frequent: Bone marrow suppression, N/V, diarrhea, edema, muscle cramps, rash, fatigue.

IRINOTECAN (Camptosar) ▶L ♀D ▶– $ varies by therapy
WARNING — Diarrhea and dehydration (may be life-threatening), bone marrow suppression (worse with radiation), orthostatic hypotension, colitis, hypersensitivity, pancreatitis. Instruct patients to report promptly diarrhea, fever, sore throat, signs of local infection, bleeding from any site, or symptoms suggestive of anemia.
ADULTS — Chemotherapy doses vary by indication. Metastatic carcinoma of the colon or rectum, in combination regimens.
PEDS — Not approved in children.
UNAPPROVED ADULTS — Non-small-cell lung cancer and small cell lung cancer, ovarian and cervical cancer.
NOTES — Enzyme-inducing drugs such as phenytoin, phenobarbital, carbamazepine, rifampin, and St John's wort decrease concentrations and possibly effectiveness. Ketoconazole is contraindicated during therapy. Atazanavir increases concentrations. Reliable contraception is recommended. Monitor CBCs. May want to withhold diuretics during active N/V. Avoid laxatives. Loperamide/fluids/electrolytes for diarrhea. Consider atropine for cholinergic symptoms during the infusion. Patients who are homozygous for the UGT1A1*28 allele are at increased risk for neutropenia. Dosage reductions may be necessary.
MOA — Topoisomerase inhibitor.
ADVERSE EFFECTS — Serious: Severe diarrhea, dehydration, bone marrow suppression, orthostatic hypotension, colitis/ileus, hypersensitivity, pancreatitis. Frequent: Diarrhea, bone marrow suppression, alopecia, N/V, rhinitis, salivation, lacrimation, miosis. Also myocardial ischemic events, elevated serum transaminases, hiccups, and megacolon have occurred.

LAPATINIB (Tykerb) ▶L ♀D ▶– $ varies by therapy
WARNING — Hepatotoxicity has been reported with lapatinib. May be severe or fatal. Decreased LVEF, QT prolongation, hepatotoxicity, interstitial lung disease, pneumonitis, severe diarrhea.
ADULTS — Chemotherapy doses vary by indication. Treatment of HER2 overexpressing Advanced or metastatic breast cancer.in combination with capecitabine, in patients who have received prior therapy including an anthracycline, a taxane, and trastuzumab. Also indicated in combination with letrozole for the treatment of postmenopausal women with hormone receptor positive metastatic breast cancer that overexpresses the HER2 receptor for whom hormonal therapy is indicated.
PEDS — Not approved in children.
FORMS — Trade only: Tabs 250 mg.
NOTES — Monitor LFTs, CBCs, and wt. Monitor for signs and symptoms of fluid retention. Increased by ketoconazole, erythromycin, itraconazole, clarithromycin. Decreased by phenytoin, carbamazepine, rifampin, phenobarbital, St. John's wort. Increases acetaminophen levels and warfarin effects. Monitor INR. Reduce dose with renal insufficiency. Reliable contraception is recommended. Modify dose for cardiac and other toxicities, severe hepatic impairment, and CYP3A4 drug interactions.
MOA — Lapatinib is a protein-tyrosine kinase inhibitor that inhibits epidermal growth factor receptor and human epidermal receptor type 2 in breast cancer cell lines.
ADVERSE EFFECTS — Serious: Diarrhea, decreased ejection fraction, QT prolongation, hepatotoxicity, interstitial lung disease, pneumonitis. Frequent: N/V, diarrhea, fatigue, plantar-palmar erythrodysesthesia, rash.

LEUCOVORIN (Wellcovorin, folinic acid) ▶gut ♀C ▶? $ varies by therapy
WARNING — Allergic sensitization.
ADULTS — Doses vary by indication. Reduction of toxicity due to folic acid antagonists (ie, methotrexate). Colorectal cancer with 5-FU. Megaloblastic anemias.
PEDS — Not approved in children.
FORMS — Generic only: Tabs 5, 10, 15, 25 mg. Injection for hospital/oncology clinic use; not intended for outpatient prescribing.
NOTES — Monitor methotrexate concentrations and CBCs.
MOA — Folic acid derivative.
ADVERSE EFFECTS — Serious: Bone marrow suppression (with 5-FU). Frequent: Stomatitis, diarrhea (with 5-FU).

LEVOLEUCOVORIN (Fusilev) ▶gut ♀C ▶? $ varies by therapy
WARNING — Allergic sensitization.
ADULTS — Doses vary by indication. Reduction of toxicity due to high-dose methotrexate for osteosarcoma.
PEDS — Not approved in children.
NOTES — Monitor methotrexate concentrations and CBCs.
MOA — Folic acid derivative.
ADVERSE EFFECTS — Serious: None. Frequent: Vomiting, stomatitis, nausea.

MITOTANE (Lysodren) ▶L ♀C ▶– $ varies by therapy
WARNING — Adrenal insufficiency, depression. Instruct patients to report promptly if N/V, loss of appetite, diarrhea, mental depression, skin rash or darkening of the skin occurs. N/V/D, alopecia.
ADULTS — Chemotherapy doses vary by indication. Adrenal cortical carcinoma, inoperable.
PEDS — Not approved in children.
FORMS — Trade only: Tabs 500 mg.
NOTES — Hold after shock or trauma; give systemic steroids. Behavioral and neurological assessments

(cont.)

ONCOLOGY: Miscellaneous

MITOTANE (cont.)
at regular intervals when continuous treatment more than 2 years. May decrease steroid and warfarin effects. Reliable contraception is recommended.
MOA — Unknown.
ADVERSE EFFECTS — Serious: Adrenal insufficiency, depression. Frequent: Anorexia, N/V, diarrhea.

NILOTINIB (*Tasigna*) ▶L ♀D ▶— $ varies by therapy
WARNING — Prolonged QT interval and sudden death, bone marrow suppression, intracranial hemorrhage, pneumonia, elevated lipase.
ADULTS — Chemotherapy doses vary by indication. Treatment of newly diagnosed adult patients with Philadelphia chromosome positive chronic myeloid leukemia (Ph+ CML in chronic phase. Treatment of chronic phase (CP) and accelerated phase (AP) Ph+ CML in adult patients resistant to or intolerant to prior therapy that included imatinib.
PEDS — Not approved in children.
FORMS — Trade only: Caps 200 mg.
NOTES — Contraindicated with hypokalemia, hypomagnesemia, or long QT syndrome. Reliable contraception is recommended. Monitor EKG, LFTs, CBCs and lipase. Increased by potent CYP450 inhibitors such as ketoconazole and decreased by CYP450 inducers such as rifampin. Avoid food at least 2 h pre dose or 1 h post dose.
MOA — Nilotinib is a protein-tyrosine kinase inhibitor that inhibits the Bcr-Abl tyrosine kinase, the constitutive abnormal tyrosine kinase created by the Philadelphia chromosome abnormality in chronic myeloid leukemia.
ADVERSE EFFECTS — Serious: Bone marrow suppression, intracranial hemorrhage, pneumonia. Frequent: Bone marrow suppression, N/V/D, rash, pruritus.

PAZOPANIB (*Votrient*) ▶L+ ♀D ▶— $$$$$
WARNING — Severe and fatal hepatotoxicty have occurred. Observe LFTs prior to and during treatment. Prolonged QT intervals and torsades de pointes have been observed. Fatal hemorrhagic events have occurred, Arterial thrombotic events have occurred and can be fatal.
ADULTS — 800 mg orally once daily without food. Treatment of advanced renal cell carcinoma.
PEDS — Not indicated in pediatrics.
FORMS — Trade only: Tabs 200 mg.
MOA — Multi-tyrosine kinase inhibitor, including VEGFR-1, VEGFR-2, VEGFR-3, PDGFR-alpha and beta, FGFR-1, FGFR-3, cKIT, Itk, Lck, and c-FMS.
ADVERSE EFFECTS — Diarrhea, hypertension, hair color changes (depigmentation), nausea, anorexia, vomiting.

PEGASPARGASE (*Oncaspar*) ▶? ♀C ▶— $ varies by therapy
WARNING — Contraindicated with previous/current pancreatitis. Hypersensitivity, including anaphylaxis. Bone marrow suppression, bleeding, hyperuricemia, hyperglycemia, hepato/nephrotoxicity, CNS toxicity, N/V/D, alopecia.
ADULTS — Chemotherapy doses vary by indication. ALL, in combination regimens.
PEDS — Chemotherapy doses vary by indication. ALL, in combination regimens.
NOTES — Monitor CBCs, LFTs, renal function, amylase, glucose and PT. Bleeding potentiated with warfarin, heparin, dipyridamole, aspirin or NSAIDs.
MOA — Unknown.
ADVERSE EFFECTS — Serious: Anaphylaxis, bone marrow suppression, bleeding, hyperglycemia, hepato/nephrotoxicity, CNS toxicity. Frequent: N/V, diarrhea, bone marrow suppression, hepatotoxicity.

PORFIMER (*Photofrin*) ▶? ♀C ▶— $ varies by therapy
WARNING — Photosensitivity, ocular sensitivity, chest pain, respiratory distress, constipation.
ADULTS — Chemotherapy doses vary by indication. Esophageal cancer. Endobronchial non-small-cell lung cancer. High-grade dysplasia in Barrett's esophagus. (all with laser therapy).
PEDS — Not approved in children.
NOTES — Avoid concurrent photosensitizing drugs.
MOA — Photosensitizer.
ADVERSE EFFECTS — Serious: Photosensitivity, ocular sensitivity, chest pain, respiratory distress. Frequent: Photosensitivity, ocular sensitivity, constipation.

RASBURICASE (*Elitek, ✦Fasturtec*) ▶L ♀C ▶— $$$$$
WARNING — May cause hypersensitivity reactions including anaphylaxis, hemolysis (G6PD-deficient patients), methemoglobinemia, interference with uric acid measurements.
ADULTS — Uric acid elevation prevention with leukemia, lymphoma, and solid tumor malignancies receiving anticancer therapy: 0.2 mg/kg IV over 30 min daily for up to 5 days.
PEDS — Uric acid elevation prevention in children (1 mo to 17 yo) with leukemia, lymphoma, and solid tumor malignancies receiving anticancer therapy: 0.2 mg/kg IV over 30 min daily for up to 5 days.
NOTES — Safety and efficacy have been established only for one 5-day treatment course. Hydrate IV if at risk for tumor lysis syndrome. Screen for G6PD deficiency in high-risk patients.
MOA — Catalyzes enzymatic oxidation of uric acid into an inactive and soluble metabolite.
ADVERSE EFFECTS — Serious: Anaphylaxis, hemolysis, methemoglobinemia, acute renal failure, arrhythmia, cardiac failure, cardiac arrest, cellulitis, cerebrovascular disorder, chest pain, convulsions, dehydration, ileus, infection, intestinal obstruction, hemorrhage, myocardial infarction, paresthesia, pancytopenia, pneumonia, pulmonary edema, pulmonary hypertension, retinal hemorrhage, rigors, thrombosis, and thrombophlebitis. Frequent: Fever, neutropenia with fever, respiratory distress, sepsis, neutropenia, mucositis, vomiting, nausea, headache, abdominal pain, constipation, diarrhea, rash.

ONCOLOGY: Miscellaneous

ROMIDEPSIN (*Istodax*) ▶L - ♀D ▶–
WARNING – QTc prolongation/ECG changes have been observed. High potential for drug interactions. Pancytopenias.
ADULTS – 14mg/m2 IV Days 1,8 and 15 of a 28 day cycle. Treatment of cutaneous T-cell lymphoma in patients who have received at least one prior systemic therapy.
PEDS – Not approved in pediatrics
FORMS – 10mg injection, powder for reconstitution.
MOA – Histone deacetylase inhibitor. Induces arrest in cell cycle at G1 and G2/M phases.
ADVERSE EFFECTS – ST-T wave changes, hypotension, fatigue, fever, pruritis, hyperglycemia, electrolyte changes, nausea, vomiting, anorexia, pancytopenias, transaminitis, weakness, infection.

SORAFENIB (*Nexavar*) ▶L ♀D ▶– $ varies by therapy
ADULTS – Chemotherapy doses vary by indication. Advanced renal cell carcinoma. Unresectable hepatocellular carcinoma.
PEDS – Not approved in children.
FORMS – Trade only: Tabs 200 mg.
NOTES – Take 1 h before or 2 h after meals for best absorption. Monitor BP. Monitor INR with warfarin. Reliable contraception is recommended. Hepatic impairment may reduce concentrations. Increases docetaxel and doxorubicin.
MOA – Angiogenesis inhibitor.
ADVERSE EFFECTS – Serious: Hemorrhage, myocardial infarction, bone marrow suppression. Frequent: Hand-foot skin reaction and rash, erythema, HTN, hemorrhage, bone marrow suppression, N/V, diarrhea, increased lipase and amylase, mucositis.

SUNITINIB (*Sutent*) ▶L ♀D ▶– $ varies by therapy
WARNING – Decrease in LVEF with possible clinical CHF, adrenal toxicity, serious and fatal GI complications, bone marrow suppression, bleeding, HTN, yellow skin discoloration, depigmentation of hair or skin, thyroid dysfunction.
ADULTS – Chemotherapy doses vary by indication. GI stromal tumors (GIST), advanced renal cell carcinoma.
PEDS – Not approved in children.
UNAPPROVED ADULTS – Treatment of advanced thyroid cancer, treatment of pancreatic neuroendocrine tumors, treatment of non-GIST soft tissue sarcomas.
FORMS – Trade only: Caps 12.5, 25, 50 mg.
NOTES – Reliable contraception is recommended. CYP3A4 inhibitors such as ketoconazole increase concentrations. CYP3A4 inducers such as rifampin and St John's wort can decrease concentrations. Increases INR in patients on warfarin. Monitor CBC.
MOA – Inhibits the intracellular phosphorylation of tyrosine kinase associated with epidermal growth factor receptor, which is expressed on the surface of normal cells and cancer cells.
ADVERSE EFFECTS – Serious: CHF, bone marrow suppression, bleeding, thyroid dysfunction. Frequent: Diarrhea, fatigue, anorexia, stomatitis, vomiting, dyspepsia, yellow skin discoloration, depigmentation of hair or skin.

TENIPOSIDE (*Vumon, VM-26*) ▶K ♀D ▶– $ varies by therapy
WARNING – Bone marrow suppression, anaphylaxis, hypotension, CNS depression, alopecia. Instruct patients to report promptly fever, sore throat, or signs of local infection.
ADULTS – Not approved in adult patients.
PEDS – Chemotherapy doses vary by indication. ALL, refractory, in combination regimens.
NOTES – Reliable contraception is recommended. Monitor CBCs, LFTs and renal function.
MOA – Mitotic Inhibitor.
ADVERSE EFFECTS – Serious: Bone marrow suppression, anaphylaxis, hypotension, CNS depression. Frequent: Mucositis, alopecia, bone marrow suppression, N/V, diarrhea.

TOPOTECAN (*Hycamtin*) ▶Plasma ♀D ▶– $ varies by therapy
WARNING – Bone marrow suppression (primary neutropenia), severe bleeding, interstitial lung disease. Instruct patients to report promptly fever, sore throat, signs of local infection, bleeding from any site, or symptoms suggestive of anemia.
ADULTS – Chemotherapy doses vary by indication. Ovarian and cervical cancer. Small cell lung cancer, relapsed.
PEDS – Not approved in children.
FORMS – Trade only: Caps 0.25, 1 mg. 4mg powder for injection.
NOTES – Reliable contraception is recommended. Monitor CBCs.
MOA – Topoisomerase inhibitor.
ADVERSE EFFECTS – Serious: Bone marrow suppression, severe bleeding. Frequent: Bone marrow suppression, N/V, diarrhea, headache.

TRETINOIN (*Vesanoid*) ▶L ♀D ▶– $ varies by therapy
WARNING – Retinoic acid-APL (RA-APL) syndrome: Fever, dyspnea, wt gain, pulmonary edema, pulmonary infiltrates and pleural/pericardial effusions, occasionally with impaired myocardial contractility and episodic hypotension, with or without leukocytosis. Reversible hypercholesterolemia/hypertriglyceridemia, increased LFTs, alopecia. Contraindicated in parabens-sensitive patients.
ADULTS – Chemotherapy doses vary by indication. Acute promyelocytic leukemia.
PEDS – Not approved in children.
UNAPPROVED PEDS – Acute promyelocytic leukemia. limited data.
FORMS – Generic/Trade: Caps 10 mg.
NOTES – Reliable contraception is recommended. Monitor CBCs, coags, LFTs, triglyceride and cholesterol levels. Ketoconazole increases levels.
MOA – Unknown.
ADVERSE EFFECTS – Serious: APL differentiation syndrome: fever, dyspnea, weight gain, pulmonary infiltrates and pleural/pericardial effusions, with or w/o leukocytosis, pseudotumor cerebri. Frequent: Reversible hyperlipidemia, headache, fever.

OPHTHALMOLOGY: Antiallergy

VORINOSTAT (*Zolinza*) ▶L ♀D ▶– $$$$$
  WARNING – PE/DVT, anemia, thrombocytopenia, QT prolongation.
  ADULTS – Chemotherapy doses vary by indication. Cutaneous T-cell lymphoma.
  PEDS – Not approved in children.
  FORMS – Trade only: Caps 100 mg.
  NOTES – Reliable contraception is recommended. Monitor CBCs, electrolytes, renal function, EKG.
  MOA – Unknown.
  ADVERSE EFFECTS – Serious: PE/DVT, anemia, thrombocytopenia, QT prolongation. Frequent: N/V/D, hyperglycemia, fatigue, chills.

OPHTHALMOLOGY: Antiallergy—Decongestants & Combinations

NOTE: Overuse can cause rebound dilation of blood vessels. Do not administer while wearing soft contact lenses. Wait 10 min after use before inserting contact lenses. On average, each mL of eye drop soln contains approximately 20 gtts. Reserve ointment formulations for bedtime use due to severe vision blurring. Most eye medications can be administered 1 gtt at a time despite common manufacturer recommendations of 1 to 2 gtts concurrently. Even a single gtt is typically more than the eye can hold, and thus a second gtt is wasteful and increases the possibility of systemic toxicity. If 2 gtts of the medication are desired separate single gtts by at least 5 min.

NAPHAZOLINE (*Albalon, All Clear, AK-Con, Naphcon, Clear Eyes*) ▶? ♀C ▶? $
  ADULTS – Ocular vasoconstrictor/decongestant: 1 to 2 gtts qid for up to 3 days.
  PEDS – Not approved for age younger than 6 yo. Give 1 to 2 gtts qid for up to 3 days for age 6 yo or older.
  FORMS – OTC Generic/Trade: Soln 0.012, 0.025% (15, 30 mL). Rx Generic/Trade: 0.1% (15 mL).
  NOTES – Avoid in patients with cardiovascular disease, HTN, narrow-angle glaucoma, children younger than 6 yo.
  MOA – Alpha-adrenergic agonist decongestant.
  ADVERSE EFFECTS – Frequent: Blurred vision, cardiovascular stimulation, dizziness, headache, nervousness, nausea, stinging, mucosal irritation, dryness, rebound dilation.

NAPHCON-A (naphazoline + pheniramine, *Visine-A*) ▶L ♀C ▶? $
  ADULTS – Ocular decongestant: 1 gtt qid prn for up to 3 days.
  PEDS – Not approved for age younger than 6 yo. Use adult dose for age 6 yo or older.
  FORMS – OTC Trade only: Soln 0.025% + 0.3% (15 mL).
  NOTES – Avoid in patients with cardiovascular disease, HTN, narrow-angle glaucoma, age younger than 6 yo.
  MOA – Antihistamine, decongestant.
  ADVERSE EFFECTS – Frequent: Dry mouth, anticholinergic effects, rebound congestion, pupillary dilation, increase in intraocular pressure.

VASOCON-A (naphazoline + antazoline) ▶L ♀C ▶? $
  ADULTS – Ocular decongestant: 1 gtt qid prn for up to 3 days.
  PEDS – Not approved for children younger than 6 yo. Use adult dose for age 6 yo or older.
  FORMS – OTC Trade only: Soln 0.05% + 0.5% (15 mL).
  NOTES – Avoid in patients with cardiovascular disease, HTN, narrow-angle glaucoma, age younger than 6 yo.
  MOA – Decongestant, antihistamine.
  ADVERSE EFFECTS – Frequent: Dry mouth, anticholinergic effects, rebound congestion.

OPHTHALMOLOGY: Antiallergy—Dual Antihistamine & Mast Cell Stabilizer

NOTE: Wait at least 10 to 15 min after use before inserting contact lenses. On average, each mL of eye drop soln contains approximately 20 gtts. Reserve ointment formulations for bedtime use due to severe vision blurring. Most eye medications can be administered 1 gtt at a time despite common manufacturer recommendations of 1 to 2 gtts concurrently. Even a single gtt is typically more than the eye can hold and thus a second gtt is both wasteful and increases the possibility of systemic toxicity. If 2 gtts of the medication are desired separate single gtts by at least 5 min.

AZELASTINE—OPHTHALMIC (*Optivar*) ▶L ♀C ▶? $$$
  ADULTS – Allergic conjunctivitis: 1 gtt bid.
  PEDS – Not approved for age younger than 3 yo. Use adult dose for age 3 yo or older.
  FORMS – Trade only: Soln 0.05% (6 mL).
  MOA – H-1 receptor antagonist, mast cell stabilizer, inhibitor of other mediators of allergic response (eg, leukotrienes).
  ADVERSE EFFECTS – Frequent: Burning, stinging, headache, somnolence, bitter taste.

EPINASTINE (*Elestat*) ▶K ♀C ▶? $$$$
  ADULTS – Allergic conjunctivitis: 1 gtt bid.
  PEDS – Not approved for age younger than 3 yo. Use adult dose for age 3 yo or older.
  FORMS – Trade only: Soln 0.05% (5 mL).
  MOA – H-1 receptor antagonist, mast cell stabilizer.
  ADVERSE EFFECTS – Frequent: Burning, pruritus, hyperemia.

OPHTHALMOLOGY: Antiallergy

KETOTIFEN—OPHTHALMIC (*Alaway, Zaditor*)
▶Minimal absorption ♀C ▶? $
ADULTS — Allergic conjunctivitis: 1 gtt in each eye q 8 to 12 h.
PEDS — Allergic conjunctivitis: 1 gtt in each eye q 8 to 12 h age older than 3 yo.
FORMS — OTC Generic/Trade: Soln 0.025% (5 mL).
MOA — H-1-receptor antagonist and mast cell stabilizer.
ADVERSE EFFECTS — Frequent: Stinging, burning, dry eyes, photophobia.

OLOPATADINE (*Pataday, Patanol*) ▶K ♀C ▶? $$$$
ADULTS — Allergic conjunctivitis: 1 gtt of 0.1% soln in each eye bid (Patanol) or 1 gtt of 0.2% soln in each eye daily (Pataday).
PEDS — Not approved for age younger than 3 yo. Use adult dose for age 3 yo or older.
FORMS — Trade only: Soln 0.1% (5 mL, Patanol), 0.2% (2.5 mL, Pataday).
NOTES — Do not administer while wearing soft contact lenses. Allow 6 to 8 h between doses.
MOA — H-1-receptor antagonist and mast cell stabilizer.
ADVERSE EFFECTS — Ocular: Frequent: Headache.

OPHTHALMOLOGY: Antiallergy—Pure Antihistamines

NOTE: Antihistamines may aggravate dry eye symptoms. Wait 10 min after use before inserting contact lenses. On average, each mL of eye drop soln contains approximately 20 gtts. Reserve ointment formulations for bedtime use due to severe vision blurring. Most eye medications can be administered 1 gtt at a time despite common manufacturer recommendations of 1 to 2 gtts concurrently. Even a single gtt is typically more than the eye can hold and thus a second gtt is both wasteful and increases the possibility of systemic toxicity. If 2 gtts of the medication are desired separate single gtts by at least 5 min.

BEPOTASTINE (*Bepreve*) ▶L (but minimal absorption) - ♀C ▶? $$$
ADULTS — Allergic conjunctivitis: 1 gtt bid.
PEDS — Not studied in children younger than 2 years.
FORMS — Trade only: Soln 1.5% (2.5, 5, 10 mL)
NOTES — Remove contact lenses prior to instillation.
MOA — Direct histamine-1-receptor antagonist.
ADVERSE EFFECTS — Frequent: Mild taste, irritation, headache.

EMEDASTINE (*Emadine*) ▶L ♀B ▶? $$$
ADULTS — Allergic conjunctivitis: 1 gtt daily to qid.
PEDS — Not approved for age younger than 3 yo. Use adult dose for age 3 yo or older.
FORMS — Trade only: Soln 0.05% (5 mL).
MOA — H-1-receptor antagonist.
ADVERSE EFFECTS — Frequent: Headache.

LEVOCABASTINE—OPHTHALMIC (*Livostin*) ▶Minimal absorption ♀C ▶? $$$
ADULTS — Allergic conjunctivitis: 1 gtt daily to qid for 2 weeks.
PEDS — Not approved for age younger than 12 yo. Use adult dose for age 12 yo or older.
FORMS — Trade only: Susp 0.05% (5, 10 mL).
NOTES — Wait 10 min after use before inserting contact lenses.
MOA — H-1-receptor antagonist.
ADVERSE EFFECTS — Frequent: Transient burning, stinging, discomfort.

OPHTHALMOLOGY: Antiallergy—Pure Mast Cell Stabilizers

NOTE: Works best as preventative agent; use continually during at risk season. Wait 10 min after use before inserting contact lenses. On average, each mL of eye drop soln contains approximately 20 gtts. Reserve ointment formulations for bedtime use due to severe vision blurring. Most eye medications can be administered 1 gtt at a time despite common manufacturer recommendations of 1 to 2 gtts concurrently. Even a single gtt is typically more than the eye can hold and thus a second gtt is both wasteful and increases the possibility of systemic toxicity. If 2 gtts of the medication are desired separate single gtts by at least 5 min.

CROMOLYN—OPHTHALMIC (*Crolom, Opticrom*) ▶LK ♀B ▶? $$
ADULTS — Allergic conjunctivitis: 1 to 2 gtts 4 to 6 times per day.
PEDS — Not approved for age younger than 4 yo. Use adult dose for age 4 yo or older.
FORMS — Generic/Trade: Soln 4% (10 mL).
NOTES — Response may take up to 6 weeks.
MOA — Prevents mast cell degranulation and release of histamine, leukotrienes and slow-reacting substance of anaphylaxis.
ADVERSE EFFECTS — Frequent: Conjunctival redness, dryness, irritation, hypersensitivity reactions.

LODOXAMIDE (*Alomide*) ▶K ♀B ▶? $$$
ADULTS — Allergic conjunctivitis: 1 to 2 gtts in each eye qid for up to 3 months.
PEDS — Not approved for age younger than 2 yo. Use adult dose for age 2 yo or older.
FORMS — Trade only: Soln 0.1% (10 mL).
NOTES — Do not administer while wearing soft contact lenses.
MOA — Mast cell stabilizer.
ADVERSE EFFECTS — Frequent: Blurred vision, eye pain, possible corneal erosion.

NEDOCROMIL—OPHTHALMIC (Alocril) ▶L ♀B ▶? $$$
  ADULTS – Allergic conjunctivitis: 1 to 2 gtts in each eye bid.
  PEDS – Children: Allergic conjunctivitis: 1 to 2 gtts bid. Not approved for age younger than 3 yo.
  FORMS – Trade only: Soln 2% (5 mL).
  NOTES – Soln normally appears slightly yellow.
  MOA – Mast cell stabilizer.
  ADVERSE EFFECTS – Frequent: Burning, irritation, stinging, conjunctival redness, photophobia.

PEMIROLAST (Alamast) ▶? ♀C ▶? $$$
  ADULTS – Allergic conjunctivitis: 1 to 2 gtts in each eye qid.
  PEDS – Not approved for age younger than 3 yo. Give 1 to 2 gtts qid for age 3 yo or older.
  FORMS – Trade only: Soln 0.1% (10 mL).
  NOTES – Decreased itching may be seen within a few days, but full effect may require up to 4 weeks.
  MOA – Mast cell stabilizer.
  ADVERSE EFFECTS – Frequent: Headache, rhinitis, cold/flu symptoms.

OPHTHALMOLOGY: Antibacterials—Aminoglycosides

NOTE: On average, each mL of eye drop soln contains approximately 20 gtts. Reserve ointment formulations for bedtime use due to severe vision blurring. Most eye medications can be administered 1 gtt at a time despite common manufacturer recommendations of 1 to 2 gtts concurrently. Even a single gtt is typically more than the eye can hold and thus a second gtt is both wasteful and increases the possibility of systemic toxicity. If 2 gtts of the medication are desired separate single gtts by at least 5 min.

GENTAMICIN—OPHTHALMIC (Garamycin, Genoptic, Gentak, ✦Diogent) ▶K ♀C ▶? $
  ADULTS – Ocular infections: 1 to 2 gtts q 2 to 4 h or ½ inch ribbon of ointment bid to tid.
  PEDS – Not approved in children.
  UNAPPROVED ADULTS – Up to 2 gtts q 1 h have been used for severe infections.
  UNAPPROVED PEDS – Ocular infections: 1 to 2 gtts q 4 h or ½ inch ribbon of ointment bid to tid.
  FORMS – Generic/Trade: Soln 0.3% (5, 15 mL) Ointment 0.3% (3.5 g tube).
  NOTES – For severe infections, use up to 2 gtts every h.
  MOA – Inhibits RNA-dependent bacterial protein synthesis.
  ADVERSE EFFECTS – Frequent: Edema, rash, pruritus, ocular irritation.

TOBRAMYCIN—OPHTHALMIC (Tobrex) ▶K ♀B ▶– $
  ADULTS – Ocular infections, mild to moderate: 1 to 2 gtts q 4 h or ½ inch ribbon of ointment bid to tid. Ocular infections, severe: 2 gtts q 1 h, then taper to q 4 h or ½ inch ribbon of ointment q 3 to 4 h, then taper to bid to tid.
  PEDS – 1 to 2 gtts q 1 to 4 h or ½ inch ribbon of ointment q 3 to 4 h or bid to tid for age 2 mo or older.
  UNAPPROVED PEDS – Ocular infections: 1 to 2 gtts q 4 h or ½ inch ribbon of ointment bid to tid.
  FORMS – Generic/Trade: Soln 0.3% (5 mL). Trade only: Ointment 0.3% (3.5 g tube).
  MOA – Inhibits RNA-dependent bacterial protein synthesis.
  ADVERSE EFFECTS – Frequent: Edema, rash, pruritus, ocular irritation.

OPHTHALMOLOGY: Antibacterials—Fluoroquinolones

NOTE: Avoid the overuse of fluoroquinolones for conjunctivitis. Ocular administration has not been shown to cause arthropathy. On average, each mL of eye drop soln contains approximately 20 gtts. Reserve ointment formulations for bedtime use due to severe vision blurring. Most eye medications can be administered 1 gtt at a time despite common manufacturer recommendations of 1 to 2 gtts concurrently. Even a single gtt is typically more than the eye can hold and thus a second gtt is both wasteful and increases the possibility of systemic toxicity. If 2 gtts of the medication are desired separate single gtts by at least 5 min.

BESIFLOXACIN (Besivance) ▶LK ♀C ▶? ?
  ADULTS – 1 gtt tid for 7 days.
  PEDS – Not approved for age less than 1 yo. Use adult dose for age 1 yo or older (solution).
  FORMS – Trade: solution 0.6% (5 mL).
  NOTES – Do not wear contacts during use.
  MOA – Inhibits DNA-gyrase in susceptible bacteria.
  ADVERSE EFFECTS – Frequent: Blurred vision, eye pain, eye irritation, eye pruritus and headache.

CIPROFLOXACIN—OPHTHALMIC (Ciloxan) ▶LK ♀C ▶? $$
  ADULTS – Corneal ulcers/ keratitis: 2 gtts q 15 min for 6 h, then 2 gtts q 30 min for 1 day; then, 2 gtts q 1 h for 1 day, and 2 gtts q 4 h for 3 to 14 days. Bacterial conjunctivitis: 1 to 2 gtts q 2 h while awake for 2 days, then 1 to 2 gtts q 4 h while awake for 5 days; or ½ inch ribbon ointment tid for 2 days, then ½ inch ribbon bid for 5 days.
  PEDS – Bacterial conjunctivitis: Use adult dose for age 1 yo or older (soln) and age 2 yo or older (ointment). Not approved below these ages.
  FORMS – Generic/Trade: Soln 0.3% (2.5, 5, 10 mL). Trade only: Ointment 0.3% (3.5 g tube).
  NOTES – May cause white precipitate of active drug at site of epithelial defect that may be confused with a worsening infection. Resolves within 2 weeks and does not necessitate discontinuation.
  MOA – Inhibits DNA-gyrase in susceptible bacteria.
  ADVERSE EFFECTS – Frequent: Headache, eye discomfort, keratopathy, burning sensation. Severe: Hypersensitivity.

OPHTHALMOLOGY: Antibacterials

GATIFLOXACIN—OPHTHALMIC (*Zymaxid*) ▶K ♀C ▶? $$$
ADULTS — Bacterial conjunctivitis: 1 to 2 gtts q 2 h while awake (up to 8 times per day on days 1 and 2), then 1 to 2 gtts q 4 h (up to 4 times per day on days 3 thru 7).
PEDS — Older than 1 yo: Adult dose. Younger than 1 yo: Not approved.
FORMS — Trade only: Soln 0.3% (5 mL).
MOA — Inhibits DNA-gyrase and topoisomerase IV in susceptible bacteria.
ADVERSE EFFECTS — Frequent: Conjunctival irritation, increased lacrimation, keratitis, papillary conjunctivitis.

LEVOFLOXACIN—OPHTHALMIC (*Iquix, Quixin*) ▶KL ♀C ▶? $$$
ADULTS — Bacterial conjunctivitis, Quixin: 1 to 2 gtts q 2 h while awake (up to 8 times per day) on days 1 and 2, then 1 to 2 gtts q 4 h (up to 4 times per day) on days 3 to 7. Bacterial conjunctivitis, Iquix: 1 to 2 gtts q 30 min to 2 h while awake and q 4 to 6 h overnight on days 1 to 3, then 1 to 2 gtts q 1 to 4 h while awake on days 4 to completion of therapy.
PEDS — Bacterial conjunctivitis, Quixin: 1 to 2 gtts q 2 h while awake (up to 8 times per day) on days 1 and 2, then 1 to 2 gtts q 4 h (up to 4 times/day) on days 3 to 7 for age older than 1 yo only. Bacterial conjunctivitis, Iquix: 1 to 2 gtts q 30 min to 2 h while awake and q 4 to 6 h overnight on days 1 to 3, then 1 to 2 gtts q 1 to 4 h while awake on days 4 to completion of therapy for age older than 6 yo only.
FORMS — Trade only: Soln 0.5% (Quixin, 5 mL), 1.5% (Iquix, 5 mL).
MOA — Inhibits DNA-gyrase in susceptible bacteria.
ADVERSE EFFECTS — Frequent: Headache, decreased vision, fever, burning, pharyngitis, photophobia. Severe: Hypersensitivity.

MOXIFLOXACIN—OPHTHALMIC (*Vigamox*) ▶LK ♀C ▶? $$$
ADULTS — Bacterial conjunctivitis: 1 gtt tid for 7 days.
PEDS — Use adult dose for age 1 yo or older, not approved for age younger than 1 yo.
FORMS — Trade only: Soln 0.5% (3 mL).
MOA — Inhibits DNA-gyrase and topoisomerase IV in susceptible bacteria.
ADVERSE EFFECTS — Frequent: Conjunctival irritation, dry eye, ocular discomfort/pain/pruritus, increased lacrimation, keratitis, conjunctivitis.

OFLOXACIN—OPHTHALMIC (*Ocuflox*) ▶LK ♀C ▶? $$
ADULTS — Corneal ulcers/keratitis: 1 to 2 gtts q 30 min while awake and 1 to 2 gtts 4 to 6 h after retiring for 2 days, then 1 to 2 gtts q 1 h while awake for 5 days, then 1 to 2 gtts qid for 3 days. Bacterial conjunctivitis: 1 to 2 gtts q 2 to 4 h for 2 days, then 1 to 2 gtts qid for 5 days.
PEDS — Bacterial conjunctivitis: Use adult dose for age 1 yo or older, not approved age younger than 1 yo.
FORMS — Generic/Trade: Soln 0.3% (5, 10 mL).
MOA — Inhibits DNA-gyrase in susceptible bacteria.
ADVERSE EFFECTS — Frequent: Ocular burning, eye discomfort. Severe: Chemical conjunctivitis/keratitis, ocular/facial edema, hypersensitivity reaction.

OPHTHALMOLOGY: Antibacterials—Other

NOTE: On average, each mL of eye drop soln contains approximately 20 gtts. Reserve ointment formulations for bedtime use due to severe vision blurring. Most eye medications can be administered 1 gtt at a time despite common manufacturer recommendations of 1 to 2 gtts concurrently. Even a single gtt is typically more than the eye can hold and thus a second gtt is both wasteful and increases the possibility of systemic toxicity. If 2 gtts of the medication are desired separate single gtts by at least 5 min.

AZITHROMYCIN—OPHTHALMIC (*Azasite*) ▶L ♀B ▶? $$$
ADULTS — Ocular infections: 1 gtt bid for 2 days, then 1 gtt daily for 5 more days.
PEDS — Ocular infections: 1 gtt bid for 2 days, then 1 gtt daily for 5 more days for age 1 yo or older.
FORMS — Trade only: Soln 1% (2.5 mL).
MOA — Inhibits RNA-dependent protein synthesis.
ADVERSE EFFECTS — Frequent: Eye irritation.

BACITRACIN—OPHTHALMIC (*AK Tracin*) ▶Minimal absorption ♀C ▶? $
ADULTS — Ocular infections: Apply ¼ to ½ inch ribbon of ointment q 3 to 4 h or bid to qid for 7 to 10 days.
PEDS — Not approved in children.
UNAPPROVED PEDS — Ocular infections: Apply ½ inch ribbon of ointment q 3 to 4 h or bid to qid for 7 to 10 days.
FORMS — Generic/Trade: Ointment 500 units/g (3.5 g tube).
MOA — Inhibits bacterial cell wall synthesis.
ADVERSE EFFECTS — Frequent: Edema of face, pain, rash, pruritus.

ERYTHROMYCIN—OPHTHALMIC (*Ilotycin, AK-Mycin*) ▶L ♀B ▶+ $
ADULTS — Ocular infections, corneal ulceration: ½ inch ribbon of ointment q 3 to 4 h or 2 to 6 times per day. For chlamydial infections: bid for 2 months or bid for the first 5 days of each month for 6 months.
PEDS — Ophthalmia neonatorum prophylaxis: ½ inch ribbon to both eyes within 1 h of birth.
FORMS — Generic only: Ointment 0.5% (1, 3.5 g tube).
MOA — Inhibits RNA-dependent protein synthesis.
ADVERSE EFFECTS — Frequent: None.

OPHTHALMOLOGY: Antibacterials

Visual Acuity Screen

```
96          20/800
873         20/400
2843   OXX  20/200
63852  XOO  20/100
87459  OXO  20/70
63925  XOX  20/50
42836 5 OXO 20/40
37425 8 XXO 20/30
9 37 8 2 6 XOO 20/25
```

Hold card in good light 14 inches from eye. Record vision for each eye separately with and without glasses. Presbyopic patients should read through bifocal glasses. Myopic patients should wear glasses only.

Pupil Diameter (mm)

. ② ③ ④ ⑤ ⑥ ⑦ ⑧ ⑨

FUSIDIC ACID—OPHTHALMIC (✦*Fucithalmic*) ▶L ♀? ▶? $
- ADULTS — Canada only. <u>Eye infections:</u> 1 gtt in both eyes q 12 h for 7 days.
- PEDS — Canada only. <u>Eye infections:</u> 1 gtt in both eyes q 12 h for 7 days for age 2 yo or older.
- FORMS — Canada trade only: gtts 1%. Multidose tubes of 3, 5 g. Single-dose preservative-free tubes of 0.2 g in a box of 12.
- MOA — Antibacterial, interferes with bacterial protein synthesis.
- ADVERSE EFFECTS — Frequent: Stinging, irritation. Severe: Hypersensitivity.

NEOSPORIN OINTMENT—OPHTHALMIC (neomycin + bacitracin + polymyxin) ▶K ♀C ▶? $
- ADULTS — <u>Ocular infections:</u> ½ inch ribbon of ointment q 3 to 4 h for 7 to 10 days or ½ inch ribbon 2 to 3 times per day for mild–moderate infection.
- PEDS — Not approved in children.
- UNAPPROVED PEDS — ½ inch ribbon of ointment q 3 to 4 h for 7 to 10 days.
- FORMS — Generic only: Ointment. (3.5 g tube).
- NOTES — Contact dermatitis can occur after prolonged use.
- MOA — Inhibits RNA-dependent protein synthesis and interferes with cell wall membranes.
- ADVERSE EFFECTS — Frequent: Topical hypersensitivity, contact dermatitis.

NEOSPORIN SOLUTION—OPHTHALMIC (neomycin + polymyxin + gramicidin) ▶KL ♀C ▶? $$
- ADULTS — <u>Ocular infections:</u> 1 to 2 gtts q 4 to 6 h for 7 to 10 days.
- PEDS — Not approved in children.
- UNAPPROVED PEDS — 1 to 2 gtts q 4 to 6 h for 7 to 10 days.
- FORMS — Generic/Trade: Soln (10 mL).
- NOTES — Contact dermatitis can occur after prolonged use.
- MOA — Inhibits RNA-dependent protein synthesis and interferes with cell wall membranes.
- ADVERSE EFFECTS — Frequent: Topical hypersensitivity, contact dermatitis, eye irritation, burning, stinging, edema, pruritus, failure to heal.

POLYSPORIN—OPHTHALMIC (polymyxin + bacitracin) ▶K ♀C ▶? $$
- ADULTS — <u>Ocular infections:</u> ½ inch ribbon of ointment q 3 to 4 h for 7 to 10 days or ½ inch ribbon bid to tid for mild–moderate infection.
- PEDS — Not approved in children.
- UNAPPROVED PEDS — <u>Ocular infections:</u> ½ inch ribbon of ointment q 3 to 4 h for 7 to 10 days.
- FORMS — Generic only: Ointment (3.5 g tube).
- MOA — Inhibits synthesis of and interferes with bacterial cell wall membranes.
- ADVERSE EFFECTS — Frequent: None.

POLYTRIM—OPHTHALMIC (polymyxin + trimethoprim) ▶KL ♀C ▶? $
ADULTS — Ocular infections: 1 to 2 gtts q 4 to 6 h (up to 6 gtts/day) for 7 to 10 days.
PEDS — Not approved age younger than 2 mo. Use adult dose for age 2 mo or older.
FORMS — Generic/Trade: Soln (10 mL).
MOA — Interferes with bacterial cell wall membranes, folate reduction.
ADVERSE EFFECTS — Frequent: None.

SULFACETAMIDE—OPHTHALMIC (*Bleph-10, Sulf-10*) ▶K ♀C ▶– $
ADULTS — Ocular infections, corneal ulceration: 1 to 2 gtts q 2 to 3 h initially, then taper by decreasing frequency as condition allows over 7 to 10 days or ½ inch ribbon of ointment q 3 to 4 h initially, then taper 7 to 10 days. Trachoma: 2 gtts q 2 h with systemic antibiotic such as doxycycline or azithromycin.
PEDS — Not approved age younger than 2 mo. Use adult dose for age 2 mo or older.
FORMS — Generic/Trade: Soln 10% (15 mL), ointment 10% (3.5 g tube). Generic only: Soln 30% (15 mL).
NOTES — Ointment may be used as an adjunct to soln.
MOA — Inhibits bacterial folic acid synthesis.
ADVERSE EFFECTS — Frequent: Irritation, stinging, burning. Severe: Stevens-Johnson syndrome, toxic epidermal necrolysis, hypersensitivity.

OPHTHALMOLOGY: Antiviral Agents

GANCICLOVIR (*Zirgan*) ▶Minimal absorption ♀C ▶? $$$$
ADULTS — Herpetic keratitis: 1 gtt 5 times per day (approximately q 3 h) until ulcer heals, then 1 gtt 3 times a day for 7 days.
PEDS — Not approved in children younger than 2 years. 2 years and older: Use adult dosing.
FORMS — Trade only: Gel 0.15% (5g).
NOTES — Do not wear contact lenses.
MOA — Inhibits DNA replication.
ADVERSE EFFECTS — Frequent: Blurred vision, eye irritation, punctate keratitis, conjunctival hyperemia.

TRIFLURIDINE (*Viroptic*) ▶Minimal absorption ♀C ▶– $$$
ADULTS — HSV keratitis: 1 gtt q 2 h to maximum 9 gtts per days. After re-epithelialization, decrease dose to 1 gtt q 4 to 6 h while awake for 7 to 14 days. Maximum of 21 days of treatment.
PEDS — Not approved age younger than 6 yo. Use adult dose for age 6 yo or older.
FORMS — Generic/Trade Soln 1% (7.5 mL).
NOTES — Avoid continuous use more than 21 days; may cause keratitis and conjunctival scarring. Urge frequent use of topical lubricants (ie, tear substitutes) to minimize surface damage.
MOA — Inhibits viral DNA replication as thymidine analog.
ADVERSE EFFECTS — Frequent: Burning, stinging.

OPHTHALMOLOGY: Corticosteroid & Antibacterial Combinations

NOTE: Recommend that only ophthalmologists or optometrists prescribe due to infection, cataract, corneal/scleral perforation, and glaucoma risk from prolonged use. Monitor intraocular pressure. Gradually taper when discontinuing. Shake suspensions well before using. On average, each mL of eye drop soln contains approximately 20 gtts. Reserve ointment formulations for bedtime use due to severe vision blurring. Most eye medications can be administered 1 gtt at a time despite common manufacturer recommendations of 1 to 2 gtts concurrently. Even a single gtt is typically more than the eye can hold and thus a second gtt is both wasteful and increases the possibility of systemic toxicity. If 2 gtts of the medication are desired separate single gtts by at least 5 min.

BLEPHAMIDE (prednisolone - ophthalmic + sulfacetamide) ▶KL ♀C ▶? $
ADULTS — Steroid-responsive inflammatory condition with bacterial infection or risk of bacterial infection: Start 1 to 2 gtts q 1 h during the days and q 2 h during the night, then 1 gtt q 4 to 8 h; or ½ inch ribbon to lower conjunctival sac 3 to 4 times/day and 1 to 2 times at night.
PEDS — Not approved in children.
FORMS — Generic/Trade: Soln/Susp (5, 10 mL), Trade only: Ointment (3.5 g tube).
MOA — Inhibits bacterial folic acid synthesis, anti-inflammatory.
ADVERSE EFFECTS — Frequent: Insomnia, nervousness, increased appetite, indigestion, local irritation, burning, stinging. Severe: Cataracts, secondary ocular infections, glaucoma, Stevens-Johnson syndrome, toxic epidermal necrolysis, hypersensitivity.

CORTISPORIN—OPHTHALMIC (neomycin + polymyxin + hydrocortisone - ophthalmic) ▶LK ♀C ▶? $
ADULTS — Steroid-responsive inflammatory condition with bacterial infection or risk of bacterial infection: 1 to 2 gtts or ½ inch ribbon of ointment q 3 to 4 h or more frequently prn.
PEDS — Not approved in children.
UNAPPROVED PEDS — 1 to 2 gtts or ½ inch ribbon of ointment q 3 to 4 h.
FORMS — Generic only: Susp (7.5 mL). Ointment (3.5 g tube).
MOA — Inhibits RNA-dependent protein synthesis, interferes with bacterial cell wall membranes, anti-inflammatory.

(cont.)

OPHTHALMOLOGY: Corticosteroid & Antibacterial Combinations

CORTISPORIN—OPHTHALMIC (cont.)
  ADVERSE EFFECTS — Frequent: None. Severe: Cataracts, secondary ocular infections, glaucoma, Stevens-Johnson syndrome, toxic epidermal necrolysis, hypersensitivity.

FML-S LIQUIFILM (prednisolone - ophthalmic + sulfacetamide) ▶KL ♀C ▶? $$
  ADULTS — Steroid-responsive inflammatory condition with bacterial infection or risk of bacterial infection: Start 1 to 2 gtts q 1 h during the days and q 2 h during the night, then 1 gtt q 4 to 8 h; or ½ inch ribbon (ointment) tid to qid initially, then daily to bid thereafter.
  PEDS — Not approved in children.
  FORMS — Trade only: Susp (10 mL).
  MOA — Anti-inflammatory.
  ADVERSE EFFECTS — Frequent: Insomnia, nervousness, increased appetite, indigestion, local irritation, burning, stinging. Severe: Cataracts, secondary ocular infections, glaucoma, Stevens-Johnson syndrome, toxic epidermal necrolysis, hypersensitivity.

MAXITROL (dexamethasone - ophthalmic + neomycin + polymyxin) ▶KL ♀C ▶? $
  ADULTS — Steroid-responsive inflammatory condition with bacterial infection or risk of bacterial infection: Ointment: Place a small amount (about ½ inch) in the affected eye 3 to 4 times per day or apply at bedtime as an adjunct with gtts. Susp: Instill 1 to 2 gtts into affected eye(s) every 3 to 4 h; in severe disease, gtts may be used hourly and tapered to discontinuation.
  PEDS — Not approved in children.
  FORMS — Generic/Trade: Susp (5 mL), ointment (3.5 g tube).
  MOA — Inhibits RNA-dependent protein synthesis, interferes with bacterial cell wall membranes, anti-inflammatory.
  ADVERSE EFFECTS — Frequent: None. Severe: Cataracts, secondary ocular infections, glaucoma, Stevens-Johnson syndrome, toxic epidermal necrolysis, hypersensitivity.

PRED G (prednisolone - ophthalmic + gentamicin) ▶KL ♀C ▶? $$
  ADULTS — Steroid-responsive inflammatory condition with bacterial infection or risk of bacterial infection: Start 1 to 2 gtts q 1 h during the days and q 2 h during the night, then 1 gtt q 4 to 8 h or ½ inch ribbon of ointment bid to qid.
  PEDS — Not approved in children.
  FORMS — Trade only: Susp (2, 5, 10 mL), ointment (3.5 g tube).
  MOA — Inhibits RNA-dependent protein synthesis, anti-inflammatory.
  ADVERSE EFFECTS — Frequent: None. Severe: Cataracts, secondary ocular infections, glaucoma, Stevens-Johnson syndrome, toxic epidermal necrolysis, hypersensitivity.

TOBRADEX (tobramycin + dexamethasone - ophthalmic) ▶L ♀C ▶? $$$
  ADULTS — Steroid-responsive inflammatory condition with bacterial infection or risk of bacterial infection: 1 to 2 gtts q 2 h for 1 to 2 days, then 1 to 2 gtts q 4 to 6 h; or ½ inch ribbon of ointment bid to qid.
  PEDS — 1 to 2 gtts q 2 h for 1 to 2 days, then 1 to 2 gtts q 4 to 6 h; or ½ inch ribbon of ointment bid to qid for age 2 yo or older.
  FORMS — Trade only (tobramycin 0.3%/dexamethasone 0.1%): Susp (2.5, 5, 10 mL), ointment (3.5 g tube).
  MOA — Inhibits RNA-dependent protein synthesis, anti-inflammatory.
  ADVERSE EFFECTS — Frequent: Eyelid itching, swelling, conjunctival erythema. Severe: Cataracts, secondary ocular infections, glaucoma.

TOBRADEX ST (tobramycin + dexamethasone - ophthalmic) ▶L ♀C ▶? $$$
  ADULTS — Steroid-responsive inflammatory condition with bacterial infection or risk of bacterial infection: 1 gtt q 2 h for 1 to 2 days, then 1 gtt q 4 to 6 h.
  PEDS — 2 yo or older: 1 gtt q 2 h for 1 to 2 days, then 1 gtt q 4 to 6 h.
  FORMS — Trade only: Tobramycin 0.3%/dexamethasone 0.05%: Susp (2.5, 5, 10 mL).
  MOA — Inhibits RNA-dependent protein synthesis, anti-inflammatory.
  ADVERSE EFFECTS — Frequent: Eyelid itching, swelling, conjunctival erythema. Severe: Cataracts, secondary ocular infections, glaucoma.

VASOCIDIN (prednisolone - ophthalmic + sulfacetamide) ▶KL ♀C ▶? $
  ADULTS — Steroid-responsive inflammatory condition with bacterial infection or risk of bacterial infection: Start 1 to 2 gtts q 1 h during the days and q 2 h during the night, then 1 gtt q 4 to 8 h; or ½ inch ribbon (ointment) tid to qid initially, then daily to bid thereafter.
  PEDS — Not approved in children.
  FORMS — Generic only: Soln (5, 10 mL).
  MOA — Inhibits bacterial folic acid synthesis, anti-inflammatory.
  ADVERSE EFFECTS — Frequent: Insomnia, nervousness, increased appetite, indigestion, local irritation, burning, stinging. Severe: Cataracts, secondary ocular infections, Stevens-Johnson syndrome, toxic epidermal necrolysis, hypersensitivity.

ZYLET (loteprednol + tobramycin) ▶LK ♀C ▶? $$$
  ADULTS — 1 to 2 gtts q 1 to 2 h for 1 to 2 days then 1 to 2 gtts q 4 to 6 h.
  PEDS — Not approved in children.
  FORMS — Trade only: Susp 0.5% loteprednol + 0.3% tobramycin (2.5, 5, 10 mL).
  MOA — Anti-inflammatory (loteprednol) and inhibits RNA-dependent bacterial protein synthesis (tobramycin).
  ADVERSE EFFECTS — Frequent: Injection, superficial punctate keratitis, ocular burning and stinging, headache. Severe: Cataracts, secondary ocular infections, glaucoma.

OPHTHALMOLOGY: Corticosteroids

NOTE: Recommend that only ophthalmologists or optometrists prescribe due to infection, cataract, corneal/scleral perforation, and glaucoma risk. Monitor intraocular pressure. Gradually taper when discontinuing. Shake susp well before using. On average, each mL of eye drop soln contains approximately 20 gtts. Reserve ointment formulations for bedtime use due to severe vision blurring. Most eye medications can be administered 1 gtt at a time despite common manufacturer recommendations of 1 to 2 gtts concurrently. Even a single gtt is typically more than the eye can hold and thus a second gtt is both wasteful and increases the possibility of systemic toxicity. If 2 gtts of the medication are desired separate single gtts by at least 5 min.

DIFLUPREDNATE (*Durezol*) ▶Not absorbed ♀C ▶? $$$$
ADULTS — 1 gtt into affected eye qid, beginning 24 h after surgery for 2 weeks, then 1 gtt into affected eye bid for 1 week, then taper based on response.
PEDS — Not approved in children.
FORMS — Trade only: Ophthalmic emulsion 0.05% (2.5, 5 mL).
NOTES — If used for more than 10 days, monitor IOP.
MOA — Anti-inflammatory.
ADVERSE EFFECTS — Frequent: Corneal edema, ciliary and conjunctival hyperemia, pain, photophobia, posterior capsule opacification, blepharitis. Severe: Cataracts, secondary ocular infections, glaucoma.

FLUOROMETHOLONE (*FML, FML Forte, Flarex*) ▶L ♀C ▶? $$
ADULTS — 1 to 2 gtts q 1 to 2 h or ½ inch ribbon of ointment q 4 h for 1 to 2 days, then 1 to 2 gtts bid to qid or ½ inch of ointment daily to tid.
PEDS — Not approved age younger than 2 yo. Use adult dose for age 2 yo or older.
FORMS — Trade only: Susp 0.1% (5, 10, 15 mL), 0.25% (2, 5, 10, 15 mL); Ointment 0.1% (3.5 g tube).
NOTES — Fluorometholone acetate (Flarex) is more potent than fluorometholone (FML, FML Forte). Use caution in glaucoma.
MOA — Anti-inflammatory.
ADVERSE EFFECTS — Frequent: Burning, blurred vision. Severe: Cataracts, secondary ocular infections, glaucoma.

LOTEPREDNOL (*Alrex, Lotemax*) ▶L ♀C ▶? $$$
ADULTS — 1 to 2 gtts qid, may increase to 1 gtt q 1 h during first weeks of therapy prn. Post-op inflammation: 1 to 2 gtts qid.
PEDS — Not approved in children.
FORMS — Trade only: Susp 0.2% (Alrex 5, 10 mL), 0.5% (Lotemax 2.5, 5, 10, 15 mL).
MOA — Anti-inflammatory.
ADVERSE EFFECTS — Frequent: Headache, rhinitis, pharyngitis, blurring of vision, chemosis, dry eyes, pruritus. Severe: Cataracts, secondary ocular infections, glaucoma.

PREDNISOLONE—OPHTHALMIC (*Pred Forte, Pred Mild, Inflamase Forte, Econopred Plus, ✦AK Tate, Diopred*) ▶L ♀C ▶? $$
ADULTS — Soln: 1 to 2 gtts (up to q 1 h during day and q 2 h at night), when response observed, then 1 gtt q 4 h, then 1 gtt tid to qid. Susp: 1 to 2 gtts bid to qid.
PEDS — Not approved in children.
FORMS — Generic/Trade: Soln, Susp 1% (5, 10, 15 mL). Trade only (Pred Mild): Susp 0.12% (5, 10 mL), Susp (Pred Forte) 1% (1 mL).
NOTES — Prednisolone acetate (Pred Mild, Pred Forte) is more potent than prednisolone sodium phosphate (AK-Pred, Inflamase Forte).
MOA — Anti-inflammatory.
ADVERSE EFFECTS — Frequent: Insomnia, nervousness, indigestion, increased appetite, hirsutism, diabetes mellitus. Severe: Cataracts, secondary ocular infections, glaucoma.

RIMEXOLONE (*Vexol*) ▶L ♀C ▶? $$
ADULTS — Post-op inflammation: 1 to 2 gtts qid for 2 weeks. Uveitis: 1 to 2 gtts q 1 h while awake for 1 week, then 1 gtt q 2 h while awake for 1 week, then taper.
PEDS — Not approved in children.
FORMS — Trade only: Susp 1% (5, 10 mL).
NOTES — Prolonged use associated with corneal/scleral perforation and cataracts.
MOA — Anti-inflammatory.
ADVERSE EFFECTS — Frequent: Blurred vision. Severe: Cataracts, secondary ocular infections, glaucoma.

OPHTHALMOLOGY: Glaucoma Agents—Beta-Blockers

NOTE: May be absorbed and cause side effects and drug interactions associated with systemic beta-blocker therapy. Use caution in cardiac conditions and asthma. Advise patients to apply gentle pressure over nasolacrimal duct for 5 min after instillation to minimize systemic absorption. On average, each mL of eye drop soln contains approximately 20 gtts. Reserve ointment formulations for bedtime use due to severe vision blurring. Most eye medications can be administered 1 gtt at a time despite common manufacturer recommendations of 1 to 2 gtts concurrently. Even a single gtt is typically more than the eye can hold and thus a second gtt is both wasteful and increases the possibility of systemic toxicity. If 2 gtts of the medication are desired separate single gtts by at least 5 min.

BETAXOLOL—OPHTHALMIC (*Betoptic, Betoptic S*) ▶LK ♀C ▶? $$
ADULTS — Chronic open angle glaucoma or ocular HTN: 1 to 2 gtts bid.
PEDS — Chronic open angle glaucoma or ocular HTN: 1 to 2 gtts bid.
FORMS — Trade only: Susp 0.25% (5, 10, 15 mL). Generic only: Soln 0.5% (5, 10, 15 mL).

(cont.)

OPHTHALMOLOGY: Glaucoma Agents

BETAXOLOL—OPHTHALMIC (cont.)
 NOTES — Selective beta-1-blocking agent. Shake susp before use.
 MOA — Inhibits beta-1 receptors to decrease aqueous fluid production.
 ADVERSE EFFECTS — Frequent: Dizziness, erythema, conjunctival hyperemia, anisocoria, keratitis, corneal staining, eye pain, vision disturbances.

CARTEOLOL—OPHTHALMIC (*Ocupress*) ▶KL ♀C ▶? $
 ADULTS — Chronic open angle glaucoma or ocular HTN: 1 gtt bid.
 PEDS — Not approved in children.
 FORMS — Generic only: Soln 1% (5, 10, 15 mL).
 NOTES — Non-selective beta-blocker but has intrinsic sympathomimetic activity.
 MOA — Inhibits beta receptors to decrease aqueous fluid production.
 ADVERSE EFFECTS — Frequent: Conjunctival hyperemia.

LEVOBUNOLOL (*Betagan*) ▶? ♀C ▶— $$
 ADULTS — Chronic open angle glaucoma or ocular HTN: 1 to 2 gtts (0.5%) daily to bid or 1 to 2 gtts (0.25%) bid.
 PEDS — Not approved in children.
 FORMS — Generic/Trade: Soln 0.25% (5, 10 mL), 0.5% (5, 10, 15 mL. Trade only: Soln 0.25% 2 mL).
 NOTES — Non-selective beta-blocker.
 MOA — Inhibits beta receptors to decrease aqueous fluid production.
 ADVERSE EFFECTS — Frequent: Stinging, burning eyes.

METIPRANOLOL (*Optipranolol*) ▶? ♀C ▶? $
 ADULTS — Chronic open angle glaucoma or ocular HTN: 1 gtt bid.
 PEDS — Not approved in children.
 FORMS — Generic/Trade: Soln 0.3% (5, 10 mL).
 NOTES — Non-selective beta-blocker.
 MOA — Nonselectively inhibits beta receptors to decrease aqueous fluid production.
 ADVERSE EFFECTS — Frequent: Transient, local discomfort.

TIMOLOL—OPHTHALMIC (*Betimol, Timoptic, Timoptic XE, Istalol, Timoptic Ocudose*) ▶LK ♀C ▶+ $$
 ADULTS — Chronic open angle glaucoma or ocular HTN: 1 gtt (0.25 or 0.5%) bid or 1 gtt of gel-forming soln (0.25 or 0.5% Timoptic XE) daily or 1 gtt (0.5% Istalol soln) daily.
 PEDS — Chronic open angle glaucoma or ocular HTN: 1 gtt (0.25 or 0.5%) of gel-forming soln daily.
 FORMS — Generic/Trade: Soln 0.25, 0.5% (5, 10, 15 mL), preservative-free soln (Timoptic Ocudose) 0.25% (0.2 mL), gel-forming soln (Timoptic XE) 0.25, 0.5% (2.5, 5 mL).
 NOTES — Administer other eye meds at least 10 min before Timoptic XE. Greatest effect if Timoptic XE is administered in the morning. Non-selective beta-blocker.
 MOA — Inhibits beta receptors to decrease aqueous fluid production.
 ADVERSE EFFECTS — Frequent: Conjunctival hyperemia.

OPHTHALMOLOGY: Glaucoma Agents—Carbonic Anhydrase Inhibitors

NOTE: Sulfonamide derivatives; verify absence of sulfa allergy before prescribing. On average, each mL of eye drop soln contains approximately 20 gtts. Reserve ointment formulations for bedtime use due to severe vision blurring. Most eye medications can be administered 1 gtt at a time despite common manufacturer recommendations of 1 to 2 gtts concurrently. Even a single gtt is typically more than the eye can hold and thus a second gtt is both wasteful and increases the possibility of systemic toxicity. If 2 gtts of the medication is desired separate single gtts by at least 5 min.

BRINZOLAMIDE (*Azopt*) ▶LK ♀C ▶? $$$
 ADULTS — Chronic open angle glaucoma or ocular HTN: 1 gtt tid.
 PEDS — Not approved in children.
 FORMS — Trade only: Susp 1% (5, 10, 15 mL).
 NOTES — Do not administer while wearing soft contact lenses. Wait 10 min after use before inserting contact lenses.
 MOA — Inhibition of carbonic anhydrase to decrease aqueous fluid production.
 ADVERSE EFFECTS — Frequent: Dermatitis, taste disturbances, transient blurred vision.

DORZOLAMIDE (*Trusopt*) ▶KL ♀C ▶— $$$
 ADULTS — Chronic open angle glaucoma or ocular HTN: 1 gtt tid.
 PEDS — Chronic open angle glaucoma or ocular HTN: 1 gtt tid.
 FORMS — Generic/Trade: Soln 2% (5, 10 mL).
 NOTES — Do not administer while wearing soft contact lenses. Keep bottle tightly capped to avoid crystal formation. Wait 10 min after use before inserting contact lenses.
 MOA — Inhibition of carbonic anhydrase to decrease aqueous fluid production.
 ADVERSE EFFECTS — Frequent: Bitter taste, ocular burning and stinging. Severe: Corneal edema in patients with low endothelial cell counts, Stevens-Johnson syndrome, and toxic epidermal necrolysis.

METHAZOLAMIDE (*Neptazane*) ▶LK ♀C ▶? $$
 ADULTS — Glaucoma: 100 to 200 mg PO initially, then 100 mg PO q 12 h until desired response. Maintenance dose: 25 to 50 mg PO (up to tid).
 PEDS — Not approved in children.
 FORMS — Generic only: Tabs 25, 50 mg.
 NOTES — Mostly metabolized in the liver thus less chance of renal calculi than with acetazolamide.
 MOA — Inhibition of carbonic anhydrase to decrease aqueous fluid production.
 ADVERSE EFFECTS — Frequent: Malaise, anorexia, diarrhea, metallic taste, polyuria, muscular weakness.

OPHTHALMOLOGY: Glaucoma Agents—Miotics

NOTE: Observe for cholinergic systemic effects (eg, salivation, lacrimation, urination, diarrhea, GI upset, excessive sweating). On average, each mL of eye drop soln contains approximately 20 gtts. Reserve ointment formulations for bedtime use due to severe vision blurring. Most eye medications can be administered 1 gtt at a time despite common manufacturer recommendations of 1 to 2 gtts concurrently. Even a single gtt is typically more than the eye can hold and thus a second gtt is both wasteful and increases the possibility of systemic toxicity. If 2 gtts of the medication are desired separate single gtts by at least 5 min.

ACETYLCHOLINE (*Miochol-E*) ▶Acetylcholinesterases ♀? ▶? $$
ADULTS – <u>Intraoperative miosis or pressure lowering:</u> 0.5 mL to 3 mL injected intraocularly.
PEDS – Not approved in children.
MOA – Stimulates cholinergic receptors to increase aqueous fluid outflow.
ADVERSE EFFECTS – Frequent: Blurred vision, miosis, headache.

CARBACHOL (*Isopto Carbachol, Miostat*) ▶? ♀C ▶? $$
ADULTS – <u>Glaucoma:</u> 1 gtt tid. <u>Intraoperative miosis or pressure lowering:</u> 0.5 mL injected intraocularly.
PEDS – Not approved in children.
FORMS – Trade only: Soln (Isopto Carbachol) 1.5, 3% (15 mL). Intraocular soln (Miostat) 0.01%.
MOA – Inhibits acetylcholinesterase resulting in cholineric stimulation to increase aqueous fluid outflow.
ADVERSE EFFECTS – Frequent: Blurred vision, miosis, headache.

ECHOTHIOPHATE IODIDE (*Phospholine Iodide*) ▶? ♀C ▶? $$$
ADULTS – <u>Glaucoma:</u> 1 gtt bid.
PEDS – <u>Accommodative esotropia:</u> 1 gtt daily (0.06%) or 1 gtt every other day (0.125%).
FORMS – Trade only: Soln 0.125% (5 mL).
NOTES – Use lowest effective dose strength. Use extreme caution if asthma, spastic GI diseases, GI ulcers, bradycardia, hypotension, recent MI, epilepsy, Parkinson's disease, history of retinal detachment. Stop 3 weeks before general anesthesia as may cause prolonged succinylcholine paralysis. Discontinue if cardiac effects noted.
MOA – Inhibits acetylcholinesterase resulting in cholineric stimulation to increase aqueous fluid outflow.
ADVERSE EFFECTS – Frequent: Blurred vision, miosis, headache. Infrequent: Iris cysts, cataracts, ocular surface scarring.

PILOCARPINE—OPHTHALMIC (*Pilopine HS, Isopto Carpine, ✦Diocarpine, Akarpine*) ▶Plasma ♀C ▶? $
ADULTS – <u>Reduction of IOP with open-angle glaucoma, acute angle-closure glaucoma, prevention of postoperative elevated IOP associated with laser surgery, induction of miosis:</u> 1 gtt up to qid or ½ inch ribbon (4% gel) at bedtime.
PEDS – <u>Glaucoma:</u> 1 gtt up to qid.
FORMS – Generic only: Soln 0.5% (15 mL), 1% (2 mL), 2% (2 mL), 3% (15 mL), 4% (2 mL), 6% (15 mL). Generic/Trade: Soln 1% (15 mL), 2% (15 mL), 4% (15 mL). Trade only (Pilopine HS): Gel 4% (4 g tube).
NOTES – Do not administer while wearing soft contact lenses. Wait at least 15 min after use before inserting contact lenses. Causes miosis. May cause blurred vision and difficulty with night vision.
MOA – Stimulates cholinergic receptors to increase aqueous fluid outflow.
ADVERSE EFFECTS – Ocular: Frequent: Blurred vision, miosis.

OPHTHALMOLOGY: Glaucoma Agents—Prostaglandin Analogs

NOTE: Do not administer while wearing soft contact lenses. Wait 10 min after use before inserting contact lenses. May aggravate intraocular inflammation. On average, each mL of eye drop soln contains approximately 20 gtts. Reserve ointment formulations for bedtime use due to severe vision blurring. Most eye medications can be administered 1 gtt at a time despite common manufacturer recommendations of 1 to 2 gtts concurrently. Even a single gtt is typically more than the eye can hold and thus a second gtt is both wasteful and increases the possibility of systemic toxicity. If 2 gtts of the medication are desired separate single gtts by at least 5 min.

BIMATOPROST (*Lumigan, Latisse*) ▶LK ♀C ▶? $$$
ADULTS – <u>Chronic open angle glaucoma or ocular HTN:</u> 1 gtt at bedtime. <u>Hypotrichosis of the eyelashes (Latisse):</u> Apply at bedtime to the skin of the upper eyelid margin at the base of the eyelashes.
PEDS – Not approved in children.
FORMS – Trade only: Soln 0.03% (Lumigan, 2.5, 5, 7.5 mL), (Latisse, 3 mL with 60 sterile, disposable applicators).
NOTES – Concurrent administration of bimatoprost for hypotrichosis and IOP-lowering prostaglandin analogs in ocular hypertensive patients may decrease the IOP-lowering effect. Monitor closely for changes in intraocular pressure.
MOA – Prostaglandin F-2 analog increases aqueous fluid outflow.
ADVERSE EFFECTS – Ocular: Frequent: Blurred vision, burning, stinging, ocular hyperemia, increased pigmentation of iris and eyelid skin, growth of eyelashes, ocular pruritus.

LATANOPROST (*Xalatan*) ▶LK ♀C ▶? $$$
ADULTS – <u>Chronic open angle glaucoma or ocular HTN:</u> 1 gtt at bedtime.
PEDS – Not approved in children.

(cont.)

LATANOPROST (cont.)
 FORMS — Trade only: Soln 0.005% (2.5 mL).
 MOA — Prostaglandin F-2 analog increases aqueous fluid outflow.
 ADVERSE EFFECTS — Ocular: Frequent: Blurred vision, burning, stinging, ocular hyperemia, increased pigmentation of iris and eyelid skin, growth of eyelashes, ocular pruritus.

TRAVOPROST (*Travatan, Travatan Z*) ▶L ♀C ▶? $$$
 ADULTS — <u>Chronic open angle glaucoma or ocular HTN:</u> 1 gtt at bedtime.
 PEDS — Not approved in children.
 FORMS — Trade only: Soln (Travatan), benzalkonium chloride-free (Travatan Z) 0.004% (2.5, 5 mL).
 NOTES — Wait 10 min after use before inserting contact lenses. Avoid if prior or current intraocular inflammation.
 MOA — Prostaglandin F-2 analog increases aqueous fluid outflow.
 ADVERSE EFFECTS — Ocular: Frequent: Conjunctival hyperemia, ocular hyperemia, increased pigmentation of iris and eyelid skin, growth of eyelashes, decreased visual acuity, eye discomfort, foreign body sensation, pain, and pruritus. Severe: Contraindicated in pregnancy, pigmentation changes.

OPHTHALMOLOGY: Glaucoma Agents—Sympathomimetics

NOTE: Do not administer while wearing soft contact lenses. Wait 10 min after use before inserting contact lenses. On average, each mL of eye drop soln contains approximately 20 gtts. Reserve ointment formulations for bedtime use due to severe vision blurring. Most eye medications can be administered 1 gtt at a time despite common manufacturer recommendations of 1 to 2 gtts concurrently. Even a single gtt is typically more than the eye can hold and thus a second gtt is both wasteful and increases the possibility of systemic toxicity. If 2 gtts of the medication are desired separate single gtts by at least 5 min.

APRACLONIDINE (*Iopidine*) ▶KL ♀C ▶? $$$$
 ADULTS — <u>Perioperative IOP elevation:</u> 1 gtt (1%) 1 hour prior to surgery, then 1 gtt immediately after surgery.
 PEDS — Not approved in children.
 FORMS — Generic/Trade: Soln 0.5% (5, 10 mL). Trade only: Soln 1% (0.1 mL).
 NOTES — Rapid tachyphylaxis may occur. Do not use long-term.
 MOA — Alpha-2-agonist decreases aqueous fluid production.
 ADVERSE EFFECTS — Frequent: Decreases night vision, distance vision alterations, lethargy, xerostomia, burning and itching eyes.

BRIMONIDINE (*Alphagan P, ❖Alphagan*) ▶L ♀B ▶? $$
 ADULTS — <u>Chronic open angle glaucoma or ocular HTN:</u> 1 gtt tid.
 PEDS — <u>Glaucoma:</u> 1 gtt tid for age older than 2 yo.
 FORMS — Trade only: Soln 0.1% (5, 10, 15 mL). Generic/Trade: Soln 0.15% (5, 10, 15 mL). Generic only: Soln 0.2% (5, 10, 15 mL).
 NOTES — Contraindicated in patients receiving MAOIs. BID dosing may have similar efficacy.
 MOA — Alpha-2-agonist decreases aqueous fluid production.
 ADVERSE EFFECTS — Frequent: Headache, drowsiness, fatigue, xerostomia, hyperemia, burning, stinging, blurring, foreign body sensation.

DIPIVEFRIN (*Propine*) ▶Eye/plasma/L ♀B ▶? $
 ADULTS — <u>Chronic open angle glaucoma or ocular HTN:</u> 1 gtt bid.
 PEDS — <u>Glaucoma:</u> 1 gtt bid.
 FORMS — Generic/Trade: Soln 0.1% (5, 10, 15 mL).
 MOA — Prodrug of epinephrine which stimulates alpha and beta adrenergic receptors to increase aqueous fluid outflow and decrease production.
 ADVERSE EFFECTS — Frequent: Headache, stinging, blurred vision, ocular pain, photophobia, conjunctivitis, local dermatitis.

OPHTHALMOLOGY: Glaucoma Agents—Combinations and Other

NOTE: On average, each mL of eye drop soln contains approximately 20 gtts. Reserve ointment formulations for bedtime use due to severe vision blurring. Most eye medications can be administered 1 gtt at a time despite common manufacturer recommendations of 1 to 2 gtts concurrently. Even a single gtt is typically more than the eye can hold and thus a second gtt is both wasteful and increases the possibility of systemic toxicity. If 2 gtts of the medication are desired separate single gtts by at least 5 min.

COMBIGAN (brimonidine + timolol) ▶LK ♀C ▶− $$$
 ADULTS — <u>Chronic open angle glaucoma or ocular HTN:</u> 1 gtt q 12 h.
 PEDS — Not approved in age younger than 2 yo.
 FORMS — Trade only: Soln brimonidine 0.2% + timolol 0.5% (5, 10 mL).
 NOTES — Do not administer while wearing soft contact lenses. Wait 10 min after use before inserting contact lenses. Contraindicated with MAOIs. See beta-blocker warnings.
 MOA — Stimulation of alpha-2 receptors and inhibition of beta-1 receptors to decrease aqueous fluid production.
 ADVERSE EFFECTS — Ocular: Frequent: Headache, drowsiness, fatigue, xerostomia, hyperemia, burning, stinging, blurring, foreign body sensation.

OPHTHALMOLOGY: Mydriatics & Cycloplegics

COSOPT (dorzolamide + timolol) ▶LK ♀D ▶− $$$
ADULTS − Chronic open angle glaucoma or ocular HTN: 1 gtt bid.
PEDS − Not approved in children.
FORMS − Generic/Trade: Soln dorzolamide 2% + timolol 0.5% (5, 10 mL).
NOTES − Do not administer while wearing soft contact lenses. Wait 10 min after use before inserting contact lenses. Not recommended if severe renal or hepatic dysfunction. Use caution in sulfa allergy. See beta-blocker warnings.
MOA − Inhibition of carbonic anhydrase and beta-1 receptors to decrease aqueous fluid production.
ADVERSE EFFECTS − Ocular: Frequent: Bitter taste, burning, stinging in eyes, allergic reaction, conjunctivitis, lid reactions. Severe: Corneal edema in patients with low endothelial cell counts, Stevens-Johnson syndrome, and toxic epidermal necrolysis.

OPHTHALMOLOGY: Macular Degeneration

PEGAPTANIB (*Macugen*) ▶Minimal absorption ♀B ▶? $$$$$
ADULTS − "Wet" macular degeneration: 0.3 mg intravitreal injection q 6 weeks.
PEDS − Not approved in children.
MOA − Selective antagonist of vascular endothelial growth factor.
ADVERSE EFFECTS − Ocular: Chamber inflammation, blurred vision, cataracts, corneal edema, reduced visual acuity, visual changes. Injection-related adverse events include: Endophthalmitis, retinal detachment, iatrogenic traumatic cataract, subconjunctival hemorrhage, and increased intraocular pressure. Severe: Anaphylaxis/anaphylactoid, angioedema.

RANIBIZUMAB (*Lucentis*) ▶Intravitreal ♀C ▶? $$$$$
ADULTS − Treatment of neovascular (wet) macular degeneration: 0.5 mg intravitreal injection every 28 days. If monthly injections not feasible, can administer every 3 months, but this regimen is less effective. Macular edema following retinal vein occlusion: 0.5 mg intravitreal injection every 28 days.
PEDS − Not approved in children.
NOTES − Increased CVA risk noted with higher doses (0.5 mg) and with prior CVA.
MOA − Binds to the receptor of VEGF-A.
ADVERSE EFFECTS − Severe: Stroke. Frequent: Eye pain, vitreous floaters, intraocular inflammation, blurred vision. Injection-related adverse events include: Endophthalmitis, retinal detachment, iatrogenic traumatic cataract, subconjunctival hemorrhage, and increased intraocular pressure.

VERTEPORFIN (*Visudyne*) ▶L/plasma ♀C ▶? $$$$$
ADULTS − Treatment of exudative age-related macular degeneration: 6 mg/m2 IV over 10 min; laser light therapy 15 min after start of infusion.
PEDS − Not approved in children.
NOTES − Severe risk of photosensitivity for 5 days; must avoid exposure to sunlight.
MOA − Laser-induced free radicals cause occlusion of abnormal vessels.
ADVERSE EFFECTS − Frequent: Injection-site irritation, blurred vision, visual field defects, decreased visual acuity (sometimes severe).

OPHTHALMOLOGY: Mydriatics & Cycloplegics

NOTE: Use caution in infants. On average, each mL of eye drop soln contains approximately 20 gtts. Reserve ointment formulations for bedtime use due to severe vision blurring. Most eye medications can be administered 1 gtt at a time despite common manufacturer recommendations of 1 to 2 gtts concurrently. Even a single gtt is typically more than the eye can hold and thus a second gtt is both wasteful and increases the possibility of systemic toxicity. If 2 gtts of the medication are desired separate single gtts by at least 5 min.

ATROPINE—OPHTHALMIC (*Isopto Atropine, Atropine Care*) ▶L ♀C ▶+ $
ADULTS − Uveitis: 1 to 2 gtts of 0.5% or 1% solution daily to qid, or ¼ inch ribbon (1% ointment) daily (up to tid. Refraction: 1 to 2 gtts of 1% solution 1 h before procedure or ⅛ to ¼ inch ribbon daily to tid.
PEDS − 1 to 2 gtts of 0.5% solution daily to tid) or ⅛ to ¼ inch ribbon daily to tid. Refraction: 1 to 2 gtts (0.5%) bid for 1 to 3 days before procedure or ⅛ inch ribbon (1% ointment) for 1 to 3 days before procedure.
UNAPPROVED PEDS − Amblyopia: 1 gtt in good eye daily.
FORMS − Generic/Trade: Soln 1% (2, 5, 15 mL). Generic only: Ointment 1% (3.5 g tube).
NOTES − Cycloplegia may last up to 5 to 10 days and mydriasis may last up to 7 to 14 days. Each drop of a 1% soln contains 0.5 mg atropine. Treat atropine overdose with physostigmine 0.25 mg every 15 min until symptoms resolve.
MOA − Anticholinergic blockage of ciliary body and iris muscles to produce loss of accommodation and pupil dilation.
ADVERSE EFFECTS − Frequent: Dry, hot skin, impaired GI motility, dry throat, xerostomia, dry eyes, blurred vision, especially reading vision, photophobia.

CYCLOPENTOLATE (*AK-Pentolate, Cyclogyl, Pentolair*) ▶? ♀C ▶? $
ADULTS − Refraction: 1 to 2 gtts (1% or 2%), repeat in 5 to 10 min prn. Give 45 min before procedure.
PEDS − May cause CNS disturbances in children. Refraction: 1 to 2 gtts (0.5%, 1%, or 2%), repeat in 5 to 10 min prn. Give 45 min before procedure.
FORMS − Generic/Trade: Soln 1% (2, 15 mL). Trade only (Cyclogyl): 0.5% (15 mL), 1% (5 mL) and 2% (2, 5, 15 mL).

(cont.)

OPHTHALMOLOGY: Non-Steroidal Anti-Inflammatories

CYCLOPENTOLATE (cont.)
- NOTES – Cycloplegia may last 6 to 24 h; mydriasis may last 1 day.
- MOA – Anticholinergic blockage of ciliary body and iris muscles to produce loss of accommodation and pupil dilation.
- ADVERSE EFFECTS – Frequent: Tachycardia, CNS effects, blurred vision, especially reading vision, increased sensitivity to light, photophobia.

HOMATROPINE (*Isopto Homatropine*) ▶? ♀C ▶? $
- ADULTS – Refraction: 1 to 2 gtts (2%) or 1 gtt (5%) in eye(s) immediately before procedure, repeat q 5 to 10 min prn. Max 3 doses. Uveitis: 1 to 2 gtts (2 to 5%) bid to tid or as often as q 3 to 4 h.
- PEDS – Refraction: 1 gtt (2%) in eye(s) immediately before procedure, repeat q 10 min prn. Uveitis: 1 gtt (2%) bid to tid.
- FORMS – Trade only: Soln 2% (5 mL), 5% (15 mL). Generic/Trade: Soln 5% (5 mL).
- NOTES – Cycloplegia and mydriasis last 1 to 3 days.
- MOA – Anticholinergic blockage of ciliary body and iris muscles to produce loss of accommodation and pupil dilation.
- ADVERSE EFFECTS – Ocular: Frequent: Blurred vision, especially reading vision, photophobia.

PHENYLEPHRINE—OPHTHALMIC (*AK-Dilate, Altafrin, Mydfrin, Refresh*) ▶Plasma, L ♀C ▶? $
- ADULTS – Ophthalmologic exams: 1 to 2 gtts (2.5%, 10%) before procedure. Ocular surgery: 1 to 2 gtts (2.5%, 10%) before surgery.
- PEDS – Not routinely used in children.
- UNAPPROVED PEDS – Ophthalmologic exams: 1 gtt (2.5%) before procedure. Ocular surgery: 1 gtt (2.5%) before surgery.
- FORMS – Rx Generic/Trade: Soln 2.5% (2, 3, 5, 15 mL), 10% (5 mL). OTC Trade only (Altafrin and Refresh): Soln 0.12% (15 mL).
- NOTES – Overuse can cause rebound dilation of blood vessels. No cycloplegia; mydriasis may last up to 5 h. Systemic absorption, especially with 10% soln, may be associated with sympathetic stimulation (eg, increased BP).
- MOA – Alpha-adrenergic and (weak) beta-adrenergic agonist to stimulate iris dilator and cause mydriasis.
- ADVERSE EFFECTS – Frequent: Reflex bradycardia, excitability, restlessness, photophobia.

TROPICAMIDE (*Mydriacyl, Tropicacyl*) ▶? ♀? ▶? $
- ADULTS – Dilated eye exam: 1 to 2 gtts (0.5%) in eye(s) 15 to 20 min before exam, repeat q 30 min prn.
- PEDS – Not approved in children.
- FORMS – Generic/Trade: Soln 0.5% (15 mL), 1% (3, 15 mL). Generic only: Soln 1% (2 mL).
- NOTES – Mydriasis may last 6 h and has weak cycloplegic effects.
- MOA – Anticholinergic blockage of iris sphincter muscle to produce pupil dilation.
- ADVERSE EFFECTS – Frequent: Tachycardia, CNS effects, blurred vision, photophobia, possible increased intraocular pressure.

OPHTHALMOLOGY: Non-Steroidal Anti-Inflammatories

NOTE: On average, each mL of eye drop soln contains approximately 20 gtts. Reserve ointment formulations for bedtime use due to severe vision blurring. Most eye medications can be administered 1 gtt at a time despite common manufacturer recommendations of 1 to 2 gtts concurrently. Even a single gtt is typically more than the eye can hold and thus a second gtt is both wasteful and increases the possibility of systemic toxicity. If 2 gtts of the medication are desired separate single gtts by at least 5 min.

BROMFENAC—OPHTHALMIC (*Xibrom*) ▶Minimal absorption ♀C, D (3rd trimester) ▶? $$$$$
- ADULTS – Post-op inflammation and pain following cataract surgery: 1 gtt bid beginning 24 h after cataract surgery for 2 weeks.
- PEDS – Not approved in children.
- FORMS – Trade only: Soln 0.09% (2.5, 5 mL).
- NOTES – Not for use with soft contact lenses. Contains sodium sulfite and may cause allergic reactions.
- MOA – Blocks prostaglandin synthesis by inhibiting cyclooxygenase.
- ADVERSE EFFECTS – Frequent: Abnormal eye sensation, conjunctival hyperemia, eye irritation, pain, pruritus, redness, headache, iritis. Severe: Keratitis, corneal thinning, erosion, ulceration, perforation.

DICLOFENAC—OPHTHALMIC (*Voltaren, ✦Voltaren Ophtha*) ▶L ♀B, D (3rd trimester) ▶? $$$
- ADULTS – Post-op inflammation following cataract surgery: 1 gtt qid for 1 to 2 weeks. Ocular photophobia and pain associated with corneal refractive surgery: 1 to 2 gtt to operative eye(s) 1 h prior to surgery and 1 to 2 gtt within 15 min after surgery, then 1 gtt qid prn for no more than 3 days.
- PEDS – Not approved in children.
- FORMS – Generic/Trade: Soln 0.1% (2.5, 5 mL).
- NOTES – Contraindicated for use with soft contact lenses.
- MOA – Blocks prostaglandin synthesis by inhibiting cyclooxygenase.
- ADVERSE EFFECTS – Frequent: Lacrimation, keratitis, increased intraocular pressure, burning, stinging. Severe: Keratitis, corneal thinning, erosion, ulceration, perforation.

FLURBIPROFEN—OPHTHALMIC (*Ocufen*) ▶L ♀C ▶? $
- ADULTS – Inhibition of intraoperative miosis: 1 gtt q 30 min beginning 2 h prior to surgery (total of 4 gtts).
- PEDS – Not approved in children.
- UNAPPROVED ADULTS – Treatment of cystoid macular edema, inflammation after glaucoma or cataract laser surgery, uveitis syndromes.

(cont.)

FLURBIPROFEN—OPHTHALMIC (cont.)
FORMS — Generic/Trade: Soln 0.03% (2.5 mL).
MOA — Blocks prostaglandin synthesis by inhibiting cyclooxygenase.
ADVERSE EFFECTS — Frequent: Transient stinging/burning. Severe: Keratitis, corneal thinning, erosion, ulceration, perforation.

KETOROLAC—OPHTHALMIC (*Acular, Acular LS*) ▶L ♀C ▶? $$$$
ADULTS — Allergic conjunctivitis: 1 gtt (0.5%) qid. Post-op inflammation following cataract surgery: 1 gtt (0.5%) qid beginning 24 h after surgery for 1 to 2 weeks. Post-op corneal refractive surgery: 1 gtt (0.4%) prn for up to 4 days.
PEDS — Not approved age younger than 3 yo. Use adult dose for age 3 yo or older.
FORMS — Generic/Trade: Soln (Acular LS) 0.4% (5 mL). Trade only: Acular 0.5% (3, 5, 10 mL), preservative-free Acular 0.5% unit dose (0.4 mL).
NOTES — Do not administer while wearing soft contact lenses. Wait 10 min after use before inserting contact lenses. Avoid use in late pregnancy.

MOA — Blocks prostaglandin synthesis by inhibiting cyclooxygenase.
ADVERSE EFFECTS — Frequent: Transient stinging/burning. Severe: Keratitis, corneal thinning, erosion, ulceration, perforation.

NEPAFENAC (*Nevanac*) ▶Minimal absorption ♀C ▶? $$$
ADULTS — Post-op inflammation following cataract surgery: 1 gtt tid beginning 24 h before cataract surgery and continued for 2 weeks after surgery.
PEDS — Not approved in children.
FORMS — Trade only: Susp 0.1% (3 mL).
NOTES — Not for use with contact lenses. Caution if previous allergy to aspirin or other NSAIDs.
MOA — A prodrug that is converted by ocular tissues to amfenac, which blocks prostaglandin synthesis by inhibiting cyclooxygenase.
ADVERSE EFFECTS — Frequent: Abnormal eye sensation, conjunctival hyperemia, eye irritation, pain, photophobia, dry eye, pruritus, redness, headache, iritis. Severe: Increased bleeding time, keratitis, corneal thinning, erosion, ulceration, perforation.

OPHTHALMOLOGY: Other Ophthalmologic Agents

ARTIFICIAL TEARS (*Tears Naturale, Hypotears, Refresh Tears, GenTeal, Systane*) ▶Minimal absorption ♀A ▶+ $
ADULTS — Ophthalmic lubricant: 1 to 2 gtts tid to qid prn.
PEDS — Ophthalmic lubricant: 1 to 2 gtts tid to qid prn.
FORMS — OTC Generic/Trade: Soln (15, 30 mL, among others).
MOA — Lubricant.
ADVERSE EFFECTS — Frequent: Mild stinging, temporary blurred vision.

CYCLOSPORINE—OPHTHALMIC (*Restasis*) ▶Minimal absorption ♀C ▶? $$$$
ADULTS — Keratoconjunctivitis sicca (chronic dry eye disease): 1 gtt in each eye q 12 h.
PEDS — Not approved in children.
FORMS — Trade only: Emulsion 0.05% (0.4 mL single-use vials).
NOTES — Wait 10 min after use before inserting contact lenses. May take 1 month to note clinical improvement.
MOA — Immunomodulator and anti-inflammatory.
ADVERSE EFFECTS — Frequent: Ocular burning.

HYDROXYPROPYL CELLULOSE (*Lacrisert*) ▶Minimal absorption ♀+ ▶+ $$$
ADULTS — Moderate–severe dry eyes: 1 insert in each eye daily. Some patients may require bid use.
PEDS — Not approved in children.
FORMS — Trade only: Ocular insert 5 mg.
NOTES — Do not use with soft contact lenses.
MOA — Lubricant.
ADVERSE EFFECTS — Frequent: Blurred vision, ocular discomfort, matting of eyelashes.

LIDOCAINE—OPHTHALMIC (*Akten*) ▶L ♀B ▶? ?
ADULTS — Do not prescribe for unsupervised use. Corneal toxicity may occur with repeated use. Local anesthetic: 2 gtts before procedure, repeat prn.
PEDS — Not approved in children.
FORMS — Generic only: Gel 3.5% (5 mL).
MOA — Ester-type local anesthetic that prevents nerve impulse initiation and potentiation through blockage of sodium ion channels.
ADVERSE EFFECTS — Ocular: Frequent: Hyperemia, corneal epithelial changes, headache, and burning.

PETROLATUM (*Lacrilube, Dry Eyes, Refresh PM, ✦Duolube*) ▶Minimal absorption ♀A ▶+ $
ADULTS — Ophthalmic lubricant: Apply ¼ to ½ inch ointment to inside of lower lid prn.
PEDS — Ophthalmic lubricant: Apply ¼ to ½ inch ointment to inside of lower lid prn.
FORMS — OTC Trade only: Ointment (3.5, 7 g) tube.
MOA — Lubricates dry eyes.
ADVERSE EFFECTS — Frequent: Blurred vision.

PROPARACAINE (*Ophthaine, Ophthetic, ✦Alcaine*) ▶L ♀C ▶? $
ADULTS — Do not prescribe for unsupervised use. Corneal toxicity may occur with repeated use. Local anesthetic: 1 to 2 gtts before procedure. Repeat q 5 to 10 min for 1 to 3 doses (suture or foreign body removal) or for 5 to 7 doses (ocular surgery).
PEDS — Not approved in children.
FORMS — Generic/Trade: Soln 0.5% (15 mL).
MOA — Amide-type local anesthetic that prevents nerve impulse initiation and potentiation through blockage of sodium ion channels.
ADVERSE EFFECTS — Ocular: Frequent: Burning, stinging.

TETRACAINE—OPHTHALMIC (*Pontocaine*) ▶Plasma ♀C ▶? $
ADULTS – Do not prescribe for unsupervised use. Corneal toxicity may occur with repeated use. Local anesthetic: 1 to 2 gtts or ½ to 1 inch in ribbon of ointment before procedure.
PEDS – Not approved in children.
FORMS – Generic only: Soln 0.5% (15 mL), unit-dose vials (0.7, 2 mL).
MOA – Ester-type local anesthetic that prevents nerve impulse initiation and potentiation through blockage of sodium ion channels.
ADVERSE EFFECTS – Ocular: Frequent: Burning, stinging, angioedema, contact dermatitis, chemosis, lacrimation, photophobia, transient stinging.

TRYPAN BLUE (*Vision Blue, Membrane Blue*) ▶Not absorbed ♀C ▶? $$
ADULTS – Aid during ophthalmic surgery by staining anterior cap: Inject into anterior chamber of eye.
PEDS – Not approved in children.
FORMS – Trade only: 0.06% (Vision Blue) ophthalmic soln (0.5 mL), 0.15% (Membrane Blue) ophthalmic soln (0.5 mL).
MOA – Acid di-azo group dye.
ADVERSE EFFECTS – Inadvertent staining of posterior lens capsule and vitreous face.

PSYCHIATRY: Antidepressants—Heterocyclic Compounds

NOTE: Gradually taper when discontinuing cyclic antidepressants to avoid withdrawal symptoms. Seizures, orthostatic hypotension, arrhythmias, and anticholinergic side effects may occur. Don't use with MAOIs. Antidepressants increase the risk of suicidal thinking and behavior in children, adolescents, and young adults; carefully weigh the risks and benefits before starting and monitor patients closely.

AMITRIPTYLINE (*Elavil*) ▶L ♀D ▶– $$
ADULTS – Depression: Start 25 to 100 mg PO at bedtime; gradually increase to usual effective dose of 50 to 300 mg/day.
PEDS – Depression, adolescents: Use adult dosing. Not approved in children younger than 12 yo.
UNAPPROVED ADULTS – Migraine prophylaxis and/or chronic pain: 10 to 100 mg/day. Fibromyalgia: 25 to 50 mg/day.
UNAPPROVED PEDS – Depression, age younger than 12 yo: Start 1 mg/kg/day PO divided tid for 3 days, then increase to 1.5 mg/kg/day. Max 5 mg/kg/day.
FORMS – Generic: Tabs 10, 25, 50, 75, 100, 150 mg. Elavil brand name no longer available; has been retained in this entry for name recognition purposes only.
NOTES – Tricyclic, tertiary amine; primarily inhibits serotonin reuptake. Demethylated to nortriptyline, which primarily inhibits norepinephrine reuptake. Usual therapeutic range is 150 to 300 ng/mL (amitriptyline + nortriptyline).
MOA – Serotonin/norepinephrine reuptake inhibitor.
ADVERSE EFFECTS – Serious: Atrial/ventricular arrhythmias, seizures, MI, CHF, stroke. Frequent: Drowsiness, dry mouth, constipation, nausea, orthostatic hypotension, dizziness, confusion, urinary retention, sexual dysfunction.

AMOXAPINE ▶L ♀C ▶– $$$
ADULTS – Rarely used; other drugs preferred. Depression: Start 25 to 50 mg PO bid to tid; increase by 50 to 100 mg bid to tid after 1 week. Usual effective dose is 150 to 400 mg/day. Max 600 mg/day.
PEDS – Not approved in children younger than 16 yo.
FORMS – Generic only: Tabs 25, 50, 100, 150 mg.
NOTES – Tetracyclic; primarily inhibits norepinephrine reuptake. Dose 300 mg/day or less may be given once daily at bed time.
MOA – Norepinephrine/serotonin reuptake inhibitor. Active metabolite is a partial dopamine receptor antagonist.
ADVERSE EFFECTS – Serious: Atrial/ventricular arrhythmias, seizures, MI, CHF, stroke, neuroleptic malignant syndrome, tardive dyskinesia. Frequent: Drowsiness, dry mouth, constipation, nausea, orthostatic hypotension, dizziness, confusion, urinary retention, sexual dysfunction, extrapyramidal side effects.

CLOMIPRAMINE (*Anafranil*) ▶L ♀C ▶+ $$$
ADULTS – OCD: Start 25 mg PO at bedtime; gradually increase over 2 weeks to usual effective dose of 150 to 250 mg/day. Max 250 mg/day.
PEDS – OCD, age 10 yo or older: Start 25 mg PO at bedtime, then increase gradually over 2 weeks to 3 mg/kg/day or 100 mg/day, max 200 mg/day. Not approved for age younger than 10 yo.
UNAPPROVED ADULTS – Depression: 100 to 250 mg/day. Panic disorder: 12.5 to 150 mg/day. Chronic pain: 100 to 250 mg/day.
FORMS – Generic/Trade: Caps 25, 50, 75 mg.
NOTES – Tricyclic, tertiary amine; primarily inhibits serotonin reuptake.
MOA – Serotonin/norepinephrine reuptake inhibitor.
ADVERSE EFFECTS – Serious: Atrial/ventricular arrhythmias, seizures, MI, CHF, stroke. Frequent: Drowsiness, dry mouth, constipation, nausea, orthostatic hypotension, dizziness, confusion, urinary retention, sexual dysfunction.

DESIPRAMINE (*Norpramin*) ▶L ♀C ▶+ $$
ADULTS – Depression: Start 25 to 100 mg PO given once daily or in divided doses. Gradually increase to usual effective dose of 100 to 200 mg/day, max 300 mg/day.
PEDS – Adolescents: 25 to 100 mg/day. Not approved in children.

(cont.)

DESIPRAMINE (cont.)
FORMS — Generic/Trade: Tabs 10, 25, 50, 75, 100, 150 mg.
NOTES — Tricyclic, secondary amine; primarily inhibits norepinephrine reuptake. Usual therapeutic range is 125 to 300 ng/mL. May cause fewer anticholinergic side effects than tertiary amines. Use lower doses in adolescents or elderly.
MOA — Norepinephrine/serotonin reuptake inhibitor.
ADVERSE EFFECTS — Serious: Atrial/ventricular arrhythmias, seizures, MI, CHF, stroke. Frequent: Drowsiness, dry mouth, constipation, nausea, orthostatic hypotension, dizziness, confusion, urinary retention, sexual dysfunction.

DOXEPIN (*Sinequan, Silenor*) ▶L ♀C ▶– $$
ADULTS — <u>Depression and/or anxiety:</u> Start 75 mg PO at bedtime. Gradually increase to usual effective dose of 75 to 150 mg/day, max 300 mg/day. <u>Insomnia (Silenor):</u> 6 mg PO 30 min before bedtime, 3 mg in age 65 yo or older.
PEDS — <u>Adolescents:</u> Use adult dosing. Not approved in children younger than 12 yo.
UNAPPROVED ADULTS — <u>Chronic pain:</u> 50 to 300 mg/day. <u>Pruritus:</u> Start 10 to 25 mg at bedtime. Usual effective dose is 10 to 100 mg/day.
FORMS — Generic/Trade: Caps 10, 25, 50, 75, 100, 150 mg. Oral concentrate 10 mg/mL.
NOTES — Tricyclic, tertiary amine; primarily inhibits norepinephrine reuptake. Do not mix oral concentrate with carbonated beverages. Some patients with mild symptoms may respond to 25 to 50 mg/day.
MOA — Norepinephrine/serotonin reuptake inhibitor.
ADVERSE EFFECTS — Serious: Atrial/ventricular arrhythmias, seizures, MI, CHF, stroke. Frequent: Drowsiness, dry mouth, constipation, nausea, orthostatic hypotension, dizziness, confusion, urinary retention, sexual dysfunction.

IMIPRAMINE (*Tofranil, Tofranil PM*) ▶L ♀D ▶– $$$
ADULTS — <u>Depression:</u> Start 75 to 100 mg PO at bedtime or in divided doses; gradually increase to max 300 mg/day.
PEDS — <u>Enuresis</u> age 6 yo or older: 10 to 25 mg/day PO given 1 h before bedtime, then increase in increments of 10 to 25 mg at 1 to 2 week intervals not to exceed 50 mg/day in 6 to 12 yo or 75 mg/day in children age older than 12 yo. Do not exceed 2.5 mg/kg/day.
UNAPPROVED ADULTS — <u>Panic disorder:</u> Start 10 mg PO at bedtime, titrate to usual effective dose of 50 to 300 mg/day. <u>Enuresis:</u> 25 to 75 mg PO at bedtime.
UNAPPROVED PEDS — <u>Depression,</u> children: Start 1.5 mg/kg/day PO divided tid; increase by 1 to 1.5 mg/kg/day q 3 to 4 d to max 5 mg/kg/day.
FORMS — Generic/Trade: Tabs 10, 25, 50 mg. Caps 75, 100, 125, 150 mg (as pamoate salt).
NOTES — Tricyclic, tertiary amine; inhibits serotonin and norepinephrine reuptake. Demethylated to desipramine, which primarily inhibits norepinephrine reuptake.
MOA — Serotonin/norepinephrine reuptake inhibitor.
ADVERSE EFFECTS — Serious: Atrial/ventricular arrhythmias, seizures, MI, CHF, orthostatic hypotension, stroke, agranulocytosis. Frequent: Drowsiness, dry mouth, constipation, nausea, dizziness, confusion, urinary retention, sexual dysfunction.

NORTRIPTYLINE (*Aventyl, Pamelor*) ▶L ♀D ▶+ $$$
ADULTS — <u>Depression:</u> Start 25 mg PO given once daily or divided bid to qid. Gradually increase to usual effective dose of 75 to 100 mg/day, max 150 mg/day.
PEDS — Not approved in children.
UNAPPROVED ADULTS — <u>Panic disorder:</u> Start 25 mg PO at bedtime, titrate to usual effective dose of 50 to 150 mg/day. <u>Smoking cessation:</u> Start 25 mg PO daily 14 days prior to quit date. Titrate to 75 mg/day as tolerated. Continue for 6 weeks or more after quit date.
UNAPPROVED PEDS — <u>Depression</u> age 6 to 12 yo: 1 to 3 mg/kg/day PO divided tid to qid or 10 to 20 mg/day PO divided tid to qid.
FORMS — Generic/Trade: Caps 10, 25, 50, 75 mg. Oral soln 10 mg/5 mL.
NOTES — Tricyclic, secondary amine; primarily inhibits norepinephrine reuptake. Usual therapeutic range is 50 to 150 ng/mL. May cause fewer anticholinergic side effects than tertiary amines. May be used in combination with nicotine replacement for smoking cessation.
MOA — Norepinephrine/serotonin reuptake inhibitor.
ADVERSE EFFECTS — Serious: Atrial/ventricular arrhythmias, seizures, MI, CHF, stroke. Frequent: Drowsiness, dry mouth, constipation, nausea, orthostatic hypotension, dizziness, confusion, urinary retention, sexual dysfunction.

PROTRIPTYLINE (*Vivactil*) ▶L ♀C ▶+ $$$$
ADULTS — <u>Depression:</u> 15 to 40 mg/day PO divided tid to qid. Maximum dose is 60 mg/day.
PEDS — Not approved in children.
FORMS — Trade only: Tabs 5, 10 mg.
NOTES — Tricyclic, secondary amine; primarily inhibits norepinephrine reuptake. May cause fewer anticholinergic side effects than tertiary amines. Dose increases should be made in the morning.
MOA — Serotonin/norepinephrine reuptake inhibitor.
ADVERSE EFFECTS — Serious: Atrial/ventricular arrhythmias, seizures, MI, CHF, stroke. Frequent: Drowsiness, dry mouth, constipation, nausea, orthostatic hypotension, dizziness, confusion, urinary retention, sexual dysfunction.

PSYCHIATRY: Antidepressants—Monoamine Oxidase Inhibitors (MAOIs)

NOTE: May interfere with sleep; avoid at bedtime dosing. Must be on tyramine-free diet throughout treatment, and for 2 weeks after discontinuation. Numerous drug interactions; risk of hypertensive crisis and serotonin syndrome with many medications, including OTC. Allow ≥2 weeks wash-out when converting from an MAOI to an SSRI (6 weeks after fluoxetine), TCA, or other antidepressant. Contraindicated with carbamazepine or oxcarbazepine. Antidepressants increase the risk of suicidal thinking and behavior in children, adolescents, and young adults; carefully weigh the risks and benefits before starting and monitor patients closely.

ISOCARBOXAZID (*Marplan*) ▶L ♀C ▶? $$$
ADULTS — Depression: Start 10 mg PO bid; increase by 10 mg q 2 to 4 days. Usual effective dose is 20 to 40 mg/day. Max 60 mg/day divided bid to qid.
PEDS — Not approved in children younger than 16 yo.
FORMS — Trade only: Tabs 10 mg.
NOTES — Requires MAOI diet.
MOA — Irreversible, nonselective monoamine oxidase inhibitor.
ADVERSE EFFECTS — Serious: Hypertensive crisis with food/drug interactions, serotonin syndrome, seizures, hepatotoxicity, agranulocytosis. Frequent: Dizziness, dry mouth, constipation, urinary retention, headache, confusion, blurred vision, weight gain.

MOCLOBEMIDE (✽*Manerix*) ▶L ♀C ▶– $$
ADULTS — Canada only. Depression: Start 300 mg/day PO divided bid after meals. May increase after 1 week to max 600 mg/day.
PEDS — Not approved in children.
FORMS — Generic/Trade: Tabs 150, 300 mg. Generic only: Tabs 100 mg.
NOTES — No dietary restrictions. Don't use with TCAs; use caution with conventional MAOIs, other antidepressants, epinephrine, thioridazine, sympathomimetics, dextromethorphan, meperidine, and other opiates. Reduce dose in severe hepatic dysfunction.
MOA — Short-acting, reversible MAOI (preferentially affects MAO-A).
ADVERSE EFFECTS — Serious: Hypertensive crisis with drug or food interactions (theoretical risk), hypotension, bradycardia. Frequent: Sleep disturbance, tremor.

PHENELZINE (*Nardil*) ▶L ♀C ▶? $$$
ADULTS — Depression: Start 15 mg PO tid. Usual effective dose is 60 to 90 mg/day in divided doses.
PEDS — Not approved in children younger than 16 yo.
FORMS — Trade only: Tabs 15 mg.
NOTES — Requires MAOI diet. May increase insulin sensitivity. Contraindicated with meperidine.
MOA — Irreversible, nonselective monoamine oxidase inhibitor.
ADVERSE EFFECTS — Serious: Hypertensive crisis with food/drug interactions, serotonin syndrome, hepatotoxicity, agranulocytosis. Frequent: Dizziness, dry mouth, constipation, urinary retention, headache, confusion, blurred vision, weight gain.

SELEGILINE—TRANSDERMAL (*Emsam*) ▶L ♀C ▶? $$$$$
ADULTS — Depression: Start 6 mg/24 h patch q 24 h. Adjust dose in 2-week intervals or more to max 12 mg/24 h.
PEDS — Not approved in children.
FORMS — Trade only: Transdermal patch 6 mg/day, 9 mg/24 h, 12 mg/24 h.
NOTES — MAOI diet is required for doses 9 mg/day or higher. Intense urges (gambling and sexual for example) have been reported. Consider discontinuing the medication or reducing the dose if these occur.
MOA — Irreversible inhibitor of MAO-B; also inhibits MAO-A when doses at least 9 mg/day are used.
ADVERSE EFFECTS — Serious: Hypertensive crisis with food/drug interactions, serotonin syndrome, orthostatic hypotension, mania/hypomania, impulse control disorders. Frequent: Application site reactions, headache, insomnia, dry mouth.

TRANYLCYPROMINE (*Parnate*) ▶L ♀C ▶– $$
ADULTS — Depression: Start 10 mg PO qam; increase by 10 mg/day at 1- to 3-week intervals to usual effective dose of 10 to 40 mg/day divided bid. Max 60 mg/day.
PEDS — Not approved in children younger than 16 yo.
FORMS — Generic/Trade: Tabs 10 mg.
NOTES — Requires MAOI diet.
MOA — Reversible, nonselective monoamine oxidase inhibitor.
ADVERSE EFFECTS — Serious: Hypertensive crisis with food/drug interactions, serotonin syndrome, seizures, hepatotoxicity, agranulocytosis. Frequent: Dizziness, dry mouth, constipation, urinary retention, headache, confusion, blurred vision, weight gain.

PSYCHIATRY: Antidepressants—Selective Serotonin Reuptake Inhibitors (SSRIs)

NOTE: Gradually taper when discontinuing SSRIs to avoid withdrawal symptoms. Observe patients for worsening depression or the emergence of suicidality, anxiety, agitation, panic attacks, insomnia, irritability, hostility, impulsivity, akathisia, mania, or hypomania, particularly early in therapy or after increases in dose. Antidepressants increase the risk of suicidal thinking and behavior in children, adolescents, and young adults; carefully weigh the risks and benefits before starting treatment and then monitor patients closely. Use of SSRIs during the third trimester of pregnancy has been associated with neonatal complications including respiratory (including persistent pulmonary HTN), GI, and feeding problems, as well as seizures and withdrawal symptoms. Balance these risks against those of withdrawal and depression for the mother. Paroxetine should be avoided throughout pregnancy. Don't use sibutramine with SSRIs. Increased risk of abnormal bleeding; use caution when combined with NSAIDs or aspirin. SSRIs have been associated with serotonin syndrome and neuroleptic malignant syndrome. Use cautiously and observe closely for serotonin syndrome if SSRI is used with a triptan or other serotonergic drugs. SSRIs and SNRIs have been associated with hyponatremia, which is often associated with SIADH. The elderly and those taking diuretics may be at increased risk.

CITALOPRAM (Celexa) ▶LK ♀C but - in third trimester ▶- $$$
ADULTS — Depression: Start 20 mg PO daily; increase by 20 mg/day at more than 1 week intervals. Usual effective dose is 20 to 40 mg/day, max 60 mg/day.
PEDS — Not approved in children.
FORMS — Generic/Trade: Tabs 10, 20, 40 mg. Oral soln 10 mg/5 mL. Generic only: Oral disintegrating tab 10, 20, 40 mg.
NOTES — Don't use with MAOIs or tryptophan.
MOA — Selective serotonin reuptake inhibitor.
ADVERSE EFFECTS — Serious: Suicidality, serotonin syndrome, neuroleptic malignant syndrome, abnormal bleeding, withdrawal reactions. Frequent: N/V, diarrhea, insomnia, drowsiness, headache, sexual dysfunction, dry mouth, anorexia, anxiety, nervousness.

ESCITALOPRAM (Lexapro, *Cipralex) ▶LK ♀C but - in 3rd trimester ▶- $$$
ADULTS — Depression, generalized anxiety disorder: Start 10 mg PO daily; may increase to max 20 mg PO daily after first week.
PEDS — Depression, adults and age 12 yo and greater: Start 10 mg PO daily. May increase to max 20 mg/day.
UNAPPROVED ADULTS — Social anxiety disorder: 5 to 20 mg PO daily.
FORMS — Generic/Trade: Tabs 5, 10, 20 mg. Trade only: Oral soln 1 mg/mL.
NOTES — Don't use with MAOIs. Doses greater than 20 mg daily have not been shown to be superior to 10 mg daily. Escitalopram is the active isomer of citalopram.
MOA — Selective serotonin reuptake inhibitor.
ADVERSE EFFECTS — Serious: Suicidality, serotonin syndrome, abnormal bleeding, withdrawal reactions. Frequent: Insomnia, ejaculatory disorders, nausea, sweating, fatigue, somnolence.

FLUOXETINE (Prozac, Prozac Weekly, Sarafem) ▶L ♀C but - in 3rd trimester ▶- $$$
ADULTS — Depression, OCD: Start 20 mg PO qam; may increase after several weeks to usual effective dose of 20 to 40 mg/day, max 80 mg/day. Depression, maintenance therapy: 20 to 40 mg/day (standard-release) or 90 mg PO once weekly (Prozac Weekly) starting 7 days after last standard-release dose. Bulimia: 60 mg PO qam; may need to titrate up to this dose slowly over several days. Panic disorder: Start 10 mg PO qam; titrate to 20 mg/day after 1 week, max 60 mg/day. Premenstrual Dysphoric Disorder (Sarafem): 20 mg PO daily given continuously throughout the menstrual cycle (continuous dosing) or 20 mg PO daily for 14 days prior to menses (intermittent dosing); max 80 mg daily.
Doses > 20 mg/day can be divided bid (in morning and at noon). Bipolar depression, olanzapine + fluoxetine: Start 5 mg olanzapine + 20 mg fluoxetine daily in the evening. Increase to usual range of 5 to 12.5 mg olanzapine plus 20 to 50 mg fluoxetine as tolerated. Treatment-resistant Depression, olanzapine + fluoxetine: Start 5 mg olanzapine + 20 mg fluoxetine daily in the evening. Increase to usual range of 5 to 20 mg olanzapine plus 20 to 50 mg fluoxetine as tolerated.
PEDS — Depression, age 7 to 17 yo: 10 to 20 mg PO qam (10 mg for smaller children), max 20 mg/day. OCD: Start 10 mg PO qam; max 60 mg/day (30 mg/day for smaller children).
UNAPPROVED ADULTS — Hot flashes: 20 mg PO daily. Posttraumatic stress disorder: 20 to 80 mg PO daily. Social anxiety disorder: 10 to 60 mg PO daily.
FORMS — Generic/Trade: Tabs 10 mg. Caps 10, 20, 40 mg. Oral soln 20 mg/5 mL. Caps (Sarafem) 10, 20 mg. Trade only: Tabs (Sarafem) 10, 15, 20 mg. Caps delayed-release (Prozac Weekly) 90 mg. Generic only: Tabs 20, 40 mg.
NOTES — Half-life of parent is 1 to 3 days and for active metabolite norfluoxetine is 6 to 14 days. Don't use with thioridazine, MAOIs, cisapride, or tryptophan; use caution with lithium, phenytoin, TCAs, and warfarin. Pregnancy exposure has been associated with premature delivery, low birth wt, and lower Apgar scores. Decrease dose with liver disease. Increases risk of mania with bipolar disorder.
MOA — Selective serotonin reuptake inhibitor.
ADVERSE EFFECTS — Serious: Suicidality, serotonin syndrome, neuroleptic malignant syndrome, SIADH, abnormal bleeding, withdrawal reactions, hypoglycemia. Frequent: N/V, diarrhea, insomnia, drowsiness, headache, sexual dysfunction, dry mouth, anorexia, anxiety, nervousness.

FLUVOXAMINE (Luvox, Luvox CR) ▶L ♀C but - in third trimester ▶- $$$$
ADULTS — OCD: Start 50 mg PO at bedtime, then increase by 50 mg/day q 4 to 7 d to usual effective dose of 100 to 300 mg/day divided bid. Max 300 mg/day. OCD and Social Anxiety Disorder (ER): Start 100 mg PO at bedtime; increase by 50 mg/day q week prn to max 300 mg/day.
PEDS — OCD (children age 8 yo or older): Start 25 mg PO at bedtime; increase by 25 mg/day q 4 to 7 d to usual effective dose of 50 to 200 mg/day divided bid. Max 200 mg/day (8 to 11 yo) or 300 mg/day (older than 11 yo). Therapeutic effect may be seen with lower doses in girls.
FORMS — Generic/Trade: Tabs 25, 50, 100 mg. Trade only: Caps extended-release 100, 150 mg.

(cont.)

FLUVOXAMINE (cont.)

NOTES – Don't use with thioridazine, pimozide, alosetron, cisapride, tizanidine, tryptophan, or MAOIs; use caution with benzodiazepines, theophylline, TCAs, and warfarin. Luvox brand not currently on US market.

MOA – Selective serotonin reuptake inhibitor.

ADVERSE EFFECTS – Serious: Suicidality, serotonin syndrome, neuroleptic malignant syndrome, SIADH, seizures, abnormal bleeding, withdrawal reactions. Frequent: N/V, diarrhea, insomnia, drowsiness, headache, sexual dysfunction, dry mouth, anorexia, anxiety, nervousness.

PAROXETINE (*Paxil, Paxil CR, Pexeva*) ▶LK ♀D ▶? $$$

ADULTS – <u>Depression:</u> Start 20 mg PO qam; increase by 10 mg/day at intervals of 1 week or more to usual effective dose of 20 to 50 mg/day, max 50 mg/day. <u>Depression, controlled-release tabs:</u> Start 25 mg PO qam; may increase by 12.5 mg/day at intervals of 1 week or more to usual effective dose of 25 to 62.5 mg/day; max 62.5 mg/day. <u>OCD:</u> Start 20 mg PO qam; increase by 10 mg/day at intervals of 1 week or more to usual recommended dose of 40 mg/day; max 60 mg/day. <u>Panic disorder:</u> Start 10 mg PO qam; increase by 10 mg/day at intervals of 1 week or more to target dose of 40 mg/day; max 60 mg/day. <u>Panic disorder, controlled-release tabs:</u> Start 12.5 mg/day; increase by 12.5 mg/day at intervals of 1 week or more to usual effective dose of 12.5 to 75 mg/day; max 75 mg/day. <u>Social anxiety disorder:</u> Start 20 mg PO qam (which is the usual effective dose); max 60 mg/day. <u>Social anxiety disorder, controlled-release tabs:</u> Start 12.5 mg PO qam; may increase at intervals of 1 week or more to max 37.5 mg/day. <u>Generalized anxiety disorder:</u> Start 20 mg PO qam (which is the usual effective dose); max 50 mg/day. <u>Posttraumatic stress disorder:</u> Start 20 mg PO qam; usual effective dose is 20 to 40 mg/day; max 50 mg/day. <u>Premenstrual dysphoric disorder (PMDD), continuous dosing:</u> Start 12.5 mg PO qam (controlled-release tabs); may increase dose after 1 week to max 25 mg qam. <u>PMDD, intermittent dosing</u> (given for 2 weeks prior to menses): Start 12.5 mg PO qam (controlled-release tabs), max 25 mg/day.

PEDS – Not recommended for use in children or adolescents due to increased risk of suicidality.

UNAPPROVED ADULTS – <u>Hot flashes related to menopause or breast cancer:</u> 20 mg PO daily (tabs), or 12.5 to 25 mg PO daily (controlled-release tabs).

FORMS – Generic/Trade: Tabs 10, 20, 30, 40 mg. Oral susp 10 mg/5 mL. Controlled-release tabs 12.5, 25 mg. Trade only: (Paxil CR) 37.5 mg.

NOTES – Start at 10 mg/day and do not exceed 40 mg/day in elderly or debilitated patients or those with renal or hepatic impairment. Paroxetine is an inhibitor of CYP2D6, and is contraindicated with thioridazine, pimozide, MAOIs, and tryptophan; use caution with barbiturates, cimetidine, phenytoin, theophylline, TCAs, risperidone, atomoxetine, and warfarin. Taper gradually after long-term use; reduce by 10 mg/day q week to 20 mg/day; continue for 1 week at this dose, and then stop. If withdrawal symptoms develop, then restart at prior dose and taper more slowly. Pexeva is paroxetine mesylate and is a generic equivalent for paroxetine HCl.

MOA – Selective serotonin reuptake inhibitor.

ADVERSE EFFECTS – Serious: Suicidality, serotonin syndrome, SIADH, hyponatremia, abnormal bleeding, withdrawal reactions. Frequent: Asthenia, nausea, diarrhea, constipation, insomnia, drowsiness, sexual dysfunction, dry mouth, anorexia, nervousness, sweating, dizziness, tremor.

SERTRALINE (*Zoloft*) ▶LK ♀C but - in third trimester ▶+ $$$

ADULTS – <u>Depression, OCD:</u> Start 50 mg PO daily; may increase after 1 week. Usual effective dose is 50 to 200 mg/day, max 200 mg/day. <u>Panic disorder, posttraumatic stress disorder, social anxiety disorder:</u> Start 25 mg PO daily; may increase after 1 week to 50 mg PO daily. Usual effective dose is 50 to 200 mg/day; max 200 mg/day. <u>Premenstrual dysphoric disorder (PMDD), continuous dosing:</u> Start 50 mg PO daily; max 150 mg/day. <u>PMDD, intermittent dosing</u> (given for 14 days prior to menses): Start 50 mg PO daily for 3 days, then increase to max 100 mg/day.

PEDS – <u>OCD,</u> age 6 to 12 yo: Start 25 mg PO daily, max 200 mg/day. <u>OCD,</u> age 13 yo or older: Use adult dosing.

UNAPPROVED PEDS – <u>Major depressive disorder:</u> Start 25 mg PO daily; usual effective dose is 50 to 200 mg/day.

FORMS – Generic/Trade: Tabs 25, 50, 100 mg. Oral concentrate 20 mg/mL (60 mL).

NOTES – Don't use with cisapride, tryptophan, or MAOIs; use caution with cimetidine, warfarin, pimozide, or TCAs. Must dilute oral concentrate before administration. Administration during pregnancy has been associated with premature delivery, low birth wt, and lower Apgar scores.

MOA – Selective serotonin reuptake inhibitor.

ADVERSE EFFECTS – Serious: Suicidality, serotonin syndrome, neuroleptic malignant syndrome, SIADH, hyponatremia, abnormal bleeding, withdrawal symptoms. Frequent: N/V, diarrhea, insomnia, drowsiness, headache, sexual dysfunction, dry mouth, anorexia, anxiety, nervousness.

PSYCHIATRY: Antidepressants—Serotonin-Norepinephrine Reuptake Inhibitors (SNRIs)

NOTE: Monitor for the emergence of anxiety, agitation, panic attacks, insomnia, irritability, hostility, impulsivity, akathisia, mania, or hypomania, and for worsening depression or the emergence of suicidality, particularly early in therapy or after increases in dose. Antidepressants increase the risk of suicidal thinking and behavior in children, adolescents, and young adults; carefully weigh the risks and benefits before starting treatment, and then monitor closely. SSRIs and SNRIs have been associated with hyponatremia, which is often associated with SIADH. The elderly and those taking diuretics may be at increased risk. Do not use with MAOIs. SNRIs have been associated with serotonin syndrome and neuroleptic malignant syndrome when used alone and especially in combination with other serotonergic drugs.

DESVENLAFAXINE (*Pristiq*) ▶LK ♀C ▶? $$$$
ADULTS – Depression: 50 mg PO daily. Max 400 mg/day.
PEDS – Not approved for use in children.
FORMS – Trade only: Tabs extended-release 50, 100 mg.
NOTES – There is no evidence that doses > 50 mg/day offer additional benefit. Reduce dose to 50 mg PO every other day in severe renal impairment (CrCl < 30 mL/min). Caution in cardiovascular, cerebrovascular, or lipid disorders. Gradually taper when discontinuing therapy to avoid withdrawal symptoms after prolonged use. Exposure to SSRIs or SNRIs during the third trimester of pregnancy has been associated with neonatal complications including respiratory, GI, and feeding problems, as well as seizures and withdrawal symptoms. Balance these risks against those of withdrawal and depression for the mother.
MOA – Selective inhibitor of serotonin and norepinephrine reuptake.
ADVERSE EFFECTS – Serious: Hypersensitivity, suicidality, serotonin syndrome, neuroleptic malignant syndrome, hypertension, hyperlipidemia, abnormal bleeding, hyponatremia, mania, seizures, narrow angle glaucoma. Frequent: Nausea, vomiting, dry mouth, constipation, diarrhea, fatigue, decreased appetite, insomnia, hyperhidrosis, headache, dizziness.

DULOXETINE (*Cymbalta*) ▶L ♀C ▶? $$$$
ADULTS – Depression: 20 mg PO bid; max 60 mg/day given once daily or divided bid. Generalized anxiety disorder: Start 30 to 60 mg PO daily, max 120 mg/day. Diabetic peripheral neuropathic pain: 60 mg PO daily, max 60 mg/day. Fibromyalgia: Start 30 to 60 mg PO daily, max 60 mg/day.
PEDS – Not approved in children.
FORMS – Trade only: Caps 20, 30, 60 mg.
NOTES – Avoid in renal insufficiency (CrCl < 30 mL/min), hepatic insufficiency, or substantial alcohol use. Don't use with thioridazine, MAOIs, or potent inhibitors of CYP1A2; use caution with inhibitors of CYP2D6. Small BP increases have been observed. Exposure during the 3rd trimester of pregnancy has been associated with neonatal complications including respiratory, GI, and feeding problems, as well as seizures, and withdrawal symptoms; balance these risks against those of withdrawal and depression for the mother.
MOA – Serotonin and norepinephrine reuptake inhibitor; also a weak inhibitor of dopamine reuptake.
ADVERSE EFFECTS – Serious: Suicidality, hypertension, seizures, hepatitis, cholestatic jaundice, serotonin syndrome, abnormal bleeding, orthostatic hypotension, hyponatremia. Frequent: N/V, dry mouth, constipation, decreased appetite, fatigue, somnolence, insomnia, sweating, dizziness, headache.

VENLAFAXINE (*Effexor, Effexor XR*) ▶LK ♀C but - in 3rd trimester ▶? $$$$
ADULTS – Depression: Start 37.5 to 75 mg PO daily (Effexor XR) or 75 mg/day divided bid to tid (Effexor). Increase in 75 mg increments q 4 d to usual effective dose of 150 to 225 mg/day, max 225 mg/day (Effexor XR) or 375 mg/day (Effexor). Generalized anxiety disorder: Start 37.5 to 75 mg PO daily (Effexor XR); increase in 75 mg increments q 4 d to max 225 mg/day. Social anxiety disorder: 75 mg PO daily (Effexor XR). Panic disorder: Start 37.5 mg PO daily (Effexor XR), may titrate by 75 mg/day at weekly intervals to max 225 mg/day.
PEDS – Not approved in children. May increase the risk of suicidality in children and teenagers.
UNAPPROVED ADULTS – Hot flashes (primarily in cancer patients): 37.5 to 75 mg/day of the extended-release form.
FORMS – Generic/Trade: Caps extended-release 37.5, 75, 150 mg. Tabs 25, 37.5, 50, 75, 100 mg. Generic only: Tabs extended-release 37.5, 75, 150, 225 mg.
NOTES – Noncyclic, serotonin-norepinephrine reuptake inhibitor (SNRI). Decrease dose in renal or hepatic impairment. Monitor for increases in BP. Don't give with MAOIs; use caution with cimetidine and haloperidol. Use caution and monitor for serotonin syndrome if used with triptans. Gradually taper when discontinuing therapy to avoid withdrawal symptoms after prolonged use. Hostility, suicidal ideation, and self-harm have been reported when used in children. Exposure during the third trimester of pregnancy has been associated with neonatal complications including respiratory, GI, and feeding problems, as well as seizures and withdrawal symptoms. Balance these risks against those of withdrawal and depression for the mother. Mydriasis and increased intraocular pressure can occur; use caution in glaucoma.
MOA – Serotonin and norepinephrine reuptake inhibitor; also a weak inhibitor of dopamine reuptake.
ADVERSE EFFECTS – Serious: Suicidality, mania/hypomania, seizures, hypertension, withdrawal symptoms, serotonin syndrome, neuroleptic malignant syndrome, interstitial lung disease and eosinophilic pneumonia, toxic epidermal necrolysis. Frequent: Drowsiness, dizziness, sexual dysfunction, anorexia, N/V, asthenia, nervousness, insomnia, diaphoresis, constipation, dry mouth, abnormal vision.

PSYCHIATRY: Antidepressants—Other

NOTE: Monitor for the emergence of anxiety, agitation, panic attacks, insomnia, irritability, hostility, impulsivity, akathisia, mania, or hypomania, and for worsening depression or the emergence of suicidality, particularly early in therapy or after increases in dose. Antidepressants increase the risk of suicidal thinking and behavior in children, adolescents, and young adults; carefully weigh the risks and benefits before starting treatment, and then monitor closely.

BUPROPION (*Wellbutrin, Wellbutrin SR, Wellbutrin XL, Aplenzin, Zyban, Buproban*) ▶LK ♀C ▶– $$$$
ADULTS — Depression: Start 100 mg PO bid (immediate-release tabs); can increase to 100 mg tid after 4 to 7 days. Usual effective dose is 300 to 450 mg/day, max 150 mg/dose and 450 mg/day. Depression, sustained-release tabs (Wellbutrin SR): Start 150 mg PO qam; may increase to 150 mg bid after 4 to 7 days, max 400 mg/day. Give the last dose no later than 5 pm. Depression, extended-release tabs (Wellbutrin XL): Start 150 mg PO qam; may increase to 300 mg qam after 4 days, max 450 mg qam. Depression, extended-release (Aplenzin): Start 174 mg PO qam; increase to target dose of 348 mg/day after 4 days or more. May increase to max dose of 522 mg/day after 4 weeks or more. Seasonal affective disorder, extended-release tabs (Wellbutrin XL): Start 150 mg PO qam in autumn; may increase after 1 week to target dose of 300 mg qam, max 300 mg/day. In the spring, decrease to 150 mg/day for 2 weeks and then discontinue. Smoking cessation (Zyban, Buproban): Start 150 mg PO qam for 3 days, then increase to 150 mg PO bid for 7 to 12 weeks. Allow 8 h between doses, with the last dose given no later than 5 pm. Max 150 mg PO bid. Target quit date should be after at least 1 week of therapy. Stop if there is no progress towards abstinence by the 7th week. Write "dispense behavioral modification kit" on first script.
PEDS — Not approved in children.
UNAPPROVED ADULTS — ADHD: 150 to 450 mg/day PO.
UNAPPROVED PEDS — ADHD: 1.4 to 5.7 mg/kg/day PO.
FORMS — Generic/Trade (for depression, bupropion HCl): Tabs 75, 100 mg. Sustained-release tabs 100, 150, 200 mg. Extended-release tabs 150, 300 mg (Wellbutrin XL). Generic/Trade (Smoking cessation): Sustained-release tabs 150 mg (Zyban, Buproban). Trade only: Extended-release (Aplenzin, bupropion hydrobromide) tabs 174, 348, 522 mg.
NOTES — Weak inhibitor of dopamine reuptake. Don't use with MAOIs. Seizures occur in 0.4% of patients taking 300 to 450 mg/day. Contraindicated in seizure disorders, eating disorders, or with abrupt alcohol or sedative withdrawal. Wellbutrin SR, Zyban, and Buproban are all the same formulation. Equivalent doses: 174 HBr = 150 mg HCl, 348 mg HBr = 300 mg HCl, 522 mg HBr = 450 mg HCl. Consider dose reductions for hepatic and renal impairment.
MOA — Norepinephrine and dopamine reuptake inhibitor.
ADVERSE EFFECTS — Serious: Suicidality, seizures, psychosis, HTN, Stevens-Johnson syndrome, rhabdomyolysis, hallucinations. Frequent: Headache, tremor, agitation, insomnia, diaphoresis, weight loss, dry mouth, nausea, constipation, dizziness.

MIRTAZAPINE (*Remeron, Remeron SolTab*) ▶LK ♀C ▶? $$
ADULTS — Depression: Start 15 mg PO at bedtime, increase after 1 to 2 weeks to usual effective dose of 15 to 45 mg/day.
PEDS — Not approved in children.
FORMS — Generic/Trade: Tabs 15, 30, 45 mg. Tabs orally disintegrating (SolTab) 15, 30, 45 mg. Generic only: Tabs 7.5 mg.
NOTES — 0.1% risk of agranulocytosis. May cause drowsiness, increased appetite, and wt gain. Don't use with MAOIs.
MOA — Presynaptic alpha-2 receptor antagonist; 5-HT2A, 5-HT-2C, and 5-HT-3 receptor antagonist; enhances norepinephrine and serotonin release.
ADVERSE EFFECTS — Serious: Suicidality, agranulocytosis, dyslipidemia, serotonin syndrome, hyponatremia. Frequent: Drowsiness, increased appetite, weight gain, dizziness, dry mouth, constipation.

NEFAZODONE ▶L ♀C ▶? $$$
WARNING — Rare reports of life-threatening liver failure. Discontinue if signs or symptoms of liver dysfunction develop. Brand name product withdrawn from the market in the United States and Canada.
ADULTS — Depression: Start 100 mg PO bid. Increase by 100 to 200 mg/day at 1 week intervals or longer to usual effective dose of 150 to 300 mg PO bid, max 600 mg/day. Start 50 mg PO bid in elderly or debilitated patients.
PEDS — Not approved in children.
FORMS — Generic only: Tabs 50, 100, 150, 200, 250 mg.
NOTES — Don't use with cisapride, MAOIs, pimozide, or triazolam; use caution with alprazolam. Many other drug interactions.
MOA — Serotonin reuptake inhibitor and 5-HT2 receptor antagonist.
ADVERSE EFFECTS — Serious: Suicidality, hepatotoxicity, liver failure. Frequent: N/V, dry mouth, constipation, drowsiness, dizziness, asthenia.

TRAZODONE (*Desyrel, Oleptro*) ▶L ♀C ▶– $
ADULTS — Depression: Start 50 to 150 mg/day PO in divided doses, increase by 50 mg/day q 3 to 4 days. Usual effective dose is 400 to 600 mg/day. Extended release: Start 150 mg PO at bedtime. May increase by 75 mg/day every 3 days to max 375 mg/day.

(cont.)

TRAZODONE (cont.)
PEDS — Not approved in children.
UNAPPROVED ADULTS — Insomnia: 50 to 100 mg PO at bedtime, max 150 mg/day.
UNAPPROVED PEDS — Depression, 6 to 18 yo: Start 1.5 to 2 mg/kg/day PO divided bid to tid; may increase q 3 to 4 days to max 6 mg/kg/day.
FORMS — Trade only: Extended release tabs (Oleptro) 150, 300 mg. Generic only: Tabs 50, 100, 150, 300 mg.
NOTES — May cause priapism. Rarely used as monotherapy for depression; most often used as a sleep aid and adjunct to another antidepressant. Use caution with CYP3A4 inhibitors or inducers.
MOA — Serotonin reuptake inhibitor and 5-HT2A receptor antagonist.

ADVERSE EFFECTS — Serious: Orthostatic hypotension, priapism, syncope. Frequent: Drowsiness, dizziness, nervousness, headache, tremor, fatigue, dry mouth, blurred vision.

TRYPTOPHAN (✦*Tryptan*) ▶K ♀? ▶? $$
ADULTS — Canada only. Adjunct to antidepressant treatment for affective disorders: 8 to 12 g/day in 3 to 4 divided doses.
PEDS — Not indicated.
FORMS — Trade only: L-tryptophan tabs 250, 500, 750, 1000 mg.
NOTES — Caution in diabetics; may worsen glycemic control.
MOA — An essential amino acid that increases serotonin synthesis in the CNS.
ADVERSE EFFECTS — Serious: Serotonin syndrome. Frequent: Drowsiness, dizziness, nausea, dry mouth.

PSYCHIATRY: Antimanic (Bipolar) Agents

LAMOTRIGINE (*Lamictal, Lamictal CD, Lamictal ODT, Lamictal XR*) ▶LK ♀C (see notes) ▶– $$$$
WARNING — Potentially life-threatening rashes (eg, Stevens-Johnson syndrome, toxic epidermal necrolysis) have been reported in 0.3% of adults and 0.8% of children, usually within 2 to 8 weeks of initiation; discontinue at first sign of rash. Drug interaction with valproate; see adjusted dosing guidelines. Recent data suggest an increased risk of suicidal ideation or behaviors with antiepileptic drugs. Monitor closely for signs of depression, anxiety, hostility, and hypomania/mania. Symptoms may develop within 1 week of initiation and risk continues through at least 24 weeks.
ADULTS — Bipolar disorder (maintenance): Start 25 mg PO daily, 50 mg PO daily if on carbamazepine or other enzyme-inducing drugs, or 25 mg PO every other day if on valproate. Increase for week 3 to 4 to 50 mg/day, 50 mg bid if on enzyme-inducing drugs, or 25 mg/day if on valproate, then adjust over week 5 to 7 to target doses of 200 mg/day, 400 mg/day divided bid if on enzyme-inducing drugs, or 100 mg/day if on valproate. See neurology section for epilepsy dosing.
PEDS — Not approved in children.
FORMS — Generic/Trade: Chewable dispersible tabs (Lamictal CD) 5, 25 mg. Tabs 25, 100, 150, 200 mg. Trade only: Orally disintegrating tabs (ODT) 25, 50, 100, 200 mg. Extended-release tabs (XR) 25, 50, 100, 200 mg.
NOTES — Drug interactions with valproate and enzyme-inducing antiepileptic drugs (ie, carbamazepine, phenobarbital, phenytoin, primidone); may need to adjust dose. May increase carbamazepine toxicity. Preliminary evidence suggests that exposure during the 1st trimester of pregnancy is associated with a risk for cleft palate and/or cleft lip. Please report all fetal exposure to the Lamotrigine Pregnancy Registry (800-336-2176) and the North American Antiepileptic Drug Pregnancy Registry (888-233-2334).
MOA — Unknown in bipolar.
ADVERSE EFFECTS — Serious: Rash (including Stevens-Johnson syndrome and toxic epidermal necrolysis), hypersensitivity reactions, blood dyscrasias, multiorgan failure. Frequent: N/V, insomnia, back pain, fatigue, rhinitis, abdominal pain, dry mouth, constipation, exacerbation of cough, pharyngitis.

LITHIUM (*Eskalith, Eskalith CR, Lithobid, ✦Lithane*) ▶K ♀D ▶– $
WARNING — Lithium toxicity can occur at therapeutic levels.
ADULTS — Acute Mania: Start 300 to 600 mg PO bid to tid; usual effective dose is 900 to 1800 mg/day. Bipolar maintenance usually 900 to 1200 mg/day titrated to therapeutic trough level of 0.6 to 1.2 mEq/L.
PEDS — Age 12 yo or older: Use adult dosing.
UNAPPROVED PEDS — Mania (age younger than 12 yo): Start 15 to 60 mg/kg/day PO divided tid to qid. Adjust weekly to achieve therapeutic levels.
FORMS — Generic/Trade: Caps 300, Extended-release tabs 300, 450 mg. Generic only: Caps 150, 600 mg, Tabs 300 mg, Syrup 300/5 mL.
NOTES — Steady state levels occur in 5 days (later in elderly or renally-impaired patients). Usual therapeutic trough levels are 1.0 to 1.5 mEq/L (acute Mania) or 0.6 to 1.2 mEq/L (maintenance). 300 mg = 8 mEq or mmol. A dose increase of 300 mg/day will increase the level by approx 0.2 mEq/L. Monitor renal and thyroid function, avoid dehydration or salt restriction, and watch closely for polydipsia or polyuria. Diuretics, ACE inhibitors, angiotensin receptor blockers, and NSAIDs may increase lithium levels (aspirin and sulindac OK). Dose-related side effects (eg, tremor, GI upset) may improve by dividing doses tid to qid or using extended-release tabs. Monitor renal function and electrolytes.
MOA — Unknown, may increase synthesis and release of serotonin and inhibit its reuptake.

(cont.)

LITHIUM (cont.)
ADVERSE EFFECTS — Serious: Seizures, ventricular arrhythmias, leukocytosis, hypothyroidism, renal failure, nephrogenic diabetes insipidus, coma, drug-induced parkinsonism. Frequent: Tremor, N/V, diarrhea, cramps, polyuria, polydipsia, rash, fatigue.

TOPIRAMATE (*Topamax*) ▶K ♀C ▶? $$$$$
WARNING — Recent data suggest an increased risk of suicidal ideation or behaviors with antiepileptic drugs. Monitor closely for signs of depression, anxiety, hostility, and hypomania/mania. Symptoms may develop within 1 week of initiation and risk continues through at least 24 weeks.
ADULTS — See neurology section.
PEDS — Not approved for psychiatric use in children; see Neurology section.
UNAPPROVED ADULTS — Bipolar disorder: Start 25 to 50 mg/day PO; titrate prn to max 400 mg/day divided bid. Alcohol dependence: Start 25 mg/day PO; titrate weekly to max 150 mg bid.
FORMS — Trade: Tabs 25, 50, 100, 200 mg. Sprinkle Caps 15, 25 mg.
NOTES — Give ½ usual adult dose to patients with renal impairment (CrCl < 70 mL/min). Cognitive symptoms, confusion, renal stones, glaucoma, and wt loss may occur. Risk of oligohidrosis and hyperthermia, particularly in children; use caution in warm ambient temperatures and/or with vigorous physical activity. Hyperchloremic, nonanion gap metabolic acidosis may occur; monitor serum bicarbonate and reduce dose or taper off if this occurs.
MOA — Unknown, but may modulate sodium channels and enhance GABA action. Weak carbonic anhydrase inhibitor.
ADVERSE EFFECTS — Serious: Angle closure glaucoma, nephrolithiasis, oligohidrosis, hyperthermia, metabolic acidosis. Frequent: Sedation, ataxia, psychomotor slowing, cognitive symptoms, confusion, diplopia, nystagmus, dizziness, depression, nervousness, weight loss, paresthesia.

VALPROIC ACID (*Depakote, Depakote ER, Stavzor, divalproex, ✦Epiject, Epival, Deproic*) ▶L ♀D ▶+ $$$$
WARNING — Fatal hepatic failure has occurred, especially in children younger than 2 yo with multiple anticonvulsants and comorbidities. Monitor LFTs frequently during first 6 months. Life-threatening pancreatitis has been reported after initial or prolonged use. Evaluate for abdominal pain, N/V, and/or anorexia and discontinue if pancreatitis occurs. May be more teratogenic than other anticonvulsants (eg, carbamazepine, lamotrigine, and phenytoin). Hepatic failure and clotting disorders have also occurred when used during pregnancy. Recent data suggest an increased risk of suicidal ideation or behaviors with antiepileptic drugs. Monitor closely for signs of depression, anxiety, hostility, and hypomania/mania. Symptoms may develop within 1 week of initiation and risk continues through at least 24 weeks.
ADULTS — Mania: Start 250 mg PO tid (Depakote or Stavzor) or 25 mg/kg once daily (Depakote ER); titrate to therapeutic level. Max 60 mg/kg/day.
PEDS — Not approved for mania in children.
UNAPPROVED PEDS — Bipolar disorder, manic or mixed phase (age older than 2 yo): Start 125 to 250 mg PO bid or 15 mg/kg/day in divided doses. Titrate to therapeutic trough level of 45 to 125 mcg/mL, max 60 mg/kg/day.
FORMS — Generic only: Syrup (Valproic acid) 250 mg/5 mL. Generic/Trade: Delayed-release tabs (Depakote) 125, 250, 500 mg. Extended-release tabs (Depakote ER) 250, 500 mg. Delayed-release sprinkle caps (Depakote) 125 mg. Trade only (Stavzor): Delayed-release caps 125, 250, 500 mg.
NOTES — Contraindicated in urea cycle disorders or hepatic dysfunction. Reduce dose in the elderly. Recommended therapeutic trough level is 50 to 125 mcg/mL for Depakote and 85 to 125 mcg/mL for Depakote ER, though higher levels have been used. Many drug interactions. Hyperammonemia, GI irritation, or thrombocytopenia may occur. Depakote ER is approximately 10% less bioavailable than Depakote. Depakote-releases divalproex sodium over 8 to 12 h (daily to qid dosing) and Depakote ER-releases divalproex sodium over 18 to 24 h (daily dosing).
MOA — Anticonvulsant; may increase GABA levels and modulate sodium channels.
ADVERSE EFFECTS — Serious: Hepatotoxicity, anaphylaxis, polycystic ovarian syndrome, bone marrow suppression, thrombocytopenia, pancreatitis, Stevens-Johnson syndrome, hyperammonemia, drug-induced parkinsonism. Frequent: N/V, diarrhea, dyspepsia, weight gain, CNS depression, drowsiness, dizziness, tremor, alopecia, rash, nystagmus.

PSYCHIATRY: Antipsychotics—First Generation (Typical)

NOTE: Antipsychotic potency is determined by affinity for D2 receptors. Extrapyramidal side effects (EPS) including tardive dyskinesia and dystonia may occur with antipsychotics. Use cautiously in patients with Parkinson's disease. High-potency agents are more likely to cause EPS and hyperprolactinemia. Can be given at bedtime, but may be divided initially to decrease side effects and daytime sedation. Antipsychotics have been associated with an increased risk of venous thromboembolism, especially early in therapy. Assess for other risk factors and monitor carefully. Off-label use for dementia-related psychosis in the elderly has been associated with increased mortality.

ANTIPSYCHOTIC RELATIVE ADVERSE EFFECTS[a]

Generation	Antipsychotic	Anticholinergic	Sedation	Hypotension	EPS	Weight Gain	Diabetes/Hyperglycemia	Dyslipidemia
1st	chlorpromazine	+++	+++	++	++	++	?	?
1st	fluphenazine	++	+	+	++++	++	?	?
1st	haloperidol	+	+	+	++++	++	0	?
1st	loxapine	++	+	+	++	+	?	?
1st	molindone	++	++	+	++	+	?	?
1st	perphenazine	++	++	+	++	+	+/?	?
1st	pimozide	+	+	+	+++	?	?	?
1st	thioridazine	++++	+++	+++	+	+++	+/?	?
1st	thiothixene	+	++	++	+++	++	?	?
1st	trifluoperazine	++	+	+	+++	++	?	?
2nd	aripiprazole	++	+	0	0	0/+	0	0
2nd	clozapine	++++	+++	+++	0	+++	+	+
2nd	olanzapine	+++	++	+	0[b]	+++	+	+
2nd	risperidone	+	++	+	+[b]	++	?	?
2nd	quetiapine	+	+++	++	0	++	?	?
2nd	ziprasidone	+	+	0	0	0/+	0	0

[a]Risk of specific adverse effects is graded from 0 (absent) to ++++ (high). ? = Limited or inconsistent comparative data. [b]EPS (EPS) are dose-related and are more likely for risperidone >6-8 mg/day/olanzapine >20 mg/day. Akathisia risk remains unclear and may not be reflected in these ratings. There are limited comparative data for aripiprazole iloperidone, paliperidone, and asenapine relative to other second generation antipsychotics.
References: Goodman & Gilman 11e p461-500, Applied Therapeutics 8e p78, APA schizophrenia practice guideline, Psychiatry Q 2002; 73:297, Diabetes Care 2004;27:596.

CHLORPROMAZINE (Thorazine) ▶LK ♀C ▶– $$$
ADULTS — Psychotic disorders: 10 to 50 mg PO bid to qid or 25 to 50 mg IM, can repeat in 1 h. Severe cases may require 400 mg IM q 4 to 6 h up to maximum of 2000 mg/day IM. Hiccups: 25 to 50 mg PO/IM tid to qid. Persistent hiccups may require 25 to 50 mg in 0.5 to 1 liter NS by slow IV infusion.
PEDS — Severe behavioral problems/psychotic disorders age 6 mo to 12 yo: 0.5 mg/kg PO q 4 to 6 h prn or 1 mg/kg PR q 6 to 8 h prn or 0.5 mg/kg IM q 6 to 8 h prn.
FORMS — Generic only: Tabs 10, 25, 50, 100, 200 mg. Generic/Trade: Oral concentrate 30 mg/mL, 100 mg/mL. Trade only: Syrup 10 mg/5 mL, Supps 25, 100 mg.
NOTES — Monitor for hypotension with IM or IV use.
MOA — Low-potency dopamine antagonist.
ADVERSE EFFECTS — Serious: Seizures, neuroleptic malignant syndrome, extrapyramidal side effects, tardive dyskinesia, QT prolongation, jaundice. Frequent: Drowsiness, nausea, dry mouth, constipation, urinary retention, hypotension, headache, hyperprolactinemia.

FLUPENTHIXOL (flupentixol, ✽Fluanxol, Fluanxol Depot) ▶? ♀? ▶– $$
ADULTS — Canada only. Schizophrenia/psychosis: Tabs initial dose: 3 mg PO daily in divided doses, maintenance 3 to 12 mg daily in divided doses. IM initial dose 5 to 20 mg IM q 2 to 4 weeks, maintenance 20 to 40 mg q 2 to 4 weeks. Higher doses may be necessary in some patients.
PEDS — Not approved in children.
FORMS — Trade only: Tabs 0.5, 3 mg.
NOTES — Relatively nonsedating antipsychotic.
MOA — High-potency dopamine receptor antagonist.
ADVERSE EFFECTS — Serious: NMS, tardive dyskinesia. Frequent: Extrapyramidal reactions, restlessness, agitation.

FLUPHENAZINE (Prolixin, ✽Modecate, Modeten) ▶LK ♀C ▶? $$$
ADULTS — Psychotic disorders: Start 0.5 to 10 mg/day PO divided q 6 to 8 h. Usual effective dose 1 to 20 mg/day. Maximum dose is 40 mg/day PO or 1.25 to 10 mg/day IM divided q 6 to 8 h. Maximum dose is 10 mg/day IM. May use long-acting formulations (enanthate/decanoate) when patients are stabilized on a fixed daily dose. Approximate conversion ratio: 12.5 to 25 mg IM/SC (depot) q 3 weeks is equivalent to 10 to 20 mg/day PO.
PEDS — Not approved in children.
FORMS — Generic/Trade: Tabs 1, 2.5, 5, 10 mg. Elixir 2.5 mg/5 mL. Oral concentrate 5 mg/mL.
NOTES — Do not mix oral concentrate with coffee, tea, cola, or apple juice.
MOA — High-potency dopamine antagonist.
ADVERSE EFFECTS — Serious: Seizures, neuroleptic malignant syndrome, agranulocytosis, aplastic anemia, extrapyramidal side effects, tardive dyskinesia, QT prolongation. Frequent: Drowsiness, nausea, dry mouth, constipation, urinary retention, hypotension, headache, hyperprolactinemia.

PSYCHIATRY: Antipsychotics

HALOPERIDOL (Haldol) ▶LK ♀C ▶– $$
ADULTS – Psychotic disorders/Tourette's: 0.5 to 5 mg PO bid to tid. Usual effective dose is 6 to 20 mg/day, maximum dose is 100 mg/day or 2 to 5 mg IM q 1 to 8 h prn. May use long-acting (depot) formulation when patients are stabilized on a fixed daily dose. Approximate conversion ratio: 100 to 200 mg IM (depot) q 4 weeks is equivalent to 10 mg/day PO haloperidol.
PEDS – Psychotic disorders age 3 to 12 yo: 0.05 to 0.15 mg/kg/day PO divided bid to tid. Tourette's or nonpsychotic behavior disorders age 3 to 12 yo: 0.05 to 0.075 mg/kg/day PO divided bid to tid. Increase dose by 0.5 mg q week to maximum dose of 6 mg/day. Not approved for IM administration in children.
UNAPPROVED ADULTS – Acute psychosis and combative behavior: 5 to 10 mg IV/IM, repeat prn in 10 to 30 min. IV route associated with QT prolongation, Torsades de Pointes, and sudden death; use ECG monitoring.
UNAPPROVED PEDS – Psychosis age 6 to 12 yo: 1 to 3 mg/dose IM (as lactate) q 4 to 8 h, max 0.15 mg/kg/day.
FORMS – Generic only: Tabs 0.5, 1, 2, 5, 10, 20 mg. Oral concentrate 2 mg/mL.
NOTES – Therapeutic range is 2 to 15 ng/mL.
MOA – High-potency dopamine antagonist.
ADVERSE EFFECTS – Serious: Seizures, neuroleptic malignant syndrome, extrapyramidal side effects, tardive dyskinesia, QT prolongation, sudden death, jaundice. Frequent: Drowsiness, nausea, dry mouth, constipation, urinary retention, hypotension, headache, hyperprolactinemia.

LOXAPINE (Loxitane, ✦Loxapac) ▶LK ♀C ▶– $$$$
ADULTS – Psychotic disorders: Start 10 mg PO bid, usual effective dose is 60 to 100 mg/day divided bid to qid. Maximum dose is 250 mg/day.
PEDS – Not approved in children.
FORMS – Generic/Trade: Caps 5, 10, 25, 50 mg.
MOA – Mid-potency dopamine antagonist.
ADVERSE EFFECTS – Serious: Seizures, neuroleptic malignant syndrome, extrapyramidal side effects, tardive dyskinesia, QT prolongation, jaundice. Frequent: Drowsiness, nausea, dry mouth, constipation, urinary retention, hypotension, headache, hyperprolactinemia.

METHOTRIMEPRAZINE (✦Nozinan) ▶L ♀? ▶? $
ADULTS – Canada only. Anxiety/analgesia: 6 to 25 mg PO per day given tid. Sedation: 10 to 25 mg bedtime. Psychoses/intense pain: Start 50 to 75 mg PO per day given in 2 to 3 doses, max 1000 mg/day. Postop pain: 20 to 40 mg PO or 10 to 25 mg IM q 8 h. Anesthesia premedication: 10 to 25 mg IM or 20 to 40 mg PO q 8 h with last dose of 25 to 50 mg IM 1 h before surgery. Limit therapy to < 30 days.
PEDS – Canada only. 0.25 mg/kg/day given in 2 to 3 doses, max 40 mg/day for child age younger than 12 yo.
FORMS – Canada only: Generic/Trade: Tabs 2, 5, 25, 50 mg.
MOA – Mid-potency dopamine antagonist.
ADVERSE EFFECTS – Serious: QT interval prolongation, neuroleptic malignant syndrome, tardive dyskinesia, orthostatic hypotension, agranulocytosis, jaundice. Frequent: Drowsiness, dry mouth, nausea, constipation, urinary retention, tachycardia, weight gain.

MOLINDONE (Moban) ▶LK ♀C ▶? $$$$$
ADULTS – Psychotic disorders: Start 50 to 75 mg/day PO divided tid to qid, usual effective dose is 50 to 100 mg/day. Maximum dose is 225 mg/day.
PEDS – Adolescents: Adult dosing. Not approved in children younger than 12 yo.
FORMS – Trade only: Tabs 5, 10, 25, 50 mg. Drug no longer manufactured and only available while current supplies last.
MOA – Mid-potency dopamine antagonist.
ADVERSE EFFECTS – Serious: Seizures, neuroleptic malignant syndrome, extrapyramidal side effects, tardive dyskinesia. Frequent: Drowsiness, nausea, dry mouth, constipation, urinary retention, hypotension, headache.

PERPHENAZINE ▶LK ♀C ▶? $$$
ADULTS – Psychotic disorders: Start 4 to 8 mg PO tid or 8 to 16 mg PO bid to qid (hospitalized patients), maximum PO dose is 64 mg/day. Can give 5 to 10 mg IM q 6 h, maximum IM dose is 30 mg/day.
PEDS – Not approved in children.
FORMS – Generic only: Tabs 2, 4, 8, 16 mg. Oral concentrate 16 mg/5 mL.
NOTES – Do not mix oral concentrate with coffee, tea, cola, or apple juice.
MOA – High-potency dopamine antagonist.
ADVERSE EFFECTS – Serious: Seizures, neuroleptic malignant syndrome, extrapyramidal side effects, tardive dyskinesia, QT prolongation, jaundice. Frequent: Drowsiness, nausea, dry mouth, constipation, urinary retention, hypotension, headache, hyperprolactinemia.

PIMOZIDE (Orap) ▶L ♀C ▶– $$$
ADULTS – Tourette's: Start 1 to 2 mg/day PO in divided doses, increase every 2 days to usual effective dose of 1 to 10 mg/day. Maximum dose is 0.2 mg/kg/day up to 10 mg/day.
PEDS – Tourette's older than 12 yo: 0.05 mg/kg PO at bedtime, increase every 3 days to maximum of 0.2 mg/kg/day up to 10 mg/day.
FORMS – Trade only: Tabs 1, 2 mg.
NOTES – QT prolongation may occur. Monitor ECG at baseline and periodically throughout therapy. Contraindicated with macrolide antibiotics, nefazodone, sertraline, citalopram, and escitalopram. Use caution with inhibitors of CYP3A4.
MOA – High-potency dopamine antagonist.
ADVERSE EFFECTS – Serious: Seizures, neuroleptic malignant syndrome, extrapyramidal side effects, tardive dyskinesia, QT prolongation, jaundice. Frequent: Drowsiness, nausea, dry mouth, constipation, urinary retention, hypotension, headache, hyperprolactinemia.

PSYCHIATRY: Antipsychotics

THIORIDAZINE (*Mellaril,* ✽*Rideril*) ▶LK ♀C ▶? $$
WARNING — Can cause QTc prolongation, torsade de pointes-type arrhythmias, and sudden death.
ADULTS — <u>Psychotic disorders:</u> Start 50 to 100 mg PO tid, usual effective dose is 200 to 800 mg/day divided bid to qid. Maximum dose is 800 mg/day.
PEDS — <u>Behavioral disorders</u> 2 to 12 yo: 10 to 25 mg PO bid to tid, maximum dose is 3 mg/kg/day.
FORMS — Generic only: Tabs 10, 15, 25, 50, 100, 150, 200 mg. Oral concentrate 30, 100 mg/mL.
NOTES — Not recommended as first line therapy. Contraindicated in patients with a history of cardiac arrhythmias, congenital long QT syndrome, or those taking fluvoxamine, propranolol, pindolol, drugs that inhibit CYP2D6 (eg, fluoxetine, paroxetine), and other drugs that prolong the QTc interval. Only use for patients with schizophrenia who do not respond to other antipsychotics. Monitor baseline ECG and potassium. Pigmentary retinopathy with doses > 800 mg/day.
MOA — Low-potency dopamine antagonist.
ADVERSE EFFECTS — Serious: Seizures, neuroleptic malignant syndrome, extrapyramidal side effects, tardive dyskinesia, QT prolongation, jaundice. Frequent: Drowsiness, nausea, dry mouth, constipation, urinary retention, hypotension, headache, hyperprolactinemia.

THIOTHIXENE (*Navane*) ▶LK ♀C ▶? $$$
ADULTS — <u>Psychotic disorders:</u> Start 2 mg PO tid. Usual effective dose is 20 to 30 mg/day, maximum dose is 60 mg/day PO.
PEDS — <u>Adolescents:</u> Adult dosing. Not approved in children younger than 12 yo.
FORMS — Generic/Trade: Caps 1, 2, 5, 10. Oral concentrate 5 mg/mL. Trade only: Caps 20 mg.
MOA — High-potency dopamine antagonist.
ADVERSE EFFECTS — Serious: Seizures, neuroleptic malignant syndrome, orthostatic hypotension, hyperglycemia, dysphagia, jaundice, dystonia. Frequent: Headache, anxiety, insomnia, N/V, light-headedness, somnolence, akathisia, constipation, weight gain.

TRIFLUOPERAZINE (*Stelazine*) ▶LK ♀C ▶− $$$
ADULTS — <u>Psychotic disorders:</u> Start 2 to 5 mg PO bid. Usual effective dose is 15 to 20 mg/day, some patients may require 40 mg/day or more. <u>Anxiety:</u> 1 to 2 mg PO bid for up to 12 weeks. Maximum dose is 6 mg/day.
PEDS — <u>Psychotic disorders</u> age 6 to 12 yo: 1 mg PO daily to bid, gradually increase to maximum dose of 15 mg/day.
FORMS — Generic/Trade: Tabs 1, 2, 5, 10 mg. Trade only: Oral concentrate 10 mg/mL.
NOTES — Dilute oral concentrate just before giving.
MOA — High-potency dopamine antagonist.
ADVERSE EFFECTS — Serious: Seizures, neuroleptic malignant syndrome, extrapyramidal side effects, tardive dyskinesia, QT prolongation, jaundice. Frequent: Drowsiness, nausea, dry mouth, constipation, urinary retention, hypotension, headache, hyperprolactinemia.

ZUCLOPENTHIXOL (✽*Clopixol, Clopixol Accuphase, Clopixol Depot*) ▶L ♀? ▶? $$$$
ADULTS — Canada only. <u>Antipsychotic.</u> Tabs: Start 10 to 50 mg PO daily, maintenance 20 to 60 mg daily. Injectable: Accuphase (acetate) 50 to 150 mg IM q 2 to 3 days, Depot (decanoate) 150 to 300 mg IM q 2 to 4 weeks.
PEDS — Not approved in children.
FORMS — Trade, Canada-only: Tabs 10, 20 mg (Clopixol).
MOA — Low-potency dopamine antagonist.
ADVERSE EFFECTS — Serious: NMS, tardive dyskinesia. Frequent: Extrapyramidal reactions, drowsiness, dizziness.

PSYCHIATRY: Antipsychotics—Second Generation (Atypical)

NOTE: Tardive dyskinesia, neuroleptic malignant syndrome, drug-induced parkinsonism, dystonia, and other extrapyramidal side effects may occur with antipsychotic medications. Atypical antipsychotics have been associated with wt gain, dyslipidemia, hyperglycemia, and diabetes mellitus; monitor closely. Off-label use for dementia-related psychosis in the elderly has been associated with increased mortality. Antipsychotics have been associated with an increased risk of venous thromboembolism, particularly early in therapy; assess for other risk factors and monitor carefully. Antipsychotics when used for schizophrenia or bipolar disorder have been associated with an increased risk of suicidal thinking and behavior. Monitor closely.

ARIPIPRAZOLE (*Abilify, Abilify Discmelt*) ▶L ♀C ▶? $$$$$
WARNING — Antipsychotics when used for schizophrenia or bipolar disorder have been associated with an increased risk of suicidal thinking and behavior. Monitor closely.
ADULTS — <u>Schizophrenia:</u> Start 10 to 15 mg PO daily. Max 30 mg daily. <u>Bipolar disorder (acute and maintenance for manic or mixed episodes):</u> Start 30 mg PO daily; reduce dose to 15 mg/day if higher dose poorly tolerated. 15 mg PO daily. May increase to 30 mg/day based on response and tolerability. <u>Agitation associated with schizophrenia or bipolar disorder:</u> 9.75 mg IM recommended. May consider 5.25 to 15 mg if indicated. May repeat in > 2 h up to max 30 mg/day. <u>Depression, adjunctive therapy:</u> Start 2 to 5 mg PO daily. Increase by 5 mg/day at intervals 1 week or more to max of 15 mg/day.
PEDS — <u>Schizophrenia,</u> 13 to 17 yo: Start 2 mg PO daily. May increase to 5 mg/day after 2 days, and to target dose of 10 mg/day after 2 more days. Max 30 mg/day. <u>Bipolar disorder (acute and maintenance for manic or mixed episodes, monotherapy or adjunctive to lithium or valproate),</u> 10 to 17 yo:

(cont.)

ARIPIPRAZOLE (cont.)

Start 2 mg PO daily. May increase to 5 mg/day after 2 days, and to target dose of 10 mg/day after 2 more days. Increase by 5 mg/day to max 30 mg/day. Irritability associated with autism: Start 2 mg PO daily. Increase by 5 mg/day as needed up to max 15 mg/day.
FORMS — Trade only: Tabs 2, 5, 10, 15, 20, 30 mg. Oral soln 1 mg/mL (150 mL). Orally disintegrating tabs (Discmelt) 10, 15, 20, 30 mg.
NOTES — Low EPS and tardive dyskinesia risk. Increase dose when used with CYP3A4 inducers such as carbamazepine. Decrease usual dose by at least half when used with CYP3A4 or CYP2D6 inhibitors such as ketoconazole, fluoxetine or paroxetine. Increase dose by ½ to 20 to 30 mg/day when used with CYP3A4 inducers such as carbamazepine. Reduce when inducer is stopped.
MOA — Dopamine-2 partial agonist, serotonin-1A partial agonist, serotoin-2A antagonist.
ADVERSE EFFECTS — Serious: Seizures, neuroleptic malignant syndrome, orthostatic hypotension, hyperglycemia, dysphagia, jaundice, suicidal thinking/behavior. Frequent: Headache, anxiety, insomnia, N/V, lightheadedness, somnolence, akathisia, constipation, weight gain.

ASENAPINE (*Saphris*) ▶L ♀C ▶–
WARNING — Antipsychotics when used for schizophrenia or bipolar disorder have been associated with an increased risk of suicidal thinking and behavior. Monitor closely.
ADULTS — Schizophrenia: Initial and maintenance, 5 mg SL bid. Max 10 mg/day. Bipolar disorder: Initial and maintenance, 10 mg SL bid. May reduce to 5 mg SL bid if needed. Max 20 mg/day.
PEDS — Not approved for use in children
FORMS — Trade: Sublingual tabs 5, 10 mg
NOTES — Must be used sublingually and not chewed or crushed.
MOA — Serotonin and dopamine receptor antagonist.
ADVERSE EFFECTS — Serious: Neuroleptic malignant syndrome, tardive dyskinesia, hyperglycemia/diabetes, syncope, orthostatic hypotension, leukopenia, neutropenia, agranulocytosis, seizures. Frequent: Akathisia, other EPS, oral hypoesthesia, somnolence, dizziness, weight gain.

CLOZAPINE (*Clozaril, FazaClo ODT*) ▶L ♀B ▶– $$$$$
WARNING — Risk of agranulocytosis is 1 to 2%, monitor WBC and ANC counts q week for 6 months, then q 2 weeks thereafter, and weekly for 4 weeks after discontinuation. Contraindicated if WBC < 3500 or ANC < 2000/mm3. Discontinue if WBC < 3000/mm3. May decrease monitoring to q 4 weeks after 12 months if WBC > 3500/mm3 and ANC > 2000/mm3. See package insert for more details. Risk of myocarditis (particularly during the first month), seizures, orthostatic hypotension, and cardiopulmonary arrest. Antipsychotics when used for schizophrenia or bipolar disorder have been associated with an increased risk of suicidal thinking and behavior. Monitor closely.
ADULTS — Severe, medically-refractory schizophrenia or schizophrenia/schizoaffective disorder with suicidal behavior: Start 12.5 mg PO daily or bid; increase by 25 to 50 mg/day to usual effective dose of 300 to 450 mg/day, max 900 mg/day. Retitrate if stopped for more than 3 to 4 days.
PEDS — Not approved in children.
FORMS — Generic/Trade: Tabs 25, 100 mg. Generic only: Tabs 12.5, 50, 200 mg. Trade only: Orally disintegrating tab (Fazaclo ODT) 12.5, 25, 100 mg (scored).
NOTES — Patients rechallenged with clozapine after an episode of leukopenia are at increased risk of agranulocytosis, and must undergo weekly monitoring for 12 months. Register all occurrences of leukopenia, discontinuation, and/or rechallenge to the Clozaril National Registry at 1-800-448-5938. Much lower risk of EPS and tardive dyskinesia than other neuroleptics. May be effective for treatment-resistant patients who have not responded to conventional agents. May cause significant wt gain, dyslipidemia, hyperglycemia, or new onset diabetes; monitor wt, fasting blood glucose, and triglycerides before initiation and at regular intervals during treatment. Excessive sedation or respiratory depression may occur when used with CNS depressants, particularly benzodiazepines. If an orally-disintegrating tab is split, then discard the remaining portion.
MOA — Dopamine receptor antagonist; 5-HT2A receptor antagonist.
ADVERSE EFFECTS — Serious: Agranulocytosis, leukopenia, seizures, hyperglycemia, diabetes, dyslipidemia, neuroleptic malignant syndrome, hepatotoxicity, QT prolongation, orthostatic hypotension, syncope, cardiopulmonary arrest, myocarditis, cardiomyopathy. Frequent: Drowsiness, weight gain, N/V, dry mouth, constipation, tachycardia, hypersalivation.

ILOPERIDONE (*Fanapt*) ▶L ♀C ▶–?
ADULTS — Schizophrenia, acute: Start 1 mg PO bid. Increase to 2 mg PO bid on day 2, then increase total daily dose by 2 mg/dose each day to usual effective range of 6 to 12 mg PO bid. Max 24 mg/day.
PEDS — Not approved in children.
FORMS — Trade: Tabs 1, 2, 4, 6, 8, 10, 12 mg.
NOTES — Dose must be titrated slowly to avoid orthostatic hypotension. Retitrate the dose if off the drug > 3 days. Reduce dose by 50% if given with strong inhibitors of CYP2D6 or CYP3A4. Avoid use with other drugs that prolong the QT interval.
MOA — Receptor antagonist; 5-HT2A receptor antagonist.
ADVERSE EFFECTS — Serious: Neuroleptic malignant syndrome, ventricular arrhythmias, tardive dyskinesia, hyperglycemia/diabetes, seizures, orthostatic hypotension. Frequent: Dizziness, dry mouth, fatigue, nasal congestion, somnolence, tachycardia, weight gain.

PSYCHIATRY: Antipsychotics

OLANZAPINE (*Zyprexa, Zyprexa Zydis, Zyprexa Relprevv*) ▶L ♀C ▶− $$$$$
WARNING − Antipsychotics when used for schizophrenia or bipolar disorder have been associated with an increased risk of suicidal thinking and behavior. Monitor closely.
ADULTS − Agitation in acute bipolar mania or schizophrenia: Start 10 mg IM (2.5 to 5 mg in elderly or debilitated patients); may repeat in after 2 h to max 30 mg/day. Schizophrenia, oral therapy: Start 5 to 10 mg PO daily. Increase weekly to usual effective dose of 10 to 15 mg/day, max 20 mg/day. Schizophrenia, extended release injection: Dose based on prior oral dose and ranges from 150 mg to 300 mg deep IM (gluteal) q 2 weeks or 300 mg to 405 mg q 4 weeks. See package insert. Bipolar disorder, maintenance treatment or monotherapy for acute manic or mixed episodes: Start 10 to 15 mg PO daily. Increase by 5 mg/day at intervals after 24 h. Clinical efficacy seen at doses of 5 to 20 mg/day, max 20 mg/day. Bipolar disorder, adjunctive therapy for acute mixed or manic episodes: Start 10 mg PO daily; usual effective dose is 5 to 20 mg/day, max 20 mg/day. Bipolar depression, olanzapine + fluoxetine: Start 5 mg olanzapine + 20 mg fluoxetine daily in the evening. Increase to usual range of 5 to 12.5 mg olanzapine plus 20 to 50 mg fluoxetine as tolerated. Treatment-resistant depression, olanzapine + fluoxetine: Start 5 mg olanzapine + 20 mg fluoxetine daily in the evening. Increase to usual range of 5 to 20 mg olanzapine plus 20 to 50 mg fluoxetine as tolerated.
PEDS − Schizophrenia and bipolar manic or mixed episodes (13-17 y.o.): Start 2.5-5 mg PO once daily. Increase to target of 10 mg/day. Max 20 mg/day.
UNAPPROVED ADULTS − Augmentation of SSRI therapy for OCD: Start 2.5 to 5 mg PO daily, max 20 mg/day. Posttraumatic stress disorder, adjunctive therapy: Start 5 mg PO daily, max 20 mg/day.
UNAPPROVED PEDS − Bipolar disorder, manic or mixed phase: Start 2.5 mg PO daily; increase by 2.5 mg/day every 3 days to max 20 mg/day.
FORMS − Trade only: Tabs 2.5, 5, 7.5, 10, 15, 20 mg. Tabs orally-disintegrating (Zyprexa Zydis) 5, 10, 15, 20 mg. Long-acting injection (Zyprexa Relprevv) 210, 300, 405 mg/vial.
NOTES − Use for acute manic episodes associated with bipolar disorder. May cause significant wt gain, dyslipidemia, hyperglycemia, or new onset diabetes; monitor wt, fasting blood glucose, and triglycerides before initiation and at regular intervals during treatment. Monitor for orthostatic hypotension, particularly when given IM. IM injection can also be associated with bradycardia and hypoventilation especially if used with other drugs that have these effects. Use caution with benzodiazepines. Use of Zyprexa Relprevv requires registration in the Zyprexa Relprevv Patient Care Program 1-877-772-9390.
MOA − Dopamine receptor antagonist; 5-HT2A receptor antagonist.
ADVERSE EFFECTS − Serious: Seizures, orthostatic hypotension, syncope, hyperglycemia, diabetes, dyslipidemia, neuroleptic malignant syndrome, extrapyramidal side effects, QT prolongation, hepatitis, suicidal thinking/behavior. Frequent: Drowsiness, weight gain, nausea, dry mouth, constipation, dizziness.

PALIPERIDONE (*Invega, Invega Sustenna*) ▶KL ♀C ▶− $$$$$
WARNING − Antipsychotics when used for schizophrenia or bipolar disorder have been associated with an increased risk of suicidal thinking and behavior. Monitor closely.
ADULTS − Schizophrenia and schizoaffective disorder (adjunctive and monotherapy: Start 6 mg PO qam. 3 mg/day may be sufficient in some. Max 12 mg/day. Extended-release injection: Start 234 mg IM (deltoid) and then 156 mg IM one week later. Recommended monthly dose 117 mg IM (deltoid or gluteal) or within range of 36-234 mg based on response.
PEDS − Not approved in children.
FORMS − Trade only: Extended-release tabs 1.5, 3, 6, 9 mg.
NOTES − Active metabolite of risperidone. For CrCl 50 to 79 mL/min start 3 mg/day with a max of 6 mg/day. For CrCl 10 to 50 mL/min start 1.5 mg/day with a max of 3 mg/day.
MOA − Dopamine receptor antagonist; 5-HT2A receptor antagonist.
ADVERSE EFFECTS − Serious: Orthostatic hypotension, syncope, QT prolongation, neuroleptic malignant syndrome, tardive dyskinesia, hyperglycemia, diabetes, stroke, extrapyramidal symptoms, suicidal thinking/behavior. Frequent: Drowsiness, salivary hypersecretion, tachycardia, akathisia, dystonia, hypertonia, parkinsonism, weight gain, dyspepsia, dizziness, headache, anxiety.

QUETIAPINE (*Seroquel, Seroquel XR*) ▶LK ♀C ▶− $$$$$
WARNING − Antipsychotics when used for schizophrenia or bipolar disorder have been associated with an increased risk of suicidal thinking and behavior. Monitor closely.
ADULTS − Schizophrenia: Start 25 mg PO bid (regular tabs); increase by 25 to 50 mg bid to tid on day 2 and 3, and then to target dose of 300 to 400 mg/day divided bid to tid on day 4. Usual effective dose is 150 to 750 mg/day, max 800 mg/day. Schizophrenia, extended-release tabs: Start 300 mg PO daily in evening, increase by up to 300 mg/day at intervals of greater than 1 day to usual effective range of 400 to 800 mg/day. Acute bipolar mania, monotherapy or adjunctive: Start 50 mg PO bid on day 1, then increase to no higher than 100 mg bid on day 2, 150 mg bid on days 3, and 200 mg bid on day 4. May increase as needed to 300 mg bid on day 5 and 400 mg bid thereafter. Usual effective dose is 400 to 800 mg/day. Acute bipolar mania, monotherapy or adjunctive, extended release: Start 300 mg PO on evening day 1, 600 mg day 2, and 400 to 800 mg/day thereafter. Bipolar depression, regular and extended release: 50 mg, 100 mg, 200 mg and 300 mg per day for Days 1-4 respectively,

(cont.)

PSYCHIATRY: Antipsychotics

QUETIAPINE (cont.)
administered at bedtime. May increase prn to 400 mg at bedtime on day 5 and 600 mg at bedtime on day 8. Bipolar maintenance: Use dose required to maintain remission of symptoms. Major depressive disorder, adjunctive to antidepressants, extended release: Start 50 mg evening of day 1, may increase to 150 mg on day 3. Max 300 mg/day.
PEDS — Schizophrenia (13 to17 yo): Start 50 mg PO day 1, 100 mg day 2, 200 mg day 3, 300 mg day 4, and 400 mg day 5 all given bid to tid. Recommended range 400 to 800 mg/day. Max 800 mg/day. Acute bipolar mania (10 to 17 yo): Start 50 mg PO day 1, 100 mg day 2, 200 mg day 3, 300 mg day 4, 400 mg day 5 all given bid to tid. Recommended range 400 to 600 mg/day. Bipolar maintenance: Use dose required to maintain remission of symptoms.
UNAPPROVED ADULTS — Augmentation of SSRI therapy for OCD: Start 25 mg PO bid, max 300 mg/day. Adjunctive for posttraumatic stress disorder: Start 25 mg daily, max 300 mg/day.
UNAPPROVED PEDS — Bipolar disorder (manic or mixed phase): Start 12.5 mg PO bid (children) or 25 mg PO bid (adolescents); max 150 mg PO tid.
FORMS — Trade only: Tabs 25, 50, 100, 200, 300, 400 mg. Extended-release tabs 50, 150, 200, 300, 400 mg.
NOTES — Eye exam for cataracts recommended q 6 months. Low risk of EPS and tardive dyskinesia. May cause significant wt gain, dyslipidemia, hyperglycemia, or new onset diabetes; monitor wt, fasting blood glucose, and triglycerides before initiation and at regular intervals during treatment. Use lower doses and slower titration in elderly patients or hepatic dysfunction. Extended-release tabs should be taken without food or after light meal.
MOA — Dopamine receptor antagonist; 5-HT2A receptor antagonist.
ADVERSE EFFECTS — Serious: Seizures, orthostatic hypotension, syncope, hyperglycemia, diabetes, dyslipidemia, neuroleptic malignant syndrome, QT prolongation, suicidal thinking/behavior. Frequent: Drowsiness, weight gain, nausea, dry mouth, constipation, dizziness.

RISPERIDONE (*Risperdal, Risperdal Consta*) ▶LK ♀C ▶– $$$$$
WARNING — Antipsychotics when used for schizophrenia or bipolar disorder have been associated with an increased risk of suicidal thinking and behavior. Monitor closely.
ADULTS — Schizophrenia: Start 2 mg/day PO given once daily or divided bid; increase by 1 to 2 mg/day at intervals of 24 h or more. Start 0.5 mg/dose and titrate by no more than 0.5 mg bid in elderly, debilitated, hypotensive, or renally or hepatically impaired patients; increases to doses greater than 1.5 mg bid should occur at intervals 1 week or more. Usual effective dose is 4 to 8 mg/day given once daily or divided bid; max 16 mg/day. Long-acting injection (Consta) for schizophrenia: Start 25 mg IM q 2 weeks while continuing oral dose for 3 weeks. May increase q 4 weeks to max 50 mg q 2 weeks. Bipolar mania: Start 2 to 3 mg PO daily; may adjust by 1 mg/day at 24 h intervals to max 6 mg/day.
PEDS — Autistic disorder irritability (5 to 16 yo): Start 0.25 mg (wt less than 20 kg) or 0.5 mg (wt 20 kg or greater) PO daily. May increase after 4 days to 0.5 mg/day (wt less than 20 kg) or 1.0 mg/day (wt 20 kg or greater). Maintain at least 14 days. May then increase at 14-day intervals or more by increments of 0.25 mg/day (wt less than 20 kg) or 0.5 mg/day (wt 20 kg or greater) to max 1.0 mg/day for wt less than 20 kg, max 2.5 mg/day for wt 20 to 44 kg or max 3.0 mg/day for wt greater than 45 kg. Schizophrenia (13 to 17 yo): Start 0.5 mg PO daily; increase by 0.5 to 1 mg/day at intervals of 24 h or more to target dose of 3 mg/day. Max 6 mg/day. Bipolar mania (10 to 17 yo): Start 0.5 mg PO daily; increase by 0.5 to 1 mg/day at intervals of 24 h or more to recommended dose of 2.5 mg/day. Max 6 mg/day.
UNAPPROVED ADULTS — Augmentation of SSRI therapy for OCD: Start 1 mg/day PO, max 6 mg/day. Adjunctive therapy for posttraumatic stress disorder: Start 0.5 mg PO at bedtime, max 3 mg/day.
UNAPPROVED PEDS — Psychotic disorders, mania, aggression: 0.5 to 1.5 mg/day PO.
FORMS — Generic/Trade: Tabs 0.25, 0.5, 1, 2, 3, 4 mg. Oral soln 1 mg/mL (30 mL). Orally disintegrating tabs 0.5, 1, 2, 3, 4 mg. Generic only: Orally disintegrating tabs 0.25 mg.
NOTES — Has a greater tendency to produce extrapyramidal side effects (EPS) than other atypical antipsychotics. EPS reported in neonates following use in third trimester of pregnancy. May cause wt gain, hyperglycemia, or new onset diabetes; monitor closely. Patients with Parkinson's disease and dementia have increased sensitivity to side effects such as EPS, confusion, falls, and neuroleptic malignant syndrome. Soln is compatible with water, coffee, orange juice, and low-fat milk; is not compatible with cola or tea. Place orally disintegrating tabs on tongue and do not chew. Establish tolerability with oral form before starting long-acting injection. Alternate injections between buttocks. May also give in deltoid.
MOA — Dopamine receptor antagonist; 5-HT2A receptor antagonist.
ADVERSE EFFECTS — Serious: Seizures, orthostatic hypotension, syncope, hyperglycemia, diabetes, neuroleptic malignant syndrome, tardive dyskinesia, extrapyramidal symptoms, QT prolongation, stroke, transient ischemic attack, suicidal thinking/behavior. Frequent: Drowsiness, insomnia, weight gain, N/V, dyspepsia, dry mouth, constipation, dizziness, orthostatic hypotension, agitation, anxiety, akathisia, tachycardia.

ZIPRASIDONE (*Geodon*) ▶L ♀C ▶– $$$$$
WARNING — May prolong QTc. Avoid with drugs that prolong QTc or in those with long QT syndrome or cardiac arrhythmias. Antipsychotics when used for schizophrenia or bipolar disorder have been

(cont.)

ZIPRASIDONE (cont.)
associated with an increased risk of suicidal thinking and behavior. Monitor closely.
ADULTS — <u>Schizophrenia:</u> Start 20 mg PO bid with food; may increase at greater than 2-day intervals to max 80 mg PO bid. <u>Acute agitation in schizophrenia:</u> 10 to 20 mg IM. May repeat 10 mg dose q 2 h or 20 mg dose q 4 h, to max 40 mg/day. <u>Bipolar mania:</u> Start 40 mg PO bid with food; may increase to 60 to 80 mg bid on day 2. Usual effective dose is 40 to 80 mg bid.
PEDS — Not approved in children.

FORMS — Trade only: Caps 20, 40, 60, 80 mg, Susp 10 mg/mL.
NOTES — Drug interactions with carbamazepine and ketoconazole.
MOA — Dopamine receptor antagonist; 5-HT2A receptor antagonist.
ADVERSE EFFECTS — Serious: Seizures, orthostatic hypotension, syncope, hyperglycemia, diabetes, dyslipidemia, neuroleptic malignant syndrome, tardive dyskinesia, extrapyramidal side effects, QT prolongation, suicidal thinking/behavior. Frequent: Drowsiness, weight gain, nausea, dry mouth, constipation, dizziness.

PSYCHIATRY: Anxiolytics/Hypnotics—Benzodiazepines—Long Half-Life (25-100 h)

NOTE: To avoid withdrawal, gradually taper when discontinuing after prolonged use. Use cautiously in the elderly; may accumulate and lead to side effects, psychomotor impairment. Sedative-hypnotics have been associated with severe allergic reactions and complex sleep behaviors including sleep driving. Use caution and discuss with patients.

BROMAZEPAM (✦*Lectopam*) ▶L ♀D ▶– $
ADULTS — Canada only. 6 to 18 mg/day PO in equally divided doses.
PEDS — Not approved in children.
FORMS — Generic/Trade: Tabs 1.5, 3, 6 mg.
NOTES — Do not exceed 3 mg/day initially in the elderly or debilitated. Gradually taper when discontinuing after prolonged use. Half-life approximately 20 h in adults but increased in elderly. Cimetidine may prolong elimination.
MOA — Benzodiazepine; enhances actions of GABA.
ADVERSE EFFECTS — Serious: Respiratory depression, dependence, withdrawal reactions. Frequent: Sedation, ataxia, depression, confusion, tinnitus, N/V.

CHLORDIAZEPOXIDE (*Librium*) ▶LK ♀D ▶– ©IV $$
ADULTS — <u>Anxiety:</u> 5 to 25 mg PO tid to qid or 25 to 50 mg IM/IV tid to qid (acute/severe anxiety). <u>Acute alcohol withdrawal:</u> 50 to 100 mg PO/IM/IV, repeat q 3 to 4 h prn up to 300 mg/day.
PEDS — <u>Anxiety,</u> age older than 6 yo: 5 to 10 mg PO bid to qid.
FORMS — Generic/Trade: Caps 5, 10, 25 mg.
NOTES — Half-life 5 to 30 h.
MOA — Enhances actions of GABA.
ADVERSE EFFECTS — Serious: Respiratory depression, dependence, withdrawal reactions, seizures. Frequent: Sedation, fatigue, ataxia, memory impairment, depression, confusion, nausea, constipation, dry mouth, rash.

CLONAZEPAM (*Klonopin, Klonopin Wafer,* ✦*Rivotril, Clonapam*) ▶LK ♀D ▶– ©IV $
ADULTS — <u>Panic disorder:</u> 0.25 mg PO bid, increase by 0.125 to 0.25 mg q 3 days to maximum dose of 4 mg/day. <u>Akinetic or myoclonic seizures:</u> Start 0.5 mg PO tid. Increase by 0.5 to 1 mg q 3 days prn. Max 20 mg/day.
PEDS — <u>Akinetic or myoclonic seizures, Lennox-Gastaut syndrome (petit mal variant), or absence seizures</u> (≤10 yo or ≤30 kg): 0.01 to 0.03 mg/kg/day PO divided bid to tid. Increase by 0.25 to 0.5 mg q 3 days prn. Max 0.1 to 0.2 mg/kg/day divided tid.
UNAPPROVED ADULTS — <u>Neuralgias:</u> 2 to 4 mg PO daily. <u>Restless legs syndrome:</u> Start 0.25 mg PO at bedtime. Max 2 mg at bedtime. <u>REM sleep behavior disorder:</u> 1 to 2 mg PO at bedtime.
FORMS — Generic/Trade: Tabs 0.5, 1, 2 mg. Orally disintegrating tabs (approved for panic disorder only) 0.125, 0.25, 0.5, 1, 2 mg.
NOTES — Half-life 18 to 50 h. Usual therapeutic range is 20 to 80 ng/mL. Contraindicated in hepatic failure or acute narrow angle glaucoma.
MOA — Enhances actions of GABA.
ADVERSE EFFECTS — Serious: Respiratory depression, CNS depression, dependence, withdrawal reactions, seizures. Frequent: Sedation, fatigue, ataxia, memory impairment, depression, confusion, nausea, constipation, dry mouth, rash.

CLORAZEPATE (*Tranxene, Tranxene SD*) ▶LK ♀D ▶– ©IV $
ADULTS — <u>Anxiety:</u> Start 7.5 to 15 mg PO at bedtime or bid to tid, usual effective dose is 15 to 60 mg/day. <u>Acute alcohol withdrawal:</u> 60 to 90 mg/day on first day divided bid to tid, gradually reduce dose to 7.5 to 15 mg/day over 5 days. Maximum dose is 90 mg/day. May transfer patients to single-dose Tabs (Tranxene-SD) when dose stabilized.
PEDS — Not approved in children younger than 9 yo.
FORMS — Generic/Trade: Tabs 3.75, 7.5, 15 mg. Trade only (Tranxene SD): Tabs extended-release 11.25, 22.5 mg.
NOTES — Half-life 40 to 50 h.
MOA — Enhances actions of GABA.
ADVERSE EFFECTS — Serious: Respiratory depression, dependence, withdrawal reactions, seizures. Frequent: Sedation, fatigue, ataxia, memory impairment, depression, confusion, nausea, constipation, dry mouth, rash.

PSYCHIATRY: Anxiolytics/Hypnotics

DIAZEPAM (*Valium, Diastat, Diastat AcuDial, ✢Vivol, E Pam, Diazemuls*) ▶LK ♀D ▶– ©IV $
ADULTS — Status epilepticus: 5 to 10 mg IV. Repeat q 10 to 15 min prn to max 30 mg. Epilepsy, adjunctive therapy: 2 to 10 mg PO bid to qid. Increased seizure activity: 0.2 to 0.5 mg/kg PR (rectal gel) to max 20 mg/day. Skeletal muscle spasm, spasticity related to cerebral palsy, paraplegia, athetosis, stiff man syndrome: 2 to 10 mg PO/PR tid to qid. 5 to 10 mg IM/IV initially, then 5 to 10 mg q 3 to 4 h prn. Decrease dose in elderly. Anxiety: 2 to 10 mg PO bid to qid or 2 to 20 mg IM/IV, repeat dose in 3 to 4 h prn. Alcohol withdrawal: 10 mg PO tid to qid for 24 h then 5 mg PO tid to qid prn.
PEDS — Skeletal muscle spasm: 0.04 to 0.2 mg/kg/dose IV/IM q 2 to 4 h. Max dose 0.6 mg/kg within 8 h. Status epilepticus, age 1 mo to 5 yo: 0.2 to 0.5 mg IV slowly q 2 to 5 min to max 5 mg. Status epilepticus, age older than 5 yo: 1 mg IV slowly q 2 to 5 min to max 10 mg. Repeat q 2 to 4 h prn. Epilepsy, adjunctive therapy, muscle spasm, and anxiety disorders, age older than 6 mo: 1 to 2.5 mg PO tid to qid; gradually increase as tolerated and needed. Increased seizure activity (rectal gel, age older than 2 yo): 0.5 mg/kg PR (2 to 5 yo), 0.3 mg/kg PR (6 to 11 yo), or 0.2 mg/kg PR (age older than 12 yo). Max 20 mg. May repeat in 4 to 12 h prn.
UNAPPROVED ADULTS — Loading dose strategy for alcohol withdrawal: 10 to 20 mg PO or 10 mg slow IV in closely monitored setting, then repeat similar or lower doses q 1 to 2 h prn until sedated. Further doses should be unnecessary due to long half-life. Restless legs syndrome: 0.5 to 4 mg PO at bedtime.
FORMS — Generic/Trade: Tabs 2, 5, 10 mg. Generic only: Oral soln 5 mg/5 mL. Oral concentrate (Intensol) 5 mg/mL. Trade only: Rectal gel (Diastat) 2.5, 5, 10, 15, 20 mg. Rectal gel (Diastat AcuDial) 10, 20 mg.
NOTES — Half-life 20 to 80 h. Respiratory and CNS depression may occur. Caution in liver disease. Abuse potential. Long half-life may increase the risk of adverse effects in the elderly. Cimetidine, oral contraceptives, disulfiram, fluoxetine, isoniazid, ketoconazole, metoprolol, propoxyphene, propranolol, and valproic acid may increase diazepam concentrations. Diazepam may increase digoxin and phenytoin concentrations. Rifampin may increase the metabolism of diazepam. Avoid combination with protease inhibitors. Diastat AcuDial is for home use and allows dosing from 5 to 20 mg in 2.5 mg increments.
MOA — Enhances actions of GABA, skeletal muscle relaxant.
ADVERSE EFFECTS — Serious: Respiratory depression, oversedation, dependence, withdrawal reactions, cardiovascular collapse (parenteral), vascular impairment or venous thrombosis (IV only), seizures. Frequent: Sedation, ataxia, CNS stimulation, depression, N/V, constipation or diarrhea, confusion, tinnitus, blurred vision.

FLURAZEPAM (*Dalmane*) ▶LK ♀X ▶– ©IV $
ADULTS — Insomnia: 15 to 30 mg PO at bedtime.
PEDS — Not approved in children age younger than 15 yo.
FORMS — Generic/Trade: Caps 15, 30 mg.
NOTES — Half-life 70 to 90 h. For short-term treatment of insomnia.
MOA — Enhances actions of GABA.
ADVERSE EFFECTS — Serious: Respiratory depression, dependence, withdrawal reactions, seizures. Frequent: Sedation, fatigue, ataxia, memory impairment, depression, confusion, nausea, constipation, dry mouth, rash.

PSYCHIATRY: Anxiolytics/Hypnotics—Benzodiazepines—Medium Half-Life (10 to 15 h)

NOTE: To avoid withdrawal, gradually taper when discontinuing after prolonged use. Sedative-hypnotics have been associated with severe allergic reactions and complex sleep behaviors including sleep driving. Use caution and discuss with patients.

ESTAZOLAM (*ProSom*) ▶LK ♀X ▶– ©IV $$
ADULTS — Insomnia: 1 to 2 mg PO at bedtime for up to 12 weeks. Reduce dose to 0.5 mg in elderly, small, or debilitated patients.
PEDS — Not approved in children.
FORMS — Generic/Trade: Tabs 1, 2 mg.
NOTES — For short-term treatment of insomnia. Avoid with ketoconazole or itraconazole; caution with less potent inhibitors of CYP3A4.
MOA — Enhances actions of GABA.
ADVERSE EFFECTS — Serious: Respiratory depression, dependence, withdrawal reactions, seizures. Frequent: Sedation, fatigue, ataxia, memory impairment, depression, confusion, nausea, constipation, dry mouth, rash.

LORAZEPAM (*Ativan*) ▶LK ♀D ▶– ©IV $
ADULTS — Anxiety: Start 0.5 to 1 mg PO bid to tid, usual effective dose is 2 to 6 mg/day. Maximum dose is 10 mg/day PO. Anxiolytic/sedation: 0.04 to 0.05 mg/kg IV/IM; usual dose 2 mg, max 4 mg. Insomnia: 2 to 4 mg PO at bedtime. Status epilepticus: 4 mg IV over 2 min. May repeat in 10 to 15 min.
PEDS — Not approved in children.
UNAPPROVED ADULTS — Alcohol withdrawal: 1 to 2 mg PO/IM/IV q 2 to 4 h prn or 2 mg PO/IM/IV q 6 h for 24 h then 1 mg q 6 h for 8 doses. Chemotherapy-induced N/V: 1 to 2 mg PO/SL/IV/IM q 6 h.
UNAPPROVED PEDS — Status epilepticus: 0.05 to 0.1 mg/kg IV over 2 to 5 min. May repeat 0.05 mg/kg for 1 dose in 10 to 15 min. Do not exceed 4 mg as single dose. Anxiolytic/Sedation: 0.05 mg/kg/dose q 4 to 8 h PO/IV, max 2 mg/dose. Chemotherapy-induced N/V: 0.05 mg/kg PO/IV q 8 to 12 h prn, max 3 mg/dose; or 0.02 to 0.05 mg/kg IV q 6 h prn, max 2 mg/dose.

(cont.)

LORAZEPAM (cont.)
FORMS — Generic/Trade: Tabs 0.5, 1, 2 mg. Generic only: Oral concentrate 2 mg/mL.
NOTES — Half-life 10 to 20 h. No active metabolites. For short-term treatment of insomnia.
MOA — Enhances actions of GABA.
ADVERSE EFFECTS — Serious: Cardiovascular collapse, hypotension, apnea (parenteral), respiratory depression, dependence, withdrawal syndrome. Frequent: Drowsiness, dizziness, ataxia, headache, confusion, memory problems, depression, paradoxical CNS stimulation.

NITRAZEPAM (✦*Mogadon*) ▶L ♀C ▶– $
ADULTS — Canada only. Insomnia: 5 to 10 mg PO at bedtime.
PEDS — Canada only. Myoclonic seizures: 0.3 to 1 mg/kg/day in 3 divided doses.
FORMS — Generic/Trade: Tabs 5, 10 mg.

NOTES — Use lower doses in elderly/debilitated patients.
MOA — Benzodiazepine with an intermediate half life.
ADVERSE EFFECTS — Serious: Dependence. Frequent: Dizziness, drowsiness, fatigue.

TEMAZEPAM (*Restoril*) ▶LK ♀X ▶– ©IV $
ADULTS — Insomnia: 7.5 to 30 mg PO at bedtime for 7 to 10 days.
PEDS — Not approved in children.
FORMS — Generic/Trade: Caps 7.5, 15, 22.5, 30 mg.
NOTES — Half-life 8 to 25 h. For short-term treatment of insomnia.
MOA — Enhances actions of GABA.
ADVERSE EFFECTS — Serious: Respiratory depression, dependence, withdrawal reactions, seizures. Frequent: Sedation, fatigue, ataxia, memory impairment, depression, confusion, nausea, constipation, dry mouth, rash.

PSYCHIATRY: Anxiolytics/Hypnotics—Benzodiazepines—Short Half-Life (< 12 h)

ALPRAZOLAM (*Xanax, Xanax XR, Niravam*) ▶LK ♀D ▶– ©IV $
ADULTS — Anxiety: Start 0.25 to 0.5 mg PO tid, may increase q 3 to 4 days to a maximum dose of 4 mg/day. Use 0.25 mg PO bid in elderly or debilitated patients. Panic disorder: Start 0.5 mg PO tid (or 0.5 to 1 mg PO daily of Xanax XR), may increase by up to 1 mg/day q 3 to 4 days to usual effective dose of 5 to 6 mg/day (3 to 6 mg/day for Xanax XR), maximum dose is 10 mg/day.
PEDS — Not approved in children.
FORMS — Generic/Trade: Tabs 0.25, 0.5, 1, 2 mg. Tabs extended-release 0.5, 1, 2, 3 mg. Orally disintegrating tab (Niravam) 0.25, 0.5, 1, 2 mg. Generic only: Oral concentrate (Intensol) 1 mg/mL.
NOTES — Half-life 12 h, but need to give tid. Divide administration time evenly during waking hours to avoid interdose symptoms. Don't give with antifungals (ie, ketoconazole, itraconazole); use caution with macrolides, propoxyphene, oral contraceptives, TCAs, cimetidine, antidepressants, anticonvulsants, paroxetine, sertraline, and others that inhibit CYP3A4.
MOA — Enhances actions of GABA.
ADVERSE EFFECTS — Serious: Respiratory depression, dependence, withdrawal reactions, seizures. Frequent: Sedation, fatigue, ataxia, memory impairment, depression, confusion, nausea, constipation, dry mouth, rash.

OXAZEPAM (*Serax*) ▶LK ♀D ▶– ©IV $$$
ADULTS — Anxiety: 10 to 30 mg PO tid to qid. Acute alcohol withdrawal: 15 to 30 mg PO tid to qid.
PEDS — Not approved in children younger than 6 yo.

UNAPPROVED ADULTS — Restless legs syndrome: Start 10 mg PO at bedtime. Max 40 mg at bedtime.
FORMS — Generic/Trade: Caps 10, 15, 30 mg. Trade only: Tabs 15 mg.
NOTES — Half-life 8 h.
MOA — Enhances actions of GABA.
ADVERSE EFFECTS — Serious: Respiratory depression, dependence, withdrawal reactions, seizures. Frequent: Sedation, fatigue, ataxia, memory impairment, depression, confusion, nausea, constipation, dry mouth, rash.

TRIAZOLAM (*Halcion*) ▶LK ♀X ▶– ©IV $
ADULTS — Hypnotic: 0.125 to 0.25 mg PO at bedtime for 7 to 10 days, maximum dose is 0.5 mg/day. Start 0.125 mg/day in elderly or debilitated patients.
PEDS — Not approved in children.
UNAPPROVED ADULTS — Restless legs syndrome: Start 0.125 mg PO at bedtime. Max 0.5 mg at bedtime.
FORMS — Generic/Trade: Tabs 0.125, 0.25 mg.
NOTES — Half-life 2 to 3 h. Anterograde amnesia may occur. Don't use with protease inhibitors, ketoconazole, itraconazole, or nefazodone; use caution with macrolides, cimetidine, and other CYP3A4 inhibitors.
MOA — Enhances actions of GABA.
ADVERSE EFFECTS — Serious: Respiratory depression, dependence, withdrawal reactions, seizures. Frequent: Sedation, fatigue, ataxia, memory impairment, depression, confusion, nausea, constipation, dry mouth, rash.

PSYCHIATRY: Anxiolytics/Hypnotics—Other

NOTE: Sedative-hypnotics have been associated with severe allergic reactions and complex sleep behaviors including sleep driving. Use caution and discuss with patients.

BUSPIRONE (*BuSpar, Vanspar*) ▶K ♀B ▶– $$$
ADULTS — Anxiety: Start 15 mg "dividose" daily (7.5 mg PO bid), increase by 5 mg/day q 2 to 3 days to usual effective dose of 30 mg/day, maximum dose is 60 mg/day.
PEDS — Not approved in children.

(cont.)

PSYCHIATRY: Anxiolytics/Hypnotics

BUSPIRONE (cont.)
FORMS — Generic/Trade: Tabs 5, 10, Dividose Tabs 15, 30 mg (scored to be easily bisected or trisected). Generic only: Tabs 7.5 mg.
NOTES — Slower onset than benzodiazepines; optimum effect requires 3 to 4 weeks of therapy. Don't use with MAOIs; caution with itraconazole, cimetidine, nefazodone, erythromycin, and other CYP3A4 inhibitors.
MOA — Serotonin 5-HT1A partial agonist.
ADVERSE EFFECTS — Serious: Parkinsonism, akathisia, dystonia, restless legs syndrome. Frequent: Drowsiness, dizziness, nausea, headache, nervousness.

CHLORAL HYDRATE (*Aquachloral Supprettes, Somnote*) ▶LK ♀C ▶+ ©IV $
ADULTS — Sedative: 250 mg PO/PR tid after meals. Hypnotic: 500 to 1000 mg PO/PR at bedtime. Acute alcohol withdrawal: 500 to 1000 mg PO/PR q 6 h prn.
PEDS — Sedative: 25 mg/kg/day PO/PR divided tid to qid, up to 500 mg tid. Hypnotic: 50 mg/kg PO/PR at bedtime, up to maximum of 1 g. Preanesthetic: 25 to 50 mg/kg PO/PR before procedure.
UNAPPROVED PEDS — Sedative: Higher than approved doses 75 to 100 mg/kg PO/PR.
FORMS — Generic only: Syrup 500 mg/5 mL, rectal supps 500 mg. Trade only: Caps 500 mg. Rectal supps: 325, 650 mg.
NOTES — Give syrup in ½ glass of fruit juice or water.
MOA — Nonselective CNS depressant.
ADVERSE EFFECTS — Serious: Leukopenia, dependence, withdrawal reactions. Frequent: N/V, diarrhea, sleepwalking.

ESZOPICLONE (*Lunesta*) ▶L ♀C ▶? ©IV $$$$
ADULTS — Insomnia: 2 mg PO at bedtime prn, max 3 mg. Elderly: 1 mg PO at bedtime prn, max 2 mg.
PEDS — Not approved for children.
FORMS — Trade only: Tabs 1, 2, 3 mg.
NOTES — Half-life is approximately 6 h. Take immediately before bedtime.
MOA — Binds to GABA-A receptors.
ADVERSE EFFECTS — Serious: chest pain. Frequent: Headache, unpleasant taste, dry mouth, dizziness, nervousness, dyspepsia, sleepdriving and other complex sleep behaviors.

RAMELTEON (*Rozerem*) ▶L ♀C ▶? $$$$
ADULTS — Insomnia: 8 mg PO at bedtime.
PEDS — Not approved for children.
FORMS — Trade only: Tabs 8 mg.
NOTES — Do not take with/after high-fat meal. No evidence of dependence or abuse liability. Inhibitors of CYP1A2, 3A4, and 2C9 may increase serum level and effect. Avoid with severe liver disease. May decrease testosterone and increase prolactin.
MOA — Melatonin receptor agonist.
ADVERSE EFFECTS — Serious: None. Frequent: Headache, somnolence, fatigue, dizziness.

ZALEPLON (*Sonata, ✽Starnoc*) ▶L ♀C ▶– ©IV $$$$
ADULTS — Insomnia: 5 to 10 mg PO at bedtime prn, maximum 20 mg.
PEDS — Not approved in children.
FORMS — Generic/Trade: Caps 5, 10 mg.
NOTES — Half-life is approximately 1 h. Useful if problems with sleep initiation or morning grogginess. For short-term treatment of insomnia. Take immediately before bedtime or after going to bed and experiencing difficulty falling asleep. Use 5 mg dose in patients with mild to moderate hepatic impairment, elderly patients, and in patients taking cimetidine. Possible drug interactions with rifampin, phenytoin, carbamazepine, and phenobarbital. Do not use for benzodiazepine or alcohol withdrawal.
MOA — Selective GABA-benzodiazepine omega-1 agonist.
ADVERSE EFFECTS — Serious: Rebound insomnia, seizures, sleepdriving, anaphylactic reactions. Frequent: Drowsiness, abdominal pain, chest pain, headache, asthenia, fatigue, photosensitivity.

ZOLPIDEM (*Ambien, Ambien CR, Zolpimist, Edluar*) ▶L ♀B ▶+ ©IV $$$$
ADULTS — Adult: Insomnia: Standard tabs:10 mg PO at bedtime; Age older than 65 yo or debilitated: 5 mg PO at bedtime. Oral spray: 10 mg PO at bedtime; Age older than 65 yo or debilitated: 5 mg PO at bedtime. Control-release tabs: 12.5 mg PO at bedtime; Age older than 65 yo or debilitated: 6.25 mg PO at bedtime.
PEDS — Not approved in children.
FORMS — Generic/Trade: Tabs 5, 10 mg. Trade only: Controlled-release tabs 6.25, 12.5 mg, oral spray 5 mg/actuation (Zolpimist), sublingual tab 5, 10 mg (Edluar).
NOTES — Half-life is 2.5 h. Ambien regular-release is for short-term treatment of insomnia characterized by problems with sleep initiation. CR is useful for problems with sleep initiation and maintenance, and has been studied for up to 24 weeks. Do not use for benzodiazepine or alcohol withdrawal. Oral spray is sprayed into the mouth over the tongue. Device must be primed with 5 pumps prior to first use or if not used for 14 days.
MOA — Selective GABA-benzodiazepine omega-1 agonist.
ADVERSE EFFECTS — Serious: Sleepdriving, abnormal thinking, behavioral changes, depression, suicidal ideation, hallucinations, anaphylaxis. Frequent: Drowsiness, dizziness, nausea, headache, nervousness, decreased daytime recall.

ZOPICLONE (*✽Imovane*) ▶L ♀D ▶– $
ADULTS — Canada only. Short-term treatment of insomnia: 5 to 7.5 mg PO at bedtime. In elderly or debilitated, use 3.75 mg at bedtime initially, and increase prn to 5 to 7.5 mg at bedtime. Maximum 7.5 mg at bedtime.
PEDS — Not approved in children.
FORMS — Generic/Trade: Tabs 5, 7.5 mg. Generic only: Tabs 3.75 mg.
NOTES — Treatment should usually not exceed 7 to 10 days without re-evaluation.

(cont.)

PSYCHIATRY: Combination Drugs

LIMBITROL (chlordiazepoxide + amitriptyline, Limbitrol DS) ▶LK ♀D ▶– ©IV $$$
ADULTS — Rarely used; other drugs preferred. Depression/Anxiety: 1 tab PO tid to qid, may increase up to 6 tabs/day.
PEDS — Not approved in children younger than 12 yo.
FORMS — Generic/Trade: Tabs 5/12.5, 10/25 mg chlordiazepoxide/amitriptyline.
MOA — Antidepressant- benzodiazepine combination.
ADVERSE EFFECTS — Serious: Seizures, arrhythmias, hypotension, agranulocytosis, dependence, withdrawal reactions, respiratory depression. Frequent: Drowsiness, dizziness, dry mouth, constipation, urinary retention, confusion, memory problems.

SYMBYAX (olanzapine + fluoxetine) ▶LK ♀C ▶– $$$$$
WARNING — Observe patients started on SSRIs for worsening depression or emergence of suicidal thoughts or behaviors in children, adolescents, and young adults, especially early in therapy or after increases in dose. Monitor for emergence of anxiety, agitation, panic attacks, insomnia, irritability, hostility, impulsivity, akathisia, mania and hypomania. Carefully weigh risks and benefits before starting and then monitor such individuals closely. The use of atypical antipsychotics to treat behavioral problems in patients with dementia has been associated with higher mortality rates. Atypical antipsychotics have been associated with wt gain, dyslipidemia, hyperglycemia, and diabetes mellitus; monitor closely.
ADULTS — Bipolar type 1 with depression and treatment-resistant depression: Start 6/25 mg PO at bedtime. Max 18/75 mg/day.
PEDS — Not approved in children younger than 12 yo.
FORMS — Trade only: Caps (olanzapine/fluoxetine) 3/25, 6/25, 6/50, 12/25, 12/50 mg.
NOTES — Efficacy beyond 8 weeks not established. Monitor wt, fasting glucose, and triglycerides before initiation and periodically during treatment. Contraindicated with thioridazine; don't use with cisapride, thioridazine, tryptophan, or MAOIs; caution with lithium, phenytoin, TCAs, aspirin, NSAIDs and warfarin. Pregnancy exposure to fluoxetine associated with premature delivery, low birth wt, and lower Apgar scores. Decrease dose with liver disease or patients predisposed to hypotension.
MOA — Olanzapine: Dopamine antagonist, serotonin 2A antagonist. Fluoxetine: Inhibits serotonin reuptake.
ADVERSE EFFECTS — Serious: Serotonin syndrome, neuroleptic malignant syndrome, hyponatremia, SIADH, seizures, hypotension, hyperglycemia/diabetes, QT prolongation, hepatitis, abnormal bleeding. Frequent: Asthenia, edema, increased appetite, peripheral edema, pharyngitis, somnolence, abnormal thinking, tremor, weight gain.

TRIAVIL (perphenazine + amitriptyline) ▶LK ♀D ▶? $$
ADULTS — Rarely used; other drugs preferred. Depression/Anxiety: 2 to 4 mg perphenazine plus 10 to 25 mg amitriptyline PO tid to qid or 4 mg perphenazine plus 50 mg amitriptyline bid. Max total per day is 16 mg perphenazine or 200 mg of amitriptyline.
PEDS — Not approved in children.
FORMS — Generic only: Tabs (perphenazine/amitriptyline) 2/10, 2/25, 4/10, 4/25, 4/50 mg.
MOA — Antidepressant-antipsychotic combination.
ADVERSE EFFECTS — Serious: Seizures, arrhythmias, hypotension, extrapyramidal side effects, neuroleptic malignant syndrome, tardive dyskinesia, corneal deposits, pigmentary retinopathy. Frequent: Dry mouth, constipation, blurred vision, photosensitivity.

PSYCHIATRY: Drug Dependence Therapy

ACAMPROSATE (*Campral*) ▶K ♀C ▶? $$$$
ADULTS — Maintenance of abstinence from alcohol: 666 mg (2 tabs) PO tid. Start after alcohol withdrawal and when patient is abstinent.
PEDS — Not approved in children.
FORMS — Trade only: Tabs delayed-release 333 mg.
NOTES — Reduce dose to 333 mg if CrCl 30 to 50 mL/min. Contraindicated if CrCl < 30 mL/min.
MOA — Unknown. Structural analogue of GABA and may restore balance to that system.
ADVERSE EFFECTS — Serious: Depression, suicidality. Frequent: Asthenia, diarrhea, anxiety, insomnia.

DISULFIRAM (*Antabuse*) ▶L ♀C ▶? $$$
WARNING — Never give to an intoxicated patient.
ADULTS — Maintenance of sobriety: 125 to 500 mg PO daily.
PEDS — Not approved in children.
FORMS — Trade only: Tabs 250, 500 mg.
NOTES — Patient must abstain from any alcohol for at least 12 h before using. Disulfiram-alcohol reaction may occur for up to 2 weeks after discontinuing disulfiram. Metronidazole and alcohol in any form (eg, cough syrups, tonics) contraindicated. Hepatotoxicity.

(cont.)

ZOPICLONE (*cont.*)
MOA — Short-acting hypnotic; structurally unrelated to benzodiazepines but shares a similar pharmacological profile to many of the benzodiazepines.
ADVERSE EFFECTS — Frequent: Taste alteration (bitter taste), anterograde amnesia, confusion, N/V, anorexia.

DISULFIRAM (cont.)
  MOA — Inhibits aldehyde dehydrogenase.
  ADVERSE EFFECTS — Serious: Angina, MI, hypotension, tachycardia, heart failure, syncope, seizures. Frequent: Rash, drowsiness, headache, impotence, rash, optic neuropathy.

NALTREXONE (ReVia, Depade, Vivitrol) ▶LK ♀C ▶? $$$$
  WARNING — Hepatotoxicity with higher than approved doses.
  ADULTS — <u>Alcohol dependence:</u> 50 mg PO daily. Extended-release injectable susp: 380 mg IM q 4 weeks or monthly. <u>Opioid dependence:</u> Start 25 mg PO daily, increase to 50 mg PO daily if no signs of withdrawal.
  PEDS — Not approved in children.
  FORMS — Generic/Trade: Tabs 50 mg. Trade only (Vivitrol): Extended-release injectable susp kits 380 mg.
  NOTES — Avoid if recent (past 7 to 10 days) ingestion of opioids. Conflicting evidence of efficacy for chronic, severe alcoholism.
  MOA — Opiate antagonist.
  ADVERSE EFFECTS — Serious: Suicidal ideation, paranoia, depression. Frequent: Insomnia, nervousness, headache, dizziness, N/V.

NICOTINE GUM (Nicorette, Nicorette DS) ▶LK ♀C ▶− $$$$
  ADULTS — <u>Smoking cessation:</u> Gradually taper 1 piece (2 mg) q 1 to 2 h for 6 weeks, 1 piece (2 mg) q 2 to 4 h for 3 weeks, then 1 piece (2 mg) q 4 to 8 h for 3 weeks. Max 30 pieces/day of 2 mg gum or 24 pieces/day of 4 mg gum. Use 4 mg pieces (Nicorette DS) for high cigarette use (more than 24 cigarettes/day).
  PEDS — Not approved in children.
  FORMS — OTC/Generic/Trade: Gum 2, 4 mg.
  NOTES — Chew slowly and park between cheek and gum periodically. May cause N/V, hiccups. Coffee, juices, wine, and soft drinks may reduce absorption. Avoid eating/drinking for 15 min before/during gum use. Available in original, orange, or mint flavor. Do not use beyond 6 months.
  MOA — Nicotine receptor agonist.
  ADVERSE EFFECTS — Serious: Atrial and ventricular arrhythmias. Frequent: Local reactions, burning, stinging, headache, insomnia, nausea, diarrhea, tachycardia, chest pain, hypertension.

NICOTINE INHALATION SYSTEM (Nicotrol Inhaler, ✣Nicorette inhaler) ▶LK ♀D ▶− $$$$$
  ADULTS — <u>Smoking cessation:</u> 6 to 16 cartridges/day for 12 weeks.
  PEDS — Not approved in children.
  FORMS — Trade only: Oral inhaler 10 mg/cartridge (4 mg nicotine delivered), 42 cartridges/box.
  MOA — Nicotine receptor agonist.
  ADVERSE EFFECTS — Serious: Atrial and ventricular arrhythmias. Frequent: Local reactions, burning, stinging, headache, insomnia, nausea, diarrhea, tachycardia, chest pain, hypertension.

NICOTINE LOZENGE (Commit, Nicorette) ▶LK ♀D ▶− $$$$$
  ADULTS — <u>Smoking cessation:</u> In those who smoke < 30 min after waking use 4 mg lozenge; others use 2 mg. Take 1 to 2 lozenges q 1 to 2 h for 6 weeks, then q 2 to 4 h in week 7 to 9, then q 4 to 8 h in week 10 to 12. Length of therapy 12 weeks.
  PEDS — Not approved in children.
  FORMS — OTC Generic/Trade: Lozenge 2, 4 mg in 48, 72, 168 count packages.
  NOTES — Allow lozenge to dissolve and do not chew. Do not eat or drink within 15 min before use. Avoid concurrent use with other sources of nicotine.
  MOA — Nicotine receptor agonist.
  ADVERSE EFFECTS — Serious: Atrial and ventricular arrhythmias. Frequent: Local reactions, headache, insomnia, nausea, diarrhea, tachycardia, chest pain, hypertension.

NICOTINE NASAL SPRAY (Nicotrol NS) ▶LK ♀D ▶− $$$$$
  ADULTS — <u>Smoking cessation:</u> 1 to 2 doses each h, each dose is 2 sprays, 1 in each nostril (1 spray contains 0.5 mg nicotine). Minimum recommended: 8 doses/day, max 40 doses/day.
  PEDS — Not approved in children.
  FORMS — Trade only: Nasal soln 10 mg/mL (0.5 mg/inhalation); 10 mL bottles.
  MOA — Nicotine receptor agonist.
  ADVERSE EFFECTS — Serious: Atrial and ventricular arrhythmias. Frequent: Local reactions, burning, stinging, headache, insomnia, nausea, diarrhea, tachycardia, chest pain, hypertension.

NICOTINE PATCHES (Habitrol, NicoDerm CQ, Nicotrol, ✣Prostep) ▶LK ♀D ▶− $$$$
  ADULTS — <u>Smoking cessation:</u> Start 1 patch (14 to 22 mg) daily and taper after 6 weeks. Total duration of therapy is 12 weeks.
  PEDS — Not approved in children.
  FORMS — OTC/Rx/Generic/Trade: Patches 11, 22 mg/24 h. 7, 14, 21 mg/24 h (Habitrol and NicoDerm). OTC/Trade: 15 mg/16 h (Nicotrol).
  NOTES — Ensure patient has stopped smoking. Dispose of patches safely; can be toxic to kids, pets. Remove opaque NicoDerm CQ patch prior to MRI procedures to avoid possible burns.
  MOA — Nicotine receptor agonist.
  ADVERSE EFFECTS — Serious: Atrial and ventricular arrhythmias. Frequent: Local reactions, burning, stinging, headache, insomnia, nausea, diarrhea, tachycardia, chest pain, hypertension.

SUBOXONE (buprenorphine + naloxone) ▶L ♀C ▶− ©III $$$$$
  ADULTS — <u>Treatment of opioid dependence:</u> Maintenance: 16 mg SL daily. Can individualize to range of 4 to 24 mg SL daily.
  PEDS — Not approved in children.
  FORMS — Trade only: SL tabs 2/0.5 mg and 8/2 mg buprenorphine/naloxone.
  NOTES — Suboxone preferred over Subutex for unsupervised administration. Titrate in 2 to 4 mg increments/decrements to maintain therapy

(cont.)

SUBOXONE (cont.)
compliance and prevent withdrawal. Prescribers must complete training and apply for special DEA number. See www.suboxone.com.
MOA — Partial opiate agonist/antagonist.
ADVERSE EFFECTS — Serious: Respiratory/CNS depression, hepatitis, dependence. Frequent: Headache, N/V, constipation, abdominal pain, sweating.

VARENICLINE (*Chantix*) ▶K ♀C ▶? $$$$
WARNING — Has been associated with the development of suicidal ideation, changes in behavior, depressed mood and attempted/completed suicides, both during treatment and after withdrawal. Unclear safety in serious psychiatric conditions.
ADULTS — Smoking cessation: Start 0.5 mg PO daily for days 1 to 3, then 0.5 mg bid days 4 to 7, then 1 mg bid thereafter. Take after meals with full glass of water. Start 1 week prior to cessation and continue for 12 weeks.
PEDS — Not approved in children.
FORMS — Trade only: Tabs 0.5, 1 mg.
NOTES — For severe renal dysfunction reduce max dose to 0.5 mg bid. For renal failure on hemodialysis may use 0.5 mg once daily if tolerated.
MOA — Nicotinic acetylcholine receptor agonist.
ADVERSE EFFECTS — Serious: Depression, suicidal thoughts, aggression, erratic behavior. Frequent: N/V, drowsiness, dreaming disturbances, insomnia, headache, abnormal dreams, constipation.

PSYCHIATRY: Stimulants/ADHD/Anorexiants

NOTE: Sudden cardiac death has been reported with stimulants and atomoxetine at usual ADHD doses; carefully assess prior to treatment and avoid if cardiac conditions or structural abnormalities. Amphetamines are associated with high abuse potential and dependence with prolonged administration. Stimulants may also cause or worsen underlying psychosis or induce a manic or mixed episode in bipolar disorder. Problems with visual accommodation have also been reported with stimulants.

ADDERALL (dextroamphetamine + amphetamine, Adderall XR) ▶L ♀C ▶− ©II $$$$
ADULTS — Narcolepsy, standard-release: Start 10 mg PO qam, increase by 10 mg q week, maximum dose is 60 mg/day divided bid to tid at 4 to 6 h intervals. ADHD, extended-release caps (Adderall XR): 20 mg PO daily.
PEDS — ADHD, standard-release tabs: Start 2.5 mg (3 to 5 yo) or 5 mg (age 6 yo or older) PO daily to bid, increase by 2.5 to 5 mg every week, max 40 mg/day. ADHD, extended-release caps (Adderall XR): If age 6 to 12 yo, then start 5 to 10 mg PO daily to a max of 30 mg/day. If 13 to 17 yo, then start 10 mg PO daily to a max of 20 mg/day. Not recommended age younger than 3 yo. Narcolepsy, standard-release: Age 6 to 12 yo: Start 5 mg PO daily, increase by 5 mg q week. Age older than 12 yo: Start 10 mg PO qam, increase by 10 mg q week, maximum dose is 60 mg/day divided bid to tid at 4 to 6 h intervals.
FORMS — Generic/Trade: Tabs 5, 7.5, 10, 12.5, 15, 20, 30 mg. Trade only: Caps, extended-release (Adderall XR) 5, 10, 15, 20, 25, 30 mg.
NOTES — Caps may be opened and the beads sprinkled on applesauce; do not chew beads. Adderall XR should be given upon awakening. Avoid evening doses. Monitor growth and use drug holidays when appropriate. May increase pulse and BP. May exacerbate bipolar or psychotic conditions.
MOA — CNS stimulant, increases norepinephrine and dopamine.
ADVERSE EFFECTS — Serious: Sudden death, seizures, psychosis, hypertension. Frequent: Appetite suppression, weight loss, insomnia, nervousness, N/V, dizziness, palpitations, tachycardia, headache.

ARMODAFINIL (*Nuvigil*) ▶L ♀C ▶? ©IV $$$$$
ADULTS — Obstructive sleep apnea/hypopnea syndrome and narcolepsy: 150 to 250 mg PO qam. Inconsistent evidence for improved efficacy of 250 mg/day dose. Shift work sleep disorder: 150 mg PO 1 h prior to start of shift.
PEDS — Not approved in children.
FORMS — Trade only: Tabs 50, 100, 150, 200, 250 mg.
NOTES — Weak inducer for substrates of CYP3A4/5 (eg, carbamazepine, cyclosporine) which may require dose adjustments. May inhibit metabolism of substrates of CYP2C19 (eg, omeprazole, diazepam, phenytoin). May reduce efficacy of oral contraceptives; consider alternatives during treatment. Reduce dose with severe liver impairment.
MOA — R-enantiomer of modafinil. Wake promoting agent – CNS stimulant.
ADVERSE EFFECTS — Serious: Rash, Stevens-Johnson syndrome, multi-organ hypersensitivity reactions, mania, psychosis, suicidal ideation. Frequent: Headache, nausea, dizziness, insomnia.

ATOMOXETINE (*Strattera*) ▶K ♀C ▶? $$$$$
WARNING — Severe liver injury and failure have been reported; discontinue if jaundice or elevated LFTs. Increases risk of suicidal thinking and behavior in children and adolescents; carefully weigh risks/benefits before starting and then monitor such individuals closely for worsening depression or emergence of suicidal thoughts or behaviors especially early in therapy or after increases in dose. Monitor for emergence of anxiety, agitation, panic attacks, insomnia, irritability, hostility, impulsivity, akathisia, mania and hypomania.
ADULTS — ADHD: Start 40 mg PO daily, then increase after more than 3 days to target of 80 mg/day divided daily to bid. Max dose 100 mg/day.
PEDS — ADHD: Children/adolescents wt 70 kg or less: Start 0.5 mg/kg daily, then increase after more than 3 days to target dose of 1.2 mg/kg/day divided

(cont.)

PSYCHIATRY: Stimulants/ADHD/Anorexiants

BODY MASS INDEX*		Heights are in feet and inches; weights are in pounds					
BMI	Class.	4' 10"	5' 0"	5' 4"	5' 8"	6' 0"	6' 4"
<19	Underweight	<91	<97	<110	<125	<140	<156
19–24	Healthy Weight	91–119	97–127	110–144	125–163	140–183	156–204
25–29	Overweight	120–143	128–152	145–173	164–196	184–220	205–245
30–40	Obese	144–191	153–204	174–233	197–262	221–293	246–328
>40	Very Obese	>191	>204	>233	>262	>293	>328

*BMI = kg/m^2 = (wt in pounds)(703)/(height in inches)^2. Anorectants appropriate if BMI ≥30 (with comorbidities ≥27); surgery an option if BMI >40 (with comorbidities 35–40). www.nhlbi.nih.gov

ATOMOXETINE (cont.)
daily to bid. Max dose 1.4 mg/kg or 100 mg/day, whichever is less. If wt greater than 70 kg use adult dose.
FORMS — Trade only: Caps 10, 18, 25, 40, 60, 80, 100 mg.
NOTES — If taking strong CYP2D6 inhibitors (eg, paroxetine or fluoxetine), use same starting dose but only increase if well-tolerated at 4 weeks and symptoms unimproved. Caution when coadministered with oral or parenteral albuterol or other beta-2 agonists, as increases in heart rate and BP may occur. May be stopped without tapering. Monitor growth. Give "Patient Medication Guide" when dispensed. Does not appear to exacerbate tics.
MOA — Selective norepinephrine reuptake inhibitor.
ADVERSE EFFECTS — Serious: Sudden death, increased blood pressure and heart rate, liver injury and failure, psychosis, mania, aggression, priapism. Frequent: N/V, dyspepsia, fatigue, decreased appetite, weight loss, dizziness, mood swings, constipation, dry mouth, insomnia, sexual dysfunction, urinary hesitancy/retention, hot flushes, dysuria, dysmenorrhea.

BENZPHETAMINE (*Didrex*) ▶K ♀X ▶? ©III $$$
WARNING — Chronic overuse/abuse can lead to marked tolerance and psychic dependence; caution with prolonged use.
ADULTS — Short-term treatment of obesity: Start with 25 to 50 mg once daily in the morning and increase if needed to 1 to 3 times daily.
PEDS — Not approved for children younger than 12 yo.
FORMS — Generic/Trade: Tabs 50 mg.
NOTES — Tolerance to anorectic effect develops within week and cross-tolerance to other drugs in class common.
MOA — CNS stimulant, increases dopamine and norepinephrine.
ADVERSE EFFECTS — Serious: Seizures, psychosis, hypertension, dependence. Frequent: Appetite suppression, weight loss, insomnia, nervousness, N/V, dizziness, palpitations, tachycardia, headache.

CAFFEINE (*NoDoz, Vivarin, Caffedrine, Stay Awake, Quick-Pep, Cafcit*) ▶L ♀B/C ▶? $
ADULTS — Fatigue: 100 to 200 mg PO q 3 to 4 h prn.
PEDS — Not approved in children younger than 12 yo, except apnea of prematurity in infants between 28 and less than 33 weeks gestational age (Cafcit): Load 20 mg/kg IV over 30 min. Maintenance 5 mg/kg PO q 24 h. Monitor for necrotizing enterocolitis.
FORMS — OTC Generic/Trade: Tabs/Caps 200 mg. Oral soln caffeine citrate (Cafcit) 20 mg/mL. OTC Trade only: Tabs extended-release 200 mg. Lozenges 75 mg.
NOTES — 2 mg caffeine citrate = 1 mg caffeine base.
MOA — CNS and cardiovascular stimulant.
ADVERSE EFFECTS — Serious: Arrhythmias, delirium, seizures, necrotizing enterocolitis. Frequent: Tremor, anxiety, twitches, headache, insomnia, N/V.

DEXMETHYLPHENIDATE (*Focalin, Focalin XR*) ▶LK ♀C ▶? ©II $$$
ADULTS — ADHD, not already on stimulants: Start 10 mg PO qam (extended-release) or 2.5 mg PO bid (immediate-release). Max 20 mg/day for immediate release and 40 mg/day for extended-release. If taking racemic methylphenidate use conversion of 2.5 mg for each 5 mg of methylphenidate.
PEDS — ADHD and age 6 yo or older and not already on stimulants: Start 5 mg PO qam (extended-release) or 2.5 mg PO bid (immediate-release), max 20 mg/day (immediate-release) or 30 mg/day (extended-release). If already on racemic methylphenidate, use conversion of 2.5 mg for each 5 mg of methylphenidate.
FORMS — Generic/Trade: Tabs, immediate-release 2.5, 5, 10 mg. Trade only: Extended-release caps (Focalin XR) 5, 10, 15, 20, 30 mg.
NOTES — Avoid evening doses. Monitor growth and use drug holidays when appropriate. May increase pulse and BP. 2.5 mg is equivalent to 5 mg racemic methylphenidate. Focalin XR caps may be opened and sprinkled on applesauce, but beads must not be chewed. May exacerbate bipolar or psychotic conditions.
MOA — CNS stimulant, increases norepinephrine and dopamine.
ADVERSE EFFECTS — Serious: Sudden death, seizures, psychosis, hypertension. Frequent: Appetite suppression, weight loss, insomnia, nervousness, N/V, dizziness, palpitations, tachycardia, headache.

PSYCHIATRY: Stimulants/ADHD/Anorexiants

DEXTROAMPHETAMINE (*Dexedrine, Dextrostat*) ▶L ♀C ▶– ©II $$$$
ADULTS — <u>Narcolepsy:</u> Start 10 mg PO q am, increase by 10 mg/day q week, max 60 mg/day divided daily (sustained-release) or bid to tid at 4 to 6 h intervals.
PEDS — <u>Narcolepsy:</u> Age 6 to 12 yo: Start 5 mg PO q am, increase by 5 mg/day q week. Age older than 12 yo: Start 10 mg PO q am, increase by 10 mg/day q week, max 60 mg/day divided daily (sustained-release) or bid to tid at 4 to 6 h intervals. <u>ADHD:</u> Age 3 to 5 yo: Start 2.5 mg PO daily, increase by 2.5 mg q week. Age 6 yo or older: Start 5 mg PO daily to bid, increase by 5 mg q week, usual max 40 mg/day divided daily to tid at 4 to 6 h intervals. Not recommended for patients younger than 3 yo. Extended-release caps not recommended for age younger than 6 yo.
FORMS — Generic/Trade: Caps extended-release 5, 10, 15 mg. Generic only: Tabs 5, 10 mg. Oral soln 5 mg/5 mL.
NOTES — Avoid evening doses. Monitor growth and use drug holidays when appropriate. May exacerbate bipolar or psychotic conditions.
MOA — CNS stimulant, increases norepinephrine and dopamine.
ADVERSE EFFECTS — Serious: Sudden death, seizures, psychosis, hypertension. Frequent: Appetite suppression, weight loss, insomnia, nervousness, N/V, dizziness, palpitations, tachycardia, headache.

DIETHYLPROPION (*Tenuate, Tenuate Dospan*) ▶K ♀B ▶? ©IV $
WARNING — Chronic overuse/abuse can lead to marked tolerance and psychic dependence; caution with prolonged use.
ADULTS — <u>Short-term treatment of obesity:</u> 25 mg PO tid 1 h before meals and mid evening if needed or 75 mg sustained-release daily at midmorning.
PEDS — Not approved for children younger than 12 yo.
FORMS — Generic/Trade: Tabs 25 mg, Tabs, extended-release 75 mg.
NOTES — Tolerance to anorectic effect develops within week and cross-tolerance to other drugs in class common.
MOA — CNS stimulant, increases dopamine and norepinephrine.
ADVERSE EFFECTS — Serious: Seizures, psychosis, hypertension, dependence. Frequent: Appetite suppression, weight loss, insomnia, nervousness, N/V, dizziness, palpitations, tachycardia, headache.

GUANFACINE (*Intuniv*) ▶LK– ♀B ▶?
ADULTS — <u>ADHD:</u> Start 1 mg PO q AM. Increase by 1 mg/week to max 4 mg/day.
PEDS — <u>ADHD</u> (6 yrs and above): Start 1 mg PO q AM. Increase by 1 mg/week to max 4 mg/day.
FORMS — Trade only: Tabs 1, 2, 3, 4 mg.
NOTES — Taper when discontinuing. Use cautiously with strong CYP3A4 inhibitors.
MOA — Selective alpha-2A adrenergic agonist.
ADVERSE EFFECTS — Serious: Hypotension, bradycardia, syncope. Frequent: Somnolence/sedation, abdominal pain, dizziness, hypotension, dry mouth, constipation, headache.

LISDEXAMFETAMINE (*Vyvanse*) ▶L ♀C ▶– ©II $$$$
ADULTS — <u>ADHD</u> Start 30 mg PO qam. May increase weekly by 10 to 20 mg/day to max 70 mg/day.
PEDS — <u>ADHD</u> ages 6 to 12 yo: Start 30 mg PO qam. May increase weekly by 10 to 20 mg/day to max 70 mg/day. Adolescents use adult dosing.
FORMS — Trade: Caps 20, 30, 40, 50, 60, 70 mg.
NOTES — May open cap and place contents in water for administration. Avoid evening doses. Monitor growth and use drug holidays when appropriate.
MOA — Prodrug of dextroamphetamine. CNS stimulant, increases norepinephrine and dopamine.
ADVERSE EFFECTS — Serious: Sudden death, seizures, psychosis, hypertension. Frequent: Appetite suppression, weight loss, insomnia, nervousness, N/V, dizziness, palpitations, tachycardia, headache, irritability, dry mouth.

METHYLPHENIDATE (*Ritalin, Ritalin LA, Ritalin SR, Methylin, Methylin ER, Metadate ER, Metadate CD, Concerta, Daytrana, ✦Biphentin*) ▶LK ♀C ▶? ©II $$
ADULTS — <u>Narcolepsy:</u> 10 mg PO bid to tid before meals. Usual effective dose is 20 to 30 mg/day, max 60 mg/day. Use sustained-release Tabs when the 8 h dosage corresponds to the titrated 8 h dosage of the conventional tabs. <u>ADHD</u> (Concerta): Start 18 to 36 mg PO qam, usual dose range 18 to 72 mg/day.
PEDS — <u>ADHD</u> age 6 yo or older: Start 5 mg PO bid before breakfast and lunch, increase gradually by 5 to 10 mg/day at weekly interval to max 60 mg/day. Sustained and extended-release: Start 20 mg PO daily, max 60 mg daily. Concerta (extended-release) start 18 mg PO qam; titrate in 9 to 18 mg increments at weekly intervals to max 54 mg/day (age 6 to 12 yo) or 72 mg/day (13 to 17 yo). Consult product labeling for dose conversion from other methylphenidate regimens. Discontinue after 1 month if no improvement observed. Transdermal patch age 6 to 17 yo: Start 10 mg/9 h, may increase at weekly intervals to max dose of 30 mg/9 h. Apply 2 h prior to desired onset and remove 9 h later. Effect may last up to 12 h after application. Must alternate sites daily.
FORMS — Trade only: Tabs 5, 10, 20 mg (Ritalin, Methylin, Metadate). Tabs extended-release 10, 20 mg (Methylin ER, Metadate ER). Tabs extended-release 18, 27, 36, 54 mg (Concerta). Caps extended-release 10, 20, 30, 40, 50, 60 mg (Metadate CD) May be sprinkled on food. Tabs sustained-release 20 mg (Ritalin SR). Caps extended-release 10, 20, 30, 40 mg (Ritalin LA). Tabs chewable 2.5, 5, 10 mg (Methylin). Oral soln 5 mg/5 mL, 10 mg/5 mL (Methylin). Transdermal patch (Daytrana) 10 mg/9 h, 15 mg/9 h, 20 mg/9 h, 30 mg/9 h. Generic only: Tabs 5, 10, 20 mg, tabs extended-release 10, 20 mg, tabs sustained-release 20 mg.
NOTES — Avoid evening doses. Avoid use with severe anxiety tension, or agitation. Monitor growth and use drug holidays when appropriate. May increase pulse and BP. Ritalin LA may be opened and sprinkled on

(cont.)

METHYLPHENIDATE (cont.)
applesauce. Apply transdermal patch to hip below beltline to avoid rubbing it off. May exacerbate bipolar or psychotic conditions.
MOA – CNS stimulant, increases norepinephrine and dopamine.
ADVERSE EFFECTS – Serious: Sudden death, seizures, psychosis, hypertension, contact sensitization (Daytrana). Frequent: Appetite suppression, weight loss, insomnia, nervousness, N/V, dizziness, palpitations, tachycardia, headache.

MODAFINIL (*Provigil, ✦Alertec*) ▶L ♀C ▶? ©IV $$$$$
WARNING – Associated with serious, life-threatening rashes in adults and children; discontinue immediately if unexplained rash.
ADULTS – <u>Narcolepsy and sleep apnea/hypopnea:</u> 200 mg PO qam. <u>Shift work sleep disorder:</u> 200 mg PO 1 h before shift.
PEDS – Not approved in children younger than 16 yo.
FORMS – Trade only: Tabs 100, 200 mg.
NOTES – May increase levels of diazepam, phenytoin, TCAs, warfarin, or propranolol; may decrease levels of cyclosporine, oral contraceptives, or theophylline. Reduce dose in severe liver impairment.
MOA – Wake-promoting agent; CNS stimulant.
ADVERSE EFFECTS – Serious: Rash, Stevens-Johnson syndrome, multi-organ hypersensitivity, leukopenia, psychosis, mania, suicidal ideation. Frequent: Insomnia, nausea, headache, nervousness, anxiety.

PHENDIMATRIZINE (*Bontril, Bontril Slow Release*) ▶K ♀C ▶? ©III $$
WARNING – Chronic overuse/abuse can lead to marked tolerance and psychic dependence; caution with prolonged use.
ADULTS – <u>Short-term treatment of obesity:</u> Start 35 mg 2 to 3 times daily 1 h before meals. Sustained-release 105 mg once in the morning before breakfast.
PEDS – Not approved in children younger than 12 yo.
FORMS – Generic/Trade: Tabs/Caps 35 mg, Caps, sustained-release 105 mg.
NOTES – Tolerance to anorectic effect develops within week and cross-tolerance to other drugs in class common.
MOA – CNS stimulant, increases dopamine and norepinephrine.
ADVERSE EFFECTS – Serious: Seizures, psychosis, hypertension, dependence. Frequent: Appetite suppression, weight loss, insomnia, nervousness, N/V, dizziness, palpitations, tachycardia, headache.

PHENTERMINE (*Adipex-P, Ionamin, Pro-Fast*) ▶KL ♀C ▶– ©IV $$
WARNING – Chronic overuse/abuse can lead to marked tolerance and psychic dependence; caution with prolonged use.
ADULTS – <u>Obesity:</u> 8 mg PO tid before meals or 1 to 2 h after meals. May give 15 to 37.5 mg PO q am or 10 to 14 h before bedtime.
PEDS – Not approved in children younger than 16 yo.
FORMS – Generic/Trade: Caps 15, 30, 37.5 mg. Tabs 37.5 mg. Trade only: Caps extended-release 15, 30 mg (Ionamin). Generic only (Pro-Fast): Caps 18.75 mg, Tabs 8 mg.
NOTES – Indicated for short-term (8–12 weeks) use only. Contraindicated for use during or within 14 days of MAOIs (hypertensive crisis).
MOA – CNS stimulant, increases norepinephrine and dopamine.
ADVERSE EFFECTS – Serious: Seizures, psychosis, hypertension. Frequent: Appetite suppression, weight loss, insomnia, nervousness, N/V, dizziness, palpitations, tachycardia, headache.

PULMONARY: Beta Agonists—Short-Acting

NOTE: Palpitations, tachycardia, tremor, lightheadedness, nervousness, headache, and nausea may occur; these effects may be more pronounced with systemic administration. Hypokalemia can occur from the transient shift of potassium into cells, rarely leading to adverse cardiovascular effects; monitor accordingly. Potential for tolerance with continued use of short-acting beta-agonists.

ALBUTEROL (*AccuNeb, Ventolin HFA, Proventil HFA, ProAir HFA, VoSpire ER, ✦Airomir, Asmavent, salbutamol*) ▶L ♀C ▶? $$
ADULTS – <u>Acute asthma:</u> MDI: 2 puffs q 4 to 6 h prn. Soln for inhalation: 2.5 mg nebulized tid to qid. Dilute 0.5 mL 0.5% soln with 2.5 mL NS. Deliver over 5 to 15 min. One 3 mL unit dose (0.083%) nebulized tid to qid. Caps for inhalation: 200 to 400 mcg inhaled q 4 to 6 h via a Rotahaler device. <u>Asthma:</u> 2 to 4 mg PO tid to qid or extended-release 4 to 8 mg PO q 12 h up to 16 mg PO q 12 h.
PEDS – <u>Acute asthma:</u> MDI: Age 4 yo or older: 1 to 2 puffs q 4 to 6 h prn. Soln for inhalation (0.5%): 2 to 12 yo: 0.1–0.15 mg/kg/dose not to exceed 2.5 mg tid to qid, diluted with NS to 3 mL. Caps for inhalation: Age 4 yo or older 200 to 400 mcg inhaled q 4 to 6 h via a Rotahaler device. <u>Asthma:</u> Tabs, syrup 6 to 12 yo: 2 to 4 mg PO tid to qid, max dose 24 mg/day in divided doses or extended-release 4 mg PO q 12 h. Syrup 2 to 5 yo: 0.1 to 0.2 mg/kg/dose PO tid up to 4 mg tid. Prevention of exercise-induced bronchospasm age 4 yo or older 2 puffs 15 to 30 min before exercise.
UNAPPROVED ADULTS – <u>COPD:</u> MDI, soln for inhalation: Use asthma dose. <u>Acute asthma:</u> MDI, soln for inhalation: Dose as above q 20 min × 3 or until improvement. Continuous nebulization: 10 to 15 mg/h until improvement. Emergency

(cont.)

PULMONARY: Beta Agonists

ALBUTEROL (cont.)
hyperkalemia: 10 to 20 mg via MDI or soln for inhalation.
UNAPPROVED PEDS – Acute asthma: Soln for inhalation: 0.15 mg/kg (minimum dose is 2.5 mg) q 20 min for 3 doses then 0.15 to 0.3 mg/kg up to 10 mg q 1 to 4 h as needed, or 0.5 mg/kg/h continuous nebulization. MDI: 4 to 8 puffs q 20 min for 3 doses then q 1 to 4 h prn. Soln for inhalation (0.5%): Age younger than 2 yo: 0.05 to 0.15 mg/kg/dose q 4 to 6 h. Syrup age younger than 2 yo: 0.3 mg/kg/24 h PO divided tid, max dose 12 mg/24 h. Prevention of exercise-induced bronchospasm: MDI: Age 4 yo or older 2 puffs 15 to 30 min before exercise.
FORMS – Trade only: MDI 90 mcg/actuation, 200 metered doses/canister. "HFA" inhalers use hydrofluoroalkane propellant instead of CFCs but are otherwise equivalent. Generic/Trade: Soln for inhalation 0.021% (AccuNeb), 0.042% (AccuNeb), and 0.083% in 3 mL vials, 0.5% (5 mg/mL) in 20 mL with dropper. Tabs extended-release 4, 8 mg (VoSpire ER). Generic only: Syrup 2 mg/5 mL. Tabs immediate-release 2, 4 mg.
NOTES – Do not crush or chew extended-release tabs. Use with caution in patients on MAOIs or cyclic antidepressants: May increase cardiovascular side effects.
MOA – Short-acting beta agonist bronchodilator.
ADVERSE EFFECTS – Serious: Hypersensitivity, paradoxical bronchospasm. Frequent: Palpitations, tachycardia, hypokalemia, tremor, lightheadedness, nervousness, headache, and nausea.

FENOTEROL (✽Berotec) ▶L ♀C ▶? $
ADULTS – Canada only. Acute asthma: MDI: 1 to 2 puffs tid to qid; maximum 8 puffs/day. Soln for nebulization: Up to 2.5 mg q 6 h.
PEDS – Not approved in children.
FORMS – Trade only: MDI 100 mcg/actuation. Soln for inhalation: 20 mL bottles of 1 mg/mL (with preservatives that may cause bronchoconstriction in those with hyperreactive airways).
MOA – Short-acting beta agonist bronchodilator.
ADVERSE EFFECTS – Serious: Hypersensitivity, paradoxical bronchoconstriction. Frequent: Tremor, hypokalemia, dizziness, headache, palpitations, tachycardia.

LEVALBUTEROL (Xopenex, Xopenex HFA) ▶L ♀C ▶? $$$
ADULTS – Acute asthma: MDI 2 puffs q 4 to 6 h prn. Soln for inhalation: 0.63 to 1.25 mg nebulized q 6 to 8 h.
PEDS – Acute asthma: MDI age 4 yo or older: 2 puffs q 4 to 6 h prn. Soln for inhalation age 12 yo or older: Use adult dose. 0.31 mg nebulized tid for age 6 to 11 yo.
FORMS – Generic/Trade: Soln for inhalation 0.31, 0.63, 1.25 mg in 3 mL and 1.25 mg in 0.5 mL unit-dose vials. Trade only: HFA MDI 45 mcg/actuation, 15 g 200/canister. "HFA" inhalers use hydrofluoroalkane propellant.

NOTES – R-isomer of albuterol. Dyspepsia may occur. Use with caution in patients on MAOIs or cyclic antidepressants; may increase cardiovascular side effects.
MOA – Short-acting beta agonist bronchodilator.
ADVERSE EFFECTS – Serious: Hypersensitivity, paradoxical bronchospasm, arrhythmias. Frequent: Palpitations, tachycardia, hypokalemia, tremor, lightheadedness, nervousness, headache, and nausea.

METAPROTERENOL (Alupent, ✽orciprenaline) ▶L ♀C ▶? $$
ADULTS – Acute asthma: MDI: 2 to 3 puffs q 3 to 4 h; max dose 12 puffs/day. Soln for inhalation: 0.2 to 0.3 mL of the 5% soln in 2.5 mL NS. 20 mg PO tid to qid.
PEDS – Acute asthma: Soln for inhalation: 0.1 to 0.3 mL of the 5% soln in 2.5 mL NS for age older than 6 yo. Tabs or syrup: 1.3 to 2.6 mg/kg/day PO in divided doses tid to qid for age 2 to 5 yo. 10 mg PO tid to qid for age 6 to 9 yo or wt less than 60 lbs, 20 mg PO tid to qid for age older than 9 yo or wt 60 lbs or greater.
UNAPPROVED PEDS – Acute asthma: MDI: 2 to 3 puffs q 3 to 4 h (up to 12 puffs/day) for age older than 6 yo. Soln for inhalation: 0.1 to 0.3 mL of the 5% soln in 2.5 mL NS q 4 to 6 h prn or q 20 min until improvement. Tabs or syrup age younger than 2 yo: 0.4 mg/kg/dose PO tid to qid.
FORMS – Trade only: MDI 0.65 mg/actuation, 14 g 200/canister. Generic/Trade: Soln for inhalation 0.4%, 0.6% in 2.5 mL unit-dose vials. Generic only: Syrup 10 mg/5 mL, Tabs 10, 20 mg.
MOA – Short-acting beta agonist bronchodilator.
ADVERSE EFFECTS – Serious: Hypersensitivity, paradoxical bronchospasm. Frequent: Palpitations, tachycardia, hypokalemia, tremor, lightheadedness, nervousness, headache, and nausea.

PIRBUTEROL (Maxair Autohaler) ▶L ♀C ▶? $$$$
ADULTS – Acute asthma: MDI: 1 to 2 puffs q 4 to 6 h. Max dose 12 puffs/day.
PEDS – Not approved in children.
UNAPPROVED PEDS – Acute asthma age 12 yo or older: Use adult dose.
FORMS – Trade only: MDI 200 mcg/actuation, 14 g 400/canister.
NOTES – Breath-actuated autohaler.
MOA – Short-acting beta agonist bronchodilator.
ADVERSE EFFECTS – Serious: Hypersensitivity. Frequent: Palpitations, tachycardia, hypokalemia, tremor, lightheadedness, nervousness, headache, and nausea.

TERBUTALINE (Brethine, ✽Bricanyl Turbuhaler) ▶L ♀B ▶– $$
ADULTS – Asthma: 2.5 to 5 mg PO q 6 h while awake. Max dose 15 mg/24 h. Acute asthma: 0.25 mg SC into lateral deltoid area; may repeat once within 15 to 30 min. Max dose 0.5 mg/4 h.
PEDS – Not approved in children.
UNAPPROVED ADULTS – Preterm labor: 0.25 mg SC q 30 min up to 1 mg in 4 h. Infusion: 2.5 to 10 mcg/

(cont.)

TERBUTALINE (*cont.*)
min IV, gradually increased to effective max doses of 17.5 to 30 mcg/min.
UNAPPROVED PEDS — <u>Asthma:</u> 0.05 mg/kg/dose PO tid, increase to max of 0.15 mg/kg/dose tid, max 5 mg/day for age 12 yo or younger, use adult dose for age older than 12 yo up to max 7.5 mg/ 24 h. <u>Acute asthma:</u> 0.01 mg/kg SC q 20 min for 3 doses then q 2 to 6 h as needed.
FORMS — Generic/Trade: Tabs 2.5, 5 mg (Brethine scored). Canada only (Bricanyl): DPI 0.5 mg/actuation, 200 per DPI.
NOTES — Give 50% normal dose in renal insufficiency; avoid in renal failure. Concomitant use with magnesium sulfate may lead to fatal pulmonary edema.
MOA — Short-acting beta agonist bronchodilator; tocolytic.
ADVERSE EFFECTS — Serious: Hypersensitivity, paradoxical bronchospasm. In labor: Pulmonary edema (with magnesium sulfate), arrhythmias, cerebral & cardiac ischemia, and increased fetal heart rate. Frequent: Palpitations, tachycardia, hypokalemia, tremor, lightheadedness, nervousness, headache, hyperglycemia, and nausea.

PULMONARY: Beta Agonists—Long-Acting

NOTE: Long-acting beta-agonists may increase the risk of asthma-related death. Use only as a second agent if inadequate control with an optimal dose of inhaled corticosteroids. Do not use for rescue therapy. Palpitations, tachycardia, tremor, lightheadedness, nervousness, headache, and nausea may occur. Decreases in serum potassium can occur, rarely leading to adverse cardiovascular effects; monitor accordingly.

ARFORMOTEROL (*Brovana*) ▶L ♀C ▶? $$$$$
ADULTS — <u>COPD:</u> 15 mcg nebulized bid.
PEDS — Not approved in children.
FORMS — Trade only: Soln for inhalation 15 mcg in 2 mL vial.
NOTES — Not for acute COPD exacerbations.
MOA — Long-acting beta agonist bronchodilator.
ADVERSE EFFECTS — Serious: Hypersensitivity, paradoxical bronchospasm. Frequent: Palpitations, tachycardia, hypokalemia, tremor, lightheadedness, nervousness, headache, and nausea.

FORMOTEROL (*Foradil, Perforomist,* ✦*Oxeze Turbuhaler*) ▶L ♀C ▶? $$$
ADULTS — <u>Chronic asthma, COPD:</u> 1 puff bid. <u>Prevention of exercise-induced bronchospasm:</u> 1 puff 15 min prior to exercise. <u>COPD:</u> 20 mcg nebulized q 12 h.
PEDS — <u>Chronic asthma,</u> age 5 yo or older: 1 puff bid. <u>Prevention of exercise-induced bronchospasm</u> age 12 yo or older: Use adult dose.
FORMS — Trade only: DPI 12 mcg, 12, 60 blisters/pack (Foradil). Soln for inhalation: 20 mcg in 2 mL vial (Perforomist). Canada only (Oxeze): DPI 6, 12 mcg 60 blisters/pack.
NOTES — Do not use additional doses for exercise if on maintenance.
MOA — Long-acting beta agonist bronchodilator.
ADVERSE EFFECTS — Serious: Hypersensitivity, paradoxical bronchospasm. Frequent: Palpitations, tachycardia, hypokalemia, tremor, insomnia, lightheadedness, nervousness, headache, and nausea.

SALMETEROL (*Serevent Diskus*) ▶L ♀C ▶? $$$$
ADULTS — <u>Chronic asthma/COPD:</u> 1 puff bid. <u>Prevention of exercise-induced bronchospasm:</u> 1 puff 30 min before exercise.
PEDS — <u>Chronic asthma</u> age 4 yo or older: 1 puff bid. <u>Prevention of exercise-induced bronchospasm:</u> 1 puff 30 min before exercise.
FORMS — Trade only: DPI (Diskus): 50 mcg, 60 blisters.
NOTES — Do not use additional doses for exercise if on maintenance. Concomitant ketoconazole increases levels and prolongs QT interval. Do not use with strong CYP3A4 inhibitors such as ritonavir, itraconazole, clarithromycin, nefazodone, etc.
MOA — Long-acting beta agonist bronchodilator.
ADVERSE EFFECTS — Serious: Hypersensitivity. Frequent: Palpitations, tachycardia, hypokalemia, tremor, lightheadedness, nervousness, headache, pharyngitis, and nausea.

PULMONARY: Combinations

ADVAIR (fluticasone - inhaled + salmeterol, **Advair HFA**) ▶L ♀C ▶? $$$$$
WARNING — Long-acting beta-agonists may increase the risk of asthma-related death; use as an adjunct only if inadequate control with an optimal dose of inhaled corticosteroids. Avoid in significantly worsening or acute asthma. Do not use for rescue therapy. Do not stop abruptly.
ADULTS — <u>Chronic asthma:</u> DPI: 1 puff bid (all strengths). MDI: 2 puffs bid (all strengths). <u>COPD maintenance:</u> DPI: 1 puff bid (250/50 only).
PEDS — <u>Chronic asthma:</u> DPI: 1 puff bid (100/50 only) for age 4 to 11 yo. Use adult dose for 12 yo or older.
UNAPPROVED ADULTS — <u>COPD:</u> 500/50, 1 puff bid.
FORMS — Trade only: DPI: 100/50, 250/50, 500/50 mcg fluticasone/salmeterol per actuation; 60 doses/DPI. Trade only (Advair HFA): MDI 45/21, 115/21, 230/21 mcg fluticasone/salmeterol per actuation; 120 doses/canister.
NOTES — See individual components for additional information. Ritonavir and other CYP3A4 inhibitors such as ketoconazole significantly increase both salmeterol and fluticasone concentrations, resulting in prolongation of QT interval (salmeterol) and systemic effects, including adrenal suppression (fluticasone). Very rare anaphylactic reaction in

(cont.)

PREDICTED PEAK EXPIRATORY FLOW (liters/min) Am Rev Resp Dis 1963; 88:644

Age (yr)	Women (height in inches)					Men (height in inches)					Child (height in inches)	
	55"	60"	65"	70"	75"	60"	65"	70"	75"	80"		
20 yr	390	423	460	496	529	554	602	649	693	740	44"	160
30 yr	380	413	448	483	516	532	577	622	664	710	46"	187
40 yr	370	402	436	470	502	509	552	596	636	680	48"	214
50 yr	360	391	424	457	488	486	527	569	607	649	50"	240
60 yr	350	380	412	445	475	463	502	542	578	618	52"	267
70 yr	340	369	400	432	461	440	477	515	550	587	54"	293

INHALER COLORS (Body then cap—Generics may differ)

Advair:	purple	Asmanex:	white/pink	Maxair Autohaler:	white/white
Advair HFA:	purple/light purple	Atrovent HFA:	clear/green	ProAir HFA:	red/white
				Proventil HFA:	yellow/orange
Aerobid:	grey/purple	Azmacort:	white/white	Pulmicort:	white/brown
Aerobid-M:	grey/green	Combivent:	clear/orange	QVAR 40 mcg:	beige/grey
Aerospan:	purple/grey			QVAR 80 mcg:	mauve/grey
Alupent:	clear/blue	Flovent HFA:	orange/peach	Serevent	
Alvesco 80 mcg:	brown/red			Diskus:	green
		Foradil:	grey/beige	Spiriva:	grey
Alvesco 160 mcg:	red/red	Intal:	white/blue	Ventolin HFA:	light blue/navy
		Maxair:	white/white	Xopenex HFA:	blue/red

ADVAIR (cont.)
patients with severe milk protein allergy. Increased risk of pneumonia in COPD.
MOA — Anti-inflammatory/long-acting beta agonist bronchodilator combination.
ADVERSE EFFECTS — Serious: Hypersensitivity, anaphylaxis, paradoxical bronchospasm, Churg-Strauss syndrome. Frequent: Thrush, dysphonia, pharyngitis, palpitations, tachycardia, tremor, lightheadedness, nervousness, headache, nausea.

COMBIVENT (albuterol + ipratropium) ▶L ♀C ▶? $$$$
ADULTS — COPD: MDI: 2 puffs qid. Max dose 12 puffs/24 h.
PEDS — Not approved in children.
FORMS — Trade only: MDI: 90 mcg albuterol/18 mcg ipratropium per actuation, 200/canister.
NOTES — Contraindicated with soy or peanut allergy. Refer to components.
MOA — Short-acting beta agonist/anticholinergic bronchodilator combination.
ADVERSE EFFECTS — Serious: Paradoxical bronchospasm. Frequent: Palpitations, tachycardia, tremor, lightheadedness, nervousness, headache, and nausea.

DUONEB (albuterol + ipratropium, ✽Combivent inhalation soln) ▶L ♀C ▶? $$$$$
ADULTS — COPD: 1 unit dose nebulized qid; may add 2 doses/day prn to max of 6 doses/day.
PEDS — Not approved in children.
FORMS — Generic/Trade: Unit dose: 2.5 mg albuterol/0.5 mg ipratropium per 3 mL vial, premixed; 30, 60 vials/carton.
NOTES — Refer to components; 3.0 mg albuterol is equivalent to 2.5 mg albuterol base.
MOA — Short-acting beta agonist/anticholinergic bronchodilator combination.
ADVERSE EFFECTS — Serious: None. Frequent: Palpitations, tachycardia, tremor, lightheadedness, nervousness, headache, nausea, dry mouth, blurred vision.

DUOVENT UDV (ipratropium + fenoterol) ▶L ♀? ▶? $$$$$
ADULTS — Canada only. Bronchospasm associated with asthma/COPD: 1 vial (via nebulizer) q 6 h prn.
PEDS — Canada only. Children age 12 yo or older: 1 vial (via nebulizer) q 6 h prn.
FORMS — Canada trade only: Unit dose vial (for nebulization) 0.5 mg ipratropium, 1.25 mg fenoterol in 4 mL of saline.
MOA — Anticholinergic and short-acting beta agonist bronchodilator.
ADVERSE EFFECTS — Serious: Hypokalemia, bronchospasm. Frequent: Dry mouth or throat, tremor.

SYMBICORT (budesonide + formoterol) ▶L ♀C ▶? $$$$
WARNING — Long-acting beta-agonists may increase the risk of asthma-related death; use as an adjunct only if inadequate control with an

(cont.)

SYMBICORT (cont.)
optimal dose of inhaled corticosteroids. Avoid in significantly worsening or acute asthma. Do not use for rescue therapy. Do not stop abruptly.
ADULTS — Chronic asthma: 2 puffs bid (both strengths). COPD: 2 puffs bid (160/4.5).
PEDS — Chronic asthma age 12 yo or older: Use adult dose.
FORMS — Trade only: MDI: 80/4.5, 160/4.5 mcg budesonide/formoterol per actuation; 120 doses/canister.
NOTES — See individual components for additional information. Ritonavir and other CYP3A4 inhibitors such as ketoconazole significantly increase budesonide concentrations, resulting in systemic effects, including adrenal suppression.
MOA — Anti-inflammatory/long-acting beta agonist bronchodilator combination.
ADVERSE EFFECTS — Serious: Hypersensitivity, anaphylaxis, paradoxical bronchospasm, Churg-Strauss syndrome. Frequent: Thrush, dysphonia, pharyngitis, palpitations, tachycardia, tremor, lightheadedness, nervousness, headache, nausea.

PULMONARY: Inhaled Steroids

NOTE: See Endocrine-Corticosteroids when oral steroids necessary. Beware of adrenal suppression when changing from systemic to inhaled steroids. Inhaled steroids are not for treatment of acute asthma; higher doses may be needed for severe asthma and exacerbations. Adjust to lowest effective dose for maintenance. Use of a DPI, a spacing device, and rinsing the mouth with water after each use may decrease the incidence of thrush and dysphonia. Pharyngitis and cough may occur with all products. Use with caution in patients with active or quiescent TB, untreated systemic fungal, bacterial, viral or parasitic infections or in patients with ocular HSV. Inhaled steroids produce small, transient reductions in growth velocity in children. Prolonged use may lead to decreases in bone mineral density and osteoporosis, thereby increasing fracture risk.

BECLOMETHASONE—INHALED (*QVAR*) ▶L ♀C ▶? $$$
ADULTS — Chronic asthma: 40 mcg: 1 to 4 puffs bid. 80 mcg: 1 to 2 puffs bid.
PEDS — Chronic asthma in 5 to 11 yo: 40 mcg 1 to 2 puffs bid.
UNAPPROVED ADULTS — Chronic asthma: NHLBI dosing schedule (puffs/day divided bid): Low dose: 2 to 6 puffs of 40 mcg or 1 to 3 puffs of 80 mcg. Medium dose: 6 to 12 puffs of 40 mcg or 3 to 6 puffs of 80 mcg. High dose: More than 12 puffs of 40 mcg or more than 6 puffs 80 mcg.
UNAPPROVED PEDS — Chronic asthma (5–11 yo): NHLBI dosing schedule (puffs/day divided bid): Low dose: 2 to 4 puffs of 40 mcg or 1 to 2 puffs of 80 mcg. Medium dose: 4 to 8 puffs of 40 mcg or 2 to 4 puffs of 80 mcg. High dose: More than 8 puffs of 40 mcg or more than 4 puffs of 80 mcg.
FORMS — Trade only: HFA MDI: 40, 80 mcg/actuation, 7.3 g 100 actuations/canister.
MOA — Steroidal anti-inflammatory.
ADVERSE EFFECTS — Serious: Adrenal suppression (high dose), hypersensitivity, bronchospasm. Frequent: Thrush, dysphonia.

BUDESONIDE—INHALED (*Pulmicort Respules, Pulmicort Flexhaler*) ▶L ♀B ▶? $$$$
ADULTS — Chronic asthma: DPI: 1 to 2 puffs daily to bid up to 4 puffs bid.
PEDS — Chronic asthma 6 to 12 yo: DPI: 1 to 2 puffs daily to bid. 12 mo to 8 yo: Susp for inhalation (Respules): 0.5 mg to 1 mg daily or divided bid.
UNAPPROVED ADULTS — Chronic asthma: NHLBI dosing schedule (puffs/day daily or divided bid): DPI: Low dose is in the range of 1 to 3 puffs of 180 mcg or 2 to 6 puffs of 90 mcg. Medium dose is in the range of 3 to 7 puffs of 180 mcg or 6 to 13 puffs of 90 mcg. High dose more than 7 puffs of 180 mcg or more than 13 puffs of 90 mcg.
UNAPPROVED PEDS — Chronic asthma (5 to 11 yo): NHLBI dosing schedule (puffs/day daily or divided bid) DPI: Low dose: 1 to 2 puffs of 180 mcg or 2 to 4 puffs of 90 mcg. Medium dose: 2 to 4 puffs of 180 mcg or 4 to 9 puffs of 90 mcg. High dose more than 4 puffs of 180 mcg or more than 9 puffs of 90 mcg. Susp for inhalation (daily or divided bid): Low dose is in the range of 0.25 to 0.5 mg for age 4 yo or younger and about 0.5 mg for age 5 to 11 yo. Medium dose more than 0.5 to 1 mg for age 4 yo or younger and 1 mg for age 5 to 11 yo. High dose more than 1 mg for age 4 yo or younger and 2 mg for age 5 to 11 yo. Some doses may be outside the package labeling.
FORMS — Trade only: DPI (Flexhaler) 90, 180 mcg powder/actuation 60, 120 doses respectively/canister, Respules 1 mg/2 mL unit dose. Generic/Trade: Respules 0.25, 0.5 mg/2 mL unit dose.
NOTES — Respules should be delivered via a jet nebulizer with a mouthpiece or face mask. CYP3A4 inhibitors such as ketoconazole, erythromycin, ritonavir, etc may significantly increase systemic concentrations, possibly causing adrenal suppression. Flexhaler contains trace amounts of milk proteins; caution with severe milk protein hypersensitivity.
MOA — Steroidal anti-inflammatory.
ADVERSE EFFECTS — Serious: Adrenal suppression (high dose), hypersensitivity, bronchospasm. Frequent: Thrush, dysphonia, headache, nausea.

CICLESONIDE—INHALED (*Alvesco*) ▶L ♀C ▶? $$$$
ADULTS — Chronic asthma MDI: 80 mcg/puff: 1 to 4 puffs bid. 160 mcg/puff: 1 to 2 puffs bid.
PEDS — Chronic asthma, age 12 yo or older: Use adult dose.
FORMS — Trade only: 80 mcg/actuation, 60 per canister. 160 mcg/actuation, 60, 120 per canister.

(cont.)

INHALED STEROIDS: ESTIMATED COMPARATIVE DAILY DOSES*

ADULTS AND CHILDREN OLDER THAN 12 yo

Drug	Form	Low Dose	Medium Dose	High Dose
beclomethasone HFA MDI	40 mcg/puff 80 mcg/puff	2–6 puffs/day 1–3 puffs/day	6–12 puffs/day 3–6 puffs/day	>12 puffs/day >6 puffs/day
budesonide DPI	90 mcg/dose 180 mcg/dose	2–6 1–3	6–13 3–7	>13 >7
budesonide	soln for nebs	-	-	-
flunisolide MDI	250 mcg/puff	2–4 puffs/day	4–8 puffs/day	>8 puffs/day
flunisolide HFA MDI	80 mcg/puff	4	5–8	>8
fluticasone HFA MDI	44 mcg/puff 110 mcg/puff 220 mcg/puff	2–6 puffs/day 1–2 puffs/day 1 puff/day	6–10 puffs/day 2–4 puffs/day 1–2 puffs/day	>10 puffs/day >4 puffs/day >2 puffs/day
fluticasone DPI	50 mcg/dose 100 mcg/dose 250 mcg/dose	2–6 inhalations/day 1–3 inhalations/day 1 inhalation/day	6–10 inhalations/day 3–5 inhalations/day 2 inhalations/day	>10 inhalations/day >5 inhalations/day >2 inhalations/day
mometasone DPI	220 mcg/dose	1	2	>2
triamcinolone MDI	75 mcg/puff	4–10 puffs/day	10–20 puffs/day	>20 puffs/day

CHILDREN (age 5 to 11 yo)

Drug	Form	Low Dose	Medium Dose	High Dose
beclomethasone HFA MDI	40 mcg/puff 80 mcg/puff	2–4 puffs/day 1–2 puffs/day	4–8 puffs/day 2–4 puffs/day	>8 puffs/day >4 puffs/day
budesonide DPI	90 mcg/dose 180 mcg/dose	2–4 1–2	4–9 2–4	>9 >4
budesonide	soln for nebs	0.5 mg 0.25–0.5 mg (0–4 yo)	1 mg >0.5–1 mg (0–4 yo)	2 mg >1 mg (0–4 yo)
flunisolide MDI	250 mcg/puff	2–3 puffs/day	4–5 puffs/day	>5 puffs/day
flunisolide HFA MDI	80 mcg/puff	2	4	≥8
fluticasone HFA MDI (0–11 yo)	44 mcg/puff 110 mcg/puff 220 mcg/puff	2–4 puffs/day 1–2 puff/day n/a	4–8 puffs/day 2–3 puffs/day 1–2 puffs/day	>8 puffs/day >4 puffs/day >2 puffs/day
fluticasone DPI	50 mcg/dose 100 mcg/dose 250 mcg/dose	2–4 inhalations/day 1–2 inhalations/day n/a	4–8 inhalations/day 2–4 inhalations/day 1 inhalation/day	>8 inhalations/day >4 inhalations/day >1 inhalation/day
mometasone DPI	220 mcg/dose	n/a	n/a	n/a
triamcinolone MDI	75 mcg/puff	4–8 puffs/day	8–12 puffs/day	>12 puffs/day

*HFA = Hydrofluoroalkane (propellant). MDI = metered dose inhaler. DPI = dry powder inhaler. Reference: http://www.nhlbi.nih.gov/guidelines/asthma/asthsumm.pdf

CICLESONIDE—INHALED (cont.)

NOTES — CYP3A4 inhibitors such as ketoconazole may significantly increase systemic concentrations, possibly causing adrenal suppression.
MOA — Steroidal anti-inflammatory.
ADVERSE EFFECTS — Serious: Adrenal suppression (high dose), hypersensitivity, bronchospasm. Frequent: Thrush, dysphonia, headache, nausea.

FLUNISOLIDE—INHALED (AeroBid, AeroBid-M, Aerospan) ▶L ♀C ▶? $$$
ADULTS — Chronic asthma: MDI: 2 puffs bid up to 4 puffs bid.
PEDS — Chronic asthma, age: 6 to 15 yo: MDI: 2 puffs bid.
UNAPPROVED ADULTS — Chronic asthma: NHLBI dosing schedule (puffs/day divided bid): Low dose: 2 to 4 puffs. Medium dose: 4 to 8 puffs. High dose: More than 8 puffs.
UNAPPROVED PEDS — Chronic asthma (5–11 yo): NHLBI dosing schedule (puffs/day divided bid): Low dose: 2 to 3 puffs. Medium dose: 4 to 5 puffs. High dose: More than 5 puffs (8 puffs or more for 80 mcg HFA).
FORMS — Trade only: MDI: 250 mcg/actuation, 100 metered doses/canister. AeroBid-M (AeroBid + menthol flavor). Aerospan HFA MDI: 80 mcg/actuation, 60, 120 metered doses/canister.
MOA — Steroidal anti-inflammatory.
ADVERSE EFFECTS — Serious: Adrenal suppression (high dose), bronchospasm. Frequent: Thrush, dysphonia.

PULMONARY: Leukotriene Inhibitors

FLUTICASONE—INHALED (*Flovent HFA, Flovent Diskus*) ▶L ♀C ▶? $$$$
ADULTS – Chronic asthma: MDI: 2 puffs bid up to 4 puffs bid. Max dose 880 mcg bid.
PEDS – Chronic asthma: 2 puffs bid of 44 mcg/puff for age 4 to 11 yo, Use adult dose for age 12 yo or older.
UNAPPROVED ADULTS – Chronic asthma: NHLBI dosing schedule (puffs/day divided bid): Low dose: 2 to 6 puffs of 44 mcg MDI. Medium dose: 2 to 4 puffs of 110 mcg MDI or 2 puffs of 220 mcg MDI. High dose: More than 4 puffs 110 mcg MDI or more than 2 puffs 220 mcg MDI.
UNAPPROVED PEDS – Chronic asthma, age 11 yo or younger: NHLBI dosing schedule (puffs/day divided bid): Low dose: 2 to 4 puffs of 44 mcg MDI. Medium dose: 4 to 8 puffs of 44 mcg MDI. 2 to 3 puffs of 110 mcg MDI. 1 to 2 puffs of 220 mcg MDI. High dose: 4 puffs or more 110 mcg MDI. 2 puffs or more 2200 mcg MDI.
FORMS – Trade only: HFA MDI: 44, 110, 220 mcg/actuation 120/canister. DPI (Diskus): 50, 100, 250 mcg/actuation delivering 44, 88, 220 mcg respectively.
NOTES – Ritonavir and other CYP3A4 inhibitors such as ketoconazole significantly increase fluticasone concentrations, resulting in systemic effects, including adrenal suppression. Increased risk of pneumonia in COPD.
MOA – Steroidal anti-inflammatory.
ADVERSE EFFECTS – Serious: Adrenal suppression (high dose), anaphylaxis, Churg-Strauss syndrome, bronchospasm. Frequent: Thrush, dysphonia, pharyngitis, headache.

MOMETASONE—INHALED (*Asmanex Twisthaler*) ▶L ♀C ▶? $$$$
ADULTS – Chronic asthma: 1 to 2 puffs qpm or 1 puff bid. If prior oral corticosteroid therapy: 2 puffs bid.
PEDS – Chronic asthma: Age 12 yo or older: Use adult dose.
UNAPPROVED ADULTS – Chronic asthma: NHLBI dosing schedule (puffs/day divided bid): Low dose: 1 puff. Medium dose: 2 puffs. High dose: More than 2 puffs.
FORMS – Trade only: DPI: 110 mcg/actuation with #30 dosage units, 220 mcg/actuation with #30, 60, 120 dosage units.
NOTES – CYP3A4 inhibitors such as ketoconazole may significantly increase concentrations.
MOA – Steroidal anti-inflammatory.
ADVERSE EFFECTS – Serious: Adrenal suppression (high dose). Frequent: Thrush, dysphonia.

TRIAMCINOLONE—INHALED (*Azmacort*) ▶L ♀C ▶? $$$$
ADULTS – Chronic asthma: MDI: 2 puffs tid to qid or 4 puffs bid. Max dose 16 puffs/day. Severe asthma: 12 to 16 puffs/day and adjust downward.
PEDS – Chronic asthma children older than 12 yo: Use adult dose. 6 to 12 yo: 1 to 2 puffs tid to qid or 2 to 4 puffs bid. Max dose 12 puffs/day.
UNAPPROVED ADULTS – Chronic asthma for age 5 to 11 yo: NHLBI dosing schedule (puffs/day divided bid): Low dose: 4 to 10 puffs. Medium dose: 10 to 20 puffs. High dose: More than 20 puffs.
UNAPPROVED PEDS – Chronic asthma: NHLBI dosing schedule (puffs/day divided bid): Low dose: 4 to 8 puffs. Medium dose: 8 to 12 puffs. High dose: More than 12 puffs.
FORMS – Trade only: MDI: 75 mcg/actuation, 240/canister. Built-in spacer.
MOA – Steroidal anti-inflammatory.
ADVERSE EFFECTS – Serious: Adrenal suppression (high dose), anaphylaxis, angioedema. Frequent: Thrush, dysphonia.

PULMONARY: Leukotriene Inhibitors

NOTE: Not for treatment of acute asthma. Abrupt substitution for corticosteroids may precipitate Churg-Strauss syndrome. Postmarket cases of agitation, aggression, anxiousness, dream abnormalities and hallucinations, depression, insomnia, irritability, restlessness, suicidal thinking and behavior (including suicide), and tremor have been reported.

MONTELUKAST (*Singulair*) ▶L ♀B ▶? $$$$
ADULTS – Chronic asthma, allergic rhinitis: 10 mg PO daily. Prevention of exercise-induced bronchoconstriction: 10 mg PO 2 h before exercise.
PEDS – Chronic asthma, allergic rhinitis: Give 5 mg PO daily for age 6 to 14 yo, give 4 mg (chew tab or oral granules) PO daily for age 2 to 5 yo. Asthma age 12 to 23 mo: 4 mg (oral granules) PO daily. Allergic rhinitis age 6 to 23 mo: 4 mg (oral granules) PO daily. Prevention of exercise-induced bronchoconstriction: Age 15 yo or older: Use adult dose.
FORMS – Trade only: Tabs 10 mg. Oral granules 4 mg packet, 30/box. Chewable tabs (cherry flavored) 4, 5 mg.
NOTES – Chewable tabs contain phenylalanine. Oral granules may be placed directly into the mouth or mixed with a spoonful of breast milk, baby formula, applesauce, carrots, rice or ice cream. If mixed with food, must be taken within 15 min. Do not mix with other liquids. Levels decreased by phenobarbital and rifampin. Dyspepsia may occur. Do not take an additional dose for exercise-induced bronchospasm if already taking other liquids chronically.
MOA – Leukotriene receptor antagonist.
ADVERSE EFFECTS – Serious: Churg-Strauss syndrome, hepatitis, anaphylaxis, angioedema, erythema nodosum, suicidal thinking, pancreatitis. Frequent: Headache, dyspepsia.

ZAFIRLUKAST (*Accolate*) ▶L ♀B ▶– $$$$
WARNING – Hepatic failure has been reported.
ADULTS – Chronic asthma: 20 mg PO bid, 1 h before meals or 2 h after meals.

(cont.)

ZAFIRLUKAST (cont.)

PEDS – Chronic asthma age 5 to 11 yo: 10 mg PO bid, 1 h before meals or 2 h after meals. Use adult dose for age 12 yo or older.
UNAPPROVED ADULTS – Allergic rhinitis: 20 mg PO bid, 1 h before meals or 2 h after meals.
FORMS – Trade only: Tabs 10, 20 mg.
NOTES – Potentiates warfarin and theophylline. Levels decreased by erythromycin and increased by high-dose aspirin. Nausea may occur. If liver dysfunction is suspected, discontinue drug and manage accordingly. Consider monitoring LFTs.
MOA – Leukotriene receptor antagonist.
ADVERSE EFFECTS – Serious: Churg-Strauss syndrome, hypersensitivity, hepatotoxicity, anaphylaxis, angioedema. Frequent: Headache, dyspepsia.

ZILEUTON (*Zyflo CR*) ▶L ♀C ▶? $$$$$
WARNING – Contraindicated in active liver disease.
ADULTS – Chronic asthma: 1200 mg PO bid.
PEDS – Chronic asthma age 12 yo or older: Use adult dose.
FORMS – Trade only: Tabs extended-release 600 mg.
NOTES – Monitor LFTs for elevation. Potentiates warfarin, theophylline, and propranolol. Dyspepsia and nausea may occur.
MOA – Leukotriene formation inhibitor.
ADVERSE EFFECTS – Serious: Hepatotoxicity, leukopenia. Frequent: Headache, dyspepsia.

PULMONARY: Other Pulmonary Medications

ACETYLCYSTEINE—INHALED (*Mucomyst*) ▶L ♀B ▶? $
ADULTS – Mucolytic nebulization: 3 to 5 mL of the 20% soln or 6 to 10 mL of the 10% soln tid to qid. Instillation, direct or via tracheostomy: 1 to 2 mL of a 10% to 20% soln q 1 to 4 h; via percutaneous intratracheal catheter: 1 to 2 mL of the 20% soln or 2 to 4 mL of the 10% soln q 1 to 4 h.
PEDS – Mucolytic nebulization: Use adult dosing.
FORMS – Generic/Trade: Soln for inhalation 10, 20% in 4, 10, 30 mL vials.
NOTES – Increased volume of liquefied bronchial secretions may occur; maintain an open airway. Watch for bronchospasm in asthmatics. Stomatitis, N/V, fever, and rhinorrhea may occur. A slight disagreeable odor may occur and should soon disappear. A face mask may cause stickiness on the face after nebulization; wash with water. The 20% soln may be diluted with NaCl or sterile water.
MOA – Mucolytic.
ADVERSE EFFECTS – Serious: Bronchospasm (asthmatics), anaphylaxis. Frequent: Stomatitis, N/V, fever, and rhinorrhea.

ALPHA-1 PROTEINASE INHIBITOR (*alpha-1 antitrypsin, Aralast, Prolastin, Zemaira*) ▶Plasma ♀C ▶? $
WARNING – Possible transmission of viruses and Creutzfeldt-Jakob disease.
ADULTS – Congenital alpha-1 proteinase inhibitor deficiency with emphysema: 60 mg/kg IV once per week.
PEDS – Not approved in children.
NOTES – Contraindicated in selected IgA deficiencies with known antibody to IgA. Hepatitis B vaccine recommended in preparation for Prolastin use.
MOA – Alpha-1 proteinase inhibitor.
ADVERSE EFFECTS – Serious: Anaphylaxis, increased LFTs. Frequent: Headache, somnolence, flu-like symptoms.

AMINOPHYLLINE (❋*Phyllocontin*) ▶L ♀C ▶? $
ADULTS – Acute asthma: Loading dose if currently not receiving theophylline: 6 mg/kg IV over 20 to 30 min. Maintenance IV infusion: Dose 0.5 to 0.7 mg/kg/h, mix 1 g in 250 mL D5W (4 mg/mL) set at rate 11 mL/h delivers 0.7 mg/kg/h for wt 70 kg patient. In patients with cor pulmonale, heart failure, liver failure, use 0.25 mg/kg/h. If currently on theophylline, each 0.6 mg/kg aminophylline will increase the serum theophylline concentration by approximately 1 mcg/mL. Maintenance: 200 mg PO bid to qid.
PEDS – Acute asthma: Loading dose if currently not receiving theophylline: 6 mg/kg IV over 20 to 30 min. Maintenance oral route age older than 1 yo: 3 to 4 mg/kg/dose PO q 6 h. Maintenance IV route for age older than 6 mo: 0.8 to 1 mg/kg/hr IV infusion.
UNAPPROVED PEDS – Neonatal apnea of prematurity: Loading dose 5 to 6 mg/kg IV/PO, maintenance: 1 to 2 mg/kg/dose q 6 to 8 h IV/PO.
FORMS – Generic only: Tabs 100, 200 mg. Oral liquid 105 mg/5 mL. Canada Trade only: Tabs controlled-release (12 h) 225, 350 mg, scored.
NOTES – Aminophylline is 79% theophylline. Administer IV infusion no faster than 25 mg/min. Multiple drug interactions (especially ketoconazole, rifampin, carbamazepine, isoniazid, phenytoin, macrolides, zafirlukast and cimetidine). Review meds before initiating treatment. Irritability, nausea, palpitations and tachycardia may occur. Overdose may be life-threatening.
MOA – Bronchodilator.
ADVERSE EFFECTS – Serious: Arrhythmias, seizures. Frequent: Irritability, nausea, palpitations, tachycardia.

BERACTANT (*Survanta*) ▶Lung ♀? ▶? $$$$$
PEDS – RDS (hyaline membrane disease) in premature infants: Specialized dosing.
MOA – Lung surfactant.
ADVERSE EFFECTS – Serious: Bradycardia, nosocomial sepsis. Frequent: Bradycardia, oxygen desaturation.

CALFACTANT (*Infasurf*) ▶Lung ♀? ▶? $$$$$
PEDS – RDS (hyaline membrane disease) in premature infants: Specialized dosing.
FORMS – Trade only: Oral susp: 35 mg/mL in 3, 6 mL vials. Preservative-free.
MOA – Lung surfactant.

(cont.)

PULMONARY: Other Pulmonary Medications

CALFACTANT *(cont.)*
ADVERSE EFFECTS — Serious: Bradycardia, cyanosis. Frequent: Cyanosis, bradycardia, airway obstruction.

CROMOLYN—INHALED *(Intal, Gastrocrom, ✦Nalcrom)*
▶LK ♀B ▶? $$$
ADULTS — <u>Chronic asthma:</u> MDI: 2 to 4 puffs qid. Soln for inhalation: 20 mg qid. <u>Prevention of exercise-induced bronchospasm:</u> MDI: 2 puffs 10 to 15 min prior to exercise. Soln for nebulization: 20 mg 10 to 15 min prior. <u>Mastocytosis:</u> 200 mg PO qid, 30 min before meals and at bedtime.
PEDS — <u>Chronic asthma</u> for age older than 5 yo using MDI: 2 puffs qid; for age older than 2 yo using soln for nebulization 20 mg qid. <u>Prevention of exercise-induced bronchospasm</u> for age older than 5 yo using MDI: 2 puffs 10 to 15 min prior to exercise, using soln for nebulization for age older than 2 yo: 20 mg 10 to 15 min prior. <u>Mastocytosis:</u> Age 2 to 12 yo: 100 mg PO qid 30 min before meals and at bedtime.
FORMS — Trade only: MDI 800 mcg/actuation, 112, 200/canister. Oral concentrate 100 mg/5 mL in 8 amps/foil pouch (Gastrocrom). Generic/Trade: Soln for nebs: 20 mg/2 mL.
NOTES — Not for treatment of acute asthma. Pharyngitis may occur. Directions for oral concentrate: 1) Break open and squeeze liquid contents of ampule(s) into a glass of water. 2) Stir soln. 3) Drink all of the liquid.
MOA — Mast cell stabilizer.
ADVERSE EFFECTS — Serious: Paradoxical bronchospasm, anaphylaxis. Frequent: Cough, pharyngitis.

DORNASE ALFA *(Pulmozyme)* ▶L ♀B ▶? $$$$$
ADULTS — <u>Cystic fibrosis:</u> 2.5 mg nebulized daily to bid.
PEDS — <u>Cystic fibrosis</u> age 6 yo or older: 2.5 mg nebulized daily to bid.
UNAPPROVED PEDS — Has been used in a small number of children as young as 3 mo with similar efficacy and side effects.
FORMS — Trade only: Soln for inhalation: 1 mg/mL in 2.5 mL vials.
NOTES — Voice alteration, pharyngitis, laryngitis, and rash may occur. Do not dilute or mix with other drugs.
MOA — Mucolytic.
ADVERSE EFFECTS — Serious: None. Frequent: Voice alteration, pharyngitis, laryngitis, and rash.

DOXAPRAM *(Dopram)* ▶L ♀B ▶? $$$
ADULTS — <u>Acute hypercapnia due to COPD:</u> 1 to 2 mg/min IV, max 3 mg/min. Maximum infusion time: 2 h.
PEDS — Not approved in children.
UNAPPROVED PEDS — <u>Apnea of prematurity unresponsive to methylxanthines:</u> Load 2.5 to 3 mg/kg over 15 min, then 1 mg/kg/h titrated to lowest effective dose. Max: 2.5 mg/kg/h. Contains benzyl alcohol; caution in neonates.
NOTES — Monitor arterial blood gases at baseline and q 30 min during infusion. Do not use with mechanical ventilation. Contraindicated with seizure disorder, severe HTN, CVA, head injury, CAD and severe heart failure.
MOA — Respiratory stimulant.
ADVERSE EFFECTS — Serious: None. Frequent: Hypertension, N/V, diarrhea, cough, dyspnea, tachypnea, tachycardia, arrhythmias, seizure, fever, and sweating.

EPINEPHRINE RACEMIC *(S-2, ✦Vaponefrin)*
▶Plasma ♀C ▶– $
ADULTS — See cardiovascular section.
PEDS — <u>Severe croup:</u> Soln for inhalation: 0.05 mL/kg/dose diluted to 3 mL with NS over 15 min prn not to exceed q 1 to 2 h dosing. Max dose 0.5 mL.
FORMS — Trade only: Soln for inhalation: 2.25% epinephrine in 15, 30 mL.
NOTES — Cardiac arrhythmias and HTN may occur.
MOA — Bronchodilator.
ADVERSE EFFECTS — Serious: Arrhythmias, cerebral hemorrhage, hypertension. Frequent: Palpitations, tachycardia, tremor, lightheadedness, nervousness, headache, and nausea.

IPRATROPIUM—INHALED *(Atrovent, Atrovent HFA)*
▶Lung ♀B ▶? $$$$
ADULTS — <u>COPD:</u> MDI (Atrovent, Atrovent HFA): 2 puffs qid; may use additional inhalations not to exceed 12 puffs/day. Soln for inhalation: 500 mcg nebulized tid to qid.
PEDS — Not approved in children younger than 12 yo.
UNAPPROVED PEDS — <u>Acute asthma:</u> MDI (Atrovent, Atrovent HFA): 1 to 2 puffs tid to qid for age 12 yo or younger. Soln for inhalation: Give 250 mcg/dose tid to qid for age 12 yo or younger: Give 250 to 500 mcg/dose tid to qid for age older than 12 yo. <u>Acute asthma:</u> Age 2 to 18 yo: 500 mcg nebulized with second and third doses of albuterol.
FORMS — Trade only: Atrovent HFA MDI: 17 mcg/actuation, 200/canister. Generic/Trade: Soln for nebulization: 0.02% (500 mcg/vial) in unit dose vials.
NOTES — Atrovent MDI is contraindicated with soy or peanut allergy; HFA not contraindicated. Caution with glaucoma, myasthenia gravis, BPH, or bladder neck obstruction. Cough, dry mouth, and blurred vision may occur.
MOA — Short-acting anticholinergic bronchodilator.
ADVERSE EFFECTS — Serious: Anaphylaxis, angioedema. Frequent: Dry mouth, blurred vision.

KETOTIFEN *(✦Zaditen)* ▶L ♀C ▶– $$
ADULTS — Not approved.
PEDS — Canada only. <u>Chronic asthma:</u> 6 mo to 3 yo: 0.05 mg/kg PO bid. Children older than 3 yo: 1 mg PO bid.
FORMS — Generic/Trade: Tabs 1 mg. Syrup 1 mg/5 mL.
NOTES — Several weeks may be necessary before therapeutic effect. Full clinical effectiveness is generally reached after 10 weeks.
MOA — Non-bronchodilator antihistamine.
ADVERSE EFFECTS — Serious: Seizures, thrombocytopenia. Frequent: Drowsiness, weight gain.

METHACHOLINE (*Provocholine*) ▶Plasma ♀C ▶? $$
WARNING — Life-threatening bronchoconstriction can result; have resuscitation capability available.
ADULTS — <u>Diagnosis of bronchial airway hyperreactivity in nonwheezing patients with suspected asthma:</u> 5 breaths each of ascending serial concentrations, 0.025 mg/mL to 25 mg/mL, via nebulization. The procedure ends when there is more than 20% reduction in the FEV1 compared with baseline.
PEDS — <u>Diagnosis of bronchial airway hyperreactivity:</u> Use adult dose.
NOTES — Avoid with epilepsy, bradycardia, peptic ulcer disease, thyroid disease, urinary tract obstruction, or other conditions that could be adversely affected by a cholinergic agent. Hold beta-blockers. Do not inhale powder.
MOA — Bronchoconstrictor.
ADVERSE EFFECTS — Serious: Respiratory/cardiac arrest, syncope. Frequent: Wheezing.

NEDOCROMIL—INHALED (*Tilade*) ▶L ♀B ▶? $$$
ADULTS — <u>Chronic asthma:</u> MDI: 2 puffs qid. Reduce dose to bid to tid as tolerated.
PEDS — <u>Chronic asthma age older than 6 yo:</u> MDI: 2 puffs qid.
FORMS — Trade only: MDI: 1.75 mg/actuation, 112/canister.
NOTES — Product to be discontinued when supplies run out. Not for treatment of acute asthma. Unpleasant taste and dysphonia may occur.
MOA — Mast cell stabilizer.
ADVERSE EFFECTS — Serious: None. Frequent: Cough, pharyngitis, bad taste.

NITRIC OXIDE (*INOmax*) ▶Lung, K ♀C ▶? $$$$
PEDS — <u>Respiratory failure with pulmonary HTN</u> in infants older than 34 weeks old: Specialized dosing.
NOTES — Risk of methemoglobinemia increases with concomitant nitroprusside or nitroglycerin.
MOA — Vasodilator.
ADVERSE EFFECTS — Serious: Methemoglobinemia. Frequent: Methemoglobinemia.

OMALIZUMAB (*Xolair*) ▶Plasma, L ♀B ▶? $$$$$
WARNING — Anaphylaxis may occur within 2 h of administration; monitor closely and be prepared to treat.
ADULTS — <u>Moderate to severe asthma with perennial allergy when symptoms not controlled by inhaled steroids:</u> 150 to 375 mg SC q 2 to 4 weeks, based on pretreatment serum total IgE level and body wt.
PEDS — <u>Moderate to severe asthma with perennial allergy:</u> Age 12 yo or older: Use adult dose.
NOTES — Not for treatment of acute asthma. Divide doses greater than 150 mg over more than 1 injection site. Monitor for signs of anaphylaxis including bronchospasm, hypotension, syncope, urticaria, angioedema.
MOA — Monoclonal antibody that inhibits IgE binding to mast cells and basophils.
ADVERSE EFFECTS — Serious: Anaphylaxis, malignancy. Frequent: Injection site reactions.

PORACTANT (*Curosurf*) ▶Lung ♀? ▶? $$$$$
PEDS — <u>RDS (hyaline membrane disease) in premature infants:</u> Specialized dosing.
MOA — Lung surfactant.
ADVERSE EFFECTS — Serious: Bradycardia, hypotension. Frequent: Bradycardia, hypotension, oxygen desaturation.

THEOPHYLLINE (*Elixophyllin, Uniphyl, Theo-24, T-Phyl, ✦Theo-Dur, Theolair*) ▶L ♀C ▶+ $
ADULTS — <u>Chronic asthma.</u> 5 to 13 mg/kg/day PO in divided doses. Max dose 900 mg/day.
PEDS — <u>Chronic asthma.</u> Initial: Age older than 1 yo and wt less than 45 kg: 12 to 14 mg/kg/day PO divided q 4 to 6 h to max of 300 mg/24 h. Maintenance: 16 to 20 mg/kg/day PO divided q 4 to 6 h to max of 600 mg/24 h. for age older than 1 yo and wt 45 kg or more: Initial: 300 mg/24 h PO divided q 6 to 8 h. Maintenance: 400 to 600 mg/24 h PO divided q 6 to 8 h. Infants age 6 to 52 weeks: [(0.2 × age in weeks) + 5] × kg = 24 h dose in mg PO divided q 6 to 8 h.
UNAPPROVED ADULTS — <u>COPD:</u> 10 mg/kg/day PO in divided doses.
UNAPPROVED PEDS — <u>Apnea and bradycardia of prematurity:</u> 3 to 6 mg/kg/day PO divided q 6 to 8 h. Maintain serum concentrations 3 to 5 mcg/mL.
FORMS — Generic/Trade: Elixir 80 mg/15 mL. Trade only: Caps: Theo-24: 100, 200, 300, 400 mg. T-Phyl: 12 Hr SR tabs 200 mg. Theolair: Tabs 125, 250 mg. Generic only: 12 Hr tabs 100, 200, 300, 450 mg, 12 Hr caps 125, 200, 300 mg.
NOTES — Multiple drug interactions (especially ketoconazole, rifampin, carbamazepine, isoniazid, phenytoin, macrolides, zafirlukast, and cimetidine). Review meds before initiating treatment. Overdose may be life-threatening.
MOA — Bronchodilator.
ADVERSE EFFECTS — Serious: Arrhythmias, seizures. Frequent: Irritability, nausea, palpitations, tachycardia.

TIOTROPIUM (*Spiriva*) ▶K ♀C ▶– $$$$
WARNING — QT prolongation has been reported.
ADULTS — <u>COPD:</u> Handihaler: 18 mcg inhaled daily.
PEDS — Not approved in children.
FORMS — Trade only: Caps for oral inhalation 18 mcg. To be used with "Handihaler" device only. Packages of 5, 30, 90 caps with Handihaler device.
NOTES — Not for acute bronchospasm. Administer at the same time each day. Use with caution in narrow-angle glaucoma, myasthenia gravis, BPH, or bladder-neck obstruction. Avoid touching opened cap. Glaucoma, eye pain, or blurred vision may occur if powder enters eyes. May increase dosing interval in patients with CrCl < 50 mL/min. Avoid if severe lactose allergy.
MOA — Long-acting anticholinergic bronchodilator.
ADVERSE EFFECTS — Serious: Anaphylaxis, angioedema, paradoxical bronchospasm, QT prolongation. Frequent: Dry mouth, cough.

TOXICOLOGY: Toxicology

ACETYLCYSTEINE (N-acetylcysteine, Mucomyst, Acetadote, ✦Parvolex) ▶L ♀B ▶? $$$$
ADULTS – <u>Acetaminophen toxicity:</u> Mucomyst: Loading dose 140 mg/kg PO or NG, then 70 mg/kg q 4 h for 17 doses. May be mixed in water or soft drink diluted to a 5% soln. Acetadote (IV): Loading dose 150 mg/kg in 200 mL of D5W infused over 60 min; maintenance dose 50 mg/kg in 500 mL of D5W infused over 4 h followed by 100 mg/kg in 1000 mL of D5W infused over 16 h.
PEDS – <u>Acetaminophen toxicity:</u> Same as adult dosing.
UNAPPROVED ADULTS – <u>Prevention of contrast-induced nephropathy:</u> 600 to 1200 mg PO bid for 2 doses before procedure and 2 doses after procedure.
FORMS – Generic/Trade: Soln 10%, 20%. Trade only: IV (Acetadote).
NOTES – May be diluted with water or soft drink to a 5% soln; use diluted soln within 1 h. Repeat loading dose if vomited within 1 h. Critical ingestion-treatment interval for maximal protection against severe hepatic injury is between 0 to 8 h. Efficacy diminishes after 8 h and treatment initiation between 15 and 24 h post ingestion yields limited efficacy. However, treatment should not be withheld, since the reported time of ingestion may not be correct. Anaphylactoid reactions usually occurs 30 to 60 min after initiating infusion. Stop infusion, administer antihistamine or epinephrine, restart infusion slowly. If anaphylactoid reactions return or severity increases, then stop treatment.
MOA – Directly combines with the toxic acetaminophen metabolite as a glutathione substitute. Antioxidant believed to attenuate ischemic renal failure.
ADVERSE EFFECTS – Serious: Hypersensitivity, anaphylaxis, angioedema, bronchoconstriction, chest tightness. Frequent: Nausea, vomiting, disagreeable odor, generalized urticaria, rash, stomatitis, fever, rhinorrhea, drowsiness, clamminess, pruritus, tachycardia, hypertension, hypotension.

CHARCOAL (activated charcoal, Actidose-Aqua, CharcoAid, EZ-Char, ✦Charcodate) ▶Not absorbed ♀+ ▶+ $
ADULTS – <u>Gut decontamination:</u> 25 to 100 g (1 to 2 g/kg or 10× the amount of poison ingested) PO or NG as soon as possible. May repeat q 1 to 4 h prn at doses equivalent to 12.5 g/h. When sorbitol is coadministered, use only with the first dose if repeated doses are to be given.
PEDS – <u>Gut decontamination:</u> 1 g/kg for age younger than 1 yo; 15 to 30 g or 1 to 2 g/kg for age 1 to 12 yo PO or NG as soon as possible. Repeat doses in children have not been established, but half the initial dose is recommended. Repeat q 2 to 6 h prn. When sorbitol is coadministered, use only with the first dose if repeated doses are to be given.
FORMS – OTC/Generic/Trade: Powder 15, 30, 40, 120, 240 g. Soln 12.5 g/60 mL, 15 g/75 mL, 15 g/120 mL, 25 g/120 mL, 30 g/120 mL, 50 g/240 mL. Susp 15 g/120 mL, 25 g/120 mL, 30 g/150 mL, 50 g/240 mL. Granules 15 g/120 mL.
NOTES – Some products may contain sorbitol to improve taste and reduce GI transit time. Chocolate milk/powder may enhance palatability for pediatric use. Not usually effective for toxic alcohols (methanol, ethylene glycol, isopropanol), heavy metals (lead, iron, bromide), arsenic, lithium, potassium, hydrocarbons, and caustic ingestions (acids, alkalis). Mix powder with 8 oz water. Greatest effect when administered < 1 h of ingestion.
MOA – Adsorbs substances therefore inhibiting GI absorption.
ADVERSE EFFECTS – Serious: Bronchiolitis obliterans, aspiration. Frequent: Vomiting, constipation, diarrhea, black stools, hypokalemia, hypernatremia.

DEFEROXAMINE (Desferal) ▶K ♀C ▶? $$$$$
ADULTS – <u>Chronic iron overload:</u> 500 to 1000 mg IM daily and 2 g IV infusion (no faster than 15 mg/kg/h) with each unit of blood or 1 to 2 g SC daily (20 to 40 mg/kg/day) over 8 to 24 h via continuous infusion pump. <u>Acute iron toxicity:</u> IV infusion up to 15 mg/kg/h (consult poison center).
PEDS – <u>Acute iron toxicity:</u> IV infusion up to 15 mg/kg/h (consult poison center).
NOTES – Contraindicated in renal failure/anuria unless undergoing dialysis.
MOA – Chelates iron in serum, ferritin, and hemosiderin.
ADVERSE EFFECTS – Serious: Cataracts, neurotoxicity-related hearing loss, hypersensitivity, hypotension, ARDS. Frequent: Visual changes (decreased acuity; impaired peripheral, night, and color vision), red urine, generalized erythema, dysuria, abdominal pain, leg cramps, tachycardia, fever, skin rash.

DIMERCAPROL (BAL in oil) ▶KL ♀C ▶? $$$$$
ADULTS – <u>Specialized dosing for arsenic, mercury, gold, and lead toxicity. Consult poison center. Mild arsenic or gold toxicity:</u> 2.5 mg/kg IM qid for 2 days, then bid for 1 day, then daily for 10 days. <u>Severe arsenic or gold toxicity:</u> 3 mg/kg IM q 4 h for 2 days, then qid for 1 day, then bid for 10 days. <u>Mercury toxicity:</u> 5 mg/kg IM initially, then 2.5 mg/kg daily to bid for 10 days. Begin therapy within 1 to 2 h of toxicity. <u>Acute lead encephalopathy:</u> 4 mg/kg IM initially, then q 4 h in combination (separate syringe) with calcium edetate for 2 to 7 days. May reduce dose to 3 mg/kg IM for less severe toxicity. Deep IM injection needed.
PEDS – Not approved in children.
UNAPPROVED PEDS – Same as adult dosing. Consult poison center.
MOA – Chelates arsenic, gold, and mercury to promote fecal and urinary excretion of the complex.
ADVERSE EFFECTS – Serious: Hemolytic anemia, HTN, tachycardia, hypersensitivity. Frequent: N/V, headache, perioral burning sensation, feeling of constriction or pain (in throat, chest or hands),

(cont.)

DIMERCAPROL (cont.)
conjunctivitis, blepharospasm, rhinorrhea, salivation, burning penis sensation, sweating, abdominal pain, injection-site irritation, painful sterile abscess, anxiety, weakness.

DUODOTE (atropine + pralidoxime) ▶K ♀C ▶? $
ADULTS — <u>Organophosphate insecticide/nerve agent poisoning, mild symptoms:</u> 1 injection in thigh. Severe symptoms: 3 injections in rapid succession (may administer through clothes).
PEDS — Not approved in children.
FORMS — Each auto-injector dose delivers atropine 2.1 mg + pralidoxime 600 mg.
MOA — Atropine is to reverse muscarinic toxicity. Pralidoxime reactives acetylcholinesterase deactivated by organophosphate nerve agents or insecticide.
ADVERSE EFFECTS — Serious: Hyperthermia, anticholinergic syndrome, myocardial ischemia. Frequent: Anticholinergic syndrome, hypertension, diplopia, dizziness.

EDETATE (EDTA, Endrate, versenate) ▶K ♀C ▶— $$$
WARNING — Beware of elevated intracranial pressure in lead encephalopathy.
ADULTS — Consult poison center. Use calcium disodium form only for lead indications. Noncalcium form (eg, Endrate) is not interchangeable and is rarely used anymore. <u>Lead toxicity:</u> 1000 mg/m2/day IM (divided into equal doses q 8 to 12 h) or IV (infuse total dose over 8 to 12 h) for 5 days. Interrupt therapy for 2 to 4 days, then repeat same regimen. Two courses of therapy are usually necessary. <u>Acute lead encephalopathy:</u> Edetate alone or in combination with dimercaprol. <u>Lead nephropathy:</u> 500 mg/m2/dose q 24 h for 5 doses (if creatinine 2 to 3 mg/dL), q 48 h for 3 doses (if creatinine 3 to 4 mg/dL), or once per week (if creatinine > 4 mg/dL). May repeat at 1 month intervals.
PEDS — Specialized dosing for lead toxicity; same as adult dosing also using calcium form. Consult poison center.
FORMS — Calcium disodium formulation used for lead poisoning, other form without calcium (eg, Endrate) is not interchangeable and rarely used anymore.
MOA — Chelates heavy metals to form complexes that undergo urinary excretion.
ADVERSE EFFECTS — Serious: Arrhythmia, renal toxicity (proteinuria, hematuria, acute tubular necrosis), hypersensitivity, transient bone marrow suppression. Frequent: Hypotension, tremor, headache, numbness, tingling, cheilosis, vomiting, anorexia, thirst, glycosuria, pain at injection site, hypercalcemia, zinc deficiency, nasal congestion, rash, increased serum transaminases, fever, chills, fatigue, malaise, myalgia, arthralgia.

ETHANOL (alcohol) ▶L ♀D ▶+ $
PEDS — Not approved in children.
UNAPPROVED ADULTS — Consult poison center. Specialized dosing for <u>methanol, ethylene glycol toxicity if fomepizole is unavailable or delayed:</u> 1000 mg/kg (10 mL/kg) of 10% ethanol (100 mg/mL) IV over 1 to 2 h then 100 mg/kg/h (1 mL/kg/h) to keep ethanol level approximately 100 mg/dL.
MOA — Prevents formation of toxic methanol metabolite formic acid by saturating alcohol dehydrogenase.
ADVERSE EFFECTS — Serious: Multiple reports with chronic use. Frequent: Acute intoxication, dehydration, numerous others with chronic use.

FLUMAZENIL (Romazicon) ▶LK ♀C ▶? $$$$
WARNING — Do not use in chronic benzodiazepine use or acute overdose with TCAs due to seizure risk.
ADULTS — <u>Benzodiazepine sedation reversal:</u> 0.2 mg IV over 15 sec, then 0.2 mg q 1 min prn up to 1 mg total dose. Usual dose is 0.6 to 1 mg. <u>Benzodiazepine overdose reversal:</u> 0.2 mg IV over 30 sec, then 0.3 to 0.5 mg q 30 sec prn up to 3 mg total dose.
PEDS — <u>Benzodiazepine sedation reversal:</u> 0.01 mg/kg up to 0.2 mg IV over 15 sec; repeat q min to max 4 additional doses.
UNAPPROVED PEDS — <u>Benzodiazepine overdose reversal:</u> 0.01 mg/kg IV. <u>Benzodiazepine sedation reversal:</u> 0.01 mg/kg IV initially (max 0.2 mg), then 0.005 to 0.01 mg/kg (max 0.2 mg) q 1 min to max total dose 1 mg. May repeat doses in 20 min, max 3 mg in 1 h.
NOTES — Onset of action 1 to 3 min, peak effect 6 to 10 min. For IV use only, preferably through an IV infusion line into a large vein. Local irritation may occur following extravasation.
MOA — Benzodiazepine receptor antagonist.
ADVERSE EFFECTS — Serious: Seizures, arrhythmia, chest pain. Frequent: Injection-site irritation, sweating, hot flashes, flushing, hypotension, hypertension, bradycardia, tachycardia, dizziness, agitation, dry mouth, tremor, insomnia, dyspnea, hyperventilation, emotional lability, confusion, dysphonia, glossitis, N/V, hiccups, visual changes, paresthesia, abnormal hearing, rigors, shivering.

FOMEPIZOLE (Antizol) ▶L ♀C ▶? $$$$$
ADULTS — Consult poison center. <u>Ethylene glycol or methanol toxicity:</u> 15 mg/kg IV (load), then 10 mg/kg IV q 12 h for 4 doses, then 15 mg/kg IV q 12 h until ethylene glycol or methanol level is below 20 mg/dL. Administer doses as slow IV infusions over 30 min. Increase frequency to q 4 h during hemodialysis.
PEDS — Not approved in children.
MOA — Inhibits alcohol dehydrogenase.
ADVERSE EFFECTS — Serious: Hypersensitivity, seizure, shock, hypotension, disseminated intravascular coagulation, multiorgan system failure. Frequent: Injection-site irritation, rash, eosinophilia, tachycardia, sinus bradycardia/tachycardia, phlebitis, phlebosclerosis, lightheadedness, nystagmus, agitation, flushing, anxiety, feeling of decreased environmental awareness, abdominal pain, diarrhea, dyspepsia, anorexia, heartburn, increases serum transaminases, anemia, pharyngitis, lymphangitis, hiccups, speech/visual disturbance, abnormal smell, blurred vision, N/V.

ANTIDOTES

Toxin	Antidote/Treatment	Toxin	Antidote/Treatment
acetaminophen	N-acetylcysteine	digoxin	**dig immune Fab**
TCAs	sodium bicarbonate	ethylene glycol	**fomepizole**
		heparin	protamine
arsenic, mercury	dimercaprol (BAL)	iron	deferoxamine
benzodiazepine	flumazenil	lead	BAL, EDTA, succimer
beta blockers	glucagon	methanol	fomepizole
calcium channel blockers	calcium chloride, glucagon	methemoglobin	methylene blue
		opioids/opiates	naloxone
cyanide	cyanide antidote kit, Cyanokit (hydroxocobalamin)	organophosphates	atropine+pralidoxime
		warfarin	**vitamin K, FFP**

HYDROXOCOBALAMIN (*Cyanokit*) ▶K ♀C ▶? $$$$$
ADULTS — Cyanide poisoning: 5 g IV over 15 min; may repeat prn.
PEDS — Not approved in children.
MOA — Binds cyanide.
ADVERSE EFFECTS — Serious: Anaphylaxis, allergy, hypertension. Frequent: None.

IPECAC SYRUP ▶Gut ♀C ▶? $
ADULTS — Emesis: 15 to 30 mL PO, then 3 to 4 glasses of water.
PEDS — AAP no longer recommends home ipecac for poisoning. Emesis, age younger than 1 yo: 5 to 10 mL, then ½–1 glass of water (controversial in children < 1 yo). Emesis, age 1 to 12 yo: 15 mL, then 1 to 2 glasses of water. May repeat dose (15 mL) if vomiting does not occur within 20 to 30 min.
FORMS — OTC Generic only: Syrup 30 mL.
NOTES — Many believe ipecac to be contraindicated in infants age younger than 6 mo. Do not use if any potential for altered mental status (eg, seizure, neurotoxicity), strychnine, beta-blocker, calcium channel blocker, clonidine, digitalis glycoside, corrosive, petroleum distillate ingestions, or if at risk for GI bleeding (coagulopathy).
MOA — Locally irritates the GI mucosa and stimulates the chemoreceptor trigger zone in the central medullary to produce vomiting.
ADVERSE EFFECTS — Serious: Cardiomyopathy (after prolonged use). Frequent: Diarrhea, coughing, choking, drowsiness, dyspepsia.

METHYLENE BLUE (*Urolene blue*) ▶K ♀C ▶? $
ADULTS — Methemoglobinemia: 1 to 2 mg/kg IV over 5 min. Dysuria: 65 to 130 mg PO tid after meals with liberal water.
PEDS — Not approved in children.
UNAPPROVED PEDS — Methemoglobinemia: 1 to 2 mg/kg/dose IV over 5 min; may repeat in 1 h prn.
FORMS — Trade only: Tabs 65 mg.
NOTES — Avoid in G6PD deficiency. May turn urine, stool, skin, contact lenses, and undergarments blue-green.
MOA — Converts methemoglobin to hemoglobin by reducing the ferric iron form of oxidized hemoglobin to ferrous form. Converts methemoglobin (Fe3+) to hemoglobin (Fe2+) by enhancing the activity of NADPH-methemoglobin reductase. Also genitourinary antiseptic and germicidal agent.
ADVERSE EFFECTS — Serious: Hypersensitivity, hemolytic anemia, cyanosis, cardiovascular abnormalities. Frequent: Photosensitivity, N/V, diarrhea, fever, bladder irritation, blue-green urine and/or stool.

PENICILLAMINE (*Cuprimine, Depen*) ▶K ♀D ▶– $$$$$
WARNING — Fatal drug-related adverse events have occurred, caution if penicillin allergy.
ADULTS — Consult poison center: Specialized dosing for copper toxicity. 750 mg to 1.5 g/day PO for 3 months based on 24 h urinary copper excretion, max 2 g/day. May start 250 mg/day PO in patients unable to tolerate.
PEDS — Specialized dosing for copper toxicity. Consult poison center.
FORMS — Trade only: Caps 125, 250 mg; Tabs 250 mg.
NOTES — Patients may require supplemental pyridoxine 25 to 50 mg/day PO. Promotes excretion of heavy metals in urine.
MOA — Chelates excess copper.
ADVERSE EFFECTS — Serious: Proteinuria, hematuria, aplastic anemia, hepatotoxicity, pancreatitis, agranulocytosis, production of insulin antibodies, thrombocytopenia, sideroblastic anemia, leukopenia, autoimmune syndromes (Goodpasture's syndrome, myasthenia gravis, pemphigus vulgaris, drug-induced lupus), hypoglycemia, hypersensitivity. Frequent: Increased serum transaminases, oral ulcers, metallic taste, rash, fever, tinnitus, neuropathy, muscle weakness, anorexia, epigastric pain.

PHYSOSTIGMINE (*Antilirium*) ▶LK ♀D ▶? $
WARNING — Discontinue if excessive salivation, emesis, frequent urination, or diarrhea. Rapid administration can cause bradycardia, hypersalivation, respiratory difficulties and seizures. Atropine should be available as an antagonist.
ADULTS — Life-threatening anticholinergic toxicity: 2 mg IV/IM, administer IV no faster than 1 mg/min. May repeat q 10 to 30 min for severe toxicity.
PEDS — Life-threatening anticholinergic toxicity: 0.02 mg/kg IM/IV injection, administer IV no faster

(cont.)

PHYSOSTIGMINE (cont.)
than, 0.5 mg/min. May repeat q 15 to 30 min until a therapeutic effect or max 2 mg dose.
UNAPPROVED ADULTS — Postanesthesia reversal of neuromuscular blockade: 0.5 to 1 mg IV/IM, administer IV no faster than 1 mg/min. May repeat q 10 to 30 min prn.
FORMS — Generic/Trade: 1 mg/mL in 2 mL ampules.
MOA — Reversible anticholinesterase agent, acts as substrate for acetylcholinesterase.
ADVERSE EFFECTS — Serious: cardiac arrest, bradycardia, hypersalivation leading to respiratory problems or convulsions. Frequent: salivation, N/V, miosis, sweating, lacrimation, bronchospasm, abdominal pain

PRALIDOXIME (*Protopam, 2-PAM*) ▶K ♀C ▶? $$$$
ADULTS — Consult poison center: Specialized dosing for organophosphate toxicity: 1 to 2 g IV infusion over 15 to 30 min or slow IV injection over 5 min or longer (max rate 200 mg/min). May repeat dose after 1 h if muscle weakness persists.
PEDS — Not approved in children.
UNAPPROVED ADULTS — Consult poison center: 20 to 40 mg/kg/dose IV infusion over 15 to 30 min.
UNAPPROVED PEDS — Consult poison center. 25 mg/kg load then 10 to 20 mg/kg/h or 25 to 50 mg/kg load followed by repeat dose in 1 to 2 h then q 10 to 12 h.
NOTES — Administer within 36 h of exposure when possible. Rapid administration may worsen cholinergic symptoms. Give in conjunction with atropine. IM or SC may be used if IV access is not available.

MOA — Reactivates cholinesterase (primarily peripherally).
ADVERSE EFFECTS — Serious: Myasthenia gravis exacerbation. Frequent: Pain at injection site, transient increase in serum transaminases, increased CK, dizziness, visual changes (blurred, diplopia, decreased accommodation), headache, drowsiness, nausea, tachycardia, increased blood pressure, hyperventilation, muscular weakness.

SUCCIMER (*Chemet*) ▶K ♀C ▶? $$$$$
PEDS — Lead toxicity 1 yo or older: Start 10 mg/kg PO or 350 mg/m2 q 8 h for 5 days, then reduce the frequency to q 12 h for 2 weeks. Not approved in children younger than 1 yo.
FORMS — Trade only: Caps 100 mg.
NOTES — Manufacturer recommends doses of 100 mg (wt 8 to 15 kg), 200 mg (wt 16 to 23 kg), 300 mg (wt 24 to 34 kg), 400 mg (wt 35 to 44 kg), and 500 mg (wt 45 kg or greater). Can open cap and sprinkle medicated beads over food, or give them in a spoon and follow with fruit drink. Indicated for blood lead levels greater than 45 mcg/dL. Allow at least 4 weeks between edetate disodium and succimer treatment.
MOA — Chelates lead to increase urinary excretion.
ADVERSE EFFECTS — Serious: Hypersensitivity, arrhythmia. Frequent: Rash, increased serum transaminases (transient), N/V, anorexia, hemorrhoids, loose stools, metallic taste, body pain, abdominal cramps, fever, flu-like syndrome, drowsiness, dizziness, paresthesia, sensorimotor neuropathy, headache, moniliasis.

UROLOGY: Benign Prostatic Hyperplasia

ALFUZOSIN (*UroXatral, ✦Xatral*) ▶KL ♀B ▶– $$$
WARNING — Postural hypotension with or without symptoms may develop within a few hours after administration. Avoid in moderate or severe hepatic insufficiency. Avoid coadministration with potent CYP3A4 inhibitors.
ADULTS — BPH: 10 mg PO daily after a meal.
PEDS — Not approved in children.
UNAPPROVED ADULTS — Promotes spontaneous passage of ureteral calculi: 10 mg PO daily usually combined with an NSAID, antiemetic and opioid of choice.
FORMS — Trade only: Tab extended-release 10 mg.
NOTES — Caution in congenital or acquired QT prolongation, and severe renal insufficiency. Intraoperative floppy iris syndrome has been observed during cataract surgery.
MOA — Selective alpha-1 receptor antagonist that increases urinary flow rate.
ADVERSE EFFECTS — Serious: Postural hypotension, chest pain, priapism, angioedema. Frequent: Dizziness, headache.

DUTASTERIDE (*Avodart*) ▶L ♀X ▶– $$$$
ADULTS — BPH: 0.5 mg PO daily with/without tamsulosin 0.4 mg PO daily.
PEDS — Not approved in children.
FORMS — Trade only: Caps 0.5 mg.
NOTES — 6 months therapy may be needed to assess effectiveness. Pregnant or potentially pregnant women should not handle caps due to fetal risk from absorption. Caution in hepatic insufficiency. Dutasteride will decrease PSA by 50%; new baseline PSA should be established after 3 to 6 months to assess potentially cancer-related PSA changes. Cap should be swallowed whole and not chewed or opened to avoid oropharyngeal irritation.
MOA — 5-alpha reductase inhibitor that decreases conversion of testosterone into dihydrotestosterone.
ADVERSE EFFECTS — Serious: Angioedema. Frequent: Impotence, decreased libido, ejaculatory dysfunction.

FINASTERIDE (*Proscar, Propecia*) ▶L ♀X ▶– $$$
ADULTS — Proscar: 5 mg PO daily alone or in combination with doxazosin to reduce the risk of symptomatic progression of BPH. Propecia: Androgenetic alopecia in men: 1 mg PO daily.
PEDS — Not approved in children.
UNAPPROVED ADULTS — Cancer prevention in "at risk" men older than 55 yo: 5 mg daily. Androgenetic alopecia in postmenopausal women (no evidence of efficacy): 1 mg PO daily.

(cont.)

UROLOGY: Bladder Agents

FINASTERIDE *(cont.)*
FORMS — Generic/Trade: Tabs 1 mg (Propecia), 5 mg (Proscar).
NOTES — Therapy for 6 to 12 months may be needed to assess effectiveness for BPH and at least 3 months for alopecia. Pregnant or potentially pregnant women should not handle crushed tabs because of possible absorption and fetal risk. Use with caution in hepatic insufficiency. Monitor PSA before therapy; finasteride will decrease PSA by 50% in patients with BPH, even with prostate cancer. Does not appear to alter detection of prostate cancer.
MOA — 5-alpha reductase inhibitor that decreases conversion of testosterone into dihydrotestosterone.
ADVERSE EFFECTS — Serious: Hypersensitivity, swelling of lips and face, breast cancer (long-term treatment). Frequent: Impotence, decreased libido, decreased ejaculatory volume, testicular pain, rash, pruritus.

TAMSULOSIN (*Flomax*) ▶LK ♀B ▶— $$$$
ADULTS — BPH: 0.4 mg PO daily 30 min after the same meal each days. If an adequate response is not seen after 2 to 4 weeks, may increase dose to 0.8 mg PO daily. If therapy is interrupted for several days, restart at the 0.4 mg dose.
PEDS — Not approved in children.
UNAPPROVED ADULTS — Promotes spontaneous passage of ureteral calculi: 0.4 mg PO daily usually combined with an NSAID, antiemetic and opioid of choice.
FORMS — Generic/Trade: Caps 0.4 mg.
NOTES — Dizziness, headache, abnormal ejaculation. Alpha-blockers are generally considered to be first-line treatment in men with more than minimal obstructive urinary symptoms. Caution in serious sulfa allergy: Rare allergic reactions reported. Intraoperative floppy iris syndrome with cataract surgery reported. Caution with strong inhibitors of CYP450 2D6 (fluoxetine) or 3A4 (ketoconazole).
MOA — Selective alpha-1 receptor antagonist that increases urinary flow rate.
ADVERSE EFFECTS — Serious: Arrhythmia, orthostatic hypotension, chest pain. Frequent: Dizziness, headache, fatigue, somnolence, edema, dyspnea, asthenia, diarrhea, dyspepsia, dry mouth, nausea, palpitations, blurred vision, abnormal ejaculation.

UROLOGY: Bladder Agents—Anticholinergics and Combinations

B&O SUPPRETTES (belladonna + opium) ▶L ♀C ▶? ©II $$$$
ADULTS — Bladder spasm: 1 suppository PR once daily or bid, max 4 doses/day.
PEDS — Not approved in children younger than 12 yo.
FORMS — Trade only: Supps 30 mg opium (15A), 60 mg opium (16A).
NOTES — Store at room temperature. Contraindicated in narrow-angle glaucoma, obstructive conditions (eg, pyloric, duodenal or other intestinal obstructive lesions, ileus, achalasia, and obstructive uropathies).
MOA — Belladonna: Inhibits the muscarinic action of acetylcholine to decrease motility in the urinary tract. Opium: Opioid agonist analgesic.
ADVERSE EFFECTS — Serious: Hypersensitivity, respiratory coma, bradycardia, hallucinations. Frequent: Dizziness, drowsiness, sedation, N/V, lightheadedness, euphoria, constipation, dry mouth, blurred vision, urinary retention, decreased sweating.

DARIFENACIN (*Enablex*) ▶LK ♀C ▶— $$$$
ADULTS — Overactive bladder with symptoms of urinary urgency, frequency and urge incontinence 7.5 mg PO daily. May increase to max dose 15 mg PO daily in 2 weeks. Max dose 7.5 mg PO daily with moderate liver impairment or when coadministered with potent CYP3A4 inhibitors (ketoconazole, itraconazole, ritonavir, nelfinavir, clarithromycin and nefazodone).
PEDS — Not approved in children.
FORMS — Trade only: Tabs extended-release 7.5, 15 mg.
NOTES — Contraindicated with uncontrolled narrow-angle glaucoma, urinary and gastric retention. Avoid use in severe hepatic impairment. May increase concentration of medications metabolized by CYP2D6.
MOA — Muscarinic receptor antagonist, inhibiting detrusor muscle contractions.
ADVERSE EFFECTS — Serious: Hypersensitivity, angioedema, hallucinations. Frequent: Dry mouth, constipation, blurred vision, dyspepsia.

FESOTERODINE (*Toviaz*) ▶plasma ♀C ▶— $$$$
ADULTS — Overactive bladder: 4 mg PO daily. Increase to 8 mg if needed. Do not exceed 4 mg daily with renal insufficiency (CrCl < 30 mL/min) or specific coadministered drugs (see Notes).
PEDS — Not approved in children.
FORMS — Trade only: Tabs extended-release 4, 8 mg.
NOTES — Contraindicated with urinary or gastric retention, or uncontrolled glaucoma. 4 mg daily max dose in renal dysfunction or with concomitant use of CYP3A4 inhibitors (eg, erythromycin, ketoconazole, itraconazole).
MOA — Muscarinic receptor antagonist to decrease bladder spasm.
ADVERSE EFFECTS — Serious: QT prolongation. Frequent: Dry mouth, constipation, headache, vertigo/dizziness, abdominal pain.

FLAVOXATE (*Urispas*) ▶K ♀B ▶ $$$$
ADULTS — Bladder spasm: 100 or 200 mg PO tid–qid. Reduce dose when improved.
PEDS — Not approved in children younger than 12 yo.
FORMS — Generic/Trade: Tabs 100 mg.
NOTES — May cause dizziness, drowsiness, blurred vision, dry mouth, N/V, urinary retention. Contraindicated in glaucoma, obstructive conditions (eg, pyloric, duodenal or other intestinal obstructive lesions, ileus, achalasia, GI hemorrhage, and obstructive uropathies).

(cont.)

UROLOGY: Bladder Agents

FLAVOXATE (cont.)
MOA – Anticholinergic that directly counteracts urinary smooth muscle contraction.
ADVERSE EFFECTS – Serious: Increased ocular pressure, eosinophilia, leukopenia. Frequent: N/V, dry mouth, nervousness, vertigo, headache, drowsiness, mental confusion, fever, blurred vision, rash, dysuria, tachycardia, disturbed eye accommodation.

OXYBUTYNIN (*Ditropan, Ditropan XL, Gelnique, Oxytrol, ✦Oxybutyn, Uromax*) ▶LK ♀B ▶? $
ADULTS – Bladder instability: 2.5 to 5 mg PO bid to tid, max 5 mg PO qid. Extended-release tabs: 5 to 10 mg PO daily same time each day, increase 5 mg/day q week to 30 mg/day. Oxytrol: 1 patch twice per week on abdomen, hips or buttocks. Gelnique: Apply contents of 1 sachet once daily to abdomen, upper arms/shoulders, or thighs. Rotate application sites.
PEDS – Bladder instability older than 5 yo: 5 mg PO bid, max dose: 5 mg PO tid. Extended-release, older than 6 yo: 5 mg PO daily, max 20 mg/day. Transdermal patch not approved in children.
UNAPPROVED ADULTS – Case reports of use for hyperhidrosis.
UNAPPROVED PEDS – Bladder instability for age less than 6 yo : 0.2 mg/kg/dose PO bid to qid.
FORMS – Generic/Trade: Tabs 5 mg. Syrup 5 mg/5 mL. Tabs extended-release 5, 10, 15 mg. Trade only: Transdermal patch (Oxytrol) 3.9 mg/day. Gelnique 10% gel, 1 g unit dose.
NOTES – May cause dizziness, drowsiness, blurred vision, dry mouth, urinary retention. Contraindicated with glaucoma, urinary retention, obstructive GU or GI disease, unstable cardiovascular status, and myasthenia gravis. Transdermal patch causes less dry mouth than oral form; avoid dose reduction by cutting. Wash hands immediately after applying Gelnique.
MOA – Anticholinergic that exerts direct antispasmodic effects and inhibits muscarinic effects on smooth muscle.
ADVERSE EFFECTS – Serious: Heat stroke, hallucinations, QT prolongation. Frequent: Somnolence, headache, dizziness, agitation, confusion, dry mouth, constipation, diarrhea, nausea, dyspepsia, blurred vision, dry eyes, asthenia, pain, rhinitis, urinary tract infection, application site reaction.

PROSED/DS (methenamine + phenyl salicylate + methylene blue + benzoic acid + hyoscyamine) ▶KL ♀C ▶? $$
ADULTS – Bladder spasm: 1 tab PO qid with liberal fluids.
PEDS – Not approved in children.
FORMS – Trade only: Tabs (methenamine 81.6 mg/phenyl salicylate 36.2 mg/methylene blue 10.8 mg/benzoic acid 9.0 mg/hyoscyamine sulfate 0.12 mg).
NOTES – May cause dizziness, drowsiness, blurred vision, dry mouth, N/V, urinary retention. May turn urine/contact lenses blue.

MOA – Combination product that decreases bladder spasm and has mild antiseptic and analgesic activity.
ADVERSE EFFECTS – Serious: Respiratory depression. Frequent: Blue urine, rash, dry mouth, flushing, urinary retention, tachycardia, dizziness, blurred vision.

SOLIFENACIN (*VESIcare*) ▶LK ♀C ▶– $$$$
ADULTS – Overactive bladder with symptoms of urinary urgency, frequency or urge incontinence: 5 mg PO daily. Max dose: 10 mg PO daily (5 mg PO daily if CrCl < 30 mL/min, moderate hepatic impairment, or concurrent ketoconazole or other potent CYP3A4 inhibitors).
PEDS – Not approved in children.
FORMS – Trade only: Tabs 5, 10 mg.
NOTES – Contraindicated with uncontrolled narrow-angle glaucoma, urinary and gastric retention. Avoid use in severe hepatic impairment. Hallucinations have been reported.
MOA – Muscarinic receptor antagonist, inhibiting detrusor muscle contractions.
ADVERSE EFFECTS – Serious: Fecal impaction, intestinal obstruction, angioedema, hallucinations, QT prolongation, torsade de pointes. Frequent: Dry mouth, constipation, blurred vision.

TOLTERODINE (*Detrol, Detrol LA, ✦Unidet*) ▶L ♀C ▶– $$$$
ADULTS – Overactive bladder: 2 mg PO bid (Detrol) or 4 mg PO daily (Detrol LA). Decrease dose to 1 mg PO bid (Detrol) or 2 mg PO daily (Detrol LA) if adverse symptoms, hepatic insufficiency, or specific coadministered drugs (see notes).
PEDS – Not approved in children.
FORMS – Trade only: Tabs 1, 2 mg. Caps extended-release 2, 4 mg.
NOTES – Contraindicated with urinary or gastric retention, or uncontrolled glaucoma. High doses may prolong the QT interval. Decrease dose to 1 mg PO bid or 2 mg PO daily (Detrol LA) in severe hepatic or renal dysfunction or with concomitant use of CYP3A4 inhibitors (eg, erythromycin, ketoconazole, itraconazole).
MOA – Muscarinic receptor antagonist to decrease bladder spasm.
ADVERSE EFFECTS – Serious: Angioedema, QT prolongation. Frequent: Dry mouth, constipation, headache, vertigo/dizziness, abdominal pain.

TROSPIUM (*Sanctura, Sanctura XR, ✦Trosec*) ▶LK ♀C ▶? $$$$
ADULTS – Overactive bladder with urge incontinence: 20 mg PO bid; give 20 mg at bedtime if CrCl < 30 mL/min. If age 75 yo or older may taper down to 20 mg daily. Extended-release: 60 mg PO qam, 1 h before food; this form not recommended with CrCl < 30 mL/min.
PEDS – Not approved in children.
FORMS – Trade only: Tabs 20 mg, Caps extended-release 60 mg.
NOTES – Contraindicated with uncontrolled narrow-angle glaucoma, urinary retention, gastroparesis.

(cont.)

TROSPIUM *(cont.)*
May cause heat stroke due to decreased sweating. Take on an empty stomach. Improvement in signs and symptoms may be seen in a week. Causes minimum CNS side effects.
MOA — Acetylcholine antagonist that reduces bladder smooth muscle tone and spasms.
ADVERSE EFFECTS — Serious: Supraventricular tachycardia, Stevens-Johnson syndrome, anaphylaxis, hypertensive crisis, rhabdomyolysis, hallucinations, delirium, heat stroke. Frequent: Dry mouth, constipation, headache, dizziness, blurred vision.

URISED (methenamine + phenyl salicylate + atropine + hyoscyamine + benzoic acid + methylene blue) ▶K ♀C ▶? $
ADULTS — <u>Dysuria:</u> 2 Tabs PO qid.
PEDS — <u>Dysuria,</u> age 6 yo or older: Reduce dose based on age and wt. Not recommended for children younger than 6 yo.
FORMS — Trade only: Tabs (methenamine 40.8 mg/phenyl salicylate 18.1 mg/atropine 0.03 mg/hyoscyamine 0.03 mg/4.5 mg benzoic acid/5.4 mg methylene blue).
NOTES — Take with food to minimize GI upset. May precipitate urate crystals in urine. Avoid use with sulfonamides. May turn urine/contact lenses blue.
MOA — Combination product that decreases bladder spasm and has mild antiseptic and analgesic activity.
ADVERSE EFFECTS — Serious: Respiratory depression. Frequent: Blue urine, rash, dry mouth, flushing, urinary retention, tachycardia, dizziness, blurred vision.

UTA (methenamine + sodium phosphate + phenyl salicylate + methylene blue + hyoscyamine) ▶KL ♀C ▶? $
ADULTS — <u>Treatment of irritative voiding/relief of inflammation, hypermotility and pain with lower UTI/relief of urinary tract symptoms caused by diagnostic procedures:</u> 1 cap PO qid with liberal fluids.
PEDS — Not recommended age less than 6 yo. Dosing must be individualized by physician for age greater than 6 yo.
FORMS — Trade only: Caps (methenamine 120 mg/sodium phosphate 40.8 mg/phenyl salicylate 36 mg/methylene blue 10 mg/hyoscyamine 0.12 mg).
NOTES — May turn urine/feces blue to blue-green. Take 2 h apart from ketoconazole. May decrease absorption of thiazide diuretics. Antacids and antidiarrheals may decrease effectiveness of methenamine.
MOA — Combination product that decreases bladder spasms and has mild antiseptic and analgesic activity.
ADVERSE EFFECTS — Serious: respiratory depression. Frequent: blue to blue-green urine/feces, tachycardia, blurred vision, dizziness, urinary retention, dry mouth, N/V.

UTIRA-C (methenamine + sodium phosphate + phenyl salicylate + methylene blue + hyoscyamine) ▶KL ♀C ▶? $$
ADULTS — <u>Treatment of irritative voiding/relief of inflammation, hypermotility and pain with lower UTI/relief of urinary tract symptoms caused by diagnostic procedures:</u> 1 cap PO qid with liberal fluids.
PEDS — Not recommended age less than 6 yo. Dosing must be individualized by physician for age greater than 6 yo.
FORMS — Trade only: Tabs (methenamine 81.6 mg/sodium phosphate 40.8 mg/phenyl salicylate 36.2 mg/methylene blue 10.8 mg/hyoscyamine 0.12 mg).
NOTES — May turn urine/feces blue to blue-green. Take 2 h apart from ketoconazole. May decrease absorption of thiazide diuretics. Antacids and antidiarrheals may decrease effectiveness of methenamine.
MOA — Combination product that decreases bladder spasms and has mild antiseptic and analgesic activity.
ADVERSE EFFECTS — Serious: Respiratory depression. Frequent: Blue to blue-green urine/feces, tachycardia, blurred vision, dizziness, urinary retention, dry mouth, N/V.

UROLOGY: Bladder Agents—Other

BETHANECHOL (*Urecholine, Duvoid, ♣Myotonachol*) ▶L ♀C ▶? $$$$
ADULTS — <u>Urinary retention:</u> 10 to 50 mg PO tid to qid or 2.5 to 5 mg SC tid to qid. Take 1 h before or 2 h after meals to avoid N/V. Determine the minimum effective dose by giving 5 to 10 mg PO initially and repeat at hourly intervals until response or to a maximum of 50 mg.
PEDS — Not approved in children.
UNAPPROVED PEDS — <u>Urinary retention/abdominal distention:</u> 0.6 mg/kg/day PO divided q 6 to 8 h or 0.12 to 0.2 mg/kg/day SC divided q 6 to 8 h.
FORMS — Generic/Trade: Tabs 5, 10, 25, 50 mg.
NOTES — May cause drowsiness, lightheadedness, and fainting. Not for obstructive urinary retention. Avoid with cardiac disease, hyperthyroidism, parkinsonism, peptic ulcer disease, and epilepsy.
MOA — Cholinergic agent that stimulates the parasympathetic nervous system to increase the strength of detrusor muscle contraction.
ADVERSE EFFECTS — Serious: Hypersensitivity, hypotension with tachycardia, bronchoconstriction. Frequent: Flushing, sense of warmth, sweating, abdominal pain, nausea, belching, diarrhea, salivation, borborygmi, lacrimation, myosis, urinary urgency, headache, malaise.

DIMETHYL SULFOXIDE (*DMSO, Rimso-50*) ▶KL ♀C ▶? $$$
ADULTS — <u>Interstitial cystitis:</u> Instill 50 mL soln into bladder by catheter and allow to remain for 15 min;

(cont.)

DIMETHYL SULFOXIDE (cont.)
expelled by spontaneous voiding. Repeat q 2 weeks until symptomatic relief is obtained; thereafter, may increase time intervals between treatments.
PEDS — Not approved in children.
NOTES — Apply analgesic lubricant gel to urethra prior to inserting the catheter to avoid spasm. May administer oral analgesics or supps containing belladonna and opium prior to instillation to reduce spasms. May give anesthesia in patients with severe interstitial cystitis and very sensitive bladders during the first, second and third treatment. May cause lens opacities and changes in refractive index; perform eye exams before and periodically during treatment. May cause a hypersensitivity reaction by liberating histamine. Monitor liver and renal function tests and CBC q 6 months. May be harmful in patients with urinary tract malignancy; can cause DMSO-induced vasodilation. Peripheral neuropathy may occur when used with sulindac. Garlic-like taste may occur within a few min of administration; odor on breath and skin may be present and remain for up to 72 h.
MOA — Has broad pharmacological properties: anti-inflammatory, antifungal activity cryoprotective effects for living cells and tissues, dissolution of collagen, nerve blockade, diuresis, cholinesterase inhibition, vasodilation, and muscle relaxation.
ADVERSE EFFECTS — Serious: Hypersensitivity, transient chemical cystitis. Frequent: Sedation, N/V, headache, dizziness, garlic-like breath, burning on urination, diarrhea, transient disturbance of color perception, photophobia, burning or aching eyes, weight loss/gain, flu syndrome, discomfort during administration.

PENTOSAN (*Elmiron*) ▶LK ♀B ▶? $$$$$
ADULTS — Interstitial cystitis: 100 mg PO tid 1 h before or 2 h after a meal.
PEDS — Not approved in children.
FORMS — Trade only: Caps 100 mg.
NOTES — Pain relief usually occurs at 2 to 4 months and decreased urinary frequency takes 6 months. May increase risk of bleeding, especially with NSAID use. Use with caution in hepatic or splenic dysfunction.
MOA — Heparin-like molecule that adheres to bladder wall mucosa and exerts anticoagulant and fibrinolytic effects and prevents irritation by buffering cell permeability.
ADVERSE EFFECTS — Serious: Thrombocytopenia, bleeding. Frequent: Alopecia, headache, rash, nausea, abdominal pain.

PHENAZOPYRIDINE (*Pyridium, Azo-Standard, Urogesic, Prodium, Pyridiate, Urodol, Baridium, UTI Relief, ✦Phenazo*) ▶K ♀B ▶? $
ADULTS — Dysuria: 200 mg PO tid after meals for 2 days.
PEDS — Dysuria in children 6 to 12 yo: 12 mg/kg/day PO divided tid for 2 days.
FORMS — OTC Generic/Trade: Tabs 95, 97.2 mg. Rx Generic/Trade: Tabs 100, 200 mg.
NOTES — May turn urine/contact lenses orange. Contraindicated with hepatitis or renal insufficiency.
MOA — Produces a topical analgesic effect on the urinary mucosa.
ADVERSE EFFECTS — Serious: Hypersensitivity, hemolytic anemia, methemoglobinemia, nephrotoxicity, hepatotoxicity. Frequent: Headache, rash, pruritus, dyspepsia, contact lens staining, urine discoloration, yellowish tinge on sclera or skin.

UROQUID-ACID NO. 2 (methenamine + sodium phosphate) ▶K ♀C ▶? $
ADULTS — Chronic/recurrent UTIs: Initial: 2 tabs PO qid with full glass of water. Maintenance: 2 to 4 tabs PO daily, in divided doses with full glass of water.
PEDS — Not approved in children.
FORMS — Trade only: Tabs methenamine mandelate 500 mg/sodium acid phosphate 500 mg.
NOTES — 83 mg sodium/tab. Thiazide diuretics, carbonic anhydrase inhibitors, antacids and urinary alkalinizing agents may decrease effectiveness. Caution with concurrent salicylates, may increase levels.
MOA — Antibacterial/urinary acidifier.
ADVERSE EFFECTS — Serious: Hematuria. Frequent: N/D/V, rash, headache, dizziness.

UROLOGY: Erectile Dysfunction

ALPROSTADIL (*Muse, Caverject, Caverject Impulse, Edex, Prostin VR Pediatric, prostaglandin E1, ✦Prostin VR*) ▶L ♀– ▶– $$$$
ADULTS — Erectile dysfunction: 1.25 to 2.5 mcg intracavernosal injection over 5 to 10 sec initially using a ½ in, 27 or 30 gauge needle. If no response, may give next higher dose after 1 h, max 2 doses/day. May increase by 2.5 mcg and then 5 to 10 mcg incrementally on separate occasions. Dose range is 1 to 40 mcg. Alternative: 125 to 250 mcg intraurethral pellet (Muse). Increase or decrease dose on separate occasions until erection achieved. Maximum intraurethral dose 2 pellets/24 h. The lowest possible dose to produce an acceptable erection should be used.
PEDS — Temporary maintenance of patent ductus arteriosus in neonates: Start 0.1 mcg/kg/min IV infusion. Reduce dose to minimal amount that maintains therapeutic response. Max dose 0.4 mcg/kg/min.
UNAPPROVED ADULTS — Erectile dysfunction intracorporeal injection: Specially formulated mixtures of alprostadil, papaverine and phentolamine. 0.10 to 0.50 mL injection.
FORMS — Trade only: Syringe system (Edex) 10, 20, 40 mcg. (Caverject) 5, 10, 20, 40 mcg. (Caverject

(cont.)

UROLOGY: Erectile Dysfunction

ALPROSTADIL (cont.)
Impulse) 10, 20 mcg. Pellet (Muse) 125, 250, 500, 1000 mcg. Intracorporeal injection of locally compounded combination agents (many variations): "Bi-mix" can be 30 mg/mL papaverine + 0.5 to 1 mg/mL phentolamine, or 30 mg/mL papaverine + 20 mcg/mL alprostadil in 10 mL vials. "Tri-mix" can be 30 mg/mL papaverine + 1 mg/mL phentolamine + 10 mcg/mL alprostadil in 5, 10, or 20 mL vials.
NOTES — Contraindicated in patients at risk for priapism, with penile fibrosis (Peyronie's disease), with penile implants, in women or children, in men for whom sexual activity is inadvisable, and for intercourse with a pregnant woman. Onset of effect is 5 to 20 min.
MOA — Relaxes trabecular smooth muscles and dilates cavernosal arteries to produce erection. Relaxes smooth muscle of the ductus arteriosus.
ADVERSE EFFECTS — Serious: Priapism, hypotension. Frequent: Penile and testicular pain, urethral discomfort (pain, burning, bleeding/spotting).

SILDENAFIL (Viagra, Revatio) ▶LK ♀B ▶- $$$$
ADULTS — Erectile dysfunction: 50 mg PO approximately 1 h (range 0.5–4 h) before sexual activity. Usual effective dose range: 25 to 100 mg. Maximum 1 dose/day. Use lower dose (25 mg) if older than 65 yo, hepatic/renal impairment, or certain coadministered drugs (see notes). Pulmonary HTN: 20 mg PO tid.
PEDS — Not approved in children.
UNAPPROVED ADULTS — Antidepressant-associated sexual dysfunction: Same dosing as above.
FORMS — Trade only (Viagra): Tabs 25, 50, 100 mg. Unscored tab but can be cut in half. Trade only (Revatio): Tabs 20 mg.
NOTES — Drug interactions with cimetidine, erythromycin, ketoconazole, itraconazole, saquinavir, ritonavir and other CYP3A4 inhibitors; use 25 mg dose. Do not exceed 25 mg/48 h with ritonavir. Doses > 25 mg should not be taken less than 4 h after an alpha-blocker. Caution if CVA, MI or other cardiovascular event within last 6 months. Do not use with itraconazole, ketoconazole, ritonavir or pulmonary veno-occlusive disease. Coadministration with CYP3A4 inducers (ie, bosentan; barbiturates, carbamazepine, phenytoin, efavirenz, nevirapine, rifampin, rifabutin) may change levels of either medication; adjust doses as needed. Use caution with CVA, MI or life-threatening arrhythmia in last 6 months; unstable angina; BP > 170/110; or retinitis pigmentosa. Contraindicated in patients taking nitrates within prior/subsequent 24 h. Caution with alpha blockers due to potential for symptomatic hypotension. There have been a few reports of sudden vision loss due to nonarteritic ischemic optic neuropathy (NAION). Patients with prior NAION are at higher risk. Sudden hearing loss, with or without tinnitus, vertigo or dizziness, has been reported. Transient global amnesia has also been reported.
MOA — Selectively inhibits phosphodiesterase-5 resulting in enhanced relaxation of penile arteries & corpus cavernosal smooth muscle; enhances erectile function by increasing penile blood flow. Relaxes pulmonary vascular smooth muscle cells resulting in vasodilation of the pulmonary vascular bed.
ADVERSE EFFECTS — Serious: MI, CVA, hypotension, syncope, cerebral thrombosis, retinal hemorrhage, vision loss (nonarteritic ischemic optic neuropathy). Frequent: Headache, flushing, dyspepsia, abnormal vision.

TADALAFIL (Cialis) ▶L ♀B ▶- $$$$
WARNING — Contraindicated with nitrates. Caution with alpha-blockers due to potential for symptomatic hypotension. There have been a few reports of sudden vision loss due to nonarteritic ischemic optic neuropathy (NAION). Patients with prior NAION are at higher risk. Retinal artery occlusion has been reported. Sudden hearing loss, with or without tinnitus, vertigo or dizziness, has been reported. Transient global amnesia.
ADULTS — Erectile dysfunction: 2.5 to 5 mg PO daily without regard to timing of sexual activity. As needed dosing: 10 mg PO prn prior to sexual activity. Optimal timing of administration unclear, but should be at least 30 to 45 min before sexual activity. May increase to 20 mg or decrease to 5 mg. Max 1 dose/day. Start 5 mg (max 1 dose/day) if CrCl 31 to 50 mL/min. Max 5 mg/day if CrCl < 30 mL/min on dialysis. Max 10 mg/day if mild to moderate hepatic impairment; avoid in severe hepatic impairment. Max 10 mg once in 72 h if concurrent potent CYP3A4 inhibitors. Pulmonary HTN: 40 mg PO daily, 20 mg if CrCl < 80 mL/min or mild to moderate hepatic impairment. Avoid with CrCl < 30 mL/min. Caution with ritonavir, see PI for specific dose adjustments.
PEDS — Not approved in children.
FORMS — Trade only (Cialis): Tabs 2.5, 5, 10, 20 mg.
NOTES — If nitrates needed give at least 48 h after the last tadalafil dose. Improves erectile function for up to 36 h. Not FDA-approved for women. Not recommended if MI in prior 90 days, angina during sexual activity, NYHA Class II or greater in prior 6 months, hypotension (< 90/50), HTN (> 170/100) or CVA in prior 6 months. Rare reports of prolonged erections. Do not use with ketoconazole or itraconazole.
MOA — Selectively inhibits phosphodiesterase-5 resulting in enhanced relaxation of penile arteries & corpus cavernosal smooth muscle; enhances erectile function by increasing penile blood flow.
ADVERSE EFFECTS — Serious: Priapism, hypotension, myocardial infarction, vision loss (nonarteritic ischemic optic neuropathy), retinal artery occlusion. Frequent: Headache, flushing, dyspepsia, back pain.

VARDENAFIL (Levitra) ▶LK ♀B ▶- $$$$
WARNING — Contraindicated with nitrates (time interval for safe administration unknown). Caution with alpha blockers due to potential for symptomatic hypotension. There have been a few reports

(cont.)

VARDENAFIL *(cont.)*
of sudden vision loss due to nonarteritic ischemic optic neuropathy (NAION). Patients with prior NAION are at higher risk. Sudden hearing loss, with or without tinnitus, vertigo or dizziness, has been reported. Seizures and seizure recurrence have been reported.
ADULTS — Erectile dysfunction: 10 mg PO 1 h before sexual activity. Usual effective dose range: 5 to 20 mg. Maximum 1 dose/day. Use lower dose (5 mg) if age 65 yo or older or moderate hepatic impairment (max 10 mg); 2.5 mg when coadministered with certain drugs (see notes). Not FDA-approved in women.
PEDS — Not approved in children.
FORMS — Trade only: Tabs 2.5, 5, 10, 20 mg.
NOTES — See the following parenthetical vardenafil dose adjustments when taken with ritonavir (max 2.5 mg/72 h); indinavir, saquinavir, atazanavir, clarithromycin, ketoconazole 400 mg daily, or itraconazole 400 mg daily (max 2.5 mg/24 h); ketoconazole 200 mg daily, itraconazole 200 mg daily, or erythromycin (max 5 mg/24 h). Avoid with alpha-blockers and antiarrhythmics, and in congenital QT prolongation. Caution if CVA, MI or other cardiovascular event within last 6 months, unstable angina, severe liver impairment, end stage renal disease or retinitis pigmentosa.
MOA — Selectively inhibits phosphodiesterase-5 resulting in enhanced relaxation of penile arteries & corpus cavernosal smooth muscle; enhances erectile function by increasing penile blood flow.
ADVERSE EFFECTS — Serious: Hypotension, syncope, myocardial infarction, priapism, vision loss (nonarteritic ischemic optic neuropathy), seizures, transient global amnesia. Frequent: Headache, flushing, rhinitis, dyspepsia.

YOHIMBINE (*Yocon, Yohimex*) ▶L ♀− ▶− $
ADULTS — No approved indications.
PEDS — No approved indications.
UNAPPROVED ADULTS — Erectile dysfunction: 1 tab PO tid. If side effects (eg, tremor, tachycardia, nervousness) occur, reduce to ½ tab tid, followed by gradual increases to 1 tab tid.
FORMS — Generic/Trade: Tabs 5.4 mg.
NOTES — Prescription yohimbine and yohimbine bark extract (see Herbal section) are not interchangeable. Contraindicated with renal disease. Avoid with antidepressant use, psychiatric disorders, the elderly, women, or ulcer history. Efficacy of therapy > 10 weeks unclear. American Urological Association does not recommend as a standard treatment due to unproven efficacy.
MOA — An alpha-2-adrenergic receptor blocker.
ADVERSE EFFECTS — Serious: Respiratory paralysis with overdose. Frequent: HTN, tachycardia, nervousness, irritability, tremor and increased motor activity.

UROLOGY: Nephrolithiasis

ACETOHYDROXAMIC ACID (*Lithostat*) ▶K ♀X ▶? $$$$
ADULTS — Chronic UTI, adjunctive therapy: 250 mg PO tid to qid for a total dose of 10 to 15 mg/kg/day. Maximum dose is 1.5 g/day. Decrease dose in patients with renal impairment to no more than 1 g/day.
PEDS — Adjunctive therapy in chronic urea-splitting UTI (eg, Proteus): 10 mg/kg/day PO divided bid to tid.
FORMS — Trade only: Tabs 250 mg.
NOTES — Do not use if CrCl < 20 mL/min. Administer on an empty stomach.
MOA — Inhibits urease and the production of ammonia by urea-splitting urinary organisms (eg, Proteus).
ADVERSE EFFECTS — Serious: Bone marrow suppression, hemolytic anemia. Frequent: Headache, rash, malaise, nervousness, anxiety, depression, vomiting, anorexia, phlebitis.

CELLULOSE SODIUM PHOSPHATE (*Calcibind*) ▶Fecal ♀C ▶+ $$$$
WARNING — Avoid in heart failure or ascites due to high sodium content.
ADULTS — Absorptive hypercalciuria Type 1 (age older than 16 yo): Initial dose with urinary calcium > 300 mg/day (on moderate calcium-restricted diet): 5 g with each meal. Decrease dose to 5 g with supper, 2.5 g with each remaining meal when calcium declines to less than 150 mg/day. Initial dose with urinary calcium 200 to 300 mg/day (controlled calcium-restricted diet): 5 g with supper, 2.5 g with each remaining meal. Mix with water, soft drink or fruit juice. Ingest within 30 min of meal.
PEDS — Do not use if age less than 16 yo.
FORMS — Trade only: Bulk powder 300 mg.
NOTES — Give concomitant supplement of 1.5 g magnesium gluconate with 15 g/day. 1 g magnesium gluconate with 10 g/day. Take magnesium supplement at least 1 h before or after each dose to avoid binding. May cause hyperparathyroidism. Long-term use may cause hypomagnesemia, hyperoxaluria, hypomagnesuria, depletion of trace metals (copper, zinc, iron); monitor calcium, magnesium, trace metals and CBC q 3 to 6 months; monitor parathyroid hormone once between the first 2 weeks and 3 months, then q 3 to 6 months thereafter. Adjust or stop treatment if PTH rises above normal. Stop when inadequate hypocalciuric response (urinary calcium of < 30 mg/5 g of cellulose sodium phosphate) occurs while patient is on moderate calcium restriction. Avoid Vitamin C supplementation since metabolized to oxalate.
MOA — Nonabsorbable ion-exchange resin. Binds to divalent cations.
ADVERSE EFFECTS — Serious: Hyperoxaluria. Frequent: Diarrhea, dyspepsia, altered taste, hypomagnesemia, hyperparathyroidism.

CITRATE (*Polycitra-K, Urocit-K, Bicitra, Oracit, Polycitra, Polycitra-LC*) ▶K ♀C ▶? $$$
ADULTS — Prevention of calcium and urate kidney stones: 1 packet in water/juice PO tid to qid with meals. 15 to 30 mL PO soln tid to qid with meals. Tabs 10 to 20 mEq PO tid to qid with meals. Max 100 mEq/day.
PEDS — Urinary alkalinization: 5 to 15 mL PO qid with meals.
FORMS — Generic/Trade: Polycitra-K packet 3300 mg potassium citrate/ea, Polycitra-K oral soln (1100 mg potassium citrate/5 mL, 480 mL). Oracit oral soln (490 mg sodium citrate/5 mL, 15, 30, 480 mL). Bicitra oral soln (500 mg sodium citrate/5 mL, 480 mL). Urocit-K wax (potassium citrate) Tabs 5, 10 mEq. Polycitra-LC oral soln (550 mg potassium citrate/500 mg sodium citrate per 5 mL, 480 mL). Polycitra oral syrup (550 mg potassium citrate/500 mg sodium citrate per 5 mL, 480 mL.
NOTES — Contraindicated in renal insufficiency, PUD, UTI, and hyperkalemia.
MOA — Increases urinary-free bases thereby increasing pH.
ADVERSE EFFECTS — Serious: Hyperkalemia. Frequent: N/V, diarrhea, dyspepsia.

UROLOGY: Other

AMINOHIPPURATE (*PAH*) ▶K ♀C ▶? $
ADULTS — Estimation of effective renal plasma flow and measurement of functional capacity of renal tubular secretory mechanism: Specialized infusion dosing available.
PEDS — Not approved in children.
NOTES — May precipitate heart failure. Patients receiving sulfonamides, procaine or thiazolsulfone may interfere with chemical color development essential for analysis. Concomitant use of probenecid my result in erroneously low effective renal plasma flow.
MOA — Chemical filtered by the glomeruli and actively secreted by the proximal tubules.
ADVERSE EFFECTS — Serious: Hypersensitivity, anaphylaxis. Frequent: Sensation of warmth or the desire to defecate or urinate during or shortly following initiation of infusion.

INDEX

2-PAM 383
3TC 46
5-aminosalicylic
   acid 228
5-Aspirin 228
5-FU
   Dermatology 139
   Oncology 315
6-MP 316
8-MOP 145
15-methyl-prostaglandin
   F2 alpha 306
292 tab 16

A

A1C Home Testing 169
A1CNow 169
A-200 143
A-spaz 223
A/T/S 137
abacavir 43, 45
abatacept 1
ABC 45
abciximab 113
Abelcet 30
Abenol 19
Abilify 357
Abilify Discmelt 357
Abraxane 325
Abreva 145
ACAM 2000 262
acamprosate 365
Acanya 135
acarbose 162
Accolate 376
Accu-Check Advantage ......
   169
Accu-Check Aviva 169
Accu-Check Compact ....
   169
Accu-Check Compact
   Plus 169
Accu-Check Complete ....
   169
Accu-Check
   Voicemate 169
Accu-Chek Active 169
Accu-Prep 226
AccuNeb 370
Accupril 89
Accuretic 107
Accutane 137
acebutolol 115
acemannan 243
Aceon 89
Acetadote 380

acetaminophen
   Analgesics 5, 6,
      .... 16–19, 21
   ENT 196, 197, 199
   Neurology 278
acetazolamide 121
acetic acid 207, 208
acetohydroxamic
   acid 389
acetylcholine 341
acetylcysteine
   Endocrine and
      Metabolic 183
   Toxicology 380
acetylcysteine—
   inhaled 377
acetylsalicylic acid
   Analgesics 5–7, 16, 18
   Cardiovascular 113
   Gastroenterology 217
Acidophilus 253
AcipHex 222
acitretin 144
Aclasta 158
Aclovate 147
acrivastine 205
ActHIB 258
Acticin 143
Actidose-Aqua 380
Actifed Cold and
   Allergy 196
Actifed Cold and
   Sinus 196
Actigall 232
Actiq 13
Activase 130
Activase rt-PA 130
activated charcoal 380
Activella 300
Actonel 158
Actonel Plus Calcium ... 158
ACTOPLUS Met 162
Actos 165
Actron 10
Acular 345
Acular LS 345
Acutrim Natural AM 245
acyclovir 40
acyclovir—topical 145
Aczone 34
Adacel 258
Adalat 120
Adalat CC 120
Adalat PA 120
Adalat XL 120
adalimumab 1

adapalene 135, 137
Adcirca 129
Adderall 367
Adderall XR 367
adefovir 53
Adenocard 94
adenosine 94
ADH 193
Adipex-P 370
Adoxa 79
adrenalin 127
Adriamycin 313
Adrucil 315
Advair 372
Advair HFA 372
Advate 238
Advicor 102
Advil 9
Aerius 193
AeroBid 375
AeroBid-M 375
Aerospan 375
Aesculus
   hippocastanum 251
Afeditab CR 120
Afinitor 322
Afluria 260
African plum tree 254
Afrin 211
agalsidase beta .... PDA
Aggrastat 114
Aggrenox 113
Agrylin 241
Airomir 370
AK Tate 339
AK Tracin 335
AK-Con 332
AK-Dilate 344
AK-Mycin 335
AK-Pentolate 343
Akarpine 341
Akineton 280
Akten 345
Akurza 138
Alamast 334
Alavert 194
Alavert D-12 196
Alaway 333
Albalon 332
albendazole 37
Albenza 37
Albumarc 131
albumin 131
Albuminar 131
albuterol 370, 373
Alcaine 345

alclometasone
   dipropionate 147
alcohol 381
aldactazide 107
Aldactone 90
Aldara 145
aldesleukin 320
Aldomet 93
Aldoril 107
Aldurazyme .... PDA
alefacept 144
alemtuzumab 320
alendronate 157
Alertec 370
Alesse 286
Aleve 11
Aleve Cold and Sinus 196
Alfenta 21
alfentanil 21
Alferon N 56
alfuzosin 383
alglucerase .... PDA
alglucosidase alfa .... PDA
Align 253
Alimta 316
Alinia 38
aliskiren 110, 111
alitretinoin 151
Alka-Seltzer 217
Alkeran 311
All Clear 332
Allegra 194
Allegra-D 12-hour 199
Allegra-D 24-hour 199
Aller-Chlor 194
Aller-Relief 194
Allerdryl 195
Allerfrim 196
Allermax 195
AllerNaze 210
Allerx 200
Alli 231
Allium sativum 249
allopurinol 172
Alluna 256
Almora 177
almotriptan 276
Alocril 334
aloe vera 243
Alomide 333
Aloprim 172
Alora 298
alosetron 229
Aloxi 213
alpha-1 antitrypsin 377

Index

alpha-1 proteinase
    inhibitor 377
alpha-galactosidase 229
Alphagan 342
Alphagan P. 342
Alphanate 238
AlphaNine SD 237
alprazolam 363
alprostadil 387
Alrex 339
Alsoy 180
Alsuma 276
Altabax 141
Altace 89
Altafrin 344
alteplase 130
Alternagel 217
Altoprev 103
altretamine 309
Alu-Cap 217
Alu-Tab 217
aluminum acetate 207
aluminum chloride 152
aluminum hydroxide
    Analgesics 5
    Gastroenterology 217,
    218
Alupent 371
Alvesco 374
alvimopan 230
amantadine 52
Amaryl 168
Amatine 128
ambenonium .... PDA
Ambien 364
Ambien CR 364
AmBisome 30
ambrisentan .... PDA
amcinonide 147
Amerge 276
amethocain .... PDA
Amevive 144
Amicar 241
Amidate 21
Amidrine 278
amifostine 317
Amigesic 8
amikacin 24
Amikin 24
amiloride 109, 123
aminocaproic acid 241
aminohippurate 390
aminolevulinic
    acid 138
aminophylline 377
aminosalicylic
    acid .... PDA
amiodarone 94
Amitiza 228
amitriptyline 346, 365
Amlactin 153
amlexanox 208
amlodipine 103,
    .... 107–110, 119

Ammonul 189
Amnesteem 137
amobarbital .... PDA
amoxapine 346
amoxicillin
    Antimicrobials 72
    Gastroenterology 220
amoxicillin-clavulanate .. 72
Amoxil 72
ampalaya 244
Amphadase .... PDA
amphetamine 367
Amphojel 217
Amphotec 30
amphotericin B
    deoxycholate 29
amphotericin B lipid
    formulations 30
ampicillin 73
ampicillin-sulbactam 73
Ampyra 278
Amrix 4
amyl nitrite .... PDA
Anacin 7
Anadrol-50 .... PDA
Anafranil 346
anagrelide 241
anakinra 1
Analpram-HC 151
Anaprox 11
Anaspaz 223
anastrozole 317
Ancef 60
Ancobon 30
Andriol 156
Andro 244
Androcur 318
Androcur Depot 318
Androderm 156
AndroGel 156
Android 156
androstenedione 244
Androxy 155
Anectine 23
Anexsia 16
Angelica sinensis 247
Angeliq 300
Angiomax 235
anhydrous glycerins 208
anidulafungin 28
Ansaid 9
Antabuse 365
Antara 106
antazoline 332
Anthemis nobilis—
    Roman chamomile 245
Anthraforte 144
anthralin 144
Anthranol 144
Anthrascalp 144
anti-inhibitor coagulant
    complex 237
Antilirium 382
Antiminth 39

antipyrine 207
antivenin—crotalidae
    immune Fab ovine
    polyvalent 263
antivenin—crotalidae
    polyvalent 263
antivenin—latrodectus
    mactans 263
Antivert 195
Antizol 381
Anusol-HC 149
Anzemet 213
Aphthasol 208
Apidra 166
Aplenzin 352
Aplisol 268
Apo-Gain 154
Apokyn 280
apomorphine 280
apraclonidine 342
aprepitant 214
Apresazide 107
Apresoline 111
Apri 286
Apriso 228
Aprodine 197
Aptivus 52
Aquachloral
    Supprettes 364
AquaMephyton 187
Aquasol E 188
AraC 315
Aralast 377
Aralen 31
Aranelle 292
Aranesp 239
Arava 3
Arcalyst .... PDA
Aredia 158
arformoterol 372
argatroban 235
Aricept 268
Arimidex 317
aripiprazole 357
Aristolochia 244
aristolochic acid 244
Aristospan 161
armodafinil 367
Armour Thyroid 182
arnica 244
Arnica montana 244
Aromasin 318
Aromaticum 246
Arranon 316
arsenic trioxide 327
Artane 280
artemether 32
Arthrotec 8
articaine 22
artichoke leaf extract ... 244
artificial tears 345
Arzerra 322
Asacol 228
Asaphen 7

Asarum 244
ascorbic acid 183,
    .... 184, 186
Ascriptin 5
asenapine 358
Aslera 247
Asmanex Twisthaler 376
Asmavent 370
asparaginase 327
Aspir-Mox 5
Aspirin 7
Assalix 257
Astelin 210
Astepro 210
astragalus 244
Astragalus
    membranaceus 244
Atacand 90
Atacand HCT 107
Atacand Plus 107
Atarax 195
Atasol 19
atazanavir 48
atenolol 110, 115
Atgam 265
Ativan 362
atomoxetine 367
atorvastatin 103
atovaquone 32, 37
atracurium 23
Atripla 42
AtroPen 96
atropine
    Cardiovascular 96
    Gastroenterology 212,
    223
    Toxicology 381
    Urology 386
Atropine Care 343
atropine—
    ophthalmic 343
Atrovent 378
Atrovent HFA 378
Atrovent Nasal Spray ... 210
Attenuvax .... PDA
ATV 48
augmented
    betamethasone
    dipropionate 147
Augmentin 72
Augmentin ES-600 72
Augmentin XR 72
Auralgan 207
auranofin 2
Avage 138
Avalide 107
Avandamet 163
Avandaryl 163
Avandia 165
Avapro 91
Avastin 321
Avaxim 258
Aveeno 154
Avelox 78

Index

Aventyl 347
avian influenza vaccine
 H5N1—inactivated
 injection 257
Aviane 286
Avinza 15
Avodart 383
Avonex 278
Axert 276
Axid 219
Axid AR 219
Aygestin 304
azacitidine 314
Azactam 81
Azasan 2
Azasite 335
azathioprine 2
azelaic acid 135
azelastine—nasal 210
azelastine—
 ophthalmic 332
Azelex 135
Azilect 282
azithromycin 67
azithromycin—
 ophthalmic 335
Azmacort 376
Azo-Standard 387
Azopt 340
Azor 107
AZT 47
aztreonam 81
Azulfidine 229
Azulfidine EN-tabs 229

B

B&O Supprettes 384
B-D Glucose 169
BabyBIG 263
Bacid 253
Baciguent 139
Bacillus of Calmette
 and Guerin 321
bacitracin
 Dermatology 139, 141
 Ophthalmology 336
bacitracin—
 ophthalmic 335
baclofen 3
Bactocill 72
Bactrim 78
Bactroban 140
BAL in oil 380
balsalazide 228
Balziva 286
banana bag 179
Banophen 195
Banzel 274
Baraclude 56
Baridium 387
barium sulfate 134
Basalgel 217
basiliximab 266
Bayer 7

Baygam 264
BayTet 266
BCG 321
BCG vaccine 257
BCNU 309
Beano 229
becaplermin 152
beclomethasone 209
beclomethasone—
 inhaled 374
Beconase AQ 209
belladonna
 Gastroenterology 222
 Urology 384
Bellergal Spacetabs 222
Bellergal-S 222
Benadryl 195
*Benadryl Allergy and
 Cold* 197
*Benadryl-D Allergy and
 Sinus* 197
benazepril 87, 109
bendamustine 309
bendroflumethiazide 108
BeneFin 255
Benefix 237
Benicar 91
Benicar HCT 108
Benoquin 154
Benoxyl 136
Bentyl 222
Bentyol 222
Benuryl 173
Benylin 196
Benylin DME 197
Benzac 136
Benzaclin 136
Benzagel 10% 136
Benzamycin 136
benzathine penicillin 70
benzocaine 207, 211
benzoic acid 385, 386
benzonatate 195
benzoyl peroxide
 135–137
benzphetamine 368
benztropine
 mesylate 280
bepotastine 333
Bepreve 333
beractant 377
Berotec 371
besifloxacin 334
Besivance 334
Beta-Val 147
Betaderm 147
Betagan 340
betahistine 283
betaine .... PDA
Betaject 159
Betaloc 116
betamethasone
 Dermatology 145, 151

Endocrine and
 Metabolic 159
betamethasone
 dipropionate 147
betamethasone valerate .....
  147
Betapace 101
Betapace AF 101
Betaseron 278
betaxolol 115
betaxolol—
 ophthalmic 339
bethanechol 386
Betimol 340
Betoptic 339
Betoptic S. 339
bevacizumab 321
bexarotene 327
Bexxar 324
bezafibrate 105
Bezalip 105
Biaxin 68
Biaxin XL 68
bicalutamide 318
bicarbonate
 Cardiovascular 96
 Gastroenterology
  .... 217, 222
Bicillin C-R 70
Bicillin L-A 70
Bicitra 390
BiCNU 309
BiDil 132
Biest .... PDA
Bifantis 253
Bifidobacteria 253
bilberry 244
Biltricide 38
bimatoprost 341
Bionect 153
BioRab 261
biotin 186
biperiden 280
Biphentin 369
Biquin durules 100
bisacodyl 227
bismuth subcitrate
 potassium 220
bismuth
 subsalicylate 211, 220
bisoprolol 111, 115
bitter melon 244
bitter orange 245
bivalirudin 235
black cohosh 245
Blenoxane 312
bleomycin 312
Bleph-10 337
blephamide 337
Blocadren 118
blood transfusion .... PDA
Bonamine 195
Bonefos 157
Bonine 195

Boniva 157
Bontril 370
Bontril Slow Release 370
Boostrix 258
boric acid 306
bortezomib 327
bosentan 128
Botox 283
Botox Cosmetic 283
botulinum toxin
 type A 283
botulinum toxin
 type B 284
botulism immune
 globulin 263
Bragantia 244
Bravelle 303
Brethine 371
Brevibloc 116
Brevicon 286
Brevicon 1/35 289
Brevital 21
Bricanyl Turbuhaler 371
brimonidine 342
brinzolamide 340
bromazepam 361
bromfenac—ophthalmic....
  344
Bromfenex 200
Bromfenex PD 200
bromocriptine 189
brompheniramine
 .... 197, 198, 200, 201
Brovana 372
buckeye 251
budesonide
 Gastroenterology 230
 Pulmonary 373
budesonide—inhaled ... 374
budesonide—nasal 209
Bufferin 5
bumetanide 122
Bumex 122
Buminate 131
bupivacaine 22, 23
Buprenex 12
buprenorphine
 Analgesics 12
 Psychiatry 366
Buproban 352
bupropion 352
Burinex 122
burn plant 243
Buscopan 223
BuSpar 363
buspirone 363
Busulfan 309
Busulfex 309
butabarbital .... PDA
butalbital 5, 6, 16
butamben 211
butenafine 141
Butisol .... PDA
butoconazole 306

butorphanol 12
butterbur 245
Byetta 169
Bystolic 117

C

C.E.S. 298
cabergoline 189
Caduet 103
Caelyx 312
Cafcit 368
Cafergot 277
Caffedrine 368
caffeine
   Analgesics 5, 6, 16, 18
   Neurology 277
   Psychiatry 368
calamine 152
Calan 121
Calcibind 389
Calciferol 184
Calcijex 183
Calcimar 189
calcipotriene 144, 145
calcitonin 189
calcitriol 183
calcium acetate 173
calcium carbonate
   Analgesics 5
   Endocrine and
     Metabolic 173
   Gastroenterology
     .... 218, 219
   OB/GYN 308
calcium chloride 174
calcium citrate 174
calcium gluconate 174
Caldolor 9
calfactant 377
CaloMist 184
Calsan 173
Caltine 189
Caltrate 173
Cambia 9
Camellia sinensis 250
Camila 304
Campath 320
Campral 365
Camptosar 329
Canasa 228
Cancidas 28
candesartan 90, 107
Candistatin
   Antimicrobials 31
   Dermatology 142
Canesten
   Antimicrobials 25
   Dermatology 141
   OB/GYN 306
Cankermelt 252
cannibis sativa L.
   extract 20
Cantil 223
Capastat .... PDA

capecitabine 314
Capex 148
Capital with Codeine
   Suspension 16
Capoten 87
Capozide 108
capreomycin .... PDA
Caprex 148
capsaicin 152
captopril 87, 108
Carac 139
Carafate 224
carbachol 341
Carbaglu .... PDA
carbamazepine 269
carbamide peroxide 207
Carbatrol 269
carbidopa 281, 282
carbidopa-levodopa 281
carbinoxamine 194, 200,
   204
Carbocaine 23
Carbodec DM 200
carboplatin 326
carboprost 306
Cardene 119
Cardene SR 119
Cardizem 120
Cardizem CD 120
Cardizem LA 120
Cardura 92
Cardura XL 92
Care 178
Care ET 178
Ceredase .... PDA
carglumic acid .... PDA
Carimune 265
carisoprodol 4, 6, 18
Carmol 40 155
Carmol HC 152
carmustine 309
Carnitor 180
carteolol—
   ophthalmic 340
Cartia XT 120
Cartilade 255
carvedilol 116
cascara 227
Casodex 318
caspofungin 28
castor oil 227
Cataflam 9
Catapres 92
Catapres-TTS 92
Cathflo 130
Caverject 387
Caverject Impulse 387
CCNU 310
Ceclor 61
Cedax 66
Cedocard SR 125
CeeNu 310
cefaclor 61
cefadroxil 60
cefazolin 60

cefdinir 64
cefditoren 64
cefepime 67
cefixime 64
Cefizox 66
cefotaxime 65
cefotetan 61
cefoxitin 61
cefpodoxime 65
cefprozil 63
ceftazidime 65
ceftibuten 66
Ceftin 63
ceftizoxime 66
ceftriaxone 66
cefuroxime 63
Cefzil 63
Celebrex 7
celecoxib 7
Celestone 159
Celestone Soluspan ... 159
Celexa 349
Cellcept 267
cellulose sodium
   phosphate 389
Celontin .... PDA
Cena-K 178
Cenestin 299
Centany 140
cephalexin 61
Ceprotin .... PDA
Ceptaz 65
Cerebyx 271
Ceredase .... PDA
Cerefolin 183
Cerefolin NAC 183
Cerezyme .... PDA
Certain Dri 152
certolizumab 230
Cerubidine 312
Cervidil 302
Cesamet 215
cesium chloride 245
Cetacaine 211
cetirizine 194, 206
Cetraxal 207
cetrorelix acetate 299
Cetrotide 299
cetuximab 321
cevimeline 208
chamomile 245
Chantix 367
CharcoAid 380
charcoal 380
Charcodate 380
chasteberry 245
Chemet 383
Cheracol D Cough 197
Cheratussin AC 200
Cheratussin DAC 200
Children's Advil Cold 197
ChiRhoStim 232
Chlor-Trimeton 194
chloral hydrate 364

chlorambucil 309
chloramphenicol 81
chlordiazepoxide ... 361, 365
chlordiazepoxide-
   clidinium 230
Chlordrine SR 200
chlorhexidine
   gluconate 208
chlorodeoxyadenosine ... 314
Chloromycetin 81
chlorophyllin copper
   complex 154
chloroprocaine .... PDA
chloroquine 31
chlorothiazide 123
chlorpheniramine 194,
   .... 196, 197, 199–201,
   203–206
chlorpromazine 355
chlorpropamide 167
chlorthalidone 108,
   .... 110, 123
chlorzoxazone 4
cholecalciferol 188
CholeRx 253
Cholestin 253
cholestyramine 101
choline magnesium
   trisalicylate 8
chondroitin 246
choriogonadotropin
   alfa 302
chorionic
   gonadotropin 302
Chrysanthemum
   parthenium 248
Ci-wu-jia 250
Cialis 388
ciclesonide 209
ciclesonide—inhaled ... 374
ciclopirox 141
Cidecin 82
cidofovir 39
cigarette .... PDA
cilazapril 87, 109
cilostazol 132
Ciloxan 334
cimetidine 218
Cimicifuga racemosa ... 245
Cimzia 230
cinacalcet 190
Cinnamomum
   Cassia 246
cinnamon 246
Cipralex 349
Cipro 75
Cipro HC Otic 207
Cipro XR 75
Ciprodex Otic 207
ciprofloxacin
   Antimicrobials 75
   ENT 207
ciprofloxacin—
   ophthalmic 334

cisapride 230
cisatracurium 23
cisplatin 326
citalopram 349
Citanest .... PDA
Citracal 174
citrate
  Gastroenterology 217
  Urology 390
Citri Lean 249
Citro-Mag 225
Citrocarbonate 217
Citrucel 225
Citrus aurantium 245
cladribine 314
Claforan 65
Claravis 137
Clarinex 193
Clarinex-D 12 hour 200
Clarinex-D 24 hour 200
Claripel 153
clarithromycin
  Antimicrobials 68
  Gastroenterology 220
Claritin 194
Claritin Hives Relief 194
Claritin RediTabs 194
Claritin-D 12 hr 197
Claritin-D 24 hr 197
Clarus 137
Clasteon 157
Clavulin 72
Clear Eyes 332
Clearasil 136
Clearasil Cleanser 138
clemastine 194
Clenia 136
Cleocin
  Antimicrobials 81
  OB/GYN 306
Cleocin T 136
clevidipine 119
Cleviprex 119
Climara 298
Climara pro 300
Clindagel 136
ClindaMax 136
clindamycin
  Antimicrobials 81
  Dermatology 135–138
clindamycin—
  topical 136
clindamycin—
  vaginal 306
Clindesse 306
Clindoxyl 137
Clinoril 11
clobazam 269
clobetasol 147
Clobex 147
clocortolone pivalate 148
Cloderm 148
clodronate 157
clofarabine 314

clofazimine 34
Clolar 314
Clomid 303
clomiphene 303
clomipramine 346
Clonapam 361
clonazepam 361
clonidine 92, 108
clonidine—epidural ..... PDA
clopidogrel 113
Clopixol 357
Clopixol Accuphase 357
Clopixol Depot 357
cloquinol 151
clorazepate 361
Clorpres 108
Clotrimaderm
  Antimicrobials 25
  Dermatology 141
  OB/GYN 306
clotrimazole
  Antimicrobials 25
  Dermatology 151
clotrimazole—
  topical 141
clotrimazole—
  vaginal 306
clozapine 358
Clozaril 358
coal tar 152
Coartem 32
Coartemether 32
cobalamin 184
cocaine .... PDA
codeine
  Analgesics 12,
  16–18
  ENT 200,
  202–205
coenzyme q10 246
Cogentin 280
Cognex .... PDA
Colace 227
Colazal 228
Colbenemid 172
colchicine 172
Colcrys 172
Cold-fX 249
colesevelam 101
Colestid 102
Colestid Flavored 102
colestipol 102
colistimethate .... PDA
colistin 207
Coly-Mycin M
  Parenteral .... PDA
Colyte 226
Combantrin 39
Combigan 342
Combipatch 300
Combivent 373
Combivent inhalation
  soln 373
Combivir 42

Combunox 16
Commiphora mukul
  extract 251
Commit 366
Compazine 216
Comtan 280
Comvax 257
Concerta 369
Condyline 146
Condylox 146
cone flower 247
Congest 298
conivaptan 190
Conray 135
Copaxone 278
Copegus 58
CoQ-10 246
Cordarone 94
Cordran 149
Cordran SP 149
Coreg 116
Coreg CR 116
Corgard 117
Coricidin HBP
  Congestion and
  Cough 197
Coricidin HBP Cough
  and Cold 197
Corlopam 111
Cormax 147
Coronex 125
Correctol 227
Cortaid 149
Cortamed 149
Cortate 149
Cortef 160
Cortenema 160
Corticaine 149
corticotropin 171
Cortifoam 149
cortisone 159
Cortisporin 150
Cortisporin Otic 207
Cortisporin TC Otic 207
Cortisporin—
  ophthalmic 337
Cortizone 149
Cortoderm 149
Cortone 159
Cortrosyn 171
Corvert 99
Corynanthe yohimbe 257
Corzide 108
Cosamin DS 250
Cosmegen 312
Cosopt 343
cosyntropin 171
Cotazym 232
cotrimoxazole 78
Coumadin 236
Covera-HS 121
Coversyl 89
Cozaar 91
Cranactin 246

cranberry 246
Crataegus
  laevigata 251
creatine 246
Creon 231, 232
Crestor 104
Crinone 305
Crixivan 50
CroFab 263
Crolom 333
cromolyn—inhaled 378
cromolyn—nasal 210
cromolyn—
  ophthalmic 333
crotamiton 143
Cryselle 286
crystalline DMSO2 252
Cubicin 82
Culturelle 253
Cuprimine 382
Curosurf 379
Cutar 152
Cutivate 149
Cutter 152
cyanocobalamin
  Endocrine and
  Metabolic 183–186
  OB/GYN 308
Cyanokit 382
Cyclen 290
Cyclessa 292
cyclobenzaprine 4
Cyclocort 147
Cyclogyl 343
Cyclomen 308
cyclopentolate 343
cyclophosphamide 310
cycloserine .... PDA
Cycloset 189
cyclosporine 266
cyclosporine—
  ophthalmic 345
Cyklokapron 243
Cymbalta 351
Cynara scolymus 244
cyproheptadine 194
cyproterone
  Dermatology 136
  Oncology 318
Cystadane .... PDA
Cystografin 134
Cystospaz 223
cytarabine 315
Cytogam 264
cytomegalovirus
  immune globulin
  human 264
Cytomel 181
Cytosar-U 315
Cytotec
  Gastroenterology 224
  OB/GYN 302
Cytovene 40
Cytoxan 310

Index

D

d-biotin 184
D.H.E. 45 277
D2T5 258
dabigatran 241
dacarbazine 310
daclizumab 267
Dacogen 315
dactinomycin 312
Dalacin 306
Dalacin C 81
Dalacin T 136
dalfampridine 278
dalfopristin 84
Dalmane 362
danazol 308
Danocrine 308
danshen 247
Dantrium 4
dantrolene 4
dapsone 34
Daptacel 258
daptomycin 82
Daraprim 39
darbepoetin 239
darifenacin 384
darunavir 49
Darvocet 16
Darvon Pulvules 15
Darvon-N 15
dasatinib 327
daunorubicin 312
DaunoXome 312
Daypro 11
Daytrana 369
DDAVP 191
DDI 46
DDrops 188
Debacterol 208
Debrox 207
Decadron 159
decitabine 315
Declomycin 79
Deconamine 201
Deconsal II 201
deet 152
deferasirox 241
deferoxamine 380
degarelix 318
dehydroepiandrosterone
  247
Delatestryl 156
delavirdine .... PDA
Delestrogen 298
Delsym 196
Deltasone 161
Demadex 122
demeclocycline 79
Demerol 14
Demser 112
Demulen 286
Denavir 146
denileukin 321
denosumab 190
Denticare 208
Depacon 275
Depade 366
Depakene 275
Depakote
  Neurology 275
  Psychiatry 354
Depakote ER
  Neurology 275
  Psychiatry 354
Depen 382
Depo-Cyt 315
Depo-Estradiol 297
Depo-Medrol 160
Depo-Provera 304
depo-subQ provera
  104 304
Depo-Testosterone 156
DepoDur 15
Deproic
  Neurology 275
  Psychiatry 354
Derma-Smoothe/FS 148
Dermalac 153
Dermasone 147
Dermatop 150
Dermazin 141
Dermolate 149
DermOtic 207
Desferal 380
desflurane .... PDA
desipramine 346
desirudin 235
desloratadine 193, 200
desmopressin 191
desogen 286
desogestrel 286, 287,
  .... 289–292, 294
Desonate 148
desonide 148
DesOwen 148
Desoxi 148
desoximetasone 148
Desoxyn .... PDA
Desquam 136
desvenlafaxine 351
Desyrel 352
Detrol 385
Detrol LA 385
devil's claw 247
Dex-4 169
Dexalone 196
dexamethasone
  Endocrine and
    Metabolic 159
  ENT 207
dexamethasone—
  ophthalmic 338
Dexasone 159
Dexatrim Natural
  Ephedrine Free 245
dexbrompheniramine
  .... 198, 203
dexchlorpheniramine
  .... 195, 205
Dexedrine 369
DexFerrum 176
Dexiron 176
dexlansoprazole 220
dexmedetomidine 21
dexmethylphenidate 368
Dexpak 159
dexrazoxane 317
dextran 132
dextroamphetamine
  .... 367, 369
dextromethorphan
  196–205
dextrose 169
Dextrostat 369
DHEA 247
DiaBeta 168
Diabinese 167
Diamicron 168
Diamicron MR 168
Diamorphine .... PDA
Diamox 121
Diamox Sequels 121
Diane-35 136
Diarr-eze 212
Diastat 362
Diastat AcuDial 362
diatrizoate 134
Diatx Zn 184
Diazemuls 362
diazepam 362
diazoxide 191
Dibenzyline 112
dibucaine 151
Dicel 201
Dicetel 232
dichloralphenazone 278
Diclectin 214
diclofenac 8, 9
diclofenac—
  ophthalmic 344
diclofenac—
  topical 138
dicloxacillin 71
dicyclomine 222
didanosine 46
Didrex 368
Didronel 157
diethylpropion 369
difenoxin 212
Differin 135
diflorasone 148
Diflucan 25
diflunisal 8
difluprednate 339
Digibind 97
Digifab 97
Digitek 97
digoxin 97
digoxin immune
  Fab 97
dihydrocodeine 18
dihydroergotamine 277
diiodohydroxyquin .... PDA
Dilacor XR 120
Dilantin 273
Dilatrate-SR 125
Dilaudid 14
Dilaudid-5 14
Diltia XT 120
diltiazem 120
Diltiazem CD 120
Diltzac 120
dimenhydrinate 214
dimercaprol 380
Dimetane-DX Cough
  Syrup 201
Dimetapp Cold and
  Allergy 197
Dimetapp Cold and
  Cough 198
Dimetapp Decongestant
  Infant Drops 206
Dimetapp Nighttime Cold
  and Congestion 198
dimethyl sulfone 252
dimethyl sulfoxide 386
dinoprostone 302
Diocarpine 341
Diodoquin .... PDA
Diogent 334
Diopred 339
Dioscorea villosa 257
Diovan 91
Diovan HCT 108
Dipentum 229
Diphen 195
Diphenhist 195
diphenhydramine 195,
  .... 197, 199, 209
diphenoxylate 212
diphtheria tetanus and
  acellular pertussis
  vaccine 258,
  .... 260, 262
diphtheria-tetanus
  toxoid 258
dipivefrin 342
Diprivan 22
Diprolene 147
Diprolene AF 147
Diprosone 147
dipyridamole 113, 114
Disalcid 8
Diskets 14
disopyramide 97
DisperMox 72
disulfiram 365
Dithranol 144
Ditropan 385
Ditropan XL 385
Diuril 123
divalproex
  Neurology 275
  Psychiatry 354
Divigel 297

Index

Dixarit 92
DLV .... PDA
DMSO 386
dobutamine 126
Dobutrex 126
docetaxel 324
docosanol 145
docusate 227, 228
dofetilide 98
dolasetron 213
Dolobid 8
Dolophine 14
Doloral 15
Doloteffin 247
Domeboro Otic 207
domperidone 214
Dona 250
donepezil 268
dong quai 247
Donnatal 223
dopamine 127
Dopram 378
Doribax 59
doripenem 59
dornase alfa 378
Doryx 79
dorzolamide 340, 343
Dostinex 189
Dovonex 144
doxapram 378
doxazosin 92
doxepin 347
doxepin—topical 153
doxercalciferol 184
Doxil 312
doxorubicin
  liposomal 312
doxorubicin
  non-liposomal 313
Doxycin 79
doxycycline 79
doxylamine
  Analgesics 17
  Gastroenterology 214
Dramamine 214
Drisdol 184
Dristan 12 Hr Nasal 211
Drithocreme 144
Drixoral Cold and
  Allergy 198
dronabinol 214
dronedarone 98
droperidol 215
drospirenone 291, 300
drotrecogin 82
Droxia 242
DRV 49
Dry Eyes 345
Drysol 152
DT 258
DTaP 258
DTIC-Dome 310
Duac 137
Duetact 163

Dulcolax 227
duloxetine 351
Duocaine 23
Duodote 381
Duolube 345
DuoNeb 373
Duovent UDV 373
Duraclon .... PDA
Duragesic 13
Duratuss 201
Duratuss GP 201
Duratuss HD 201
Durdrin 278
Durezol 339
Duricef 60
dutasteride 383
Duvoid 386
Dyazide 108
Dynacin 80
DynaCirc 119
DynaCirc CR 119
Dynapen 71
Dyrenium 123
Dytan 195

E

E Pam 362
E-mycin 68
E. angustifolia 247
E. pallida 247
E. purpurea 247
Ebixa 269
EC-Naprosyn 11
echinacea 247
Echinacin Madaus 247
EchinaGuard 247
echothiophate iodide 341
econazole 142
Econopred Plus 339
Ecotrin 7
Ecstacy .... PDA
eculizumab .... PDA
ED Spaz 223
Edecrin 122
edetate 381
Edex 387
Edluar 364
edrophonium 279
EDTA 381
EES 69
efavirenz 42, 44
Effer-K 178
Effexor 351
Effexor XR 351
Effient 114
Efidac/24 206
eflornithine 153
Efudex 139
EFV 44
EGb 761 249
Elaprase .... PDA
Elavil 346
Eldepryl 283
elderberry 247

Eldopaque 153
Eldoquin 153
Eldoquin Forte 153
Electropeg 226
Elestat 332
Elestrin 297
eletriptan 276
Eleutherococcus
  senticosus 250
Elidel 146
Eligard 319
Elimite 143
Elitek 330
Elixophyllin 379
Ellence 313
Elmiron 387
Elocom 150
Elocon 150
Eloxatin 326
Elspar 327
eltrombopag .... PDA
Eltroxin 181
Emadine 333
Emcyt 318
emedastine 333
Emend 214
Emetrol 215
EMLA 153
Emo-Cort 149
Empirin 7
Empirin with Codeine 16
Emsam 348
Emtec 18
emtricitabine 42, 43, 46
Emtriva 46
Enablex 384
enalapril 87, 109, 111
enalaprilat 87
Enbrel 1
Enca 80
Endantadine 52
Endocet 18
Endocodone 15
Endodan 18
Endometrin 305
Endrate 381
Enduron 124
Enemeez 227
Enemol 226
Enfamil 180
enflurane .... PDA
enfuvirtide 43
Engerix-B 259
Enjuvia 299
Enlon 279
enoxaparin 233
Enpresse 292
entacapone 280, 282
entecavir 56
Entereg 230
Entex LA 201
Entex liquid 201
Entex PSE 202
Entocort EC 230

Entonox .... PDA
Entozyme 231
Entrophen 7
Entsol 211
Enulose 225
Epaxal 258
ephedra 248
Ephedra sinica 248
ephedrine 127
Epiduo 137
Epifoam 151
Epiject 354
epinastine 332
epinephrine 127
epinephrine racemic 378
EpiPen 127
EpiPen Jr 127
EpiQuin Micro 153
epirubicin 313
Epitol 269
Epival
  Neurology 275
  Psychiatry 354
Epivir 46
Epivir-HBV 46
eplerenone 90
epoetin alfa 239
Epogen 239
epoprostenol 129
Eprex 239
eprosartan 91, 110
eptifibatide 114
Epzicom 43
Equalactin 225
Equetro 269
Eraxis 28
Erbitux 321
ergocalciferol 184
Ergomar .... PDA
ergotamine
  Gastroenterology 222
  Neurology 277
erlotinib 328
Errin 304
Ertaczo 142
ertapenem 59
Ery-Tab 68
Erybid 68
Eryc 68
Erycette 137
Eryderm 137
Erygel 137
Eryped 69
Erysol 137
Erythrocin IV 69
Erythromid 68
erythromycin base
  Antimicrobials 68
  Dermatology 136
erythromycin ethyl
  succinate 69
erythromycin
  lactobionate 69

Index

erythromycin—
  ophthalmic 335
erythromycin—
  topical 137
escitalopram 349
Esclim 298
Esgic 5
Esidrix 124
Eskalith 353
Eskalith CR 353
esmolol 116
esomeprazole 220
Esoterica 153
Estalis 300
estazolam 362
esterified estrogens 297,
  .... 300, 301
Estrace 297, 298
Estraderm 298
estradiol 297, 300, 301
estradiol .... PDA
estradiol acetate 297
estradiol acetate
  vaginal ring 297
estradiol cypionate 297
estradiol gel 297
estradiol topical
  emulsion 297
estradiol transdermal
  patch 298
estradiol transdermal
  spray 298
estradiol vaginal ring ... 298
estradiol vaginal tab 298
estradiol valerate 298
Estradot 298
estramustine 318
Estrasorb 297
Estratest 300
Estratest H.S. 300
Estring 298
estriol .... PDA
Estrogel 297
estrogen vaginal
  cream 298
estrogens
  conjugated 298, 301
estrogens synthetic
  conjugated A 299
estrogens synthetic
  conjugated B 299
estrone .... PDA
estropipate 299
Estrostep FE 292
eszopiclone 364
etanercept 1
ethacrynic acid 122
ethambutol 34
ethanol 381
ethinyl estradiol
  Dermatology 136
  OB/GYN 285–294, 301
ethinyl estradiol
  transdermal 296

ethinyl estradiol
  vaginal ring 296
ethionamide .... PDA
ethosuximide 270
ethotoin .... PDA
Ethrane .... PDA
ethynodiol 286, 287, 292
Ethyol 317
Etibi 34
etidronate 157
etodolac 9
etomidate 21
etonogestrel 294, 296
Etopophos 328
etoposide 328
ETR 45
etravirine 45
Euflex 318
Euglucon 168
Eulexin 318
Eurax 143
Euthyrox 181
Evamist 298
evening primrose oil 248
Everolimus 322
Evista 305
Evithrom 243
Evoclin 136
Evoxac 208
Evra 296
Ex-Lax 227
Excedrin Migraine 6
Exelon 268
Exelon Patch 268
exemestane 318
exenatide 169
Exforge 108
Exforge HCT 108
Exjade 241
Exsel 155
Extina 142
EZ-Char 380
ezetimibe 105
Ezetrol 105

F

Fabrazyme .... PDA
Factive 77
Factor IX 237
Factor VIIA 237
Factor VIII 238
famciclovir 41
famotidine 218, 219
Famvir 41
Fanapt 358
Fangchi 244
Fansidar 32
Fareston 320
Faslodex 318
Fasturtec 330
fat emulsion 179
FazaClo ODT 358
febuxostat 172
Feen-a-Mint 227

Feiba NF 237
Feiba VH 237
Feiba VH Immuno 237
felbamate 270
Felbatol 270
Feldene 11
felodipine 109, 119
Femaprin 245
Femara 319
Femcon FE 286
FemHRT 301
Femizol-M 307
FemPatch 298
Femring 297
Femtrace 297
fenofibrate 106
fenofibric acid 106
fenoldopam 111
fenoprofen .... PDA
fenoterol 371, 373
fentanyl 13
Fentora 13
fenugreek 248
Feosol 175
Fer-in-Sol 175
Feraheme 175
Fergon 175
Feridex 134
Ferodan 175
Ferrex 150 176
ferric gluconate
  complex 174
Ferrlecit 174
ferrous fumarate
  287–289,
  .... 292, 293
ferrous gluconate 175
ferrous sulfate 175
Fertinex 303
ferumoxides 134
ferumoxsil 134
ferumoxytol 175
fesoterodine 384
feverfew 248
Fexicam 11
Fexmid 4
fexofenadine 194, 199
fiber—dietary .... PDA
Fiberall 225
FiberCon 225
Fibricor 106
Fidelin 247
filgrastim 240
Finacea 135
finasteride 383
Finevin 135
Fioricet 6
Fioricet with Codeine 16
Fiorinal 6
Fiorinal C-1/2 16
Fiorinal C-1/4 16
Fiorinal with Codeine ... 16
fish oil 180
FK 506 267

Flagyl 84
Flagyl ER 84
Flamazine 141
Flarex 339
Flavocoxid 248
Flavoxate 384
Flebogamma 265
flecainide 98
Flector 9
Fleet 225, 227
Fleet enema 226
Fleet EZ-Prep 226
*Fleet Mineral Oil
  Enema* 228
Fleet Pain Relief 151
Fleet Phospho-Soda .. 226
Fletcher's Castoria 227
Flexeril 4
Flixonase 149
Flixotide 149
Flo-Pred 161
Flolan 129
Flomax 384
Flonase 210
Florastor 253
Florazole ER 84
Florinef 160
Flovent Diskus 376
Flovent HFA 376
Floxin 76
Floxin Otic 208
floxuridine 315
Fluanxol 355
Fluanxol Depot 355
Fluarix 260
fluconazole 25
flucytosine 30
Fludara 315
fludarabine 315
fludrocortisone 160
FluLaval 260
Flumadine 53
flumazenil 381
flumethasone 151
FluMist 260
flunarizine 278
flunisolide 210
flunisolide—inhaled 375
fluocinolone 148, 155
fluocinolone—
  ophthalmic .... PDA
fluocinolone—otic 207
fluocinonide 148
Fluor-A-Day 176
Fluor-I-Strip .... PDA
Fluor-I-Strip AT .... PDA
fluorescein .... PDA
fluoride 176
fluorometholone 339
Fluoroplex 139
fluorouracil 315
fluorouracil—topical 139
Fluothane .... PDA
Fluotic 176

Index

fluoxetine 349, 365
fluoxymesterone 155
flupenthixol 355
Flupentixol 355
fluphenazine 355
flurandrenolide 149
flurazepam 362
flurbiprofen 9
flurbiprofen—
 ophthalmic 344
flutamide 318
*Fluticasone—
 inhaled* 376
fluticasone—nasal 210
fluticasone—topical 149
fluvastatin 103
Fluviral 260
Fluvirin 260
fluvoxamine 349
Fluzone 260
FML 339
FML Forte 339
FML-S Liquifilm 338
Focalin 368
Focalin XR 368
folate Folvite 185
Folgard 185
Folgard Rx 185
folic acid
 Endocrine and
  Metabolic 184–186
 OB/GYN 308
folinic acid 329
Follistim AQ 303
*Follistim-Antagon
 Kit* 299
follitropin alfa 303
follitropin beta 303
Folotyn 316
Foltx 185
fomepizole 381
fondaparinux 234
food .... PDA
Foradil 372
Forane .... PDA
formoterol 372, 373
formulas—infant 180
Formulex 222
Fortamet 170
Fortaz 65
Forteo 193
Fortical 189
Fosamax 157
Fosamax Plus D 157
fosamprenavir 49
Fosaprepitant 214
Fosavance 157
foscarnet 40
Foscavir 40
fosfomycin 83
fosinopril 88, 109
fosphenytoin 271
fospropofol 21
Fosrenol 180

FPV 49
FreeStyle Flash 169
FreeStyle Freedom 169
*FreeStyle Freedom
 Lite* 169
FreeStyle Lite 169
French maritime pine
 tree bark 254
Frisium 269
Froben 9
Froben SR 9
Frova 276
frovatriptan 276
FSH 303
FSH and LH 303
FTC 46
Fucidin 139
Fucidin H 150
Fucithalmic 336
FUDR 315
Ful-Glo .... PDA
fulvestrant 318
Fulvicin 30
Fungizone 29
Furadantin 84
furosemide 122
fusidic acid 150
fusidic acid—
 ophthalmic 336
fusidic acid—
 topical 139
Fusilev 329
Fuzeon 43

G

G-CSF 240
G115 250
gabapentin 271
Gabitril 274
gadobenate 134
gadodiamide 134
gadopentetate 134
gadoteridol 134
gadoversetamide 134
galantamine 268
gallium 191
galsulfase .... PDA
Galzin 179
Gamastan 264
gamma
 hydroxybutyrate 284
Gammagard 265
Gammaplex 265
Gamunex 265
ganciclovir
 Antimicrobials 40
 Ophthalmology 337
Gani-Tuss NR 202
ganirelix 299
Ganite 191
Garamycin
 Antimicrobials 24
 Dermatology 139
 Ophthalmology 334

garcinia 249
Garcinia cambogia 249
Gardasil 260
garlic supplements 249
Gas-X 224
Gastrocrom 378
Gastrografin 134
GastroMARK 134
gatifloxacin—
 ophthalmic 335
Gaviscon 217
gefitinib 328
Gelclair 208
Gelnique 385
gemcitabine 316
gemfibrozil 107
gemifloxacin 77
Gemzar 316
Gengraf 266
Genisoy 256
Genoptic 334
Genotropin 192
Gentak 334
gentamicin
 Antimicrobials 24
 Ophthalmology 338
gentamicin—
 ophthalmic 334
gentamicin—topical 139
GenTeal 345
Gentran 132
Geodon 360
GHB 284
GI cocktail 223
ginger 249
ginkgo biloba 249
Ginkgold 249
Ginkoba 249
Ginsana 250
ginseng—American 249
ginseng—Asian 250
ginseng—Siberian 250
glatiramer 278
Gleevec 328
Gliadel 309
gliclazide 168
glimepiride 163, 168
glipizide 164, 168
GlucaGen 169
glucagon 169
Glucobay 162
Gluconorm 167
Glucophage 170
Glucophage XR 170
glucosamine 250
glucose home testing .. 169
Glucotrol 168
Glucotrol XL 168
Glucovance 164
Glumetza 170
glutamine .... PDA
Glutose 169
glyburide 164, 168
glycerin 225

GlycoLax 226
glycopyrrolate 230
Glycyrrhiza glabra 252
Glycyrrhiza uralensis ... 252
Glynase PresTab 168
Glyquin 153
Glysennid 227
Glyset 162
GM-CSF 241
gold sodium
 thiomalate 2
goldenseal 250
GoLytely 226
gonadotropins 303
Gonal-F 303
Gonal-F RFF Pen 303
Goody's Extra Strength
 Headache Powder 6
Goserelin 318
gramicidin 336
granisetron 213
grape seed extract 250
grapefruit juice .... PDA
Gravol 214
green goddess 223
green tea 250
Grifulvin V 30
Gris-PEG 31
griseofulvin 30
griseofulvin
 ultramicrosize 31
guaiacolsulfonate 203
guaifenesin 196–206
Guaifenex DM 202
Guaifenex PSE 202
Guaitex II SR/PSE 202
guanabenz 92
guanfacine
 Cardiovascular 93
 Psychiatry 369
guarana 251
guggul 251
guggulipid 251
Guiatuss 196
Guiatuss AC 202
Guiatuss PE 198
Guiatussin DAC 202
Gynazole 306
Gyne-Lotrimin 306
Gynodiol 297

H

H-BIG 264
H.P. Acthar Gel 171
Habitrol 366
haemophilus B
 vaccine 257, 258, 262
halcinonide 149
Halcion 363
Haldol 356
HalfLytely 226
Halfprin 7
halobetasol
 propionate 149

Index

halofantrine ....PDA
Halog.............................149
haloperidol 356
Halotestin.....................155
halothane.....................PDA
Halotussin AC...............202
Halotussin DAC 203
Harpadol 247
Harpagophytum
  procumbens 247
Havrix..........................258
hawthorn 251
HCE50 251
hCG..............................302
HCTZ 124
Healthy Woman 256
HeartCare....................251
Hectorol.......................184
helidac 220
Helixate 238
Hemabate....................306
Hemofil M 238
HepaGam B 264
Hepalean.....................235
heparin........................235
hepatitis A vaccine......258,
 262
hepatitis B immune
  globulin 264
hepatitis B vaccine 257,
  ....259, 260, 262
Hepsera.........................53
Heptovir........................46
Herceptin.....................324
heroin..........................PDA
Hespan 132
hetastarch...................132
Hexabrix 135
Hexalen 309
Hexit............................143
Hextend 132
HibTITER.....................258
Hicon...........................182
Hiprex..........................PDA
Histinex HC..................203
histrelin.......................319
Histussin D..................203
Histussin HC 203
Hizentra.......................265
homatropine
  ENT 203
  Ophthalmology 344
honey..........................251
horse chestnut seed
  extract......................251
HP-Pac........................220
huang qi......................244
huckleberry.................244
Humalog......................166
Humalog Mix 50/50 165
Humalog Mix 75/25 165
human growth
  hormone 192

human papillomavirus
  recombinant
  vaccine.....................260
Humate P.....................238
Humatrope 192
Humibid DM 203
Humibid LA..................203
Humira 1
Humulin 50/50.............165
Humulin 70/30.............165
Humulin N....................165
Humulin R....................166
Hyalgan 20
hyaluronate 20
hyaluronic acid 153
hyaluronidase..............PDA
Hycamtin.....................331
Hycoclear Tuss............203
Hycodan 203
Hycort..........................149
Hycotuss.....................204
Hyderm 149
hydralazine... 107, 111, 132
HydraSense 211
Hydrastis canadensis ..250
Hydrea 242
hydrochlorothiazide
  ....107–111, 124
hydrochlorothiazide......107
Hydrocil.......................225
hydrocodone
  Analgesics............16–19
  ENT...................201, 203,
  ....204, 206
hydrocortisone
  Dermatology ... 150, 154
  Endocrine and
    Metabolic 160
  ENT...................207, 208
hydrocortisone—
  ophthalmic 337
hydrocortisone
  acetate 149, 152
hydrocortisone
  butyrate 149
hydrocortisone
  probutate 150
hydrocortisone
  valerate 150
hydrocortisone—
  topical 149
HydroDiuril 124
Hydromorph Contin.....14
hydromorphone............14
hydroquinone........153, 155
Hydroval 150
hydroxocobalamin 382
hydroxychloroquine........3
hydroxyprogesterone
  caproate 304
hydroxypropyl
  cellulose 345
hydroxyurea 242
hydroxyzine 195

Hylan GF-20 20
hymenoptera venom 268
hyoscine 223
hyoscyamine
  Gastroenterology 223
  Urology 385, 386
Hyosol..........................223
Hyospaz.......................223
Hypaque 134
HyperHep B..................264
Hypericum
  perforatum 255
HyperRAB S/D..............266
HyperRHO S/D.............308
Hyperstat.....................191
Hypertet.......................266
Hyphanox......................26
Hypocol.......................255
Hypotears....................345
Hytone.........................149
Hytrin 94
Hytuss.........................196
Hyzaar.........................108

I

ibandronate.................157
ibritumomab 322
Ibudone 16
ibuprofen
  Analgesics......... 9, 16, 19
  ENT...........................197
ibutilide.........................99
Idamycin 313
idarubicin....................313
idursulfase..................PDA
IDV 50
Ifex 310
ifosfamide...................310
iloperidone 358
iloprost 129
Ilotycin 335
imatinib 328
Imdur 125
imiglucerase ....PDA
imipenem-cilastatin......60
imipramine 347
imiquimod 145
Imitrex.........................276
Immucyst
  Immunology 257
  Oncology..................321
immune globulin—
  intramuscular 264
immune globulin—
  intravenous 265
immune globulin—
  subcutaneous..........265
Immunine VH..............237
Immunoprin....................2
Imodium......................212
Imodium AD................212
Imodium Multi-Symptom
  Relief 212
Imogam Rabies-HT......266

Imovane 364
Imovax Rabies............261
Implanon.....................294
Imuran............................2
inamrinone..................127
Inapsine 215
Increlex.......................191
indapamide.................124
Inderal.........................118
Inderal LA....................118
Inderide.......................109
Indigo Carmine............PDA
indigotindisulfonate.....PDA
indinavir........................50
Indium DTPA...............PDA
Indocid-P.D.A..................9
Indocin 9
Indocin IV.......................9
Indocin SR......................9
indomethacin 9
Infanrix........................258
Infasurf........................377
InFed 176
Infergen57
Inflamase Forte 339
infliximab 1
influenza vaccine—
  inactivated
  injection 260
influenza vaccine—live
  intranasal 260
Infufer..........................176
INH 35
Inhibace........................87
inhibace plus 109
InnoPran XL................118
INOmax........................379
Inspra............................90
Insta-Glucose.............169
insulin—injectable
  combinations 165
insulin—injectable
  intermediate/
  long-acting 165
insulin—injectable
  short/rapid-acting.....166
Intal 378
Integrilin 114
Intelence 45
interferon alfa-2A........322
interferon alfa-2B 56
interferon alfa-n3.........56
interferon alfacon-1 56
interferon beta-1A.......278
interferon beta-1B.......278
interleukin-2 320
IntestiFlora 253
Intralipid 179
Intron A 56
Intropin 127
Intuniv.........................369
Invanz 59
Invega 359
Invega Sustenna 359

Index

Inversine 112
Invirase 51
iodixanol 135
iodoquinol .... PDA
Iodotope 182
iohexol 135
Ionamin 370
IONSYS 13
iopamidol 135
Iopidine 342
iopromide 135
Iosat 181
iothalamate 135
ioversol 135
ioxaglate 135
ioxilan 135
ipecac syrup 382
IPOL 261
ipratropium 373
ipratropium—
  inhaled 378
ipratropium—
  nasal 210
Iprivask 235
Iquix 335
irbesartan 91, 107
Iressa 328
irinotecan 329
iron dextran 176
iron polysaccharide ... 176
iron sucrose 177
Isentress 44
ISMO 125
isocarboxazid 348
isoflurane .... PDA
isometheptene 278
Isomil 180
isoniazid 35–37
isopropyl alcohol 208
isoproterenol 99
Isoptin SR 121
Isopto Atropine 343
Isopto Carbachol 341
Isopto Carpine 341
Isopto Homatropine ... 344
Isordil 125
isosorbide
  dinitrate 125, 132
isosorbide mononitrate ....
  125
isosulfan blue .... PDA
Isotamine 35
isotretinoin 137
Isovue 135
isoxsuprine 133
isradipine 119
Istalol 340
Istodax 331
Isuprel 99
itraconazole 26
ivermectin 37
ixabepilone 324
Ixempra 324

J

Jantoven 236
Janumet 164
Januvia 171
Japanese encephalitis
  vaccine 260
JE-Vax 260
Jin Fu Kang 244
Jolivette 304
Junel 287
Junel FE 287

K

K 178
K+10 178
K+8 178
K-Dur 178
K-G Elixir 178
K-Lease 178
K-Lor 178
K-Lyte 178
K-Lyte Cl 178
K-Norm 178
K-Phos 178
K-Tab 178
K-vescent 178
Kabikinase 131
Kadian 15
Kaletra 50
kanamycin .... PDA
Kantrex .... PDA
Kaochlor 178
Kaon 178
Kaon Cl 178
Kaopectate 211
*Kaopectate Stool
  Softener* 227
Kapidex 220
karela 244
Kariva 287
kava 252
Kay Ciel 178
Kayexalate 192
Kaylixir 178
Keflex 61
Kelnor 287
Kemstro 3
Kenalog
  Dermatology 150
  Endocrine and
    Metabolic 161
Kenalog in Orabase ... 150
Kepivance 317
Keppra 272
Keppra XR 272
Kerlone 115
Ketalar 21
ketamine 21
Ketek 85
ketoconazole 26
ketoconazole—
  topical 142
Ketoderm 142
ketoprofen 10
ketorolac 10
ketorolac—
  ophthalmic 345
ketotifen 378
ketotifen—
  ophthalmic 333
kidrolase 327
Kineret 1
Kinlytic 131
Kira 255
Klaron 138
Klean-Prep 226
Klonopin 361
Klonopin Wafer 361
Klor-con 178
*Klorvess
  Effervescent* 178
Klotrix 178
Koate 238
Kogenate 238
Kolyum 178
kombucha tea 252
Kondremul 228
Konsyl 225
Konsyl Fiber 225
Korean red ginseng ... 250
Kristalose 225
Ku-Zyme 231
Ku-Zyme HP 232
Kuvan .... PDA
Kwai 249
Kwellada-P 143
Kyolic 249
Kytril 213

L

L-glutamine .... PDA
L-methylfolate 183, 186
L-Thyroxine 181
labetalol 116
Lac-Hydrin 153
lacosamide 271
Lacrilube 345
Lacrisert 345
Lactaid 231
lactase 231
lactic acid 153
Lactinex 253
Lactobacillus 253
lactulose 225
Lamictal
  Neurology 271
  Psychiatry 353
Lamictal CD
  Neurology 271
  Psychiatry 353
Lamictal ODT
  Neurology 271
  Psychiatry 353
Lamictal XR 353
Lamisil
  Antimicrobials 31
  Dermatology 142
Lamisil AT 142
lamivudine 42, 43, 46
lamotrigine
  Neurology 271
  Psychiatry 353
Lamprene 34
Lanoxicaps 97
Lanoxin 97
lanreotide .... PDA
lansoprazole 220, 221
Lansoyl 228
lanthanum carbonate ... 180
Lantus 165
Lanvis 317
lapatinib 329
Lariam 33
laronidase .... PDA
Lasix 122
latanoprost 341
Latisse 341
Lectopam 361
Leena 292
leflunomide 3
Legalon 253
lenalidomide 322
Lenoltec 18
leopard's bane 244
lepirudin 236
Lescol 103
Lescol XL 103
Lessina 287
Letairis .... PDA
Letrozole 319
leucovorin 329
Leukeran 309
Leukine 241
Leuprolide 319
Leustatin 314
levalbuterol 371
Levaquin 77
Levatol 118
Levbid 223
Levemir 165
levetiracetam 272
Levitra 388
Levlen 287
Levlite 287
Levo-Dromoran 14
Levo-T 181
levobunolol 340
levocabastine—
  nasal 211
levocabastine—
  ophthalmic 333
levocarnitine 180
levocetirizine 195
levodopa 282
levofloxacin 77
levofloxacin—
  ophthalmic 335
Levolet 181
levoleucovorin 329
levonorgestrel ... 286–289,
  .... 291–294, 300

Index

levonorgestrel 1S............ 294
Levophed....................... 128
Levora............................ 287
levorphanol 14
Levothroid..................... 181
levothyroxine 181, 182
Levoxyl.......................... 181
Levsin............................ 223
Levsinex........................ 223
Levulan Kerastick........... 138
Lexapro......................... 349
Lexiva.............................. 49
Lexxel............................ 109
LI-160............................ 255
Lialda............................ 228
Librax............................ 230
Librium.......................... 361
licorice 252
Lidemol 148
Lidex.............................. 148
Lidex-E........................... 148
lidocaine 99
lidocaine—Local
  anesthetic 23
lidocaine—local
  anesthetic 23
lidocaine—topical
 153–155
lidocaine—local
  anesthetic 23
lidocaine—
  ophthalmic 345
lidocaine—topical 153
lidocaine—viscous 208
Lidoderm...................... 153
Limbitrol........................ 365
Limbitrol DS 365
Limbrel.......................... 248
Lincocin.......................... 83
Lincomycin..................... 83
lindane.......................... 143
linezolid.......................... 83
Lioresal 3
liothyronine 181, 182
Liotrix............................ 182
Lipidil EZ....................... 106
Lipidil Micro 106
Lipidil Supra 106
Lipitor........................... 103
Lipofen.......................... 106
Lipolysar....................... 255
Liposyn......................... 179
Liqui-Doss..................... 228
liraglutide 170
lisdexamfetamine.......... 369
lisinopril......... 88, 110, 111
Lithane.......................... 353
lithium........................... 353
Lithobid......................... 353
Lithostat........................ 389
Livalo............................ 104
LiveBac 253
Livostin......................... 333
Livostin Nasal Spray..... 211

LMX............................... 153
Lo/Ovral........................ 288
Locacorten Vioform....... 151
LoCHOLEST................... 101
LoCHOLEST Light.......... 101
Locoid........................... 149
Locoid Lipocream 149
Lodosyn........................ 281
lodoxamide................... 333
Loestrin........................ 288
Loestrin 24 FE 288
Loestrin FE 288
Lomine 222
Lomotil.......................... 212
lomustine 310
Loniten 112
Loperacap 212
loperamide 212
Lopid............................ 107
lopinavir-ritonavir 50
Lopressor..................... 116
Lopressor HCT.............. 109
Loprox.......................... 141
loratadine..... 194, 196, 197
lorazepam 362
Lorcet............................. 17
Lortab............................. 17
losartan.............. 91, 108
Loseasonique 288
Losec............................ 221
Lotemax........................ 339
Lotensin.......................... 87
Lotensin HCT................ 109
loteprednol 338, 339
Lotrel............................ 109
Lotriderm...................... 151
Lotrimin AF........... 141, 142
Lotrimin Ultra................ 141
Lotrisone 151
Lotronex....................... 229
lovastatin............. 102, 103
Lovaza.......................... 180
Low-Ogestrel................ 288
Loxapac........................ 356
loxapine........................ 356
Loxitane........................ 356
Lozide........................... 124
Lozol............................. 124
LPV/r.............................. 50
lubiprostone................. 228
Lucentis........................ 343
Ludiomil....................... PDA
lumefantrine 32
Lumigan........................ 341
Luminal......................... 273
Lunesta......................... 364
Lupron.......................... 319
Lupron Depot............... 319
Lupron Depot-Ped........ 319
Luride........................... 176
Lusedra.......................... 21
Lustra........................... 153
Lutera........................... 288
lutropin alfa.................. 303

Luveris.......................... 303
Luvox............................ 349
Luvox CR 349
Luxiq foam 147
Lybrel 288
Lymphazurin................ PDA
lymphocyte immune
  globulin.................... 265
Lyrica 274
Lysodren...................... 329
Lysteda......................... 243

M

M-M-R II....................... 260
M-Zole.......................... 307
M.O.S............................. 15
ma huang..................... 248
Maalox.......................... 217
MabCampath 320
Macrobid 84
Macrodantin.................. 84
Macrodex..................... 132
Macugen 343
mafenide 139
Mag-200 178
Mag-Ox 400.................. 178
magaldrate................... 218
Maganate..................... 177
Magic Mouthwash........ 209
Maglucate.................... 177
Magnacet....................... 17
magnesium carbonate
  Analgesics.................... 5
  Gastroenterology 217
magnesium chloride..... 177
magnesium citrate 225
magnesium gluconate.. 177
magnesium hydroxide
  Analgesics.................... 5
  Gastroenterology ....
    217–219, 226
magnesium oxide
  Analgesics.................... 5
  Endocrine and
    Metabolic................ 178
magnesium sulfate 178
Magnevist 134
Magtrate 177
Malarone....................... 32
malathion..................... 143
Maltodextrin................. 208
Manchurian or
  Kargasok tea 252
Mandelamine............... PDA
Manerix 348
mangafodipir 134
mannitol....................... 284
Mantoux....................... 268
maprotiline.................. PDA
maraviroc 42
Marcaine........................ 22
marijuana .... PDA
Marinol......................... 214
Marplan........................ 348

Marvelon 286, 290
Matricaria recutita—
  German chamomile... 245
Matulane...................... 311
Mavik.............................. 89
Maxair Autohaler.......... 371
Maxalt........................... 276
Maxalt MLT................... 276
Maxeran 215
Maxidone....................... 17
Maxiflor 148
Maxilene....................... 153
Maximum Strength
  Pepcid AC................. 218
Maxipime....................... 67
Maxitrol........................ 338
Maxivate....................... 147
Maxzide........................ 109
Maxzide-25................... 109
MD-Gastroview............ 134
MDMA.......................... PDA
measles mumps &
  rubella vaccine.....260, 261
measles vaccine........... PDA
Mebaral........................ PDA
mebendazole.................. 38
mecamylamine............. 112
mecasermin 191
mechlorethamine 311
Meclicot........................ 195
meclizine...................... 195
meclofenamate 10
Medihoney 251
Medispaz...................... 223
Medivert....................... 195
Medrol.......................... 160
medroxyprogesterone
  ....301, 304
medroxyprogesterone—
  injectable 304
mefenamic acid 10
mefloquine 33
Mefoxin.......................... 61
Megace......................... 304
Megace ES.................... 304
Megacillin....................... 70
megestrol..................... 304
Melaleuca
  alternifolia 256
melaleuca oil................ 256
Melanex........................ 153
melatonin..................... 252
Mellaril......................... 357
meloxicam..................... 10
melphalan.................... 311
memantine................... 269
Membrane Blue............ 346
Menactra...................... 260
Menest......................... 297
Meni-D 195
meningococcal
  vaccine..................... 260
Menjugate.................... 260
Menofem 245

Index

Menomune-A/C/Y/W-135 260
Menopur 303
Menostar 298
menotropins 303
Mentax 141
Mentha x piperita oil 253
mepenzolate 223
meperidine 14
mephobarbital .... PDA
Mephyton 187
mepivacaine 23
Mepron 37
mequinol 155
mercaptopurine 316
meropenem 60
Merrem IV 60
Mersyndol with Codeine 17
Meruvax II .... PDA
mesalamine 228
Mesasal 228
mesna 317
Mesnex 317
Mestinon 279
Mestinon Timespan 279
mestranol 289, 290
Metadate CD 369
Metadate ER 369
Metadol 14
Metaglip 164
Metamucil 225
Metanx 186
metaproterenol 371
Metastron 326
metaxalone 4
metformin 162–164, 170
methacholine 379
methadone 14
Methadose 14
methamphetamine ...... PDA
methazolamide 340
methenamine 385–387
methenamine hippurate .... PDA
methenamine mandelate .... PDA
Methergine 306
methimazole 181
Methitest 156
methocarbamol 5
methohexital 21
methotrexate 3
methotrimeprazine 356
methoxsalen 145
methscopolamine
 ENT 200
 Gastroenterology 224
methsuximide .... PDA
methyclothiazide 124
methylaminolevulinate ... 139
methylcellulose 225
methylcobalamin .. 183, 186
methyldopa 93, 107

methylene blue
 Toxicology 382
 Urology 385, 386
methylenedioxymetham- phetamine .... PDA
methylergonovine 306
Methylin 369
Methylin ER 369
methylnaltrexone 231
methylphenidate 369
methylprednisolone 160
methylsulfonylmethane 252
methyltestosterone
 Endocrine and Metabolic 156
 OB/GYN 300, 301
metipranolol 340
metoclopramide 215
metolazone 124
Metopirone 171
metoprolol 109, 116
Metozolv ODT 215
MetroCream 139
MetroGel 139
MetroGel-Vaginal 307
MetroLotion 139
metronidazole
 Antimicrobials 84
 Gastroenterology 220
metronidazole— topical 139
metronidazole— vaginal 307
Metvix 139
Metvixia 139
metyrapone 171
metyrosine 112
Mevacor 103
mexiletine 99
Mexitil 99
Miacalcin 189
micafungin 29
Micardis 91
Micardis HCT 109
Micardis Plus 109
Micatin 142
miconazole 307
miconazole—topical 155
miconazole—buccal 27
miconazole—topical 142
Micort-HC Lipocream 149
Micozole 307
MICRhoGAM 308
Micro-K 178
Micro-K LS 178
microgestin fe 289
Micronor 304
Microzide 124
Midamor 123
midazolam 21
midodrine 128
Midrin 278
Mifeprex 308

mifepristone 308
MIG-99 248
miglitol 162
miglustat .... PDA
Migquin 278
Migra-Lief 248
Migranal 277
MigraSpray 248
Migratine 278
Migrazone 278
mild and strong silver protein 256
Milk of Magnesia 226
milk thistle 253
milnacipran 284
milrinone 128
Min-Ovral 287, 289
mineral oil 228
Minestrin 1/20 288
Minipress 93
Minirin 191
Minitran 126
Minizide 109
Minocin 80
minocycline 80
Minox 154
minoxidil 112
Minoxidil for Men 154
minoxidil—topical 154
Miochol-E 341
Miostat 341
MiraLax 226
Mirapex 281
Mirapex ER 281
Mircette 289
mirtazapine 352
misoprostol
 Analgesics 8
 Gastroenterology 224
misoprostol- OB 302
mitomycin 313
Mitomycin-C 313
mitotane 329
mitoxantrone 313
MMRV 261
Moban 356
Mobic 10
Mobicox 10
moclobemide 348
modafinil 370
Modecate 355
Modeten 355
Modicon 289
Moduret 109
Moduretic 109
moexipril 89, 110
Mogadon 363
molindone 356
mometasone— inhaled 376
mometasone—nasal 210
mometasone—topical ... 150
Momordica charantia 244

Monarc-M 238
Monascus purpureus 255
Monazole 307
Monistat 307
Monistat 1-Day 307
monobenzone 154
Monoclate P 238
Monocor 115
Monodox 79
monogyna 251
Monoket 125
Mononessa 289
Mononine 237
Monopril 88
Monopril HCT 109
montelukast 376
Monurol 83
Morinda citrifolia 253
morphine 15
Motilium 214
Motofen 212
Motrin 9
Movana 255
Moviprep 226
Moxatag 72
moxifloxacin 78
moxifloxacin— ophthalmic 335
Mozobil 242
MS Contin 15
MSIR 15
MSM 252
Mu Tong 244
Mucaine 217
Mucinex 196
mucinex d 198
Mucinex DM 198
Mucomyst
 Pulmonary 377
 Toxicology 380
Multaq 98
MultiHance 134
multivitamins 186
mumps vaccine .... PDA
Mumpsvax .... PDA
mupirocin 140
Murine Ear 207
Muse 387
Mustargen 311
Mutamycin 313
MVC 42
MVI 186
Myambutol 34
Mycamine 29
Mycelex
 Antimicrobials 25
 Dermatology 141
Mycelex 7 306
Mycelex-3 306
Mycobutin 35
Mycolog II 151
mycophenolate mofetil 267

Mycostatin
   Antimicrobials............ 31
   Dermatology.............. 142
   OB/GYN 307
Mydfrin................... 344
Mydriacyl................ 344
Myfortic.................. 267
Mylanta
   ENT 209
   Gastroenterology 218
Mylanta Children's 173
Myleran 309
Mylicon 224
Myobloc 284
Myocet...................... 312
Myochrysine................. 2
Myotonachol............... 386
Myozyme....................PDA
Mysoline................... 274
Mytelase....................PDA

N

N-acetyl-5-
   methoxytryptamine.... 252
N-acetylcysteine 380
n-n-diethyl-m-toluamide......
   152
NABI-HB 264
nabilone 215
nabumetone 11
nadolol 108, 117
Nadopen-V 70
nafarelin 299
nafcillin........................ 71
naftifine 142
Naftin......................... 142
Naglazyme..................PDA
nalbuphine 12
Nalcrom...................... 378
Nalfon ....PDA
naloxone
   Analgesics.................. 19
   Psychiatry................ 366
naltrexone 366
Namenda..................... 269
Namenda XR 269
naphazoline 332
Naphcon..................... 332
Naphcon-A 332
NapraPac 11
Naprelan 11
Naprosyn 11
naproxen
   Analgesics................. 11
   ENT........................ 196
   Neurology 277
naratriptan................... 276
Narcan 19
Nardil 348
Naropin ....PDA
Nasacort AQ............... 210
Nasacort HFA.............. 210
NaSal 211
NasalCrom 210

Nasalide..................... 210
Nasarel...................... 210
Nascobal 184
Nasonex..................... 210
natalizumab................. 279
nateglinide.................. 167
Natrecor 133
Navane....................... 357
Navelbine 325
Nebcin 25
nebivolol 117
NebuPent..................... 38
Necon 289
Necon 1/50 289
Necon 10/11 285
Necon 7/7/7................ 293
nedocromil—inhaled ... 379
nedocromil—
   ophthalmic 334
nefazodone.................. 352
nelarabine................... 316
nelfinavir...................... 51
Nemasol Sodium ....PDA
Nembutal 22
Neo-Fradin 231
Neo-Synephrine
   Cardiovascular.......... 128
   ENT......................... 211
neomycin
   Dermatology 140,
   .... 141, 150
   ENT........................ 207
   Ophthalmology
   336–338
neomycin—oral 231
Neoprofen...................... 9
Neoral........................ 266
Neosar....................... 310
Neosporin Cream......... 140
Neosporin ointment...... 141
Neosporin ointment—
   ophthalmic............. 336
Neosporin solution—
   ophthalmic............. 336
neostigmine 279
Neovisc....................... 20
nepafenac 345
Nephrocap 186
Nephrovite 186
Neptazane................... 340
Nesacaine ....PDA
nesiritide.................... 133
NESP 239
nettle root................... 253
Neulasta..................... 240
Neumega 240
Neupogen 240
Neupro....................... 282
Neurontin 271
Neutra-Phos............... 178
Nevanac 345
nevirapine.................... 45
Nexavar 331
Nexium 220

NFV 51
niacin
   Cardiovascular
   .... 102, 104
   Endocrine and
     Metabolic.............. 186
Niacinamide................ 184
Niacor........................ 186
Niaspan...................... 186
Niastase..................... 237
nicardipine.................. 119
NicoDerm CQ.............. 366
Nicolar....................... 186
Nicorette.................... 366
Nicorette DS............... 366
Nicorette inhaler......... 366
nicotine gum 366
nicotine inhalation
   system 366
nicotine lozenge 366
nicotine nasal
   spray 366
nicotine patches........... 366
Nicotinic acid 186
Nicotrol...................... 366
Nicotrol Inhaler........... 366
Nicotrol NS 366
Nidazol 84
nifedipine.................... 120
Niferex...................... 176
Niferex-150 176
Nilandron 320
nilotinib....................... 330
Nilstat
   Antimicrobials.......... 31
   Dermatology 142
   OB/GYN 307
nilutamide................... 320
Nimbex 23
nimodipine 284
Nimotop..................... 284
Nipent 316
Niravam 363
nisoldipine 120
nitazoxanide.................. 38
nitisinone...................PDA
Nitoman 284
nitrazepam 363
nitric oxide 379
Nitro-BID 125
Nitro-Dur................... 126
nitrofurantoin............... 84
nitroglycerin intravenous
   infusion 125
nitroglycerin
   ointment................ 125
nitroglycerin spray........ 126
nitroglycerin
   sublingual 126
nitroglycerin sustained
   release 126
nitroglycerin
   transdermal 126
Nitrolingual................. 126

NitroMist 126
Nitropress................... 112
nitroprusside................ 112
NitroQuick 126
Nitrostat.................... 126
nitrous oxide..............PDA
Nix............................ 143
nizatidine.................... 219
Nizoral
   Antimicrobials........... 26
   Dermatology 142
NoDoz........................ 368
Nolvadex.................... 305
noni 253
Nor-Q.D. 304
Nora-BE..................... 304
Norco 17
Norcuron..................... 24
Nordette 289
Norditropin 192
Norditropin NordiFlex.... 192
Norelgestromin............ 296
norepinephrine............. 128
norethindrone.......285–290,
   .... 292, 293, 300,
   .... 301, 304
Norflex 5
norfloxacin.................... 76
Norgesic 6
norgestimate.........289–291,
   .... 293, 294, 301
norgestrel..... 286, 288, 290
Norinyl 1+35............... 289
Norinyl 1+50............... 289
Noritate 139
Noroxin 76
Norpace....................... 97
Norpace CR 97
Norpramin.................. 346
Nortrel 290
nortrel 7/7/7 293
nortriptyline................. 347
Norvasc..................... 119
Norvir 51
Nostrilla 211
Novafed A................... 204
Novamoxin................... 72
Novantrone 313
Novarel 302
Novasen 7
Novasoy..................... 256
Novocain ....PDA
Novolin 70/30............. 165
Novolin N................... 165
Novolin R................... 166
NovoLog..................... 166
Novolog Mix 50/50....... 165
Novolog Mix 70/30....... 165
NovoRapid................. 166
NovoSeven................. 237
NovoSeven RT 237
Novothyrox................. 181
Noxafil 27
Nozinan 356

Index

Nplate 242
Nu-Iron 150 176
Nubain 12
Nucynta 20
NuLev 223
NuLytely 226
Numby Stuff 153
Nupercainal 151
Nuprin 9
Nursoy 180
Nutramigen Lipil 180
NutreStore .... PDA
Nutropin 192
Nutropin AQ 192
Nutropin Depot 192
Nuvaring 296
Nuvigil 367
NVP 45
Nyaderm
  Antimicrobials 31
  Dermatology 142
  OB/GYN 307
nystatin
  Antimicrobials 31
  Dermatology 151
nystatin—topical 142
nystatin—vaginal 307
Nytol 195

O

oatmeal 154
Ocean 211
Octagam 265
Octostim 191
octreotide 231
Ocufen 344
Ocuflox 335
Ocupress 340
Oenothera biennis 248
Oesclim 298
Ofatumumab 322
Off 152
ofloxacin 76
ofloxacin—
  ophthalmic 335
ofloxacin—otic 207
Ogen 299
Ogestrel 290
olanzapine 359, 365
Oleptro 352
olmesartan 91, 107,
  .... 108, 110
olopatadine 333
olopatadine—nasal 211
olsalazine 229
Olux 147
omalizumab 379
omega 3 fatty acids 180
omega-3-acid ethyl
  esters 180
omeprazole 221, 222
Omnaris 209
Omnicef 64
Omnipaque 135

Omniscan 134
Omnitrope 192
Oncaspar 330
Oncotice
  Immunology 257
  Oncology 321
Oncovin 325
ondansetron 213
OneTouch Ultra 169
OneTouch UltraMin 169
Onglyza 171
Ontak 321
Onxol 325
Opana 15
Ophthaine 345
Ophthetic 345
opium
  Gastroenterology 212
  Urology 384
opium tincture 212
oprelvekin 240
Oprisine 2
Opticrom 333
OptiMARK 134
Optipranolol 340
Optiray 135
Optivar 332
Oracea 79
Oracit 390
Oracort 150
OraDisc A 208
Oramorph SR 15
Orap 356
Orapred 161
Orapred ODT 161
oraquix 23
Oravig 27
Orazinc 179
orciprenaline 371
Orencia 1
Oretic 124
Orfadin .... PDA
Orgalutran 299
orlistat 231
orphenadrine 5, 6
Ortho Evra 296
Ortho Novum 10/11 285
Ortho Tri-Cyclen 293
Ortho Tri-Cyclen LO 293
Ortho-Cept 290
Ortho-Cyclen 290
Ortho-Est 299
Ortho-Novum 1/35 290
Ortho-Novum 1/50 290
Ortho-novum 7/7/7 293
Orthovisc 20
Orudis 10
Orudis KT 10
Orudis SR 10
Oruvail 10
Orvaten 128
Os-Cal 173
oseltamivir 53
Osmitrol 284

Osmoprep 226
Osteoforte 184
others 214
Ovcon-35 290
OVCON-50 290
Ovide 143
Ovidrel 302
Ovol 224
ovral 290
oxacillin 72
oxaliplatin 326
Oxandrin 156
oxandrolone 156
oxaprozin 11
oxazepam 363
oxcarbazepine 273
Oxeze Turbuhaler 372
oxiconazole 142
Oxilan 135
Oxistat 142
Oxizole 142
oxprenolol 117
Oxsoralen-Ultra 145
Oxyacantha 251
oxybate 284
Oxybutyn 385
oxybutynin 385
Oxycocet 18
Oxycodan 18
oxycodone 15–18
OxyContin 15
OxyFAST 15
OxyIR 15
oxymetazoline 211
oxymetholone .... PDA
oxymorphone 15
oxytocin 302
Oxytrol 385
Oyst-Cal 173

P

P.C.E. 68
Pacerone 94
Pacis 321
paclitaxel 325
PAH 390
Palgic 194
Palgic DS 204
palifermin 317
paliperidone 359
palivizumab 57
palonosetron 213
pamabrom 21
Pamelor 347
pamidronate 158
Pamine 224
Pamine Forte 224
Panadol 19
Panafil 154
Panax ginseng 250
Panax
  quinquefolius L. 249
Pancrease 232
pancreatin 231

Pancreaze 232
Pancrecarb 232
pancrelipase 232
pancuronium 23
Pandel 150
panitumumab 323
Panixine DisperDose 61
Panretin 151
Pantoloc 221
pantoprazole 221
pantothenic acid
  .... 184, 186
papain 154
papaverine 133
para-aminosalicylic
  acid .... PDA
paracetamol 19
Parafon Forte DSC 4
Paraplatin 326
Parcopa 281
paregoric 212
paricalcitol 187
Pariet 222
Parlodel 189
Parnate 348
paromomycin 38
paroxetine 350
Parvolex 380
PAS .... PDA
Paser .... PDA
Pataday 333
Patanase 211
Patanol 333
Paullinia cupana 251
Pausinystalia
  yohimbe 257
Pavulon 23
Paxil 350
Paxil CR 350
pazopanib 330
PCO 250
PediaCare Infants'
  Decongestant
  Drops 206
Pediapred 161
pediarix 260
Pediatrix 19
Pediazole 69
Pediotic 207
PedvaxHIB 258
Peg-Intron 57
Peg-Lyte 226
Peganone .... PDA
pegaptanib 343
pegaspargase 330
Pegasys 57
pegfilgrastim 240
peginterferon alfa-2a 57
peginterferon alfa-2b 57
pegvisomant192
pemetrexed 316
pemirolast 334
Penbritin 73
penbutolol 118

Index

penciclovir ... 146
penicillamine ... 382
penicillin G ... 70
penicillin v ... 70
Penlac ... 141
Pentam ... 38
pentamidine ... 38
Pentasa ... 228
pentazocine ... 12, 18
pentetate indium ... PDA
pentobarbital ... 22
Pentolair ... 343
pentosan ... 387
pentostatin ... 316
Pentothal ... 22
pentoxifylline ... 133
Pepcid ... 218
Pepcid AC ... 218
Pepcid Complete ... 219
peppermint oil ... 253
Peptic Relief ... 219
Pepto-Bismol ... 211
Percocet ... 18
Percocet-demi ... 18
Percodan ... 18
Percolone ... 15
Perforomist ... 372
Pergonal ... 303
Peri-Colace ... 228
Periactin ... 194
Peridex ... 208
perindopril ... 89
Periogard ... 208
Periostat ... 79
Perlane ... 153
permethrin ... 143
perphenazine ... 356, 365
Persantine ... 114
Petadolex ... 245
Petasites hybridus ... 245
Petaforce ... 245
pethidine ... 14
petrolatum ... 345
Pexeva ... 350
PGE1
  Gastroenterology ... 224
  OB/GYN ... 302
PGE2 ... 302
Pharmorubicin ... 313
Phazyme ... 224
Phenazo ... 387
phenazopyridine ... 387
phendimatrizine ... 370
phenelzine ... 348
Phenergan ... 216
Phenergan VC ... 204
Phenergan VC w/ codeine ... 204
Phenergan with Codeine ... 204
Phenergan/ Dextromethorphan ... 204
Pheniramine ... 332

phenobarbital
  Gastroenterology ... 222, 223
  Neurology ... 273
phenoxybenzamine ... 112
phentermine ... 370
phentolamine ... 112
Phenyl salicylate ... 385, 386
phenylephrine ... 196-199, 201, 203-206
phenylephrine— intravenous ... 128
phenylephrine— nasal ... 211
phenylephrine— ophthalmic ... 344
Phenytek ... 273
phenytoin ... 273
Phoslax ... 226
PhosLo ... 173
Phospholine Iodide ... 341
phosphorated carbohydrates ... 215
phosphorus ... 178
Photofrin ... 330
Phrenilin ... 6
Phyllocontin ... 377
physostigmine ... 382
Phyto Joint ... 247
phytonadione ... 187
Phytosoya ... 256
pilocarpine ... 209
pilocarpine— ophthalmic ... 341
Pilopine HS ... 341
pimecrolimus ... 146
pimozide ... 356
Pin-X ... 39
pinaverium ... 232
pindolol ... 118
Pinworm ... 39
pioglitazone ... 162, 163, 165
Piper methysticum ... 252
piperacillin ... 74
piperacillin- tazobactam ... 74
piperonyl butoxide ... 143, 144
pirbuterol ... 371
piroxicam ... 11
pitavastatin ... 104
Pitocin ... 302
Pitressin ... 193
plague vaccine ... 261
Plan B ... 294
Plan B One-Step ... 294
Plaquenil ... 3
Plasbumin ... 131
plasma ... PDA
plasma protein fraction ... 132
Plasmanate ... 132

Plasmatein ... 132
Platinol-AQ ... 326
Plavix ... 113
Plendil ... 119
plerixafor ... 242
Pletal ... 132
Pliagis ... 154
Pneumo 23 ... 261
pneumococcal 23-valent vaccine ... 261
pneumococcal 7-valent conjugate vaccine ... 261
Pneumovax ... 261
Podocon-25 ... 146
Podofilm ... 146
podofilox ... 146
Podofin ... 146
podophyllin ... 146
Polaramine ... 195
policosanol ... 253
polio vaccine ... 260, 261
Polocaine ... 23
poly-l-lactic acid ... 154
polycarbophil ... 225
Polycitra ... 390
Polycitra-K ... 390
Polycitra-LC ... 390
polyethylene glycol ... 226
polyethylene glycol with electrolytes ... 226
polymyxin
  Dermatology ... 140, 141, 150
  ENT ... 207
  Ophthalmology .. 336-338
Polyphenon E ... 250
Polysporin ... 141
Polysporin— ophthalmic ... 336
Polytar ... 152
polythiazide ... 109
Polytopic ... 141
Polytrim— ophthalmic ... 337
Ponstan ... 10
Ponstel ... 10
Pontocaine346
poractant ... 379
porfimer ... 330
Portia ... 291
posaconazole ... 27
Potaba ... PDA
potassium ... 178
potassium iodide ... 181
potassium p-aminobenzoate ... PDA
Power-Dophilus ... 253
PPD ... 268
Pradaxa ... 241
Pralatrexate ... 316
pralidoxime ... 381, 383
pramipexole ... 281
pramlintide ... 170
pramosone ... 154

Pramox HC ... 154
pramoxine ... 151, 154
prandimet ... 164
Prandin ... 167
Prasterone ... 247
prasugrel ... 114
Pravachol ... 104
pravastatin ... 104
praziquantel ... 38
prazosin ... 93, 109
Precedex ... 21
Precose ... 162
Pred Forte ... 339
Pred G ... 338
Pred Mild ... 339
prednicarbate ... 150
prednisolone ... 161
prednisolone— ophthalmic ... 337, 338
prednisone ... 161
Prefest ... 301
pregabalin ... 274
Pregnyl ... 302
Prelone ... 161
Premarin ... 298
Premesis-RX ... 308
Premphase ... 301
Premplus ... 301
Prempro ... 301
Prepidil ... 302
Pressyn AR ... 193
Pretz ... 211
Prevacid
  Analgesics ... 11
  Gastroenterology ... 221
Prevalite ... 101
Prevex-HC ... 149
previfem ... 291
Prevnar ... 261
PrevPac ... 220
Prezista ... 49
Prialt ... PDA
Priftin ... 36
prilocaine
  Anesthesia ... 23
  Dermatology ... 153
Prilosec ... 221
Primacor ... 128
Primadophilus ... 253
primaquine ... 33
Primaxin ... 60
primidone ... 274
Primsol ... 86
Principen ... 73
Prinivil ... 88
Prinzide ... 110
Priorix ... 260
Pristiq ... 351
Privigen ... 265
Pro-Banthine ... 224
Pro-Fast ... 370
ProAir HFA ... 370
ProAmatine ... 128
probenecid ... 172, 173

Index

Probiotica..................... 253
probiotics..................... 253
procainamide............... 100
procaine....................... PDA
procaine penicillin.... 70, 71
procarbazine................ 311
Procardia..................... 120
Procardia XL................ 120
Prochieve..................... 305
prochlorperazine........... 216
Procrit......................... 239
Proctocream HC........... 149
Proctofoam HC............. 151
Proctofoam NS............. 151
procyanidolic
   oligomers.................. 250
Prodium....................... 387
Prodium Plain.............. 225
Progest........................ PDA
progesterone gel........... 305
progesterone in oil........ 305
progesterone
   micronized................ 305
progesterone vaginal
   insert....................... 305
Proglycem.................... 191
Prograf........................ 267
proguanil....................... 32
Prohance..................... 134
Prolastin..................... 377
Proleukin.................... 320
Prolia.......................... 190
Prolixin....................... 355
Proloprim..................... 86
Promacta.................... PDA
Promensil................... 254
promethazine
   ENT.......................... 204
   Gastroenterology........ 216
Prometrium................. 305
Pronestyl..................... 100
Propaderm.................. 147
propafenone................ 100
Propanthel.................. 224
propantheline.............. 224
proparacaine............... 345
Propasi HP.................. 303
Propecia..................... 383
Propine....................... 342
propofol....................... 22
propoxyphene..... 15, 16, 19
propranolol......... 109, 118
Propulsid.................... 230
Propyl Thyracil............ 182
propylene glycol........... 208
propylthiouracil............ 182
ProQuad..................... 261
ProQuin XR.................. 75
Proscar....................... 383
Prosed/DS.................. 385
Prosobee.................... 180
ProSom...................... 362
prostaglandin E1.......... 387
Prostep...................... 366

Prostigmin................... 279
Prostin E2................... 302
Prostin VR................... 387
Prostin VR Pediatric..... 387
protamine.................... 242
protein C concentrate... PDA
Protenate.................... 132
Protonix...................... 221
Protopam.................... 383
Protopic...................... 146
protriptyline................. 347
Protropin..................... 192
Protylol....................... 222
Proventil HFA............... 370
Provera....................... 304
Provigil....................... 370
Provocholine................ 379
Prozac........................ 349
Prozac Weekly............. 349
prussian blue............... PDA
Pseudo-Chlor............... 204
pseudoephedrine.... 196–206
Pseudofrin................... 206
Psorcon E................... 148
Psyllium...................... 225
PTU............................ 182
Pulmicort Flexhaler....... 374
Pulmicort Respules...... 374
Pulmozyme.................. 378
Puregon...................... 303
Purinethol................... 316
PVF-K........................... 70
pycnogenol.................. 254
pygeum africanum....... 254
Pylera......................... 220
pyrantel........................ 39
pyrazinamide........... 35, 37
pyrethrins............. 143, 144
Pyridiate..................... 387
Pyridium..................... 387
pyridostigmine............. 279
pyridoxal phosphate..... 186
pyridoxine
   Endocrine and
      Metabolic......... 183–187
   Gastroenterology........ 214
   OB/GYN.................... 308
pyrilamine................... 205
pyrimethamine......... 32, 39
PZA.............................. 35

Q

Quadramet.................. 326
Qualaquin..................... 33
Quasense.................... 291
Quelicin........................ 23
Questran..................... 101
Questran Light............. 101
quetiapine................... 359
Quick-Pep................... 368
quinapril............... 89, 107
quinidine..................... 100
quinine......................... 33
quinupristin.................. 84

Quixin......................... 335
QVAR.......................... 374

R

R&C............................ 143
RabAvert..................... 261
rabeprazole................. 222
rabies immune globulin
   human..................... 266
rabies vaccine.............. 261
Rabies Vaccine
   Adsorbed................. 261
Radiogardase............... PDA
RAL.............................. 44
rally pack.................... 180
raloxifene.................... 305
raltegravir..................... 44
ramelteon.................... 364
ramipril........................ 89
Ranexa....................... 133
ranibizumab................ 343
Raniclor........................ 61
ranitidine.................... 219
ranolazine................... 133
Rapamune.................. 267
rasagiline.................... 282
rasburicase................. 330
Razadyne.................... 268
Razadyne ER............... 268
Reactine..................... 194
Rebetol........................ 58
Rebif.......................... 278
Reclast....................... 158
reclipsen..................... 291
Recombinate............... 238
Recombivax HB............ 259
recothrom................... 243
red clover................... 254
red clover isoflavone
   extract..................... 254
red wine..................... PDA
red yeast rice.............. 255
Redoxon..................... 183
ReFacto...................... 238
Refludan..................... 236
Refresh....................... 344
Refresh PM................. 345
Refresh Tears.............. 345
Regitine...................... 112
Reglan........................ 215
Regonal...................... 279
Regranex.................... 152
Rejuva-A..................... 138
Relafen........................ 11
Relenza........................ 53
Relistor....................... 231
Relpax........................ 276
Remeron..................... 352
Remeron SolTab........... 352
Remicade...................... 1
Remifemin................... 245
remifentanil.................. 22
Reminyl...................... 268
Remodulin................... 130

Renagel...................... 180
Renedil....................... 119
Reno-60...................... 134
Reno-DIP.................... 134
RenoCal...................... 134
Renografin.................. 134
Renova....................... 138
Renvela...................... 180
ReoPro....................... 113
repaglinide........... 164, 167
Repel......................... 152
Repronex.................... 303
Requip....................... 282
Requip XL................... 282
Rescriptor................... PDA
Resectisol................... 284
reserpine...................... 94
RespiGam.................... 266
Restasis..................... 345
Restoril....................... 363
Restylane.................... 153
retapamulin................. 141
Retavase..................... 130
reteplase.................... 130
Retin-A....................... 138
Retin-A Micro.............. 138
Retisert...................... PDA
Retisol-A..................... 138
Retrovir........................ 47
Revatio
   Cardiovascular.......... 129
   Urology.................... 388
ReVia......................... 366
Revlimid..................... 322
Reyataz........................ 48
Rheomacrodex............. 132
Rheumatrex................... 3
Rhinalar...................... 210
Rhinocort Aqua............ 209
RHO immune
   globulin................... 308
RhoGAM..................... 308
Rhophylac.................. 308
Rhotral....................... 115
Ribasphere................... 58
ribavirin—inhaled.......... 58
ribavirin—oral............... 58
riboflavin............. 183, 184,
                        186, 188
RID............................ 144
Ridaura......................... 2
Rideril........................ 357
rifabutin....................... 35
Rifadin......................... 36
Rifamate....................... 36
rifampin................. 36, 37
rifapentine.................... 36
Rifater......................... 37
rifaximin....................... 84
rilonacept................... PDA
Rilutek....................... 284
riluzole....................... 284
Rimactane.................... 36
rimantadine.................. 53

Index

rimexolone 339
Rimostil 254
Rimso-50 386
Riomet 170
Riopan 218
risedronate 158
Risperdal 360
Risperdal Consta 360
risperidone 360
Ritalin 369
Ritalin LA 369
Ritalin SR 369
ritonavir 51
Rituxan 323
rituximab 323
rivastigmine 268
Rivotril 361
rizatriptan 276
Robaxin 5
Robaxin-750 5
Robinul 230
Robinul Forte 230
Robitussin 196
Robitussin AC 205
Robitussin CF 198
Robitussin Cough 196
Robitussin DAC 205
Robitussin DM 198
Rocaltrol 183
Rocephin 66
rocuronium 23
Rofact 36
Roferon-A 322
Rogaine 154
Rogaine Extra
  Strength 154
Rogitine 112
Rolaids 218
Romazicon 381
Romidepsin 331
romiplostin 242
Rondec 205
Rondec DM 205
Rondec Infant Drops ... 205
ropinirole 282
ropivacaine .... PDA
Rosasol 139
rosiglitazone 163, 165
Rosula 137
Rosula NS 138
rosuvastatin 104
Rotarix 261
RotaTeq 261
rotavirus vaccine 261
rotigotine 282
Rowasa 228
Roxanol 15
Roxicet 18
Roxicodone 15
Rozerem 364
RSV immune
  globulin 266
RTV 51
RU-486 308

rubella vaccine .... PDA
Rubex 313
Rubini 247
Rufen 9
rufinamide 274
Rylosol 101
Ryna-12 S 205
Rynatan 205
Rynatan pediatric
  suspension 205
Rythmodan 97
Rythmodan-LA 97
Rythmol 100
Rythmol SR 100
Ryzolt 20

S

S-2 378
S-Adenosylmethionine ... 255
S.A.S. 229
Sabril 275
Saccharomyces
  boulardii 253
Saint John's Wort 255
Saizen 192
Salagen 209
Salazopyrin En-tabs 229
salbutamol 370
Salflex 8
salicin 257
Salicis cortex 257
salicylic acid 138
saline nasal spray 211
Salix alba 257
salmeterol 372
Salofalk 228
salsalate 8
Salvia miltiorrhiza 247
SAM-e 255
samarium 153 326
Sambucol 247
Sambucus nigra 247
sammy 255
Samsca 193
Sanctura 385
Sanctura XR 385
Sancuso 213
Sandimmune 266
Sandostatin 231
Sandostatin LAR 231
Sans-Acne 137
Saphris 358
sapropterin .... PDA
saquinavir 51
Sarafem 349
sargramostim 241
Sativex 20
Savella 284
saw palmetto 255
saxagliptin 171
Scopace 216
scopolamine 216, 223
Sculptra 154

SeaMist 211
Seasonale 291
Seasonique 291
Secobarbital .... PDA
Seconal .... PDA
SecreFlo 232
secretin 232
Sectral 115
Sedapap 6
Select 1/35 289
selegiline 283
selegiline—
  transdermal 348
selenium sulfide 155
Selsun 155
Selzentry 42
Semprex-D 205
senna 227, 228
sennosides 228
Senokot 227
Senokot-S 228
SenokotXTRA 227
Sensipar 190
Sensorcaine 22
Septocaine 22
Septra 78
Serax 363
Serc 283
Serenoa repens 255
Serevent Diskus 372
Seromycin .... PDA
Serophene 303
Seroquel 359
Seroquel XR 359
Serostim 192
Serostim LQ 192
Serpasil 94
sertaconazole 142
sertraline 350
sevelamer 180
Seville orange 245
Sevoflurane .... PDA
Sevorane .... PDA
shark cartilage 255
Sibelium 278
Siladryl 195
sildenafil
  Cardiovascular 129
  Urology 388
Silenor 347
Silvadene 141
silver ion 256
silver—colloidal 256
Silybum marianum 253
silymarin 253
simcor 104
simethicone 212, 218,
  224
Similac 180
Simulect 266
simvastatin 104, 105
sinecatechins 146
Sinemet 281
Sinemet CR 281

Sinequan 347
Singulair 376
Sinupret 247
sirolimus 267
sitagliptin 164, 171
Skelaxin 4
Skelid 158
Sl. 178
Slo-Niacin 186
Slow FE 175
Slow-Fe 175
Slow-Mag 177
Slow-Trasicor 117
smallpox vaccine 262
smoking .... PDA
sodium benzoate 189
sodium iodide I-131 ... 182
Sodium Iodide I-131
  Therapeutic 182
sodium
  phenylacetate 189
sodium phosphate
  Gastroenterology 226
  Urology 386, 387
sodium polystyrene
  sulfonate 192
sodium valproate 275
Solag 155
Solage 155
Solaquin 153
Solaraze 138
solifenacin 385
Soliris .... PDA
Solodyn 80
Soltamox 305
Solu-Cortef 160
Solu-Medrol 160
Solugel 136
Soma 4
Soma Compound 6
Soma Compound with
  Codeine 18
somatropin 192
Somatuline Depot ..... PDA
Somavert 192
Sominex 195
Somnote 364
Sonata 364
sorafenib 331
sorbitol 227
Soriatane 144
sotalol 101
Sotret 137
soy 256
Soyalac 180
Spacol 223
Spasdel 223
Spectracef 64
Spiriva 379
spironolactone 90, 107
Sporanox 26
sprintec 291
Sprycel 327
SQV 51

Index

SSD 141
SSKI 181
Stadol 12
Stadol NS 12
Stalevo 282
standardized extract
    WS 1442—Crataegutt
    novo 251
starch 151
Starlix 167
Starnoc 364
Statex 15
Stavzor
    Neurology 275
    Psychiatry 354
Stay Awake 368
Stelara 145
Stelazine 357
Stemetil 216
Sterapred 161
stevia 256
Stevia rebaudiana 256
Stieprox shampoo 141
Stieva-A 138
Stimate 191
stinging nettle 253
Strattera 367
Streptase 131
streptokinase 131
streptomycin 24
streptozocin 311
Striant 156
Stridex Pads 138
Stromectol 37
strontium-89 326
Sublimaze 13
Suboxone 366
Subutex 12
succimer 383
succinylcholine 23
sucralfate
    ENT 209
    Gastroenterology 224
Sudafed 206
Sudafed 12 Hour 206
Sudafed PE 206
Sufenta 22
sufentanil 22
Sular 120
Sulcrate 224
Sulf-10 337
Sulfacet-R 138
sulfacetamide
    Dermatology ... 136–138
    Ophthalmology 337, 338
sulfacetamide—
    ophthalmic 337
sulfacetamide—
    topical 138
sulfadiazine 78
Sulfadoxine 32
Sulfamylon 139
sulfasalazine 229

Sulfatrim 78
sulfisoxazole 69
sulfonated phenolics 208
sulfur 136–138
sulfuric acid 208
sulindac 11
sumatriptan 276, 277
Sumycin 80
sunitinib 331
sunscreen .... PDA
Supartz 20
Supeudol 15
Supprelin LA 319
Suprane .... PDA
Suprax 64
Supro 256
Surfak 227
Surgam 11
Surgam SR 11
Surmontil .... PDA
Surpass 173
Survanta 377
Sustiva 44
Sutent 331
Swim-Ear 208
Symax 223
symbicort 373
symbyax 365
Symlin 170
Symlinpen 170
Symmetrel 52
Synacort 149
Synacthen 171
Synagis 57
Synalar 148
Synalgos-DC 18
Synarel 299
Synera 155
Synercid 84
Synphasic 293
Syntest D.S. 301
Syntest H.S. 301
Synthroid 181
Synvisc 20
Syprine .... PDA
Systane 345

T

T-20 43
t-PA 130
T-Phyl 379
T3 181
T4 181
Tabloid 317
Taclonex 145
tacrine .... PDA
tacrolimus 267
tacrolimus—topical 146
tadalafil
    Cardiovascular 129
    Urology 388
Tagamet 218
Tagamet HB 218
Talacen 18

Talwin NX 12
Tambocor 98
Tamiflu 53
Tamofen 305
Tamone 305
tamoxifen 305
tamsulosin 384
Tanacetum
    parthenium L. 248
Tanafed DMX 205
Tapazole 181
tapentadol 20
Tarabine 315
Tarceva 328
Targretin 327
Tarka 110
TARO-sone 147
Tarsum 152
Tasigna 330
Tasmar .... PDA
Tavist ND 194
Tavist-1 194
Taxol 325
Taxotere 324
tazarotene 138
Tazicef 65
Tazocin 74
Tazorac 138
Taztia XT 120
Td 258
Tdap 258
TDF 47
tea tree oil 256
Tears Naturale 345
Tebrazid 35
Tecnal 6
Tecnal C-1/2 16
Tecnal C-1/4 16
tegaserod 232
Tegens 244
Tegretol 269
Tegretol XR 269
Tegrin 152
Tegrin-HC 149
Tekturna 111
Tekturna HCT 110
telavancin 85
telbivudine 59
telithromycin 85
telmisartan 91, 109, 110
Telzir 49
temazepam 363
Temodal 311
Temodar 311
Temovate 147
temozolomide 311
Tempra 19
temsirolimus 323
tenecteplase 131
Tenex 93
teniposide 331
tenofovir 42, 43, 47
tenoretic 110
Tenormin 115

Tensilon 279
Tenuate 369
Tenuate Dospan 369
Terazol 307
terazosin 94
terbinafine 31
terbinafine—topical 142
terbutaline 371
terconazole 307
teriparatide 193
Tesalin 245
Teslascan 134
Tessalon 195
Tessalon Perles 195
Testim 156
Testopel 156
testosterone 156
Testred 156
Testro AQ 156
tetanus immune
    globulin 266
tetanus toxoid 262
tetrabenazine 284
tetracaine
    Dermatology ... 154, 155
    ENT 211
tetracaine—
    ophthalmic 346
tetracycline
    Antimicrobials 80
    Gastroenterology 220
Tev-Tropin 192
Teveten 91
Teveten HCT 110
thalidomide 323
Thalitone 123
Thalomid 323
Theo-24 379
Theo-Dur 379
Theolair 379
Theophylline 379
TheraCys 321
Theroxidil Extra
    Strength 154
thiamine 184, 186, 188
thiethylperazine 216
thioguanine 317
Thiola .... PDA
thiopental 22
Thioplex 311
Thioridazine 357
thiotepa 311
thiothixene 357
Thisylin 253
thonzonium 207
Thorazine 355
Thrombin-JMI 243
thrombin—topical 243
Thyro-Tabs 181
Thyrogen .... PDA
Thyroid USP 182
thyroid—desiccated 182
Thyrolar 182
Thyrosafe 181

Thyroshield 181
thyrotropin alfa .... PDA
tiagabine 274
Tiamol 148
tiaprofenic acid 11
Tiazac 120
ticarcillin-clavulanate 74
Tice BCG
   Immunology 257
   Oncology 321
Ticlid 114
ticlopidine 114
Tigan 216
tigecycline 85
Tikosyn 98
Tilade 379
tiludronate 158
Timentin 74
timolol
   Cardiovascular 118
   Ophthalmology 342,
                            343
timolol—ophthalmic ... 340
Timoptic 340
Timoptic Ocudose 340
Timoptic XE 340
Tinactin 143
Tindamax 39
tinidazole 39
tinzaparin 234
tioconazole 307
tiopronin .... PDA
tiotropium 379
tipranavir 52
tirofiban 114
Tirosint 181
tizanidine ....:.............. 5
TNKase 131
tobacco .... PDA
TOBI 25
TobraDex 338
TobraDex ST 338
tobramycin
   Antimicrobials 25
   Ophthalmology 338
tobramycin—
   ophthalmic 334
Tobrex 334
tocopherol 188
Tofranil 347
Tofranil PM 347
tolazamide 167
tolbutamide 167
tolcapone .... PDA
Tolectin 11
Tolinase 167
tolmetin 11
tolnaftate 143
tolterodine 385
tolvaptan 193
Topamax
   Neurology 274
   Psychiatry 354
Topicort 148

Topicort LP 148
Topilene Glycol 147
topiramate
   Neurology 274
   Psychiatry 354
Toposar 328
topotecan 331
Toprol-XL 116
Topsyn 148
Toradol 10
Torecan 216
toremifene 320
Torisel 323
torsemide 122
tositumomab 324
Totect 317
Toviaz 384
tpa 130
TPV 52
Tracleer 128
tracrium 23
Tramacet 6
tramadol 6, 20
Trandate 116
trandolapril 89, 110
tranexamic acid 243
Transderm-Scop 216
Transderm-V 216
Tranxene 361
Tranxene SD 361
tranylcypromine 348
Trasicor 117
trastuzumab 324
Travatan 342
Travatan Z 342
travoprost 342
trazodone 352
Treanda 309
Trecator .... PDA
trefoil 254
Trelstar Depot 320
Trental 133
treprostinil 130
treprostinil sodium 130
tretinoin
   Dermatology 138, 155
   Oncology 331
tretinoin—topical 138
Trexall 3
treximet 277
Tri-Cyclen 293
Tri-Legest 293
Tri-Legest FE 293
Tri-Levlen 293
Tri-Luma 155
Tri-Nasal 210
Tri-Norinyl 293
Tri-Previfem 294
Tri-Sprintec 294
Triaderm 150
triamcinolone
   Dermatology 151
   Endocrine and
      Metabolic 161

triamcinolone—
   vitreous .... PDA
triamcinolone—
   inhaled 376
triamcinolone—
   nasal 210
triamcinolone—
   topical 150
Triaminic Chest and
   Nasal Congestion 199
Triaminic Cold and
   Allergy 199
Triaminic Cough and
   Sore Throat 199
Triaminic Day Time
   Cold and Cough 199
Triaminic Flu Cough
   and Fever 199
Triaminic Night Time
   Cold and Cough 199
Triaminic Oral Infant
   Drops 206
triamterene 108, 109,
                             123
Trianal 6
Triatec 18
triavil 365
Triazide 109
triazolam 363
Tribenzor 110
TriCor 106
Tridesilon 148
Tridil 125
trientine .... PDA
Triesence .... PDA
Triest .... PDA
trifluoperazine 357
trifluridine 337
Trifolium pratense 254
Triglide 106
Trigonelle foenum-
   graecum 248
trihexyphenidyl 280
TriHibit 262
Trikacide 84
Trileptal 273
TriLipix 106
Trilisate 8
TriLyte 226
trimethobenzamide 216
trimethoprim 86
trimethoprim-
   sulfamethoxazole 78
trimipramine .... PDA
Trimox 72
trimethoprim 337
trinessa 293
Trinipatch 126
Trinovin 254
Triostat 181
Tripacel 258
Tripedia 258
Triphasil 293
triprolidine 196, 197

triptorelin 320
Triquilar 292
Trisenox 327
Trivaris 161
Trivora-28 294
Trizivir 43
Tropicacyl 344
tropicamide 344
Trosec 385
trospium 385
Trusopt 340
Truvada 43
trypan blue 346
Tryptan 353
tryptophan 353
Tuberculin PPD 268
Tubersol 268
Tucks 151
Tucks Hemorrhoidal
   Ointment 151
Tucks Suppositories 151
Tuinal .... PDA
Tums 173
Tuss-HC 206
Tussicaps 206
Tussionex 206
Twinject 127
Twinrix 262
Twynsta 110
Tygacil 85
Tykerb 329
Tylenol 19
Tylenol with Codeine 18
tylox 18
Typherix 262
Typhim Vi 262
typhoid vaccine—
   inactivated injection . 262
typhoid vaccine—live
   oral 262
tyramine-rich foods ..... PDA
Tysabri 279
Tyvaso 130
Tyzeka 59

U

ubiquinone 246
Uloric 172
Ultane .... PDA
Ultiva 22
Ultracet 6
Ultradol 9
Ultram 20
Ultram ER 20
Ultraquin 153
Ultrathon 152
Ultravate 149
Ultravist 135
Unasyn 73
Unidet 385
Uniphyl 379
Uniretic 110
Unisom Nighttime
   Sleep Aid 214

Index

Unithroid 181	Vaqta 258	vinblastine 325	**W**
Univasc 89	vardenafil 388	Vincasar 325	
UP446 248	varenicline 367	vincristine 325	warfarin 236
urea 152, 154, 155	varicella vaccine 261, 263	vinorelbine 325	Wartec 146
Urecholine 386	varicella-zoster immune	Viokase 232	Welchol 101
Urex .... PDA	globulin 266	Viracept 51	Wellbutrin 352
Urised 386	Varilrix 263	Viramune 45	Wellbutrin SR 352
Urispas 384	Varivax 263	Virazole 58	Wellbutrin XL 352
Urocit-K 390	VariZIG 266	Viread 47	Wellcovorin 329
Urodol 387	Vascoray 135	Virilon 156	Westcort 150
urofollitropin 303	Vaseretic 111	Viroptic 337	white petrolatum 155
Urogesic 387	Vasocidin 338	Visicol 226	wild yam 257
urokinase 131	Vasocon-A 332	Visine-A 332	willow bark
Urolene blue 382	Vasodilan 133	Vision Blue 346	extract 257
Uromax 385	vasopressin 193	Visipaque 135	Winpred 161
Uromitexan 317	Vasotec 87	Visken 118	WinRho SDF 308
Uroquid-Acid No. 2 387	Vaxigrip 260	Vistaril 195	witch hazel 151
UroXatral 383	VCR 325	Vistide 39	wolf's bane 244
URSO 232	Vectibix 323	Visudyne 343	Women's Rogaine 154
URSO Forte 232	vecuronium 24	vitamin A 188	Women's Tylenol
ursodiol 232	Veetids 70	Vitamin A Acid	Menstrual Relief 21
Urtica dioica radix 253	Velban 325	Cream 138	Wycillin 71
ustekinumab 145	Velcade 327	vitamin B1 188	Wygesic 19
UTA 386	Velivet 294	vitamin B12 184	Wytensin 92
UTI Relief 387	Venastat 251	vitamin B2 188	**X**
Utira-C 386	venlafaxine 351	vitamin B3 186	
V	Venofer 177	vitamin B6 187	Xalatan 341
	Ventavis 129	vitamin C 183	Xanax 363
Va-Zone 278	Ventolin HFA 370	vitamin D2 184	Xanax XR 363
vaccinia vaccine 262	VePesid 328	vitamin D3 188	Xatral 383
Vaccinium	Veramil 121	vitamin E 188	Xeloda 314
macrocarpon 246	Veramyst 210	vitamin K 187	Xenazine 284
Vaccinium myrtillus 244	verapamil 110, 121	Vitex agnus castus	Xenical 231
Vagifem 298	Verdeso 148	fruit extract 245	Xibrom 344
Vagistat-1 307	Veregen 146	Vitis vinifera L. 250	Xifaxan 84
valacyclovir 41	Verelan 121	Vivactil 347	Xigris 82
Valcyte 40	Verelan PM 121	Vivaglobulin 265	Xodol 19
valerian 256	Vermox 38	Vivarin 368	Xolair 379
Valeriana officinalis 256	Versed 21	Vivelle 298	Xolegel 142
valganciclovir 40	Versel 155	Vivelle Dot 298	Xopenex 371
Valium 362	Versenate 381	Vivitrol 366	Xopenex HFA 371
valproic acid	verteporfin 343	Vivol 362	Xuezhikang 255
Neurology 275	Vesanoid 331	Vivotif Berna 262	Xylocaine
Psychiatry 354	Vesicare 385	VLB 325	Anesthesia 23
valrubicin 314	Vetch 244	VM-26 331	Cardiovascular 99
valsartan 91, 108, 110	Vexol 339	Voltaren	Dermatology 153
Valstar 314	Vfend 27	Analgesics 9	ENT 208
Valtaxin 314	Viactiv 173	Dermatology 138	Xylocard 99
Valtrex 41	Viagra 388	Ophthalmology 344	Xyntha 238
Valtropin 192	Vibativ 85	Voltaren Ophtha 344	Xyrem 284
Valturna 110	Vibra-Tabs 79	Voltaren Rapide 9	Xyzal 195
Vancenase 209	Vibramycin 79	Voltaren XR 9	**Y**
Vancenase AQ Double	Vicks Sinex 211	voriconazole 27	
Strength 209	Vicks Sinex 12 Hr. 211	vorinostat 332	Yasmin 291
Vancocin 86	Vick's 44 Cough 196	Vosol HC 208	YAZ 291
vancomycin 86	Vicodin 18	VoSpire ER 370	yellow fever
Vandazole 307	Vicoprofen 19	Votrient 330	vaccine 263
Vaniqa 153	Victoza 170	VP-16 328	YF-Vax 263
Vanos 148	Vidaza 314	VSL#3 253	Yocon 389
Vanspar 363	Videx 46	Vumon 331	Yodoxin .... PDA
Vantas 319	Videx EC 46	Vusion 155	yohimbe 257
Vantin 65	vigabatrin 275	Vytorin 105	yohimbine 389
Vaponefrin 378	Vigamox 335	Vyvanse 369	Yohimex 389
Vaprisol 190	Vimpat 271	VZIG 266	

Z

Zaditen 378
Zaditor 333
zafirlukast 376
zaleplon 364
Zanaflex 5
zanamivir 53
Zanosar 311
Zantac 219
Zantac 150 219
Zantac 75 219
Zantac Efferdose 219
Zarontin 270
Zaroxolyn 124
Zavesca .... PDA
ZDV 47
ZE 339 245
ZeaSorb AF 142
Zebeta 115
Zegerid 222
Zelapar 283
Zelnorm 232
Zemaira 377
Zemplar 187
Zemuron 23
Zenapax 267
Zenpep 232
Zephrex-LA 206
Zestoretic 111
Zestril 88
Zetia 105
Zevalin 322
Zhibituo 255
Ziac 111
Ziagen 45
Ziana 138
ziconotide .... PDA
zidovudine 42, 43, 47
zileuton 377
Zinacef 63
zinc acetate 179
zinc oxide
  Dermatology 155
  Endocrine and
    Metabolic 184
zinc sulfate 179
Zincate 179
Zinecard 317
Zingiber officinale 249
Zingo 153
ziprasidone 360
Zipsor 9
Zirgan 337
Zithromax 67
Zmax 67
Zocor 105
Zofran 213
Zoladex 318
zoledronic acid 158
Zolinza 332
zolmitriptan 277
Zoloft 350
zolpidem 364
Zolpimist 364
Zometa 158
Zomig 277
Zomig ZMT 277
Zonalon 153
Zonegran 276
zonisamide 276
zopiclone 364
Zorbtive 192
Zorcaine 22
Zorprin 7
Zostavax 263
zoster vaccine—live ... 263
Zostrix 152
Zostrix-HP 152
Zosyn 74
Zovia 292
Zovirax
  Antimicrobials 40
  Dermatology 145
zuclopenthixol 357
Zyban 352
Zydone 19
Zyflo CR 377
Zylet 338
Zyloprim 172
Zymaxid 335
Zyprexa 359
Zyprexa Relprevv 359
Zyprexa Zydis 359
Zyrtec 194
Zyrtec-D 206
Zyvox 83
Zyvoxam 83

APPENDIX

ADULT EMERGENCY DRUGS (selected)

ALLERGY	diphenhydramine (*Benadryl*): 50 mg IV/IM. epinephrine: 0.1–0.5 mg IM (1:1000 solution), may repeat after 20 minutes. methylprednisolone (*Solu-Medrol*): 125 mg IV/IM.
HYPERTENSION	esmolol (*Brevibloc*): 500 mcg/kg IV over 1 minute, then titrate 50–200 mcg/kg/min. fenoldopam (*Corlopam*): Start 0.1 mcg/kg/min, titrate up to 1.6 mcg/kg/min. labetalol (*Normodyne*): Start 20 mg slow IV, then 40–80 mg IV q10 min prn up to 300 mg total cumulative dose. nitroglycerin (*Tridil*): Start 10–20 mcg/min IV infusion, then titrate prn up to 100 mcg/min. nitroprusside (*Nipride*): Start 0.3 mcg/kg/min IV infusion, then titrate prn up to 10 mcg/kg/min.
DYSRHYTHMIAS / ARREST	adenosine (*Adenocard*): PSVT (not A-fib): 6 mg rapid IV & flush, preferably through a central line or proximal IV. If no response after 1–2 minutes, then 12 mg. A third dose of 12 mg may be given prn. amiodarone (*Cordarone, Pacerone*): V-fib or pulseless V-tach: 300 mg IV/IO; may repeat 150 mg just once. Life-threatening ventricular arrhythmia: Load 150 mg IV over 10 min, then 1 mg/min × 6 h, then 0.5 mg/min × 18 h. atropine: 0.5 mg IV, repeat prn to maximum of 3 mg. diltiazem (*Cardizem*): Rapid A-fib: bolus 0.25 mg/kg or 20 mg IV over 2 min. May repeat 0.35 mg/kg or 25 mg 15 min after 1st dose. Infusion 5–15 mg/h. epinephrine: 1 mg IV/IO q 3–5 minutes for cardiac arrest. [1:10,000 solution]. lidocaine (*Xylocaine*): Load 1 mg/kg IV, then 0.5 mg/kg q 8–10 min prn to max 3 mg/kg. Maintenance 2 g in 250 mL D5W (8 mg/mL) at 1–4 mg/min drip (7–30 mL/h).
PRESSORS	dobutamine (*Dobutrex*): 2–20 mcg/kg/min. 70 kg: 5 mcg/kg/min with 1 mg/mL concentration (eg, 250 mg in 250 mL D5W) = 21 mL/h. dopamine (*Intropin*): Pressor: Start at 5 mcg/kg/min, increase prn by 5–10 mcg/kg/min increments at 10 min intervals, max 50 mcg/kg/min. 70 kg: 5 mcg/kg/min with 1600 mcg/mL concentration (eg, 400 mg in 250 mL D5W) = 13 mL/h. Doses in mcg/kg/min: 2–4 = (traditional renal dose, apparently ineffective) dopaminergic receptors; 5–10 = (cardiac dose) dopaminergic and beta1 receptors; >10 = dopaminergic, beta1, and alpha1 receptors. norepinephrine (*Levophed*): 4 mg in 500 mL D5W (8 mcg/mL) at 2–4 mcg/min. 22.5 mL/h = 3 mcg/min. phenylephrine (*Neo-Synephrine*): Infusion for hypotension: 20 mg in 250 mL D5W (80 mcg/mL) at 40–180 mcg/min (35–160 mL/h).
INTUBATION	etomidate (*Amidate*): 0.3 mg/kg IV. methohexital (*Brevital*): 1–1.5 mg/kg IV. propofol (*Diprivan*): 2.0–2.5 mg/kg IV. rocuronium (*Zemuron*): 0.6–1.2 mg/kg IV. succinylcholine (*Anectine*): 1 mg/kg IV. Peds (<5 yo): 2 mg/kg IV. thiopental (*Pentothal*): 3–5 mg/kg IV.
SEIZURES	diazepam (*Valium*): 5–10 mg IV, or 0.2–0.5 mg/kg rectal gel up to 20 mg PR. fosphenytoin (*Cerebyx*): Load 15–20 "phenytoin equivalents" per kg either IM, or IV no faster than 100–150 mg/min. lorazepam (*Ativan*): 0.05–0.15 mg/kg up to 3–4 mg IV/IM. phenobarbital: 200–600 mg IV at rate ≤60 mg/min; titrate prn up to 20 mg/kg. phenytoin (*Dilantin*): 15–20 mg/kg up to 1000 mg IV no faster than 50 mg/min.

CARDIAC DYSRHYTHMIA PROTOCOLS (for adults and adolescents)

Chest compressions ~100/min. Ventilations 8–10/min if intubated; otherwise 30:2 compression/ventilation ratio. Drugs that can be administered down ET tube (use 2–2.5 × usual dose): epinephrine, atropine, lidocaine, naloxone, vasopressin*.

V-Fib, Pulseless V-Tach
Airway, oxygen, CPR until defibrillator ready
Defibrillate 360 J (old monophasic), 120–200 J (biphasic), or with AED
Resume CPR × 2 minutes (5 cycles)
Repeat defibrillation if no response
Vasopressor during CPR:
- Epinephrine 1 mg IV/IO q 3–5 minutes, or
- Vasopressin* 40 units IV to replace 1st or 2nd dose of epinephrine

Rhythm/pulse check every ~2 minutes
Consider antiarrhythmic during CPR:
- Amiodarone 300 mg IV/IO; may repeat 150 mg just once
- Lidocaine 1.0–1.5 mg/kg IV/IO, then repeat 0.5–0.75 mg/kg to max 3 doses or 3 mg/kg
- Magnesium sulfate 1–2 g IV/IO if suspect torsades de pointes

Asystole or Pulseless Electrical Activity (PEA)
Airway, oxygen, CPR
Vasopressor (when IV/IO access):
- Epinephrine 1 mg IV/IO q3–5 minutes, or
- Vasopressin* 40 units IV/IO to replace 1st or 2nd dose of epinephrine

Consider atropine 1 mg IV/IO for asystole or slow PEA. Repeat q 3–5 min up to 3 doses.
Rhythm/pulse check every ~2 minutes
Consider 6 H's: hypovolemia, hypoxia, H+ acidosis, hyper / hypokalemia, hypoglycemia, hypothermia
Consider 5 T's: Toxins, tamponade-cardiac, tension pneumothorax, thrombosis (coronary or pulmonary), trauma

Bradycardia, <60 bpm and Inadequate Perfusion
Airway, oxygen, IV
Prepare for transcutaneous pacing; don't delay if advanced heart block
Consider atropine 0.5 mg IV; may repeat q 3–5 min to max 3 mg
Consider epinephrine (2–10 mcg/min) or dopamine (2–10 mcg/kg/min)
Prepare for transvenous pacing

Tachycardia with Pulses
Airway, oxygen, IV
If unstable and heart rate >150 bpm, then synchronized cardioversion
If stable narrow-QRS (<120 ms):
- Regular: Attempt vagal maneuvers. If no success, adenosine 6 mg IV, then 12 mg prn (may repeat × 1)
- Irregular: Control rate with diltiazem or beta blocker (caution in CHF or severe obstructive pulmonary disease).

If stable wide-QRS (>120 ms):
- Regular and suspect V-tach: Amiodarone 150 mg IV over 10 min; repeat prn to max 2.2 g/24 h. Prepare for elective synchronized cardioversion.
- Regular and suspect SVT with aberrancy: adenosine as per narrow-QRS above.
- Irregular and A-fib: Control rate with diltiazem or beta blocker (caution in CHF/ severe obstructive pulmonary disease).
- Irregular and A-fib with pre-excitation (WPW): Avoid AV nodal blocking agents; consider amiodarone 150 mg IV over 10 minutes.
- Irregular and torsades de pointes: magnesium 1–2 g IV load over 5–60 minutes, then infusion.

bpm=beats per minute; CPR=cardiopulmonary resuscitation; ET=endotracheal; IO=intraosseous; J=Joules; ms=milliseconds; WPW=Wolff-Parkinson-White. Sources: *Circulation* 2005; 112, suppl IV; *NEJM 2008;359:21-30 (demonstrated no benefit over epinephrine and worse long-term neurological outcomes).

Antiviral Drugs for Influenza A	Treatment* (Duration of 5 days)	Prevention (Duration of 10 days post-exposure)
OSELTAMIVIR (*Tamiflu*)		
Adults and adolescents age 13 years and older		
	75 mg PO bid	75 mg PO once daily
Children, 1 year of age and older[†]		
Body weight ≤15 kg	30 mg PO bid	30 mg PO once daily
Body weight >15 to 23 kg	45 mg PO bid	45 mg PO once daily
Body weight >23 to 40 kg	60 mg PO bid	60 mg PO once daily
Body weight >40 kg	75 mg PO bid	75 mg PO once daily
Infants, newborn to 11 months of age[†,‡]		
Age 3 to 11 months old	3 mg/kg/dose PO bid	3 mg/kg/dose PO once daily
Age younger than 3 months old[¶]	3 mg/kg/dose PO bid	Not for routine prophylaxis in infants <3 mo
ZANAMIVIR (*Relenza*)[§]		
Adults and children (age 7 years and older for treatment, age 5 years and older for prophylaxis)		
	10 mg (two 5-mg inhalations) bid	10 mg (two 5-mg inhalations) once daily

Adapted from http://www.cdc.gov/h1n1flu/recommendations.htm

*Start treatment as soon as possible; benefit is greatest when started within 2 days of symptom onset. Hospitalized patients with severe infection might require treatment for longer than 5 days.

[†]A dosing syringe with graduations of 30, 45, and 60 mg is provided with *Tamiflu* oral suspension. The 75 mg dose can be measured by combining 30 mg and 45 mg. For infants less than 1 year old, a different oral syringe must be used to measure the dose. The concentration of oseltamivir differs between commercial *Tamifu* suspension (12 mg/mL) and pharmacist-compounded suspension (15 mg/mL). Capsules can be opened and mixed with sweetened fluids to mask bitter taste. Make sure units of measure on dosing instructions match dosing device provided.

[‡]Oseltamavir is not FDA-approved for use in infants less than 1 year old. An Emergency Use Authorization for use in infants expired in June 2010.

[¶]This dose is not intended for premature infants. Immature renal function may lead to slow clearance and high concentrations of oseltamivir in this age group.

[§]Zanamivir should not be used by patients with underlying pulmonary disease. Do not attempt to use *Relenza* in a nebulizer or ventilator; lactose in the formulation may cause the device to malfunction.

NOTES

NOTES

Stay Connected with Tarascon Publishing!

Monthly Dose eNewsletter
—Tarascon's Monthly eNewsletter

Stay up-to-date and subscribe today at: www.tarascon.com

Written specifically with Tarascon customers in mind, the Tarascon Monthly Dose will provide you with new drug information, tips and tricks, updates on our print, mobile and online products as well as some extra topics that are interesting and entertaining.

Sign up to receive the Tarascon Monthly Dose Today! Simply register at www.tarascon.com.

You can also stay up-to-date with Tarascon news, new product releases, and relevant medical news and information on Facebook, Twitter page, and our Blog.

STAY CONNECTED

Facebook: www.facebook.com/tarascon
Twitter: @JBL_Medicine
Blog: portfolio.jblearning.com/medicine